Nursing Theorists

and Their Work

Nursing Theorists

and Their Work

Seventh Edition

Martha Raile Alligood, PhD, RN, ANEF
Professor and Director, PhD program
College of Nursing
East Carolina University
Greenville, North Carolina

Ann Marriner Tomey, PhD, RN, FAAN
Professor Emeritus
College of Nursing, Health and Human Services
Indiana State University
Terre Haute, Indiana

MOSBY

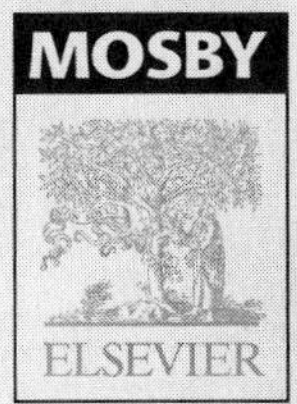

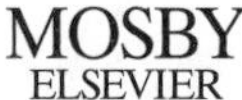

3251 Riverport Lane
Maryland Heights, Missouri 63043

NURSING THEORISTS AND THEIR WORK, SEVENTH EDITION ISBN: 978-0-323-05641-0

Notice

Neither the Publisher nor the Authors assume any responsibility for any loss or injury and/or damage to persons or property arising out of or related to any use of the material contained in this book. It is the responsibility of the treating practitioner, relying on independent expertise and knowledge of the patient, to determine the best treatment and method of application for the patient.

The Publisher

Library of Congress Cataloging-in-Publication Data

Nursing theorists and their work / [edited by] Martha Raile Alligood,
Ann Marriner Tomey. -- 7th ed.
p. ; cm.
Includes bibliographical references and index.
ISBN 978-0-323-05641-0 (pbk. : alk. paper) 1. Nursing--Philosophy.
2. Nursing models. I. Alligood, Martha Raile. II. Marriner-Tomey, Ann,
1943-
[DNLM: 1. Nursing Theory. 2. Models, Nursing. 3. Nurses--Biography.
4. Philosophy, Nursing. WY 86 N9738 2010]
RT84.5.N9 2010
610.7301--dc22

2009020629

Acquisitions Editor: Yvonne Alexopoulos
Developmental Editor: Heather Bays
Publishing Services Manager: Hemamalini Rajendrababu
Project Manager: Srikumar Narayanan
Designer: Charlie Seibel

Printed in United States of America

Last digit is the print number: 9 8 7 6 5 4 3 2

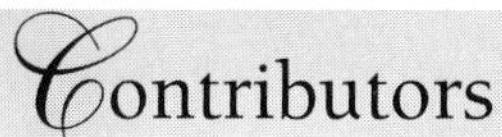

Contributors

Herdis Alvsvåg, RN, Cand Polit
Associate Professor
Department of Education and Health Promotion
University of Bergen
Bergen, Norway;
Associate Professor II
Bergen Deaconess University College
Bergen, Norway

Donald E. Bailey, Jr., PhD, RN
Associate Professor
School of Nursing
Duke University
Durham, North Carolina

Barbara Banfield, RN, PhD
Farmington Hills, Michigan

Violeta A. Berbiglia, EdD, MSN, RN
Associate Professor, Retired
The University of Texas Health Science Center at San Antonio School of Nursing
San Antonio, Texas;
Educational Consultant
Helotes, Texas;
Faculty
Friendship Bridge to Vietnam
Evergreen, Colorado;
Co-Editor
Self-Care, Dependent-Care, and Nursing
St. Louis, Missouri

Sue Marquis Bishop, PhD, RN, FAAN
Professor and Dean Emerita
College of Health and Human Services
University of North Carolina, Charlotte
Charlotte, North Carolina

Debra A. Bournes, RN, PhD
Director of Nursing
New Knowledge and Innovation
University Health Network
Toronto, Canada

Vigdis Elisabeth Brekke, Cand Polit
Associate Professor
Haraldsplass Deaconess University College
Ulriksdal, Bergen, Norway

Nancy Brookes, PhD, RN, MSc (A), CPMHN (C)
Nurse Scholar
Royal Ottawa Health Care Group
Royal Ottawa Mental Health Centre
Ottawa, Ontario, Canada

Janet Witucki Brown, PhD, RN, CNE
Associate Professor
College of Nursing
University of Tennessee
Knoxville, Tennessee

Karen A. Brykczynski, RN, FNP, DNSc, FAANP
Professor
School of Nursing at Galveston
The University of Texas Medical Branch
Galveston, Texas

Sherrilyn Coffman, DNS, RN
Professor
School of Nursing
Nevada State College
Henderson, Nevada

Doris D. Coward, PhD, RN
Associate Professor, Retired
School of Nursing
The University of Texas at Austin
Austin, Texas

Thérèse Dowd, PhD, RN, CHTP
Associate Professor
College of Nursing
The University of Akron
Akron, Ohio

Nellie S. Droes, DNSc, RN
Associate Professor
College of Nursing
East Carolina University
Greenville, North Carolina

Margaret E. Erickson, PhD, RN, CNS, AHN-BC
Executive Director
American Holistic Nurses' Certification Corporation
Cedar Park, Texas

Bjørn Inge Follevaag, RN
Translator
Bergen, Norway

Barbara T. Freese, RN, EdD, FRCNA
Professor Emeritus
School of Nursing
Lander University
Greenwood, South Carolina

Mary E. Gunther, RN, MSN, PhD
Assistant Professor
College of Nursing
University of Tennessee
Knoxville, Tennessee

Sonya R. Hardin, PhD, RN, CCRN, APRN
Associate Professor
Department of Adult Health Nursing
School of Nursing
College of Health and Human Services
University of North Carolina, Charlotte
Charlotte, North Carolina

Patricia A. Higgins, PhD, RN
Assistant Professor
Francis Payne Bolton School of Nursing
Case Western Reserve University
Cleveland, Ohio

Bonnie Holaday, DNS, RN, FAAN
Professor and Director, Graduate Studies
School of Nursing and Institute on Family and Neighborhood Life
Clemson University
Clemson, South Carolina

Eun-Ok Im, PhD, MPH, RN, CNS, FAAN
Professor and La Quinta Motor Inns Inc. Centennial Professor
School of Nursing
The University of Texas at Austin
Austin, Texas

D. Elizabeth Jesse, PhD, RN, CNM
Associate Professor
College of Nursing
East Carolina University
Greenville, North Carolina

Lisa Kitko, RN, PhD(c), CCRN,
Doctoral Candidate
School of Nursing
The Pennsylvania State University
University Park, PA

Theresa G. Lawson, MS, APRN, BC, FNP
Instructor
Department of Nursing
Lander University
Greenwood, South Carolina

Lisbet Lindholm, RN, PhD
Associate Professor
Department of Caring Science
Faculty of Social and Caring Sciences
Åbo Academy University
Vaasa, Finland

Unni Å. Lindström, PhD, RN
Professor
Department of Caring Science
Faculty of Social and Caring Sciences
Åbo Academy University
Vaasa, Finland

Chin-Fang Liu, PhD, RN
Assistant Professor
Nursing Department
Chang Gung Institute of Technology
Taiwan;
Assistant Professor
College of Nursing
Kaohsiung Medical University
Taiwan;
Professional Registered Nurse
Department of Nursing
Kaohsiung Medical University
Taiwan

M. Katherine Maeve, PhD, RN
Nurse Researcher
Charlie Norwood VAMC
Augusta, Georgia

Marilyn R. McFarland, PhD, RN, FNP, BC, CTN
Associate Professor of Nursing and Family Nurse Practitioner
Urban Health and Wellness Center
University of Michigan
Flint, Michigan

Molly Meighan, RNC, PhD
Professor Emerita
Division of Nursing
Carson-Newman College
Jefferson City, Tennessee

Patricia R. Messmer, PhD, RN-BC, FAAN
Director
Patient Care Services Research
Children's Mercy Hospital and Clinics
Kansas City, Missouri

Gail J. Mitchell, RN, BScN, MScN, PhD
Associate Professor
York University
Toronto, Ontario, Canada

Janice Penrod, PhD, RN
Associate Professor of Nursing
School of Nursing and of Humanities
College of Medicine;
Associate Director
Penn State Hartford Center for Geriatric Nursing Excellence
Coordinator
Doctoral Programs in Nursing
The Pennsylvania State University
University Park, Pennsylvania

Susan A. Pfettscher, DNSc, RN
Retired
Bakersfield, California

Kenneth D. Phillips, PhD, RN
Professor and Associate Dean for Research and Evaluation
College of Nursing
The University of Tennessee
Knoxville, Tennessee

Marie E. Pokorny, PhD, RN
Professor and Acting Associate Dean of Graduate Programs
Department of Graduate Nursing Science
College of Nursing
East Carolina University
Greenville, North Carolina

Marguerite J. Purnell, PhD, RN, AHN-BC
Assistant Professor
Christine E. Lynn College of Nursing
Florida Atlantic University
Boca Raton, Florida

Teresa J. Sakraida, PhD, RN
Assistant Professor
College of Nursing
University of Colorado, Denver
Aurora, Colorado

Karen Moore Schaefer, PhD, RN
Associate Chair and Associate Professor
Department of Nursing
College of Health Professions
Temple University
Philadelphia, Pennsylvania

Kirsten Costain Schou, PhD
Freelancer
Heggedal, Norway

Ann M. Schreier, PhD, RN
Associate Professor
School of Nursing
East Carolina University
Greenville, North Carolina

Carrie J. Scotto, PhD, RN
Assistant Professor
College of Nursing
University of Akron
Akron, Ohio

Christina L. Sieloff, PhD, RN, NE, BC
Associate Professor
College of Nursing
Montana State University
Billings, Montana

Janet L. Stewart, PhD, RN
Assistant Professor
Department of Health Promotion and Development
School of Nursing
University of Pittsburgh
Pittsburgh, Pennsylvania

Danuta M. Wojnar, PhD, RN, MEd, IBCLC
Assistant Professor
College of Nursing
Seattle University
Seattle, Washington

Joan E. Zetterlund, PhD, RN
Professor Emerita of Nursing
School of Nursing
North Park University
Chicago, Illinois

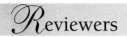

Reviewers

Mary Curtis, PhD, APRN-BC
Director
Nursing Program
Maryville University
St. Louis, Missouri

Debra Miles, EdD, MSN, RN
Associate Professor
School of Nursing
Gardner-Webb University
Boiling Springs, North Carolina

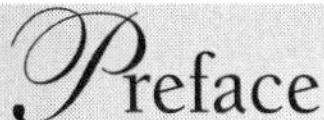

Preface

This book is a tribute to the nursing theorists. It identifies major thinkers in nursing, reviews some of their important ideas, lists their publications, and points the reader to those who have used the works and written about it in their own theoretical publications.

Chapter 1 introduces the text with a brief history of nursing theory, its significance, and the framework for analysis of the theoretical works included. Other chapters in Unit I discuss the history and philosophy of science, logical reasoning, and the process of theory development. Ten works from earlier editions of *Nursing Theorists and Their Work* are discussed briefly in Chapter 5 as nursing theorists of historical significance. They are Peplau; Henderson; Abdellah; Wiedenbach; Hall; Travelbee; Barnard; Adam; Roper, Logan, Tierney, and Orlando.

The philosophies of Nightingale, Watson, Ray, Benner, Martinsen, and Eriksson are presented in Unit II. Unit III includes nursing models by Levine, Rogers, Orem, King, Neuman, Roy, and Johnson. The work of Boykin and Schoenhofer begins Unit IV on nursing theory, followed by a new chapter about Meleis. Also included in Unit IV are the works of Pender; Leininger; Newman; Parse; Erickson, Tomlin, and Swain; and the Husteds. Unit V presents the middle range theoretical works of Mercer; Mishel; Reed; Wiener and Dodd; Eakes, Burke and Hainsworth; Barker; Kolcaba; Beck; Swanson; Ruland and Moore. Unit VI addresses the state of the art and science of nursing theory from the perspective of the philosophy of nursing science, the expansion of theory development, and the global nature and use of nursing theoretical works around the world.

The work of each theorist is presented with a framework using the following headings to facilitate uniformity and comparison among the theorists and their works:

- Credentials and background
- Theoretical sources for theory development
- Use of empirical data
- Major concepts and definitions
- Major assumptions
- Theoretical assertions
- Logical form
- Acceptance by the nursing community
- Further development
- Critique of the work
- Summary
- Case study based on the work
- Critical thinking activities
- Points for further study
- References and bibliographies

The works of nurse theorists from all over the world are included, and works by some of the international theorists have been translated into English. *Nursing Theorists and Their Work* has been translated into numerous languages for nursing students in other parts of the world.

Nurses and students at all stages of their education will be interested in learning about nursing theory and nurse theorist works from around the world. Those who are just beginning their nursing education, such as associate degree and baccalaureate students, will be interested in the concepts, definitions, and theoretical assertions, graduate students, those at the masters and doctoral levels, will be more interested in the logical form, acceptance by the nursing community, the theoretical sources for theory development, and the use of empirical data. The references and extensive bibliographies are particularly useful to graduate students for locating primary and secondary sources. These resources augment the websites specific to the theorist. The following comprehensive websites are excellent resources with information about theory resources and links to the individual theorists featured in this book:

- Nursing Theory link page, Clayton College and State University, Department of Nursing: *http://www.healthsci.clayton.edu/eichelberger/nursing.htm*
- Nursing Theory page, Hahn School of Nursing and Health Science, University of San Diego: *http://www.sandiego.edu/academics/nursing/theory/*
- A comprehensive collection of nursing theory media, *The Nurse Theorists: Portraits of Excellence, Vol. I and Vol. II and Nurse Theorists: Excellence in Action: http://www.fitne.net/*

The theorists and the theoretical works presented stimulated phenomenal growth in the nursing literature and enriched our professional lives by guiding nursing research, education, administration, and practice. This growth continues as we analyze and synthesize their work, generate new ideas, and develop new theory and applications for education in the discipline and for quality care in the profession.

Acknowledgments

We are thankful to the theorists for critiquing the original and many subsequent chapters about themselves to keep the content current and accurate. Rather than an omission of the text, Paterson and Zderad requested their work not be included.

We are grateful to the librarians who have helped us locate obscure information and to the other people working behind the scenes over the years with previous editions. It was in the third edition that Martha Raile Alligood joined Ann Marriner Tomey, to reorder the chapters, serve as a contributing author, and edit for consistency with the new organization of the text. Dr. Tomey then recommended Dr. Alligood to Mosby-Elsevier to design and coedit *Nursing Theory: Utilization and Application* with her and, based on Alligood's expertise in nursing theory, invited her to become coeditor and contributing author to future editions of this text, *Nursing Theorists and Their Work.*

We would like to thank the publishers at Mosby-Elsevier for their guidance and assistance through the years to bring us to this seventh edition. The external reviews requested by Mosby-Elsevier editors have contributed to the successful development of each new edition. The chapter authors who over the years have contributed their expert knowledge of the theorists and their work continue to make a most valuable contribution.

Martha Raile Alligood
Ann Marriner Tomey

I would like to recognize and thank Ann Marriner Tomey for her vision to develop the first and successive editions of this book. Her mentorship, wisdom, and collegial friendship have been special to me in my professional career. Most of all her dedication to this work has been valuable to the discipline and the profession of nursing. I wish her a very restful retirement.

Martha Raile Alligood

Contents

UNIT I

Evolution of Nursing Theories

1 **Introduction to Nursing Theory: Its History, Significance, and Analysis, 3**
Martha Raile Alligood

2 **History and Philosophy of Science, 16**
Sonya R. Hardin and Sue Marquis Bishop

3 **Logical Reasoning, 26**
Sonya R. Hardin and Sue Marquis Bishop

4 **Theory Development Process, 36**
Sonya R. Hardin and Sue Marquis Bishop

5 **Nursing Theorists of Historical Significance, 50**
Marie E. Pokorny

Hildegard E. Peplau
Virginia Henderson
Faye Glenn Abdellah
Ernestine Wiedenbach
Lydia Hall
Joyce Travelbee
Kathryn E. Barnard
Evelyn Adam
Nancy Roper, Winifred W. Logan, and Alison J. Tierney
Ida Jean (Orlando) Pelletier

UNIT II

Philosophies

6 **Florence Nightingale: Modern Nursing, 71**
Susan A. Pfettscher

7 **Jean Watson: Watson's Philosophy and Theory of Transpersonal Caring, 91**
D. Elizabeth Jesse

8 **Marilyn Anne Ray: Theory of Bureaucratic Caring, 113**
Sherrilyn Coffman

9 **Patricia Benner: Caring, Clinical Wisdom, and Ethics in Nursing Practice, 137**
Karen A. Brykczynski

10 **Kari Martinsen: Philosophy of Caring, 165**
Herdis Alvsvåg

11 **Katie Eriksson: Theory of Caritative Caring, 190**
Unni Å. Lindström, Lisbet Lindholm, and Joan E. Zetterlund

UNIT **III**

Nursing Models

12 **Myra Estrin Levine: The Conservation Model, 225**
Karen Moore Schaefer

13 **Martha E. Rogers: Unitary Human Beings, 242**
Mary E. Gunther

14 **Dorothea E. Orem: Self-Care Deficit Theory of Nursing, 265**
Violeta A. Berbiglia and Barbara Banfield

15 **Imogene M. King: Conceptual System and Middle Range Theory of Goal Attainment, 286**
Christina L. Sieloff and Patricia R. Messmer

16 **Betty Neuman: Systems Model, 309**
Barbara T. Freese and Theresa G. Lawson

17 **Sister Callista Roy: Adaptation Model, 335**
Kenneth D. Phillips

18 **Dorothy Johnson: Behavioral System Model, 366**
Bonnie Holaday

UNIT **IV**

Nursing Theories

19 **Anne Boykin and Savina O. Schoenhofer: The Theory of Nursing as Caring: A Model for Transforming Practice, 393**
Marguerite J. Purnell

20 **Afaf Ibrahim Meleis: Transition Theory, 416**
Eun-Ok Im

21 **Nola J. Pender: Health Promotion Model, 434**
Teresa J. Sakraida

22 **Madeleine M. Leininger: Culture Care Theory of Diversity and Universality, 454**
Marilyn R. McFarland

23 **Margaret A. Newman: Health as Expanding Consciousness, 480**
Janet Witucki Brown

24 **Rosemarie Rizzo Parse: Humanbecoming, 503**
Gail J. Mitchell and Debra A. Bournes

25 **Helen C. Erickson, Evelyn M. Tomlin, Mary Ann P. Swain: Modeling and Role-Modeling, 536**
Margaret E. Erickson

26 **Gladys L. Husted and James H. Husted: Symphonological Bioethical Theory, 560**
Carrie J. Scotto

UNIT **V**

Middle Range Theories

27 **Ramona T. Mercer: Maternal Role Attainment—Becoming a Mother, 581**
Molly Meighan

28 **Merle H. Mishel: Uncertainty in Illness Theory, 599**
Donald E. Bailey, Jr., and Janet L. Stewart

29 **Pamela G. Reed: Self-Transcendence Theory, 618**
Doris D. Coward

30 **Carolyn L. Wiener and Marylin J. Dodd: Theory of Illness Trajectory, 638**
Janice Penrod, Lisa Kitko, and Chin-Fang Liu

31 **Georgene Gaskill Eakes, Mary Lermann Burke, and Margaret A. Hainsworth: Theory of Chronic Sorrow, 656**
Ann M. Schreier and Nellie S. Droes

32 **Phil Barker: The Tidal Model of Mental Health Recovery, 673**
Nancy Brookes

33 **Katharine Kolcaba: Theory of Comfort, 706**
Thérèse Dowd

34 **Cheryl Tatano Beck: Postpartum Depression Theory, 722**
M. Katherine Maeve

35 **Kristen M. Swanson: Theory of Caring, 741**
Danuta M. Wojnar

36 **Cornelia M. Ruland and Shirley M. Moore: Peaceful End of Life Theory, 753**
Patricia A. Higgins

UNIT **VI**

Future of Nursing Theory

37 **State of the Art and Science of Nursing Theory, 765**
Martha Raile Alligood

UNIT

I

Evolution of Nursing Theories

- *Searching for substantive knowledge led nurse scholars to recognize the need for theories to guide nursing research and professional practice.*
- *Nursing followed a path from concepts to conceptual frameworks to models to theories, and finally to middle range theory, in this era of theory utilization.*
- *Nursing history demonstrates the significance of theory for nursing as a division of education (the discipline) and a specialized field of practice (the profession).*
- *Knowledge of the theory development process is basic to a personal understanding of the theoretical works of the discipline.*
- *Theory analysis begins the process by exploring for a decision making guide to be used in nursing research or practice.*
- *Analysis facilitates learning through systematic review, critical thinking, and reflection on theoretical works of the discipline.*

CHAPTER

1

Introduction to Nursing Theory: Its History, Significance, and Analysis

Martha Raile Alligood

"The systematic accumulation of knowledge is essential to progress in any profession... however theory and practice must be constantly interactive. Theory without practice is empty and practice without theory is blind" (Cross, 1981, p. 110).

This text is designed to introduce the reader to nursing theorists and their work. Nursing theory has become a major theme over the past 50 years, stimulating phenomenal growth and vast expansion of nursing education and literature. Selected nursing theorists are presented in this text to expose students to a broad range of nurse theorists and different types of theoretical works. Many nurses of early eras delivered excellent care to patients; however, much of what was known about nursing was passed on through vocational education that was focused on skillful completion of functional tasks. Whereas many of these practices seemed effective, they were not tested nor used uniformly. Developing nursing knowledge on which to base nursing practice was a major goal put forth by leaders of the nursing profession in the twentieth century, as nurses sought to improve practice and to gain recognition of nursing as a profession. The history of nursing clearly documents sustained efforts put forth toward the goal of developing a substantive body of nursing knowledge to guide nursing practice (Alligood, 2006a; Bixler & Bixler, 1959; Chinn & Kramer, 2008; George, 2002; Johnson & Webber, 2004; McEwen & Wills, 2006; Meleis, 2007; Parker, 2006).

In this chapter, the reader is introduced to nursing theory under three major headings: history, significance, and analysis. A brief history of the movement of nursing from vocation to profession describes the search for nursing substance that led to this exciting time in nursing history, linking the theory era with nursing as an academic discipline and a practice profession. Although sustained efforts were put forth by nurse leaders in the first half of the twentieth century to attain recognition of nursing as a profession, it was in the second half of the twentieth century that leaders realized the necessity for conceptual and theoretical frameworks for the development of substantive nursing knowledge and the path to professional nursing practice (Batey, 1977; Hardy, 1978). Development of nursing knowledge was a significant force during this period; the baccalaureate degree began to be accepted more

---

Previous authors: Martha Raile Alligood, Elizabeth Chong Choi, Juanita Fogel Keck, and Ann Marriner Tomey.

widely as the first educational level for professional nursing, and nursing attained nationwide recognition and acceptance as an academic discipline in higher education. Nurse researchers worked to develop and clarify a substantive body of nursing knowledge with goals of improving the quality of patient care, providing a professional style of practice, and being recognized as a profession. Nursing history provides the context for understanding the significance of nursing theory for professional nursing practice in the theory utilization era. The history and significance of nursing theory lead logically into analysis, the final section of this chapter. Analysis of nursing theoretical works and of their role in knowledge development is presented as an essential process of critical reflection required for acquisition of knowledge. Criteria for analysis of the works of theorists are presented, along with a brief discussion of how each criterion contributes to our understanding of theory (Chinn & Kramer, 2008).

HISTORY OF NURSING THEORY

The history of professional nursing began with Florence Nightingale. It was Nightingale who envisioned nurses as a body of educated women at a time when women were neither educated nor employed in public service. Following her service of organizing and caring for the wounded in Scutari, during the Crimean War, her vision and establishment of a School of Nursing at St. Thomas' Hospital in London marked the birth of modern nursing. Nightingale's pioneering activities in nursing practice and subsequent writings describing nursing education became a guide for establishing nursing schools in the United States at the beginning of the twentieth century (Kalisch & Kalisch, 2003; Nightingale, 1859/1969). Nursing began with a strong emphasis on practice, but throughout the century, nurses worked toward the development of nursing as a profession through successive periods recognized as historical eras (Alligood, 2006a).

The curriculum era addressed the question of what prospective nurses should study to learn how to be a nurse. In this era, the emphasis was on what courses nursing students should take, with the goal of arriving at a standardized curriculum (Alligood, 2006a). By the mid-1930s, a standardized curriculum had been published. However, it was also in this era that the idea of moving nursing education from hospital-based diploma programs into colleges and universities emerged. Even so, it was the middle of the century before this goal began to be acted upon in many states (Kalisch & Kalisch, 2003).

As nurses increasingly sought degrees in higher education, a research emphasis era, as it is deemed, began to emerge. This era came about as more and more nurses embraced higher education and arrived at a common understanding of the scientific age, that is, that research is the path to new nursing knowledge. Nurses began to participate in research, and research courses began to be included in the nursing curricula of many developing graduate programs (Alligood, 2006a).

The research era and the graduate education era developed in tandem. Master's degree programs in nursing emerged to meet the public need for nurses with specialized clinical nursing education. Many of these programs included a nursing research course. It was also in this era that most nursing master's programs began to include courses in concept development or nursing models that introduced students to early nursing theorists and the knowledge development process (Alligood, 2006a).

The theory era was a natural outgrowth of the research and graduate education eras. As our understanding of research and knowledge development increased, it soon became obvious that research without theory produced isolated information, and that it was research and theory together that produced nursing science (Batey, 1977; Fawcett, 1978; Hardy, 1978). In the early years of the theory era, doctoral education in nursing flourished with an emphasis on theory development.

In the theory utilization era, emphasis was placed on middle range theory for theory-based nursing practice, as well as on theory development (Alligood & Tomey, 1997, 2002, 2006; Batey, 1977; Chinn & Kramer, 2008; Fawcett, 2005; Tomey & Alligood, 2006).

Each era addressed nursing knowledge in a unique way that contributed to and is observable in the history of nursing. Within each era, the pervading question "What is the nature of the knowledge that is needed for the practice of nursing?" seems to have been addressed at the level of understanding that prevailed at that time (Alligood, 2006a).

Nightingale's (1859/1969) vision of nursing has been practiced for more than a century, and theory development in nursing has evolved rapidly over the past 5 decades, leading to the recognition of nursing as an academic discipline with a substantive body of knowledge (Alligood, 2006a, 2006b; Alligood & Tomey, 2006; Chinn & Kramer, 2008; Fawcett, 2005; Tomey & Alligood, 2006; Walker & Avant, 2005). In the mid-1800s, Nightingale wrote that nursing knowledge is distinct from medical knowledge. She described a nurse's proper function as putting the patient in the best condition for nature (God) to act upon him or her. She proposed that care of the sick is based on knowledge of persons and their surroundings—a different knowledge base than that used by physicians in their practice. Despite this early edict from Nightingale in the 1850s, it was 100 years later, during the 1950s, that the nursing profession began to engage in serious discussion about the need to develop, articulate, and test nursing theory (Alligood, 2006d; Alligood, 2004; Chinn & Kramer, 2008; Meleis, 2007; Walker & Avant, 2005). Until the emergence of nursing as a science in the 1950s, nursing practice was based on principles and traditions that had been passed on through an apprenticeship model of education and hospital-kept procedure manuals (Alligood, 2002a; Kalisch & Kalisch, 2003).

Although some nursing leaders aspired for nursing to be recognized as a profession and become an academic discipline, nursing practice continued to reflect its vocational heritage more than a professional vision. The transition from vocation to profession included successive eras of history as nurses searched for a body of substantive knowledge on which to base nursing practice. The curriculum era emphasized course selection and content for nursing programs and gave way to the research era, which focused on learning the research process and meeting the long-range goal of acquiring substantive knowledge to guide nursing practice.

In the mid-1970s, an evaluation of the first 25 years of the journal *Nursing Research* revealed that nursing studies lacked conceptual connections and theoretical frameworks (Batey, 1977). An awareness of the need for concept and theory development coincided with two other significant milestones in the evolution of nursing theory. One was the standardization of curricula for nursing master's education provided by the National League for Nursing accreditation criteria for baccalaureate and higher degree programs, and the second was the decision that doctoral education for nurses should be in nursing (Alligood, 2006a). The nursing theory era, coupled with an awareness of nursing as a profession and as an academic discipline in its own right, emerged from debates and discussions in the 1960s regarding the proper direction and appropriate discipline for nursing knowledge development. The explosive proliferation of nursing doctoral programs and nursing theory literature substantiated that nursing doctorates should be in nursing (Nicoll, 1986, 1992, 1997; Reed, Shearer, & Nicoll, 2003; Reed & Shearer, 2008). In the 1970s, nursing continued to make the transition from vocation to profession as more and more nurses asked, "Will nursing be other-discipline based or be nursing based?" The history records the answer, "Nursing practice needs to be based on nursing science" (Alligood, 2006a; Fawcett, 1978; Nicoll, 1986). It is as Meleis (2007) noted, "theory is not a luxury in the discipline of nursing . . . but an integral part of the nursing lexicon in education, administration, and practice" (p. 4).

The 1980s was a period of major developments in nursing theory characterized as a transition from the pre-paradigm to the paradigm period (Fawcett, 1984; Hardy, 1978). The prevailing nursing paradigms (models) provided perspectives for nursing practice, administration, education, research and further theory development. In the 1980s, Fawcett's seminal proposal of four global nursing concepts presented a nursing metaparadigm that served as an organizing structure for existing nursing frameworks, and introduced a way of grouping what previously had been viewed as individual theoretical works (Fawcett, 1978, 1984, 1993). Classifying the nursing models as paradigms within a metaparadigm of the concepts *person, environment, health*, and *nursing* systematically united the nursing theoretical works for the discipline. This system clarified and improved comprehension of a knowledge development process by embedding the theorists' works in a larger context, thus facilitating understanding of the growth of nursing science from a paradigm perspective (Alligood & Tomey, 2006; Fawcett, 2005). The body of nursing science and research, education, administration, and practice continues to expand through nursing scholarship. Podium presentations at national and international conferences, newsletters, journals, and books written by communities of scholars associated with the various nursing models and theories describe a theoretical basis for practice and research presenting their scholarship on a selected model or theory from a paradigm perspective (Alligood, 2004; Alligood & Tomey, 2006; Fawcett, 2005; Parker, 2006).

These observations of nursing theory development bring Kuhn's (1970) description of normal science to life. His philosophy of science clarifies our understanding of the evolution of nursing theory through paradigm science. It is important historically that it was individual efforts that led to the first theory as nurse leaders in various areas of the country published their works, which later came to be viewed collectively within a systematic structure of knowledge (Fawcett, 1984, 2000, 2005). Theory development emerged as a product of professional scholarship and growth among nurse leaders, administrators, educators, and practitioners who sought higher education. These leaders recognized limitations of theory from other disciplines to describe, explain, or predict nursing outcomes, and they labored to establish a scientific basis for nursing management, curricula, practice, and research. The use of theory to convey an organizing structure and meaning for these processes led to the convergence of ideas that resulted in what is recognized today as the *nursing theory era* (Alligood, 2006b; Alligood & Tomey, 2006; Nicoll, 1986, 1992, 1997; Reed, Shearer & Nicoll, 2003; Reed & Shearer, 2008).

The accomplishments of normal science opened the theory utilization era as emphasis shifted to theory application in nursing practice, education, administration, and research (Alligood, 2006c; Wood & Alligood, 2006). The theory utilization era restored balance between research and practice for knowledge development in the discipline of nursing. The reader is referred to the fourth edition *Nursing Theory: Utilization & Application* (Alligood, 2010, in press) for case applications and discussion of utilization of nursing theoretical works in practice.

This brief history provides a context for your study of the nursing theorists and their work. The theory era continues with emphasis on development and use of nursing theory to produce evidence for professional practice. Particular utility of middle range theories to guide the thought and action of nursing practice is noted (Alligood, 2006c; Alligood & Tomey, 2006; Fawcett, 2005; Peterson, 2008; Smith & Leihr, 2008). Therefore, preparation for practice in the profession of nursing requires knowledge of the theoretical works of the discipline.

The theoretical works presented in this text are frameworks that have been organized into four types. Box 1-1 lists the theorists included in each type. The four types, although somewhat arbitrary, reflect a certain level of abstraction or the preference of the theorist.

The first type is nursing philosophy. Philosophy sets forth the meaning of nursing phenomena through analysis, reasoning, and logical presentation. Early works that pre-date the nursing theory era contributed to knowledge development by providing direction or a basis for subsequent developments. Later works reflect contemporary human science and its methods (Alligood, 2006b; Chinn & Kramer, 2008; Meleis, 2007). Selected works classified as nursing philosophies are presented in Unit II, Chapters 6 through 11.

Box 1-1 *Types of Nursing Theoretical Works*

NURSING PHILOSOPHIES

Nightingale
Watson
Ray
Benner
Martinsen
Eriksson

NURSING CONCEPTUAL MODELS

Levine
Rogers
Orem
King
Neuman
Roy
Johnson

NURSING THEORIES

Boykin and Schoenhofer
Meleis
Pender
Leininger
Newman
Parse
Erickson, Tomlin, and Swain
Husted and Husted

MIDDLE RANGE NURSING THEORIES

Mercer
Mishel
Reed
Wiener and Dodd
Eakes, Burke, and Hainsworth
Barker
Kolcaba
Beck
Swanson
Ruland and Moore

A second type, nursing conceptual models, comprises nursing works by the theorists who also are referred to as pioneers in nursing (Chinn & Kramer, 2008; Fawcett, 2005; Meleis, 2007). Fawcett (2005) explains, "A conceptual model provides a distinct frame of reference for its adherents . . . that tells them how to observe and interpret the phenomena of interest to the discipline" (p. 16). The nursing models are comprehensive and define the metaparadigm concepts—person, environment, health, and nursing—according to their framework (Fawcett, 2005; Tomey & Alligood, 2006). Many nursing conceptual models include theories that the theorists have explicitly derived from them, and some models have implicit theories within them. Theories differ from models in that they propose a direction or action that is testable (Alligood & Tomey, 2006). An example of theory derived from a nursing model is seen in Roy's work, wherein a theory of the person as an adaptive system is derived from her Adaptation Model. The highly abstract level of the theory (sometimes referred to as grand theory) in this example facilitates the derivation from it of many middle range theories that are specific to nursing practice (Alligood, 2006d). Works classified as nursing models are discussed in Unit III, Chapters 12 through 18.

The third type, nursing theory, is derived from nursing philosophies, conceptual models, or more abstract nursing theories, or from works of other disciplines (Tomey & Alligood, 2006). A work that is classified as a nursing theory is developed from some conceptual framework and is more specific than the framework. Theories may be specific to a particular aspect or setting of nursing practice. For example, Meleis's transition theory (Chapter 20) is specific to aspects of the patient's life process in health and illness. Nursing theories are presented in Unit IV, Chapters 19 through 26.

The fourth type, middle range theory, has an even more specific focus and is more concrete than nursing theory in its level of abstraction (Alligood 2006b, 2006d; Chinn & Kramer, 2008; Fawcett, 2005). Therefore, middle range theories are more precise, with a focus on answering specific nursing practice questions. They specify such factors as the age group of the patient, the family situation, the health condition, the location of the patient, and, most important the action of the nurse (Alligood, 2006c). Middle range theories address the specifics of nursing situations within the perspective of the model or theory from which they are derived (Alligood, 2006b, 2006c, 2006d; Fawcett, 2005). Middle range theories in the nursing literature have been developed inductively as well as deductively. Selected middle range theories are presented in Unit V, Chapters 27 through 36. Table 1-1 presents an example of theoretical knowledge at each level of abstraction within a knowledge structure.

SIGNIFICANCE OF NURSING THEORY

At the beginning of the twentieth century, nursing was neither an academic discipline nor a profession. The accomplishments of the past century have led to the recognition of nursing in both areas. Although these terms (*discipline* and *profession*) are interrelated and some use them interchangeably, important differences between them should be noted. Each has a specific meaning that is important to understand, as noted here:

- A **discipline** is specific to academia and refers to a branch of education, a department of learning, or a domain of knowledge (Donaldson & Crowley, 1978; Orem, 2001; Styles, 1982). A **profession** refers to a specialized field of practice, founded upon the theoretical structure of the science or knowledge of that discipline and accompanying practice abilities (Donaldson & Crowley, 1978; Orem, 2001; Styles, 1982).

The achievements of the profession over the past century were highly relevant to nursing science development, but they did not come easily. History shows that many nurses pioneered the various causes and challenged the status quo with creative ideas for both the health of people and the development of nursing. Their achievements ushered in this exciting time when nursing became recognized as both an academic discipline and a profession (Fitzpatrick, 1983; Kalisch & Kalisch, 2003; Meleis, 2007). This section addresses the significance of theoretical works for the discipline and the profession of nursing. Nursing theoretical works represent the most comprehensive presentation of systematic nursing knowledge; therefore, nursing theoretical works are vital to the future of both the discipline and the profession of nursing.

Significance for the Discipline

Nurses entered baccalaureate and higher degree programs in universities during the last half of the twentieth century, and the goal of developing knowledge as a basis for nursing practice began to be realized. University baccalaureate programs proliferated,

Table 1-1 *Knowledge Structure Levels with Examples*

Structure Level	Example
Metaparadigm	Person, environment, health, and nursing
Philosophy	Nightingale
Conceptual models	Neuman's systems model
Theory	Neuman's theory of optimal client stability
Middle range theory	Maintaining optimal client stability with structured activity (body recall) in a community setting for healthy aging.

Data from Alligood, M. R., & Tomey, A. M. (2006). *Nursing theory: Utilization & application* (3rd ed.). St. Louis: Mosby; and Fawcett, J. (2005). *Contemporary nursing knowledge: Conceptual models of nursing and nursing theories* (2nd ed.). Philadelphia: F. A. Davis.

master's programs in nursing were developed, and a national standardized curriculum was realized through the accreditation process. As was mentioned earlier in this chapter, nursing passed through eras of gradual development (Alligood, 2006a). Nursing leaders offered different perspectives on the development of nursing science. Some advocated nursing as an applied science and others proclaimed nursing as a basic science (Donaldson & Crowley, 1978; Johnson, 1959; Rogers, 1970). History provides evidence of the consensus that was reached; nursing research became essential content in master's curricula, and interest in nursing doctoral programs was on the increase.

In 1977, after *Nursing Research* had been published for 25 years, studies were reviewed comprehensively, and strengths and weaknesses were reported in the journal that year. Batey (1977) called attention to the importance of nursing conceptualization in the research process and the role of a conceptual framework in the design of research for the production of science. This emphasis led into the theory development era that moved nursing toward the goal of developing nursing knowledge to guide nursing practice. At that time, nursing theoretical works began to be published (Johnson, 1968, 1974; King, 1971; Levine, 1969; Neuman, 1974; Orem, 1971; Rogers, 1970; Roy, 1970). Soon after, Fawcett (1978) presented her double helix metaphor, now a classic, on the interdependent relationship of theory and research. It was also at about this time that nursing scholars such as Henderson, Nightingale, Orlando, Peplau, and Wiedenbach were recognized for the relevant nature of their earlier theoretical writings. These early works were developed by educators as frameworks to structure curriculum content or guide course content in nursing programs. Similarly, Orlando's (1961, 1972) theory was derived from the report of an early nationally funded research project designed to study nursing practice.

When the Nurse Educator Nursing Theory Conference was held in New York City in 1978, the major theorists were brought together on the same stage for the first time. Most of them began their presentations by stating that they were not theorists. Although our understanding of the significance of these works for nursing was limited at the time, many in the audience seemed to be aware of the significance of the event. After the first few introductions, the audience just laughed at the theorists' denial of being theorists and quickly became silent and listened carefully as the theorists described the theoretical work they had developed for curricula, research, or practice.

Also noteworthy, Donaldson and Crowley (1978) presented the keynote address at the Western Commission of Higher Education in Nursing Conference in 1977, just as their nursing doctoral program was about to open. They reopened the discussion of the nature of nursing science and the nature of knowledge needed for the discipline and the profession. The published version of their keynote address became a classic reference for use by students in considering nursing as a discipline and recognizing the difference between the discipline and the profession. These speakers called for both basic and applied research, asserting that knowledge was vital to nursing as both a discipline and a profession. They stated that the discipline and the profession are inextricably linked, and failure to recognize and separate them from each other anchors nursing in a vocational rather than a professional view.

Soon after this, nursing conceptual frameworks began to be required as frameworks for curricula in nursing programs and to be recognized as nursing conceptual models that address the major and most vital concepts (metaparadigm) of nursing. The creative conceptualization of a nursing metaparadigm and a conceptual-theoretical structure of nursing knowledge clarified the related nature of the collective works of the major nursing theorists as conceptual frameworks and paradigms of nursing. This approach organized nursing theoretical works into a system of theoretical knowledge, although developed by theorists at different times and in different parts of the country. Each nursing conceptual model was classified on the basis of its performance in relation to a set of analysis and evaluation criteria (Fawcett, 1984). Enhanced understanding of the separate nursing works collectively under a metaparadigm umbrella fostered recognition of nursing theoretical works as a body of nursing knowledge. In short, the significance of theory for the discipline of nursing is that the discipline is dependent upon theory for its continued existence, that is, we can be a vocation or we can be a discipline with a professional style of theory-based practice. The theoretical works have taken nursing to higher levels of education and practice as nurses have moved from the functional focus, or what the nurse does, to a knowledge focus, or what nurses know and how they use what they know to guide their thinking and decision making while concentrating on the patient. Nursing continues to be practiced at numerous levels, including as a vocation and as a profession.

Frameworks and theories are structures about human beings and their health that provide nurses with a perspective of the patient that is characteristic of professional practice. Professionals provide public service in a practice that is focused on those whom they serve. The nursing process is used in practice, but the primary focus is the patient, or human being. Knowledge of persons, health, and environment forms the basis for recognition of nursing as a discipline, and this knowledge is taught to those who enter the profession. Every discipline or field of knowledge includes theoretical knowledge. Therefore, nursing as an academic discipline depends on the existence of nursing knowledge. For those entering the profession, this knowledge is basic for their practice in the profession. Kuhn (1970), a noted philosopher of science, stated, "The study of paradigms . . . is what mainly prepares the student for membership in the particular scientific community with which he [or she] will later practice" (p. 11). This is important to all nurses, but it is particularly important to those who are entering the profession because "in the absence of a paradigm . . . all of the facts that could possibly pertain to the development of a given science are likely to seem equally relevant" (Kuhn, 1970, p. 15). Finally, with regard to the priority of paradigms, Kuhn states, "By studying them and by practicing with them, the members of their corresponding community learn their trade" (Kuhn, 1970, p. 43). Master's students apply and test theoretical knowledge in their nursing practice. Doctoral students who are studying to become nurse scientists develop nursing theory, test theory, and contribute nursing science by conducting theory-based and theory-generating research studies.

Significance for the Profession

Not only is theory essential for the existence of nursing as an academic discipline, it is also vital to the practice of professional nursing. Recognition as a profession was a less urgent issue as the twentieth century ended because nurses had made consistent progress toward professional status through the century. Higher degree nursing is recognized as a profession today. Throughout much of the twentieth century, the criteria for a profession were used as a guide for development. Nursing was the subject of numerous studies by sociologists who used the criteria for a profession. Bixler and Bixler (1959) published a set of criteria tailored to nursing in the *American Journal of Nursing*. These criteria set forth that a profession:

1. Utilizes in its practice a well-defined and well-organized body of specialized knowledge [that] is on the intellectual level of the higher learning
2. Constantly enlarges the body of knowledge it uses and improves its techniques of education and service through use of the scientific method
3. Entrusts the education of its practitioners to institutions of higher education
4. Applies its body of knowledge in practical services vital to human and social welfare
5. Functions autonomously in the formulation of professional policy and thereby in the control of professional activity
6. Attracts individuals with intellectual and personal qualities of exalting service above personal gain who recognize their chosen occupation as a life work
7. Strives to compensate its practitioners by providing freedom of action, opportunity for continuous professional growth, and economic security (pp. 1142-1146)

These criteria have historical value for enhancing our understanding of the developmental path that nurses followed. For example, a knowledge base that is well defined, organized, and specific to the discipline was formalized during the last half of the twentieth century, but this knowledge is not static. Rather, it continues to grow in relation to the profession's goals for the human and social welfare of the society that nurses serve. So although the body of knowledge is important, the theories and research are vital to the discipline and the profession, so that new knowledge continues to be generated. The application of nursing knowledge in practice is a criterion that is currently at the forefront, with emphasis on accountability for nursing practice, theory-based evidence for nursing practice, and the growing recognition of middle range theory for professional nursing practice (Alligood & Tomey, 2006).

In the last decades of the twentieth century, in anticipation of the new millennium, ideas targeted toward moving nursing forward were published. Styles (1982) described a distinction between a collective nursing profession and the individual professional nurse and called for internal developments for a new endowment based on ideals and beliefs of nursing. Her premise was that the profession needed a new, positive approach for the future that was devoid of past problems, if progress in professional development was to continue. Similarly, Fitzpatrick (1983) presented a historical chronicle of twentieth century achievements that led to the professional status of nursing. Both Styles (1982) and Fitzpatrick (1983) referenced a detailed history specific to the development of nursing as a profession. In this text, nursing is recognized as a profession, and emphasis is placed on the relationship between nursing theoretical works and achievement of status as a profession. Similarities and differences have been noted in sets of criteria used to evaluate the status of professions; however, all require the development and use of a body of knowledge that is foundational to the practice of the given profession (Styles, 1982).

As individual nurses grow in their professional status, the use of substantive knowledge for theory-based evidence for nursing is a quality that is characteristic of their practice. This commitment to theory-based evidence for practice is beneficial to patients in that it guides systematic, knowledgeable care. It serves the profession as nurses are recognized for the contributions they make to the healthcare of society. As was noted previously in relation to the discipline of nursing, the development of knowledge is an important activity for nurse scholars to pursue. It is important that nursing continue to be recognized and respected as a scholarly discipline that contributes to the health of society. Finally, and most important, nursing theory is a tool to be used for the reasoning, critical thinking, and decision making required for quality nursing practice because of the following:

> Nursing practice settings are complex, and the amount of data (information) confronting nurses is virtually endless. Nurses must analyze a vast amount of information about each patient and decide what to do. A theoretical approach helps practicing nurses not to be overwhelmed by the mass of information and to progress through the nursing process in an orderly manner. Theory enables them to organize and understand what happens in practice, to analyze patient situations critically for clinical decision making; to plan care and propose appropriate nursing interventions; and to predict patient outcomes from the care and evaluate its effectiveness (Alligood, 2004, p. 247).

Professional practice requires a systematic approach that is focused on the patient, and the theoretical works provide just such perspectives of the patient. The theoretical works presented in this text are examples of those various perspectives. Philosophies of nursing, conceptual models of nursing, nursing theories, and middle range theories provide the nurse with a view of the patient and a guide for data processing, evaluation of evidence, and decisions regarding action to take in practice (Alligood & Tomey, 2006; Chinn & Kramer, 2008; Fawcett, 2005).

With the background of the history and significance of nursing theory for the discipline and the profession, along with the introduction to levels of abstraction of various types of theory within a structure of nursing knowledge, as considered so far in this chapter, we now turn to the topic of analysis of theory, a systematic process for the critical reflection of nursing theoretical works (Chinn & Kramer, 2008).

ANALYSIS OF THEORY

Analysis of theory is the process that is carried out to acquire knowledge of the theoretical work. Analysis is an important process, and it is the first step in applying nursing theoretical works to education, research, administration, or practice. Analysis, critique, and evaluation are methods used to study nursing theoretical works critically. The criteria for analysis of each theoretical work included in this text are clarity, simplicity, generality, empirical precision or accessibility, and the importance of derivable consequences (Chinn & Kramer, 2008). This process is useful for learning about the works and is especially essential for nurse scientists who intend to test, expand, or extend the works. When nurse scientists consider their research interests in the context of one of the theoretical works, areas for further development are discovered through the processes of critique, analysis, and critical reflection. Therefore, analysis is an important process for learning, for developing research projects, and for expanding the science associated with the theoretical works of nursing in the future. Understanding a theoretical framework is vital to applying it in your practice.

Clarity

> How clear is this theory? (Chinn & Kramer, 2008, p. 237)

Clarity and consistency are reviewed in terms of semantics and structure. The meaning of terms speaks to definition, and meaning and structure speak to logic and the consistent and complete use of these terms in the theory. Analysis begins as the major concepts and subconcepts and their definitions are identified. Words have multiple meanings within and across disciplines; therefore, a word should be defined carefully and specifically to the framework (philosophy, conceptual model, or theory) within which it is developed. Diagrams and examples facilitate clarity and consistency. The logical development and type of structure used should be clear, and assumptions should be stated clearly and be consistent with the goal of the theory (Chinn & Kramer, 2008; Reynolds, 1971; Walker & Avant, 2005). Reynolds (1971) speaks to intersubjectivity and says, "There must be shared agreement of the definitions of concepts and relationships between concepts within a theory" (p. 13). Hardy (1978) refers to meaning and logical adequacy and says, "Concepts and relationships between concepts must be clearly identified and valid" (p. 106). Ellis (1968) called it "the criterion of terminology" used to evaluate theory and addresses "the danger of lost meaning when terms are borrowed from other disciplines and used in a different context" (p. 221). Walker and Avant (2005) assert that the logical adequacy of a theory comes from the logical structure of the concepts and statements proposed in the theory.

Simplicity

> How simple is this theory? (Chinn & Kramer, 2008, p. 237)

Simplicity has been highly valued in nursing theory development. Chinn and Kramer (2008) called for simple forms of theory, such as middle range, to guide practice. A theory should be sufficiently comprehensive, presented at a level of abstraction to provide guidance, and have as few concepts as possible with simplistic relations to aid clarity. Reynolds (1971) contends, "the most useful theory provides the greatest sense of understanding" (p. 135). Walker and Avant (2005) suggest that parsimony is elegant in its simplicity, yet broad in content.

Generality

> How general is this theory? (Chinn & Kramer, 2008, p. 237)

The generality of a theory speaks to the scope of concepts and the purpose within the theory. Ellis

(1968) stated, "The broader the scope, the greater the significance of the theory" (p. 129).

The generality of a theoretical work varies by how abstract or concrete it is (Fawcett, 2005).

The significance of abstraction has become better understood in recent years as doctoral students and nurse scientists have come to understand that abstract frameworks are useful for the development of middle range theories. Rogers' (1986) Theory of Accelerating Change is an example of an abstract theory from which numerous middle range theories have been generated.

Empirical Precision

> How accessible is this theory? (Chinn & Kramer, 2008, p. 237)

Empirical precision is linked to the testability and ultimate use of a theory, and it refers to the "extent that the defined concepts are grounded in observable reality" (Hardy, 1978, p. 144). Reynolds (1971) evaluates empirical relevance if "anyone [is] able to examine the correspondence between a particular theory and the objective empirical data" (p. 18). He notes that other scientists should be able to evaluate and verify results by themselves. Walker and Avant (2005) evaluate precision based on the theory's capacity to generate hypotheses and be useful to scientists in adding to the body of knowledge. Chinn and Kramer (2008) discuss accessibility in the context of empirical indicators, clearly bringing the concepts to the level for practice application.

Derivable Consequences

> How important is this theory? (Chinn & Kramer, 2008, p. 237)

A parallel can be drawn between outcome and importance. If research, theory, and practice are to be related meaningfully, then nursing theory should lend itself to research testing, and research testing should lead to knowledge that guides practice. Nursing theory guides research and practice, generates new ideas, and differentiates the focus of nursing from that of other professions (Chinn & Kramer, 2008). Ellis (1968) indicates that to be considered useful, "it is essential for theory to develop and guide practice... theories should reveal what knowledge nurses must, and should, spend time pursuing" (p. 220).

You will see these five criteria for the analysis of theory—clarity, simplicity, generality, empirical precision, and derivable consequences—as they are used for critical reflection of each theoretical work in Chapters 6 through 36. These broad criteria are sufficient for analysis of theoretical works, whether they are applied to works at the level of abstraction of philosophies, conceptual models, theories, or middle range theories.

SUMMARY

This chapter presented an introduction to nursing theory with discussion of its history, significance, and analysis. A nurse increases professional power when using theoretical knowledge as a systematic guide for critical thinking and decision making. Nurses who use theory to structure their practice improve the quality of care as they sort patient data quickly, decide on the nursing action needed, and deliver care with an expectation of the outcome. They are able to discuss with other health professionals how they structure their practice. Theory contributes to achievement of professional autonomy by guiding practice, education, and research within the profession. Considering nursing practice in a theory context helps students develop analytical skills and critical thinking ability and clarify their values and assumptions, and it provides a guide for practice, education, and research (Alligood & Tomey, 2006; Chinn & Kramer, 2008; Fawcett, 2005; Meleis, 2007; Tomey & Alligood, 2006).

Globally nurses are recognizing the rich heritage of the works of the nursing theorists, that is, the philosophies, conceptual models, theories, and middle range theories of nursing. The contributions of the theorists present nursing as a discipline and provide knowledge structure for further development. Models and theories guide theory-based research for evidence-based practice. Debates about which model is best have given way to recognition of the diversity of nursing values that each model represents. Today, we see more and more clarification of the theoretical works as they are used by more and more nurses as framework for theory-based practice. Most important, the philosophies, models, theories, and middle range theories are used in nursing education, administration, research, and practice.

Recognition of normal science from the theoretical works has occurred in this era. The scholarship of the past 3 decades has resulted in an expanded volume of nursing literature around the philosophies, models, theories, and middle range theories that also has improved qualitatively. As more nurses have acquired higher education, understanding of nursing theoretical works has expanded. Use of theory by nurses has dramatically increased knowledge development, and the benefit of improved quality of nursing practice has emerged (Alligood, 2006a; Chinn & Kramer, 2008; George, 2002; Johnson & Webber, 2004; McEwen & Wills, 2006; Parker, 2006).

POINTS FOR *Further Study*

- The Nursing Theory Page at Hahn School of Nursing, University of San Diego at: http://www.sandiego.edu/ACADEMICS/nursing/theory
- http://www.nursingtheory.net
- Clayton State University, School of Nursing, Nursing Theory Link Page at: http://nursing.clayton.edu/eichenberger/nursing
- Donaldson, S. K., & Crowley, D. M. (1978). The discipline of nursing. *Nursing Outlook, 26*(2), 1113-1120.
- Fawcett, J. (1984). The metaparadigm of nursing: Current status and future refinements. *Image: The Journal of Nursing Scholarship, 16*, 84-87.
- Kalisch, P. A., & Kalisch, B. J. (2003). *American nursing in history* (4th ed.). Philadelphia: Lippincott Williams & Wilkins.

REFERENCES

Alligood, M. R. (2006a). The nature of knowledge needed for nursing practice. In M. R. Alligood & A. M. Tomey (Eds.), *Nursing theory: Utilization & application* (3rd ed., pp. 3-15). St. Louis: Mosby.

Alligood, M. R. (2006b). Models and theories in nursing practice. In M. R. Alligood & A. M. Tomey (Eds.), *Nursing theory: Utilization & application* (3rd ed., pp. 17-42). St. Louis: Mosby.

Alligood, M. R. (2006c). Models and theories: Critical thinking structures. In M. R. Alligood & A. M. Tomey (Eds.), *Nursing theory: Utilization & application* (3rd ed., pp. 43-65). St. Louis: Mosby.

Alligood, M. R. (2006d). Areas for further development of theory-based nursing practice. In M. R. Alligood & A. M. Tomey (Eds.), *Nursing theory: Utilization & application* (3rd ed., pp. 487-497). St. Louis: Mosby.

Alligood, M. R. (2004). Nursing theory: The basis for professional nursing practice. In K. K. Chitty (Ed.), *Professional nursing: Concepts and challenges* (4th ed., pp. 271-298). Philadelphia: W. B. Saunders.

Alligood, M. R., & Tomey, A. M. (Eds.). (1997). *Nursing theory: Utilization & application.* St. Louis: Mosby.

Alligood, M. R., & Tomey, A. M. (Eds.). (2002). *Nursing theory: Utilization & application* (2nd ed.). St. Louis: Mosby.

Alligood, M. R., & Tomey, A. M. (Eds.). (2006). *Nursing theory: Utilization & application* (3rd ed.). St. Louis: Mosby.

Batey, M. V. (1977). Conceptualization: Knowledge and logic guiding empirical research. *Nursing Research, 26*(5), 324-329.

Bixler, G. K., & Bixler, R. W. (1959). The professional status of nursing. *American Journal of Nursing, 59*(8), 1142-1146.

Chinn, P. L., & Kramer, M. K. (2008). *Integrated knowledge development in nursing* (7th ed.). St. Louis: Elsevier-Mosby.

Cross, K. P. (1981). *Adults as learners.* Washington DC: Jossey-Bass, a subsidiary of John Wiley & Sons.

Donaldson, S. K., & Crowley, D. M. (1978). The discipline of nursing. *Nursing Outlook, 26*(2), 1113-1120.

Ellis, R. (1968). Characteristics of significant theories. *Nursing Research, 27*(5), 217-222.

Fawcett, J. (1978). The relationship between theory and research: A double helix. *ANS Advances in Nursing Science, 1*(1), 49-62.

Fawcett, J. (1984). The metaparadigm of nursing: Current status and future refinements. *Image: The Journal of Nursing Scholarship, 16*, 84-87.

Fawcett, J. (1993). *Analysis and evaluation of: Nursing theories.* Philadelphia: FA Davis.

Fawcett, J. (2000). *Contemporary nursing knowledge: Conceptual models of nursing and nursing theories.* Philadelphia: F. A. Davis.

Fawcett, J. (2005). *Contemporary nursing knowledge: Conceptual models of nursing and nursing theories* (2nd ed.). Philadelphia: F. A. Davis

Fitzpatrick, M. L. (1983). *Prologue to professionalism.* Bowie, MD: Robert J. Brady.

George, J. (2002). *Nursing theories* (5th ed.). Upper Saddle River, NJ: Prentice-Hall.

Hardy, M. E. (1978). Perspectives on nursing theory. *ANS Advances in Nursing Science, 1*(1), 27-48.

Johnson, B., & Webber, P. (2004). *An introduction to theory and reasoning in nursing* (2nd ed.). Philadelphia: J. B. Lippincott.

Johnson, D. (1959). The nature of a science of nursing. *Nursing Outlook, 7*, 291-294.

Johnson, D. (1968). One conceptual model for nursing. Unpublished paper presented at Vanderbilt University, Nashville, TN.

Johnson, D. (1974, Sept/Oct). Development of the theory: A requisite for nursing as a primary health profession. *Research Nursing, 23*, 372-377.

Kalisch, P. A., & Kalisch, B. J. (2003). *American nursing in history* (4th ed.). Philadelphia: Lippincott Williams & Wilkins.

King, I. (1971). *Toward a theory of nursing.* New York: John Wiley.

Kuhn, T. S. (1970). *The structure of scientific revolutions.* Chicago: University of Chicago Press.

Levine, M. (1969). *Introduction to clinical nursing.* Philadelphia: F. A. Davis.

McEwen, M., & Wills, E. (2006). *Theoretical basis of nursing* (2nd ed.). Philadelphia: Lippincott Williams & Wilkins.

Meleis, A. (2007). *Theoretical nursing: Development and progress* (4th ed.). Philadelphia: Lippincott Williams & Wilkins.

Neuman, B. (1974). The Betty Neuman health systems model: A total person approach to patient problems. In J. P. Riehl & C. Roy (Eds.), *Conceptual models for nursing practice* (pp. 94-114). New York: Appleton-Century-Crofts.

Nicoll, L. (1986). *Perspectives on nursing theory.* Boston: Little, Brown.

Nicoll, L. (1992). *Perspectives on nursing theory* (2nd ed.). Philadelphia: J. B. Lippincott.

Nicoll, L. (1997). *Perspectives on nursing theory* (3rd ed.). Philadelphia: J. B. Lippincott.

Nightingale, F. (1969). *Notes on nursing: What it is and what it is not.* New York: Dover. (Originally published 1859.)

Orem, D. (1971). *Nursing: Concepts of practice.* St. Louis: Mosby.

Orem, D. (2001). *Nursing: Concepts of practice* (6th ed.). St. Louis: Mosby.

Orlando, I. (1961). *The dynamic nurse-patient relationship.* New York: G. P. Putnam's Sons.

Orlando, I. (1972). *The discipline and teaching of nursing process.* New York: G. P. Putnam's Sons.

Parker, M. (2006). *Nursing theory and nursing practice* (2nd ed.). Philadelphia: F. A. Davis.

Peterson, S. (2008). *Middle-range theories: Applications to nursing research* (2nd ed.). Philadelphia: Lippincott Williams & Wilkins.

Reed, P., & Shearer, N. (2008). *Perspectives on nursing theory* (5th ed.). New York: Lippincott Williams & Wilkins.

Reed, P., Shearer, N., & Nicoll, L. (2003). *Perspectives on nursing theory* (4th ed.). Philadelphia: Lippincott Williams & Wilkins.

Reynolds, P. D. (1971). *A primer for theory construction.* Indianapolis: Bobbs-Merrill.

Rogers, M. E. (1970). *An introduction to the theoretical basis of nursing.* Philadelphia: F. A. Davis.

Rogers, M. E. (1986). Science of unitary human beings. In V. Malinski (Ed.), *Explorations on Martha Rogers' science of unitary human beings.* Norwalk, CT: Appleton-Century-Crofts.

Roy, C. (1970). Adaptation: A conceptual framework for nursing. *Nursing Outlook, 18*, 42-45.

Smith, M., & Leihr, P. (2008). *Middle range theory for nursing* (2nd ed.). New York: Springer Publishing.

Styles, M. M. (1982). *On nursing: Toward a new endowment.* St. Louis: Mosby.

Tomey, A. M., & Alligood, M. R. (2006). *Nursing theorists and their work* (6th ed.). St. Louis: Mosby.

Walker, L. O., & Avant, K. C. (2005). *Strategies for theory construction in nursing* (4th ed.). Norwalk, CT: Appleton Lange.

Wood, A. F., & Alligood, M. R. (2006). Nursing models: Normal science for nursing practice. In M. R. Alligood and A. M. Tomey (Eds.) *Nursing theory: Utilization & application,* 3rd ed. (pp. 17-42). St. Louis: Mosby-Elsevier.

CHAPTER 2

History and Philosophy of Science

Sonya R. Hardin and Sue Marquis Bishop

"The study of paradigms…is what mainly prepares the student for membership in the particular scientific community with which he [she] will later practice (p. 11). In the absence of a paradigm…all the facts that could possibly pertain to the development of a given science are likely to seem equally relevant" (Kuhn, 1970, p. 15).

Modern science was established over 400 years ago as an intellectual activity to formalize given phenomena of interest in an attempt to describe, explain, predict, or control states of affairs in nature. Scientific activity has persisted because it has improved quality of life and has satisfied human needs for creative work, a sense of order, and the desire to understand the unknown (Bronowski, 1979; Gale, 1979; Piaget, 1970). The development of nursing science has evolved since the 1960s as a pursuit to be understood as a scientific discipline. Because it is a scientific discipline, the unique contribution of nursing to the care of patients, families, and communities is acknowledged.

HISTORICAL VIEWS OF THE NATURE OF SCIENCE

To formalize the science of nursing, basic questions must be considered, such as "What is science, knowledge, and truth?" and "What methods produce scientific knowledge?" These are philosophical questions. The term *epistemology* is concerned with the theory of knowledge in philosophical inquiry. The particular philosophical perspective selected to answer these questions will influence how scientists perform scientific activities, how they interpret outcomes, and even what they regard as science and knowledge (Brown, 1977). Although philosophy has been documented as an activity for 3000 years, formal science is a relatively new human pursuit (Brown, 1977; Foucault, 1973). Scientific activity only recently has become the object of investigation.

Two competing philosophical foundations of science, rationalism and empiricism, have evolved in the era of modern science with several variations. Gale (1979) labeled these alternative epistemologies as centrally concerned with the power of reason and the power of sensory experience. Gale noted similarities in the divergent views of science in the time of the classical Greeks. For example, Aristotle believed that advances in biological science would occur through systematic observation of objects and events in the natural world, whereas Pythagoras believed that knowledge of the natural world would

Previous author: Sue Marquis Bishop.

result from mathematical reasoning (Brown, 1977; Gale, 1979).

As the discipline has developed, nursing science has been characterized by two branching philosophies of knowledge. Various terms are used to describe these stances, including empiricist and interpretive, mechanistic and holistic, quantitative and qualitative, and deductive and inductive forms of science. Understanding the nature of these philosophical stances facilitates an appreciation of what each form contributes to nursing knowledge.

Rationalism

Rationalist epistemology (scope of knowledge) emphasizes the importance of *a priori* reasoning as the appropriate method for advancing knowledge. *A priori* reasoning utilizes deductive logic by reasoning from the cause of an effect or by generalizing to a particular instance. An example in nursing is to reason that appendicitis (cause) will result in pain (effect). The scientist in this tradition approaches the task of scientific inquiry by developing a systematic explanation (theory) of a given phenomenon (Gale, 1979). This conceptual system is analyzed by addressing the logical structure of the theory and the logical reasoning involved in its development. Theoretical assertions derived by deductive reasoning then are subjected to experimental testing to corroborate the theory. Reynolds (1971) labeled this approach the *theory-then-research strategy.* If research findings fail to correspond to the theoretical assertions, additional research is conducted, or modifications are made in the theory and additional tests are devised; otherwise, the theory is discarded in favor of an alternative explanation (Gale, 1979; Zetterberg, 1966). Popper (1962) argued that science would evolve more rapidly through the process of conjectures and refutations by devising research in an attempt to refute new ideas. For example, his point is simple: You can never prove that all individuals with appendicitis have pain because there might be one individual who presents with no pain. A single person with appendicitis who does not have pain disproves the theory that *all* individuals with appendicitis have pain. From Popper's perspective, "research consists of generating general hypotheses and then attempting to refute them" (Lipton, 2005, p. 1263).

The rationalist view is most clearly evident in the work of Einstein, the theoretical physicist, who made extensive use of mathematical equations in developing his theories. The theories that Einstein constructed offered an imaginative framework, which has directed research in numerous areas (Calder, 1979). As Reynolds (1971) noted, if someone believes that science is a process of inventing descriptions of phenomena, the appropriate strategy for theory construction is the theory-then-research strategy. In Reynolds' view, "as the continuous interplay between theory construction (invention) and testing with empirical research progresses, the theory becomes more precise and complete as a description of nature and, therefore, more useful for the goals of science" (p. 145).

Empiricism

The empiricist view is based on the central idea that scientific knowledge can be derived only from sensory experience. Francis Bacon (Gale, 1979) received credit for popularizing the basis for the empiricist approach to inquiry. Bacon believed that scientific truth was discovered through generalization of observed facts in the natural world. This approach, called the *inductive method,* is based on the idea that the collection of facts precedes attempts to formulate generalizations, or as Reynolds (1971) called it, the *research-then-theory strategy.* One of the best examples that can be used to demonstrate this form of logic in nursing has to do with formulating a differential diagnosis. Formulating a differential diagnosis requires collecting facts, then devising a list of possible theories to explain the facts.

The strict empiricist view is reflected in the work of the behaviorist Skinner. In a 1950 paper, Skinner asserted that advances in the science of psychology could be expected if scientists would focus on the collection of empirical data. He cautioned against drawing premature inferences and proposed a moratorium on theory building until additional facts were collected. Skinner's (1950) approach to theory construction was clearly inductive. His view of science and the popularity of behaviorism have been credited with influencing psychology's shift in emphasis from the building of theories to the gathering of facts between the 1950s and 1970s (Snelbecker, 1974). The difficulty with the inductive mode of inquiry is that the world presents an infinite number of possible observations and, therefore, the scientist must bring ideas to her experiences to decide what to observe and what to exclude (Steiner, 1977). Although Skinner disclaimed to be developing a theory in his early writings, Bixenstine (1964) noted, "Skinner is startlingly creative in applying the conceptual elements of his, let's be frank, theory to a wide variety of issues, ranging from training pigeons in the guidance of missiles, to developing teaching machines, to constructing a model society" (p. 465).

EARLY TWENTIETH CENTURY VIEWS OF SCIENCE AND THEORY

During the first half of this century, philosophers focused on the analysis of theory structure, whereas scientists focused on empirical research (Brown, 1977). Minimal interest was seen in the history of science, the nature of scientific discovery, or the similarities between the philosophical view of science and the scientific methods (Brown, 1977). *Positivism,* a term first used by Comte, emerged as the dominant view of modern science (Gale, 1979). Modern logical positivists believed that empirical research and logical analysis were two approaches that would produce scientific knowledge. Logical positivists hailed the system of symbolic logic, published from 1910 to 1913 by Whitehead and Russell, as an appropriate approach to discovering truth (Brown, 1977).

The logical empiricists offered a more lenient view of logical positivism and argued that theoretical propositions (a proposition affirms or denies something) must be tested through observation and experimentation (Brown, 1977). This perspective is rooted in the idea that empirical facts exist independently of theories and offer the only basis for objectivity in science (Brown, 1977). In this view, objective truth exists independently of the researcher, and the task of science is to discover it. The empiricist view shares similarities with Aristotle's view of biological science and Bacon's inductive method as the true method of scientific inquiry (Gale, 1979). This view of science often is presented in research method courses as the single orthodox view of the scientific enterprise, and it is taught in the following manner: "The scientist first sets up an experiment; observes what occurs . . . reaches a preliminary hypothesis to describe the occurrence; runs further experiments to test the hypothesis [and] finally corrects or modifies the hypothesis in light of the results" (Gale, 1979, p. 13).

The increasing use of computers, which permit the analysis of large data sets, may have contributed to the acceptance of the positivist approach to modern science (Snelbecker, 1974). However, in the 1950s, the literature began to reflect an increasing challenge to the positivist view, thereby ushering in a new view of science (Brown, 1977).

EMERGENT VIEWS OF SCIENCE AND THEORY IN THE LATE TWENTIETH CENTURY

In the latter years of the twentieth century, several authors presented analyses that challenged the positivist position, thus offering the basis for a new perspective on science (Brown, 1977; Foucault, 1973; Hanson, 1958; Kuhn, 1962; Toulmin, 1961). Foucault (1973) published his analysis (first published in French in 1966) of the *epistemology* (knowledge) of human sciences from the seventeenth to the nineteenth century. His major thesis stated that empirical knowledge was arranged in different patterns at a given time and in a given culture. Over time, he found changes in the focus of inquiry in what was regarded by scholars as scientific knowledge and in how knowledge was organized. Further, he concluded that humans only recently emerged as objects of study. Schutz (1967), in his *Phenomenology of the Social World,* argued that scientists seeking to understand the social world could not cognitively know an external world that is independent of their own life experiences. Phenomenology as set forth by Edmund Husserl (1859-1938) proposed that the objectivism of science precluded adequate apprehension of the world (Husserl, 1931, 1970). A phenomenological approach reduces observations or text to the meanings of phenomena, independent of their particular occasions. This approach typically focuses on the lived meaning of experiences.

In 1977, Brown argued an intellectual revolution in philosophy that emphasized that the history of science was replacing formal logic as the major analytical tool in the philosophy of science. One of the major perspectives in the new philosophy emphasized science as a process of continuing research rather than as a product focused on findings. In this emergent epistemology, emphasis shifted to understanding scientific discovery and process as theories change over time.

Empiricists view phenomena objectively, collect data, and analyze them to inductively propose a theory (Brown, 1977). This form is based on the position that objective truth exists in the world, waiting to be discovered. Brown (1977) set forth a new epistemology to challenge the empiricist view, proposing that theories play a significant role in determining what the scientist observes and how it is interpreted. The following story, related to Marquis Bishop by her grandmother, illustrates Brown's premise that observations are concept laden, that is, an observation is influenced by values and ideas in the mind of the observer:

> A husband and wife are sitting by the fire silently watching their firstborn son asleep in the cradle. The mother looks at her infant son and imagines him learning to talk and then to walk. She continues her reverie by imagining him playing with friends, coming home from school, and then going to college. She ends her daydreaming by visualizing him elected president of the United States. She smiles and glances up at her husband, who also had been staring intently at their son. "What are you thinking, honey?" The husband replies, "I was just thinking that I can't imagine how anyone could build a fine cradle like this, sell it for $24.95, and still make a profit."

Brown (1977) presented the example of a chemist and a child walking together past a steel mill. The chemist perceived the odor of sulfur dioxide, and the child smelled rotten eggs. Both observers in the example responded to the same observation but with distinctly different interpretations. In studying family dynamics, students may analyze videotapes of family therapy sessions to learn different approaches to family situations. Novice students tend to focus on the content of family interaction (what one member says to another) or the behaviors of individual family members. After studying a system view of families focused on patterned transactions among family members, students recognize and describe transactions among family members that they did not perceive when first viewing the videotapes. For example, the son withdraws when his parents argue, or the wife grits her teeth when her husband speaks. Concepts and theories set up boundaries and specify pertinent phenomena for reasoning about specific patterns. For example, a social network concept may be more fruitful for studying social relations than the group concept in some instances, because it focuses attention on a more complex set of relationships that are beyond the boundaries of any one setting (Bishop, 1984; Irving, 1977). These examples represent different ideas that can emerge from each person.

If scientists perceive patterns in the empirical world based on their pre-supposed theories, how can new patterns ever be perceived or new discoveries become formulated? Gale (1979) answered by proposing that the scientist is able to perceive forceful intrusions from the environment that challenge his or her *a priori* mental set, thereby introducing questions regarding the current theoretical perspective. Therefore, Brown (1977) maintained that a pre-supposed theoretical framework influences perception; however, theories are not the single determining factor of the scientist's perception. Brown identified the following three different views of the relationship between theory and observation:

1. Scientists are merely passive observers of occurrences in the empirical world. Observable data consist of objective truth waiting to be discovered.
2. Theories structure what the scientist perceives in the empirical world.
3. Pre-supposed theories and observable data interact in the process of scientific investigation (Brown, 1977, p. 298).

Brown's argument for an interactionist's perspective coincides with the scientific consensus in the study of pattern recognition of how humans process information. The following distinct mini-theories have directed research efforts in this area: (1) the data-driven, or bottom-up, theory and (2) the conceptually driven, or top-down, theory (Norman, 1976). In the former, cognitive expectations (what is known or ways of organizing meaning) are used to select input and process incoming information from the environment. The second theory asserts that incoming data are perceived as unlabeled input and are analyzed as raw data with increasing levels of complexity until all data are classified. Current research evidence suggests that human pattern recognition progresses through an interaction of both data-driven and conceptually driven processes, and it uses sources of information in currently organized, cognitive categories and in stimuli from the sensory environment. The interactionist's perspective is clearly reflected in Piaget's theory of human cognitive functioning:

> Piagetian man actively selects and interprets environmental information in the construction of his own knowledge, rather than passively copying the information just as it is presented to his senses. While paying attention to and taking account of the structure of the environment during knowledge seeking, Piagetian man reconstrues and reinterprets that environment [according to] his own mental framework . . . The mind neither copies the world . . . nor does it ignore the world [by] creating a private mental conception of it out of whole cloth. The mind meets the environment in an extremely active, self-directed way (Flavell, 1977, p. 6).

If the thesis is accepted that objective truth does not exist and science is an interactive process between invented theories and empirical observations, how are scientists to determine truth and scientific knowledge? In the new epistemology, science is viewed as an ongoing process. Much importance is given to the idea of consensus among scientists. As Brown (1977) concluded, it is a myth that science can establish final truths. Tentative consensus based on reasoned judgments about available evidence is the most that can be expected. In this view, scientific knowledge is what the community of scientists in any given historical era regard as scientific knowledge. Current consensus among scientists determines the truth of a given theoretical statement by concluding whether or not it presents an adequate description of reality (Brown, 1977). This consensus is possible through the collaboration of many scientists as they make their work available for public review and debate, and as they build upon previous inquiries (Randall, 1964). "The individual (scientist) introduces ideas, the scientific community appraises them" by its objective criteria (Randall, 1964, p. 59).

In any given era and in any given discipline, science is structured by an accepted set of pre-suppositions that define the phenomena for study and define appropriate methods for data collection and interpretation (Brown, 1977; Foucault, 1973; Kuhn, 1962). These pre-suppositions set the boundaries for scientific enterprise in a particular field. In Brown's view of the transactions between theory and empirical observation:

> Theory determines what observations are worth making and how they are to be understood, and observation provides challenges to accepted theoretical structures. The continuing attempt to produce a coherently organized body of theory and observation is the driving force of research, and the prolonged failure of specific research projects leads to scientific revolutions (Brown, 1977, p. 167).

The presentation and acceptance of a revolutionary theory may alter existing pre-suppositions and theories, thereby creating a different set of boundaries and procedures. The result is a new set of problems or a new way of interpreting observations, that is, a new picture of the world (Kuhn, 1962). In this view of science, emphasis must be placed on ongoing research rather than on established findings. According to Kuhn, science progresses from a pre-science, then to a normal science, then to a crisis, then to a revolution, and then to a new normal science. Once normal science develops, the process begins again when a crisis erupts and leads to revolution, and a new normal science emerges once again (Kuhn, 1970; Nyatanga, 2005). This is what Kuhn refers to as a paradigm shift in scientific development within a discipline.

INTERDEPENDENCE OF THEORY AND RESEARCH

Traditionally, theory building and research have been presented to students in separate courses. Often, this separation has caused problems for students in understanding the nature of theories and in comprehending the relevance of research efforts (Winston, 1974). Acceptance of the positivist view of science may have influenced the sharp distinction between theory and research methods (Gale, 1979). Although theory and research can be viewed as distinct operations, they are regarded more appropriately as interdependent components of the scientific process (Dubin, 1978). In constructing a theory, the theorist must be knowledgeable about available empirical findings and must be able to take these into account, because theory is, in part, concerned with organizing and formalizing available knowledge of a given phenomenon. The theory is subject to revision if hypotheses fail to correspond with empirical findings, or the theory may be abandoned in favor of an alternative explanation that accounts for the new information (Brown, 1977; Dubin, 1978; Kuhn, 1962).

In contemporary theories of science, the scientific enterprise has been described as a series of phases, with an emphasis on the discovery and verification (or acceptance) phases (Gale, 1979; Giere, 1979). According to Gale, these phases are concerned primarily with the presentation and testing of new ideas. New ways of thinking about phenomena or new data are introduced to the scientific community during the discovery phase. During this time, the focus is on presenting a persuasive argument to show that the new conceptions represent an improvement over previous conceptions (Gale, 1979). Verification is characterized by the scientific community's efforts to critically analyze and test the new conceptions in an attempt to refute them. The new views then are subjected to testing and analysis (Gale, 1979). However, Brown (1977) argued that discovery and verification could not be viewed as distinct phases, because the scientific community does not usually accept a new conception until it has been subjected to significant testing. Only then can it be accepted as a new discovery.

In any scientific discipline, it is not appropriate to judge a theory on the basis of authority, faith, or intuition; it should be judged on the basis of scientific consensus (Randall, 1964). For example, if a specific nursing theory is deemed acceptable, this judgment should not be made because a respected nursing leader advocates the theory. Personal feelings, such as "I like this theory" or "I don't like this theory," do not provide a valid basis for judgment. The theory should be judged acceptable on the basis of logical and on conceptual or empirical grounds. The scientific community makes these judgments (Gale, 1979).

The advancement of science is thus a collaborative endeavor in which many researchers evaluate and build on the work of others. Theories, procedures, and findings from empirical studies must be made available for critical review by scientists for evidence to be cumulative. The same procedures can be used to support or refute a given analysis or finding. A theory is accepted when scientists agree that it provides a description of reality that captures the phenomenon of available research findings (Brown, 1977). The acceptance of a scientific hypothesis depends on appraisal of the coherence of theory, which involves questions of logic, and on correspondence of the theory, which involves efforts to relate the theory to observable phenomena through research (Steiner, 1978). Gale (1979) labeled these criteria as epistemological and metaphysical concerns.

The consensus regarding the correspondence of the theory, therefore, is not based on a single study. Repeated testing is crucial. The study must be replicated under the same conditions, and the theoretical assertions must be explored under different conditions or with different measures. Consensus, therefore, is based on accumulated evidence (Giere, 1979). When the theory does not appear to be supported by research, the scientific community does not necessarily reject it. Rather than agreeing that a problem exists with the theory itself, the community may make judgments about the validity or the reliability of the measures used in testing the theory, or about the appropriateness of the research design. These possibilities are considered when all attempts to test a given theory are evaluated critically.

Scientific consensus is necessary in three key areas for any given theory as follows: (1) agreement on the boundaries of the theory, that is, the phenomenon it addresses and the phenomena it excludes (criterion of coherence); (2) agreement on the logic used in constructing the theory to enhance understanding from a similar perspective (criterion of coherence); and (3) agreement that the theory fits the data collected and analyzed through research (criterion of correspondence) (Brown, 1977; Dubin, 1978; Steiner, 1977, 1978). Essentially, consensus in these three areas constitutes an agreement among scientists to "look at the same 'things,' to do so in the same way, and to have a level of confidence certified by an empirical test" (Dubin, 1978, p. 13). Therefore, the theory must be capable of being operationalized to test it against reality. Retroductive (abductive reasoning), deductive, and inductive forms of reasoning may be used as science progresses by building theoretical descriptions and explanations of reality, attempting to account for available findings, deriving testable hypotheses, and evaluating theories from the perspective of new empirical data (Steiner, 1978).

Most research may be considered within the category that Kuhn (1962) called *normal science.* Scientific inquiry in normal science involves testing a given theory, developing new applications of a theory, or extending a given theory. Occasionally, a new theory with different assumptions is developed that could replace previous theories. Kuhn (1962) described this as revolutionary science and explained the theory with different pre-suppositions as a revolutionary theory. A change in the accepted presuppositions creates a set of boundaries and procedures that suggest a new set of problems or a new way of interpreting observations (Kuhn, 1962).

In the social and behavioral sciences, challenges to the assumptions underlying accepted methods of experimental design, measurement, and statistical analysis emphasize the search for universal laws and emphasize the use of procedures for random assignment of subjects across contexts. Mishler (1979) argued that, in studying behavior, scientists should develop methods and procedures that are dependent on context for meaning rather than eliminating context by searching for laws that hold across contexts. This critique of the methods and assumptions of research is emerging from phenomenological and ethnomethodological theorists, who view the scientific process from a very different paradigm (Bowers, 1992; Hudson, 1972; Mishler, 1979; Pallikkathayil & Morgan, 1991).

The proper focus of research is not to attempt to support a theory or hypothesis, but rather to refute a given hypothesis (Popper, 1962). Repeated failed attempts at refutation lend support for the theory and acceptance of the theory by the scientific community (Dubin, 1978). However, emphasis is always placed on ongoing research rather than on established findings (Brown, 1977). In the future, new information or a new, compelling way of viewing the same evidence may lead to a reappraisal of the theory. One previously accepted theory is abandoned for another theory if it fails to correspond with empirical findings, or if it does not present clear direction for further research. The scientific community judges the selected alternative theory to account for available data and to suggest additional lines of inquiry (Brown, 1977).

Popper observed that refutations of a given theory frequently are viewed as a failure of the theorist or the theory. In his view, "Every refutation should be regarded as a great success; not merely as a success of the scientist who refuted the theory, but also of the scientist who created the refuted theory and who thus . . . suggested, if only indirectly, the refutation experiment" (Popper 1962, p. 243).

There is neither a single science nor a single scientific method. Several sciences, each with unique phenomena and structure and methods for inquiry, are known (Springagesh & Springagesh, 1986). However, the commonality among sciences concerns the scientists' efforts to separate truth from speculation to advance knowledge (Snelbecker, 1974). In questions regarding the structure of knowledge in a given science, the consensus of scientists in the discipline decides what is to be regarded as scientific knowledge and appropriate methods of inquiry (Brown, 1977; Gale, 1979).

Consensus has emerged in the field of nursing that the knowledge base for nursing practice is incomplete, and that the development of a scientific base for nursing practice is a high priority for the discipline. The postpositivist and interpretive paradigms have achieved a degree of acceptance in nursing as paradigms for guiding knowledge development (Ford-Gilboe, Campbell, & Berman, 1995). Postpositivism focuses on discovery of patterns that may describe, explain, or predict phenomena. It rejects the older, traditional positivist views of an ultimate objective knowledge that is observable only through the senses (Ford-Gilboe et al., 1995; Weiss, 1995). The interpretive paradigm tends to promote understanding by addressing the meanings of the participants' social interactions that emphasize situation, context, and the multiple cognitive constructions that individuals create from everyday events (Ford-Gilboe et al., 1995). A critical paradigm for knowledge development in nursing also has been described as an emergent, postmodern paradigm that provides the framework for inquiries about the interaction between social, political, economic, gender, and cultural factors and the experiences of health and illness (Ford-Gilboe et al., 1995). A broad conception of postmodernism includes the particular philosophies that challenge the "objectification of knowledge," such as phenomenology, hermeneutics, feminism, critical theory, and poststructuralism (Omery, Kasper, & Page, 1995).

The various sciences are at different stages of development. Physics, with the exception of mathematics, is considered the most exacting of the sciences; the life sciences, such as botany, are not as well developed scientifically; the social sciences are even less developed. Until the late 1950s, use of the term *nursing science* in the literature was uncommon. The philosophy of nursing has been developing over a 150-year period; however, Fry (1999) concluded that philosophical inquiry is still a recent development in nursing that is not yet well defined in nursing. She cited the following evidence of increasing interest and productivity in the philosophy of nursing as a field of inquiry:

1. Establishment of the Institute for Philosophical Nursing Research at the University of Alberta in the 1980s
2. Increased publication of articles and books on nursing philosophy
3. Establishment of the journal *The Philosophy of Nursing*

It has been argued that evolutionary changes associated with the information age are changing nurses' views of possible realities and are creating a philosophical shift in nursing (Carper, 1978; Silva, Sorrell, & Sorrell, 1995). This shift was viewed as a transfer from a focus on an exclusive, philosophical emphasis on epistemological questions about knowing to a focus on ontological questions about meaning, being, and reality (Silva et al., 1995). More recently, explosive development of graduate nursing education and increased numbers of nursing doctoral programs have been proposed to be associated with shifts in the philosophy of nursing science, nurses' ontological concerns, and increased attention to the art of nursing (Alligood, 2002).

Compared with other developing sciences, nursing science is in the early stages of scientific development. However, as we begin the twenty-first century, there is abundant evidence that a greater number of nurse scholars are actively engaged in the advancement of knowledge for the discipline of nursing through research and scholarly dialogue. This can be seen in the emergence of middle range theories that utilize inductive and deductive theories, as well as synthesis of theories from different disciplines (Peterson & Bredow, 2004; Sieloff & Frey, 2007; Smith & Liehr, 2003). This new century of nursing scholarship by nurse scientists and scholars explores nursing phenomena of interest and provides evidence for quality, advanced practice.

SCIENCE AS A SOCIAL ENTERPRISE

The process of scientific inquiry may be viewed as a social enterprise (Mishler, 1979). In Gale's words, "Human beings do science" (1979, p. 290). Therefore, it might be anticipated that social, economic, or political factors may influence the scientific enterprise (Brown, 1977). For example, the popularity of certain ideologies may influence how phenomena are viewed and what problems are selected for study (Hudson, 1972). In addition, the availability of funds for research in a specified area may increase research activity in that area. Science does not depend on the personal characteristics or persuasions of any given scientist or group of scientists, but it is powerfully self-correcting within the community of scientists (Randall, 1964). Science progresses by "reasoned judgments on the part of scientists and through debate within the scientific community" (Brown, 1977, p. 167). The dialogue within the discipline of nursing continues to evolve toward increased respect for each approach that elicits new understanding of a phenomenon. The use of a single paradigm or multiple paradigms or the creation of a merged paradigm from many paradigms is debated in relationship to advancements in the epistemology of nursing.

POINTS FOR *Further Study*

- *100 Basic Philosophical Terms* at: http://www.str.org/site/News2?page=NewsArticle&id=5493
- *Kant's Philosophy of Science* at: http://plato.stanford.edu/entries/kant-science/
- *Karl Popper* at: http://www.cscs.umich.edu/~crshalizi/notabene/popper.html
- *Edmund Husserl* at: http://plato.stanford.edu/entries/husserl/
- *Phenomenology* at: http://plato.stanford.edu/entries/phenomenology/
- *Abductive reasoning* at: http://user.uni-frankfurt.de/~wirth/inferenc.htm

REFERENCES

Alligood, M. R. (2002). A theory of the art of nursing discovered in Rogers' Science of Unitary Human Beings, *International Journal for Human Caring, 6*(2), 55-60.

Bishop, S. M. (1984). Perspectives on individual-family-social network interrelations. *Interrelational Journal of Family Therapy, 6*(2), 124-135.

Bixenstine, E. (1964). Empiricism in latter-day behavioral science. *Science, 145*, 465.

Bowers, L. (1992). Ethnomethodology I: An approach to nursing research. *International Journal of Nursing Studies, 29*(1), 59-67.

Bronowski, J. (1979). *The visionary eye: Essays in the arts, literature and science.* Cambridge, MA: MIT Press.

Brown, H. (1977). *Perception, theory and commitment: The new philosophy of science.* Chicago: University of Chicago Press.

Calder, N. (1979). *Einstein's universe.* New York: Viking.

Carper, B. (1978). Fundamental patterns of knowing in nursing. *ANS Advances in Nursing Science, 1*(1), 13-23.

Dubin, R. (1978). *Theory building.* New York: Free Press.

Flavell, J. H. (1977). *Cognitive development.* Englewood Cliffs, NJ: Prentice-Hall.

Ford-Gilboe, M., Campbell, J., & Berman, H. (1995). Stories and numbers: Coexistence without compromise. *ANS Advances in Nursing Science, 18*(1), 14-26.

Foucault, M. (1973). *The order of things: An archaeology of the human sciences.* New York: Vintage Books.

Fry, S. (1999). The philosophy of nursing. *Scholarly Inquiry for Nursing Practice: An International Journal, 13*(1), 5-15.

Gale, G. (1979). *Theory of science: An introduction to the history, logic and philosophy of science.* New York: McGraw-Hill.

Giere, R. N. (1979). *Understanding scientific reasoning.* New York: Holt, Rinehart, & Winston.

Hanson, N. R. (1958). *Patterns of discovery.* Cambridge, MA: Cambridge University Press.

Hudson, L. (1972). *The cult of the fact.* New York: Harper & Row.

Husserl, E. (1931). *Ideas: General introduction to pure phenomenology.* W. R. Boyce Gibson, trans. New York: Humanities Press.

Husserl, E. (1970). *The crisis of European sciences and transcendental phenomenology.* David Carr, trans. Evanston, IL: Northwestern University Press.

Irving, H. W. (1977). Social networks in the modern city. *Social Forces, 55,* 867-880.

Kuhn, T. S. (1962). *The structure of scientific revolutions.* Chicago: University of Chicago Press.

Kuhn, T. S. (1970). *The structure of scientific revolutions* (3rd ed.). Chicago: University of Chicago Press.

Lipton, P. (2005). The Medawar lecture 2004. The truth about science. *Philosophical Transactions of The Royal Society, 360,* 1259-1269.

Mishler, E. G. (1979). Meaning in context: Is there any other kind? *Harvard Educational Review, 49,* 1-19.

Norman, D. A. (1976). *Memory and attention: An introduction to human information processing.* New York: John Wiley & Sons.

Nyatanga, L. (2005). Nursing and the philosophy of science. *Nurse Education Today, 25*(8), 670-674.

Omery, A., Kasper, C. E., & Page, G. G. (1995). *In search of nursing science.* Thousand Oaks, CA: Sage Publications.

Pallikkathayil, L., & Morgan, S. (1991). Phenomenology as a method for conducting clinical research. *Applied Nursing Research, 4*(4), 195-200.

Peterson, S. J., & Bredow, T. S. (2004). *Middle range theories: Application to nursing research.* Philadelphia: Lippincott Williams & Wilkins.

Piaget, J. (1970). *The place of the sciences of man in the system of sciences.* New York: Harper & Row.

Popper, K. (1962). *Conjectures and refutations.* New York: Basic Books.

Randall, J. H. (1964). *Philosophy: An introduction.* New York: Barnes & Noble.

Reynolds, P. (1971). *A primer in theory construction.* Indianapolis, IN: Bobbs-Merrill.

Schutz A. (1967). *The phenomenology of the social world.* Evanston, IL: Northwestern University Press.

Sieloff, C. L. & Frey, M. A. (Eds.) (2007). *Middle range theory development using King's conceptual system.* New York: Springer Publishing Co.

Silva, M. C., Sorrell, J. M., & Sorrell, C. D. (1995). From Carper's patterns of knowing to ways of being: An ontological philosophical shift in nursing. *ANS Advances in Nursing Science, 18*(1), 1-13.

Skinner, B. F. (1950). Are theories of learning necessary? *Psychological Review, 57,* 193-216.

Smith, M. J., & Liehr, P. R. (2003). *Middle range theory for nursing.* New York: Springer Publishing Co.

Snelbecker, G. (1974). *Learning theory, instructional theory, and psychoeducational design.* New York: McGraw-Hill.

Springagesh, K., & Springagesh, S. (1986). Philosophy and scientific approach. *Contemporary Philosophy, 11*(6), 18-20.

Steiner, E. (1977). *Criteria for theory of art education.* Unpublished monograph presented at Seminar for Research in Art Education, Philadelphia.

Steiner, E. (1978). *Logical and conceptual analytic techniques for educational researchers.* Washington, DC: University Press.

Toulmin, S. (1961). *Foresight and understanding.* New York: Harper & Row.

Weiss, S. J. (1995). Contemporary empiricism. In A. Omery, C. E. Kasper, & G. G. Page (Eds.), *In search of nursing science.* Thousand Oaks, CA: Sage Publications.

Winston, C. (1974). *Theory and measurement in sociology.* New York: John Wiley & Sons.

Zetterberg, H. L. (1966). *On theory and verification in sociology.* Totowa, NJ: Bedminster Press.

CHAPTER

3

Logical Reasoning

Sonya R. Hardin and Sue Marquis Bishop

"Like most other words, deduction and induction have common meanings related to, but different from their meaning within systems of logic" (Chinn & Kramer, 2008, p. 215).

Logic is a branch of philosophy that concerns analysis of inferences and arguments. An inference involves forming a conclusion that is based on some evidence. Although the common meaning of *argument* implies a disagreement, in logic, an argument consists of a conclusion and its supportive evidence, such that the premises justify the conclusion. The evidence supporting a conclusion may involve one or more theoretical statements, or premises. Tools of logic permit the analysis of reasoning from the premises to the conclusion (Pospesel, 1974).

Inference describes a systematic form of reasoning that progresses from scientific discovery to a conclusion (Davis, 2006). Whether the conclusion is true requires scientific methods to conduct research studies for truth and explanation of phenomena. Scientists create theories for the purpose of explanation (Gustafsson, 2006).

A theory may be developed through deductive, inductive, or retroductive (abductive) reasoning. The internal coherence of a theory is assessed by the criterion of logical development. This analysis assesses whether the development of the series of theoretical statements in the theory follows a logical form of reasoning. Traditionally, deductive and retroductive approaches have been presented as systematic procedures for devising theory. Although in-depth discussion of the forms of reasoning is beyond the scope of this chapter, it is important to understand the basic differences between the forms of reasoning, so one can follow how a given theorist chose to approach theory building and proceed with evaluation of coherence of the theory.

DEDUCTION

Deduction is the form in which specific conclusions are inferred from more general premises or assertions. Reasoning proceeds from general assertions to specific conclusions. A theory that is developed deductively follows a process with a sequence of premises called *axioms,* that is, statements or propositions that derive from broader premises. The concluding statement is an unknown that leads to theoretical prediction and formation of hypotheses to be

Previous author: Sue Marquis Bishop.

tested empirically. A very basic deductive example is as follows:

1. If A were true, then B would be true.
2. A is true.
3. Therefore B is true (Steiner, 1978).

In logical analysis, letters may be substituted for concepts to keep the emphasis of the analysis focused on the form of argument. The examples below illustrate the process of deductive reasoning.

Example A

Premise 1: *All victims of abuse have low self-esteem.* **(From published research)**

Premise 2: *Jennifer and Tom are victims of abuse.* **(Verified clinically)**

Conclusion: *The nurse would anticipate Jennifer and Tom to have low self-esteem.*

Example B

Premise 1: *All patients with heart failure have low oxygen saturation, crackles in the lungs, shortness of breath, and peripheral edema.* **(From published research)**

Premise 2: *Mrs. Morris, a 54-year-old female, is admitted to the telemetry unit with a diagnosis of heart failure.* **(Verified clinically)**

Conclusion: *The nurse can expect Mrs. Morris to have low oxygen saturation, crackles in the lungs, shortness of breath, and peripheral edema.*

In Examples A and B, the conclusions follow or are deduced from general premises of what is known. Deductive reasoning is based on what is known, and the conclusion represents something yet to be verified in clinical research. Only information presented in the premises is presented in the conclusion. Usually, a number of premises in a proposal lead to the conclusion.

In the nursing literature, you may find the deductive form, whereby authors present their logic for deriving a theory from a nursing model (particularly a middle range theory). This process of premises and conclusions, performed in sequence and clearly labeled, is included more often in dissertations. Once deductive reasoning is learned, it is possible to identify and label the premises and conclusions when reading narrative text (Salmon, 1973). Salmon suggests certain words or phrases as clues that indicate specific statements presented as premises or conclusions. Terms that often precede a premise are connecting words such as *since, for*, and *because.* Terms that often precede a conclusion are *therefore, consequently, hence, so*, and *it follows that* (Salmon, 1973).

A nursing theory example developed through the use of deductive logic is the Roy Adaptation Model. Roy used Helson's (1964) adaptation-level theory as the general premise for her nursing model. Helson presented the behavioral response (of the eye) to stimuli in modes of adaptation to changes in the environment. He labeled stimuli with three classes of cues: focal, contextual, and organic. Working from Helson's premises about adaptation, Roy developed the premise for her theory of the person as an adaptive system and her adaptation model. Tsai (2003) utilized the Roy Adaptation Model to develop a middle range theory of caregiver stress by selecting concepts and specifying their relationships in the context of caregivers and the chronically ill (a full discussion of Roy's theoretical work can be found in Chapter 17 of this text). Example C displays deductive reasoning as used in the Roy Adaptation Theory.

Example C

Premise: *Responses to stimuli represent modes of adaptation to the environment.*

Premise: *Persons experience and respond to stimuli.*

Conclusion: *Therefore persons adapt to their environment.*

The argument may be evaluated in at least two different ways as follows: (1) The validity of the conclusion may be assessed as to whether it logically follows the premises, and (2) the content of the premises may be assessed in terms of the truth or falsity of the statements (Pospesel, 1974). So if you look at example C, the argument can be evaluated by asking these questions: Are the premises true statements? Is the conclusion valid? Do the premises support the conclusion?

The validity of a deductive argument refers to the logic involved in reasoning from the premises to the conclusion, to ensure that, if the premises are true, the conclusion must be true (Pospesel, 1974; Salmon, 1973; Steiner, 1978). A deductive argument may contain all true statements, or one or more false statements, and it may be considered valid or invalid. This judgment is made on the basis of whether the conclusion is supported by the premises.

Example D

Premise: *All victims of abuse have low self-esteem.*
Premise: *Justin has low self-esteem.*
Conclusion: *Therefore Justin is a victim of abuse.*

Although Justin may be the victim of abuse, the truth or falsity of the conclusion or of any of the statements is not an issue when the validity of an argument is evaluated. In Example D, the premises do not present any supportive evidence that Justin is a victim of abuse. Further, the premises do not assert that only victims of abuse have low self-esteem. Justin's low self-esteem could be the result of other antecedents or causes, such as he may have significant physical deformities and poor social support that negatively influenced his social development. The conclusion therefore goes beyond the explicit and implicit information in the premises. This is not a valid argument. Compare the reasoning in Examples A and B and C with that in Example D. *Validity* refers to the form of the deductive argument, and *truth* refers to the content of a given theoretical statement. Therefore, it is inappropriate to label a single theoretical statement as valid or to label an argument as true (Salmon, 1973).

In a valid deductive argument, if the premises are true, the conclusion must be true. This combination is marked *(R)* in Figure 3-1. It is impossible for the conclusion to be false. This combination is marked *(S)* in Figure 3-1. However, if one or more of the premises is false, two outcomes are possible: The conclusion may be either true or false.

Example E presents a deductively valid argument that illustrates how false premises may lead to a false conclusion. This combination is marked *(X)* in Figure 3-1.

Example E

Premise: *The golf ball is larger than the tennis ball.* **(False)**
Premise: *The tennis ball is larger than the basketball.* **(False)**
Conclusion: *Therefore the golf ball is larger than the basketball.* **(False)**

As Figure 3-1 suggests and as Example E illustrates, it is possible that a valid argument can lead to one or more false premises and a true conclusion. This combination is marked *(Y)* in Figure 3-1.

Example F

Premise: *The tennis ball is larger than the basketball.* **(False)**
Premise: *The basketball is larger than the golf ball.* **(True)**
Conclusion: *Therefore the tennis ball is larger than the golf ball.* **(True)**

It may be helpful to study Examples E and F to understand how conclusions derive from the information given in the premises. In science, deductive arguments are a powerful form of reasoning to derive new conclusions in that they explicate implied information. The derived conclusion then is subjected to hypotheses and empirical testing to

		The conclusion is:	
		True	False
If the premises are:	All true	Necessary (R)	Impossible (S)
	Not all true	Possible (Y)	Possible (X)

(R) If the premises are true, it *necessarily follows* that the conclusion be true.
(S) If the premises are true, it is therefore *impossible* for the conclusion to be false.
(Y), (X) If one or more of the premises are false, it is *possible* the conclusion may be *either* true or false.

Figure 3-1 Potential Outcomes of a Valid Deductive Argument. (From Giere, R. N. [1979]. *Understanding scientific reasoning.* [pp. 37-38]. New York: Holt, Rinehart & Winston. Reprinted with permission of Wadsworth, an imprint of Wadsworth Group, a division of Thomson Learning.)

determine whether what was logically concluded corresponds with research findings.

The use of deductive reasoning in a clinical discipline such as nursing requires one to move from the de-contextualized world (an isolated laboratory) to a real life situation (a clinical setting), where one is influenced by emotional and social factors (Smorti, 2008). Human science is an inexact science for this very reason, and the possibility of invalid deductive logic exists. For example, if one believes as a true statement that every patient with hypothyroidism has an abnormal TSH (thyroid-stimulating hormone) test, how does one explain a patient with a normal TSH with hypothyroidism? Use of a universal law to explain patient situations is flawed. Elements of uncertainty in all healthcare decisions require providers to use probability and other forms of reasoning such as inductive reasoning (Soltani & Moayyeri, 2007).

INDUCTION

Induction is a form of logical reasoning in which a generalization is induced from a number of specific, observed instances. Inductive reasoning is not as clearly developed as deductive reasoning (Pospesel, 1974). The form of the inductive argument is as follows:

1. A is true of $b_1, b_2 \ldots b_n$.
2. $b_1, b_2 \ldots b_n$ are some members of class B.
3. Therefore A is true of all members of class B (Steiner, 1978).

The inductive form is based on the assumption that members of any given class share common characteristics. Therefore, what is true for any randomly selected member of the class is accepted as true for all members of the class (Steiner, 1978). Suppose a sample of abuse victims has been selected for study. Example G presents an argument in the inductive form that may be developed on the basis of this hypothetical study.

EXAMPLE G

Premise: *Victims of abuse who have been observed have low self-esteem.*

Conclusion: *All victims of abuse have low self-esteem.*

In another study, a sample of the population of fathers and their newborns has been selected for study. Fathers selected for the study live in the southern city of Charlotte, North Carolina, and are white collar professionals and Asian. Example H presents an argument in the inductive form that may be developed on the basis of a father-newborn pair study of bonding.

EXAMPLE H

Premise: *Every father in the study developed a strong loving bond with his newborn within 2 weeks of birth.*

Conclusion: *All new fathers develop a strong loving bond with their newborns within 2 weeks of birth.*

The premise in Example H states observations from a number of instances, that is, a limited number of subjects and limited to one ethnic, regional, and socioeconomic group. The conclusion states a generalization that extends beyond these observations to the entire class of fathers and their newborns.

The inductive generalization may be stated in terms of a mathematical quantity (Salmon, 1973). For example, assume a researcher surveys a sample of 400 nurses to learn their opinions about whether nurses should establish independent private practices. Results indicate that 60% of those nurses support independent private practice activities in nursing. The inductive statement may be stated as follows.

EXAMPLE I

Premise: *Sixty percent of nurses in the sample support independent private practice activities in nursing.*

Conclusion: *Sixty percent of all nurses support independent private practice activities in nursing.*

The inductive argument can have true premises and still produce a false conclusion. Unlike the deductive argument, if the premises are true, the conclusion must be true. An inductive conclusion based on limited or biased evidence clearly can lead to a fallacious argument and perhaps a false conclusion (Salmon, 1973). Suppose the argument in Example H was developed through one observational study with five middle-class Asian fathers from a city in the Midwest. The conclusion that all fathers develop a strong and loving bond with their newborns within 2 weeks may or may not be true. In any case, this conclusion is not warranted on the basis of a limited number of observed instances. The evidence in this case is insufficient to justify the conclusion about all fathers in America or in the world, or even about middle-class, Midwest, or Asian families.

Even if the sample size is appropriately sufficient (as in Example I), the sample may be biased. Assume that the sample of nurses in Example I was drawn from nursing faculty at large research universities. The opinions of this select group of nurses may be expected to differ in some respects from, and may not reflect the opinions of, all nurses or even of nursing faculty in all schools of nursing. Consideration of a number of factors in selecting representative samples can help avoid the introduction of bias into observations. This reasoning serves as the basis for the random selection of subjects in research projects. Descriptive and inferential statistics are used to characterize the sample of the population and to help with decisions about the strength of the evidence (Giere, 1979). The inductive inference has been termed the *statistical inference* (Steiner, 1978; Weiner, 1958).

In inductive arguments, the inferred conclusion goes beyond the implicit and explicit information in the premises. In Example H, not all fathers and newborns had been observed. Rather, the conclusion is inferred on the basis of selected instances. In a deductive argument, the conclusion can be considered true if the argument is structured so that implicit information in the premises is made explicit (Salmon, 1973). Conversely, the inductive argument goes beyond the information in the premises. Rather, the inductive argument expands upon the presented information. Giere (1979) has noted that induction permits justification of scientific conclusions that may not be verified with the use of deductive reasoning, because they contain information beyond the premises. Whereas deductive arguments are considered valid or invalid, inductive reasoning is viewed in terms of degrees of strength and the probability that the premises lead to a given conclusion (Salmon, 1973). The inferred conclusion may be determined to have low, medium, or high probability (Salmon, 1973). Statistical procedures are used in making these judgments.

In Example A, the conclusion can be false only if one or more of the premises are false, that is, if all victims of abuse do not have low self-esteem, or if Jennifer and Tom are not victims of abuse. If these premises are true, the conclusion must be true. However, in Example G, reasoning suggests that all victims of abuse have low self-esteem. The premises state that only selected victims of abuse have been observed. The premises may lend some support for the conclusion. That victims of abuse without low self-esteem were not observed may be considered evidence, but this fact will not preclude the possibility that a victim with high self-esteem may not be observed in the future (Salmon, 1973). Factors from other studies such as severity of abuse, age at abuse, length of time victim was abused, and subsequent environmental supports, for example, may theoretically change or further specify the assertions to be made about abuse victims.

Whereas deductive arguments are considered to preserve truth, inductive arguments are a form of logic used to explore and uncover new information (Giere, 1979; Salmon, 1973). Scientific generalizations about instances not observed in the present and projections about the future are examples. Although this form of reasoning is useful in advancing science, the very nature of induction may introduce error into the scientific process (Gramling, Lambert, & Pursley-Crotteau, 1998). Even if the premises were accurate, the accuracy of the conclusion cannot be confirmed. In Giere's view, if the premises are assumed to be true, then "the difference between a good inductive argument and a valid deductive argument is that the deductive argument guarantees the truth of its conclusion while the inductive argument guarantees only an appropriately high probability of its conclusion" (1979, pp. 37-38).

Within a human science such as nursing, the use of inductive logic is the norm for the clinician at the bedside. A clinician makes decisions based on the evidence, weighing the degrees of strength of the evidence in the choice of an intervention or the best path to take. Much of evidence-based practice has been designed to standardize care according to the strength of success in an intervention. Theories often are conceptualized initially through an understanding of individual experiences.

Nurse theorists such as Watson and Benner (Chapters 7 & 9, respectively, in this text) used inductive reasoning in developing their theoretical works. Margaret Newman (Chapter 23 in this text) is an example of a work that clearly used both types of reasoning. In her earlier work, she deductively proposed and studied time, space, and consciousness of patterning at particular instances in the life process. Experiences of patients with respect to time informed her how individuals use space and are bound in time. After building on the early foundational work, her theory of Health as Expanding Consciousness subsequently has been expanded through numerous inductive studies and developments.

RETRODUCTION*

Whereas deduction and induction may explicate and evaluate ideas, retroduction generates ideas (Steiner, 1977). *Retroductive reasoning* is an approach to theoretical inquiry that uses analogy as a method for devising theory. Retroduction is also referred to as *abductive reasoning.* In 1878, Charles Peirce described three kinds of reasoning as constituting the major steps of inquiry: (1) retroduction, (2) deduction, and (3) induction, as cited in Steiner (1978). According to Steiner (1978), Peirce viewed retroductive reasoning as the first stage in the search for understanding of a surprising phenomenon, in which a viewpoint that offers a possible explanation is identified. Peirce stated that once a viewpoint was identified that held the promise of explaining an observed phenomenon, deductive reasoning was used to develop the explanation. Peirce considered the final stage of inquiry in terms of induction and focused on checking out the devised hypotheses in experience (Steiner, 1978). Steiner† further developed a theory models approach, using retroductive inference as a method for devising theory. Following is the form of the retroductive inference:

1. The surprising fact, C, is observed.
2. If A were true, C would be a matter of course.
3. Therefore there is reason to suspect that A is true, because no other hypothesis better explains C (Steiner, 1976).

An analysis of the preceding form reveals that theory models (or retroductive inference) diagram the steps of the theory but do not establish truth. Rather, it functions to trigger ideas about selected phenomena that can be developed and tested further. The theory model is useful for devising theory in a field that has few available theories; an innovation to advance knowledge by graphically describing selected observations (Steiner, 1978; Walker & Avant, 2005).

The retroductive theorist may approach the development of a *wanted theory* by identifying a *source theory* in another field that has potential for developing the wanted theory. The theory models approach uses analogy and metaphor between two sets of similar phenomena. This requires that the theorist possess considerable creativity and intuitive knowledge of the phenomena of interest (Steiner, 1976). The theory models approach is represented as follows (Steiner, 1977; Steiner, 1978).

Theory 1 →	*Theory model* →	*Theory 2*
(Source theory)		(Wanted theory)

Therefore, theory models are not models of, but models for, devising representations of selected phenomena (Steiner, 1976). The theory model is essentially a metamodel, which serves as a model for developing theory (Steiner, 1977). To devise a theory using retroductive inference, the theorist seeks out a source theory to form a theory model. The wanted theory is devised from this theory model. The source

*This discussion of retroduction has been adapted from the work of Elizabeth Steiner (Steiner, 1977; Steiner, 1978; Stevens, 1979; Tsai, 2003).

†Elizabeth Steiner's earlier work on theory models was published under her married name of Maccia (Maccia, Maccia, & Jewett, 1963; Norman, 1976).

theory is selected on the basis of a similarity in structure, form, or relationships between the two sets of phenomena (Steiner, 1978). The selected source theory is perceived to present ideas that may be useful for developing a theory about the observations of interest. These ideas are selected from theory 1 and transformed into a point of view or a theory model that will serve as the framework for developing theory 2. This approach is based on the assumption that new conjectures, or ideas, in a given field may be devised from conjectures and theories in other fields (Maccia & Maccia, 1966; Maccia et al., 1963; Steiner, 1978). The ideas selected from theory 1 for the theory model may involve any combination of concepts, hypothesized relationships, and theory structures. The viewpoint presented by the theory model is used to develop theory 2 by adding content to the theory model and by altering concepts and relationships to fit the phenomenon of interest for theory 2. It should be clear that this process of theory building is not borrowing a theory from one field and applying it unchanged to another (Steiner, 1976). The retroductive inference theory-building process, then, may result in a new theory. For example, one could take a theory of the chronic cycle in patients and draw a parallel relationship to a similar cycle in homeless persons by comparing and establishing the similar pattern in their characteristics, resulting in a new theory of homeless persons.

The theory model approach is not considered reductive or derived because theory 1 is not equivalent to theory 2 (Maccia et al., 1963; Steiner, 1977; Steiner, 1978; Walker & Avant, 2005). This approach is not considered deductive either, because theory 2 was not developed by deduction from theory 1. The hypotheses in theory 2 cannot be derived from theory 1 (Steiner, 1977, 1978). A theory devised by this method must meet the criteria for adequacy of a theory (Steiner, 1977, 1978). The new theory is evaluated in terms of its correspondence with available scientific nursing literature, and hypotheses can be tested empirically through research (Smorti, 2008).

The use of analogy to develop theory was a common occurrence in the development of early scientific fields. In Sigmund Freud's time, the machine model was popular. Freud used the notion of machine operations to develop his theoretical assertions about psychological tension-reduction relationships in his theory of psychosexual development. Three or more decades ago, basic texts in human anatomy and physiology used the telephone switchboard as an analogy for explaining brain function. The computer is used often as a model for contemplating the brain and for developing theories of human information processing (Norman, 1976; Shepherd, 1974). In nursing, Fawcett (2005) has noted the inadequacy of mechanistic models for nursing science.

Stevens (1979) proposed that nursing research had little impact on nursing practice because the research was based on categories and characteristics in borrowed theories. In this instance, the problem was not as much that the theory was borrowed, but that it was applied unchanged to nursing studies of phenomena that were presented in a different context. Whereas, theories in other fields may suggest a possible framework for addressing nursing phenomena, a borrowed theory has to be reformulated into nursing, that is, the borrowed theory must be analyzed and synthesized to represent appropriate categories and characteristics for application within the discipline of nursing.

The derivation strategy of Walker and Avant (2005) for theory construction draws from the theory models approach that Steiner developed. Walker and Avant (2005) present examples of the derivation strategy that clearly illustrate how to reformulate concepts, theoretical statements, and theories from other fields to the discipline of nursing. Similarly, Villarruel, Bishop, Simpson, Jemmott, and Fawcett (2001) emphasized the need for systematic analysis of borrowed theories to contextualize the theory in nursing, and to examine whether it adequately describes, explains, or predicts nursing phenomena.

The Modeling and Role Modeling Theory (Erickson, Tomlin, & Swain, 2002) presented in chapter 25 of this text and the Symphonological Bioethical Theory discussed in Chapter 26 of this text are examples of theories that utilized retroductive reasoning. Both propose models to explain their approach to phenomena. Gordon, Morton, and Brooks (2005) reported on the use of abductive reasoning (retroduction) and inferred that the Tidal Model of Mental Health Recovery (Chapter 32 of this text) resulted in provision of improved quality of care to patients, as well as enhanced nurse satisfaction.

Another example, Dalton (2003), used a modified version of theory derivation to develop a theory of triadic collaborative decision making in nursing practice. She selected aspects of a dyadic theory of nurse-patient decision making and added additional key concepts and relationships from nursing practice (e.g., family caregiver) to expand the theory model to a triadic theory of decision making. The inclusion of the family caregiver concept introduced other elements that required additional information from the literature about the family caregiver and the relationship of the caregiver with the patient and the nurse (e.g., concepts about caregivers and coalition formation among participants in the model). The resulting theory of client-nurse-family caregiver collaborative decision making then was analyzed for its correspondence with the literature. Aspects of this derived theory have been subjected to initial testing (Dalton, 2003). Nursing middle range theories may resemble abduction or retroduction in that they introduce new clinical detail; however, they are not retroductive in that they are developed deductively and directly from a nursing model to which they are linked linguistically. They contain clinical details; however, they present clear propositions and relationship statements that are drawn deductively from a nursing conceptual model. In the earliest phase of her work, Tsai (2003), mentioned earlier, presented an example of a middle range theory that may have used retroduction; she clearly anchored her middle range theory as a formulation by using Roy's Adaptation Model.

However, Gramling and colleagues (1998) provided a good example of the use of retroduction with the goal of developing a theoretical model of stressors and coping in young women. Aspects of the Lazarus and Folkman transactional theory of coping were selected, and aspects of women's development from the literature were incorporated into the model. The resulting framework guided a qualitative study of 26 women, and these findings reported a new model of coping for young women. The theory models approach (retroductive inference) permits the translation and expansion of ideas within the milieu of nursing and may result in the development of a new nursing theory. A nursing theory devised by this method may be developed further with the use of deductive strategies as it is subjected to rigorous analysis for congruence with the existing research literature and rigorous testing in empirical studies. In conclusion, Table 3-1 presents for your review a summary of deductive, inductive, and retroductive forms of reasoning.

Table 3-1 Deduction, Induction, and Retroduction Summary

Type	Question	Techniques	Definition	Example	Question
Deduction	Given that the premises are true, what other propositions may be inferred as necessary conclusions from the premises?*	Logical and conceptual analysis*	(1) If A were true, then B would be true (2) A is true (3) Therefore B is true†	*Premises:* All victims of abuse have low self-esteem Mary and Tom are victims of abuse *Conclusion:* Mary and Tom have low self-esteem	*Explicates and derives further truth:* If premises are true, establishes truth of something else by derivation‡

Continued

Table 3-1 Deduction, Induction, and Retroduction Summary—cont'd

Type	Question	Techniques	Definition	Example	Question
Induction	Given that the premises are true, what is the strength of the link between them and the conclusion?*	Logical and conceptual analysis based on statistical analysis‡§	(1) A is true of $b_1, b_2 \ldots b_n$ (2) $b_1, b_2 \ldots b_n$ are some members of class B (3) Therefore A is true of all members of class B†	*Premise:* $b_1, b_2 \ldots b_n$ victims of abuse who have been observed have low self-esteem *Conclusion:* All victims of abuse have low self-esteem	*Evaluates and expands information:* Based on probability of observed cases Does not establish truth Establishes probability of certainty, strength of evidence New data may change conclusion‖
Retroduction	Given a surprising observation, what explanation would result in the expectation that the observation would be a matter of course?*	Logical and conceptual analysis‡	(1) The surprising fact, C, is observed (2) But if A were true, C would be a matter of course (3) Therefore there is reason to expect that A is true†	*Proposition 1:* The role of expecting a reward determines a relation between student and teacher that establishes a path for influence of the teacher on the student‖ *Proposition 2:* The role of expecting care and comfort determines a relation between patient and nurse that establishes a path for influence of the nurse on the patient	*Originates ideas:* Does not establish truth Suggests lines of thought worthy of exploration and testing‡

*Steiner, 1976.
†Steiner, 1977.
‡Steiner, 1978.
§Stevens, 1979.
‖Giere, 1979.
¶Maccia et al., 1963.

POINTS FOR *Further Study*

- Deduction and Induction Reasoning Comparison Diagram at: http://www.socialresearchmethods.net/kb/dedind.php
- Chinn, P. L., & Kramer, M. K. (2008). *Integrated theory and knowledge development in nursing* (7th ed., pp. 214-216). St. Louis: Mosby-Elsevier.
- Abductive Reasoning at: http://user.uni-frankfurt.de/~wirth/inferenc.htm

REFERENCES

Chinn, P. L., & Kramer, M. K. (2008). *Integrated theory and knowledge development in nursing* (7th ed.). St. Louis: Mosby-Elsevier.

Dalton, J. M. (2003). Development and testing of the theory of collaborative decision-making in nursing practice for triads. *Journal of Advanced Nursing, 41*(1), 22-33.

Davis, R. H. (2006). Strong inference: rationale or inspiration? *Perspectives in Biology and Medicine, 49*(2), 238-250.

Erickson, H., Tomlin, E. M., & Swain, M. A. P. (2002). *Modeling and role-modeling: A theory and paradigm for nursing.* Englewood Cliffs, NJ: Prentice Hall.

Fawcett, J. (2005). *Analysis and evaluation of contemporary nursing knowledge* (2nd ed.). Philadelphia: FA Davis.

Giere, R. N. (1979). *Understanding scientific reasoning.* New York: Holt, Rinehart, & Winston.

Gordon, W., Morton, T., & Brooks, G. (2005). Launching the Tidal Model: Evaluating the evidence. *Journal of Psychiatric & Mental Health Nursing, 12*(6), 703-712.

Gramling, L. F., Lambert, V. A., & Pursley-Crotteau, S. (1998). Coping in young women: Theoretical retroduction. *Journal of Advanced Nursing, 28*(5), 1082-1091.

Gustafsson, B. (2006). The philosophy of science from a nursing-scientific perspective. *Theoria, Journal of Nursing Theory, 15*(4), 31-41.

Helson, H. (1964). *Adaptation level theory.* New York, NY: Harper & Row.

Maccia, E. S., & Maccia, G. (1966). *Construction of educational theory derived from three educational theory models* (Project No. 5-0638). Washington, DC: U.S. Department of Health, Education, and Welfare.

Maccia, E. S., Maccia, G., & Jewett, R. (1963). *Construction of educational theory models* (Cooperative Research Project No. 1632). Washington, DC: Office of Education, U.S. Department of Health, Education, and Welfare.

Norman, D. A. (1976). *Memory and attention: An introduction to human information processing.* New York: John Wiley & Sons.

Pospesel, H. (1974). *Propositional logic.* Englewood Cliffs, NJ: Prentice Hall.

Salmon, W. C. (1973). *Logic.* Englewood Cliffs, NJ: Prentice Hall.

Shepherd, G. M. (1974). *The synaptic organization of the brain.* New York: Oxford University Press.

Smorti, A. (2008). Everyday life reasoning, possible worlds and cultural processes. *Integrative Psychological & Behavioral Science, 42*(2), 224-232.

Soltani, A., & Moayyeri, A. (2007). Deterministic versus evidence-based attitude towards clinical diagnosis. *Journal of Evaluation in Clinical Practice, 13*(4), 533-537.

Steiner, E. (1976). *Logical and conceptual analytic techniques for educational researchers.* Unpublished paper presented at the American Educational Research Association, San Francisco.

Steiner, E. (1977). *Criteria for theory of art education.* Unpublished paper presented at the Seminar for Research in Art Education, Philadelphia.

Steiner, E. (1978). *Logical and conceptual analytic techniques for educational researchers.* Washington, DC: University Press.

Stevens, B. (1979). *Nursing theory: Analysis, application, evaluation.* Boston: Little, Brown.

Tsai, P. (2003). A middle-range theory of caregiver stress. *Nursing Science Quarterly, 16*(2), 137-145.

Villarruel, A. M., Bishop, T. L., Simpson, E. M., Jemmott, L. S., & Fawcett, J. (2001). Borrowed theories, shared theories, and the advancement of nursing knowledge. *Nursing Science Quarterly, 14*(2), 158-163.

Walker, L. O., & Avant, K. C. (2005). *Strategies for theory construction in nursing.* Norwalk, CT: Appleton & Lange.

Weiner, P. (1958). *Values in universe of chance.* New York: Doubleday.

CHAPTER

4

Theory Development Process

Sonya R. Hardin and Sue Marquis Bishop

"Nursing's potential for meaningful human service rests on the union of theory and practice for its fulfillment" (Rogers, 1970, p. viii).

Theory development in nursing is an essential component of nursing scholarship undertaken to advance the knowledge of the discipline. Nursing theories that clearly set forth an understanding of nursing phenomena guide scholarly development of the science of nursing practice through research. Once a nursing theory addressing a phenomenon of interest has been proposed, several considerations follow, such as its completeness and logic, internal consistency, and correspondence with empirical findings, and whether it has been defined operationally for testing. Analyses of this nature lead logically to further development of the theory. Scientific evidence accumulates through repeated rigorous research that supports or refutes theoretical assertions and guides modifications or extensions of the theory. Nursing theory development is not a mysterious activity, but a scholarly endeavor that is pursued systematically. Rigorous development of nursing theories, then, is a high priority for the future of the discipline and the practice of the profession of nursing.

It is important to understand the concept of *systematic development* because approaches to construction of theory differ. One aspect that they have in common is that they approach theory development in a precise, systematic manner, making the stages of development explicit. The nurse who systematically devises a theory of nursing and publishes it for the nursing community to review and debate engages in a process that is essential to advancement of theory development. As scholarly work is published in the literature, nurse theoreticians and researchers review and critique the adequacy of the logical processes used in the development of the theory with fresh eyes in relation to practice and available research findings.

THEORY COMPONENTS

Development of theory requires an understanding of selected scholarly terms, definitions, and assumptions, so that scholarly review and analysis may occur. Attention is given to terms and defined meanings to enhance understanding of the theory development process that was used. Therefore, the clarity of terms and their scientific utility and value to the discipline are important considerations in the process.

Hage (1972) identified six theory components and specified the contributions that they make

Previous author: Sue Marquis Bishop.

to theory (Table 4-1). Three categories of theory for these components are presented as a basis for understanding the function of each element in the theory-building process.

Concepts and Definitions

Concepts, the building blocks of theories, classify the phenomena of interest (Kaplan, 1964). It is crucial that concepts are considered within the theoretical system in which they are embedded and from which they derive their meaning, because concepts may have different meanings in various theoretical systems. Scientific progress is based on critical review and testing of a researcher's work by the scientific community.

Concepts may be abstract or concrete. Abstract concepts are constructed mentally independent of a specific time or place, whereas concrete concepts are experienced directly and relate to a particular time or place (Chinn & Kramer, 2008; Hage, 1972; Reynolds, 1971).

Abstract Concepts	Concrete Concepts
Social system	The Marquis family 2 South Surgery Floor Memorial Hospital Nurse-patient-family caregiver
Debate	Obama-McCain Debate
Telemetry	Electrocardiogram, Holter monitor
Loss of relationship	Divorce, widowhood
Nurse competency	Cultural, nasogastric tube placement, medication administration

The Marquis family, the surgery unit, the hospital, and the nurse-patient-family caregiver are examples of concrete concepts of the abstract concept, social system; the other examples illustrate the abstract to concrete difference. In a given theoretical system, the

Table 4-1 *Theory Components and Their Contributions to the Theory*

Theory Components	Contributions to the Theory
CONCEPTS AND DEFINITIONS	
Concepts	Describe and classify phenomena
Theoretical definitions of concept	Establish meaning
Operational definitions of concept	Provide measurement
RELATIONAL STATEMENTS	
Theoretical statements	Relate concepts to one another; permit analysis
Operational statements	Relate concepts to measurements
LINKAGES AND ORDERING	
Linkages of theoretical statements	Provide rationale for why theoretical statements are linked; add plausibility
Linkages of operational statements	Provide rationale for how measurement variables are linked; permit testability
Organization of concepts and definitions into primitive and derived terms	Eliminates overlap (tautology)
Organization of statements and linkages into premises and derived hypotheses and equations	Eliminates inconsistency

Modified from Hage, J. (1972). *Techniques and problems in theory construction in sociology.* New York: John Wiley & Sons.

definition, characteristics, and functioning of a social system clarify more specific instances, such as the nurse-patient-family caregiver social system.

Concepts may be classified as *discrete* or *continuous concepts.* This system of labels differentiates types of concept that specify categories of phenomena. A discrete concept identifies categories or classes of phenomena, such as patient, nurse, health, or environment. A student can become a nurse or can choose another profession, but he or she cannot become a partial nurse. Phenomena identified as belonging to, or not belonging to, a given class or category may be called *nonvariable concepts.* Sorting phenomena into nonvariable, discrete categories conveys the assumption that the associated reality is captured by the classification (Hage, 1972). The amount or degree of the variable is not an issue.

Theories may be used as a series of nonvariable discrete concepts (and subconcepts) that can be used to build typologies. Typologies are systematic arrangements of concepts within a given category. For example, a typology on marital status could be partitioned into marital statuses in which a population is classified as married, divorced, widowed, or single. These discrete categories could be partitioned further to permit the classification of an additional variable in this typology. A typology of marital status and gender is shown in Table 4-2. Participants are of one gender or the other; no degree of how much they adhere to this is shown in this discrete category. If the illustration is taken further, the typology can be partitioned while the discrete concept of children is added. Participants would be classified for gender and marital status, and as *having or not having children.*

A *continuous concept,* on the other hand, permits classification of dimensions or gradations of a phenomenon, indicating degree of marital conflict. Marital couples may be classified, with a range representing degrees of marital conflict in their relationships.

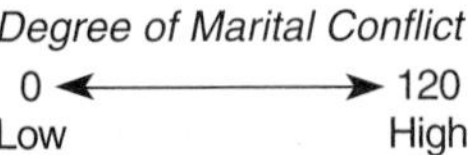

Other continuous concepts that may be used to classify couples might include extent of communication, number of shared activities, and number of children. Examples of continuous concepts used to classify patients include degree of temperature, level of anxiety, and age. Another example is how nurses conceptualize pain as a continuous concept, when they ask patients to rate their pain on a scale from 0 to 10 so they can better understand their pain threshold or pain experience.

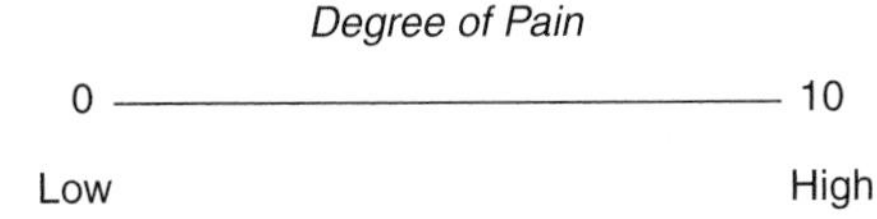

Continuous concepts are not expressed in either/or terms but rather in *degrees on a continuum.* The use of variable concepts on a continuum tends to focus on one dimension but does so without assuming that a single dimension captures all of the reality of the phenomenon. Additional dimensions may be devised to measure additional aspects of the phenomenon. Instruments may measure a concept and may have subscales that measure discrete concepts related to the overall concept. Variable concepts, such as ratio of

Table 4-2 Typology of Marital Status and Gender

	MARITAL STATUS			
Participants	**Single**	**Married**	**Divorced**	**Widowed**
Male	15	75	23	6
Female	25	72	41	13
Total	40	147	64	19

professional to nonprofessional staff, communication flow, or ratio of registered nurses to patients, are used to characterize healthcare organizations. Although nonvariable concepts are useful in classifying phenomena in theory development, Hage (1972) points out major breakthroughs in several disciplines as the focus shifted from nonvariable to variable concepts, because variable concepts permit scoring of the full range of variation of the phenomenon.

The development of concepts, then, permits description and classification of phenomena (Hage, 1972). The labeled concept specifies boundaries for selecting phenomena for observation and for reasoning about the phenomena of interest. New concepts may focus attention on new phenomena or may facilitate thinking about phenomena in a different way (Hage, 1972). Scholarly analysis of the concepts in nursing theories is a critical beginning step in the process of theoretical inquiry. The concept process continues to flourish, with many examples given in the nursing literature. See Table 4-3 for references to analyses carried out using different approaches.

Concept analysis is an important beginning step in the process of theory development undertaken to develop a conceptual definition. It is crucial that concepts are defined clearly to reduce ambiguity in the given concept or set of concepts. To eliminate perceived differences in meaning, explicit definitions are necessary. As the theory develops, theoretical and operational definitions provide the theorist's meaning of the concept and the basis for empirical indicators. For example, Spear and Kulbok (2004) published a concept analysis of the autonomy of adolescents, in which autonomy was defined theoretically as independence or self-governance during the adolescent years. The concept of autonomy was operationalized as an active, individualized, holistic, contextual, and developmental process–oriented state of being.

Theories are tested in reality; therefore the concepts must be linked to operational definitions that relate the concepts to observable phenomena specifying empirical indicators. See Table 4-4 for examples of concepts and their theoretical definitions and operational definitions. These linkages are vital to the logic of the theory, its observation, and its measurement.

Relational Statements

Statements in a theory may state definitions or relations among concepts. Whereas definitions provide descriptions of the concept, relational statements

Table 4-3 *Examples of Published Concept Analyses with Different Approaches*

Concept	Approach	Author
Spirituality	Chinn & Kramer (2008)	Buck (2006)
Readiness to change	Chinn & Kramer (2008)	Dalton & Gottlieb (2003)
Facilitation	Morse (1995)	Harvey, et al. (2002)
Ethical sensitivity	Morse (1995)	Weaver, Morse, & Mitcham (2008)
Self-management of child and adolescent type I diabetes	Rodgers (1989)	Schilling, Grey, & Knafl (2002)
Risk	Rodgers (1989)	O'Byrne (2008)
Symptom perception	Schwartz-Barcott & Kim (2000)	Posey (2006)
Being sensitive	Schwartz-Barcott & Kim (2000)	Sayers & de Vries (2008)
Authenticity	Walker & Avant (2005)	Starr (2008)
Competency	Walker & Avant (2005)	Scott Tilley (2008)

Table 4-4 Examples of Theoretical and Operational Definitions

Concept	Theoretical Definition	Operational Definition
Body temperature	Homeothermic range of one's internal environment maintained by the thermoregulatory system of the human body	Degree of temperature measured by oral thermometer taken for 1 minute under the tongue
Heart failure	Inadequate cardiac function to meet circulatory demands*	Stage of heart failure is measured by the New York Heart Association (NYHA) classification†
Spirituality	A pan-dimensional awareness of the mutual human/environmental field process (integrality) as a manifestation of higher frequency patterning (resonancy) associated with innovative, increasingly creative and diverse (helicy) experiences‡	Score on the Spiritual Inventory Belief Scale (SIBS), an instrument that measures a person's spirituality in the search for meaning and purpose§ The SIBS consists of four subscales: 1) Internal/fluid 2) Humility/personal application 3) External/meditative 4) External/ritual‖

*Hussey & Hardin, 2003.
†AHA, 2004.
‡Malinski, 1994.
§Hatch, Burg, Naberhaus, & Hellmich, 1998.
‖Hardin, Hussey, & Steele, 2003.

propose relationships between and among two or more concepts. Concepts are the building blocks of theory, and theoretical statements are the chains that link the blocks to build theory. Concepts must be connected with one another in a series of theoretical statements to devise a nursing theory.

In connections between variables, one variable may be proposed to influence a second. In this case, the first variable may be viewed as the antecedent or determinant (independent) and the second as the consequent or resultant (dependent) variable (Giere, 1997). Zetterberg (1966) concluded that the development of two-variate theoretical statements could be an important intermediate step in the development of a theory. These statements can be reformulated later as the theory evolves, or as new information becomes available. An example of an antecedent and a consequence is explained by looking at the concept of autonomy in which the antecedents of autonomy were identified as experience, education, ability to prioritize, ability to discriminate, self-discipline, and acceptance of responsibility; consequences are identified with accountability. These antecedents and consequences were developed from the literature (Keenan, 1999).

Theoretical assertions are a necessary or sufficient condition, or both. These labels characterize conditions that help explain the nature of the relationship between two variables in theoretical statements. For example, a relational statement expressed as a sufficient condition could be the following: If nurses react with approval of patients' self-care behaviors *(NA)*, patients increase their efforts in self-care activities *(PSC)*. This is a type of compound statement that links antecedent and consequent variables. The statement does not assert the truth of the antecedent.

Rather, the assertion is made that if the antecedent is true, then the consequence is true (Giere, 1979). In addition, no assertion appears in the statement to explain why the antecedent is related to the consequence. In symbolic notation form, the statements may be expressed as follows:

NA ——→ *PSC*
(Antecedent/determinant ——→ Consequent/resultant)

A sufficient condition asserts that one variable results in the occurrence of another variable. It does not claim that it is the only variable that can result in the occurrence of the other variable. This statement asserts that nurse approval of a patient's self-care behaviors is sufficient for the occurrence of the patient's self-care activities. However, patient assumption of self-care activities resulting from other factors, such as the patient's health status and personality variables, is not ruled out. Other antecedent conditions may be sufficient for the patient's assumption of self-care activities.

A statement in the form of a necessary condition asserts that one variable is required for the occurrence of another variable. For example:

If patients are motivated to get well (WM = wellness motivation), then they will adhere to their prescribed treatment regimen (AR).

WM ——→ *AR*

This means that adherence to a treatment regimen *(AR)* never occurs unless wellness motivation *(WM)* occurs. It is not asserted that patients' adherence to the treatment regimen stems from their wellness motivation. However, it is asserted that if the wellness motivation is absent, patients will not assume strict adherence to their treatment regimens. The wellness motivation is a necessary, but not a sufficient, condition for the occurrence of this consequence.

The term *if* generally is used to introduce a sufficient condition, whereas *only if* and *if . . . then* are used to introduce necessary conditions (Giere, 1979). Usually, conditional statements are not both necessary and sufficient. However, it is possible for a statement to express both conditions. In such instances, the term *if and only if* is used to imply that conditions are both necessary and sufficient for one another. In this case, (1) the consequence never occurs in the absence of the antecedent, and (2) the consequence always occurs when the antecedent occurs (Giere, 1979). It should be noted that not all conditional statements are causal. For example, "If this month is November, then the next month is December," does not assert that November causes December to occur; rather, the sequence of months suggests that December follows November (Dubin, 1978; Giere, 1979).

Giere (1997) further differentiates deterministic models from probabilistic models in his discussion of causal statements. Theoretical statements from a deterministic model assert that the presence or absence of one variable determines the presence or absence of a second variable. The probabilistic model is another approach that views humans as complex social and environmental phenomena best conceptualized from a probability framework. Probabilistic statements generally are based on statistical data and assert relationships between variables that do not occur in every instance, but are likely to occur based on some estimate of probability. As an example, it has been asserted that a lack of exercise may lead to obesity, a growing national health problem. It is clear that a lack of exercise *(LE)* does not always lead to obesity, because not all couch potatoes become medically obese *(MO)*. However, the probability of developing medical obesity *(PMO)* may be increased for persons who routinely avoid exercise at least to some degree of probability. In symbolic notation:

IF LE ——→ *P MO*

Relational statements that assert connections between variables provide for analysis and establish a basis for explanation and prediction (Hage, 1972).

Linkages and Ordering

Specification of linkages is a vital part of the development of theory (Hage, 1972). Although theoretical statements assert connections between concepts, the rationale for the stated connections must be developed and presented clearly. The development of theoretical linkages provides an explanation of why the variables are connected in a certain manner; that is, the theoretical reason for particular relationships (Hage, 1972). Operational linkages contribute testability to the theory by specifying how measurement variables are connected (Hage, 1972). Operational definitions specify the measurability of the concepts, and operational linkages provide the testability of the assertions. It is the operational linkages that contribute a perspective for understanding the nature of the relationship between concepts, so one can know whether the relationship between the concepts is negative or positive, linear or curvilinear (Hage, 1972).

A theory may be considered fairly complete if it presents the concepts, definitions, statements, and linkages. Complete development of a theory, however, requires organization of the concepts, definitions, relational statements, and linkages into premises and hypotheses (Hage, 1972). As the theory evolves, concepts and theoretical statements are developed, thereby establishing a logical organization of the theory components. The conceptual arrangement of statements and linkages into premises reveals any areas of inconsistency (Hage, 1972). Premises (or axioms) are the more general assertions from which hypotheses are derived. It generally is agreed that conceptual ordering of theoretical statements and their linkages is indicated when the theory contains a logical list of theoretical statements.

Reynolds (1971) describes three forms for organizing theory: *set-of-laws*, *axiomatic*, and *causal process*. Each is a different conceptual approach to organization with different limitations.

The *set-of-laws* approach organizes findings from available research in an area of particular interest from the literature for evaluation. Findings are evaluated and sorted into the categories of laws, empirical generalizations, and hypotheses based on the degree of research evidence supporting each assertion (Reynolds, 1971). Limitations to the set-of-laws approach to theory building have been noted.

First, the nature of research requires a focus on the relationships between a limited set of variables; therefore, attempts to develop a set-of-laws theory from statements of findings may result in a lengthy number of statements that assert relationships between but limited to two or more variables. This lengthy set of generalizations may be difficult to organize and interrelate. Second, for research to be conducted, concepts must be defined operationally so they are measurable. Therefore, the empirical findings selected from the reports may not include some of the theoretical concepts necessary for proper application (Foster, 1997).

Reynolds (1971) concluded that the set-of-laws form provides for classification of phenomena or prediction of relationships between selected variables; however, it does not enhance understanding or advance science because it is based on what is already known. Finally, Reynolds (1971) notes that each statement in the set-of-laws form is considered to be independent, in that the various statements have not been interrelated into a system of description and explanation or have not evolved from an organized conceptual model or framework (Figure 4-1). Each statement must be tested because the statements are not interrelated, and one statement does not provide support for another statement. This set of laws may be useful for beginning theory development; however, research efforts must be more extensive.

The *axiomatic form* of theory organization is an interrelated, logical system. Specifically, an axiomatic theory consists of explicit definitions, a set of concepts, a set of existence statements, and a set of relationship statements arranged in hierarchical order (Reynolds, 1971). The concepts may include abstract, intermediate, and concrete concepts. The set of existence statements describe situations wherein the theory is applicable. Statements that delineate the boundaries describe the scope of the theory (Dubin, 1978; Hage, 1972; Reynolds, 1971). Relational statements consist of axioms and propositions. Abstract, theoretical statements, or axioms, are at the top of the hierarchy of relational statements. The other propositions are developed through logical deduction from the axioms or from research findings in the literature (Figure 4-2). This results in a highly interrelated, explanatory system.

Set-of-Laws Form

Laws (overwhelming empirical support)
1.
2.
3.

Empirical generalizations (some empirical support)
1.
2.
3.
4.

Hypotheses (no empirical support)
1.
2.
3.
4.
5.

Figure 4-1 Set-of-laws Form. (From Reynolds, P. [1971]. *A primer in theory construction.* Indianapolis, IN: Bobbs-Merrill. Used with permission from Allyn & Bacon, a division of Pearson Education.)

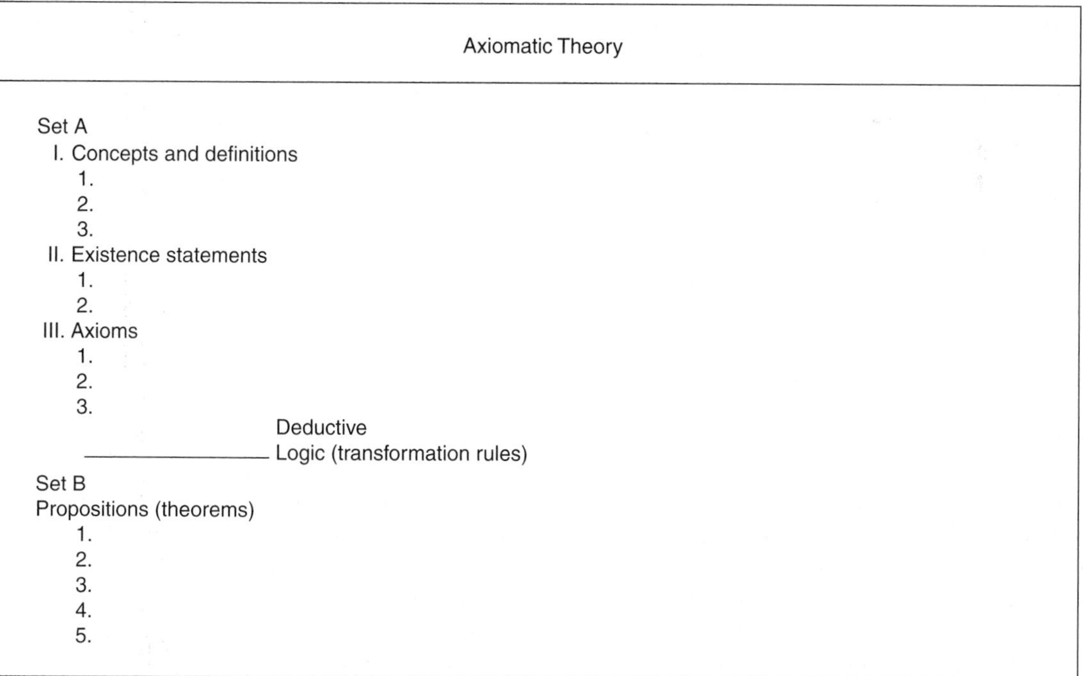

Axiomatic Theory
Set A
I. Concepts and definitions
1.
2.
3.
II. Existence statements
1.
2.
III. Axioms
1.
2.
3.
Deductive
Logic (transformation rules)
Set B
Propositions (theorems)
1.
2.
3.
4.
5.

Figure 4-2 Axiomatic Theory Represented in Schematic Form. (Developed from Werkmeister, W. [1959]. Theory construction and the problem of objectivity. In L. Gross [Ed.], *Symposium of sociological theory.* Evanston, IL: Row, Peterson, & Co. [schemata]; and Reynolds, P. [1971]. *A primer in theory construction.* Indianapolis, IN: Bobbs-Merrill [terminology].)

Axiomatic theorists avoid the problem of contradictory axioms by using a conceptual system with a few broad axioms from which a set of propositions are derived. The seven nursing conceptual models in this text are examples of frameworks with broad axioms from which theory may be developed. As science progresses and new empirical data known, the general axioms may be modified or extended. Some of the nursing theories and middle range theories developed with the use of a nursing conceptual model as their broad axioms are examples of the type of extension that is described here. However, these additions must be consistent with the logical system of the model and should not include contradictions in the theory, or the theory would be rejected (Schlotfeldt, 1992). New theories also may subsume portions of previous theories as special cases (Brown, 1977). Einstein's theory of relativity incorporating Newton's law of gravitation is a classic example. Axiomatic theories are less common in the social and behavioral sciences, but they are clearly evident in the fields of physics and mathematics.

Development of theories in axiomatic form has several advantages (Reynolds, 1971; Salmon, 1973). First, because theory is a set of interrelated statements in which some statements derive from others, only concepts to be measured must be operationally defined (Reynolds, 1971). This allows the theorist to incorporate highly abstract and less measurable concepts in providing the explanation. The interrelated axiomatic system also may be more efficient for explanation than are a lengthy number of theoretical statements in the set-of-laws form. In addition, empirical support for a single theoretical statement may be based on findings of support from earlier research, thereby permitting less extensive research than the requirement to test each statement in the set-of-laws form. In certain instances, the axiomatic theory may be organized in a causal process form to enhance understanding and substantiate findings.

The distinguishing feature of the *causal process* form of theory development is the theoretical statements that specify causal mechanisms between independent and dependent variables. This form of theory organization consists of a set of concepts, a set of definitions, a set of existence statements, and a set of theoretical statements that specify a causal process (Reynolds, 1971). Concepts include abstract and concrete ideas. Existence statements function as they do in axiomatic theories to describe the scope conditions of the theory, that is, the assumed situations in which the theory applies (Dubin, 1978; Hage, 1972; Reynolds, 1971). Causal statements specify the hypothesized effects of one variable upon one or more other variables for testing. In complex causal processes, feedback loops and paths of influence through several variables are hypothesized in a set of interrelated causal statements (Mullins, 1971; Nowak, 1975). Reynolds (1971) concludes that the causal process form of theory provides for testing an explanation of the process of how events happen. He identified several advantages of the causal process form of organization. First, similar to axiomatic theory, it provides for highly abstract, theoretical concepts. Second, again similar to axiomatic theory, this form permits more efficient research testing with its interrelated theoretical statements. Finally, the causal process statements provide a sense of understanding of the phenomenon of interest that is not possible with other forms. This is a highly developed form of theory development that builds successively on previous research findings in the researcher's area of research with extensive theory building and testing over time. Figure 4-3 displays a causal model for testing a theory of active coping. The broken lines show the direction of expected linkage. The dotted lines indicate potential new relationships. The arrows indicate the direction of cause that is predicted in the hypotheses of the study. The numbers along the lines identify previous studies that lend support for the relationships that are proposed.

CONTEMPORARY ISSUES IN NURSING THEORY DEVELOPMENT

Theoretical Boundaries and Levels to Advance Nursing Science

Since Fawcett's (1984) seminal proposal of the four metaparadigm concepts—person, environment, health, and nursing—general agreement has been reached

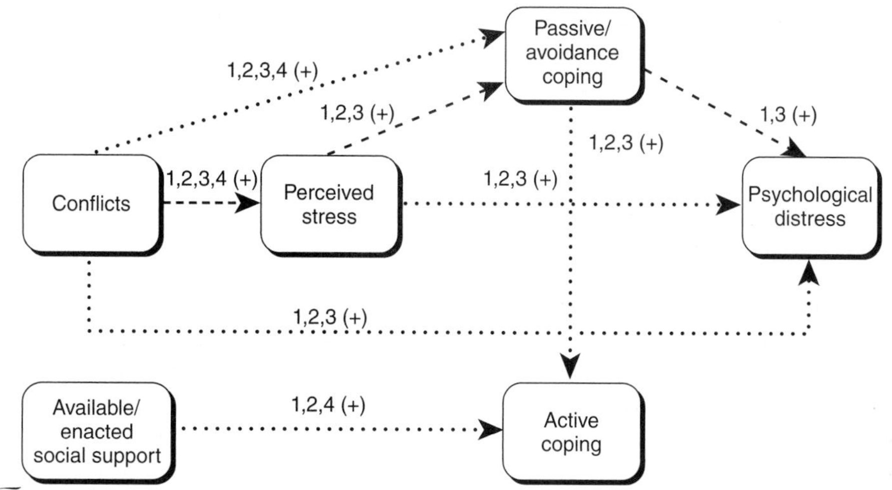

Figure 4-3 Causal Model of Active Coping. (From Ducharme, F., Ricard, N., Duquette, A., & Lachance, I. [1998]. Empirical testing of a longitudinal model derived from the Roy Adaptation Model. *Nursing Science Quarterly, 11*[4], 149-159.)

among nursing scholars such that the proposed framework now is used without reference to the author for the development of nursing science. In general, a metaparadigm should specify the broad boundaries of the phenomenon of concern within a discipline, for example, to set nursing apart from other disciplines, such as medicine, clinical exercise physiology, or sociology. Fawcett (2005) proposes that a metaparadigm defines the totality of phenomena inherent in the discipline in a parsimonious way and is perspective-neutral and international in scope. Her definition of perspective-neutral is that the metaparadigm concepts reflect nursing but not any particular nursing conceptual model or paradigm. This criterion is illustrated clearly in that the nursing models and paradigms include the metaparadigm concepts but define each in distinctly different ways. This supports their generic nature as broad metaparadigm concepts that have specificity within each conceptual theory or paradigm. It is important to grasp the significance of Fawcett's point. Because the metaparadigm is the highly philosophical level in the structure of knowledge, models and theories define the terms specifically within each of their works, and differences among them is anticipated. Thorne and colleagues (1998) proposed that it was not productive to continue metaparadigm debates about which conceptual system should define these concepts, but that each conceptual model is labeled as a nursing conceptual model because it clearly addresses each of the metaparadigm concepts, although from different philosophical perspectives. Scholarly debates are expected to continue among doctoral students and communities of scholars engaged in scholarship and inquiry. Discussions within the nursing discipline and approaches to nursing knowledge are anticipated as nurses address dynamic social obligations, the tentativeness of theory, and new developments as the discipline advances (Monti & Tingen, 1999).

Viewing the metaparadigm from different cultural perspectives enhances our understanding and expands our ideas as the discipline develops globally. For example, the work conducted by Kao, Reeder, Hsu, and Cheng (2006) proposes a Chinese view of the Western nursing paradigm through the lens of Confucianism and Taoism. The concept of person is more than a biopsychosocial spiritual being and is also responsibility bound. Health includes the flow of qi, yin-yang, and the five phases—wood, water, fire, metal, and earth. The challenge in knowledge development is to learn how to consider nursing phenomena through many lenses and to enhance the development of knowledge and improve the nursing of people around the globe.

In the discipline of nursing, the earlier focus on theory development has evolved to an emphasis on theory utilization with the development and use of middle range theories focused at the practice level (Acton, Irvin, Jensen, Hopkins, & Miller, 1997; Good, 1998; Im & Meleis, 1999; Lawson, 2003; Liehr & Smith, 1999; Smith & Liehr, 2008). *Situation-specific theories* (the term preferred by Meleis, 2007) are applicable to a nursing problem or a specific group of patients. An integrative approach to situation-specific theories is summarized as involving four broad interrelated steps: (1) checking assumptions for theory development, (2) exploring the phenomenon through multiple sources, (3) theorizing, and (4) reporting/validating (Im, 2005, 2006).

Middle range theory was described very early in the nursing literature by a sociologist (Merton, 1967). He proposed that it focused on specific phenomena (rather than attempting to address a broader range of phenomena) and comprised hypotheses with two or more concepts linked together in a conceptual system. Today in the nursing literature, many middle range theories have been developed qualitatively from practice observations and interviews and quantitatively from nursing conceptual models or theories. Middle range theory is pragmatic at the practice level and contains specific aspects about the practice situation as follows:

- The situation or health condition involved
- Client population or age group
- Location or area of practice (such as community)
- Action of the nurse or the intervention

It is these specifics that make middle range theory so applicable to nursing practice (Alligood, 2006, p. 488). Therefore, the development of middle range theory facilitates conceptions of relationships between theory, nursing practice, and patient outcomes in focused areas. In 1996, Lenz (in Liehr & Smith, 1999) identified the following six approaches for devising middle range theories:

1. Inductive approach through research
2. Deductive approach from grand nursing theories
3. Integration of nursing and non-nursing theories
4. Derivative (retroductive) approach from non-nursing theories
5. Theories devised from guidelines for clinical practice
6. Synthesis approach from research findings

Liehr and Smith (1999) reviewed 10 years of nursing literature on middle range theories from 1985 and 1995 and listed 22 middle range theories that could be categorized as five approaches to theory building.

The nursing literature abounds with a range of different approaches to middle range theory building and development. The recent nursing literature emphasizes the importance of relating middle range theories to broader nursing theories and paradigms and continuing to pursue empirical testing and the replication of studies to advance nursing knowledge. Fahs, Morgan, and Kalman (2003) have called for replication of research studies to ensure that nursing scholars can provide "a (reliable) research-to-practice link"... that (provides) "safe, effective, quality care to consumers" (p. 70). Middle range theories essentially have grown over the past 10 years with textbooks no in their second editions (Peterson, 2008; Sieloff & Frey, 2007; Smith & Liehr, 2008) and being taught at the graduate level of education in theory-based practice.

Numerous authors have proposed criteria to be used in evaluating theories (Chinn & Kramer, 2008; Fawcett, 2005; Meleis, 2007; Parker, 2006). These criteria reflect the importance of nursing knowledge to the future of the discipline, as well as the diversity of approaches. Is the theory relevant, significant, or functional to the discipline of nursing? Chapter 1 presents the criteria used for analysis of theory in this text (Chinn & Kramer, 2008).

Nursing Theory, Practice, and Research

Theory-testing research may lead one nursing theory to fall aside as a new theory is developed that explains nursing phenomena more adequately. Therefore, it is critical that theory-testing research continue for advancement of the discipline. Nursing scholars have presented criteria for evaluating theory-testing research in nursing (Acton, Irvin, & Hopkins, 1991; Silva, 1986). These criteria emphasize the importance of using a nursing framework to design the purpose and focus of the study, to derive hypotheses, and to relate the significance of the findings back to nursing. In addition to the need for more rigorous theory-testing research in nursing, nursing scholars and practitioners call for increased attention to the relationships among theory, research, and practice. Their recommendations include the following:

- Continue developing nursing theories relevant to nurses' specialty practice
- Promote collaboration between scientists and practitioners (Lorentzon, 1998)
- Encourage nurse researchers to communicate research findings to practitioners
- Increase efforts to relate middle range theories to nursing paradigms
- Increase emphasis on clinical research
- Increase the use of nursing theories for theory-based practice and clinical decision making

(See Chinn & Kramer, 2008; Cody, 1999; Hoffman & Bertus, 1991; Liehr & Smith, 1999; Lutz, Jones, & Kendall, 1997; Reed, 2000; and Sparacino, 1991.)

Within education, some use one theory to guide the nursing curriculum; however, others utilize a framework of the metaparadigm. Malinski (2000) and others have urged increased attention to nursing theory–based research and strengthening of nursing theory–based curricula, especially in master's and doctoral programs.

Regarding the use of nursing knowledge in clinical practice, Cody asserted, "It is a professional nurse's ethical responsibility to utilize the knowledge base of her or his discipline" (1997, p. 4). In 1992, in the first issue of the journal *Clinical Nursing Research*, Schlotfeldt stated the following:

> It will be nursing's clinical scholars . . . that will identify the human phenomena that are central to nurses' practice . . . and that provoke consideration of the practice problems about which knowledge is needed but is not yet available. It is nursing's clinical scholarship that must be depended on to generate promising theories for testing that will advance nursing knowledge and ensure nursing's continued essential services to humankind (1992, p. 9).

In summary, contemporary nursing scholars are emphasizing the following in theory-building processes:

- Continued development of theoretical inquiry in nursing
- Continued scholarship with middle range theories and situation-specific theories, including efforts to relate to nursing theories and paradigms
- Greater attention to synthesis of nursing knowledge
- Development of stronger nursing theory-research-practice linkages

The discipline of nursing has developed into an understanding of the relationships among theory, practice, and research that no longer separates them into distinct categories. Rather, their complementary interrelationships foster the development of new understanding about practice as theory is used to guide practice and as practice innovations drive new middle range theory. Similarly, nurse scientists have reached new understandings of the relationship of theory to research as quantitative study reports include explicit descriptions of their frameworks and qualitative researchers interpret their findings in the context of nursing frameworks. The complementary nature of these relationships is fostering a new era of nursing science growth. So the chapter concludes as it began. Emphasis on theory is important because theory development in nursing is an essential component of nursing scholarship conducted to advance the knowledge of the discipline.

POINTS FOR *Further Study*

- Webber, P. B. (2008). Yes, Virginia, nursing does have laws. *Nurse Science Quarterly, 21*(1), 68-73.

Classic References

- Dubin, R. (1978). *Theory building.* New York: Free Press.
- Hage, J. (1972). *Techniques and problems of theory construction in sociology.* New York: John Wiley & Sons.

- Kaplan, A. (1964). *The conduct of inquiry: Methodology for behavioral science.* New York: Chandler.
- Mullins, N. (1971). *The art of theory: Construction and use.* New York: Harper & Row.
- Wilson, J. (1969) *Thinking with concepts.* Cambridge: Cambridge University Press.

REFERENCES

Acton, G., Irvin, B., & Hopkins, B. (1991). Theory-testing research: Building the science. *ANS Advances in Nursing Science, 14*(1), 52-61.

Acton, G., Irvin, B., Jensen, B., Hopkins, B., & Miller, E. (1997). Explicating middle-range theory through methodological diversity. *ANS Advances in Nursing Science, 19*(3), 78-85.

Alligood, M. R. (2006). Areas for further development of theory-based nursing practice. In M. R. Alligood & A. M. Tomey (Eds.). *Nursing theory: Utilization & application* (3rd ed., pp. 487-497). St. Louis: Mosby.

American Heart Association (AHA). (2004). *Diagnosing heart disease.* Dallas: AHA. Retrieved April 26, 2004 from: http://www.americanheart.org/presenter. jhtml?identifier=330

Brown, H. (1977). *Perception, theory and commitment: The new philosophy of science.* Chicago: University of Chicago Press.

Buck, H. (2006). Spirituality: Concept analysis and model development. *Holistic Nursing Practice, 20*(6), 288-292.

Chinn, P., & Kramer, M. (2008). *Integrated theory and knowledge development in nursing.* St. Louis: Mosby.

Cody, W. (1997). Of tombstones, milestones, and gem-stones: A retrospective and prospective on nursing theory. *Nursing Science Quarterly, 10*(1), 3-5.

Cody, W. (1999). Middle range theories: Do they foster the development of nursing science? *Nursing Science Quarterly, 12*(1), 9-14.

Dalton, C., & Gottlieb, L. N. (2003). The concept of readiness to change. *Journal of Advanced Nursing, 42*(2), 108-117.

Dubin, R. (1978). *Theory building.* New York: Free Press.

Ducharme, F., Ricard, N., Duquette, A., & Lachance, I. (1998). Empirical testing of a longitudinal model derived from the Roy Adaptation Model, *Nursing Science Quarterly, 11*(4), 149-159.

Fahs, P. S., Morgan, L. L., & Kalman, M. (2003). A call for replication. *Journal of Nursing Scholarship, 35*(1), 67-72.

Fawcett, J. (1984). The metaparadigm of nursing: Present status and future refinements. *Image: The Journal of Nursing Scholarship, 16*(3), 84-87.

Fawcett, J. (2005). *Analysis and evaluation of contemporary nursing knowledge: Nursing models and theories* (2nd ed.). Philadelphia: F. A. Davis.

Foster, L. (1997). Addressing epistemologic and practical issues in multimethod research: A procedure for conceptual triangulation. *Advances in Nursing Science, 20*(2), 1-12.

Giere, R. N. (1979). *Understanding scientific reasoning.* New York: Holt, Rinehart, & Winston.

Giere, R. N. (1997). *Understanding scientific reasoning* (4th ed.). Fort Worth, TX: Harcourt, Brace College Publishers.

Good, M. (1998). Middle range theory of acute pain management: Use in research. *Nursing Outlook, 46,* 120-124.

Hage, J. (1972). *Techniques and problems of theory construction in sociology.* New York: John Wiley & Sons.

Hardin, S. R., Hussey, L. C., & Steele, L. (2003). Spirituality as integrality among chronic heart failure patients: A pilot study. *Visions: The Journal of Rogerian Nursing Science, 11*(1), 43-53.

Harvey, G., Loftus-Hills, A., Rycroft-Malone, J., Titchen, A., Kitson, A., McCormack, B., et al. (2002). Getting evidence into practice: The role and function of facilitation. *Journal of Advanced Nursing, 37*(6), 577-588.

Hatch, R. L., Burg, M. A., Naberhaus, D. S., & Hellmich, L. K. (1998). The Spiritual Involvement and Beliefs Scale: Development and testing of a new instrument. *Journal of Family Practice, 46,* 6.

Hoffman, A., & Bertus, P. (1991). Theory and practice: Bridging scientists' and practitioners' roles. *Archives of Psychiatric Nursing, 7*(1), 2-9.

Hussey, L. C., & Hardin, S. R. (2003). Sex-related differences in heart failure. *Heart & Lung, 32*(4), 215-225.

Im, E. (2005). Development of situation-specific theories. *Advances in Nursing Science, 28*(2), 137-151.

Im, E. (2006). A situation-specific theory of Caucasian cancer patients' pain experience. *Advances in Nursing Science, 29*(3), 232-244.

Im, E., & Meleis, A. (1999). Situation-specific theories: Philosophical roots, properties and approach. *ANS Advances in Nursing Science, 22*(2), 11-24.

Kao, H., Reeder, F., Hsu, M. & Cheng, S. (2006). A Chinese view of the Western nursing metaparadigm. *Journal of Holistic Nursing 24*(2), 92-101.

Kaplan, A. (1964). *The conduct of inquiry: Methodology for behavioral science.* New York: Chandler.

Keenan, J. (1999). A concept analysis of autonomy. *Journal of Advanced Nursing, 29*(3), 556-562.

Lawson, L. (2003). Becoming a success story: How boys who have molested children talk about treatment. *Journal of Psychiatric and Mental Health Nursing, 10,* 259-268.

Liehr, P., & Smith, M. J. (1999). Middle range theory: Spinning research and practice to create knowledge for the new millennium. *ANS Advances in Nursing Science, 21*(4), 81-91.

Lorentzon, M. (1998). The way forward: Nursing research or collaborative health care research? *Journal of Advanced Nursing, 27,* 675-676.

Lutz, K., Jones, K., & Kendall, J. (1997). Expanding the praxis debate: Contributions to clinical inquiry. *ANS Advances in Nursing Science, 20*(2), 13-22.

Malinski, V. (1994). Spirituality: A pattern manifestation of the human/environment mutual process. *Visions: The Journal of Rogerian Science, 2*(1), 12-18.

Malinski, V. (2000). Research-based evaluation of conceptual models of nursing. *Nursing Science Quarterly, 13*(2), 103-110.

Meleis, A. (2007). *Theoretical nursing: Development and progress.* (4th ed.). Philadelphia: Lippincott Williams & Wilkins.

Merton, R. K. (1967). *On theoretical sociology.* New York: Free Press.

Monti, E., & Tingen, M. (1999). Multiple paradigms of nursing science. *ANS Advances in Nursing Science, 21*(4), 64-80.

Morse, J. (1995). Exploring the theoretical basis of nursing using advanced techniques of concept analysis. *Advances in Nursing Science, 17,* 31-46.

Mullins, N. (1971). *The art of theory: Construction and use.* New York: Harper & Row.

Nowak, S. (1975). Causal interpretations of statistical relationships in social research. In H. Blalock (Ed.), *Quantitative sociology: International perspectives on mathematical and statistical modeling.* New York: Academic Press.

O'Byrne, P. (2008). The dissection of risk: A conceptual analysis. *Nursing Inquiry, 15*(1), 30-39.

Parker, M. E. (2006). *Nursing theories & nursing practice.* (2nd ed.). Philadelphia: F. A. Davis.

Peterson, S. J. (2008). *Middle range theories: Application to nursing research.* (2nd ed.). Philadelphia, PA: Lippincott Williams & Wilkins.

Posey, A. (2006). Symptom perception: A concept exploration. *Nursing Forum, 41*(3), 113-124.

Reed, P. (2000). Nursing reformation: Historical reflections and philosophic foundations. *Nursing Science Quarterly, 13*(2), 129-136.

Reynolds, P. (1971). *A primer in theory construction.* Indianapolis, IN: Bobbs-Merrill.

Rodgers, B. L. (1989). Concept analysis, the development of knowledge: The evolutionary cycle. *Journal of Advanced Nursing, 14,* 330-335.

Rogers, M. E. (1970). An introduction to the theoretical basis of nursing. Philadelphia: F. A. Davis.

Salmon, W. D. (1973). *Logic.* Englewood Cliffs, NJ: Prentice Hall.

Sayers, K., & de Vries, K. (2008). A concept development of 'being sensitive' in nursing. *Nursing Ethics, 15*(3), 289-303.

Schilling, L. S., Grey, M., & Knafl, K. A. (2002). The concept of self-management of type I diabetes in children and adolescents: An evolutionary concept analysis. *Journal of Advanced Nursing, 37*(1), 87-99.

Schlotfeldt, R. (1992). Why promote clinical nursing scholarship? *Clinical Nursing Research, 1*(1), 5-8.

Schwartz-Barcott, D., & Kim, H. S. (2000). An expansion and elaboration of the hybrid model of concept development. In B. L. Rodgers & K. A. Knafl (Eds.), *Concept development in nursing* (2nd ed., pp. 129-160). Philadelphia: Saunders.

Scott Tilley, D. (2008). Competency in nursing: a concept analysis. *Journal of Continuing Education in Nursing, 39*(2), 58-64.

Sieloff, C., & Frey, M. A. (2007). *Middle range theory development using King's conceptual system.* New York: Springer.

Silva, M. (1986). Research testing nursing theory: State of the art. *ANS Advances in Nursing Science, 9*(10), 1-11.

Smith, M. J., & Liehr, P. (2008). *Middle range theory for nursing* (2nd ed.). New York: Springer.

Sparacino, P. (1991). The reciprocal relationship between practice and theory. *Clinical Nurse Specialist, 5*(3), 138.

Spear, H., & Kulbok, P. (2004). Autonomy and adolescence: A concept analysis. *Public Health Nursing, 21*(2), 144-152.

Starr, S. (2008). Authenticity: A concept analysis. *Nursing Forum, 43*(2), 55-62.

Thorne, S., Canam, C., Dahinten, S., Hall, W., Henderson, A., & Kirkham, S. R. (1998). Nursing's metaparadigm concepts: Disimpacting the debates. *Journal of Advanced Nursing, 27,* 1257-1268.

Walker, L., & Avant, K. (2005). *Strategies for theory construction in nursing.* (4th ed.). Upper Saddle River, NJ: Prentice Hall.

Weaver, K., Morse, J., & Mitcham, C. (2008). Ethical sensitivity in professional practice: Concept analysis. *Journal of Advanced Nursing, 62*(5), 607-618.

Werkmeister, W. (1959). Theory construction and the problem of objectivity. In L. Gross (Ed.), *Symposium of sociological theory.* Evanston, IL: Row, Peterson, & Co.

Wilson, J. (1969) *Thinking with concepts.* Cambridge: Cambridge University Press.

Zetterberg, H. L. (1966). *On theory and verification in sociology.* New York: John Wiley & Sons.

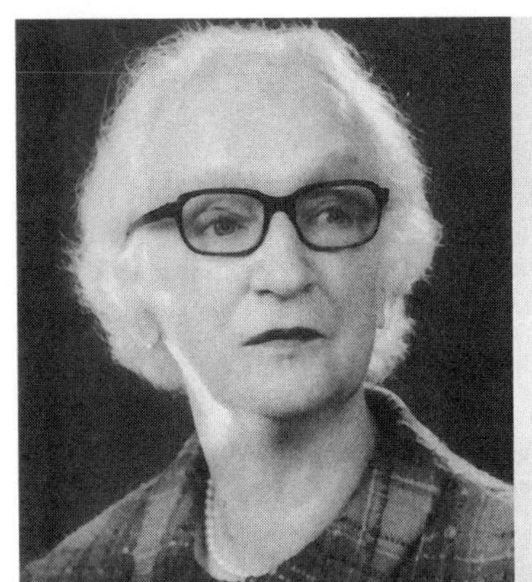

CHAPTER 5

Hildegard E. Peplau

1909-1999

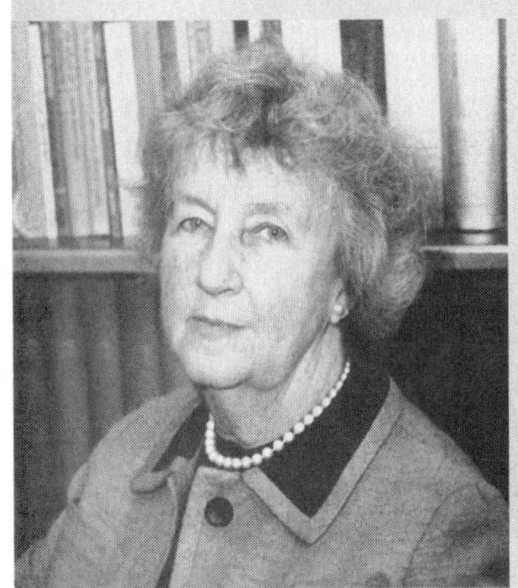

Virginia Henderson

1897-1996

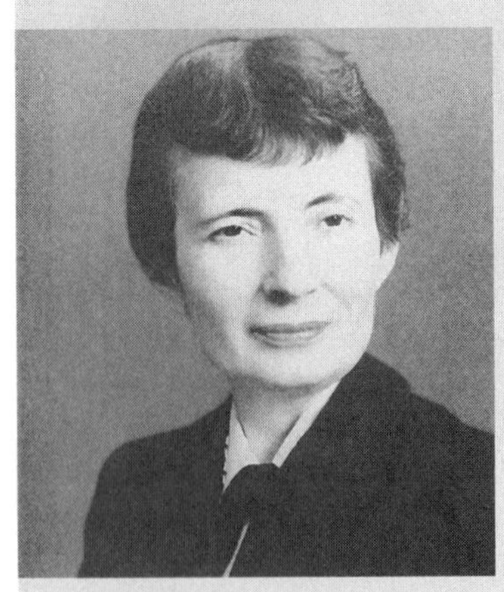

Faye Glenn Abdellah

1919-present

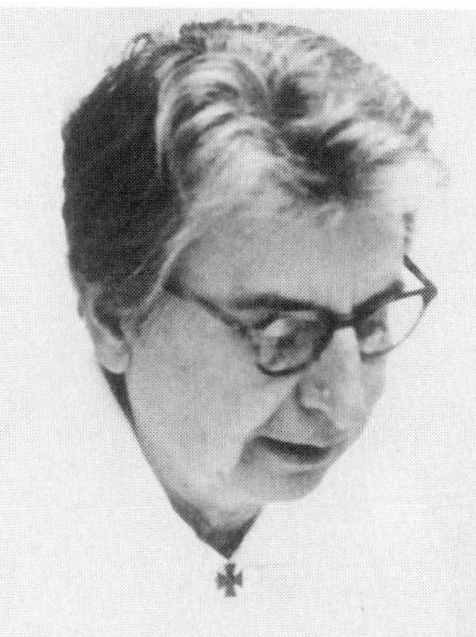

Ernestine Wiedenbach

1900-1996

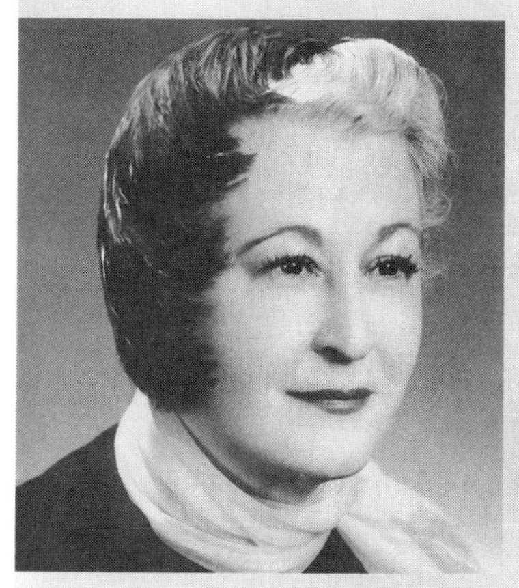

Lydia Hall

1906-1969

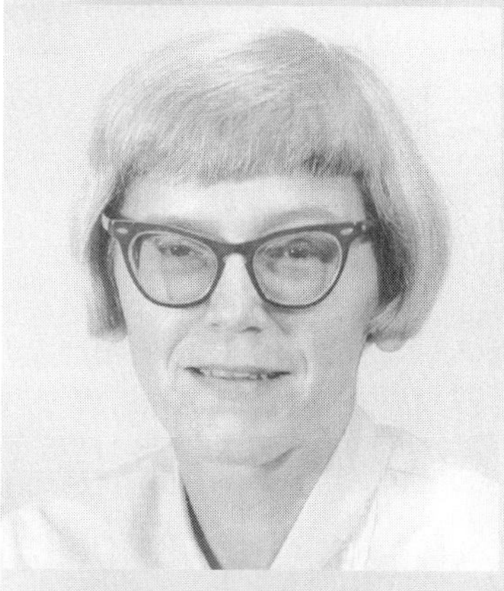

Photo Credit: Louisiana State University Health Sciences Center, School of Nursing, New Orleans, LA.

Joyce Travelbee

1926-1973

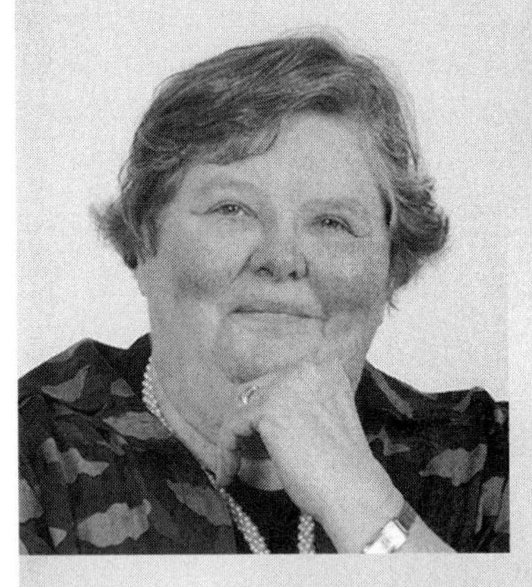

Kathryn E. Barnard

1938-present

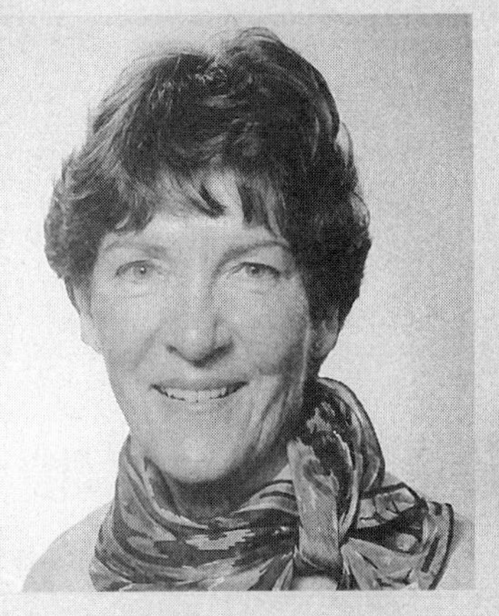

Evelyn Adam

1929-present

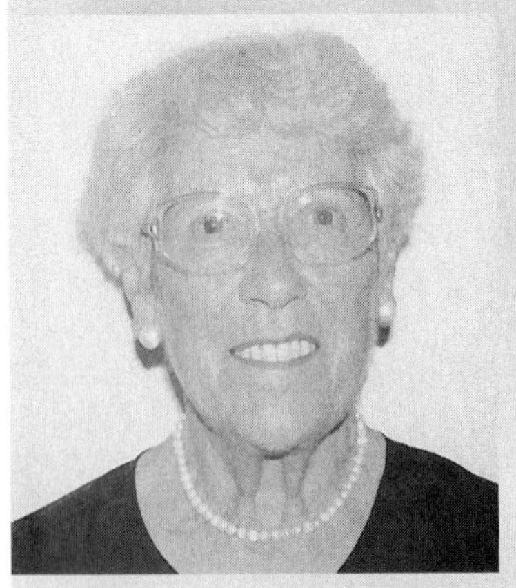

Nancy Roper

1918-2004

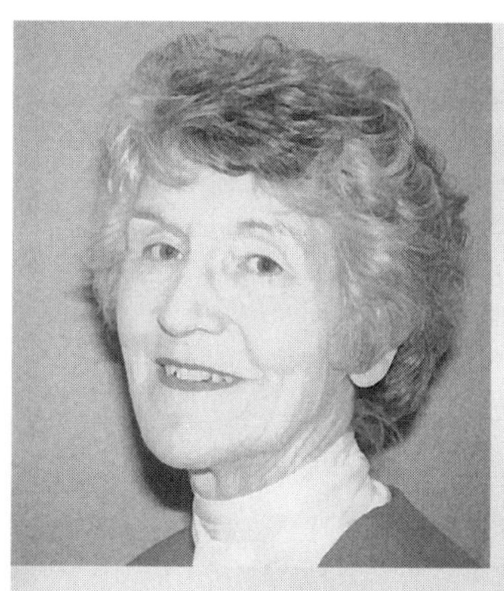

Winifred W. Logan

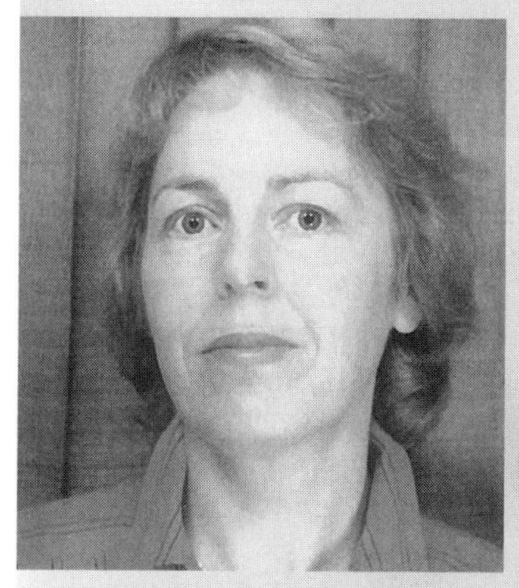

Alison J. Tierney

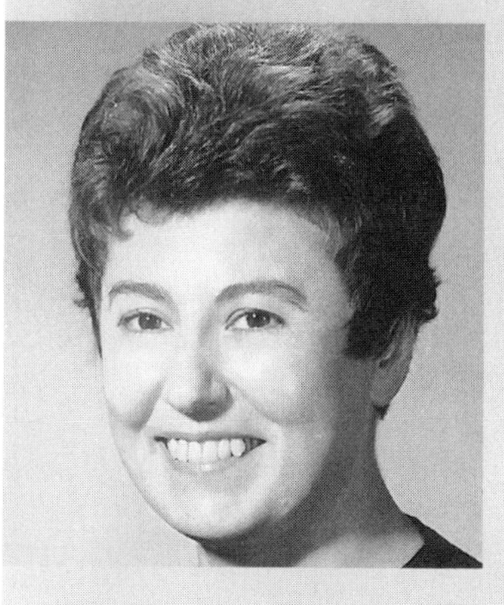

Ida Jean (Orlando) Pelletier

1926-2007

Nursing Theorists of Historical Significance

Marie. E. Pokorny

"The idea of nursing, historically rooted in the care of the sick and in the provision of nurturance for those vulnerable to ill health, is foundational to the profession" (Wolf, 2006, p. 301).

HILDEGARD E. PEPLAU

Theory of Interpersonal Relations

Hildegard E. Peplau has been described as the mother of psychiatric nursing because her theoretical and clinical work led to the development of the distinct specialty field of psychiatric nursing. Her scope of influence in nursing includes her contributions as a psychiatric nursing expert, educator, author, and nursing leader and theorist.

Peplau provided major leadership in the professionalization of nursing. She served as Executive Director and later as President of the American Nurses Association. She promoted professional standards and regulation through credentialing. She taught the first classes for graduate psychiatric nursing students at Teachers College, Columbia University, where she stressed the importance of nurses' ability to understand their own behavior so they can help others identify perceived difficulties. Her seminal book, *Interpersonal Relations in Nursing* (1952), described the importance of the nurse-patient relationship as a "significant, therapeutic interpersonal process" (p. 16) and is considered by many to be the first nursing theory textbook since Nightingale's work in the 1850s. She identified four phases of the nurse-patient relationship: orientation, identification, exploitation, and resolution (Figure 5-1).

Peplau diagrammed changing aspects of nurse-patient relationships (Figure 5-2) and proposed and described the following six nursing roles: stranger, resource person, teacher, leader, surrogate, and counselor (Figure 5-3). In addition, she discussed four psychobiological experiences that compel destructive or constructive responses, as follows: needs, frustrations, conflicts, and anxieties.

Peplau's experiences with professionals from psychiatry, medicine, education, and sociology influenced her view of what a profession is and does and what it should be (Sills, 1998). Her work

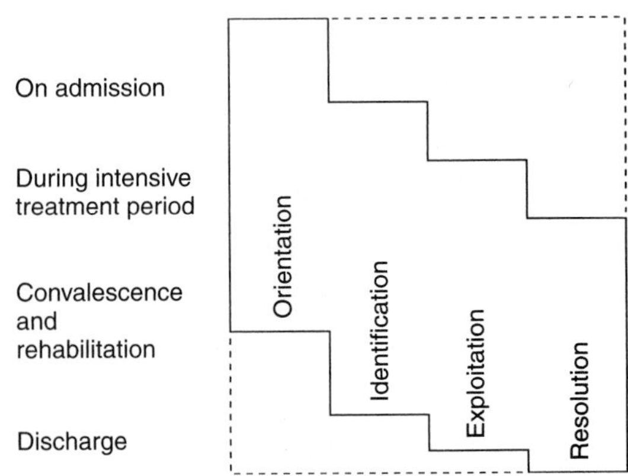

Figure 5-1 Overlapping Phases in Nurse-Patient Relationships. (From Peplau, H. E. [1952]. *Interpersonal relations in nursing*. New York: G. P. Putnam's Sons.)

Previous author: Ann Marriner Tomey.

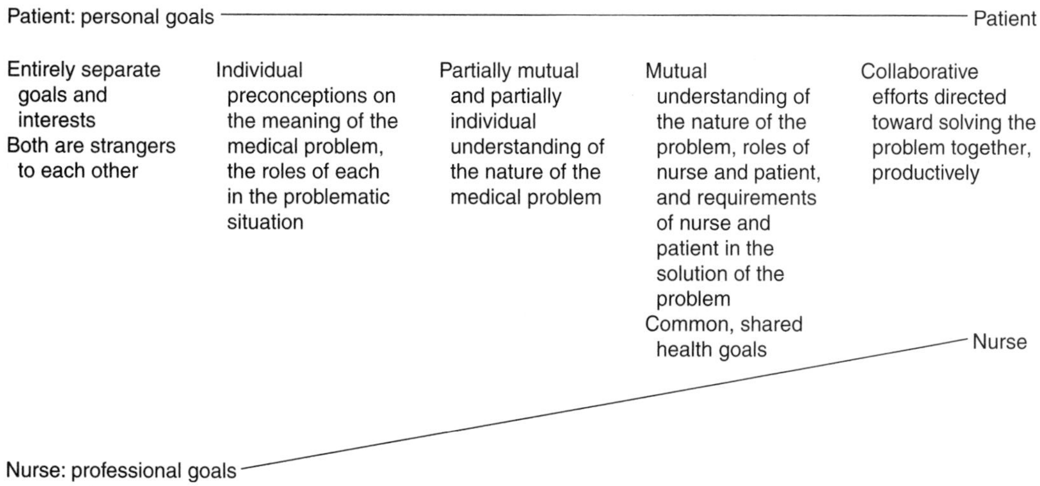

Patient: personal goals				Patient
Entirely separate goals and interests Both are strangers to each other	Individual preconceptions on the meaning of the medical problem, the roles of each in the problematic situation	Partially mutual and partially individual understanding of the nature of the medical problem	Mutual understanding of the nature of the problem, roles of nurse and patient, and requirements of nurse and patient in the solution of the problem Common, shared health goals	Collaborative efforts directed toward solving the problem together, productively
Nurse: professional goals				Nurse

Figure 5-2 **Continuum Showing Changing Aspects of Nurse-Patient Relationships.** (From Peplau, H. E. [1952]. *Interpersonal relations in nursing.* New York: G. P. Putnam's Sons.)

Nurse:	Stranger	Unconditional Surrogate mother		Counselor Resource person Leadership Surrogate: Mother Sibling	Adult person
Patient:	Stranger	Infant	Child	Adolescent	Adult person
Phases in nursing relationship:	Orientation ——	Identification ——			
		Exploitation ——			
	——				Resolution

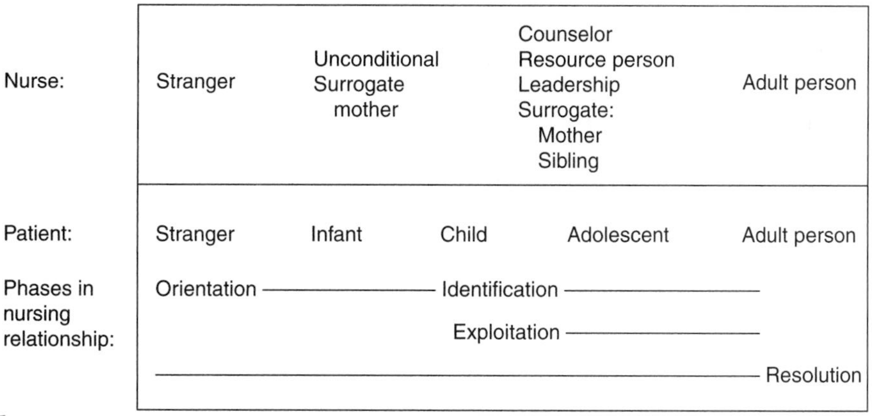

Figure 5-3 **Phases and Changing Roles in Nurse-Patient Relationships.** (From Peplau, H. E. [1952]. *Interpersonal relations in nursing.* New York: G. P. Putnam's Sons.)

was influenced by Freud, Maslow, and Sullivan's interpersonal relationship theories, and by the contemporaneous psychoanalytical model. She borrowed the psychological model to synthesize her Theory of Interpersonal Relations (Haber, 2000). Peplau's work is specific to the nurse-patient relationship and is categorized as a theory for the practice of nursing.

VIRGINIA HENDERSON

Definition of Nursing

Virginia Henderson viewed the patient as an individual who requires help toward achieving independence and completeness or wholeness of mind and body. She envisioned the practice of nursing as independent from the practice of physicians and acknowledged her interpretation of the nurse's function as a synthesis of many influences. Her work is based on (1) that of Thorndike, an American psychologist, (2) her student experiences with the Henry House Visiting Nurse Agency, (3) her experience in rehabilitation nursing, and (4) Orlando's conceptualization of deliberate nursing action (Henderson, 1964; Orlando, 1961).

Henderson emphasized the art of nursing and identified 14 proposed basic human needs on which nursing care is based. Her contributions include defining nursing, delineating autonomous nursing functions, stressing goals of interdependence for the patient, and creating self-help concepts. Her self-help concepts influenced the works of Abdellah and Adam (Abdellah, Beland, Martin, & Matheney, 1960; Adam, 1980, 1991).

Henderson made extraordinary contributions to nursing during her 60 years of service as a nurse, teacher, author, and researcher, and she published extensively throughout those years. Henderson wrote three books that have become nursing classics: *Textbook of the Principles and Practice of Nursing* (1955), *Basic Principles of Nursing Care* (1960), and *The Nature of Nursing* (1966). Her major contribution to nursing research, an 11-year Yale-sponsored Nursing Studies Index Project, resulted in a four-volume annotated index to nursing's biographical, analytical, and historical literature from 1900 to 1959.

In 1958, the nursing service committee of the International Council of Nurses (ICN) asked her to describe her concept of nursing. This now historical definition, published by ICN in 1961, represented her final crystallization on the subject:

> The unique function of the nurse is to assist the individual, sick or well, in the performance of those activities contributing to health or its recovery (or to peaceful death) that he would perform unaided if he had the necessary strength, will, or knowledge; and to do this in such a way as to help him gain independence as rapidly as possible (Henderson, 1964, p. 63).

Henderson's definition of nursing was adopted subsequently by ICN and disseminated widely; it continues to be used worldwide.

In *The Nature of Nursing: A Definition and Its Implications for Practice, Research, and Education*, Henderson (1966) identified 14 basic needs upon which nursing care is based (Box 5-1). In addition, she identified three levels of nurse-patient relationships in which the nurse acts as the following: (1) a substitute for the patient, (2) a helper to the patient, and (3) a partner with the patient.

The nurse through the interpersonal process must in a sense get "inside the skin" of each of her patients in order to know what help is needed (Harmer and

Box 5-1 Henderson's 14 Needs

1. Breathe normally.
2. Eat and drink adequately.
3. Eliminate body wastes.
4. Move and maintain desirable postures.
5. Sleep and rest.
6. Select suitable clothes; dress and undress.
7. Maintain body temperature within a normal range by adjusting clothing and modifying the environment.
8. Keep the body clean and well groomed and protect the integument.
9. Avoid dangers in the environment and avoid injuring others.
10. Communicate with others in expressing emotions, needs, fears, or opinions.
11. Worship according to one's faith.
12. Work in such a way that there is a sense of accomplishment.
13. Play or participate in various forms of recreation.
14. Learn, discover, or satisfy the curiosity that leads to normal development and health, and use the available health facilities.

From Henderson, V. A. (1991). *The nature of nursing: Reflections after 25 years* (pp. 22-23). New York: National League for Nursing Press.

Henderson, 1955, p. 5). Although she believed that the functions of nurses and physicians overlap, Henderson asserted that the nurse works in interdependence with other health professionals and with the patient; she used wedges of a pie graph to illustrate the relative contributions of members of the healthcare team. In *The Nature of Nursing: Reflections after 25 Years*, Henderson (1991) added addenda to each chapter of the 1966 edition to present changes in her views and to discuss her opinions. Henderson's work may be viewed as a philosophy of the purpose and function of nursing.

FAYE GLENN ABDELLAH

Twenty-One Nursing Problems

Faye Glenn Abdellah is recognized as a leader in the development of nursing research and nursing as a profession within the Public Health Service (PHS) and as an international expert on health problems. She has been active in professional associations devoted to nursing and has been a prolific author, with more than 150 publications to her credit. In her 40-year career as a Commissioned Officer in the U.S. Public Health Service (1949-1989), she served as the Chief Nurse Officer from 1970 to 1987 and was the first nurse to achieve the rank of a two-star Flag Officer (Abdellah, 2004). Abdellah was the first woman and nurse Deputy Surgeon General (1982-1989). After retirement, she founded the only federal graduate school of nursing. Abdellah considers her greatest accomplishment being able to "play a role in establishing a foundation for nursing research as a science" (p. iii). Her book, *Patient-Centered Approaches to Nursing,* emphasizes the science of nursing and has elicited changes throughout nursing curricula. Her work, which is based on the problem-solving method, serves as a vehicle for delineating nursing (patient) problems as the patient moves toward a healthy outcome.

Abdellah views nursing as both an art and a science that molds the attitude, intellectual competencies, and technical skills of the individual nurse into the desire and ability to help individuals cope with their health needs, whether they are ill or well. Although she believes that nursing actions are carried out under general or specific medical direction, she formulated 21 nursing problems based on a review of nursing research studies (Box 5-2). She used Henderson's 14 basic human needs (see Box 5-1) and nursing research to establish the classification of nursing problems.

Her work differs from that of Henderson in that Abdellah's problems are formulated in terms of nursing-centered services, which are used to determine the patient's needs. Her contribution to nursing theory development consists of a systematic analysis of research reports conducted to formulate the 21 nursing problems that served as an early guide for comprehensive nursing care. The typology of her 21 nursing problems first appeared in the 1960 edition of *Patient-Centered Approaches to Nursing* (Abdellah et al., 1960). It evolved into *Preparing for Nursing Research in the 21st Century: Evolution, Methodologies, and Challenges* (Abdellah & Levine, 1994). The 21 nursing problems have progressed to a second-generation development of patient problems and patient outcomes, instead of nursing problems and nursing outcomes. Abdellah's work reflects a problem-centered approach or philosophy of nursing. Those who wish to explore Abdellah's papers will be assisted by this website: http://www.nlm.nih.gov/hmd/manuscripts/ead/abdellah.html

ERNESTINE WIEDENBACH

The Helping Art of Clinical Nursing

Ernestine Wiedenbach is known for her work in theory development and maternal infant nursing. She developed her theory when she was teaching maternity nursing at the School of Nursing, Yale University. Wiedenbach taught with Ida Orlando at Yale and wrote with philosophers Dickoff and James a classic work on theory in a practice discipline that still is used today among those studying the evolution of nursing theory (Dickoff, James, & Wiedenbach, 1968). Wiedenbach's work grew as the result of 40 years of experience in the clinical and teaching setting. She directed the major curriculum in maternal and

Box 5-2 *Abdellah's Typology of 21 Nursing Problems*

1. To maintain good hygiene and physical comfort
2. To promote optimal activity: exercise, rest, sleep
3. To promote safety through prevention of accident, injury, or other trauma and through prevention of the spread of infection
4. To maintain good body mechanics and prevent and correct deformity
5. To facilitate the maintenance of a supply of oxygen to all body cells
6. To facilitate the maintenance of nutrition for all body cells
7. To facilitate the maintenance of elimination
8. To facilitate the maintenance of fluid and electrolyte balance
9. To recognize the physiologic responses of the body to disease conditions—pathologic, physiologic, and compensatory
10. To facilitate the maintenance of regulatory mechanisms and functions
11. To facilitate the maintenance of sensory function
12. To identify and accept positive and negative expressions, feelings, and reactions
13. To identify and accept interrelatedness of emotions and organic illness
14. To facilitate the maintenance of effective verbal and nonverbal communication
15. To promote the development of productive interpersonal relationships
16. To facilitate progress toward achievement and personal spiritual goals
17. To create or maintain a therapeutic environment
18. To facilitate awareness of self as an individual with varying physical, emotional, and developmental needs
19. To accept the optimum possible goals in the light of limitations, physical and emotional
20. To use community resources as an aid in resolving problems that arise from illness
21. To understand the role of social problems as influencing factors in the cause of illness

From Abdellah, F. G., Beland, I. L., Martin, A., & Matheney, R. V. (1960). *Patient-centered approaches to nursing.* New York: Macmillan. Reprinted with the permission of Scribner, a division of Simon & Schuster.

newborn health nursing when the Yale School of Nursing established a master's degree program (Kaplan & King, 2000) and is the author of books used widely in nursing education. Her definition of nursing reflects her nurse-midwife background. She stated the following: "People may differ in their concept of nursing, but few would disagree that nursing is nurturing or caring for someone in a motherly fashion" (Wiedenbach, 1964, p. 1).

Wiedenbach's orientation is a philosophy of nursing that guides the nurse's action in the art of nursing. Wiedenbach specified four elements of clinical nursing: (1) philosophy, (2) purpose, (3) practice, and (4) art. She postulated that clinical nursing is directed toward meeting the patient's perceived need for help. Her vision of nursing reflects the period when considerable emphasis was placed on the art of nursing. She followed Orlando's theory of deliberate rather than automatic nursing and incorporated the steps of the nursing process. In her book (1964), *Clinical Nursing: A Helping Art,* Wiedenbach outlines nursing steps in sequence.

Wiedenbach proposes that nurses identify patients' need for help in the following ways:

1. Observing behaviors consistent or inconsistent with their comfort
2. Exploring the meaning of their behavior
3. Determining the cause of their discomfort or incapability
4. Determining whether they can resolve their problems or have a need for help

Following this, the nurse administers the help needed (Figure 5-4) and validates that the need for help was met (Figure 5-5) (Wiedenbach, 1964). Wiedenbach's work may be considered a philosophy of the art of nursing.

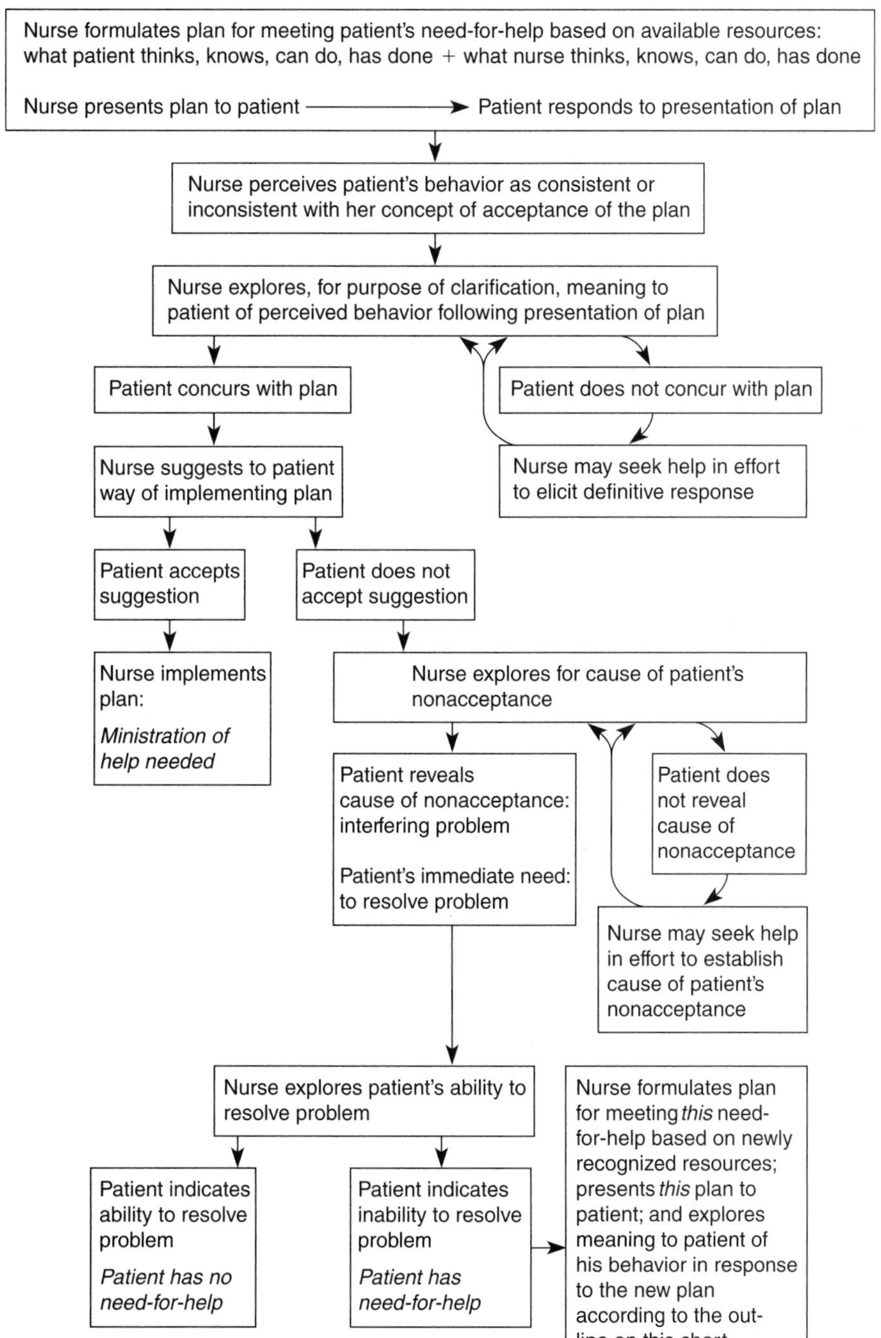

Figure 5-4 **Ministration of Help.** (From Wiedenbach, E. [1964]. *Clinical nursing: A helping art* [p. 61]. New York: Springer.)

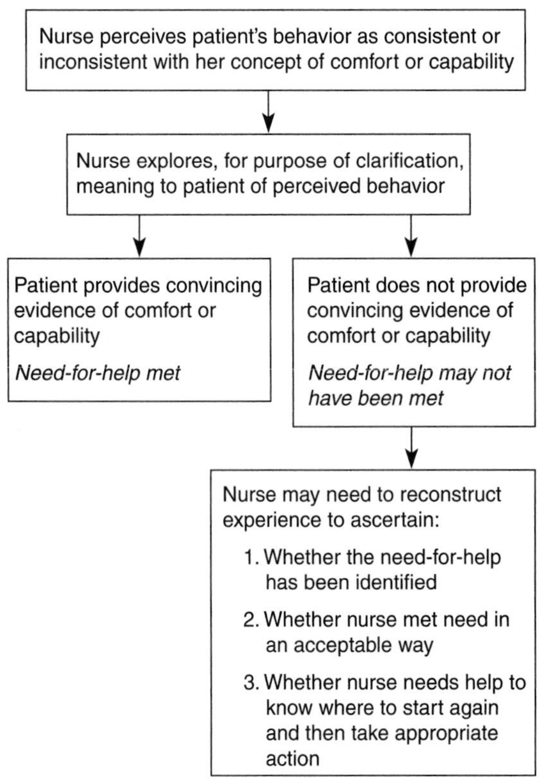

Figure 5-5 Validation that the Need for Help was Met. (From Wiedenbach, E. [1964]. *Clinical nursing: A helping art* [p. 62]. New York: Springer.)

LYDIA HALL

Core, Care, and Cure Model

Lydia Hall was a rehabilitation nurse who used her philosophy of nursing to establish the Loeb Center for Nursing and Rehabilitation at Montefiore Hospital in New York and served as administrative director of the Loeb Center from the time of its opening in 1963 until her death in 1969. In the 1960s, she published more than 20 articles about the Loeb Center and her theories of long-term care and chronic disease control. In 1964, Hall's work was presented in "Nursing: What Is It?" in *The Canadian Nurse.* In 1969, it was discussed in "The Loeb Center for Nursing and Rehabilitation" in the *International Journal of Nursing Studies.* In her innovative work at the Loeb Center, Hall argued that a need exists in society for the provision of hospital beds grouped into units that focus on the delivery of therapeutic nursing. The Loeb plan has been seen in many ways as similar to what later emerged as "primary nursing" (Wiggins, 1980).

An evaluation study of the Loeb Center for Nursing published in 1975 revealed that those admitted to the nursing unit when compared with those in a traditional unit were readmitted less often, were more independent, had a higher post-discharge quality of life, and were more satisfied with their hospital experience (Hall, Alfano, Rifkin, & Levine, 1975).

Using three interlocking circles to represent aspects of the patient, Hall proposed that nursing functions differ. The care circle represents the patient's body, the cure circle represents the disease that affects the patient's physical system, and the core circle represents the inner feelings and management of the person (Figure 5-6). The three circles change in size and overlap in relation to the patient's phase in the disease process. A nurse functions in all three circles but to different degrees. For example, in the care phase, the nurse gives hands-on bodily care to the patient in relation to activities of daily living

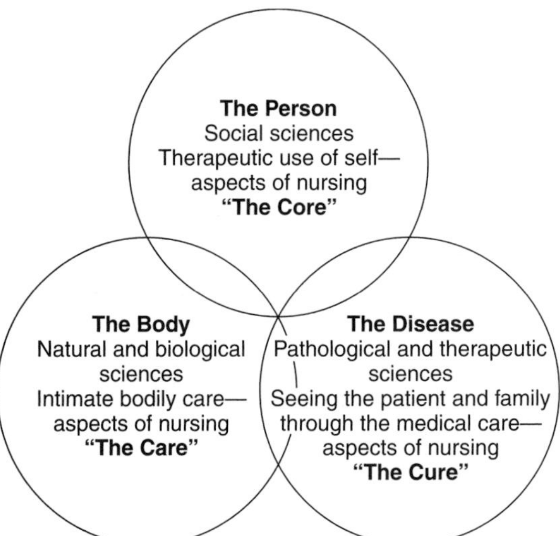

Figure 5-6 Core, Care, and Cure Model. (From Hall, L. [1964]. Nursing: What is it? *The Canadian Nurse, 60*[2], 151.)

such as toileting and bathing. In the cure phase, the nurse applies medical knowledge to treatment of the person, and in the core phase, the nurse addresses the social and emotional needs of the patient for effective communication and a comfortable environment (Touhy & Birnbach, 2001). Nurses also share the circles with other providers. Lydia Hall's theory was used to show improvement in patient-nurse communication, self-growth, and self-awareness in patients whose heart failure was managed in the home setting (McCoy, Davidhizar, & Gillum, 2007).

Hall believed that professional nursing care hastened recovery, and that as less medical care was needed, more professional nursing care and teaching were necessary. Hall stressed the autonomous function of nursing. Her conceptualization encompasses adult patients who have passed the acute stage of illness. The goal for the patient is rehabilitation and success in self-actualization and self-love. Her contribution to nursing theory was the development and use of her philosophy of nursing care at the Loeb Center in New York. She also recognized professional nurses and encouraged them to make a contribution to patient outcomes. Hall's work may be viewed as a philosophy of nursing.

JOYCE TRAVELBEE

Human-to-Human Relationship Model

Joyce Travelbee presented her Human-to-Human Relationship Theory in her book, *Interpersonal Aspects of Nursing* (1966, 1971). She published predominantly in the mid-1960s and died in 1973 at a relatively young age. She proposed that the goal of nursing was to assist an individual, family, or community to prevent or cope with the experiences of illness and suffering and, if necessary, to find meaning in these experiences, with the ultimate goal being the presence of hope (Travelbee, 1966, 1971). She discussed her theory with Victor Frankel (1963), whom she credits along with Rollo May (1953) for influencing her thinking (Meleis, 2007). Travelbee's work was conceptual, and she wrote about illness, suffering, pain, hope, communication, interaction, empathy, sympathy, rapport, and therapeutic use of self. She proposed that nursing was accomplished through human-to-human relationships that began with (1) the original encounter, which progressed through stages of (2) emerging identities, (3) developing feelings of empathy and, later, (4) sympathy, until (5) the nurse and the patient attained rapport in the final stage (Figure 5-7). Travelbee believed that it was as important to sympathize as it was to empathize if the nurse and the patient were to develop a *human-to-human* relationship (Travelbee, 1964). She was explicit about both the patient's and the nurse's spirituality, observing the following:

> "It is believed the spiritual values a person holds will determine, to a great extent, his perception of illness. The spiritual values of the nurse or her philosophical beliefs about illness and suffering will determine the degree to which he or she will be able to help ill persons find meaning, or no meaning, in these situations" (Travelbee, 1971, p. 16).

Travelbee's theory extended the interpersonal relationship theories of Peplau and Orlando, but her unique synthesis of their ideas differentiated her work in terms of the therapeutic human relationship between nurse and patient. Travelbee's emphasis on caring stressed empathy, sympathy, rapport, and the emotional aspects of nursing (Travelbee, 1963, 1964). Rich (2003) revisited Travelbee's argument on the value of sympathy in nursing and updated it with a reminder that compassion is central to holistic nursing care. Travelbee's work is categorized as a nursing theory.

KATHRYN E. BARNARD

Child Health Assessment

Kathryn E. Barnard is an active researcher, educator, and consultant who has published extensively since the mid-1960s about improving the health of infants and their families. She began her work by studying mentally and physically handicapped children and adults, moved into studying the activities of the well child, and then expanded her work to include methods of evaluating the growth and development of

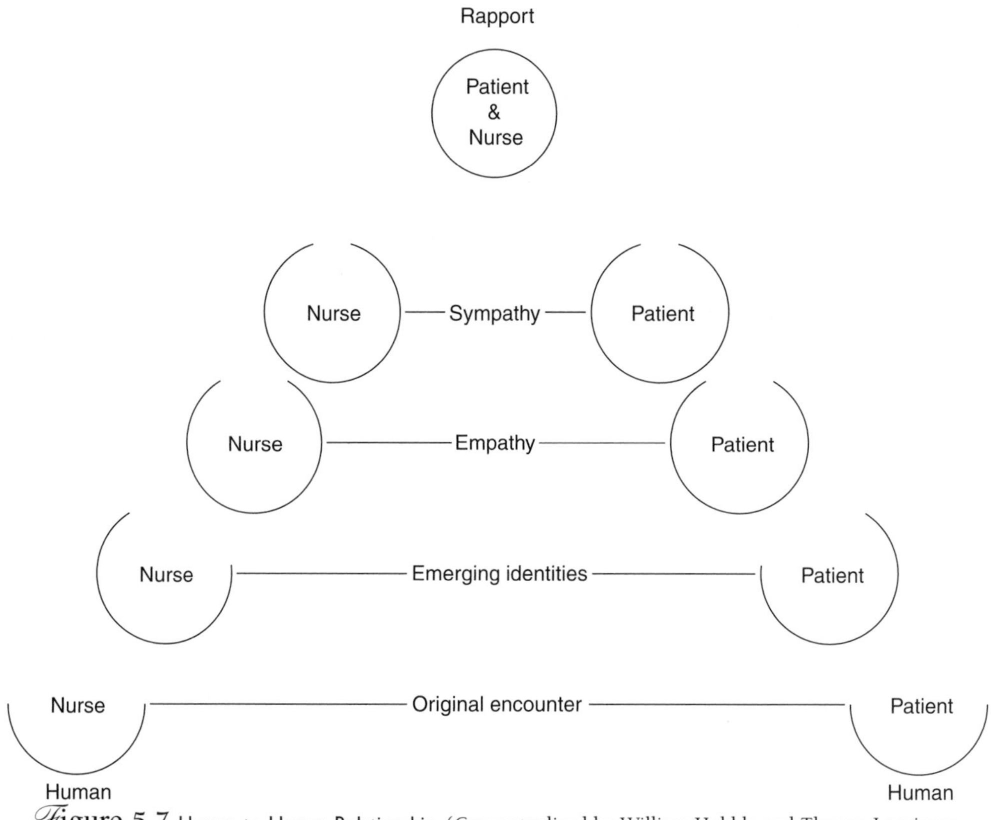

Figure 5-7 **Human-to-Human Relationship.** (Conceptualized by William Hobble and Theresa Lansinger, based on Joyce Travelbee's writings.)

children and mother-infant relationships, and how the environment can influence the course of development for children and families (Barnard, 2004). She is the founder of the Nursing Child Assessment Satellite Training Project (NCAST), which provides healthcare workers around the globe with guidelines for assessing infant development and parent-child interactions.

Although Barnard never intended to develop theory, the longitudinal nursing child assessment study provided the basis for her Child Health Assessment Interaction Theory (Figure 5-8). Barnard (1978) proposed that the individual characteristics of each member influence the parent-infant system, and that adaptive behavior modifies those characteristics to meet the needs of the system. Barnard's theory borrows from psychology and human development and focuses on mother-infant interaction with the environment. Her theory is based on scales designed to measure the effects of feeding, teaching, and environment (Kelly & Barnard, 2000). With continual research, she has refined the theory and has provided a close link to practice that has transformed the way that healthcare providers evaluate children in light of the parent-child relationship. Her model of mother-child interaction was used to study community problems that affect health disparities (Reifsnider, Gallagher, & Forgione, 2005). She models the role of researcher in clinical practice as she engages in theory development in practice for the advancement of nursing science. Barnard's work is a theory of nursing.

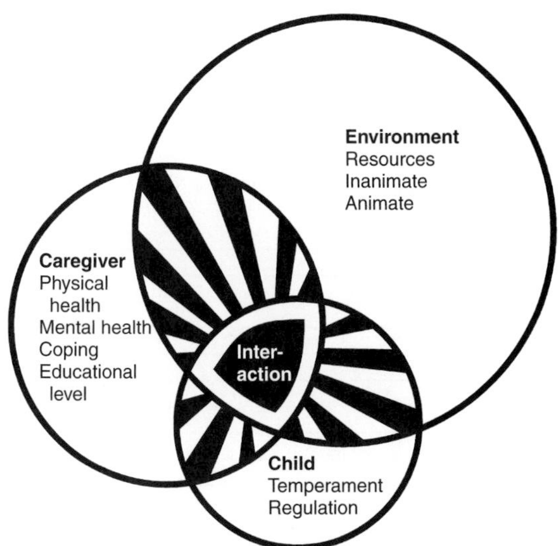

Figure 5-8 Child Health Assessment Model. (From Sumner, G., & Spietz, A. [Eds.]. [1994]. *NCAST caregiver/parent-child interaction teaching manual* [p. 3]. Seattle: NCAST Publications, University of Washington School of Nursing.)

EVELYN ADAM

Conceptual Model for Nursing

Evelyn Adam is a Canadian nurse who started publishing in the mid-1970s. Much of her work focuses on the development of models and theories on the concept of nursing (1983, 1987, 1999). She uses a model that she learned from Dorothy Johnson. In her book, *To Be a Nurse* (1980), she applies Virginia Henderson's definition of nursing to Johnson's model and identifies the assumptions, beliefs, and values, as well as major units. In the latter category, she includes the goal of the profession, the beneficiary of the professional service, the role of the professional, the source of the beneficiary's difficulty, the intervention of the professional, and the consequences. She expanded her work in a 1991 second edition. Adam's work is a good example of using a unique basis of nursing for further expansion. Adam's argument for a need for an ideological framework in nursing was described in a health telematics education conference (Tallberg, 1997). She has contributed to theory development with clear explanation of earlier works. Adam's work is a theory of nursing.

NANCY ROPER, WINIFRED W. LOGAN, AND ALISON J. TIERNEY

A Model for Nursing Based on a Model of Living

Nancy Roper is described as a practical theorist who produced a simple nursing theory, "which actually helped bedside nurses" (Dopson, 2004; Scott, 2004). After 15 years as a principal tutor in a school of nursing in England, Nancy Roper began her career as a full-time book writer during the 1960s and published several popular textbooks, including *Principles of Nursing* (1967). She investigated the concept of an identifiable "core" of nursing for her MPhil research study, published in a monograph titled *Clinical Experience in Nurse Education* (1976). This work served as the basis for her later work with theorists Winifred Logan and Alison Tierney. She authored *The Elements of Nursing* in 1980, 1985, and 1990. The trio collaborated in the fourth and most recent edition of *The Elements of Nursing: A Model for Nursing Based on a Model of Living* (1996). During the 1970s, they conducted research to discover the core of nursing, based on a Model of Living (Figure 5-9). This occurred in response to the use of qualifiers for naming nursing practice according to the ideas of medical practice. Three decades of study of the elements of nursing by Roper evolved into a model for nursing with five main factors that influenced activities of living (ALs) (Figure 5-10 and Table 5-1).

Rather than revising the fourth edition of their textbook, these theorists prepared a monograph (Roper, Logan, & Tierney, 2000) about the model titled *The Roper-Logan-Tierney Model of Nursing: Based on Activities of Living,* without application of the model. Holland, Jenkins, Solomon, and Whittam (2003) explored the use of the Roper-Logan-Tierney Model of Nursing. They used case studies and exercises about adult patients with a variety of health problems in acute care and community-based settings to help students develop problem-solving skills.

In the Model of Nursing, the ALs include maintaining a safe environment, communicating,

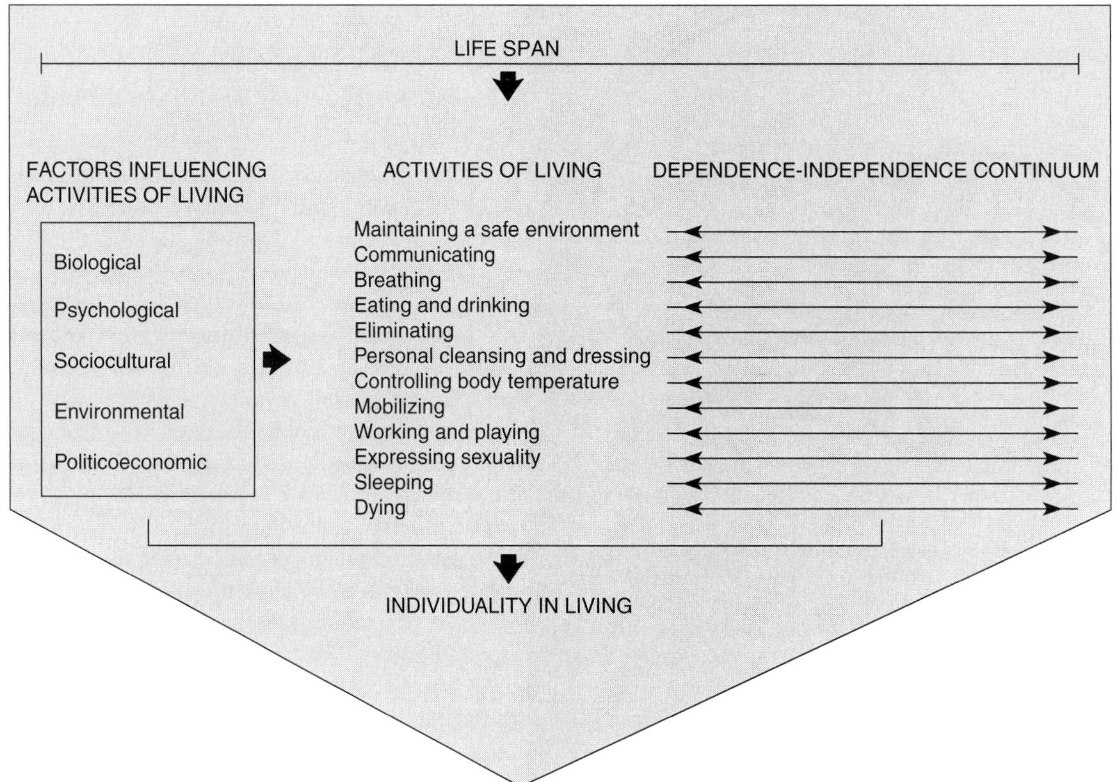

Figure 5-9 Diagram of the Model of Living. (From Roper, N., Logan W. W., & Tierney, A. J. [1996]. *The elements of nursing: A model for nursing based on a model of living* [4th ed., p. 20]. Edinburgh: Churchill Livingstone.)

breathing, eating and drinking, eliminating, personal cleansing and dressing, controlling body temperature, mobilizing, working and playing, expressing sexuality, sleeping, and dying. Life span ranges from birth to death, and the dependence-independence continuum ranges from total dependence to total independence. The five groups of factors that influence the ALs are biological, psychological, sociocultural, environmental, and politicoeconomic. Individuality of living is the way in which the individual attends to the ALs in regard to the individual's place in the life span, on the dependence-independence continuum, and as influenced by biological, psychological, sociocultural, environmental, and politicoeconomic factors.

In the Model of Nursing, the five components can be used to describe the individual in relation to maintaining health, preventing disease, coping during periods of sickness and rehabilitation, coping positively during periods of chronic ill health, and coping when dying. Individualizing nursing is accomplished by using the process of nursing, which involves four phases: (1) assessing, (2) planning, (3) implementing, and (4) evaluating. The process is simply a method of logical thinking, and it should be used with an explicit nursing model. The patient's individuality in living must be borne in mind during all four phases of the process. This model has been used as a guide for nursing practice, research, and education.

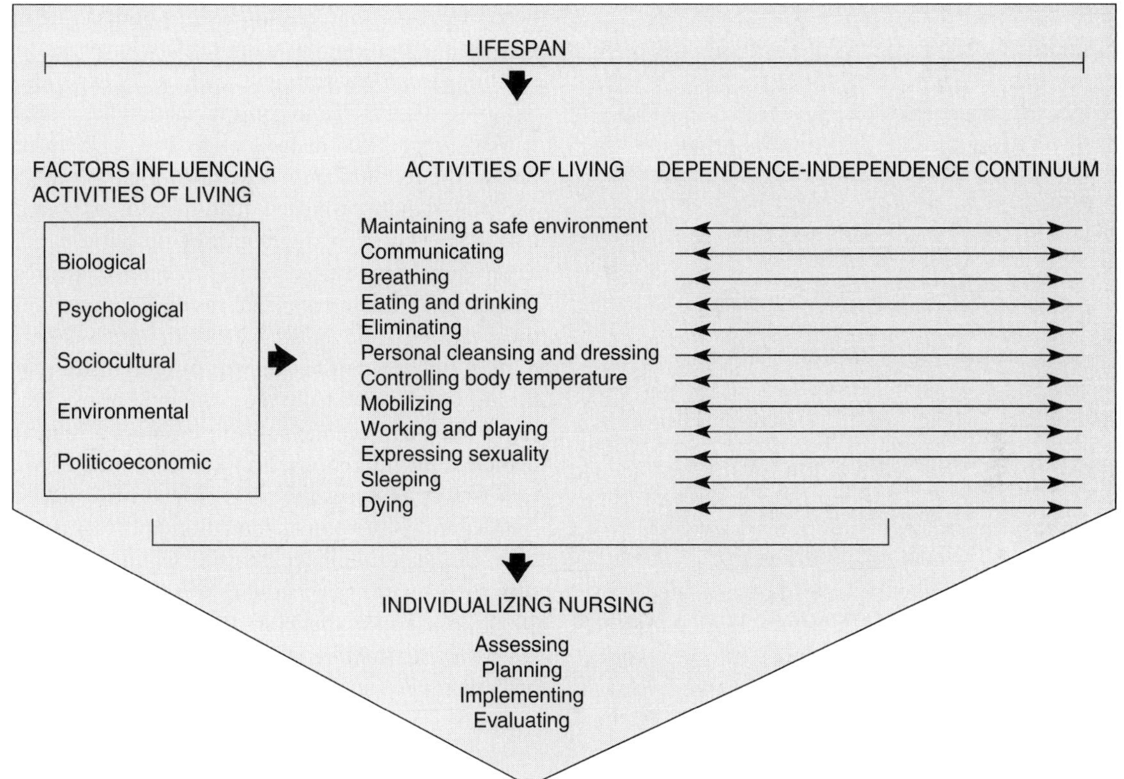

Figure 5-10 Diagram of the Model for Nursing. (From Roper, N., Logan, W. W., & Tierney, A. J. [1996]. *The elements of nursing: A model for nursing based on a model of living* [4th ed., p. 34]. Edinburgh: Churchill Livingstone.)

IDA JEAN (ORLANDO) PELLETIER

Nursing Process Theory

Ida Jean Orlando developed her theory from a study that she conducted at Yale University School of Nursing on integrating mental health concepts into a basic nursing curriculum. This study was carried out by observing and participating in experiences with patients, students, nurses, and instructors and was derived inductively from field notes for this study. Orlando analyzed the content of 2000 nurse-patient contacts and created her theory based on analysis of these data (Schmieding, 1993). Meleis (2007) has noted, "... Orlando was one of the early thinkers in nursing who proposed that patients have their own meanings and interpretations of situations and therefore nurses must validate their inferences and analyses with patients before drawing conclusions..." (p. 347). The foundation for her theory was published *in The Dynamic Nurse-Patient Relationship* (1961), which was an outcome of this project. The purpose of her book was to contribute to concern about the nurse-patient relationship, the nurse's professional role and identity, and the knowledge development distinct to nursing (Schmieding, 1993). In 1990, the National League for Nursing (NLN) reprinted Orlando's 1961 publication. In the preface to the NLN edition, Orlando states the following: "If I had been more courageous in 1961, when this book was first written, I would have proposed it

Table 5-1 Comparison of the Main Concepts in the Model of Living and the Model for Nursing

Model of Living	Model for Nursing
12 ALs	12 ALs
Life span	Life span
Dependence-independence continuum	Dependence-independence continuum
Factors influencing the ALs	Factors influencing the ALs
Individuality in living	Individualizing nursing

From Roper, N., Logan, W. W., & Tierney, A. J. (1996). *The elements of nursing: A model for nursing based on a model for living* (4th ed., p. 33). Edinburgh: Churchill Livingstone.

as 'nursing process theory' instead of as a 'theory of effective nursing practice'" (Orlando, 1990, p. vii).

She continued to develop and refine her work, and in her second book, *The Discipline and Teaching of Nursing Process: An Evaluative Study* (1972), she redefined and renamed deliberative nursing process as nursing process discipline.

Orlando's nursing theory stresses the reciprocal relationship between patient and nurse. What the nurse and the patient say and do affects them both. Orlando (1961) views the professional function of nursing as finding out and meeting the patient's immediate need for help. This function is fulfilled when the nurse finds out and meets a patient's immediate need for help. She was one of the first nursing leaders to identify and emphasize the elements of nursing process and the critical importance of the patient's participation in the nursing process. Orlando's theory focuses on how to produce improvement in the patient's behavior. Evidence of relieving the patient's distress is seen as positive changes in the patient's observable behavior. Orlando may have facilitated the development of nurses as logical thinkers (Nursing Theories Conference Group & George, 1980).

According to Orlando (1961), persons become patients who require nursing care when they have needs for help that cannot be met independently because they have physical limitations, have negative reactions to an environment, or have an experience that prevents them from communicating their needs. Patients experience distress or feelings of helplessness as the result of unmet needs for help (Orlando, 1961). Orlando proposed that there is a positive correlation between the length of time the patient experiences unmet needs and the degree of distress. Therefore, immediacy is emphasized throughout her theory. In Orlando's view, when individuals are able to meet their own needs, they do not feel distress and do not require care from a professional nurse. Practice guided by Orlando's theory employs a reflexive principle for inference testing (Schmieding, 2006a). Orlando emphasizes that it is crucial for nurses to share their perceptions, thoughts, and feelings so they can determine whether their inferences are congruent with the patient's need (Schmieding, 2006b). Orlando's theory remains one of the most effective practice theories and is especially helpful to new nurses as they begin their practice.

POINTS FOR *Further Study*

- Travelbee, J. (1971). *Interpersonal aspects of nursing* (2nd ed.). Philadelphia: F. A. Davis.
- Roper, N., Logan, W. W., & Tierney, A. J. (1996). *The elements of nursing: A model for nursing based on a model for living* (4th ed.). Edinburgh: Churchill Livingstone.
- Orlando, I. J. (1990). *The dynamic nurse-patient relationship: Function, process, and principles* (Pub. No. 15-2341). New York: National League for Nursing.
- Orlando interview: Nursing process discipline (n.d.). In *Nurse theorists: Portraits of excellence, Volume I* (video). Athens, Ohio: Fitne, Inc.
- Peplau, H. (1952). *Interpersonal relations in nursing.* New York: G. P. Putnam's Sons.
- Peplau Interview: Interpersonal relations in nursing. (n.d.). In *Nurse theorists: Portraits of excellence, Volume I* (video). Athens, Ohio: Fitne, Inc.
- Schmieding, N. (2006a). Orlando's nursing process

theory and nursing practice. In M. R. Alligood & A. M. Tomey (Eds.). *Nursing Theory: Utilization & application* (3rd ed., pp. 335-361). St. Louis: Mosby.

- Schmieding, N. J. (2006b). Ida Jean Orlando (Pelletier): Nursing process theory. In A. M. Tomey & M. R. Alligood (Eds.). *Nursing theorists and their work* (6th ed., pp. 431-451). St. Louis: Mosby.
- Barnard, K. E. (2004). Welcome and Opening Plenary. Proceedings from AMCHP '04: *Mental health—Promoting a new paradigm for MCH public health practice.* Transcript available at: http://128.248.232.90/archives/mchb/amchp2004/p1/transcripts/session09f.htm
- Kaplan, D., & King, C. (2000). *Guide to the Ernestine Wiedenbach papers.* Retrieved from: http://webtext.library.yale.edu/xml2html/mssa.1647.con.html#top

REFERENCES

Abdellah, F. G. (2004). Interview with Rear Admiral Faye Glenn Abdellah. Interview by Captain Melvin Lessing. *Military Medicine. 169*(11):iii-xi.

Abdellah, F. G., Beland, I. L., Martin, A., & Matheney, R. V. (1960). *Patient-centered approaches to nursing.* New York: Macmillan.

Abdellah, F. G., & Levine, E. (1994). *Preparing for nursing research in the 21st century: Evolution, methodologies, challenges.* New York: Springer.

Adam, E. (1980). *To be a nurse.* Philadelphia: W. B. Saunders.

Adam, E. (1983). Frontiers of nursing in the 21st century: Development of models and theories on the concept of nursing. *Journal of Advanced Nursing, 8,* 41-45.

Adam, E. (1987). Nursing theory: What it is and what it is not. *Nursing papers. Perspectives in Nursing, 19,* 5-14.

Adam, E. (1991). *To be a nurse* (2nd ed.). Montreal: W. B. Saunders Company Canada.

Adam, E. (1999). Conceptual models. *Canadian Journal of Nursing Research, 30,* 103-114.

Barnard, K. E. (1978). *Nursing child assessment and training: Learning resource manual.* Seattle: University of Washington.

Barnard, K. E. (2004). Welcome and Opening Plenary. Proceedings from AMCHP '04: *Mental health—Promoting a new paradigm for MCH public health practice.* Transcript available at: http://128.248.232.90/archives/mchb/amchp2004/p1/transcripts/session09f.htm

Dickoff, J. James, P., & Wiedenbach, E. (1968). Theory in a practice discipline, part II: Practice oriented research. *Nursing Research, 17*(6), 545-554.

Dopson, L. (2004, October 15). Obituary: Nancy Roper. *The Independent.* Retrieved from: http://www.independent.co.uk

Frankel, V. (1963). *Man's search for meaning: An introduction to logotherapy.* New York: Washington Square Press.

Haber, J. (2000). Hildegard E. Peplau: The psychiatric nursing legacy of a legend. *Journal of the American Psychiatric Nurses Association, 6,* 56-62.

Hall, L. E. (1964, Feb.). Nursing: What is it? *The Canadian Nurse, 60,* 150-154.

Hall, L. E. (1969). The Loeb Center for nursing and rehabilitation. *International Journal of Nursing Studies, 6,* 81-95.

Hall, L. E., Alfano G. J., Rifkin E., & Levine H. S. (1975). *Longitudinal effects of an experimental nursing process (final report).* New York: Loeb Center for Nursing and Rehabilitation.

Henderson, V. (1955). *Textbook of the principles and practice of nursing,* 5th ed. New York: Macmillan. (Note: earlier editions were Harmer & Henderson).

Henderson, V. (1960). *Basic principles of nursing care.* London: International Council of Nurses.

Henderson, V. (1964). The nature of nursing. *American Journal of Nursing, 64,* 62-68.

Henderson, V. (1966). *The nature of nursing: A definition and its implications for practice, research, and education.* New York: Macmillan.

Henderson, V. A. (1991). *The nature of nursing: Reflections after 25 years.* New York: National League for Nursing Press.

Holland, K., Jenkins, J., Solomon, J., & Whittam, S. (2003). *Applying the Roper-Logan-Tierney Model in practice.* Edinburgh: Churchill Livingstone.

Kaplan, D., & King, C. (2000). *Guide to the Ernestine Wiedenbach papers.* Retrieved from: http://webtext.library.yale.edu/xml2html/mssa.1647.con.html#top

Kelly, J. F., & Barnard, K. E. (2000). Assessment of parent-child interaction: Implications for early intervention. In S. Shonkoff & S. J. Meisels (Eds.), *Handbook of early childhood intervention* (pp. 258-289). Cambridge: Cambridge University Press.

May, R. (1953). *Man's search for himself.* New York: W. W. Norton.

Meleis, A. (2007). *Theoretical nursing: Development and progress* (4th ed.). Philadelphia: Lippincott Williams & Wilkins.

McCoy, M. L., Davidhizar, R., & Gillum, D. R. (2007). A correlational pilot study of home health nurse management of heart failure patients and hospital readmissions. *Home Health Care Management and Practice, 19,* 392-396.

National Library of Medicine. (1988). *Finding aid to the Faye Glenn Abdellah papers, 1952-1989.* (NIH Collection No. MS C 424). Bethesda, MD: National Library of Medicine. Retrieved from: http://www.nlm.nih.gov/hmd/manuscripts/ead/abdellah.html

Nursing Theories Conference Group, & George, J. B. (Chairperson). (1980). *Nursing theories: The base for professional practice.* Englewood Cliffs, NJ: Prentice-Hall.

Orlando, I. J. (1961). *The dynamic nurse-patient relationship: Function, process and principles of professional nursing practice.* New York: G. P. Putnam's Sons.

Orlando, I. J. (1972). *The discipline and teaching of nursing process: An evaluative study.* New York: G. P. Putnam's Sons.

Orlando, I. J. (1990). *The dynamic nurse-patient relationship: Function, process, and principles* (Pub. No. 15-2341). New York: National League for Nursing.

Peplau, H. E. (1952). *Interpersonal relations in nursing.* New York: G. P. Putnam's Sons.

Reifsnider, E., Gallagher, M., & Forgione, B. (2005). Using ecological models in research on health disparities. *Journal of Professional Nursing, 21*, 216-222.

Rich, K. (2003) Revisiting Joyce Travelbee's question: What's wrong with sympathy?. *Journal of the American Psychiatric Association, 9*(6):202-205.

Roper, N. (1967). *Principles of nursing.* Edinburgh: Churchill Livingstone.

Roper, N. (1976). *Clinical experience in nurse education* (Research monograph). Edinburgh: Churchill Livingstone.

Roper, N. (1980). *The elements of nursing: A model for nursing.* Edinburgh: Churchill Livingstone.

Roper, N. (1985). *The elements of nursing: A model for nursing* (2nd ed.). Edinburgh: Churchill Livingstone.

Roper, N. (1990). *The elements of nursing: A model for nursing based on a model of living* (3rd ed.). Edinburgh: Churchill Livingstone.

Roper, N., Logan, W. W., & Tierney, A. J. (1996). *The elements of nursing: A model for nursing based on a model for living* (4th ed.). Edinburgh: Churchill Livingstone.

Roper, N., Logan, W. W, & Tierney, A. J. (2000). *The Roper-Logan-Tierney model of nursing: Based on activities of living.* Edinburgh: Churchill Livingstone.

Schmieding, N. J. (1993). *Ida Jean Orlando: A nursing process theory.* Newbury Park, CA: Sage Publications.

Schmeiding, N. (2006a). Orlando's nursing process theory and nursing practice. In M. R. Alligood and A. M. Tomey (Eds.), *Nursing theory: Utilization & application* (3rd ed., pp. 335-361). St. Louis: Mosby.

Schmieding, N. J. (2006b). Ida Jean Orlando (Pelletier): Nursing process theory. In A. M. Tomey & M. R. Alligood (Eds.), *Nursing theorists and their work* (6th ed., pp. 431-451). St. Louis: Mosby.

Scott, H. (2004). Nancy Roper (1918-2004): A great nursing pioneer. *British Journal of Nursing, 19*, 1121.

Sills, G. M. (1998). Peplau and professionalism: The emergence of the paradigm of professionalization. *Journal of Psychiatric and Mental Health Nursing, 5*, 167-171.

Tallberg, M. (1997). Supporting the nursing process—An aim for education in nursing informatics. In Mantas J. (ed.), *Health telematics education: Studies in health technology and informatics*, vol 41 (pp. 291-296). Amsterdam: IOS Press.

Touhy, T. A., & Birnbach, N. (2001). Lydia Hall, The care, core, cure model. In M. E. Parker (Ed.), *Nursing theories and nursing practice* (pp. 135-137). Philadelphia: F. A. Davis.

Travelbee, J. (1963). What do we mean by rapport? *The American Journal of Nursing, 63*, 70-72.

Travelbee, J. (1964). What's wrong with sympathy? *American Journal of Nursing, 64*, 68-71.

Travelbee, J. (1966). *Interpersonal aspects of nursing.* Philadelphia: F. A. Davis.

Travelbee, J. (1971). *Interpersonal aspects of nursing* (2nd ed.). Philadelphia: F. A. Davis.

Wiedenbach, E. (1964). *Clinical nursing: A helping art.* New York: Springer.

Wiggins, R. L. (1980). Lydia Hall's place in the development of theory of nursing. *Image: Journal of Nursing Scholarship, 12*, 10-12.

Wolf, K. A. (2006). Advancing the profession. In L. C. Andrist, P. K. Nicholas, & K. A. Wolf (Eds.), *A history of nursing ideas* (pp. 301-304). Sudbury, MA: Jones & Bartlett Publishers.

UNIT

II

Philosophies

- *Nursing philosophy sets forth the meaning of nursing phenomena through analysis, reasoning, and logical argument.*
- *Philosophies contribute to nursing knowledge by providing direction for the discipline, forming a basis for professional scholarship and leading to new theoretical understandings.*
- *Nursing philosophies represent early works pre-dating the theory era, as well as contemporary works of a philosophical nature.*
- *Philosophies are works that provide broad understanding that advances the discipline and its professional application.*

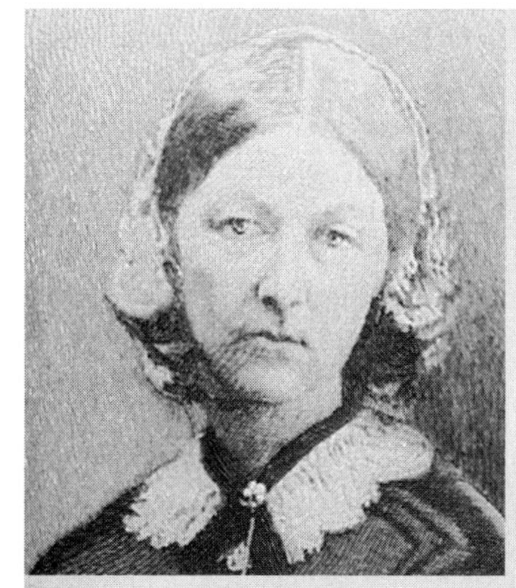

CHAPTER 6

Florence Nightingale

1820-1910

Modern Nursing

Susan A. Pfettscher

"Recognition of nursing as a professional endeavor distinct from medicine began with Nightingale" (Chinn & Kramer, 2008, p. 30).

CREDENTIALS AND BACKGROUND OF THE THEORIST

Florence Nightingale, the founder of modern nursing, was born on May 12, 1820, in Florence, Italy, while her parents were on an extended European tour; she was named after her birthplace. The Nightingales were a well-educated, affluent, aristocratic Victorian family with residences in Derbyshire (Lea Hurst their primary home) and Hampshire (Embley Park). This latter residence was near London, allowing the family to participate in London's social seasons.

Although the extended Nightingale family was large, the immediate family included only Florence Nightingale and her older sister, Parthenope. During her childhood, Nightingale's father educated her more broadly than other girls of the time. Her father and others tutored her in mathematics, languages, religion, and philosophy (influences on her lifework). Although she participated in the usual Victorian aristocratic activities and social events during her adolescence, Nightingale developed the sense that her life should become more useful. In 1837, Nightingale wrote about her "calling" in her diary: "God spoke to me and called me to his service" (Holliday & Parker, 1997, p. 41). The nature of her calling was unclear to her for some time. After she understood that she was called to become a nurse, she was able to complete her nursing training in 1851 at Kaiserwerth, Germany, a Protestant religious community with a hospital facility. She was there for approximately 3 months, and at the end, her teachers declared her trained as a nurse.

After her return to England, Nightingale was employed to examine hospital facilities, reformatories,

Previous authors: Susan A. Pfettscher, Karen R. de Graff, Ann Marriner Tomey, Cynthia L. Mossman, and Maribeth Slebodnik.

and charitable institutions. Only 2 years after completing her training (in 1853), she became the superintendent of the Hospital for Invalid Gentlewomen in London.

During the Crimean War, Nightingale received a request from Sidney Herbert (a family friend and the Secretary of War) to travel to Scutari, Turkey, with a group of nurses to care for wounded British soldiers. She arrived there in November of 1854, accompanied by 34 newly recruited nurses who met her criteria for professional nursing—young, middle-class women with a basic general education. To achieve her mission of providing nursing care, she needed to address the environmental problems that existed, including the lack of sanitation and the presence of filth (few chamber pots, contaminated water, contaminated bed linens, and overflowing cesspools). In addition, the soldiers were faced with exposure, frostbite, louse infestations, wound infections, and opportunistic diseases as they recovered from their battle wounds (Thomas, 1993).

Nightingale's work in improving these deplorable conditions made her a popular and revered person to the soldiers, but the support of physicians and military officers was less enthusiastic. She was called The Lady of the Lamp, as immortalized in the poem "Santa Filomena" (Longfellow, 1857), because she made ward rounds during the night, providing emotional comfort to the soldiers. In Scutari, Nightingale became critically ill with Crimean fever, which might have been typhus or brucellosis and which may have affected her physical condition for years afterward.

After the war, Nightingale returned to England to great accolades, particularly from the royal family (Queen Victoria), the soldiers who had survived the Crimean War, their families, and the families of those who died at Scutari. She was awarded funds in recognition of this work, which she used to establish schools for nursing training at St. Thomas' Hospital and King's College Hospital in London. Within a few years, the Nightingale School began to receive requests to establish new schools at hospitals worldwide, and Florence Nightingale's reputation as the founder of modern nursing was established (Lobo, 1995).

Nightingale devoted her energies not only to the development of nursing as a vocation (profession), but even more to local, national, and international societal issues, in an attempt to improve the living environment of the poor and to create social change (Isler, 1970). She continued to concentrate on army sanitation reform, the functions of army hospitals, sanitation in India, and sanitation and healthcare for the poor in England. Her writings, *Notes on Matters Affecting the Health, Efficiency, and Hospital Administration of the British Army Founded Chiefly on the Experience of the Late War* (Nightingale, 1858a), *Notes on Hospitals* (Nightingale, 1858b), and *Report on Measures Adopted for Sanitary Improvements in India from June 1869 to June 1870* (Nightingale, 1870), reflect her continuing concern about these issues.

Shortly after her return to England, Nightingale confined herself to her residence in London, citing her continued ill health. Until age 80, she wrote between 15,000 and 20,000 letters to friends, acquaintances, allies, and opponents. Her strong, clear written word conveyed her beliefs, observations, and desire for change in healthcare and in society. Through these writings, she was able to influence issues in the world that concerned her. When necessary and when her health allowed, she received powerful persons as visitors in her home to maintain dialogue, plot strategies to support causes, and carry out her work.

During her lifetime, Nightingale's work was recognized through the many awards she received from her own country and from many others. She was able to work into her 80s until she lost her vision; she died in her sleep on August 13, 1910, at age 90.

Modern biographers and essayists have attempted to analyze Nightingale's lifework through her family relationships, notably with her parents and sister. Film dramatizations have focused frequently and inaccurately on her personal relationships with family and friends. Although her personal and public life holds great intrigue for many, these retrospective analyses often are very negative and harshly critical or overly positive in their descriptions of this Victorian leader and founder of modern nursing.

Many biographies have been written to describe Nightingale's life and work. Cook (1913) wrote the first original and comprehensive biography of Nightingale, which was based on her written papers but may have been biased by her family's involvement in and oversight of this project. It remains the most positive biography written. Shortly thereafter, Strachey (1918) described her negatively as arrogant and manipulative in his book, *Eminent Victorians.* O'Malley (1931) wrote a more positive biography that focused on her life from 1820 to 1856; however, the second volume, which would have described the rest of her life and activities, was never published. Woodham-Smith's book (1951) chronicled her entire life and was drawn primarily from original documents made available by her family. This is the biography with which most Americans are familiar; it has endured as the definitive biography of Nightingale's life, and although it is more balanced, it maintains a positive tone. In 1982, F. B. Smith (1982) wrote *Florence Nightingale: Reputation and Power*, which is critical of Nightingale's character and her work. Most recently, Small (1998) published yet another Nightingale biography titled *Florence Nightingale: Avenging Angel.* Although he is critical of specific aspects of her character and work, he is more balanced in his presentation. He notes that Nightingale's life "is better documented than perhaps any previous life in history" because of the vast quantity of family and personal papers that remain available today (Small, 2000). His concerns and disagreements with other biographers have been noted in reviews (Small, 2008). Small continues to study Nightingale and updates his website with additional information about the Crimean War and Nightingale. The controversy and intrigue about Nightingale's role, her status, and her confined lifestyle continue; a London newspaper recently reported on newly found letters related to the conflicts Nightingale had with Sir John Hall (chief British army medical officer in the Crimea) (Kennedy, 2007). Perhaps in this current time, one might consider a diagnosis of post-traumatic stress disorder (PTSD).

An Internet search reveals thousands of sites that provide various articles, resources, and commentaries about Nightingale. Clearly, the world still is fascinated by this unique woman.

The nursing community in the United States remains similarly fascinated by the life and work of Nightingale. During their professional careers, Kalisch and Kalisch (1983a, 1983b, 1987) published several critiques of media portrayals that provide a better understanding of the many histories of Florence Nightingale; their techniques may provide methods of analyzing more recent publications and events for persons interested in studying Nightingale's life and work. Dossey's (2000) comprehensive book, *Florence Nightingale: Mystic, Visionary, Healer*, provides the reader with another in-depth history and interpretation of Nightingale's personal life and work. Using quotes from Nightingale's own writings (diaries and letters) and from those of people with whom she interacted and corresponded during her lifetime, Dossey focused on interpreting the spiritual nature of her being and her lifework, creating yet another way of looking at her. In an introduction/prelude to her descriptions of spirituality for nurses' lives based on Nightingale's writings, Macrae (2001) explores Nightingale's personal spirituality as she interprets it after review of writings and documents. Lorentzon (2003) more recently has provided a review and analysis of letters written between Nightingale and one of her former students that clearly demonstrate her role as mentor.

Finally, all of Nightingale's surviving writings are in the process of being published as *The Collected Works of Florence Nightingale.* To date, ten of the sixteen volumes have been published under the leadership of sociologist Lynn McDonald (McDonald, 2001-present). This large project and other newly discovered/released documents will continue to spawn articles and books that will explore, interpret, and speculate on her life and work.

THEORETICAL SOURCES FOR THEORY DEVELOPMENT

Many factors influenced the development of Nightingale's philosophy of nursing. Her personal, societal, and professional values and concerns all were integral to the development of her beliefs. She combined her individual resources with societal and professional resources available to her to produce change.

As noted, Nightingale's education was an unusual one for a Victorian girl. Her tutelage by her well-educated, intellectual father in subjects such as mathematics and philosophy provided her with knowledge and conceptual thinking abilities that were unique for women of her time. Although her parents initially opposed her desire to study mathematics, they relented and allowed her to receive additional tutoring from well-respected mathematicians. Her aunt Mai, a devoted relative and companion, described her as having a great mind; this is not a description that was used at the time for Victorian women, but it is one that was accepted for Nightingale. It remains unknown whether or not Nightingale was a genius who would have been a great leader and thinker under any circumstance, or whether her unique, formal education and social status were necessary for this to occur at the time. Would Nightingale become such a leader if born today? What would nursing be today if she had not been born at that time and in that place?

The Nightingale family's aristocratic social status provided her with easy access to people of power and influence. Many were family friends, such as Stanley Herbert, who remained an ally and staunch supporter until his death. Nightingale learned to understand the political processes of Victorian England through the experiences of her father during his short-lived political career and through his continuing role as an aristocrat involved in the political and social activities of his community. She most likely relied on this foundation and on her own experiences as she waged political battles for her causes.

Nightingale also recognized the societal changes of her time and their impact on the health status of individuals. The industrial age had descended upon England, creating new social classes, new diseases, and new social problems. Dickens' social commentaries and novels provided English society with scathing commentaries on healthcare and the need for health and social reform in England. In the novel, *Martin Chuzzlewit* (Dickens, 1987), Dickens' portrayal of Sairey Gamp as a drunken, untrained nurse provided society with an image of the horrors of Victorian nursing practice. Nightingale's alliance with Dickens undoubtedly influenced her definitions of nursing and healthcare and her theory for nursing; that relationship also provided her with a forum for expressing her views about social and healthcare issues (Dossey, 2000; Kalisch & Kalisch, 1983a; Woodham-Smith, 1951).

Similar dialogues with political leaders, intellectuals, and social reformers of the day (John Stuart Mill, Benjamin Jowett, Edwin Chadwick, and Harriet Marineau) advanced Nightingale's philosophical and logical thinking, which is evident in her philosophy and theory of nursing (Dossey, 2000; Kalisch & Kalisch, 1983a; Woodham-Smith, 1951). These dialogues likely inspired her to strive to change the things she viewed as unacceptable in the society in which she lived. No other nursing leader could better exemplify Chinn and Kramer's statement that "When individual, professional, or societal values change, the potential exists for creating fundamental change in knowledge and practice" (2008, p. 69).

Finally, Nightingale's religious affiliation and beliefs were especially strong sources for her nursing theory. Reared as a Unitarian, her belief that action for the benefit of others is a primary way of serving God served as the foundation for defining her nursing work as a religious calling. In addition, the Unitarian community strongly supported education as a means of developing divine potential and helping people move toward perfection in their lives and in their service to God. Nightingale's faith provided her with personal strength throughout her life and with the belief that education was a critical factor in establishing the profession of nursing. Also, religious conflicts of the time, particularly between the Anglican and Catholic Churches in the British Empire, may have led to her strongly held belief that nursing could and should be a secular profession (Dossey, 2000; Helmstadter, 1997; Nelson, 1997; Woodham-Smith, 1951). Despite her strong religious beliefs and her acknowledgment of her calling, this was not a requirement for her nurses.

Indeed, her opposition to the work of the nuns in Crimea (she reported that they were proselytizing) escalated the conflict to the level of involvement of the Vatican (Dossey, 2000; Woodham-Smith, 1951). As parish nursing has seen a resurgence in the United States and missionary work by nurses continues throughout the world, Nelson's review of pastoral care in the nineteenth century provides an interesting historical view of the role of religious service in nursing (Nelson, 1997).

MAJOR CONCEPTS & DEFINITIONS

Nightingale's theory focused on the environment. Although Nightingale never used the term *environment* in her writing, she did define and describe in detail the concepts of ventilation, warmth, light, diet, cleanliness, and noise—components of surroundings that have come to be known as environment in discussions of her work.

Although Nightingale defined concepts precisely, she did not distinguish aspects of the patient's environment as physical, emotional, or social. When reading *Notes on Nursing* (Nightingale, 1969) and her other writings, one can easily identify an emphasis on the physical environment. In the context of the specific issues she identified and struggled to improve and correct in various settings (war-torn environment and workhouses) during her time, this emphasis appears to be most appropriate (Gropper, 1990). Her concern about healthy surroundings involved hospital settings in Crimea and England, but it also extended to the public in their private homes and to the physical living conditions of the poor. She believed that healthy surroundings were necessary for proper nursing care. Her theoretical work on five essential components of environmental health (pure air, pure water, efficient drainage, cleanliness, and light) is as relevant today as it was 150 years ago.

Proper ventilation for the patient seemed to be of greatest concern to Nightingale; her charge to nurses was to "keep the air he breathes as pure as the external air, without chilling him" (Nightingale, 1969, p. 12). Notwithstanding her rejection of the germ theory (newly developed at the time), Nightingale's emphasis on proper ventilation indicates that she seemed to recognize this environmental component as a source of disease and recovery. In addition to discussing ventilation in the room or home, Nightingale provided a description for measuring the patient's body temperature through palpation of extremities to check for heat loss (Nightingale, 1969). The nurse was instructed to manipulate the environment continually to maintain ventilation and patient warmth by using a good fire, opening windows, and properly positioning the patient in the room.

The concept of light was also of importance in Nightingale's theory. In particular, she identified direct sunlight as a particular need of patients. She noted that "light has quite as real and tangible effects upon the human body . . . Who has not observed the purifying effect of light, and especially of direct sunlight, upon the air of a room?" (Nightingale, 1969, pp. 84-85). To achieve the beneficial effects of sunlight, nurses were instructed to move and position patients to expose them to sunlight.

Cleanliness as a concept is another critical component of Nightingale's environmental theory (Nightingale, 1969). In this regard, she specifically addressed the patient, the nurse, and the physical environment. She noted that a dirty environment (floors, carpets, walls, and bed linens) was a source of infection through the organic matter it contained. Even if the environment was well ventilated, the presence of organic material created a dirty area; therefore, appropriate handling and disposal of bodily excretions and sewage were required to prevent contamination of

Continued

MAJOR CONCEPTS & DEFINITIONS—cont'd

the environment. Finally, Nightingale advocated bathing patients on a frequent, even daily, basis at a time when this practice was not the norm. She required that nurses also bathe daily, that their clothing be clean, and that they wash their hands frequently (Nightingale, 1969). This concept held special significance for individual patient care, and it was critically important in improving the health status of the poor who were living in crowded, environmentally inferior conditions with inadequate sewage and limited access to pure water (Nightingale, 1969).

Nightingale included the concepts of quiet and diet in her environmental theory. The nurse was required to assess the need for quiet and to intervene as needed (Nightingale, 1969). Noise created by physical activities in the areas around a patient's room was to be avoided because it could harm the patient.

Nightingale was also concerned about the patient's diet (Nightingale, 1969). She instructed nurses to assess not only dietary intake, but also the meal schedule and its effect on the patient. She believed that patients with chronic illness could be starved to death unintentionally, and that intelligent nurses were those who were successful in meeting their patients' nutritional needs.

Another component of Nightingale's writing was a description of petty management (Nightingale, 1969). She pointed out that the nurse was in control of the environment both physically and administratively. The nurse was to control the environment to protect the patient from both physical and psychological harm, for example, the nurse should protect the patient from receiving upsetting news, from seeing visitors who could negatively affect recovery, and from experiencing sudden disruptions of sleep. In addition, Nightingale recognized that pet visits (small animals) might be of comfort to the patient. Nightingale believed that the nurse remained in charge of the environment, even when she was not physically present, because she should oversee others who worked in her absence.

USE OF EMPIRICAL EVIDENCE

Nightingale's reports describing health and sanitary conditions in the Crimea and in England identify her as an outstanding scientist and empirical researcher. Her expertise as a statistician is evident in the reports that she generated throughout her lifetime on the varied subjects of healthcare, nursing, and social reform.

Nightingale's carefully collected information that illustrated the efficacy of her hospital nursing system and organization during the Crimean War is perhaps her best-known work. Her report of her experiences and collected data was submitted to the British Royal Sanitary Commission in *Notes on Matters Affecting the Health, Efficiency, and Hospital Administration of the British Army Founded Chiefly on the Experience of the Late War* (Nightingale, 1858a). This Commission had been organized in response to Nightingale's charges of poor sanitary conditions. The data in this report provided a strong argument in favor of her proposed reforms in the Crimean hospital barracks. According to Cohen (1984), she created the polar area diagram to represent dramatically the extent of needless death in British military hospitals in the Crimea. In this article, Cohen summarized the work of Nightingale as both a researcher and a statistician by noting that "she helped to pioneer the revolutionary notion that social phenomena could be objectively measured and subjected to mathematical analysis" (1984, p. 128). Palmer (1977) described Nightingale's research skills as including recording, communicating, ordering, coding, conceptualizing, inferring, analyzing, and synthesizing. The observation of social phenomena at both individual and systems levels was especially important to Nightingale and served as the basis of her writings. Nightingale emphasized the concurrent use of observation and performance of tasks in the education of nurses and expected them to continue to use both of these activities in their work.

MAJOR ASSUMPTIONS

Nursing

Nightingale believed that every woman, at one time in her life, would be a nurse in the sense that nursing is being responsible for someone else's health. Nightingale's book *Notes on Nursing* was published originally in 1859, to provide women with guidelines for caring for their loved ones at home and to give advice on how to "think like a nurse" (Nightingale, 1969, p. 4). Trained nurses, however, were to learn additional scientific principles to be applied in their work and were to be more skilled in observing and reporting patients' health status while providing care as the patient recovered.

Person

In most of her writings, Nightingale referred to the person as a *patient.* Nurses performed tasks to and for the patient and controlled the patient's environment to enhance recovery. For the most part, Nightingale described a passive patient in this relationship. However, specific references are made to the patient performing self-care when possible and, in particular, being involved in the timing and substance of meals; thus, the patient was not totally viewed as a passive individual. The nurse was instructed to ask the patient about his or her preferences, which reveals the belief that Nightingale saw each patient as an individual. However, Nightingale (1969) emphasized that the nurse was in control of and responsible for the patient's environment and, by default, was in control of some personal choices and behaviors. One can infer from her writings, particularly those about the soldiers in Crimea, that Nightingale had respect for persons of various backgrounds and was not judgmental about social worth. Indeed, her conviction about the need for secular nurses supports her respect for persons without judgment of their religious beliefs.

Health

Nightingale defined *health* as being well and using every power (resource) to the fullest extent in living life. Additionally, she saw disease and illness as a reparative process that nature instituted when a person did not attend to health concerns. Nightingale envisioned the maintenance of health through prevention of disease via environmental control and social responsibility. What she described led to public health nursing and the more modern concept of health promotion. She distinguished the concept of health nursing as different from nursing a sick patient to enhance recovery, and from living better until peaceful death. Her concept of health nursing exists today in the role of district nurses and health workers in England and in other countries where lay healthcare workers are used to maintain health and teach people how to prevent disease and illness. Her concept of health nursing is a model employed by many public health agencies and departments in the United States.

Environment

Nightingale's concept of environment emphasized that nursing was "to assist nature in healing the patient. This was to be accomplished by managing the internal and external environments in an assistive way—in a way that was consistent with the laws of nature" (Chinn & Kramer, 2008, p. 31). Little, if anything, in the patient's world is excluded from her definition of environment. Her admonition to nurses, both those providing care in the home and trained nurses in hospitals, was to create and maintain a therapeutic environment that would enhance the comfort and recovery of the patient. Her treatise on rural hygiene includes an incredibly specific description of environmental problems and their results, as well as practical solutions to these problems for households and communities (Halsall, 1997).

Nightingale's assumptions and understanding about the environmental conditions of the day were most relevant to her philosophy. She believed that sick poor people would benefit from environmental improvements that would affect both their bodies and their minds. She believed that nurses could be instrumental in changing the social status of the poor by improving their physical and psychological living conditions.

Many aristocrats of the time were unaware of the living conditions of the poor, not unlike current societal behaviors. Nightingale's mother, however, had visited and provided care to poor families in the communities surrounding their estates; Nightingale accompanied her on these visits as a child and continued them when she was older. Thus Nightingale's understanding of physical environments and their effect on health status was acquired through first-hand observation and experience beyond her own comfortable living situation.

THEORETICAL ASSERTIONS

Nightingale believed that disease was a reparative process; disease was nature's effort to remedy a process of poisoning or decay, or it was a reaction against the conditions in which a person was placed. Although these concepts seem ridiculous today, they were more scientific than the prevailing ones of the time (e.g., disease as punishment). Nightingale did not provide a definition of nature. She often capitalized the word *nature* in her writings, thereby suggesting that it was synonymous with God. Her Unitarian religious beliefs would support this view of God as nature. However, when she used the word *nature* without capitalization, it is unclear whether or not the intended meaning is different and perhaps synonymous with an organic pathological process. Nightingale believed that the role of nursing was to prevent an interruption of the reparative process and to provide optimal conditions for its enhancement, thus ensuring the patient's recovery.

Nightingale was totally committed to nursing education (training). Although she wrote *Notes on Nursing* (1969) for all women, her primary treatise was that women were to be trained specifically to provide care for the sick person, and that nurses who provide preventive healthcare (public health nursing) require even more training. Nightingale (1969) believed that nurses needed to be excellent observers of their patients and the environment; observation was an ongoing activity for trained nurses. In addition, she believed that nurses needed to use common sense, coupled with observation, perseverance, and ingenuity, in their nursing practice. Finally, Nightingale believed that people desired good health, that they would cooperate with the nurse and nature to allow the reparative process to occur, and that they would alter their environment to prevent disease.

Although Nightingale has been maligned or ridiculed often for not embracing the germ theory, she very clearly understood the concept of contagion and contamination through organic materials from the patient and the environment. Many of her observations are consistent with the concepts of infection and the germ theory, for example, she embraced the concept of vaccination against various diseases. Small (2008) argues that Nightingale did indeed believe in a germ theory but not in the one that suggests that that disease germs cause inevitable infection. Such a theory was antithetical to her belief that sanitation and good hygiene could prevent infection. Her belief that appropriate manipulation of the environment would prevent disease underlies modern sanitation activities.

Nightingale did not explicitly discuss the caring behaviors of nurses. She wrote very little about interpersonal relationships, except as they influence the patient's reparative processes. She did describe the phenomenon of being called to nursing and the need for commitment to nursing work. From the perspectives of Victorian England and her religious beliefs, these descriptions may describe a caring component of her nursing theory. Her own example of nursing practice in the Crimea provides evidence of caring behaviors. These include her commitment to observing her patients at night, a new concept and practice; sitting with them during the dying process; standing beside them during surgical procedures; writing letters for them; and providing reading materials, including a reading room, during their recuperation. Finally, she wrote letters to their families following soldiers' deaths.

Nightingale believed that nurses should be moral agents. She addressed their professional relationship with their patients; she instructed them on the principle of confidentiality and advocated for care for the poor to improve their health and social situations. In addition, she commented on patient decision making, a component of a relevant modern ethical concept. Nightingale (1969) called for concise and clear decision making by the nurse and physician regarding the patient, noting that indecision (irresolution) or changing the mind is more harmful to the patient than the patient's having to make a decision.

LOGICAL FORM

Nightingale used inductive reasoning to extract laws of health, disease, and nursing from her observations and experiences. Her childhood education, particularly in philosophy and mathematics, may have contributed to her logical thinking and inductive reasoning abilities. For example, her observations of the conditions in the Scutari hospital led her to conclude that the contaminated, dirty, dark environment led to disease. Not only could she prevent disease from flourishing in such an environment, but she recognized that disease prevention would be achieved through environmental controls. From her own nursing training, her brief experience as a superintendent in London, and her experiences in the Crimea, she was able to make observations and establish principles for nursing training and patient care (Nightingale, 1969).

ACCEPTANCE BY THE NURSING COMMUNITY

Practice

Nightingale's nursing principles remain the foundation of nursing practice today. The environmental aspects of her theory (ventilation, warmth, quiet, diet, and cleanliness) remain integral components of nursing care. As nurses practice in the twenty-first century, these concepts continue to be relevant; in fact, they have increased relevance as a global society faces new issues of disease control. Although modern sanitation and water treatment have controlled traditional sources of disease fairly successfully in the United States, contaminated water due to environmental changes or to the introduction of uncommon contaminants remains a health issue in many communities. Global travel has altered dramatically the actual and potential spread of disease more rapidly than ever anticipated. In addition, modern sanitation, adequate water treatment, and recognition and control of other methods of disease transmission remain challenges for nurses worldwide.

New environmental concerns have been created by modern architecture (e.g., sick-building syndrome); nurses need to ask whether modern, environmentally controlled buildings meet Nightingale's principle of good ventilation. On the other hand, controlled environments increasingly protect the public from second-hand cigarette smoke, toxic gases, auto emissions, and other environmental hazards. Disposal of these wastes, including toxic waste, and the use of chemicals in this modern society challenge professional nurses and other healthcare professionals to reassess the concept of a healthy environment (Butterfield, 1999; Gropper, 1990; Michigan Nurses Association (MNA), 1999; Sessler, 1999; Shaner, 1998).

In healthcare facilities, the ability to control room temperature for an individual patient often is increasingly difficult. This same environment may create great noise through activities and the technology (equipment) used to assist the patient's reparative process. Nurses are looking in a scholarly way at these problems as they continue to affect patients and the healthcare system (McCarthy, Ouimet, & Daun, 1991; McLaughlin, McLaughlin, Elliott, & Campalani, 1996; MNA, 1999; Pope, 1995).

Monteiro (1985) provided the American public health community with a comprehensive review of Nightingale's work as a sanitarian and a social reformer, reminding them of the extent of her impact on healthcare in various settings and her concern about poverty and sanitation issues. Although other disciplines in the United States have increasingly addressed such issues, it is clear that nurses and nursing have an active role in providing direct patient care and in becoming involved in the social and political arenas to ensure healthy environments for all citizens.

McPhaul and Lipscomb (2005) have applied Nightingale's environmental principles to practice in occupational health nursing. These nurse specialists have increasingly recognized current environmental health problems at local, regional, and global levels. Modern changes in travel, migration, and the physical environments are causing health problems for many.

Infectious diseases (e.g., HIV, TB, West Nile virus) are examples of these changes. In addition, nurses are confronted by an epidemic of toxic substances and nosocomial infections and the development of resistant organisms (e.g., MRSA) in their patient care environments; first-line prevention measures of handwashing and environmental cleanliness harken back to Nightingale's original environmental theory and principles. Other problems created by environmental changes and pollution might astound Nightingale but probably would be approached by her in a typically aggressive fashion for control. As healthcare systems and providers struggle to promote patient safety through prevention of infection in healthcare facilities, this work can be framed in these words of Florence Nightingale: "It seems a strange principle to enunciate, as the very first requirement, in a hospital that it should Do the Sick No Harm" (Vincent, 2005).

Although some of Nightingale's rationales have been modified or disproved by medical advances and scientific discovery, many of her concepts and portions of her theory have endured the tests of time and technological advances. In reading and interpreting Nightingale's Victorian writings, remembering the uniqueness of her early life, and considering the sociopolitical nature of the era, it is clear that much of her theory remains relevant for nursing today. Concepts from Nightingale's writings, from political commentary to scholarly research, continue to be cited in the nursing literature.

Several authors have analyzed recently Nightingale's petty management concepts and actions, again identifying some of the timelessness and universality of her management style (Decker & Farley, 1991; Henry, Woods, & Nagelkerk, 1990; Monteiro, 1985; Nightingale, 1969; Ulrich, 1992). Lorentzon (2003) has focused specifically on Nightingale's role as a mentor to a former student in her review and analysis of letters written between her and her former student Rachel Williams. This analysis provides a review of mentoring approaches based on Nightingale's theories; her comments on management as offered to Rachel Williams might stimulate good discussion about the needs of nurses today for mentoring and professional development. Lannon (2007) and Narayanasamy and Narayanasamy (2007) based their examinations of nursing staff and leadership development on Nightingale's statements about the essential need for continued learning in nursing practice. These authors then outline methods for achieving continued learning.

Finally, several writers have analyzed Nightingale's role in the suffrage movement, especially in the context of feminist theory development. Although she has been criticized for not actively participating in this movement, Nightingale indicated in a letter to John Stuart Mill that she could do work for women in other ways (Woodham-Smith, 1951). Although she supported the principle of political power for women, she did not feel that she had time to participate actively in this movement. Her essay titled *Cassandra* (1852) appears to reflect great support for the concept that is now known as *feminism.* Scholars continue to assess and analyze her role and position in the feminist movement of this modern era (Dossey, 2000; Hektor, 1994; Holliday & Parker, 1997; Welch, 1990).

Education

Nightingale's principles of nursing training (instruction in scientific principles and practical experience for the mastery of skills) provided a universal template for early nurse training schools, beginning with St. Thomas' Hospital and King's College Hospital in London. Using the Nightingale model of nurse training, the following three experimental schools were established in the United States in 1873 (Ashley, 1976):

1. Bellevue Hospital in New York
2. New Haven Hospital in Connecticut
3. Massachusetts Hospital in Boston

The influence of this training system and of many of its principles is still evident in today's nursing programs. Although Nightingale advocated independence of the nursing school from a hospital to ensure that students would not become involved in the hospital's labor pool as part of their training, American nursing schools were unable to achieve such independence for many years (Ashley, 1976). Nightingale (Decker & Farley, 1991) believed that the art of nursing could not be measured by licensing examinations, but she used testing methods, including case studies (notes), for nursing probationers at St. Thomas' Hospital.

Clearly, Nightingale understood that good practice could result only from good education. This message resounds throughout her writings on nursing. Nightingale historian Joanne Farley responded to a modern nursing student by noting that "Training is to teach a nurse to know her business . . . Training is to enable the nurse to act for the best . . . like an intelligent and responsible being" (Decker & Farley, 1991, pp. 12-13). It is difficult to imagine what the care of sick human beings would be like if Nightingale had not defined the educational needs of nurses and established these first schools.

Research

Nightingale's interest in scientific inquiry and statistics continues to define the scientific inquiry used in nursing research. She was exceptionally efficient and resourceful in her ability to gather and analyze data; her ability to represent data graphically was first identified in the polar diagrams, the graphical illustration style that she invented (Agnew, 1958; Cohen, 1984). Her empirical approach to solving problems of healthcare delivery is obvious in the data that she often included in her numerous reports and letters.

When Nightingale's writings are defined and analyzed as theory, they are seen to lack the complexity and testability of modern nursing theories. However, concepts that Nightingale identified have served as the basis for current research, which adds to modern nursing science and practice. Most notable is her focus on the surroundings (environment) and its importance to nursing. Her concepts serve as the basis of continued analysis and nursing research throughout the world; they are cited frequently to support current nursing practices.

Finally, it is interesting to note that Nightingale used brief case studies, possible exemplars, to illustrate a number of the concepts that she discussed in *Notes on Nursing* (1969). Scholarly nurses have refined this technique for inclusion in texts and research; such a style thus had an auspicious beginning in nursing education and literature.

FURTHER DEVELOPMENT

Nightingale's philosophy and theory of nursing are stated clearly and concisely in *Notes on Nursing* (1969), Nightingale's most widely known work. In this writing, she provides guidance for care of the sick and in so doing clarifies what nursing is and what it is not. The content of the text seems most amenable to theory analysis. Nightingale organized the chapters of this text by concept; however, in continued discussion, these concepts appear as they relate to the topic of subsequent chapters.

Hardy (1978) proposed that Nightingale formulated a grand theory that explains the totality of behavior. As knowledge of nursing theory has developed, Nightingale's work has come to be recognized as a philosophy of nursing. Although some formulations have been tested, most often principles are derived from anecdotal situations to illustrate their meaning and support their claims. Her work has been discussed as a theory, and it is clear that Nightingale's premises have provided a foundation for the development of both nursing practice and current nursing theories. Tourville and Ingalls (2003) described her as the trunk of the living tree of nursing theories.

CRITIQUE

Simplicity

Nightingale's work contains the following three major relationships:

1. Environment to patient
2. Nurse to environment
3. Nurse to patient

She believed that the environment was the main factor that created illness in a patient and regarded disease as "the reactions of kindly nature against the conditions in which we have placed ourselves" (Nightingale, 1969, p. 56). Nightingale recognized the potential harmfulness of an environment, and she emphasized the benefit of a good environment in preventing disease.

The nurse's practice includes manipulation of the environment in a number of ways to enhance patient recovery. Elimination of contamination and contagion and exposure to fresh air, light, warmth, and quiet were identified as elements to be controlled or manipulated in the environment. Nightingale began to develop relationships between some of these elements in her discussions of contamination and ventilation, light and patient position in the room, cleanliness and darkness, and noise and patient stimulation. She also described the relationship between the sickroom and the rest of the house and the relationship between the house and the surrounding neighborhood. Nightingale recognized the need to manipulate the environment to prevent disease, as evidenced by her discussion of the homes of the poor, the workhouses, and preventing exposure of children to measles.

The nurse-patient relationship may be the least well defined in Nightingale's writings. Yet cooperation and collaboration between the nurse and patient is suggested in her discussions of a patient's eating patterns and preferences, the comfort of a beloved pet to the patient, protection of the patient from emotional distress, and conservation of energy while the patient is allowed to participate in self-care. Finally, it is interesting to note that Nightingale discussed the concept of observation extensively, including its use to guide the care of patients and to measure improvement or lack of response to nursing interventions. This aspect of training and practice suggests the origins of the nursing process (Ulrich, 1992).

Nurses are increasingly recognizing the role of observation and measurement of outcomes as an essential component of nursing practice. Burnes Bolton and Goodenough (2003), Erlen (2007), Robb, Mackie, & Elcock (2007), and Weir-Hughes (2007) all have written about measurement of patient outcomes and methods of quality improvement based on nurse observation and have attributed this modern component of nursing practice to Nightingale's original research (observation and patient outcomes) in the Crimea.

Nightingale provided a descriptive, explanatory theory rather than one of prediction. Its environmental focus along with its epidemiological components had predictive potential, but Nightingale never tested the theory in that manner. It is unclear whether Nightingale intended to develop a theory of nursing. She did intend to define the science and art of nursing and to provide general rules along with explanations that would result in good nursing care for patients. Thus her objective of setting forth general rules for the practice and development of nursing was met through this simple theory.

Generality

Nightingale's theories have been used to provide general guidelines for all nurses since she introduced them more than 150 years ago. Although some activities that she described are no longer relevant, the universality and timelessness of her concepts remain pertinent. The relation concepts (nurse, patient, and environment) remain applicable in all nursing settings today. Therefore they meet the criterion of generality.

Empirical Precision

Concepts and relationships within Nightingale's theory frequently are stated implicitly and are presented as truths rather than as tentative, testable statements. In contrast to her quantitative research on mortality performed in the Crimea, Nightingale advised nurses that their practice should be based on their observations and experiences rather than on systematic, empirical research. If she were addressing the development of the art of nursing, her admonitions would be amenable to study via qualitative or phenomenological research methods.

Derivable Consequences

To an extraordinary degree, Nightingale's writings direct the nurse to take action on behalf of the patient and the nurse. These directives encompass the areas of practice, research, and education. Her principles that attempt to shape nursing practice are the most specific. She urges nurses to provide physicians with "not your opinion, however respectfully given, but your facts" (Nightingale, 1969, p. 122). Similarly, she advised that "if you cannot get the habit of observation one way or other, you had better give up being a nurse, for it is not your calling, however kind and anxious you may be" (Nightingale, 1969, p. 113). Her encouragement for a measure of independence and precision previously unknown in nursing still may guide and motivate nurses today as the profession continues to evolve.

Nightingale's view of humanity was consistent with her theories of nursing. She believed in a creative, universal humanity with the potential and ability for growth and change (Dossey, 2000; Hektor, 1994; Palmer, 1977). Deeply religious, she viewed nursing as a means of doing the will of her God. Perhaps it is because she viewed nursing as a divine calling that she relegated the patient to a relatively passive role with his or her wants and needs provided for by the nurse. The zeal and self-righteousness that come from being a reformer might explain some of her beliefs and the practices that she advocated. Finally, the period and place in which she lived, Victorian England, must be considered and understood if one is to better understand and interpret her views.

Nightingale's basic principles of environmental manipulation and psychological care of the patient can be applied in contemporary nursing settings. Although her rejection of the germ theory and her inability to recognize a unified body of nursing knowledge that is testable (rather than relying only on personal observation and experience) have subjected her to some criticism and ridicule, other parts of her theory and her activities are relevant to the professional identity and practice of nursing.

As one reads *Notes on Nursing,* sentences and observations made by Nightingale can have great significance for the world of nursing today. Vidrine, Owen-Smith, and Faulkner (2002) have identified one of these observations as the guiding theory for their work with equine-facilitated group psychotherapy: "a small pet animal is often an excellent companion for the sick, for long chronic cases especially" (Nightingale, 1969, p. 102). Although a horse may not qualify as a "small animal in the sickroom," these authors have found that their therapy is successful with their patients. After reading this statement several times in *Notes on Nursing,* this writer believes that the modern programs of pet therapy instituted in various acute and chronic patient care settings should be attributed to Florence Nightingale rather than to those who are taking credit for "discovering" the beneficial effects of pet therapy. Indeed, Nightingale is a testament to her own theory; it is reported that she had 60 cats over her lifetime (she was chronically ill for much of her adult life and lived to age 90).

SUMMARY

Florence Nightingale is a unique figure in the history of the world. No other woman has been and still is revered as an icon by so many people in so many diverse geographical locations around the globe. Few other figures continue to stimulate such interest in, controversy about, and interpretation of their lives and work. The nursing profession continues to embrace her as the founder of modern nursing.

Nightingale defined the professional skills, behaviors, and knowledge required for nursing. Remnants of those descriptions serve the nursing profession well today, although their origins probably are not known or remembered by most of today's nurses.

Because of scientific and social changes that have occurred in the world, some of her observations have been rejected, only to find after closer analysis that her underlying beliefs, philosophy, and observations continue to be valid. Nightingale did not consciously attempt to develop what is considered a theory of nursing; she provided the first definitions from which nurses could develop theory and the conceptual models and frameworks that inform professional nursing today. Her lifework (professional career) embodies the current definition of all nurses as clinicians, researchers, educators, and leaders. Other professionals increasingly identify her as their matriarch—mathematicians revere her for her work as an outstanding statistician, and epidemiologists, public health professionals, and lay healthcare workers trace the origins of their disciplines to her descriptions of people who perform health promotion and disease prevention; sociologists acknowledge her leadership role in defining communities and their social ills, and in working to correct problems of society as a way of improving the health of its members.

Nurses, both students and practitioners, would be wise to become familiar with her original writings and to review the many books and documents that are increasingly available. If you have read *Notes on Nursing* before, rereading it can reveal new and inspirational ideas and can provide a brief look at her wry sense of humor. The logic and common sense that are embodied in her writings can serve to stimulate productive thinking for the individual nurse and the nursing profession. Reading the work that is becoming available now can expand our thinking and horizons beyond the narrow aspects of our nursing careers and professions. To emulate the life of Nightingale is to become a good citizen and leader in the community, the country, and the world. It is only right that Nightingale should continue to be recognized as the brilliant and creative founder of modern nursing and its first nursing theorist. What would Nightingale say about nursing today? Whatever she would say, she probably would provide an objective, logical, and revealing analysis and critique.

Case Study

You are caring for an 82-year-old woman who has been hospitalized for several weeks for burns that she sustained on her lower legs during a cooking accident. Before the time of her admission, she lived alone in a small apartment. She reported on admission that she has no surviving family. Her support system appears to be other elders who live in her neighborhood. Because of transportation difficulties, most of them are unable to visit frequently. One of her neighbors has reported that she is caring for the patient's dog, a Yorkshire terrier. As you care for this lady, she begs you to let her friend bring her dog to the hospital. She says that none of the other nurses have listened to her about such a visit. As she asks you about this, she begins to cry and tells you that they have never been separated. You recall that the staff discussed their concern about this woman's well-being during report that morning. They said that she has been eating very little and seems to be depressed. Based on Nightingale's work, identify specific interventions that you would provide in caring for this patient.

1. Describe what action, if any, you would take regarding her request to see her dog. Discuss the theoretical basis of your decision and action based on your understanding of Nightingale's work.
2. Describe and discuss what nursing diagnoses you would make and what interventions you would initiate to address her nutritional status and emotional well-being.
3. As this patient's primary nurse, identify and discuss the planning that you would undertake regarding her discharge from the hospital. Identify members of the discharge team and their roles in this process. Describe how you would advocate for this patient based on Nightingale's observations and descriptions of the role of the nurse.

CRITICAL THINKING *Activities*

1. Using Nightingale's concepts of ventilation, light, noise, and cleanliness, analyze the setting in which you are practicing nursing or working as an employee or student.
2. As you participate in a nursing outcome or continuous quality improvement project in your work setting, describe how Nightingale may have defined the problem and approached its analysis.
3. Your community is at risk for a specific type of natural disaster (e.g., tornado, flood, hurricane, earthquake). Using Nightingale's principles and observations about the environment, develop an emergency plan for one of these events.
4. Your community has reported an outbreak of an airborne infection (e.g., *Legionella* infection [Legionnaire's disease], histoplasmosis, coccidioidomycosis [valley fever]). Identify Nightingale's theories and commentaries that apply to this situation in regard to infection, the work required by healthcare professionals, and its societal influence on the health of citizens. Analyze the similarities between her theories and current practices.

POINTS FOR *Further Study*

- Nightingale, F. (1969). *Notes on nursing: What it is and what it is not.* New York: Dover.
- *Florence Nightingale: The nurse theorists: Portraits of excellence,* The Helene Fuld Health Trust (1990), Studio Three Productions, a division of Samuel Merritt College, Oakland, CA. (Video/DVD available from Fitne, Inc., Athens, Ohio.)
- McDonald, L. (Ed.). (2001-present). *The collected works of Florence Nightingale.* Ontario, Canada: Wilfred Laurier University Press. Retrieved July 26, 2008, from: http://www.sociology.uoguelph.ca/fnightingale
- The Florence Nightingale Museum. Retrieved July 26, 2008, from: http://www.florence-nightingale.co.uk

REFERENCES

Agnew, L. R. (1958). Florence Nightingale, statistician. *American Journal of Nursing, 58,* 644.

Ashley, J. A. (1976). *Hospitals, paternalism, and the role of the nurse.* New York: Teachers College Press.

Burnes Bolton, L., & Goodenough, A. (2003). A Magnet nursing service approach to nursing's role in quality improvement. *Nursing Administration Quarterly, 27*(4), 344-354.

Butterfield, P. (1999). Integrating environmental health into clinical nursing. *Journal of the New York State Nurses Association, 30*(1), 24-27.

Chinn, P., & Kramer, M. (2008). *Theory and nursing: A systematic approach.* St. Louis: Mosby.

Cohen, I. B. (1984). Florence Nightingale. *Scientific American, 250*(3), 128-137.

Cook, E. T. (1913). *The life of Florence Nightingale.* London: Macmillan.

Decker, B., & Farley, J. K. (1991, May/June). What would Nightingale say? *Nurse Educator, 16*(3), 12-13.

Dickens, C. (1987). *Life and adventures of Martin Chuzzlewit.* London: New Oxford Press.

Dossey, B. M. (2000). *Florence Nightingale: Mystic, visionary, healer.* Springhouse, PA: Springhouse Corporation.

Erlen, J. A. (2007). Patient safety, error reduction, and ethical practice. *Orthopaedic Nursing, 26*(2), 130-133.

Gropper, E. I. (1990). Florence Nightingale: Nursing's first environmental theorist. *Nursing Forum, 25*(3), 30-33.

Halsall, P. (1997). *Modern history sourcebook: Florence Nightingale: Rural hygiene.* Retrieved from: http://www.fordham.edu/halsall/mod/nightingale-rural.html

Hardy, M. (1978). Perspectives on nursing theory. *ANS Advances in Nursing Science, 1,* 37-48.

Hektor, M. (1994). Florence Nightingale and the women's movement: Friend or foe? *Nursing Inquiry, 1*(1), 38-45.

Helmstadter, C. (1997). Doctors and nurses in the London teaching hospitals: Class, gender, religion, and professional expertise, 1850-1890. *Nursing History Review, 5,* 161-167.

Henry, B., Woods, S., & Nagelkerk, J. (1990). Nightingale's perspective of nursing administration. *Nursing and Health Care, 11*(4), 200-206.

Holliday, M. E., & Parker, D. L. (1997). Florence Nightingale, feminism and nursing. *Journal of Advanced Nursing, 28,* 483-488.

Isler, C. (1970). *Florence Nightingale: Rebel with a cause.* Oradell, NY: Medical Economics.

Kalisch, B. J., & Kalisch, P. A. (1983a, April). Heroine out of focus: Media images of Florence Nightingale. Part I: Popular biographies and stage productions. *Nursing and Health Care, 4*(4), 181-187.

Kalisch, B. J., & Kalisch, P. A. (1983b, May). Heroine out of focus: Media images of Florence Nightingale. Part II: Film, radio, and television dramatizations. *Nursing and Health Care, 4*(5), 270-278.

Kalisch, P. A., & Kalisch B. J. (1987). *The changing image of the nurse.* Menlo Park, CA: Addison-Wesley.

Kennedy, M. (2007). *Angel of mercy or power-crazed meddler? Unseen letters challenge view of pioneer nurse.* Retrieved from: http://www.guardian.co.uk/uk/2007/sep/03/health.healthandwellbeing/print

Lannon, S. L. (2007). Leadership skills beyond the classic: Professional development classes for the staff nurse. *The Journal of Continuing Education in Nursing, 38*(1), 17-21.

Lobo, M. L. (1995). Florence Nightingale. In J. B. George (Ed.), *Nursing theories: The base for professional nursing practice.* Norwalk, CT: Appleton & Lange.

Longfellow, H. W. (1857). Santa Filomena. *Atlantic Monthly, 1*(1), 22-23.

Lorentzon, M. (2003). Florence Nightingale as "mentor of matrons": Correspondence with Rachel Williams at St. Mary's Hospital. *Journal of Nursing Management, 11*, 266-274.

Macrae, J. A. (2001). *Nursing as a spiritual practice: A contemporary application of Florence Nightingale's views.* New York: Springer Publishing.

McCarthy, D. O., Ouimet, M. E., & Daun, J. M. (1991, May). Shades of Florence Nightingale: Potential impact of noise stress on wound healing. *Holistic Nursing Practice, 5*(4), 39-48.

McDonald, L. (Ed.). (2001-present). *The collected works of Florence Nightingale.* Ontario, Canada: Wilfred Laurier University Press.

McLaughlin, A., McLaughlin, B., Elliott, J., & Campalani, G. (1996). Noise levels in a cardiac surgical intensive care unit: A preliminary study conducted in secret. *Intensive and Critical Care Nursing, 12*(4), 226-230.

McPhaul, K. M., & Lipscomb, J. A. (2005). Incorporating environmental health into practice. *American Association of Occupational Health Nursing (AAOHN) Journal, 53*(1), 31-36.

Michigan Nurses Association (MNA). (1999). Nursing practice: Moving toward environmentally responsible health care. *Michigan Nurse, 72*(1), 8-9.

Monteiro, L. A. (1985, Feb.). Florence Nightingale on public health nursing. *American Journal of Public Health, 75*, 181-186.

Narayanasamy, A., & Narayanasamy, M. (2007). Advancing nursing development and progression in nursing. *British Journal of Nursing, 16*(7), 384-388.

Nelson, S. (1997). Pastoral care and moral government: Early nineteenth century nursing and solutions to the Irish question. *Journal of Advanced Nursing, 26*, 6-14.

Nightingale, F. (1852). *Cassandra.* [Unpublished essay.]

Nightingale, F. (1858a). *Notes on matters affecting the health, efficiency, and hospital administration of the British army founded chiefly on the experience of the late war. Presented by request to the Secretary of State for War.* London: Harrison & Sons.

Nightingale, F. (1858b). *Notes on hospitals: Being two papers read before the National Association for the Promotion of Social Science, at Liverpool, in October* 1858. *With evidence given to the Royal Commissioner on the state of the army in 1857.* London: John W. Park and Son.

Nightingale, F. (1871). *Report on measures adopted for sanitary improvements in India, from June 1870 to June 1871.* London: George Edward Eye and William Spottiswoode.

Nightingale, F. (1969). *Notes on nursing: What it is and what it is not.* New York: Dover.

O'Malley, I. B. (1931). *Life of Florence Nightingale, 1820-1856.* London: Butterworth.

Palmer, I. S. (1977). Florence Nightingale: Reformer, reactionary, researcher. *Nursing Research, 26*, 84-89.

Pope, D. S. (1995). Music, noise, and the human voice in the nurse-patient environment. *Image: The Journal of Nursing Scholarship, 27*, 291-295.

Robb, E., Mackie, S., & Elcock, K. (2007). Monitoring quality. *Nursing Management, 14*(5), 22-26.

Sessler, A. (1999). Doing more than doing no harm: Nursing professionals turn their attention to the environment. *On-Call, 2*(4), 20-23.

Shaner, H. (1998). Pollution prevention for nurses: Minimizing the adverse environmental impact of healthcare delivery. *Vermont Registered Nurse, 64*(4), 9-11.

Small, H. (1998). *Avenging angel.* New York: St. Martin's Press.

Small, H. (2000). *Florence Nightingale's 20th century biographies.* Paper originally presented to the Friends of Florence Nightingale Museum, London. Retrieved July 26, 2008, from: http://www.florence-nightingale-avenging-angel.co.uk/biograph.htm

Small, H. (2008). *Florence Nightingale, avenging angel.* Retrieved July 26, 2008, from: http://www.florence-nightingale-avenging-angel.co.uk/Nightingale.html

Smith, F. B. (1982). *Florence Nightingale: Reputation and power.* New York: St. Martin.

Strachey, L. (1918). *Eminent Victorians.* London: Chatto & Windus.

Thomas, S. P. (1993). The view from Scutari: A look at contemporary nursing. *Nursing Forum, 28*(2), 19-24.

Tourville, C., & Ingalls, K. (2003). The living tree of nursing theories. *Nursing Forum, 38*(3), 21-30.

Ulrich, B. T. (1992). *Leadership and management according to Florence Nightingale.* Norwalk, CT: Appleton & Lange.

Vidrine, M., Owen-Smith, P., & Faulkner, P. (2002). Equine-facilitated group psychotherapy: Applications for therapeutic vaulting. *Issues in Mental Health Nursing, 23*, 587-603.

Vincent, C. (2005). *Patient safety.* London: Churchill Livingstone Elsevier.

Weir-Hughes, D. (2007). Reviewing nursing diagnoses. *Nursing Management, 14*(5), 32-35.

Welch, M. (1990, June). Florence Nightingale: The social construction of a Victorian feminist. *Western Journal of Nursing Research, 12*, 404-407.

Woodham-Smith, C. (1951). *Florence Nightingale.* New York: McGraw-Hill.

BIBLIOGRAPHY

Primary Sources

Books

Nightingale, F. (1911). *Letters from Miss Florence Nightingale on health visiting in rural districts.* London: King.

Nightingale, F. (1954). *Selected writings* [Compiled by Lucy R. Seymer]. New York: Macmillan.

Nightingale, F. (1957). *Notes on nursing.* Philadelphia: J. B. Lippincott. [Originally published 1859.]

Nightingale, F. (1969). *Notes on nursing: What it is and what it is not.* New York: Dover.

Nightingale, F. (1974). *Letters of Florence Nightingale in the history of nursing archive.* Boston: Boston University Press.

Nightingale, F. (1976). *Notes on hospitals.* New York: Gordon.

Nightingale, F. (1978). *Notes on nursing.* London: Duckworth.

Nightingale, F. (1992). *Notes on nursing.* Philadelphia: J. B. Lippincott. [Commemorative edition with commentaries by contemporary nursing leaders.]

Journal Articles*

Nightingale, F. (1930, July). Trained nursing for the sick poor. *International Nursing Review, 5*, 426-433.

Nightingale, F. (1954, May). Maternity hospital and midwifery school. *Nursing Mirror, 99*, ix-xi, 369.

Nightingale, F. (1954). The training of nurses. *Nursing Mirror, 99*, iv-xi.

Secondary Sources

Books

Aiken, C. A. (1915). *Lessons from the life of Florence Nightingale.* New York: Lakeside.

Aldis, M. (1914). *Florence Nightingale.* New York: National Organization for Public Health Nursing.

Andrews, M. R. (1929). *A lost commander.* Garden City, NY: Doubleday.

Baly, M. E. (1986). *Florence Nightingale: The nursing legacy.* New York: Methuen.

*All published posthumously.

Barth, R. J. (1945). *Fiery angel: The story of Florence Nightingale.* Coral Gables, FL: Glade House.

Bishop, W. J. (1962). *A bio-bibliography of Florence Nightingale.* London: Dawson's of Pall Mall.

Boyd, N. (1982). *Three Victorian women who changed their world.* New York: Oxford.

Bull, A. (1985). *Florence Nightingale.* North Pomfret, VT: David and Charles.

Bullough, V. L., Bullough, B., & Stanton, M. P. (Eds.). (1990). *Florence Nightingale and her era: A collection of new scholarship.* New York: Garland.

Calabria, M., & Macrae, J. (Eds.). (1994). *Suggestions for thought by Florence Nightingale: Selections and commentaries.* Philadelphia: University of Pennsylvania Press.

Collins, D. (1985). *Florence Nightingale.* Milford, MI: Mott Media.

Columbia University Faculty of Medicine and Department of Nursing. (1937). *Catalogue of the Florence Nightingale collection.* New York: Author.

Cook, E. T. (1913). *The life of Florence Nightingale.* London: Macmillan.

Cook, E. T. (1941). *A short life of Florence Nightingale.* New York: Macmillan.

Cope, Z. (1958). *Florence Nightingale and the doctors.* Philadelphia: J. B. Lippincott.

Cope, Z. (1961). *Six disciples of Florence Nightingale.* New York: Pitman.

Davies, C. (1980). *Rewriting nursing history.* London: Croom Helm.

Dossey, B. M. (2000). *Florence Nightingale: Mystic, visionary, healer.* Springhouse, PA: Springhouse.

Editors of RN. (1970). *Florence Nightingale: Rebel with a cause.* Oradell, NJ: Medical Economics.

French, Y. (1953). *Six great Englishwomen.* London: H. Hamilton.

Goldie, S. (1987). *I have done my duty: Florence Nightingale in the Crimea War, 1854-1856.* London: Manchester University Press.

Goldsmith, M. L. (1937). *Florence Nightingale: The woman and the legend.* London: Hodder and Stoughton.

Gordon, R. (1979). *The private life of Florence Nightingale.* New York: Atheneum.

Hall, E. F. (1920). *Florence Nightingale.* New York: Macmillan.

Hallock, G. T., & Turner, C. E. (1928). *Florence Nightingale.* New York: Metropolitan Life Insurance Co.

Herbert, R. G. (1981). *Florence Nightingale: Saint, reformer, or rebel?* Melbourne, FL: Krieger.

Holmes, M. (n.d.). *Florence Nightingale: A cameo lifesketch.* London: Woman's Freedom League.

Huxley, E. J. (1975). *Florence Nightingale.* London: Putnam.

Hyndman, J. A. (1969). *Florence Nightingale: Nurse to the world.* Cleveland, OH: World Publishing.

Keele, J. (Ed.). (1981). *Florence Nightingale in Rome.* Philadelphia: American Philosophical Society.

Lammond, D. (1935). *Florence Nightingale.* London: Duckworth.

Macrae, J. A. (2001). *Nursing as a spiritual practice: A contemporary application of Florence Nightingale's views.* New York: Springer Publishing.

Miller, B. W. (1947). *Florence Nightingale: The lady with the lamp.* Grand Rapids, MI: Zondervan.

Miller, M. (1987). *Florence Nightingale.* Minneapolis: Bethany House.

Mosby, C. V. (1938). *Little journey to the home of Florence Nightingale.* New York: C. V. Mosby.

Muir, D. E. (1946). *Florence Nightingale.* Glasgow: Blackie and Son.

Nash, R. (1937). *A sketch for the life of Florence Nightingale.* London: Society for Promoting Christian Knowledge.

O'Malley, I. B. (1931). *Life of Florence Nightingale, 1820-1856.* London: Butterworth.

Pollard, E. (1902). *Florence Nightingale: The wounded soldiers' friend.* London: Partridge.

Presbyterian Hospital School of Nursing. (1937). *Catalogue of the Florence Nightingale collection.* New York: Author.

Quiller-Couch, A. T. (1927). *Victor of peace.* New York: Nelson.

Quinn, V., & Prest, J. (Eds.). (1987). *Dear Miss Nightingale: A selection of Benjamin Jowett's letters to Florence Nightingale, 1860-1893.* Oxford: Clarendon Press.

Rappe, E. C. (1977). *God bless you, my dear Miss Nightingale.* Stockholm: Almqvist och Wiksell.

Sabatini, R. (1934). *Heroic lives.* Boston: Houghton.

Saint Thomas's Hospital. (1960). *The Nightingale training school: St. Thomas's Hospital, 1860-1960.* London: Author.

Selanders, L. C. (1993). *Florence Nightingale: An environmental adaptation theory.* Newbury Park, CA: Sage Publications.

Seymer, L. R. (1951). *Florence Nightingale.* New York: Macmillan.

Shor, D. (1987). *Florence Nightingale.* Lexington, NH: Silver.

Small, H. (1998). *Avenging angel.* New York: St. Martin's Press.

Smith, F. B. (1982). *Florence Nightingale: Reputation and power.* New York: St. Martin's Press.

Stark, M. (1979). *Introduction to Cassandra: An essay by Florence Nightingale.* Old Westbury, NY: Feminist Press.

Stephenson, G. E. (1924). *Some pioneers in the medical and nursing world.* Shanghai: Nurses's Association of China.

Strachey, L. (1918). *Eminent Victorians.* London: Chatto & Windus.

Tooley, S. A. (1905). *The life of Florence Nightingale.* New York: Macmillan.

Turner, D. (1986). *Florence Nightingale.* New York: Watts.

Vicinus, M., & Nergaard, B. (1990). *Ever yours, Florence Nightingale.* Cambridge, MA: Harvard University Press.

Wilson, W. G. (1940). *Soldier's heroine.* Edinburgh: Missionary Education Movement.

Woodman-Smith, C. (1983). *Florence Nightingale.* New York: Atheneum.

Woodham-Smith, C. B. (1951). *Florence Nightingale, 1820-1910.* New York: McGraw-Hill.

Woodham-Smith, C. B. (1951). *Lonely crusader: The life of Florence Nightingale, 1820-1910.* New York: Whittlesey House.

Woodham-Smith, C. B. (1956). *Lady-in-chief.* London: Methven.

Woodham-Smith, C. B. (1977). *Florence Nightingale, 1820-1910.* London: Collins.

Unpublished Dissertations

Hektor, L. M. (1992). *Nursing, science, and gender: Florence Nightingale and Martha E. Rogers.* [Unpublished doctoral dissertation, University of Miami, Miami.]

Newton, M. E. (1949). *Florence Nightingale's philosophy of life and education.* [Unpublished doctoral dissertation, Stanford University, Stanford, CA.]

Selanders, L. C. (1992). *An analysis of the utilization of power by Florence Nightingale.* [Unpublished doctoral dissertation, Western Michigan University, Kalamazoo, MI.]

Tschirch, P. (1992). *The caring tradition: Nursing ethics in the United States, 1890-1915.* [Unpublished doctoral dissertation, The University of Texas at Galveston, Graduate School of Biomedical Science, Galveston, TX.]

Journal Articles

A criticism of Miss Florence Nightingale. (1907, Feb.). *Nursing Times, 3,* 89.

Address by the Archbishop of York. (1970, May). Florence Nightingale. *Nursing Times, 66,* 670.

Address given at fiftieth anniversary of founding by Florence Nightingale of first training school for nurses at St. Thomas's Hospital, London, England. (1911, Feb.). *American Journal of Nursing, 11,* 331-361.

A passionate statistician. (1931, May). *American Journal of Nursing, 31,* 566.

Attewell, A. (1998). Florence Nightingale's relevance to nurses. *Journal of Holistic Nursing, 16,* 281-291.

Baly, M. (1986, June). Shattering the Nightingale myth. *Nursing Times, 82*(24), 16-18.

Baly, M. E. (1969, Jan.). Florence Nightingale's influence on nursing today. *Nursing Times, 65*(Suppl.), 1-4.

Barber, E. M. (1935, July). A culinary campaign. *Journal of the American Dietetic Association, 11,* 89-98.

Barber, J. A. (1999). Concerning our national honour: Florence Nightingale and the welfare of Aboriginal Australians. *Collegian: Journal of the Royal College of Nursing Australia, 6*(1), 36-39.

Barker, E. R. (1989, Oct.). Caregivers as casualties: War experiences and the postwar consequences for both Nightingale- and Vietnam-era nurses. *Western Journal of Nursing Research, 11,* 628-631.

Barritt, E. R. (1973). Florence Nightingale's values and modern nursing education. *Nursing Forum, 12*, 7-47.

Berentson, L. (1982, April/May). Florence Nightingale: Change agent. *Registered Nurse, 6*(2), 3, 7.

Bishop, W. J. (1957, May). Florence Nightingale's letters. *American Journal of Nursing, 57*, 607.

Bishop, W. J. (1960, May). Florence Nightingale's message for today. *Nursing Outlook, 8*, 246.

Blanc, E. (1980, May). Nightingale remembered: Reflections on times past. *California Nurse, 75*(10), 7.

Blanchard, J. R. (1939, June). Florence Nightingale: A study in vocation. *New Zealand Nursing Journal, 32*, 193-197.

Boylen, J. O. (1974, April). The Florence Nightingale-Mary Stanley controversy: Some unpublished letters. *Medical History, 18*(2), 186-193.

Bridges, D. C. (1954, April). Florence Nightingale centenary. *International Nurses Review, 1*, 3.

Brow, E. J. (1954, April). Florence Nightingale and her international influence. *International Nursing Review, 1*, 17-19.

Brown, E. (2000). Nightingale's values live on. *Kai Tiaki: Nursing New Zealand, 6*(3), 31.

Carlisle, D. (1989, Dec.). A nightingale sings: Florence Nightingale: Unknown details of her life story. *Nursing Times, 85*(50), 38-39.

Charatan, F. B. (1990, Feb.). Florence Nightingale: The most famous nurse in the world. *Today's OR Nurse, 12*(2), 25-30.

Cherescavich, G. (1971, June). Florence, where are you? *Nursing Clinics of North America, 6*, 217-223.

Choa, G. H. (1971, May). Speech by Dr. the Hon. G. H. Choa at the Florence Nightingale Day Celebration on Wednesday, 12th May, 1971, at City Hall, Hong Kong. *Nursing Journal, 10*, 33-34.

Clayton, R. E. (1974, April). How men may live and not die in India: Florence Nightingale. *Australian Nurses Journal, 2*, 10-11.

Coakley, M. L. (1989, Winter). Florence Nightingale: A one-woman revolution. *Journal of Christian Nursing, 6*, 20-25.

Cohen, S. (1997). Miss Loane, Florence Nightingale, and district nursing in late Victorian Britain. *Nursing History Review, 5*, 83-103.

de Guzman, G. (1935, July). Florence Nightingale. *Filipino Nurse, 10*, 10-14.

Dennis, K. E., & Prescott, P. A. (1985, Jan.). Florence Nightingale: Yesterday, today, and tomorrow. *ANS Advances in Nursing Science, 7*(2), 66-81.

de Tornayay, R. (1976, Nov./Dec.). Past is prologue: Florence Nightingale, *Pulse, 12*(6), 9-11.

Dwyer, B. A. (1937, Jan.). The mother of our modern nursing system. *Filipino Nurse, 12*, 8-10.

Florence Nightingale: Rebel with a cause. (1970, May). *Registered Nurse, 33*, 39-55.

Florence Nightingale: The original geriatric nurse. (1980, May). *Oklahoma Nurse, 25*(4), 6.

Gibbon, C. (1997). The influence of Florence Nightingale's image on Liverpool nurses 1945-1995. *International History of Nursing Journal, 2*(3), 17-26.

Gordon, J. E. (1972, Oct.). Nurses and nursing in Britain. 21. The work of Florence Nightingale. I. For the health of the army. *Midwife Health Visitor and Community Nurse, 8*, 351-359.

Gordon, J. E. (1972, Nov.). Nurses and nursing in Britain. 22. The work of Florence Nightingale. II. The establishment of nurse training in Britain. *Midwife Health Visitor and Community Nurse, 8*, 391-396.

Gordon, J. E. (1973, Jan.). Nurses and nursing in Britain. 23. The work of Florence Nightingale. III. Her influence throughout the world. *Midwife Health Visitor and Community Nurse, 9*, 17-22.

Hoole, L. (2000). Florence Nightingale must remain as nursing's icon. *British Journal of Nursing, 4*, 189.

Ifemesia, C. C. (1976, July/Sept.). Florence Nightingale (1820-1910). *Nigerian Nurse, 8*(3), 26-34.

Kelly, L. Y. (1976, Oct.). Our nursing heritage: Have we renounced it? (Florence Nightingale). *Image: The Journal of Nursing Scholarship, 8*(3), 43-48.

Large, J. T. (1985, May). Florence Nightingale: A multifaceted personality. *Nursing Journal of India, 76*(5), 110, 114.

LeVasseur, J. (1998). Student scholarship: Plato, Nightingale, and contemporary nursing. *Image: The Journal of Nursing Scholarship, 30*, 281-285.

Light, K. M. (1997). Florence Nightingale and holistic philosophy. *Journal of Holistic Nursing, 15*(1), 25-40.

Macmillan, K. (1994, April/May). Brilliant mind gave Florence her edge: Florence Nightingale. *Registered Nurse, 6*(2), 29-30.

Macrae, J. (1995, Spring). Nightingale's spiritual philosophy and its significance for modern nursing. *Image: The Journal of Nursing Scholarship, 27*, 8-10.

McDonald, L. (1998). Florence Nightingale: Passionate statistician. *Journal of Holistic Nursing, 16*, 267-277.

Monteiro, L. A. (1985, Nov.). Response in anger: Florence Nightingale on the importance of training for nurses. *Journal of Nursing History, 1*(1), 11-18.

Rabstein, C. (2000). Patron saint or has-been? Role models: Is Florence Nightingale holding us back? *Nursing, 30*(1), 8.

Selanders, L. C. (1998). Florence Nightingale: The evolution and social impact of feminist values in nursing. *Journal of Holistic Nursing, 16*(2), 227-243.

Selanders, L. C. (1998). The power of environmental adaptation: Florence Nightingale's original theory for nursing practice. *Journal of Holistic Nursing, 16*, 247-263.

Sparacino, P. S. A. (1994, March). Clinical practice: Florence Nightingale: A CNS role model. *Clinical Nurse Specialist, 8*(2), 64.

Stronk, K. (1997). Florence Nightingale: Mother of all nurses. *Journal of Nursing Jocularity, 7*(2), 14.

Ulrich, B. T. (1999). Continuing education. Still so much to do: The legacy of Florence Nightingale. *Nurse Week, 12*(25), 10-12.

Watson, J. (1998). Reflections: Florence Nightingale and the enduring legacy of transpersonal human caring. *Journal of Holistic Nursing, 16*, 292-294.

Welch, M. (1986, April). Nineteenth-century philosophic influences on Nightingale's concept of the person. *Journal of Nursing History, 1*(2), 3-11.

Wheeler, W., & Walker, M. (1999, May). Florence: Death of an icon: Florence Nightingale. *Nursing Times, 95*(19), 24-26.

Widerquist, J. G. (1992, Jan./Feb.). The spirituality of Florence Nightingale. *Nursing Research, 41*, 49-55.

Widerquist, J. G. (1997). Sanitary reform and nursing: Edwin Chadwick and Florence Nightingale. *Nursing History Review, 5*, 149-160.

Williams, B. (2000). Florence Nightingale: A relevant heroine for nurses today? *California Nurse, 96*(1), 9, 27.

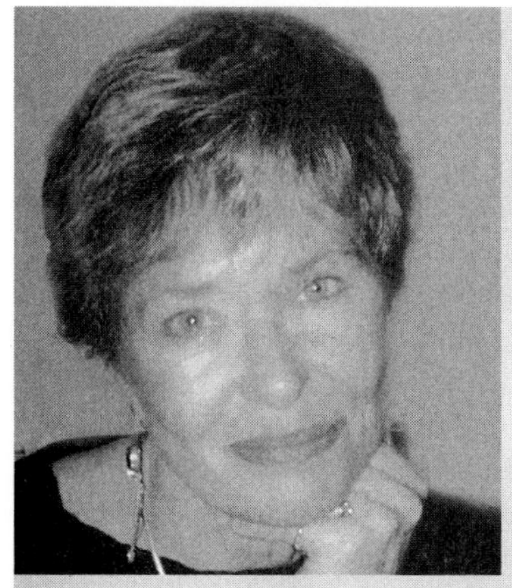

CHAPTER

7

Jean Watson

1940-present

Watson's Philosophy and Theory of Transpersonal Caring

D. Elizabeth Jesse

"The nursing profession, and each nurse within it, is invited to consider/reconsider: How do we walk through life? How do we get our footing to bring the artistry of caring and global caritas consciousness into our lives, our work, and our world?" (Watson, 2006a, p. 296)

CREDENTIALS AND BACKGROUND OF THE THEORIST

Margaret Jean Harman Watson, PhD, RN, AHN-BC, FAAN, was born in southern West Virginia and grew up during the 1940s and 1950s in the small town of Welch, West Virginia, in the Appalachian Mountains. As the youngest of eight children, she was surrounded by an extended family–community environment.

Watson attended high school in West Virginia and then the Lewis Gale School of Nursing in Roanoke, Virginia. After graduation in 1961, she married her husband, Douglas, and moved west to his native state of Colorado. Douglas, whom Watson describes not only as her physical and spiritual partner, but also as her best friend, died in 1998. She has two grown daughters, Jennifer (born in 1963) and Julie (born in 1967), and five grandchildren. She continues to live in Boulder, Colorado.

After moving to Colorado, Watson continued her nursing education and graduate studies at the University of Colorado. She earned a baccalaureate degree in nursing in 1964 at the Boulder campus, a master's degree in psychiatric–mental health nursing in 1966 at the Health Sciences campus, and a

Previous authors: Ruth M. Neil, Ann Marriner Tomey, Tracey J. F. Patton, Deborah A. Barnhart, Patricia M. Bennett, Beverly D. Porter, and Rebecca S. Sloan. These authors wish to thank Dr. Jean Watson for her ongoing inspiration and support, along with her review of the content of this chapter for accuracy and her assistance in updating the references and bibliography.

doctorate in educational psychology and counseling in 1973 at the Graduate School, Boulder campus. After Watson completed her doctoral degree, she joined the School of Nursing faculty of the University of Colorado Health Sciences Center in Denver, where she has served in both faculty and administrative positions. In 1981 and 1982, she pursued international sabbatical studies and diverse learning experiences in New Zealand, Australia, India, Thailand, and Taiwan; in 2005, she took a sabbatical for a walking pilgrimage in the Spanish El Camino.

In the 1980s, Watson and colleagues established the Center for Human Caring at the University of Colorado, the nation's first interdisciplinary center committed to using human caring knowledge that forms the moral and scientific basis for clinical practice, scholarship, and administration and leadership (Watson, 1986). During the center's existence, Watson and others sponsored clinical, educational, and community scholarship activities and projects in human caring. These activities involved national and international scholars in residence, as well as international connections with colleagues around the world, such as Australia, Brazil, Canada, Korea, Japan, New Zealand, United Kingdom, Scandinavia, Thailand, and Venezuela, among others. Activities such as these continue at the University of Colorado's International Certificate Program in Caring-Healing, where Watson offers her theory courses for doctoral students.

At the University of Colorado School of Nursing, Watson has served as chairperson and assistant dean of the undergraduate program. She was involved in early planning and implementation of the nursing PhD program and served as coordinator and director of the PhD program between 1978 and 1981. Watson was appointed dean of the University of Colorado School of Nursing and Associate Director of Nursing Practice at University Hospital from 1983 to 1990. During her deanship, she was instrumental in the development of a post baccalaureate nursing curriculum in human caring, health, and healing that led to a Nursing Doctorate (ND), a professional clinical doctoral degree. In 2005, this ND program was converted to the Doctor of Nursing Practice (DNP) degree.

During her career, Watson has been active in many community programs, such as founder and member of the Board of Boulder County Hospice, and numerous other collaborations with area healthcare facilities. Watson has received several research and advanced education federal grants and awards and numerous university and private grants and extramural funding for her faculty and administrative projects and scholarships in human caring.

The University of Colorado School of Nursing honored her as a distinguished professor of nursing in 1992. She received six honorary doctoral degrees from universities in the United States and three Honorary Doctorates in international universities, including Göteborg University in Sweden, Luton University in London, and the University of Montreal in Quebec, Canada. In 1993, she received the National League for Nursing (NLN) Martha E. Rogers Award, which recognizes nurse scholars' significant contributions to advancing nursing knowledge and knowledge in other health sciences. Between 1993 and 1996, Watson served as a member of the Executive Committee and the Governing Board, and as an officer for the NLN, and was elected president from 1995 to 1996. In 1997, NLN awarded her an honorary lifetime certificate as a holistic nurse. Finally, in 1999, she assumed the nation's first Murchison-Scoville Endowed Chair of Caring Science and currently is a distinguished professor of nursing.

In 1998, she was recognized as a Distinguished Nurse Scholar by New York University, and in 1999, she received the Fetzer Institute's national Norman Cousins Award in recognition of her commitment to developing, maintaining, and exemplifying relationship-centered care practices (Watson, personal communication, August 14, 2000).

Watson is a Distinguished and/or Endowed Lecturer at national universities, including Boston College, Catholic University, Adelphi University, Columbia University-Teachers College, State University of New York, and at universities and scholarly meetings in numerous foreign countries. Her international activities also include an International Kellogg Fellowship in Australia (1982), a Fulbright Research and Lecture Award to Sweden and other parts of Scandinavia (1991), and a lecture tour in the United Kingdom (1993). She has been involved in international projects and has received invitations to New Zealand, India, Thailand, Taiwan, Israel, Japan, Venezuela, Korea, and other places.

Watson is featured in at least 20 nationally distributed audio tapes, videotapes, and/or CDs on nursing theory, a few of which are listed in Points for Further Study at the end of the chapter.

Jean Watson has authored 10 books, shared in authorship of five books, and has written countless articles in nursing journals. The following publications reflect the evolution of her theory of caring from her ideas about the philosophy and science of caring.

Her first book, *Nursing: The Philosophy and Science of Caring* (1979), was developed from her notes for an undergraduate course taught at the University of Colorado. Yalom's 11 curative factors stimulated Watson's thinking about her 10 carative factors, described as the organizing framework for her book (Watson, 1979), "central to nursing" (p. 9), and a moral ideal. Watson's early work embraced the 10 carative factors, but her ideas have evolved to include "caritas" that make explicit connections between caring and love (Watson, personal correspondence, 2004). Her first book was reprinted in 1985 and subsequently was translated into Korean and French.

Her second book, *Nursing: Human Science and Human Care—A Theory of Nursing*, published in 1985 and reprinted in 1988 and 1999, addressed some conceptual and philosophical problems in nursing. Watson (1985) hopes her work will help nurses develop a meaningful moral and philosophical base for practice, and that others will join her to "elucidate the human care process in nursing, preserve the concept of the person in our science, and better our contribution to society" (Watson, 1988, p. ix). Her second book has been translated into Chinese, German, Japanese, Korean, Swedish, Norwegian, Danish, and probably other languages by now.

Her third book, *Postmodern Nursing and Beyond* (1999), was presented as a model to bring nursing practice into the twenty-first century. Watson describes two personal life-altering events that contributed to her writing. In 1997, she experienced an accidental injury that resulted in the loss of her left eye. Soon after, in 1998, her husband died. Watson states that she is "attempting to integrate these wounds into my life and work. One of the gifts through the suffering was the privilege of experiencing and receiving my own theory through the care from my husband and loving nurse friends and colleagues" (Watson, personal communication, August 31, 2000). This third book has been translated into Portuguese and Japanese. *Instruments for Assessing and Measuring Caring in Nursing and Health Sciences* (2002) is a collection of 21 instruments used to assess and measure caring. This text received the *American Journal of Nursing* Book of the Year Award.

Her fifth and latest book, *Caring Science as Sacred Science* (2005), describes her personal journey to enhance understanding about caring science, spiritual practice, the concept and practice of care, and caring-healing work. This book leads the reader through thought-provoking experiences and the sacredness of nursing by emphasizing deep inner reflection and personal growth, communication skills, use of self-transpersonal growth, and attention to both caring science and healing through forgiveness, gratitude, and surrender. It received *AJN*'s 2005 Book of the Year Award.

THEORETICAL SOURCES

Watson's work has been called a philosophy, blueprint, ethic, paradigm, worldview, treatise, conceptual model, framework, and theory (Watson, 1996). This chapter uses the terms *theory* and *framework* interchangeably. To develop her theory, Watson (1988) defines theory as "an imaginative grouping of knowledge, ideas, and experience that are represented symbolically and seek to illuminate a given phenomenon" (p. 1). She states further, "It (Human Science) is a theory because it helps me 'to see' more broadly (clearly)" (p. 1). Watson draws heavily on the sciences and the humanities, providing a phenomenological, existential, and spiritual orientation. She acknowledges philosophical and intellectual guidance from feminist theory, metaphysics, phenomenology, quantum physics, wisdom traditions, perennial philosophy, and Buddhism (Watson, 1995, 1997, 1999, 2005). In addition to traditional nursing knowledge, she cites as background for her theory nursing philosophies and theorists, including Nightingale, Henderson, Leininger, Peplau, Rogers, and Newman, and the work of Gadow, a nursing philosopher and healthcare ethicist (Watson, 1985, 1997, 2005). She describes a close connection with "Nightingale's sense of 'calling,' guided by a deep sense of commitment and a covenantal ethic of human service" (Watson, 2007a).

Watson reports that she was influenced in her earlier work by Western and Eastern worldviews and by philosophers such as Carl Rogers, Maslow, Heidegger, Erickson, Kierkegaard, Selye, Lazarus, Rumi, Whitehead, de Chardin, Sartre, and Thich Naht Hanh (Watson, 1996).

Watson attributes her emphasis on the interpersonal and transpersonal qualities of congruence, empathy, and warmth to the views of Carl Rogers and more recent writers of transpersonal psychology. Watson points out that Carl Rogers' phenomenological approach, with his view that nurses are not here to manipulate and control others but rather to understand, was profoundly influential at a time when "clinicalization" (therapeutic control and manipulation of the patient) was considered the norm (Watson, personal communication, August 31, 2000). In her latest book, *Caring Science as Sacred Science,* Watson (2005) describes the wisdom of French philosopher, Emmanuael Levinas (1969), and Danish philosopher, Knud Løgstrup (1995), which is foundational to her work.

Watson explains that concepts, defined as building blocks of theory (Watson, 1988), bring new meaning to the paradigm of nursing and were "derived from clinically inducted, empirical experiences, combined with my philosophical, intellectual and experiential background; thus my early work emerged from my own values, beliefs, and perceptions about personhood, life, health, and healing . . . " (Watson, 1997, p. 49). Watson's main concepts include the 10 carative factors (see box below or Table 7-1), and transpersonal healing and transpersonal caring relationship, caring moment, caring occasion, caring healing modalities, caring consciousness, caring consciousness energy, and phenomenal file/unitary consciousness. Watson expanded the carative factors to a closely related concept, *caritas,* a Latin word that means to "cherish, to appreciate, to give special attention, if not loving attention." As carative factors evolved within an expanding perspective, and as her ideas and values evolved, Watson offered a translation of the original carative factors into clinical caritas processes that suggested open ways in which they could be considered (Table 7-1).

Watson (1999) describes a "Transpersonal Caring Relationship" as foundational to her theory; it is a "special kind of human care relationship—a union with another person—high regard for the whole person and their being-in-the-world" (p. 63).

MAJOR CONCEPTS & DEFINITIONS

ORIGINAL 10 CARATIVE FACTORS

Watson bases her theory for nursing practice on the following 10 carative factors. Each has a dynamic phenomenological component that is relative to the individuals involved in the relationship as encompassed by nursing. The first three interdependent factors serve as the "philosophical foundation for the science of caring" (Watson, 1979, pp. 9-10). As Watson's ideas and values have evolved, she has translated the 10 carative factors into caritas processes. Caritas processes include a decidedly spiritual dimension and overt evocation of love and

MAJOR CONCEPTS & DEFINITIONS—cont'd

caring (Watson, 2007a). (See Table 7-1 [p. 97] for the original carative factors and for caritas process interpretation.)

1. **Formation of a Humanistic altruistic System of Values**
   Humanistic and altruistic values are learned early in life but can be influenced greatly by nurse educators. This factor can be defined as satisfaction through giving and extension of the sense of self (Watson, 1979).
2. **Instillation of Faith-Hope**
   This factor, incorporating humanistic and altruistic values, facilitates the promotion of holistic nursing care and positive health within the patient population. It also describes the nurse's role in developing effective nurse-patient interrelationships and in promoting wellness by helping the patient adopt health-seeking behaviors (Watson, 1979).
3. **Cultivation of Sensitivity to Self and to Others**
   The recognition of feelings leads to self-actualization through self-acceptance for both the nurse and the patient. As nurses acknowledge their sensitivity and feelings, they become more genuine, authentic, and sensitive to others (Watson, 1979).
4. **Development of a Helping-Trust Relationship**
   The development of a helping-trust relationship between the nurse and patient is crucial for trans-personal caring. A trusting relationship promotes and accepts the expression of both positive and negative feelings. It involves congruence, empathy, non-possessive warmth, and effective communication. Congruence involves being real, honest, genuine, and authentic. Empathy is the ability to experience and, thereby, understand the other person's perceptions and feelings and to communicate those understandings. Non-possessive warmth is demonstrated by: a moderate speaking volume, a relaxed open posture, and facial expressions that are congruent with other communications. Effective communication has cognitive, affective, and behavior response components (Watson, 1979).
5. **Promotion and Acceptance of the Expression of Positive and Negative Feelings**
   The sharing of feelings is a risk-taking experience for both nurse and patient. The nurse must be prepared for either positive or negative feelings. The nurse must recognize that intellectual and emotional understandings of a situation differ (Watson, 1979).
6. **Systematic Use of the Scientific Problem-Solving Method for Decision Making**
   Use of the nursing process brings a scientific problem-solving approach to nursing care, dispelling the traditional image of a nurse as the doctor's handmaiden. The nursing process is similar to the research process in that it is systematic and organized (Watson, 1979).
7. **Promotion of Interpersonal Teaching-Learning**
   This factor is an important concept for nursing in that it separates caring from curing. It allows the patient to be informed and shifts the responsibility for wellness and health to the patient. The nurse facilitates this process with teaching-learning techniques that are designed to enable patients to provide self-care, determine personal needs, and provide opportunities for their personal growth (Watson, 1979).
8. **Provision for Supportive, Protective, and Corrective Mental, Physical, Sociocultural, and Spiritual Environment**
   Nurses must recognize the influence that internal and external environments have on the health and illness of individuals. Concepts relevant to the internal environment include the mental and spiritual well-being and

Continued

MAJOR CONCEPTS & DEFINITIONS—cont'd

sociocultural beliefs of an individual. In addition to epidemiological variables, other external variables include comfort, privacy, safety, and clean, aesthetic surroundings (Watson, 1979).

9. **Assistance with Gratification of Human Needs**
   The nurse recognizes the biophysical, psychophysical, psychosocial, and intrapersonal needs of self and patient. Patients must satisfy lower-order needs before attempting to attain higher-order needs. Food, elimination, and ventilation are examples of lower-order biophysical needs, whereas activity, inactivity, and sexuality are considered lower-order psychophysical needs. Achievement and affiliation are higher-order psychosocial needs. Self-actualization is a higher-order intrapersonal-interpersonal need (Watson, 1979).
10. **Allowance for Existential-Phenomenological Forces**
    Phenomenology describes data of the immediate situation that help people understand the phenomena in question. Existential psychology is a science of human existence that uses phenomenological analysis. Watson considers this factor difficult to understand. It is included to provide a thought-provoking experience leading to a better understanding of the self and others.

    Watson believes that nurses have the responsibility to go beyond the 10 carative factors and to facilitate patients' development in the area of health promotion through preventive health actions. This goal is accomplished by teaching patients personal changes to promote health, providing situational support, teaching problem-solving methods, and recognizing coping skills and adaptation to loss (Watson, 1979).

USE OF EMPIRICAL EVIDENCE

Watson's research into caring incorporates empiricism, but it emphasizes methods that begin with nursing phenomena rather than with the natural sciences (Leininger, 1979). She has used human science, empirical phenomenology, and transcendent phenomenology in her work. She has investigated new languages, such as metaphor and poetry, to communicate, convey, and elucidate human caring and healing (Watson, 1987, 2005). In her inquiry and writing, she increasingly incorporates her conviction that a sacred relationship exists between humankind and the universe (Watson, 1997, 2005).

MAJOR ASSUMPTIONS

Watson calls for joining of science with humanities so that nurses will have a strong liberal arts background and will understand other cultures as a requisite for using Caring Science and a mind-body-spiritual framework. She believes that study of the humanities expands the mind and enhances thinking skills and personal growth. Watson compares the current status of nursing with the mythological Danaides, who attempted to fill a broken jar with water, only to see water flow through the cracks. Until nursing merges theory and practice through the combined study of the sciences and the humanities, Watson believes that similar cracks will be evident in the scientific basis of nursing knowledge (Watson, 1981, 1997).

Most recently, Watson describes assumptions for a Transpersonal Caring Relationship extending to multidisciplinary practitioners:

- Moral commitment, intentionality, and caritas consciousness by the nurse protect, enhance, and potentiate human dignity, wholeness, and healing, thereby allowing a person to create or co-create his/her own meaning for existence.

Table 7-1 Carative Factors and Caritas Process

Carative Factors	Caritas Process
1. "The formation of a humanistic-altruistic system of values"	"Practice of loving-kindness and equanimity within the context of caring consciousness"
2. "The instillation of faith-hope"	"Being authentically present and enabling and sustaining the deep belief system and subjective life-world of self and one being cared for"
3. "The cultivation of sensitivity to one's self and to others"	"Cultivation of one's own spiritual practices and transpersonal self going beyond the ego self"
4. "Development of a helping-trust relationship" became "development of a helping-trusting, human caring relation" (in 2004 Watson website)	"Developing and sustaining a helping trusting authentic caring relationship"
5. "The promotion and acceptance of the expression of positive and negative feelings"	"Being present to, and supportive of, the expression of positive and negative feelings as a connection with deeper spirit and self and the one-being-cared for"
6. "The systematic use of the scientific problem solving method for decision making" became "systematic use of a creative problem solving caring process" (in 2004 Watson website)	"Creative use of self and all ways of knowing as part of the caring process; to engage in the artistry of caring-healing practices"
7. "The promotion of transpersonal teaching-learning"	"Engaging in genuine teaching-learning experience that attends to unity of being and meaning, attempting to stay within others' frame of reference"
8. "The provision of supportive, protective, and (or) corrective mental, physical, societal, and spiritual environment"	"Creating healing environment at all levels (physical as well as nonphysical, subtle environment of energy and consciousness, whereby wholeness, beauty, comfort, dignity, and peace are potentiated)"
9. "The assistance with gratification of human needs"	"Assisting with basic needs, with an intentional caring consciousness, administering 'human care essentials,' which potentiate alignment of mind body spirit, wholeness, and unity of being in all aspects of care"
10. "The allowance for existential-phenomenological forces" became "allowance for existential-phenomenological-spiritual forces" (in 2004 Watson website)	"Opening and attending to spiritual-mysterious and existential dimensions of one's own life-death; soul care for self and the one-being-cared for"

From Watson, J. (1979). *Nursing: The philosophy and science of caring* (pp. 9-10). Boston: Little, Brown & Co. (for original carative factors); and Watson, J. (2004). *Theory of human caring* (website). Denver, CO: Jean Watson/University of Colorado School of Nursing. Retrieved January 25, 2008, from: http://hschealth.uchsc.edu/son/faculty/jw_evolution.htm (for caritas processes and revised carative factors).

- The conscious will of the nurse affirms the subjective and spiritual significance of the patient while seeking to sustain caring in the midst of threat and despair—biological, institutional, or otherwise. The result is honoring of an I-Thou Relationship rather than an I-It Relationship.
- The nurse seeks to recognize, accurately detect, and connect with the inner condition of spirit of another through genuine presence and by being centered in the caring moment; actions, words, behaviors, cognition, body language, feelings, intuition, thoughts, senses, the energy field, and so

forth, all contribute to the transpersonal caring connection.

- The nurse's ability to connect with another at this transpersonal spirit-to-spirit level is translated via movements, gestures, facial expressions, procedures, information, touch, sound, verbal expressions, and other scientific, technical, aesthetic, and human means of communication, into nursing human art/acts or intentional caring-healing modalities.
- The caring-healing modalities within the context of transpersonal caring/caritas consciousness potentiate harmony, wholeness, and unity of being by releasing some of the disharmony, that is, the blocked energy that interferes with natural healing processes; thus the nurse helps another through this process to access the healer within, in the fullest sense of Nightingale's view of nursing.
- Ongoing personal and professional development and spiritual growth, as well as personal spiritual practice, assist the nurse in entering into this deeper level of professional healing practice, allowing for awakening to a transpersonal condition of the world and fuller actualization of the "ontological competencies" necessary at this level of advanced practice of nursing.
- The nurse's own life history, previous experiences, opportunities for focused study, having lived through or experienced various human conditions, and having imagined others' feelings in various circumstances are valuable teachers for this work; to some degree, the knowledge and consciousness needed can be gained through work with other cultures and study of the humanities (art, drama, literature, personal story, narratives of illness journeys, etc.), along with exploration of one's own values, deep beliefs, and relationship with self, others, and one's world.
- Other facilitators are personal growth experiences such as psychotherapy, transpersonal psychology, meditation, bioenergetics work, and other models for spiritual awakening.
- Continuous growth for developing and maturing within a transpersonal caring model is ongoing. The notion of health professionals as wounded healers is acknowledged as part of the necessary growth and compassion called forth within this theory/philosophy (Watson, 2006b).

THEORETICAL ASSERTIONS

Nursing

According to Watson (1988), the word *nurse* is both noun and verb. To her, nursing consists of "knowledge, thought, values, philosophy, commitment, and action, with some degree of passion" (p. 53). Nurses are interested in understanding health, illness, and the human experience; promoting and restoring health; and preventing illness. Her theory calls upon nurses to go beyond procedures, tasks, and techniques used in practice settings, coined as the "trim" of nursing, in contrast to the "core" of nursing, meaning those aspects of the nurse-patient relationship resulting in a therapeutic outcome that are included in the transpersonal caring process (Watson, 2005; Watson, 2007). Using the original and evolving 10 carative factors, the nurse provides care to various patients. Each carative factor and, more recently, the clinical caritas processes describe the caring process of how a patient attains or maintains health or dies a peaceful death. Conversely, Watson describes *curing* as a medical term that refers to the elimination of disease (Watson, 1979). As Watson's work has evolved, she has increased her focus on the human care process and the transpersonal aspects of caring-healing in a Transpersonal Caring Relationship (1999, 2005).

Watson's evolving work continues to make explicit that humans cannot be treated as objects and humans cannot be separated from self, other, nature, and the larger universe. The caring-healing paradigm is located within a cosmology that is both metaphysical and transcendent with the co-evolving human in the universe. She asks others to be open to possibility and to put away assumptions of self and others, to learn again, and to "see" using all of one's senses. The context calls for a "sense of reverence and sacredness with regard to life and all living things. It incorporates both art and science, as they are also being redefined, acknowledging a convergence between the two" (Watson, 2007, para. 14).

Personhood (Human Being)

Watson uses interchangeably the terms *human being, person, life, personhood,* and *self.* She views the person as "a unity of mind/body/spirit/nature" (1996, p. 147), and she describes that "personhood is tied to notions that one's soul possess a body that is not confined by objective time and space . . . " (Watson, 1988, p. 45). Watson states, "I make the point to use mind, body, soul or unity within an evolving emergent world view-connectedness of all, sometimes referred to as Unitary Transformative Paradigm-Holographic thinking. It is often considered dualistic because I use the *three* words 'mind, body, soul.' I do it intentionally to connote and make explicit spirit/metaphysical—which is silent in other models" (Watson, personal communication, April 12, 1994).

Health

Originally, Watson's (1979) definition of *health* was derived from the World Health Organization as, "The positive state of physical, mental, and social well-being with the inclusion of three elements: (1) a high level of overall physical, mental, and social functioning; (2) a general adaptive-maintenance level of daily functioning; (3) the absence of illness (or the presence of efforts that lead to its absence)" (p. 220). Later, she defined *health* as "unity and harmony within the mind, body, and soul"; it is associated with the "degree of congruence between the self as perceived and the self as experienced" (Watson, 1988, p. 48). Watson (1988) stated further, "illness is not necessarily disease; [instead it is a] subjective turmoil or disharmony within a person's inner self or soul at some level of disharmony within the spheres of the person, for example, in the mind, body, and soul, either consciously or unconsciously (p. 47)." "While illness can lead to disease, illness and health are [a] phenomenon that is not necessarily viewed on a continuum. Disease processes can also result from genetic, constitutional vulnerabilities and manifest themselves when disharmony is present. Disease in turn creates more disharmony" (Watson, 1985, 1988, p. 48).

Environment

In the original ten carative factors, Watson speaks to the nurse's role in the environment as "attending to supportive, protective, and or corrective mental, physical, societal, and spiritual environments" (Watson, 1979, p. 10). In her later work, she describes that "healing spaces can be used to help others transcend illness, pain, and suffering," and she emphasizes that environment and person are connected: "when the nurse enters the patient's room, a magnetic field of expectation is created" (Watson, 2003, p. 200). She also has a broad view of environment: "the caring science is not only for sustaining humanity, but also for sustaining the planet . . . Belonging is to an infinite universal spirit world of nature and all living things; it is the primordial link of humanity and life itself, across time and space, boundaries and nationalities" (Watson, 2003, p. 305).

LOGICAL FORM

The framework is presented in a logical form. It contains broad ideas and addresses health-illness phenomena. Watson's definition of *caring* as opposed to *curing* delineates nursing from medicine. This concept is helpful in classifying the body of nursing knowledge as a separate science.

Since 1979, the development of the theory has been toward clarifying the person of the nurse and the person of the patient. Another emphasis has been on existential-phenomenological and spiritual factors. Her current work (2005) reminds us of the "spirit-filled dimensions of caring work and caring knowledge" (p. x).

Watson's theory has foundational support from theorists in other disciplines, such as Rogers, Erikson, and Maslow. She is adamant in her support for nursing education that incorporates holistic knowledge from many disciplines and integrates the humanities, arts, and sciences. She believes that the increasingly complex requirements of the healthcare system and patient needs require nurses to have a broad, liberal education. The ideals, content, and theory of liberal education must be integrated into professional nursing education (Sakalys & Watson, 1986).

Watson recently has incorporated dimensions of a postmodern paradigm shift throughout her theory of transpersonal caring. Modern theoretical underpinnings have been associated with concepts such as steady-state maintenance, adaptation, linear interaction, and problem-based nursing practice. The postmodern approach moves beyond this point; the redefining of such a nursing paradigm leads to a more holistic, humanistic, open system, wherein harmony, interpretation, and self-transcendence are the emerging directions reflected in this epistemological shift. Watson (1999) believes that nursing must be challenged to construct and co-construct ancient and new knowledge toward an ever-evolving humanity of possibilities to further clarify nursing for a new era. "The theory evolution has tended to place greater emphasis on transpersonal caring, intentionality, caring consciousness, and the caring field" (Watson, personal communication, August 21, 2000).

APPLICATION BY THE NURSING COMMUNITY

Practice

Attending Nurse Caring Model (ANCM)

Watson's theory is being validated in a variety of outpatient, inpatient, and community health clinical settings, and with various populations. Watson and Foster (2003) described an exemplary application of theory to practice; the Attending Nurse Caring Model (ANCM) is a unique pilot project in a Denver children's hospital that is modeled after the "Attending" Physician Model. However, unlike a medical/cure model, the ANCM is concerned with the nursing care model. "It is constructed as a Nursing-Caring Science, theory-guided, evidence based, collaborative practice model for applying it to the conduct and oversight of pain management on a 37-bed, post surgical unit" (Watson & Foster, 2003, p. 363). Nurses who participate in the project learn about Watson's caring theory, carative factors, caring consciousness, intentionality, and caring-healing practices. The mission of ANCM is to have a continuous caring relationship with children in pain and their families. ANCM is made visible in a caring-healing presence throughout the hospital. (See Watson's website [http://www.watsoncaringscience.org] for additional examples of Watson's theory in practice and further information about clinical agencies that use Watson's work, such as Miami Baptist Hospital, Resurrection Health System [Chicago], Denver Veterans Administration Hospital and Children's Hospital [Denver], Inova Health System [Virginia], Baptist Central Hospital [Kentucky], Elmhurst Hospital [New York], Pascak Valley Hospital [New Jersey], Sarasota Memorial Hospital and Tampa Memorial Hospital [Florida], and Scripps Memorial Hospital [California], among others.)

Administration/Leadership

Watson's theory calls for administrative practices and business models to embrace caring (Watson, 2006c), even in a healthcare environment of increased acuity levels of hospitalized individuals, short hospital stays, increasing complexity of technology, and rising expectations in the "task" of nursing. These challenges call for solutions that address healthcare system reform at a deep and ethical level, and that would enable nurses to follow their own professional practice model rather than short-term solutions, such as increasing numbers of beds, sign-on bonuses, and/or relocation incentives for nurses. Many hospitals seeking Magnet status, such as Central Baptist Hospital in Lexington, Kentucky, are meeting these challenges by using Watson's Theory of Human Caring for administrative change. This and other examples of caring administrative practices are described at her website and in her recent article, "Caring Theory as an Ethical Guide to Administrative Practices" (Watson, 2006c).

Education

Watson's writings focus on educating graduate nursing students and providing them with ontological (study of conceptions of reality and the nature of being), ethical, and epistemological bases for their praxis, along with research directions. Watson has been active in curriculum planning at the University of Colorado.

Her caring framework has been taught in numerous baccalaureate nursing curricula, including Bellarmine College in Louisville, Kentucky; Assumption College in Worcester, Massachusetts; Indiana State University in Terre Haute; and Florida Atlantic University in Boca Raton. In addition, these concepts now are used widely in nursing programs in Australia, Sweden, Finland, and the United Kingdom.

Research

Qualitative, naturalistic, and phenomenological methods are relevant to the study of transpersonal caring and to the development of nursing as a human science and art (Watson, 2005). Watson acknowledges that combination qualitative-quantitative inquiry may be useful. There is a growing body of national and international research that tests, expands, and evaluates the theory. Watson (2005) recognizes that Swanson's exemplar research contributes to Caring Science knowledge, including a middle range theory of caring (Swanson, 1991), a study (Swanson, 1999) on the effects of caring for women who miscarried, and a meta-analysis of 130 studies in caring knowledge. Smith (2004) published a review of 40 research studies that specifically used Watson's theory. Persky, Nelson, Watson, and Bent's (2008) study (n = 170) is one of few that have used a quantitative approach to determine the attributes of a "Caritas nurse" as part of an effort to initiate Relationship-Based Care (RBC) at New York Presbyterian Hospital/Columbia University Medical Center. Watson's book, *Caring Science as Sacred Science* (2005), outlines possibilities for future "caring" research, stating, "exploratory, observational studies, triangulated with qualitative inquiry, provide the most appropriate starting point for discerning the impact of healing relationship on selected outcomes" (pp. 154-155).

FURTHER DEVELOPMENT

Watson's most recent writings present guidelines for development, along with goals, instruments, and directions for further development of the theory of human caring.

CRITIQUE

Clarity

Watson, a spirit/poet/artist of nursing, uses nontechnical, sophisticated, fluid, and evolutionary language to artfully describe her concepts, such as caring-love, carative factors, and caritas. Paradoxically, abstract and simple concepts such as caring-love can be the most difficult to practice, yet practicing and experiencing these concepts leads to greater understanding of Caring Science (2005). At times, lengthy phrases (e.g., "symbiotic relationship between humankind-technology-nature") (Watson, 1999, p. xiv) and sentences must be read more than once to convey meaning. Her increasing inclusion of metaphors, personal reflections, artwork, and poetry make her complex concepts more tangible and more aesthetically appealing. She continues to refine her theory and recently has revised the original carative factors, which she now describes as caritas processes. Critics of Watson's work have concentrated on the use of undefined or changing/shifting definitions and terms and her focus on the psychosocial rather than the pathophysiological aspects of nursing. Watson (1985) addresses the last critique in her first book, *Nursing: The Philosophy and Science of Caring* (1979, 1988); in the preface of her second book, *Nursing: Human Science and Human Care—A Theory of Nursing* (1985), and in her latest book, *Caring Science as Sacred Science* (Watson, 2005), she defines her intent to describe the core rather than the trim of nursing. With this focus, the framework is not limited to any nursing specialty. Table 7-1 outlines the evolution of Watson's thinking.

Simplicity

Watson draws on a number of disciplines to formulate her theory. To understand the theory as it is presented, the reader does best by being familiar with the broad subject matter. This theory is viewed as complex when the existential-phenomenological nature of her work is considered, in part because many nurses have a limited liberal arts background and baccalaureate nursing curricula have limited integration of liberal arts. Although some consider her theory complex, others find it easy to understand and to apply in practice. The theory is more about being than about doing, and it must be internalized thoroughly by the nurse if it is to be actualized in practice.

Generality

Watson's theory seeks to provide a moral and philosophical basis for nursing. The scope of the framework encompasses all aspects of the health-illness phenomenon. In addition, the theory addresses aspects of preventing illness and experiencing a peaceful death, thereby increasing its generality. The carative factors that Watson described provide important guidelines for nurse-patient interactions; however, some critics have stated that their generality is limited by the emphasis placed on psychosocial rather than physiological aspects of caring.

Another characteristic of the theory is that it does not furnish explicit direction about what to do to achieve authentic caring-healing relationships. Nurses who want concrete guidelines may not feel secure when trying to rely on this theory alone. Some suggest that it would take too much time to incorporate the caritas into practice, and others purport that the emphasis on Watson's personal growth gives her latest book (2005) an "idiosyncratic quality that while appealing to some may not appeal to others" (Drummond, 2005, p. 218).

Empirical Precision

Although the framework is difficult to study empirically, Watson draws heavily on widely accepted work from other disciplines. This solid foundation strengthens her views. Watson describes her theory as descriptive; she acknowledges the evolving nature of the theory and welcomes input by others. The theory does not lend itself easily to research conducted through traditional scientific methods. However, in her recent book, *Caring Science and Sacred Science* (2005), Watson provides research guidelines, design recommendations, and a table of potential instruments for caring research.

Derivable Consequences

Watson's theory continues to provide a useful and important metaphysical orientation for the delivery of nursing care. Watson's theoretical concepts, such as use of self, patient-identified needs, the caring process, and the spiritual sense of being human, may help nurses and their patients to find meaning and harmony in a period of increasing complexity. Watson's rich and varied knowledge of philosophy, the arts, the human sciences, and traditional science and traditions, joined with her prolific ability to communicate, has enabled professionals in many disciplines to share and recognize her work.

SUMMARY

Jean Watson began developing her theory while assistant dean of the undergraduate program, and it evolved into early planning and implementation of the nursing PhD program at the University of Colorado. Her first book started as class notes that emerged from teaching in an innovative, integrated curriculum. She became coordinator and director of the PhD program when it was initiated in 1978 and served until 1981. While serving as Dean of the University of Colorado School of Nursing, she was instrumental in the development of a post baccalaureate nursing curriculum in human caring that would lead to a career professional clinical doctoral degree (ND). This curriculum was implemented in 1990 and had been a national demonstration program until 2005, when it was merged into the Doctor of Nursing Practice (DNP) degree. Watson initiated the Center for Human Caring, the nation's first interdisciplinary center, with a commitment to develop and use knowledge of human caring for practice and scholarship and became the nation's first Endowed Chair in Caring Science. She worked from Yalom's 11 curative factors to formulate her 10 carative factors. She modified the 10 factors slightly over time and developed the caritas processes, which have a spiritual dimension and use a more fluid and evolutionary language. She added spiritual aspects and believes that the core of nursing is seen in those nurse-patient relationships that result in a therapeutic outcome.

Case Study

The following case study was adapted from Valerie Taylor's (2008) clinical example for a presentation in Advanced Nursing Synthesis for the Nurse-Midwifery Concentration, East Carolina University College of Nursing (reprinted with permission).

You are a recently graduated master's prepared nurse-midwife working in a small 100-bed hospital, and you are committed to applying Watson's theory to practice by building a nurse-midwife-patient relationship resulting in therapeutic outcomes. Because you are new, you are slowly promoting the theory with staff, co-midwives and physicians. Today you are excited and challenged to integrate Watson's theory into your midwifery care of Maria, a 23-year-old Hispanic female, gravida 4 para, TPAL 4004 (meaning term, preterm, abortion, and live births in her pregnancy history), who presents in labor at 39 weeks gestation. She transfers into your group's practice from the health department at 36 weeks, is self-pay, and receives Maternity Medicaid when she presents in labor. She cannot speak English and uses her husband, Daniel, as an interpreter, who states that he could read and write but that she cannot. She and Daniel have moved to the area for factory work, so they have little social support from family and friends, and Maria stays home caring for their three children. Maria's sister-in-law is caring for their three children while Maria is in the hospital. Although they are Catholic, they do not presently belong to a church. Her medical history is unremarkable and her prenatal history normal. Her first two children were delivered in Mexico, and her last child was delivered a year ago at another hospital in the United States.

As the nurse-midwife caring for Maria, Watson's theory leads me to view Maria and her family holistically, wherein the body, mind, and soul are interrelated. I remember to incorporate the carative factors, caring consciousness, intentionality, and caring-healing practices, and to go beyond procedures, tasks, and techniques to create a mentally, physically, and spiritually healing environment, while assisting with basic needs. Watson's theory helps me realize the importance of being authentically present and developing and sustaining a helping, trusting, caring relationship with Maria and her husband. At 0045 today, I attend Maria for her spontaneous vaginal delivery of a healthy infant girl, Lilia, who has an Apgar score of 8 and 9. Maria's labor is uneventful, although she is treated for group B infection. After the delivery, I place Lilia on Maria's abdomen for skin-to-skin touch and help Maria with positioning for breastfeeding. Maria and Daniel gaze at Lilia as she latches on for the first breastfeeding. After initial bonding, infant Lilia is transported to the newborn nursery; her exam is normal and without problems. When the nurses note that Lilia has not wet a diaper in over 6 hours, the neonatologist determines that Lilia has a kidney problem, and she has to be transported to the Level III regional hospital for additional tests and evaluation.

From your initial plan of care, you know how important it is to maintain a reciprocal dialogue among the interpreter, obstetrician, neonatologist, nursing staff, and social worker. You stand close as the neonatologist explains to Maria and her husband, through the interpreter, that Lilia will receive exemplary care at the tertiary hospital. Maria is tearful and her husband appears stressed as the interpreter translates that their newborn is being prepared for immediate transport to the regional hospital for specialized assessment and care. Maria is stable and her postpartum course is normal with the exception of her anxiety related to the unknowns of Lilia's condition, separation from her newborn, delayed breastfeeding, and language barriers that prevent a better understanding of events pertaining to her and Lilia's care.

You let the theory guide you as you assess Maria's stress/anxiety related to her separation from her newborn, fear of her newborn's prognosis, inability to breastfeed, language barriers, and financial concerns. You know that if Maria does not have skin-to-skin touch, impairment of bonding may lead to oxytocin suppression and delays in milk production. Her stress and lack of rest also can hinder her normal recovery from a spontaneous vaginal delivery and may lead to blood loss and delayed involution. Engorgement or decreased lactogenesis may occur as the result of infrequent or interrupted breastfeeding. Maria has limited family support, with the exception of her sister-in-law, who lives 3 hours away; she lacks a friend network because of her immigration from Mexico, and she has no support group to support coping. Although Maria has a Christian belief system, she has no church affiliation at this time for spiritual guidance/support or fellowship of members. You know that Watson's caring theory and carative factors/caritas can potentiate successful outcomes and an optimum state of health for Maria, her husband, and their newborn daughter.

After the routine postpartum exam, you address Maria's biophysical needs for rest and her emotional concerns. You encourage the neonatologist and nursery staff to let the parents bond with Lilia before her transport. Then you consult the hospital chaplain for visitation and request a Spanish-speaking priest and a hospital interpreter to be available for patient teaching for instructions and early discharge after her 24-hour stay. You speak with the social worker since she can be a liaison between mother and newborn during Lilia's transport. Throughout the care of Maria, Daniel, and Lilia, you facilitate a practice of loving kindness among the caregiving staff to achieve continuous culturally sensitive care, as that guides your practice. You know that the nurse-midwife–patient relationship has resulted in a therapeutic outcome because Maria and Daniel report feeling some comfort after speaking to the priest and the nurses at the tertiary care hospital. Maria is able to rest the previous night, and her postpartum examination is normal. Maria now has a breast pump, and the staff nurses explain its use. The social workers have arranged transportation for Maria and Daniel to visit their newborn at the Level III hospital after they are discharged today. Maria has spoken to her sister-in-law, and she will continue to care for the children for several more days. Maria and Daniel tell you how grateful they feel that you have been their nurse-midwife throughout their experience.

Valerie G. Taylor, MSN, CNM
Hickory, North Carolina

CRITICAL THINKING *Activities*

On the basis of the original and evolving 10 carative assumptions, Watson's theory provides a framework on which nurses can establish a precedent of collaboration to assist the patient in gaining control, knowledge, and health. The following exercises demonstrate critical and reflective thinking from the perspective of Watson's theory:

1. Review your values and beliefs to ascertain how Watson's 10 carative/caritas assumptions fit with your own personal philosophy of caring in relation to the patient, environment, health, and nursing.
2. Develop a mission statement with your teammates, integrating your shared beliefs about basing your practice on using the science of caring. Revisit this periodically, and discuss how your values and beliefs are evolving.
3. Think of a time in your life when you felt that someone truly cared for you. Then think of a time when you demonstrated care for another person. (These events can be health-care related or not.) Then identify the major characteristics of those interactions.
4. Make a list of caring behaviors from your own thoughts. Then look at *Instruments for Assessing and Measuring Caring in Nursing and Health Science* (Watson, 2002) and make a list of caring behaviors from these instruments. Compare and contrast the lists.
5. Begin to create a work culture that nurtures you and your co-workers. Plan a time and place to meditate for 10 minutes each week, while sitting in a chair, softly closing your eyes, and listening to quiet music or in silence. Reflect on ways to feel compassionate, intentional, calm, and peaceful during your everyday clinical practice.

POINTS FOR *Further Study*

- Watson, J. (1989). *The nurse theorists: Portraits of excellence* [Videotape, CD, DVD]. New York: Helene Fuld Health Trust. Available from Fitne, Inc., at: http://www.fitne.net/
- Watson, J. (1989). *Theories at work* [Videotape]. New York: National League for Nursing.
- Watson, J. (2005). Sequence on caring in education. On *Student-centered learning in nursing education* [CD]. Baltimore: Laureate Education, Inc.
- Watson, J. (2005). A caring moment. On *Care for the journey: Messages & music for sustaining the heart of healthcare* [CD]. Larkspur, CA: Companion Arts.
- Watson, J. (2005). *Caring science as sacred science.* Philadelphia: F. A. Davis.
- University of Colorado's International Certificate Program and selected in-resident studies with Dr. Watson are noted on: http://www2.uchsc.edu/son/caring/content
- Jesse, D. E. (2006). Watson's philosophy in nursing practice. In M. R. Alligood & A. M. Tomey: *Nursing theory: Utilization & application* (3rd ed., pp. 97-121). St. Louis: Mosby, Inc.
- An updated list of caring theory publications is available through the University of Colorado School of Nursing website at: http://hschealth.uchsc.edu/son/faculty/jw_caritaspractice.htm

REFERENCES

Drummond, J. (2005). Caring science as sacred science. [Book review.] *Nursing Philosophy, 6,* 218-220.

Jesse, D. E. (2006). Watson's philosophy in nursing practice. In M. R. Alligood & A. M. Tomey (Eds.), *Nursing theory: Utilization & application* (3rd ed., pp. 97-121). St. Louis: Mosby, Inc.

Leininger, M. (1979). Preface. In J. Watson (Ed.), *Nursing: The philosophy and science of caring.* Boston: Little, Brown.

Levinas, E. (1969). *Totality and infinity.* (A. Lingis, Trans.) Pittsburgh, PA: Duquesne University.

Løgstrup, K. E. (1995). *Metaphysics,* vol 1. Milwaukee: Marquette University.

Persky, G. J., Nelson, J. W., Watson, J., & Bent, K. (2008). Creating a profile of a nurse effective in caring. *Nursing Administration Quarterly, 32*(1), 15-20.

Sakalys, J. A., & Watson, J. (1986). Professional education: Post-baccalaureate education for professional nursing. *Journal of Professional Nursing, 2*(2), 91-97.

Smith, M. (2004). Review of research related to Watson's theory of caring. *Nursing Science Quarterly, 17*(1), 13-25.

Swanson, K. (1991). Empirical development of a middle range theory of caring. *Nursing Research, 40*(3), 161-166.

Swanson, K. (1999). What is known about caring in nursing science: A literary meta-analysis. In A. S. Hinshaw, S. Feetham, & J. Shaver (Eds.). *Handbook of clinical nursing research* (pp. 31-60). Thousands Oaks, CA: Sage.

Watson, J. (1979). *Nursing: The philosophy and science of caring.* Boston: Little, Brown.

Watson, J. (1981). Nursing's scientific quest. *Nursing Outlook, 29,* 413-416.

Watson, J. (1985). *Nursing: Human science and human care—A theory of nursing.* Norwalk, CT: Appleton-Century-Crofts.

Watson, J. (1986, Dec.). The dean speaks out: Center for human caring established. *The University of Colorado School of Nursing News,* 1-6.

Watson, J. (1987). Nursing on the caring edge: Metaphorical vignettes. *ANS Advances in Nursing Science, 10*(1), 10-18.

Watson, J. (1988). *Nursing: Human science and human care—A theory of nursing.* New York: National League for Nursing.

Watson, J. (1995). Post modernism and knowledge development in nursing. *Nursing Science Quarterly, 8*(2), 60-64.

Watson, J. (1996). Watson's theory of transpersonal caring. In P. J. Walker & B. Neuman (Eds.), *Blueprint for use of nursing models: Education, research, practice and administration* (pp. 141-184). New York: National League for Nursing Press.

Watson, J. (1997). The theory of human caring: Retrospective and prospective. *Nursing Science Quarterly, 10*(1), 49-52.

Watson, J. (1999). *Postmodern nursing and beyond.* Edinburgh: Churchill Livingstone.

Watson, J. (2002). *Instruments for assessing and measuring caring in nursing and health sciences.* New York: Springer.

Watson, J. (2003). Caring science: Belonging before being as ethical cosmology. *Nursing Science Quarterly, 18*(4), 304-305.

Watson, J. (2005). *Caring science as sacred science.* Philadelphia: F. A. Davis.

Watson, J. (2006a). Walking pilgrimage as caritas action in the world. *Journal of Holistic Nursing, 24*(4), 289-296.

Watson, J. (2006b). Transpersonal caring and the caring moment defined. Retrieved January 26, 2008, from: http://www2.uchsc.edu/son/caring/content/transpersonal.asp

Watson, J. (2006c). Caring theory as an ethical guide to administrative and clinical practices. *Nursing Administration Quarterly, 30*(1), 48-55.

Watson, J. (2007a). Theory evolution. Retrieved January 25, 2008, from: http://www2.uchsc.edu/son/caring/content/evolution.asp

Watson, J., & Foster, R. (2003). The attending nurse caring model: Integrating theory, evidence, and advanced caring-healing therapeutics for transforming professional practice. *Journal of Clinical Nursing, 12,* 360-365.

BIBLIOGRAPHY

Primary Sources

Books

Bevis, E. O., & Watson, J. (1989). *Toward a caring curriculum: A new pedagogy for nursing.* New York: National League for Nursing.

Bevis, E. O., & Watson, J. (2000, reprinted). *Toward a caring curriculum: A new pedagogy for nursing.* Sudbury, MA: Jones & Bartlett.

Chinn, P., & Watson, J. (Eds.). (1994). *Art and aesthetics of nursing.* New York: National League for Nursing.

Leininger, M., & Watson, J. (Eds.). (1990). *The caring imperative in education.* New York: National League for Nursing.

Taylor, R., & Watson, J. (Eds.). (1989). *They shall not hurt: Human suffering and human caring.* Boulder, CO: University Press of Colorado.

Watson, J. (1979, reprinted 1985 by University Press of Colorado). *Nursing: The philosophy and science of caring.* Boston: Little, Brown. [Translated into French.]

Watson, J. (1985, reprinted 1988. reprinted by NLN & Bartlett, 1999). *Nursing: Human science and human care.* Norwalk, CT: Appleton-Century-Crofts. [Translated into Japanese, Swedish, Chinese, Korean, German, Norwegian, and Danish.]

Watson, J. (1985). *Nursing: The philosophy and science of caring* [2nd printing]. Boulder, CO: University Press of Colorado.

Watson, J. (1988). *Nursing: Human science and human care* [2nd printing]. New York: National League for Nursing. [Translated into Japanese, 1990.]

Watson, J. (Ed.). (1994). *Applying the art and science of human caring.* New York: National League for Nursing.

Watson, J. (1999). *Postmodern nursing and beyond.* Edinburgh, Scotland: Churchill Livingstone/W. B. Saunders. [Translated into Japanese, 2001.]

Watson, J. (2002). *Instruments for assessing and measuring caring in nursing and health sciences.* New York: Springer. [AJN Book of the Year Award, 2002. Japanese translation in print.]

Watson, J. (2005). *Caring science as sacred science.* Philadelphia: F. A. Davis. (AJN Book of the Year Award, 2005.)

Watson, J., Jones, W., & Levin, J. (Eds.). (1999). *Essentials of complementary alternative medicine.* Philadelphia: Lippincott Williams & Wilkins.

Watson, J., & Ray, M. (Eds.). (1988). *The ethics of care and the ethics of cure: Synthesis in chronicity.* New York: National League for Nursing.

Chapters and Monographs

Watson, J. (1980). Self losses. In F. Bower (Ed.), *Nursing and the concept of loss* (pp. 51-84). New York: Wiley.

Watson, J. (1981). Some issues related to a science of caring for nursing practice. In M. Leininger (Ed.), *Caring: An essential human need* (pp. 61-67). Proceedings from National Caring Conference, University of Utah. Thorofare, NJ: Charles B. Slack.

Watson, J. (1982). The nurse-client relationship. In L. Sonstegard, K. Kowalski, & B. Jennings (Eds.), *Women's health care* (pp. 45-56). New York: Grune & Stratton.

Watson, J. (1983). Delivery and assurance of quality health care: A rights based foundation. In R. Luke, J. Krueger, & R. Madrow (Eds.), *Organization and change in health care quality assurance* (pp. 13-19). Rockville, MD: Aspen Systems.

Watson, J. (1985). Reflection on different methodologies for the future of nursing. In M. Leininger (Ed.), *Qualitative research methods in nursing* (pp. 343-349). Orlando, FL: Grune & Stratton.

Watson, J. (1987). The dream curriculum. In National League for Nursing (Ed.), *Patterns in nursing: Strategic planning for nursing education* (pp. 91-104). New York: Author.

Watson, J. (1988). A case study: Curriculum in transition. In National League for Nursing (Ed.), *Curriculum revolution: Mandate for change* (pp. 1-8). New York: Author.

Watson, J. (1988). Introduction. In J. Watson & M. Ray (Eds.), *The ethics of care and the ethics of cure: Synthesis in chronicity* (pp. 1-3). New York: National League for Nursing.

Watson, J. (1988). The professional doctorate as an entry level into practice. In National League for Nursing (Ed.), *Perspectives* (pp. 41-47). New York: Author.

Watson, J. (1989). Human caring and suffering: A subjective model for health sciences. In R. Taylor & J. Watson (Eds.), *They shall not hurt* (pp. 125-135). Boulder, CO: University Press of Colorado.

Watson, J. (1989). Watson's philosophy and theory of human caring in nursing. In J. Riehl-Sisca (Ed.), *Conceptual models for nursing practice* (3rd ed.; pp. 219-236). Norwalk, CT: Appleton & Lange.

Watson, J. (1990). Transformation in nursing: Bring care back to health care. In National League for Nursing (Ed.), *Curriculum revolution: Redefining the student-teacher relationship* (pp. 15-20). New York: National League for Nursing.

Watson, J. (1990). Transpersonal caring: A transcendent view of person, health, and healing. In M. Parker (Ed.),

Nursing theories in practice (pp. 277-288). New York: National League for Nursing.

Watson, J. (1992). Notes on nursing: Guidelines for caring then and now. In F. Nightingale (Ed.), *Notes on nursing.* Philadelphia: J. B. Lippincott.

Watson, J. (1994). A frog, a rock, a ritual: An eco-caring cosmology. In E. Schuster & C. Brown (Eds.), *Caring and environmental connection.* New York: National League for Nursing.

Watson, J. (1994). Anthology on art and esthetics. In J. Watson & P. Chinn (Eds.), *Art and aesthetics as passage between centuries.* New York: National League for Nursing.

Watson, J. (1994). Introduction. In J. Watson (Ed.), *Applying the art and science of human caring* (pp. 1-10). New York: National League for Nursing.

Watson, J. (1994). Overview of caring theory. In J. Watson (Ed.), *Applying the art and science of human caring.* New York: National League for Nursing.

Watson, J. (1994). Poeticizing as truth through language. In P. L. Chinn & J. Watson (Eds.), *Art and aesthetics in nursing* (pp. 3-17). New York: National League for Nursing.

Watson, J. (1995). Into the future. In O. Slevin & L. Basford (Eds.), *Theory and practice of nursing: An integrated approach to patient care* (2nd ed.). Cheltenham, UK: Nelson Thornes.

Watson, J. (1996). Art, caring, spirituality, and humanity. In E. Farmer (Ed.), *Exploring the spiritual dimension of care* (pp. 29-40). Wiltshire, England: Mark Allen.

Watson, J. (1996). Artistry and caring: Heart and soul of nursing. In D. Marks-Maran & P. Rose (Eds.), *Reconstructing nursing: Beyond art and science* (pp. 54-63). London: Bailliere Tindall Ltd. (Division of Harcourt Brace).

Watson, J. (1996). Beyond art and science. In D. Marks-Maran & P. Rose (Eds.), *Reconstructing nursing: Beyond art and science.* London: Bailliere Tindall.

Watson, J. (1996). Nursing, caring-healing paradigm. In D. Pesat (Ed.), *Capsules of comments in psychiatric nursing.* St. Louis: Mosby.

Watson, J. (1996). Poeticizing as truth on nursing inquiry. In J. Kikuchi, H. Simmons, & D. Romyn (Eds.), *Truth on nursing inquiry* (pp. 125-138). Thousand Oaks, CA: Sage.

Watson, J. (1996). Watson's theory of transpersonal caring. In P. J. Walker & B. Neuman (Eds.), *Blueprint for use of nursing models: Education, research, practice and administration* (pp. 141-184). New York: National League for Nursing Press.

Watson, J. (1999). Postmodern nursing and beyond. In N. Chaska (Ed.), *The nursing profession: Nursing theories and nursing practice* (pp. 343-354). Philadelphia: F. A. Davis.

Watson, J. (2000). *Monograph of instruments for measuring and assessing caring.* New York: Springer Publishing.

Watson, J. (2000). Postmodern nursing and beyond. In N. L. Chaska (Ed.), *The nursing profession: Tomorrow's vision and beyond* (pp. 299-308). Thousand Oaks, CA: Sage.

Watson, J. (2001). Jean Watson: Theory of human caring. In M. E. Parker (Ed.), *Nursing theories and nursing practice* (pp. 344-354). Philadelphia: F. A. Davis.

Watson, J. (2002). Illuminating the spiritual journey: Jean Watson tells her story. In P. Burkhardt & M. G. Nagai-Jackson (Eds.), *Spirituality: Living our connectedness* (pp. 181-186). New York: Delmar.

Watson, J. (2006). Jean Watson's Theory of Human Caring. In M. Parker (Ed.), *Nursing theories and nursing practice* (2nd ed., pp. 295-301). Philadelphia: F. A. Davis.

Watson, J., & Bevis, E. (1990). Coming of age for a new age. In N. L. Chaska (Ed.), *The nursing profession: Turning points* (pp. 100-105). St. Louis: Mosby.

Journal Articles

Carozza, V., Congdon, J. A., & Watson, J. (1978, Nov.). An experimental educationally sponsored pilot internship program. *Journal of Nursing Education, 17,* 14-20.

Fawcett, J., Watson, J., Neuman, B., & Hinton-Walker, P. (2001). On missing theories and evidence. *Journal of Nursing Scholarship, 33*(2), 115-119.

Krysl, M., & Watson, J. (1988, Jan.). Poetry on caring and addendum on center for human caring. *ANS Advances in Nursing Science, 10*(2), 12-17.

Persky, G. J., Nelson, J. W., Watson, J., & Bent, K. (2008). Creating a profile of a nurse effective in caring. *Nursing Administration Quarterly, 32*(1), 15-20.

Quinn, J., Smith, M., Swanson, K., Ritenbaugh, C., & Watson, J. (2003). The healing relationship in clinical nursing: Guidelines for research. *Journal of Alternative Therapies, 9*(3), A65-A79.

Sakalys, J., & Watson, J. (1985, Sep/Oct.). New directions in higher education: A review of trends. *Journal of Professional Nursing, 1*(5), 293-299.

Sakalys, J., & Watson, J. (1986, Mar./Apr.). Professional education: Post-baccalaureate education for professional nursing. *Journal of Professional Nursing, 2*(2), 91-97.

Watson, J. (1980). [Response to review of *Nursing: Philosophy and science of caring.*] *Western Journal of Nursing Research, 2*(2), 514-515.

Watson, J. (1980). [Review of the book *Nursing: Philosophy and science of caring.*] *Western Journal of Nursing Research, 2*(2), 514-515.

Watson, J. (1980). [Review of the book *Starting point: An introduction to the dialectic of existence.*] *Western Journal of Nursing Research, 2*(3), 637-638.

Watson, J. (1981). Conceptual systems of students and practicing nurses. *Western Journal of Nursing Research, 3*(2), 172-192.

Watson, J. (1981). Nursing's scientific quest. *Nursing Outlook, 29*(7), 413-416.

Watson, J. (1981, Aug.). Professional identity crisis—Is nursing finally growing up? *American Journal of Nursing, 81*, 1488-1490.
Watson, J. (1981). Response to conceptual systems, students, practitioner. *Western Journal of Nursing Research, 3*(2), 197-198.
Watson, J. (1981, reprinted 1983). The lost art of nursing. *Nursing Forum, 20*(3), 244-249.
Watson, J. (1982, Aug.). Traditional v. tertiary: Ideological shifts in nursing education. *The Australian Nurses Journal, 12*(2), 44-46.
Watson, J. (1983, Fall). Commentary on instructor directed research model. *Western Journal of Nursing Research, 5*(4), 310-311.
Watson, J. (1987, Oct.). Nursing on the caring edge: Metaphorical vignettes. *ANS Advances in Nursing Science, X*(1), 10-18.
Watson, J. (1987). [Review of the book *Health as expanding consciousness.*] *Journal of Professional Nursing, 3*(5), 315.
Watson, J. (1987). [Review of the book *Practical psychotherapy.*] *Journal of Psychosocial Nursing and Mental Health Services, 25*(3), 42.
Watson, J. (1988). Human caring as moral context for nursing education. *Nursing and Health Care, 9*(8), 422-425.
Watson, J. (1988). New dimensions of human caring theory. *Nursing Science Quarterly, 1*(4), 175-181.
Watson, J. (1988). Of nurses, women and the devaluation of caring. [Review of the book *Images of Nurses: Perspectives for history, art, and literature.*] *Medical Humanities Review, 2*(2), 60-62.
Watson, J. (1988). Response to caring and practice: Construction of the nurses' world. *Scholarly Inquiry for Nursing Practice: An International Journal, 2*(3), 217-221.
Watson, J. (1989). Caring theory. *Journal of Japan Academy of Nursing Science, 9*(2), 29-37.
Watson, J. (1989, Oct.). Keynote address: Caring theory. *Journal of Japan Academy of Nursing Science, 9*(2), 9-37.
Watson, J. (1990). Caring knowledge and informed moral passion. *ANS Advances in Nursing Science, 13*(1), 15-24.
Watson, J. (1990). Caring knowledge and informed moral passion. *ANS Advances in Nursing Science, 15*(1), 13-24.
Watson, J. (1990). Reconceptualizing nursing ethics: A response. *Scholarly Inquiry for Nursing Practice: An International Journal, 4*(3), 219-221.
Watson, J. (1990). The moral failure of the patriarchy. *Nursing Outlook, 28*(2), 62-66.
Watson, J. (1991). From revolution to renaissance. *Revolution: Journal of Nurse Empowerment, 1*(1), 94-100.
Watson, J. (1991). Robb, Dock, and Nutting: I wish I'd been there. *Nursing and Health Care, 12*(4), 210.
Watson, J. (1992). Response to caring, virtue, theory, and a foundation for nursing ethics. *Scholarly Inquiry for Nursing Practice: An International Journal, 6*(2), 169-171.
Watson, J. (1992, Summer). Response to caring, virtue through a foundation for nursing ethics: A response to Pamela Salsberry. *Scholarly Inquiry for Nursing Practice: An International Journal, 6*(2), 169-171.
Watson, J. (1993). Dr. Jean Watson with E. Henderson—An interview. *Alberta Association of Registered Nurses Newsletter, 49*(6), 10-12.
Watson, J. (1993). Should NPs, CNMs, and CNAs, etc., add graduate credentials? *Open Mind, 2*(3), 2.
Watson, J. (1994). Guest editorial. *Nursing Praxis in New Zealand, 9*(1), 2-5.
Watson, J. (1994). Have we arrived or are we on our way out? Promises, possibilities, and paradigms. [Invited editorial.] *Image: The Journal of Nursing Scholarship, 26*(2), 86.
Watson, J. (1995). Advanced nursing practice and what might be. *Journal of Nursing and Health Care, 16*(2), 78-83.
Watson, J. (1995). A Fulbright in Sweden: Runes, academics, archetypal motifs, and other things. *Image: The Journal of Nursing Scholarship, 27*(1), 71-75.
Watson, J. (1995). A yearning for new debates. *NLN Update, 1*(3), 6-8.
Watson, J. (1995). Nursing's caring-healing model as an exemplar for alternative medicine. *Journal of Alternative Therapies in Health and Medicine, 1*(3), 64-69.
Watson, J. (1995). Postmodernism and knowledge development in nursing. *Nursing Science Quarterly, 8*(2), 60-64.
Watson, J. (1995). President's message: Challenges and summons from within and without. *Journal of Nursing and Health Care, 16*(6), 340.
Watson, J. (1995). President's message: Visioning on: Toward action transformation. *Journal of Nursing and Health Care, 16*(5), 290.
Watson, J. (1995). [Review of the book *Healing power of aromatherapy.*] *Journal of Alternative Therapies in Health and Medicine, 1*(3), 64-69.
Watson, J. (1996). President's message: From discipline specific to "inter" to "multi" to "transdisciplinary" health care education and practice. *Journal of Nursing and Health Care, 17*(2), 90-91.
Watson, J. (1996, May). [Review of the book *Healing nutrition.*] *Journal of Alternative Therapies in Health and Medicine, 2*(3), 91.
Watson, J. (1996, May). The wait, the wonder, the watch: Caring in a transplant unit. *Journal of Clinical Nursing, 5*(3), 199-200.
Watson, J. (1996). United States of America: Can nursing theory and practice survive? *International Journal of Nursing Practice, 2*(4), 241-243.
Watson, J. (1997). From the mountaintop to the marsh/fens: Punting on the River Cam. [Guest editorial.] *Journal of Clinical Nursing, 6*(1), 3-4.
Watson, J. (1997). The future of nursing-scholarship. *Image: The Journal of Nursing Scholarship, 29*(2), 117.

Watson, J. (1997). The theory of human caring: Retrospective and prospective. *Nursing Science Quarterly, 10*(1), 49-52.

Watson, J. (1998). Nightingale and the enduring legacy of transpersonal human caring. *Journal of Holistic Nursing, 16*(2), 292.

Watson, J. (1999, Spring). Aesthetic expressions of caring: Private psalms—Surrendering to the sacred. Personal professional reflections on caring and healing. *International Journal of Human Caring, 3*(3), 34.

Watson, J. (2000). Leading via caring-healing: The fourfold way toward transformative leadership. *Nursing Administration Quarterly, 25*(1), 1-6.

Watson, J. (2000). Philosophical perspectives in home care: Reconsidering caring. *Journal of Geriatric Nursing, 21*(6), 330-331.

Watson, J. (2000). Reconsidering caring in the home. *Journal of Geriatric Nursing, 21*(6), 330-333.

Watson, J. (2000). Via negative: Considering caring by way of non-caring. *Australian Journal of Holistic Nursing, 7*(1), 4-8.

Watson, J. (2001). Post-hospital nursing: Shortages, shifts, and script. *Nursing Administration Quarterly, 25*(3), 77-82.

Watson, J. (2002). Caring and healing our living and dying. *The International Nurse, 14*(2), 4-5.

Watson, J. (2002). Holistic nursing and caring: A values-based approach. *Journal of Japan Academy of Nursing Science, 22*(2), 69-74.

Watson, J. (2002). Intentionality and caring-healing consciousness: A theory of transpersonal nursing. *Holistic Nursing Journal, 16*(4), 12-19.

Watson, J. (2002). Metaphysics of virtual caring communities. *International Journal of Human Caring, 6*(1).

Watson, J. (2002, Spring). Nursing: Seeking its source and survival. [Guest editorial.] *ICU Nursing Web Journal, Spring*(9), 1-7. Retrieved June 7, 2004, from: http://www.nursing.gr/J.W.editorial.pdf

Watson, J. (2003). Love and caring: Ethics of face and hand. *Nursing Administration Quarterly, 27*(3), 197-202.

Watson, J. (2004). Caritas and communitas: An ethic for caring science. *Journal Japan Academy of Nursing Science, 24*(3), 66-67.

Watson, J. (2004). The relational core of nursing practice as partnership. [Invited commentary.] *Journal of Advanced Nursing, 47*(3).

Watson, J. (2004). Caritas and communitas: An ethic for caring science. *Journal Japan Academy of Nursing Science*, 24(1), 66-71.

Watson, J. (2005). Caring for our future: An interview with Jean Watson. [Interview by Carla Mariano.] *Beginnings (American Holistic Nurses' Association), 25*(3), 1, 12-14.

Watson, J. (2005). Caring science: Belonging before being as ethical cosmology. Nursing Science Quarterly, 18(4), 304-305.

Watson, J. (2005). Commentary on Shattell, M. (2004) Nurse-patient interaction: A review of the literature. *Journal of Clinical Nursing*, 14, 530-532.

Watson, J. (2005). What, may I ask, is happening to nursing knowledge and professional practices? What is nursing thinking at this turn in human history? Journal of Clinical Nursing, 14(8), 913-914.

Watson, J. (2005). Current issues and haunting concerns for survival of nursing profession. *Japanese* Journal of Nursing Science, 30(11), 50-53.

Watson, J. (2005). Love and caring. [Reprinted.] *Alternative Journal of Nursing*, 9. Available at: www.altjn.com

Watson, J. (2005). *An overview of Watson's theory of human caring.* Tokyo, Japan: Bulletin of Japanese Red Cross University College of Nursing.

Watson, J. (2006). Frontline and backstage caring: American nurse/world-wide nurses. *American Nurse Today*, 1(1), 24-28.

Watson, J. (2006). Carative factors—Caritas processes guide to professional nursing. *Danish Clinical Nursing Journal*, 20(3), 21-27.

Watson, J. (2006). Can an ethic of caring be maintained? *Journal of Advanced Nursing*, 54(3), 257-259.

Watson, J. (2006). Caring theory as an ethical guide to administrative and clinical practices. *JONAS Healthcare Law, Ethics and Regulation, 8*(3), 87-93.

Watson, J. (2006). Caring theory as an ethical guide to administrative and clinical practices. *Nursing Administration Quarterly, 30*(1), 48-55.

Watson, J. (2006). Walking pilgrimage as caritas action in the world. *Journal of Holistic Nursing, 24*(4), 289-296.

Watson, J. (2007). Theoretical questions and concerns: Response from a caring science framework. *Nursing Science Quarterly, 20*(1), 13-15.

Watson, J. Bauer, R., & Biley, F. (2002). Bavarian nursing secret: An inside view. *Reflections on Nursing Leadership: Sigma Theta Tau International Magazine, 28*(1), 26-28.

Watson, J., Biley, F. C., & Biley, A. M. (2001). Aesthetics, postmodern nursing, complementary therapies and more: An Internet dialogue. *Theoria: Journal of Nursing Theory, 10*(3), 13-16.

Watson, J., Biley, F. C., & Biley, A. M. (2002). Aesthetics, postmodern nursing, complementary therapies, and more: An Internet dialogue. *Complementary Therapies in Nursing and Midwifery, 8*, 81-83.

Watson, J., & Foster, R. (2003). The Attending Nurse Caring Model: Integrating theory, evidence, and advanced caring-healing therapeutics for transforming professional practice. *Journal of Clinical Nursing, 12*, 360-365.

Watson, J., & Phillips, S. (1992). A call for educational reform: Colorado nursing doctorate model as exemplar. *Nursing Outlook, 40*, 20-26.

Watson, J., & Smith, M. C. (2002). Caring science and the science of unitary human beings: A trans-theoretical discourse for nursing knowledge development. *Journal of Advanced Nursing, 7*(5), 452-461.

Secondary Sources

Book

Brencick, J., & Webster, G. (1999). *Philosophy of nursing.* Albany, NY: State University of New York.

Chapters and Monographs

Burns, P. (1991). Elements of spirituality and Watson's theory of transpersonal caring: Expansion of focus. In P. L. Chinn (Ed.), *Anthology of caring* (pp. 141-153). New York: National League for Nursing.

Duffy, J. R. (1992). The impact of nursing caring on patient outcomes. In D. Gaut (Ed.), *The presence of caring in nursing* (pp. 113-136). New York: National League for Nursing.

Fawcett, J. (2000). Watson's theory of human caring. In J. Fawcett (Ed.), *Analysis and evaluation of contemporary nursing knowledge: Nursing models and theories* (pp. 657-687). Philadelphia: F. A. Davis.

Jesse, E. (2006). Watson's philosophy in nursing practice. In M. R. Alligood & A.M. Tomey (Eds.). *Nursing theory: Utilization & application* (3rd ed., pp. 97-121). St. Louis: Mosby, Inc.

Jesse, E. (2006). La filosofia di Watson nella pratica informieristica. In M. R. Alligood & A. M. Tomey, *La teoria del nursing* (3rd ed., pp. 91-115). [C. Calamandrei, Italian translation.] Milano, Italy: McGraw-Hill.

McGraw, M. J. (2003). Watson's philosophy in nursing practice. In M. R. Alligood & A. M. Tomey, *Nursing theory: Utilization & application* (3rd ed., pp. 97-121). St. Louis: Mosby, Inc.

Morris, D. L. (1998). Watson's human care model. In J. J. Fitzpatrick (Ed.), *Encyclopedia of Nursing Research* (pp. 593-595). New York: Springer.

Neil, R. M. (1990). Watson's theory of caring in nursing: The rainbow of and for people living with AIDS. In M. E. Parker (Ed.), *Nursing theories in practice* (pp. 289-301). New York: National League for Nursing.

Neil, R. M. (1995). Evidence in support of basing a nursing center on nursing theory: The Denver nursing project in human caring. In B. Murphy (Ed.), *Nursing centers: The time is now* (pp. 33-46). New York: National League for Nursing.

Neil, R. M. (2003). Philosophy and science of caring. In A. M. Tomey & M. R. Alligood, *Nursing theorists and their work* (6th ed., pp. 91-115). St. Louis: Mosby, Inc.

Nyberg, J. (1994). Implementing Watson's theory of caring. In J. Watson (Ed.), *Applying the art and science of human caring* (pp. 53-61). New York: National League for Nursing.

Woodward, T. K. (2006). Application of Jean Watson's Theory of Human Caring. In M. Parker (Ed.), *Nursing theories and nursing practice* (2nd ed., pp. 302-308). Philadelphia: F. A. Davis.

Journal Articles

Bent, K. N. (1999). The ecologies of community caring. *ANS Advances in Nursing Science, 21*, 29-36.

Biley, A. (2000). [Review of the book *Postmodern nursing and beyond.*] *Journal of Clinical Nursing, 9*, 649-653.

Burchiel, R. N. (1995). The Watson theory of human care applied to ASPO/Lamaze perinatal education. *Journal of Perinatal Education, 6*(1), 43-47.

Coates, C. J. (1997). The caring efficacy scale: Nurses' self-reports of caring in practice settings. *Advanced Practice Nursing Quarterly, 3*(1), 53-59.

Eddins, B. B., & Riley-Eddins, E. A. (1997). Watson's theory of human caring: The twentieth century and beyond. *Journal of Multicultural Nursing and Health, 3*, 30-35.

Falk, R., & Adeline, R. (2000). Watson's philosophy, science and theory of human caring as a conceptual framework for guiding community health nursing practice. *ANS Advances in Nursing Science, 23*(2), 34-50.

Fawcett, J. (2002). The nurse theorists: 21st century updates—Jean Watson. *Nursing Science Quarterly, 15*(3), 214-219.

From, M. A. (1995). Utilizing the home setting to teach Watson's theory of human caring. *Nursing Forum, 30*, 5-11.

Horrigan, B. (2000). Regions hospital opens holistic nursing unit. *Alternative Therapies, 6*(4), 92-93.

Jensen, K. P., Back-Pettersson, S. R., & Segesten, K. M. (1993). The caring moment and the green-thumb phenomenon among Swedish nurses. *Nursing Science Quarterly, 6*, 98-104.

Kilby, J. W. (1997). Case study: Transpersonal caring theory in perinatal loss. *Journal of Perinatal Education, 6*(2), 45-50.

Marck, B. B. (1995). Watson's theory of caring: A model for implementation in practice. *Journal of Nursing Care Quality, 9*(4), 43-54.

McNamara, S. A. (1995). Perioperative nurses' perceptions of caring practices. *AORN Journal 61*(377), 380-385.

Mullaney, J. A. (2000, June). The lived experience of using Watson's actual caring occasion to treat depressed women. *Journal of Holistic Nursing, 18*(2), 129-142.

Nelson-Marten, P., Hecomovich, K., & Pangle, M. (1998). Caring theory: A framework for advanced practice nursing. *Advanced Practice Nursing Quarterly, 4*, 70-77.

Norred, C. (2000). Minimizing preoperative anxiety with alternative caring-healing therapies. *AORN Journal, 72*(3), 1-4.

Nyman, C. S., & Lutzen, K. (1999). Caring needs of patients with rheumatoid arthritis. *Nursing Science Quarterly, 12*(2), 164-169.
Perry, B. (1997). Beliefs of eight exemplary nurses related to Watson's nursing theory. *Canadian Oncology Nursing Journal, 8*(2), 97-101.
Ray, M. A. (1997). Consciousness and the moral ideal: A transcultural analysis of Watson's theory of transpersonal caring. *Advanced Practice Nursing Quarterly, 3*, 25-31.
Saewyc, E. (2000, June). Nursing theories of caring. *Journal of Holistic Nursing, 18*(2), 109-113.
Schindel-Martin, L. (1991). Using Watson's theory to explore the dimensions of adult polycystic kidney disease. *American Nephrology Nurses' Association Journal, 18*, 493-496.
Schroeder, C. (1993). Nursing's response to the crisis of access, costs, and quality in health care. *ANS Advances in Nursing Science, 16*(1), 1-20.
Schroeder, C., & Maeve, M. K. (1992). Nursing care partnerships at the Denver nursing project in human caring: An application and extension of caring theory in practice. *ANS Advances in Nursing Science, 15*(2), 25-38.
Smith, M. C. (1997). Nursing theory-guided practice: Practice guided by Watson's theory. The Denver nursing project in human caring. *Nursing Science Quarterly, 10*, 56-58.
Swanson, K. M. (1991). Empirical development of a middle range theory of caring. *Nursing Research, 40*, 161-166.
Updike, P., Cleveland, M. J., & Nyberg, J. (2000). Complementary caring-healing practices of nurses caring for children with life-challenging illnesses and their families: A pilot project with case reports. *Alternative Therapies, 6*(4), 108-112.
Walker, C. A. (1996). Coalescing the theories of two nurse visionaries: Parse and Watson. *Journal of Advanced Nursing, 24*, 988-996.
Ward, S. (1998). Caring and healing in the 21st century. *MCN Journal 23*(4), 210-215.

Dissertation Abstracts

Bauman, R.A. (2003). The lived experience of nurses providing futile care to critically ill newborns and infants. [Masters' dissertation, Southern Connecticut State University, 2003.] *ProQuest Digital Dissertations Database*, AAT1412197.
Bishop, M. E. (1994). Nurses' knowledge and attitude related to organ donation. [Masters' dissertation, Grand Valley State University, 1994.] *ProQuest Digital Dissertations Database*, AAT1359750.
Brencick, J. M. (1997). Universality and singularity: A philosophy of nursing. [Doctoral dissertation, University of Colorado Health Sciences Center, 1997.] *ProQuest Digital Dissertations Database*, AAT 9804624.
Carson, E. M. (2002). A comparison of evidence of Watson's carative factors in performance appraisals for medical surgical registered nurses in the state of Illinois. [Doctoral dissertation, Northern Illinois University, 2002.] *ProQuest Digital Dissertations Database*, AAT3064619.
Covington, H. (2002). Caring presence: Journey toward a mutual goal. [Doctoral dissertation, University of Colorado Health Sciences Center, 2002.] *ProQuest Digital Dissertations database*, AAT3069581.
Darling, A. A. (1997). A qualitative study of caring within the human-animal bond in adults living with chronic illness. [Masters' dissertation, D'Youville College, 1997.] *ProQuest Digital Dissertations database*, AAT1386773.
Dechairo, A. E. (2000). Quality patient outcomes through nursing case management in acute care hospitals. [Doctoral dissertation, University of California, Los Angeles, 2000.] *ProQuest Digital Dissertations database*, AAT9973201.
Disparti, J. (1991). Ethics education in baccalaureate nursing programs: Instructional strategies for an ethic of care. [Doctoral dissertation, Columbia University Teachers College, 1991.] *ProQuest Digital Dissertations database*, AAT9136375.
Donohue, M. A. (1991). The lived experience of stigma in individuals with AIDS: A phenomenological investigation. [Doctoral dissertation, Adelphi University, 1991.] *ProQuest Digital Dissertations database*, AAT9216862.
Guana, M. C. (1998). An exploration of the carative beliefs and behavior of female emergency room nurses: A study of caring in theory and practice. [Doctoral dissertation, University of Maryland, College Park, 1998.] *ProQuest Digital Dissertations database*, AAT9836404.
Hoopfer, D. L. (1998). Advancing an integrated ethic for nursing. [Doctoral dissertation, University of Alberta {Canada}, 1998.] *ProQuest Digital Dissertations database*, AATNQ34779.
Lomas, L. E. (1996). Patient advocacy: Shared vulnerability and personal integrity. [Masters' dissertation, Florida Atlantic University, 1996.] *ProQuest Digital Dissertations database*, AAT1380867.
McCarthy, M. P. (1992). A relational ontology: The interplay of transcendence, spirituality, and community. [Doctoral dissertation, University of Colorado Health Sciences Center, 1992.] *ProQuest Digital Dissertations database*, AAT9238380.
Moore, M. L. (2002). What are the perceptions of caring and non-caring behaviors in the primary care setting? [Masters' dissertation, University of Nevada, Reno, 2002.] *ProQuest Digital Dissertations database*, AAT1410206.
Running, A. F. (1992). Visit as a method of existential inquiry in nursing: Stories of health from the oldest old. [Doctoral dissertation, University of Colorado Health Sciences Center, 1992.] *ProQuest Digital Dissertations database*, AAT9230874.

Ryan, M. S. (1997). Comparison of the meaning of death for persons with cancer and persons with AIDS at the end of life. [Masters' dissertation, The University of Arizona, 1997.] *ProQuest Digital Dissertations database,* AAT1385732.

Sellers, S. C. (1991). A philosophical analysis of conceptual models of nursing. [Doctoral dissertation, Iowa State University, 1991.] *ProQuest Digital Dissertations database,* AAT9126248.

Sitzman, K. L. (2001). Effective ergonomic teaching for positive client outcomes. [Masters' dissertation, University of Utah College of Nursing, 2001.] *ProQuest Digital Dissertations database,* AAT1402808.

Tretton, J. L. (1999). Caring behaviors of nurses as perceived by patients and nurses. [Masters' dissertation, University of Nevada, Reno, 1999.] *ProQuest Digital Dissertations database,* AAT1395234.

Tuttle, S. B. (1997). Patient perceptions of nurse behaviors as indicators of caring. [Masters' dissertation, Grand Valley State University, 1997.] *ProQuest Digital Dissertations database,* AAT1384254.

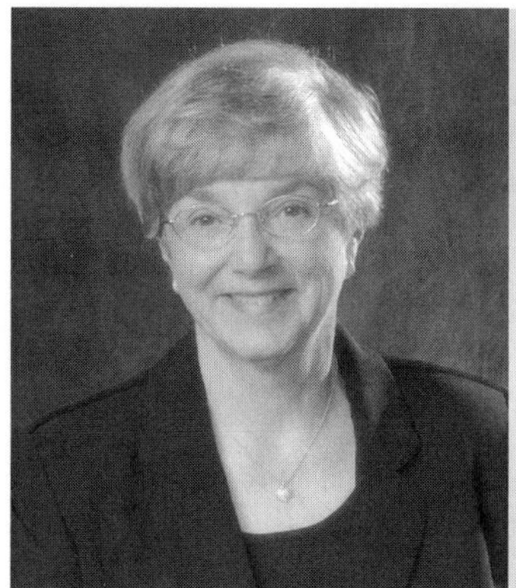

Photo credit: M. Dauley, Artistic Images, Littleton, CO.

CHAPTER

8

Marilyn Anne Ray

1938-present

Theory of Bureaucratic Caring

Sherrilyn Coffman

"Improved patient safety, infection control, reduction in medication errors, and overall quality of care in complex bureaucratic health care systems cannot occur without knowledge and understanding of spiritual-ethical caring, compassion and right action for all patients and professionals" (M. Ray, personal communication, April 13, 2008).

CREDENTIALS OF THE THEORIST

Marilyn Anne (Dee) Ray was born in Hamilton, Ontario, Canada, and grew up in a family of six children. When Ray was 15, her father became seriously ill, was hospitalized, and almost died. A nurse saved his life. Marilyn decided that she would become a nurse so that she could help others and perhaps save their lives, too.

In 1958, Marilyn Ray graduated from St. Joseph Hospital School of Nursing, Hamilton, and left for Los Angeles, California. She worked at the University of California, Los Angeles Medical Center on a number of units, including obstetrics and gynecology, emergency department, and cardiac and critical care with adults and children. In Southern California, she enjoyed meeting new friends from different cultures and cared for children from vulnerable populations. While working with people of diverse cultures, particularly African Americans and Latinos, Ray began to see how important cultures were in the development of people's views about nursing and the world.

In 1965, Ray returned to school for her BSN and MSN in Maternal-Child Nursing at the University of Colorado, School of Nursing. This is where she met Dr. Madeleine Leininger, who was the first nurse anthropologist and the Director of the Federal Nurse-Scientist program. Through her mentorship, Leininger profoundly influenced Ray's life. Ray took a special interest in her first courses on nursing and anthropology, including childhood and culture. She studied organizations as small cultures, and her research project in graduate school involved the study of a children's hospital as a small culture. While being educated at the University of Colorado, Ray worked in organizations and practiced with children and adults in critical care and renal dialysis, and in occupational health nursing with family-centered care.

In the mid-1960s, Ray became a citizen of the United States. Shortly afterward, in 1967, she joined and was commissioned as an officer in the United States Air Force Reserve, Nurse Corps (and Air National Guard). She graduated as a flight nurse from the School of Aerospace Medicine at Brooks Air Force Base, San Antonio, Texas, and served as an aeromedical evacuation nurse. She cared for combat casualties and other patients onboard various types of aircraft during the Viet Nam war. Since that time, Ray has served longer than 30 years in different positions in the Air Force—flight nurse, clinician, administrator, educator, and researcher—and held the rank of colonel for longer than 10 years. Her interest in space nursing stimulated her to attend the program for educators at Marshall Space Flight Center in Huntsville, Alabama. She remains a charter member of the Space Nursing Society. In 1990, she was the first nurse to go to the Soviet Union with the Aerospace Medical Association, when the former USSR opened its space operations to American space engineers and physicians. Ray was called to active duty during the First Persian Gulf War in 1991, at which time she was assigned to Eglin Air Force Base, Valparaiso, Florida, where she orchestrated discharge planning and later conducted research in the emergency department.

Ray is the recipient of a number of medals, including Air Force commendation medals for nursing education and research developments received during her Air Force career. Most notably, in 2000 she received the Federal Nursing Services Essay Award from the Association of Military Surgeons of the United States for research on the impact of TRICARE/Managed Care on Total Force Readiness. This award recognized her accomplishments as a participant in a research program on economics and the nurse-patient relationship that received nearly $1 million in funding from the TriService Military Nursing Research Council. In 2008, she was awarded the TriService Nursing Research Program Coin for excellence in nursing research.

Ray's first teaching positions were held at the University of California San Francisco and the University of San Francisco in undergraduate nursing education. At that time, she was on the faculty of nursing at the University of California San Francisco with Drs. Barney Glaser and Anselm Strauss, authors of the grounded theory method. This association intensified her interest in qualitative research approaches. She continued to be intrigued by the study of nursing as a culture and had opportunities to teach students from various American and Asian cultures. During the summer of 1971, she traveled to Mexico with colleagues to study anthropology and health. She acknowledges how much she learned about aboriginal peoples and their fascinating life ways from the people of a small village.

During the years 1973 to 1977, Ray returned to Canada to be with her family. She joined the nursing faculty at McMaster University in Hamilton, Ontario, and taught in the family nurse practitioner program. In this position, Ray again had the opportunity to integrate culture and health into the curriculum. This was an exciting time, because the McMaster University Health Sciences Center was initiating evidence-based teaching, education, and practice. Ray completed a Master of Arts in Cultural Anthropology at McMaster University and studied human relationships, decision making and conflict, and the hospital as an organizational culture. Her clinical work in neonatal intensive care was completed at that time at McMaster University Health Sciences Center.

Ray was thrilled when she received a letter from Leininger asking whether she would be interested in applying for the first transcultural nursing doctoral program in the United States. At the University of Utah, where she studied with her mentor Dr. Leininger, Ray met wonderful colleagues who have taken their places in the history of nursing through their research and scholarly work, especially Drs. Joyceen Boyle, Joan Uhl-Pierce, Kathryn McCance, and Janice Morse. Ray's doctoral dissertation (1981a) was a study on caring in the complex hospital organizational culture. From this research, the Theory of Bureaucratic Caring, which is the focus of this chapter, emerged.

During her doctoral studies, Ray married James L. Droesbeke, whom she credits as her inspiration and friend, and the love of her life. He was a constant source of support and help to her over the course of her career until his untimely death from cancer in 2001. He remains a significant spiritual influence in her personal and professional life. After completing her doctorate in 1981, Ray rejoined the University of Colorado School of Nursing. At the University of Colorado, Ray had the good fortune to work with Dr. Jean Watson, who developed and advanced the theory and practice of human caring in nursing. With Watson and several other scholars, Ray founded the International Association for Human Caring, which awarded her its Lifetime Achievement Award in 2008. In the 1980s, Dr. Max van Manen from the University of Alberta was her mentor in phenomenology and hermeneutic human science research methods. At the University of Colorado, Ray continued her study and teaching of phenomenology and other qualitative research approaches with Dr. Francelyn Reeder and directed the dissertation work of Dr. Alice Davidson, focusing on the new sciences of complexity.

In 1989, Ray accepted an appointment as the Christine E. Lynn Eminent Scholar at Florida Atlantic University, College of Nursing, a position that she held until 1994. Her appointment as the first in-residence eminent scholar was made through the efforts of Dr. Anne Boykin, Dean of the College of Nursing, who advanced nursing as caring in the curriculum and in research. Florida Atlantic University developed the Center for Caring, which has housed caring memorabilia since the inception of the International Association for Human Caring in 1977. Ray also held the position of Yingling Visiting Scholar Chair at Virginia Commonwealth University, School of Nursing, from 1994 to 1995, and was a visiting professor at the University of Colorado from 1989 to 1999. Ray has been a visiting professor at universities in Australia, New Zealand, and Thailand, promoting and advancing the teaching and research of human caring (Ray 1994b, 2000; Ray & Turkel, 2000). She authored several theoretical and research publications in transcultural caring, transcultural ethics, and caring inquiry while serving as an eminent scholar and visiting professor.

Ray continues as Professor Emeritus at Florida Atlantic University, Christine E. Lynn College of Nursing, Boca Raton, Florida, where she is a part-time faculty member in the PhD program and a faculty mentor. Ray's interest in transcultural nursing remains a common theme in her research, teaching, and practice. With Dr. Sherrilyn Coffman, she completed a grounded theory research study of high-risk pregnant African American women (Coffman & Ray, 1999, 2002). Learning more about vulnerable populations gave Ray a deeper understanding of the needs of these populations, particularly equal access to healthcare and the importance of caring communities. Ray held the position of vice president of Floridians for Health Care (universal healthcare) from 1998 to 2000. She has been a Certified Trans-cultural Nurse since 1988 and is a member of the International Transcultural Nursing Society. She has made international presentations on transcultural caring and ethics in such countries as China, Saudi Arabia, and England. In 1984, Ray was awarded the Leininger Transcultural Nursing Award, which is given for excellence in transcultural nursing. In 2005, she was named a Transcultural Nursing Scholar by the International Transcultural Nursing Society. Ray has served on the review boards of the *Journal of Transcultural Nursing* and *Qualitative Health Research,* and she is writing a book on transcultural caring dynamics in nursing and health (Ray, in press).

Ray's research interests continue to focus on nurses, nurse administrators, and patients in critical care and intermediate care, and in nursing administration in complex hospital organizational cultures. She has developed a program of research with Dr. Marian Turkel with federal funding from the TriService Nursing Research Program, to study the nurse-patient relationship as an economic resource (Turkel & Ray, 2000, 2001, 2003). These studies have focused on the impact of caring relationships on patient and economic outcomes in complex organizations. With Turkel, Ray has published in the areas of complex caring relational theory, organizational transformation through caring and ethical choice making, instrument development on organizational caring, economic and political caring, and caring organization creation. Involvement in the PhD program at Florida Atlantic University has given Ray opportunities to continue to influence complex organizations and to create caring organizations and environments in local, national, and global contexts. Her contributions to nursing education were recognized in 2005, when she was awarded an honorary degree from Nevada State College in Henderson, Nevada. In 2007, she received the Distinguished Alumna Award from the University of Utah College of Nursing, Salt Lake City, Utah.

THEORETICAL SOURCES

Ray's interest in caring as a topic of nursing scholarship was stimulated by her work with Leininger, beginning in 1968, which focused on transcultural nursing and ethnographic-ethnonursing research methods. She used ethnographic methods in combination with phenomenology to generate substantive and formal grounded theories, resulting in the overarching Theory of Bureaucratic Caring (Ray, 1981a, 1984, 1989, 1994b). This formal theory focuses on nursing in complex organizations, such as hospitals. What distinguishes organizations as cultures is their foundation in anthropology, or the study of how people behave in communities and the significance or meaning of work life (Louis, 1985). Organizational cultures are viewed as social constructions, which are formed symbolically through meaning in interaction (Smircich, 1985).

Ray's work (1981b, 1989; Moccia, 1986) was influenced by the philosophy of Hegel, who posited the interrelationship between thesis, antithesis, and synthesis. In Hegel's philosophy, the thesis of being and the antithesis or its opposite, non-being, arenegated and then reconciled emerging into a unitive force of becoming. In Ray's theory, the thesis of caring (humanistic, spiritual, and ethical) and the antithesis of bureaucracy (technological, economic, political, and legal) are reconciled and synthesized into the unitive force, bureaucratic caring. The synthesis, as a process of becoming, is a transformation. This process continues to repeat itself—thesis, antithesis, synthesis—always changing, emerging, and transforming.

As she revisited and continued to develop her formal theory, Ray (2001, 2006) discovered that her study findings fit well with explanations from chaos theory, quantum physics' contribution to the science of complexity. Chaos theory describes simultaneous order and disorder, and order within disorder (the edge of chaos). An underlying order or interconnectedness exists in apparently random events (Briggs & Peat, 1984). Mathematical studies, from which chaos theory originated, have shown that what may seem random is actually part of a larger pattern. Application of this theory to organizations demonstrates that within a state of chaos, the system is held within boundaries that are well ordered (Wheatley, 1999). Furthermore, chaos is necessary for new creative ordering. The creative process as described by Briggs & Peat in chaos theory is as follows:

> . . . when we enter the vital turbulence of life, we realize that, at bottom, everything is always new. Often we have simply failed to notice this fact. When we're being creative, we take notice. (1999, p. 30)

Ray compares change in complex organizations with this creative process and challenges nurses to step back and renew their perceptions of everyday events, to discover the embedded meanings. This is particularly important during organizational change.

Complexity is a more general concept than chaos and focuses on wholeness or holonomy (the whole is in the part and the part in the whole). Complex systems, such as organizations, have a great many agents interacting with each other in multiple ways. As a result, these systems are dynamic and always changing. Systems behave in nonlinear fashion because they do not react proportionately to inputs.

Small inputs can have large effects and may create different effects at different times. For example, a simple intervention such as asking a colleague for help with a procedure may be accommodated easily or may be seen as unreasonable on a busy day. This makes the behavior of complex systems impossible to predict (Vicenzi, White, & Begun, 1997). Nevertheless, this chaos exists only because the entire system is holistic. Briggs and Peat (1999, pp. 156-157) describe this "chaotic wholeness" as "full of particulars, active and interactive, animated by nonlinear feedback and capable of producing everything from self-organized systems to fractal self-similarity to unpredictable chaotic disorder." These ideas are influential in Ray's ongoing development of bureaucratic caring theory, which suggests that multiple system inputs are interconnected with caring in the whole of the organizational culture. Nurses involved in small group work can apply these ideas by broadening the scope of information utilized in decision making, while considering all possible relevant factors.

Ray's reflection on the Theory of Bureaucratic Caring as holographic was influenced by the historic revolution that was taking place in science based on the new holographic worldview (Ray, 2001, 2006). The discovery of interconnectedness between apparently unrelated subatomic events has intrigued scientists. In experiments, electrons were found to lose their individual properties as they spun, charged, and changed from matter to energy to meet the requirements of the whole. In this process, the electrons did not remain as parts; they were drawn together by a process of internal connectedness. Scientists concluded that systems possess the capacity to self-organize; therefore, attention is shifting away from describing parts and instead is focusing on the totality as an actual process (Wheatley, 1999). The conceptualization of the hologram portrays how every structure interpenetrates and is interpenetrated by other structures—so the part is the whole, and the whole is reflected in every part (Talbot, 1991).

The hologram has provided scientists with a new way of understanding order. Bohm conceptualized the universe as a kind of giant, flowing hologram (Talbot, 1991). He asserted that our day-to-day reality is really an illusion, like a holographic image. Bohm termed our conscious level of existence *explicate,* or unfolded order, and the deeper layer of reality of which humans are usually unaware *implicate,* or enfolded order. In the Theory of Bureaucratic Caring, Ray compares the healthcare structures of political, legal, economic, educational, physiological, social-cultural, and technological with the explicate order and spiritual-ethical caring with the implicate order. An example related to healthcare might focus on a case manager's decisions about obtaining resources for a client's care in the home. At first glance, explicate structures such as the legal managed care contract or the physical needs of the client might appear to provide enough information. However, through the case manager's caring relationship with the client, more implicate issues, such as the client's values and desires, may emerge. In truth, each nursing situation involves endless enfolding and unfolding of information that may be viewed as explicate and implicate order, and all is important to consider in the decision making process.

Making things work in a healthcare organizational system requires knowledge and understanding of bureaucracy, which is rigid, and the complexity of change. Bureaucracy and complexity may seem like the antithesis of each other, but in reality, the *structure* of bureaucracy (illuminating the political, economic, legal, and technological systems in organizations) works in conjunction with the *complex relational process* of networks to co-create patterns of human behavior and patterns of caring. Both bureaucracy and complexity influence the ways in which diverse participants describe and intuitively live out their life world experience in the system. No one thing or person in a system is independent; rather, they are interdependent. The system is holographic where the whole and the part are intertwined. Thus, bureaucracy and complexity co-create and transform each other. The Theory of Bureaucratic Caring is a representation of the relatedness of system and caring factors.

Major Concepts & Definitions

The theoretical processes of awareness of viewing truth, or seeing the good of things (caring), and of communication are central to the theory. The dialectic of spiritual-ethical caring (the implicate order) in relation to the surrounding structures of political, legal, economic, educational, physiological, social-cultural, and technological (the explicate order) illustrates that everything is interconnected with caring and the system within a macrocosm of the whole culture. In the model (see Figure 8-2), everything is infused with spiritual-ethical caring (the center) by integrative and relational connection to the structures of organizational life. Spiritual-ethical caring involves qualitatively different processes, such as political, economic, and technological ones.

The interconnectedness of concepts led Ray to reflect upon the Theory of Bureaucratic Caring as a holographic theory (Ray, 2001, 2006). *Holography* means that everything is a whole in one context and a part in another—each part being in the whole and the whole being in the part (Talbot, 1991). Spiritual-ethical caring is both a part and a whole. Likewise every part secures its meaning from each of the parts, which also can be considered wholes.

CARING

Caring is defined as a complex, transcultural, relational process grounded in an ethical, spiritual context. Caring is the relationship between charity and right action, between love as compassion in response to suffering and need and justice or fairness in terms of what ought to be done. Caring occurs within a culture or society, including personal culture, hospital organizational culture, and societal and global culture (M. Ray, personal communication, March 27, 2002).

SPIRITUAL-ETHICAL CARING

Spirituality involves creativity and choice and is revealed in attachment, love, and community. The ethical imperatives of caring join with the spiritual and are related to moral obligations to others. This means never treating people as a means to an end or as an end in themselves but rather as beings with the capacity to make choices. Spiritual-ethical caring for nursing focuses on how facilitation of choices for the good of others can or should be accomplished (Ray, 1989, 1997a).

EDUCATIONAL

Formal and informal educational programs, use of audiovisual media to convey information, and other forms of teaching and sharing information are examples of educational factors related to the meaning of caring (Ray, 1981a, 1989).

PHYSICAL

Physical factors are related to the physical state of being, including biological and mental patterns. Because the mind and body are interrelated, each pattern influences the other (Ray, 2001, 2006).

SOCIAL-CULTURAL

Examples of social and cultural factors are ethnicity and family structures; intimacy with friends and family; communication; social interaction and support; understanding interrelationships, involvement, and intimacy; and structures of cultural groups, community, and society (Ray, 1981a, 1989, 2001, 2006).

LEGAL

Legal factors related to the meaning of caring include responsibility and accountability; rules and principles to guide behaviors, such as policies and procedures; informed consent; rights to privacy; malpractice and liability issues; client, family, and professional rights; and the practice of defensive medicine and nursing (Ray, 1981a, 1989).

Continued

MAJOR CONCEPTS & DEFINITIONS—cont'd

TECHNOLOGICAL

Technological factors include nonhuman resources, such as the use of machinery to maintain the physiological well-being of the patient, diagnostic tests, pharmaceutical agents, and the knowledge and skill needed to utilize these resources (Ray, 1987, 1989). Also included with technology are computer-assisted practice and documentation (M. Ray, personal communication, June 16, 2004).

ECONOMIC

Factors related to the meaning of caring include money, budget, insurance systems, limitations, and guidelines imposed by managed care organizations, and, in general, allocation of scarce human and material resources to maintain the economic viability of the organization (Ray, 1981a, 1989). Caring as an interpersonal resource should be considered, as well as goods, money, and services (Turkel & Ray, 2000, 2001, 2003).

POLITICAL

Political factors and the power structure within healthcare administration influence how nursing is viewed in healthcare and include patterns of communication and decision making in the organization; role and gender stratification among nurses, physicians, and administrators; union activities, including negotiation and confrontation; government and insurance company influences; uses of power, prestige, and privilege; and, in general, competition for scarce human and material resources (Ray, 1989).

USE OF EMPIRICAL EVIDENCE

The Theory of Bureaucratic Caring was generated from qualitative research involving health professionals and clients in the hospital setting. This research focused on caring in the organizational culture and first appeared in the doctoral dissertation in 1981, and in other literature in 1984 and 1989. The purpose of the dissertation study was to generate a theory of the dynamic structure of caring in a complex organization. The methodss used were grounded theory, phenomenology and ethnography to elicit the meaning of caring to study participants.

The grounded theory approach is a qualitative research method that uses a systematic set of procedures to develop an inductive theory of a social process. The aim of the researcher is to construct what the participants see as their social reality (Strauss & Corbin, 1990). This process results in the evolution of substantive theory (caring data generated from experience) and formal theory (integrated synthesis of caring and bureaucratic structures).

Ray spent longer than 7 months in the field studying caring in all areas of a hospital, from nursing practice to materials management to administration, including nursing administration. More than 200 respondents participated in the purposive and convenience sample. The principal question asked was "What is the meaning of caring to you?" Through dialogue, caring evolved from in-depth interviews, participant observation, caregiving observation, and documentation in field notes (Ray, 1989).

Ray's discovery of bureaucratic caring began as a substantive theory and evolved to a formal theory. The substantive theory emerged as Differential Caring, revealing that the meaning of caring differentiates itself by its context. Dominant caring dimensions vary in terms of areas of practice or hospital units. For example, an intensive care unit has a dominant value of technological caring (i.e., monitors, ventilators, treatments, and pharmacotherapeutics), and an oncology unit has a value of a more intimate, spiritual caring (i.e., family focused, comforting, compassionate). Staff nurses value caring in relation to patients, and administrators value caring as more system related, such as safeguarding when the economic well-being of the hospital.

The formal Theory of Bureaucratic Caring symbolized a dynamic structure of caring. This structure emerges from the dialectic between the thesis of caring as humanistic (social, education, ethical, and religious-spiritual structures) and the antithesis of caring as bureaucratic (economic, political, legal, and technological structures). The dialectic of caring in relation to various structures illustrates that everything is interconnected with caring, and the organizational system is a macrocosm of the whole of culture.

The evolution of Ray's theory is illustrated in Figure 8-1, which contains diagrams of the bureaucratic caring structure published in 1981 and 1989. In the original grounded theory (see Figure 8-1, *A*), political and economic structures occupied a larger dimension to illustrate their increasing influence on the nature of institutional caring (Ray, 1981a). Subsequent research conducted in intensive care and intermediate care units (Ray, 1989) emphasized the differential nature of caring, as seen through its competing structures of political, legal, economic, technological-physiological, spiritual-religious, ethical, and educational-social elements (see Figure 8-1, *B*). Ray's work was one of the first to focus on caring in the high-technology area of critical care, and her research was truly innovative. In her 1987 article on technological caring, Ray noted that "critical care nursing is intensely human, moral, and technocratic" (p. 172). Ray encouraged other researchers to study this area to enhance nursing's understanding of the advantages and limitations of technology in critical care. The *Dimensions of Critical Care Nursing* journal presented Ray their Researcher of the Year award for her groundbreaking work.

With continued reflection and analysis of her work, combined with research on the economics

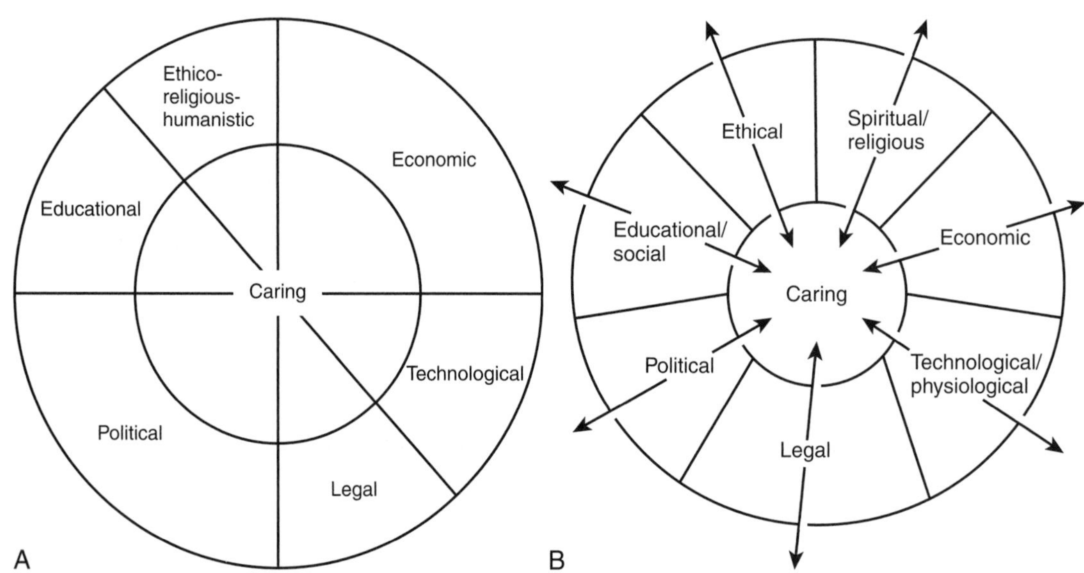

Figure 8-1 **A, The Original Grounded Theory of Bureaucratic Caring.** (From Ray, M. A. [1981a]. A study of caring within an institutional culture. *Dissertation Abstracts International,* 42[06]. [University Microfilm No. 8127787.].) **B, Subsequent Grounded Theory Revealing Differential Caring.** (From Parker, M. E. [2006]. *Nursing theories and nursing practice* [3rd ed.]. Philadelphia: F. A. Davis. Graphics redrawn from originals by J. Castle and B. Jensen, Nevada State College, Henderson, NV.)

of the nurse-patient relationship, Ray began to illuminate the ethical-spiritual realm of nursing (Figure 8-2) (Ray, 2001). Spiritual-ethical caring became a dominant modality because of discoveries that focused on the nurse-patient relationship. Qualitatively different systems, such as political, economic, social-cultural, and physiological, when viewed as open and interactive, are whole and operate through the choice making of nurses (Davidson & Ray, 1991; Ray, 1994a). Spiritual-ethical caring suggests how choice making for the good of others can be accomplished in nursing practice.

Ray's research reveals that in complex organizations, nursing as caring is practiced and lived out at the margin between the humanistic-spiritual dimension and the systemic dimension. These findings are consistent with worldviews from the science of complexity, which propose that phenomena that are antithetical actually coexist (Briggs & Peat, 1999; Ray, 1998). Thus, technological and humanistic systems exist together. Complexity theory explains why there is a resolution of the paradox between differing systems (thesis and antithesis) represented in the synthesis or the Theory of Bureaucratic Caring.

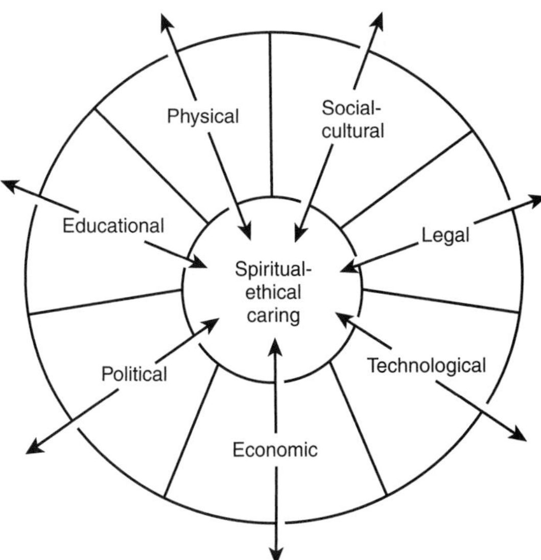

Figure 8-2 The Holographic Theory of Bureaucratic Caring. (From Parker, M. E. [2006]. *Nursing theories and nursing practice* [3rd ed.]. Philadelphia: F. A. Davis. Graphics redrawn from originals by J. Castle and B. Jensen, Nevada State College, Henderson, NV.)

In summary, the Theory of Bureaucratic Caring emerged using a grounded theory methodology, blended with phenomenology and ethnography. The initial theory was examined using the philosophy of Hegel. The theory was revisited in 2001 after continuing research, and findings were examined in light of the science of complexity and chaos theory, resulting in the holographic Theory of Bureaucratic Caring (see Figure 8-2).

MAJOR ASSUMPTIONS

Nursing

Nursing is holistic, relational, spiritual, and ethical caring that seeks the good of self and others in complex community, organizational, and bureaucratic cultures. Dwelling more deeply with the nature of caring reveals that the foundation of spiritual caring is love. Through knowledge of the inner mystery of the inspirational life within, love calls forth a responsible ethical life that enables the expression of concrete actions of caring in the lives of nurses. As such, caring is cultural and social. Transcultural caring encompasses beliefs and values of compassion or love and justice or fairness, which find significance in the social realm, where relationships are formed and transformed. Transcultural caring serves as a unique lens through which human choices are seen, and understanding in health and healing emerges. Thus, through compassion and justice, nursing strives toward excellence in the activities of caring through the dynamics of complex cultural contexts of relationships, organizations, and communities (M. Ray, personal communication, May 25, 2004).

Person

A person is a spiritual and cultural being. Persons are created by God, the Mystery of Being, and they engage co-creatively in human organizational and transcultural relationships to find meaning and value (M. Ray, personal communication, May 25, 2004).

Health

Health provides a pattern of meaning for individuals, families, and communities. In all human societies, beliefs and caring practices about illness and health are central features of culture. Health is not simply the consequence of a physical state of being. People construct their reality of health in terms of biology, mental patterns, characteristics of their image of the body, mind, and soul, ethnicity and family structures, structures of society and community (political, economic, legal, and technological), and experiences of caring that give meaning to lives in complex ways. The social organization of health and illness in society (the healthcare system) determines the way that people are recognized as sick or well. It determines how health professionals view health and illness, and how individuals view health and illness. Health is related to the way that people in a cultural group or organizational culture or bureaucratic system construct reality and give or find meaning (Helman, 1997; M. Ray, personal communication, May 25, 2004).

Environment

Environment is a complex spiritual, ethical, ecological, and cultural phenomenon. This conceptualization of environment embodies knowledge and conscience about the beauty of life forms and symbolic (representational) systems or patterns of meaning. These patterns are transmitted historically and are preserved or changed through caring values, attitudes, and communication. Functional forms identified in the social structure or bureaucracy (i.e., political, legal, technological, and economic) play a role in facilitating understanding of the meaning of caring, cooperation, and conflict in human cultural groups and complex organizational environments. Nursing practice in environments embodies the elements of the social structure and spiritual and ethical caring patterns of meaning (M. Ray, personal communication, May 25, 2004).

THEORETICAL ASSERTIONS

Person, nursing, environment, and health are integrated into the structure of the Theory of Bureaucratic Caring. The theory implies a dialectical relationship (thesis, antithesis, synthesis) between humans (person and nurse), the dimension of spiritual-ethical caring, and the structural (nursing, environment) dimensions of the bureaucracy or organizational culture (technological, economic, political, legal, and social). For Ray, the dialectic of caring and bureaucracy is synthesized into a theory of bureaucratic caring. Bureaucratic caring, the synthetic margin between the human and structural dimensions, is where nurses, patients, and administrators integrate person, nursing, health, and environment.

Theoretical assertions within the Theory of Bureaucratic Caring are as follows:

1. *The meaning of caring is highly differential, depending on its structures* (social-cultural, educational, political, economic, physical, technological, legal). The substantive theory of Differential Caring discovered that caring in nursing is contextual and is influenced by organizational structure or culture. The meaning of *caring* is varied in the emergency department, intensive care unit, oncology unit, and other areas of the hospital. The meaning of caring is influenced further by the role and position that a person holds. For example, patients primarily express the need for human care, while physicians' descriptions are predominantly in the technical sphere. The meaning of caring emerged as differential because no one definition or meaning of caring was identified (Ray, 1989). The theoretical statement that describes the substantive theory of Differential Caring is formulated as:

   > In a hospital, differential caring is a dynamic social process that emerges as a result of the various values, beliefs, and behaviors expressed about the meaning of caring. Differential Caring relates to competing [cooperating] educational, social, humanistic, religious/spiritual, and ethical forces as

> well as political, economic, legal, and technological forces within the organizational culture that are influenced by the social forces within the dominant American [world] culture (Ray, 1989, p. 37).

2. *Caring is bureaucratic, as well as spiritual/ethical,* given the extent to which its meaning can be understood in relation to the organizational structure (Ray, 1989, 2001, 2006). In the theoretical model (see Figure 8-2), everything is infused with spiritual-ethical caring by its integrative and relational connection to the structures of organizational life (e.g., political, educational). Spiritual-ethical caring is both a part and a whole, just as each of the organizational structures is both part and whole. Every part secures its purpose and meaning from the other parts. Understanding spiritual-ethical caring in the bureaucratic organizational system as a complex, holographic formation facilitates improvement in patient outcomes and transformation for human environment well-being (M. Ray, personal communication, April 13, 2008).
3. *Caring is the primordial construct and consciousness of nursing.* Spiritual-ethical caring and the organizational structures in Figure 8-2, when integrated, open, and interactive, are whole and must operate by conscious choice. Nurses' choice making occurs with the interest of humanity at heart, utilizing ethical principles as the compass in deliberations. Ray (2001) states, "Spiritual-ethical caring for nursing does not question whether or not to care in complex systems, but intimates how sincere deliberations and ultimately the facilitation of choices for the good of others can or should be accomplished" (p. 429).

LOGICAL FORM

The formal Theory of Bureaucratic Caring was induced primarily by comparative analysis and insight into the whole of the experience. Review of the literature on nursing, philosophy, social processes, and organizations was combined with the substantive theory titled Differential Caring that Ray discovered through ethnography, phenomenology, and grounded theory research. These ideas were integrated and analyzed through a process that was inductive and logical. It was inductive by building on the data from the substantive theory and the literature. It was logical by drawing upon the philosophical argument of Hegel's dialectic (Moccia, 1986; Ray, 1989) and complexity science to synthesize caring and bureaucracy to a new theoretical formulation (Ray, 2001).

ACCEPTANCE BY THE NURSING COMMUNITY

Practice

The Theory of Bureaucratic Caring has direct application for nursing. In the clinical setting, staff nurses are challenged to integrate knowledge, skills, and caring all at once (Turkel, 2001). This synthesis of behaviors and knowledge reflects the holistic nature of the Theory of Bureaucratic Caring. At the edge of chaos, contemporary issues such as inflation of healthcare costs serve as the catalyst for change within corporate healthcare organizations. The ethical component embedded in spiritual-ethical caring (see Figure 8-2) addresses nurses' moral obligations to others. Ray (2001) emphasizes that "transformation can occur even in the businesslike atmosphere of today if nurses reintroduce the spiritual and ethical dimensions of caring. The deep values that underlie choice to do good for the many will be felt both inside and outside organizations" (p. 429).

Deborah McCray-Stewart, a correction health service administrator at Telfair State Prison in Helena, Georgia, described how nurses in correctional healthcare settings integrate the Theory of Bureaucratic Caring into the framework of their practice (D. McCray-Stewart, personal communication, April 5, 2008). Nurses in corrections have the responsibility of caring for a very complex special population. They must understand this culture, see prisoners as human beings, and have the ability to communicate, educate, and rehabilitate this population in the area of healthcare. Their effectiveness results from incorporating the sociocultural, physical, educational, legal, and ethical dimensions of caring theory into daily practice. In the economic and political areas of the correctional system, nurses struggle with the same issues as nurses in a hospital system, such as decreasing healthcare costs while providing quality care. Economic strategies include conducting health services at the facility level as opposed to transporting patients to a hospital. Radiology, laboratory, and telemedicine are being introduced into the system rapidly, requiring nurses to be cross-trained to work in all areas. Unlike other systems that are driven by managed care, the government must provide a constitution of care for this special population.

Ray has addressed the interface of diverse cultures within the healthcare system. The Transcultural Communicative Caring Tool provides guidelines to help nurses understand the needs, adversity, problems, and questions of people that arise in culturally dynamic healthcare situations (Ray & Turkel, 2000). The dimensions of this tool are as follows:

1. Compassion
2. Advocacy
3. Respect
4. Interaction
5. Negotiation
6. Guidance

Administration

Ray's research has shown that nurses, patients, and administrators value the caring intentionality that is co-created in the nurse-patient or administrator-nurse relationship. By creating ethical caring relationships, administrators and staff can transform the work environment (Ray, Turkel, & Marino, 2002). The Theory of Bureaucratic Caring suggests that organizations fostering ethical choices, respect, and trust will become the successful organizations of the future.

Miller (1995) summarized the work of Ray and other theorists and encouraged nurse executives to examine their daily caring skills and to use these skills in administrative practice. Nyberg studied with Ray and acknowledged the impact of Ray's ideas in her own book, *A Caring Approach in Nursing Administration* (Nyberg, 1998). In her book, Nyberg urged nurse administrators to create a more caring and compassionate system, while still being accountable for organizational management, costs, and economic forces. Turkel and Ray's (2003) study conducted with U.S. Air Force personnel resulted in dissemination of findings and increased awareness of issues between civilian and military policy makers.

Karen O'Brien, Director of Public Health Nursing in Denver, Colorado, described how public health nurse consultants developed an orientation for new nurses by incorporating the core principles of Ray's Theory of Bureaucratic Caring (O'Brien, direct communication, April 12, 2008). The orientation curriculum includes the components of legal, technological, economic, and spiritual/ethical influences on caring for whole populations. Nurses are encouraged to use the political and economic dimensions of the theory to guide their practice. Complex governmental environments offer opportunity for trusted public health nurses to influence policy that affects the health of the public. The Theory of Bureaucratic Caring provides a framework by which a nurse can view the whole population and all its components to understand the ways in which nursing can influence health outcomes.

At the National University of Colombia in Bogota, Colombia, Professor Olga J. Gomez and her nursing students studied Ray's Theory of Bureaucratic Caring, focusing on the hospital nursing administration role (Gomez, personal communication, April 5, 2008). As they studied the paradox between the concepts of human caring and economics, the students developed a framework for phenomenological research. They explored the perceptions of executive nurses about the relationships between human care, economics, and control of health costs. One outcome of the study was recognition of the importance of working together in university and practice settings for empowerment and satisfaction of clients within the managed hospital environment.

Education

The theory is useful in nursing education in terms of its broad focus on caring in nursing and its conceptualization of the healthcare system. The holographic theory combines differentiation of structures within a holistic framework. Discussion of the structures or forces within complex organizations (e.g., legal, economic, social-cultural) provides an overview of factors involved in nursing situations. Infusion of these structures with spiritual-ethical caring emphasizes the moral imperatives and the choice making of nurses.

When developing a new baccalaureate nursing program at Nevada State College, the faculty was particularly drawn to the theory because of its description of the dimensions relevant to nursing within a philosophy of caring. The conceptual framework of the new nursing program combined Ray's Theory of Bureaucratic Caring with theoretical ideas from Watson (1985) and Johns (2000). Figure 8-3 depicts the ways in which nurses and clients interact in the healthcare system and how reflection on practice influences this process.

A description of the conceptual framework, as illustrated in Figure 8-3, is as follows:

> . . . the holographic theory of caring recognizes the interconnectedness of all things, and that everything is a whole in one context and a part of the

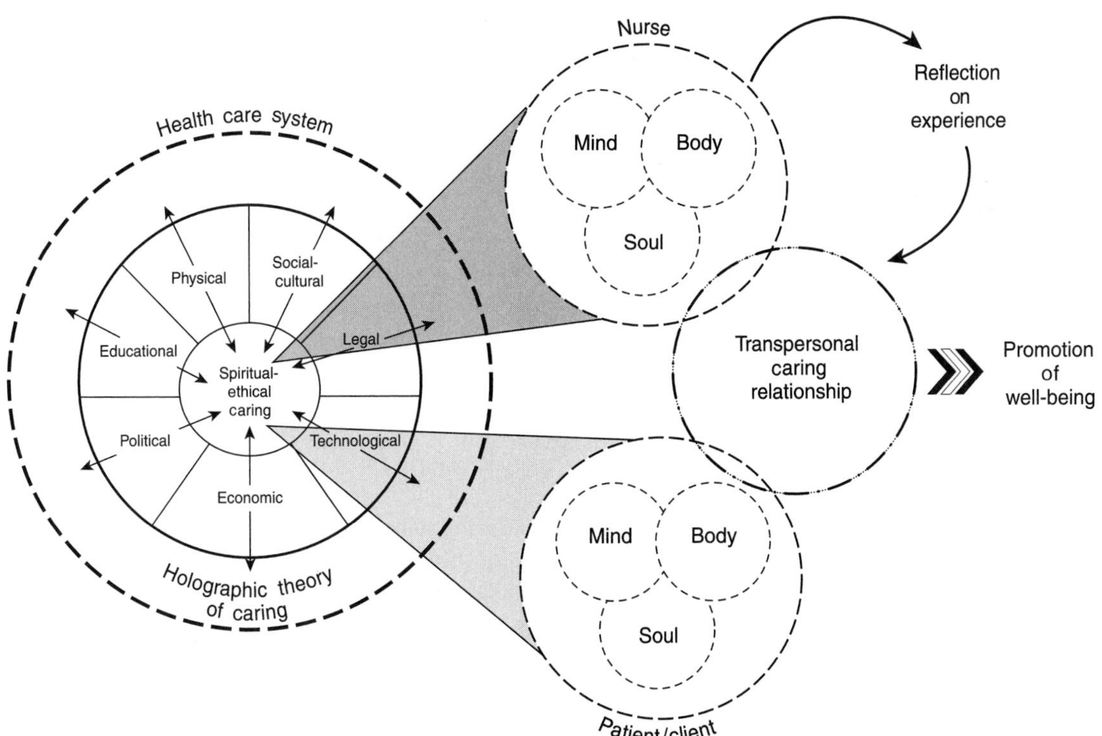

Figure 8-3 Nevada State College Nursing Organizing Framework. (Reprinted with permission of Nevada State College, Department of Nursing, Henderson, NV, 2003. Graphics redrawn from original by J. Castle, Nevada State College, Henderson, NV.)

> whole in another context. Spiritual-ethical caring, the focus for communication, infuses all nursing phenomena, including physical, social-cultural, legal, technological, economic, political, and educational forces. The arrows reflect the dynamic nature of spiritual-ethical caring by the nurse and the forces that influence the changing structure of the health care system. These forces impact both the client/patient and the nurse (Nevada State College, 2003, p. 2).

While in the healthcare system, the client-patient and the nurse come together in a dynamic transpersonal caring relationship (Watson, 1985). This means that the nurse, through communication, views the person as having the capacity to make choices. Through reflection on experience, the nurse assesses which force has the most influence on the nursing situation (Johns, 2000). The nurse draws upon empirical, ethical, and personal knowledge to inform and influence the aesthetic response to the patient. Through the nurse's caring activities within the transpersonal relationship, the goal of nursing can be achieved—the promotion of well-being through caring (Nevada State College, 2003).

The Theory of Bureaucratic Caring is being used to guide curriculum development in the master's program in nursing administration at Florida Atlantic University (Turkel, 2001). Structures from the theory, including ethical, spiritual, economic, technological, legal, political, and social, serve as a framework for exploration of current healthcare issues. Students are challenged to analyze the contemporary economic structure of healthcare from the perspective of caring. Caring within the healthcare delivery system is a key concept in nursing courses.

Research

From her research that resulted in the Theory of Bureaucratic Caring, Ray developed a phenomenological-hermeneutic approach that has continued to guide her studies (Ray, 1985, 1991, 1994b). This research approach is particularly significant because it is grounded in the philosophy of humanism and caring, and encourages nurses to utilize phenomenological hermeneutics through the lens of caring. The evolution of Ray's research methods began with ethnography-ethnonursing, grounded theory, and phenomenology, culminating in Caring Inquiry and Complex Caring Dynamics approaches. These approaches consist of the generation of data by inquiry into the meaning of participants' life-world and relational experiences. Interviews and narrative discourse are the primary methods of data generation in these approaches. In Caring Inquiry, an ontology of caring is a part of the approach, in that Complex Caring Dynamics includes qualitative data generation and analysis, as well as complex quantitative research data collection and analysis techniques. The researcher dwells on the essential meanings of phenomena and through further reflection facilitates the interpretation of interview data, transforming data into interpretative themes and meta-themes. The ultimate goals are to capture the unity of meaning and to synthesize meanings into a theory.

Based on the Theory of Bureaucratic Caring, Ray and Turkel have developed a program of research focusing on nursing in complex organizations. These studies have further explored the meaning of caring and the nature of nursing among hospital nurses, administrators, and clients-patients. A TriService Nursing Research Program grant supported extensive research on nursing as an economic resource. Table 8-1 outlines publications that describe this ongoing program.

FURTHER DEVELOPMENT

Development of the Theory of Bureaucratic Caring is ongoing in Ray's program of research and scholarship. Her work is a synthesis of nursing science, ethics, philosophy, complexity science, economics, and organizational management. In *Nursing Science Quarterly,* Ray described her most recent program of research as sponsored by the TriService Nursing Research program (Turkel & Ray, 2001). It included instrument development and psychometric testing

Table 8-1 Research Publications Related to the Theory of Bureaucratic Caring

Year	Citation	Research Focus and Findings
1981	Ray, M.A. Study of caring within an institutional culture. *Dissertation Abstracts International, 42*(06). (University Microfilms No. 8127787.)	The dissertation analyzed the meaning of caring expressions and behaviors among 192 participants in a hospital culture. The substantive theory of Differential Caring and the formal Theory of Bureaucratic Caring were abstracted.
1984	Ray, M. The development of a classification system of institutional caring. In M. Leininger (Ed.), *Care: The essence of nursing and health.* Thorofare, NJ: Slack.	The discussion examines the construct of caring within the cultural context of the hospital. The classification system included cultural caring symbols of psychological, practical, interactional, and philosophical factors.
1987	Ray, M. Technological caring: A new model in critical care. *Dimensions in Critical Care Nursing, 6*(3), 166-173.	This phenomenological study examined the meaning of caring to critical care unit nurses. The study showed that ethical decisions, moral reasoning, and choice undergo a process of growth and maturation.
1989	Ray, M.A. The theory of bureaucratic caring for nursing practice in the organizational culture. *Nursing Administration Quarterly, 13*(2), 31-42.	Caring within the organizational culture was the focus of the study. It describes the substantive theory of Differential Caring and the formal Theory of Bureaucratic Caring. With caring at the center of the model, the study included ethical, spiritual-religious, economic, technological-physiological, legal, political, and educational-social structures.
1989	Valentine, K. Caring is more than kindness: Modeling its complexities. *Journal of Nursing Administration, 19*(11), 28-34.	Nurses, patients, and corporate health managers provided quantitative and qualitative data to define caring. Data were organized using the categorization schema developed by Ray (1984).
1993	Ray, M.A. A study of care processes using total quality management as a framework in a USAF regional hospital emergency service and related services. *Military Medicine, 158*(6), 396-403.	This descriptive study investigated access to care processes in a military regional hospital emergency service using a total quality management framework. The study lends support to the need for a decentralized, coordinated healthcare system with greater authority and control given to local commands.
1997	Ray, M. The ethical theory of existential authenticity: The lived experience of the art of caring in nursing administration. *Canadian Journal of Nursing Research, 29*(1), 111-126.	Existential authenticity was uncovered as the unity of meaning of caring by nurse administrators. This was described as an ethic of living and caring for the good of nursing staff members and the good of the organization.
1998	Ray, M.A. A phenomenologic study of the interface of caring and technology in intermediate care: Toward a reflexive ethics for clinical practice. *Holistic Nursing Practice, 12*(4), 69-77.	This phenomenological study examined the meaning of caring for technologically dependent patients. Results revealed that vulnerability, suffering, and the ethical situations of moral blurring and moral blindness were the dynamics of caring for these patients.

Continued

Table 8-1 Research Publications Related to the Theory of Bureaucratic Caring—cont'd

Year	Citation	Research Focus and Findings
2000	Turkel, M., & Ray, M. Relational complexity: A theory of the nurse-patient relationship within an economic context. *Nursing Science Quarterly, 13*(4), 307-313.	The formal theory of Relational Complexity illuminated that the caring relationship is complex and dynamic, is both process and outcome, and is a function of both economic and caring variables; that, as a mutual process, is lived all at once as relational and system self-organization.
2001	Ray, M., & Turkel, M. Impact of TRICARE/managed care on total force readiness. *Military Medicine, 166*(4), 281-289.	A phenomenological study was conducted to illuminate the life world descriptions of experiences of USAF active duty and reserve personnel with managed care in the military and civilian healthcare systems. The research illuminated the need for policy change to better meet the healthcare needs of these USAF personnel and their families.
2001	Turkel, M., & Ray, M. Relational complexity: From grounded theory to instrument theoretical testing. *Nursing Science Quarterly, 14*(4), 281-287.	The article describes a series of studies that examined the relationships among caring, economics, cost, quality, and the nurse-patient relationship. The results of theory testing revealed relational caring as a process and the strongest predictor of the outcome:–relational self-organization that is aimed at well-being.
2002	Ray, M., Turkel, M., & Marino, F. The transformative process for nursing in workforce redevelopment. *Nursing Administration Quarterly, 26*(2), 1-14.	Relational self-organization is a shared, creative response to a continuously changing and interconnected work environment. Strategies of respecting, communicating, maintaining visibility, and engaging in participative decision making are the transformative processes leading to growth and transformation.
2003	Turkel, M. A journey into caring as experienced by nurse managers. *International Journal for Human Caring, 7*(1), 20-26.	The purpose of this phenomenological study was to capture the meaning of caring as experienced by nurse managers. Essential themes that emerged were growth, listening, support, intuition, receiving gifts, and frustration.
2003	Turkel, M., & Ray, M. A process model for policy analysis within the context of political caring. *International Journal for Human Caring, 7*(3), 17-25.	This phenomenological study illuminated the experiences of USAF personnel with managed care in the military and civilian healthcare systems. A model outlining the process of policy analysis was generated.

USAF, U.S. Air Force.

of the original Nurse-Patient Relationship Resource Analysis Tool, now referred to as the Relational Caring Questionnaire (Professional Form) and the Relational Caring Questionnaire (Patient Form). These tools are Likert-type questionnaires for healthcare professionals (nurses and non-nurses and nurse-administrators) and patients. They measure the nurse-patient relationship as an administrative and interpersonal resource. The Professional and Patient Relational Caring Questionnaires are to be included in Watson's forthcoming 2nd edition on the assessment and measurement of caring (Watson, 2009). These tools will help researchers link the non-economic (interpersonal) resources of caring with the administrative system resources (including economic/budgetary procedures). The tools are being translated into Swedish and are being tested. This interdisciplinary research is at the cutting edge in nursing and will lead to enhanced understanding of the concepts and relationships outlined in the Theory of Bureaucratic Caring.

CRITIQUE

Clarity

The major structures, spiritual-religious, ethical, technological-physiological, social, legal, economic, political, and educational, are defined clearly in Ray's 1989 publication. These definitions are consistent with definitions commonly used by practicing nurses. They have semantic consistency in that concepts are used in ways consistent with their definitions (Chinn & Kramer, 2004). Most terms did not change from the 1989 article to the 2001 publication; however, some concepts combined or separated as Ray's development of the theory evolved. Therefore, for this chapter, currently used terms were clarified with the theorist. Furthermore, the formal definitions of the terms *spiritual-ethical caring, social-cultural, physical,* and *technological,* as they relate to the theory, are published for the first time in this chapter.

The diagram presented in Figure 8-2 enhances clarity. The interrelationship of spiritual-ethical caring with the other structures and the openness of the system are depicted by the organization of concepts and the dynamic arrows. Ray's description (2001, pp. 428-429) of the theory assists the reader in imaging the theory relationships as holographic.

Simplicity

Ray's theory simplifies the dynamics of complex bureaucratic organizations. From numerous descriptions of the inductive grounded theory study, Ray derived the integrative concept of spiritual-ethical caring and the seven interrelated concepts of physical, social-cultural, legal, technological, economic, political, and educational structures. Given the complexity of bureaucratic organizations, the number of concepts is minimal.

Generality

The Theory of Bureaucratic Caring is a philosophy that addresses the nature of nursing as caring. Alligood (2006) notes, "Philosophies set forth the meaning of nursing and nursing phenomena through reasoning and logical presentation of ideas" (p. 46). Ray's theory addresses questions such as, What is the nature of caring in nursing? And, What is the nature of nursing practice as caring? Philosophies are broad and propose general ideas about how the profession of nursing fulfills "its moral obligation to society" (Alligood, p. 45). The Theory of Bureaucratic Caring proposes that nurses are choice makers guided by spiritual-ethical caring, in relation to legal, economic, technological, and other structures.

The Theory of Bureaucratic Caring provides a unique view of healthcare organizations and of how nursing phenomena interrelate as wholes and parts of the system. Concepts were derived logically from inductive research. Ray's analysis incorporated ideas from complexity science. The conceptualization of the healthcare system as holographic emphasizes the holistic nature of concepts and relationships. As nurses in all areas of practice study these new conceptualizations, they may be led to question the cause and effect stance of older linear ideas. Therefore, the Theory of Bureaucratic Caring has the potential to change the paradigm or way of thinking of practicing nurses.

Empirical Precision

Because the Theory of Bureaucratic Caring is generated using grounded theory and has undergone continued revisions based largely on research, empirical precision is high with concepts grounded in observable reality. The theory corresponds directly to the research data that are summarized in published reports (Ray, 1981a, 1981b, 1984, 1987, 1989, 1997b, 1998).

Ray, Turkel, and colleagues use this theory in a program of research into the nurse-patient relationship as an economic resource (Ray, 1998; Ray, et al., 2002; Turkel, 2003; Turkel & Ray, 2000, 2001, 2003). These studies provide guidance for nursing practice and enhance nurses' understanding of the dynamics of healthcare organizations. Ray (2001) proposes that bureaucratic caring theory culminates "in a vision for understanding the deeper reality of nursing life" (p. 426).

Derivable Consequences

The issues that confront nurses today include economic constraints in the managed care environment and the effects of these constraints (e.g., staffing ratios) on the nurse-patient relationship. These are the very issues that the Theory of Bureaucratic Caring addresses. Nurses in administrative, research, and clinical roles can use the political and economic dimensions of the theory as a framework to inform their practice. This theory is relevant to the contemporary work world of nurses.

Ray and Turkel have generated middle range theories through their program of research based on the Theory of Bureaucratic Caring. The Theory of Existential Authenticity was uncovered by Ray (1997b) as the unity of meaning for nurse-administrator caring art, and more recently was adapted by Sorbello (2008). Nurse administrators described an ethic of living caring for the good of their staff nurses and for the good of the organization. Relational (Caring) Complexity focuses on the nurse-patient relationship within an economic context (Turkel & Ray, 2000, 2001). Study data show that relational caring between administrators, nurses, and patients are the strongest predictor of relational self-organization aimed at well-being. Relational self-organization is a shared, creative response that involves growth and transformation (Ray, et al., 2002). Transformative processes that can lead to relational self-organization include respecting, communicating, maintaining visibility, and engaging in participative decision making in the workplace. Finally, Ray's work emphasizes the need for reflexive ethics for clinical practice, to enhance understanding of how deep values and moral interactions shape ethical decisions (Ray, 1998).

SUMMARY

The Theory of Bureaucratic Caring challenges participants in nursing to think beyond their usual frame of reference and envision the world more holistically, while considering the universe as a hologram. Appreciation of the interrelatedness of persons, environments, and events is key to an understanding of this theory. The theory provides a unique view of how healthcare organizations and nursing phenomena interrelate as wholes and parts in the system. Unique constructs within Ray's theory include technological and economic caring.

The theory was derived inductively and was synthesized through further reflection and analysis. Ray acknowledges the influences of the philosophy of Hegel, chaos theory, complexity science, and the holographic worldview. Theory development by Ray's colleagues and other scholars continues. Ray challenges nurses to envision the spiritual and ethical dimensions of caring, so insights from the Theory of Bureaucratic Caring may inform nurses to use their creativity and imagination to transform the work world.

Case Study

Mrs. Smith was a 73-year-old widow who lived alone with no significant social support. She had been suffering from emphysema for several years and had had frequent hospitalizations for respiratory problems. On the last hospital admission, her pneumonia quickly progressed to organ failure. Death appeared to be imminent, as she went in and out of consciousness, alone in her hospital room. The medical-surgical nursing staff and the Nursing Director focused on making her end-of-life period as comfortable as possible. Based on discussions with unit staff, the Nursing Director reorganized patient assignments. Over the next few hours, a staff member who had volunteered her assistance provided personal care for Mrs. Smith. With help from her team, the nurse turned, bathed, and suctioned

Mrs. Smith. She quietly sang hymns in her room, creating a peaceful environment that expressed caring for her and calmed the nursing unit staff. Mrs. Smith died with caring persons at her bedside, and the unit staff felt comforted that she had not died alone.

1. What caring behaviors prompted the nursing staff to approach the Nursing Director for help with this situation?
2. What issues (ethical, spiritual, legal, social-cultural, economic) from the structure of the Theory of Bureaucratic Caring influenced this situation?
3. How did the Nursing Director balance these issues? What considerations went into her decision making?
4. What interrelationships are evident between persons in this environment, that is, how were staff, patient, and administrators connected in this situation?

CRITICAL THINKING *Activities*

1. Read the book, *The Spirit Catches You and You Fall Down* by Anne Fadiman (1998). This is the story of a 3-month-old infant diagnosed with epilepsy and the cultural differences experienced by her Laotian refugee parents and American healthcare personnel. Although social-cultural forces were predominant in this situation, what other structures or forces were important in this story (see Figure 8-2)? What were the meanings of this child's seizure disorder to the family and to the professional staff? Using insights gained from the Theory of Bureaucratic Caring, describe alternative approaches to transcultural care in this situation.
2. Think back on a problem that you encountered in a clinical practice situation. What structures (social-cultural, legal, political, physical, educational, economic, technological) within the healthcare system were involved? How were these structures or issues interrelated? Would envisioning these structures holographically (each as a whole and as a part of a whole) change your perception of the situation and your nursing approaches?
3. How does the Theory of Bureaucratic Caring enlarge your views about a complex organization where you work? Describe how staff members' interactions with each other reflect caring. Is caring different for staff in different clinical roles and work areas? What decisions and choices reflecting spiritual-ethical caring occur regularly in each setting?

POINTS FOR *Further Study*

- Ray, M. (in press). *Transcultural caring dynamics in nursing and health care.* Philadelphia: F.A. Davis.
- International Association for Human Caring, at: www.humancaring.org
- New England Complex Systems Institute, Cambridge, MA, at: www.necsi.org
- Florida Atlantic University, Christine E. Lynn College of Nursing, Boca Raton, FL, at: www.fau.edu
- Santa Fe Institute, Santa Fe, NM, at: www.santafe.edu
- Plexus Institute, Allentown, NJ, at: www.plexusinstitute.org

REFERENCES

Alligood, M. R. (2006). Philosophies, models, and theories: Critical thinking structures. In M. R. Alligood & A. M. Tomey (Eds.), *Nursing theory: Utilization & application* (3rd ed., pp. 43-65). St. Louis: Mosby.

Briggs, J., & Peat, F. D. (1984). *Looking glass universe: The emerging science of wholeness.* New York: Simon & Schuster.

Briggs, J., & Peat, F. D. (1999). *Seven life lessons of chaos: Spiritual wisdom from the science of change.* New York: Harper Collins.

Chinn, P. L., & Kramer, M. K. (2004). *Integrated knowledge development in nursing.* St. Louis: Mosby.

Coffman, S., & Ray, M. A. (1999). Mutual intentionality: A theory of support processes in pregnant African American women. *Qualitative Health Research, 9*(4), 479-492.

Coffman, S., & Ray, M. A. (2002). African American women describe support processes during high-risk pregnancy and postpartum. *Journal of Obstetric, Gynecologic, and Neonatal Nursing, 31*(5), 536-544.

Davidson, A., & Ray, M. (1991). Studying the human-environment phenomenon using the science of complexity. *ANS Advances in Nursing Science, 14*(2):73-87.

Fadiman, A. (1998). *The spirit catches you and you fall down.* New York: Farrar, Straus, & Giroux.

Helman, C. (1997). *Culture, health and illness* (3rd ed.). Oxford, UK: Butterworth-Heinemann.

Johns, C. (2000). *Becoming a reflective practitioner.* Oxford, UK: Blackwell Science.

Louis, M. (1985). An investigator's guide to workplace culture. In P. Frost, L. Moore, M. Louis, L. C. Lundberg, & J. Martin (Eds.), *Organizational culture* (pp. 73-93). Beverly Hills, CA: Sage.

Miller, K. (1995). Keeping the care in nursing care: Our biggest challenge. *Journal of Nursing Administration, 25*(11), 29-32.

Moccia, P. (1986). *New approaches to theory development* (Pub. No. 15-1992). New York: National League for Nursing.

Nevada State College. (2003, August 19). *Nursing organizing framework.* Henderson, NV: Author.

Nyberg, J. J. (1998). *A caring approach in nursing administration.* Niwot, CO: University Press of Colorado.

Ray, M. (1981a). A study of caring within an institutional culture. *Dissertation Abstracts International, 42*(06). (University Microfilms No. 8127787.)

Ray, M. (1981b). A philosophical analysis of caring within nursing. In M. Leininger (Ed.), *Caring: An essential human need* (pp. 25-360). Thorofare, NJ: Slack.

Ray, M. (1984). The development of a classification system of institutional caring. In M. Leininger (Ed.), *Care: The essence of nursing and health* (pp. 95-112). Thorofare, NJ: Slack.

Ray, M. (1987). Technological caring: A new model in critical care. *Dimensions in Critical Care Nursing, 6*(3), 166-173.

Ray, M. (1989). The Theory of Bureaucratic Caring for nursing practice in the organizational culture. *Nursing Administration Quarterly, 13*(2), 31-42.

Ray, M. (in press). *Transcultural caring dynamics in nursing and health care.* Philadelphia: F. A. Davis.

Ray, M. A. (1985). A philosophical method to study nursing phenomena. In M. Leininger (Ed.), *Qualitative research methods in nursing* (pp. 81-92). New York: Grune & Stratton.

Ray, M. A. (1991). Caring inquiry: The esthetic process in the way of compassion. In D. Gaut & M. Leininger (Eds.), *Caring: The compassionate healer* (pp. 181-189). New York: National League for Nursing Press.

Ray, M. A. (1994a). Complex caring dynamics: A unifying model for nursing inquiry. *Theoretic and Applied Chaos in Nursing, 1*(1), 23-32. (Journal renamed *Complexity and Chaos in Nursing.*)

Ray, M. A. (1994b). The richness of phenomenology: Philosophic, theoretic, and methodologic concerns. In J. Morse (Ed.), *Critical issues in qualitative research methods* (pp. 116-135). Newbury Park, CA: Sage.

Ray, M. A. (1997a). Consciousness and the moral ideal: A transcultural analysis of Watson's theory of transpersonal caring. *Advanced Practice Nursing Quarterly, 3*(1):25-31.

Ray, M. A. (1997b). The ethical theory of existential authenticity: The lived experience of the art of caring in nursing administration. *Canadian Journal of Nursing Research, 29*(1), 111-126.

Ray, M. A. (1998). A phenomenologic study of the interface of caring and technology: A new reflexive ethics in intermediate care. *Holistic Nursing Practice, 12*(4), 71-79.

Ray, M. A. (2000). Transcultural assessment of older adults. In S. Garratt & S. Koch (Eds.), *Assessing older people: A practical guide for health professionals.* Sydney, Australia: MacLennan & Petty.

Ray, M. A. (2001). The Theory of Bureaucratic Caring. In M. Parker (Ed.), *Nursing theories and nursing practice* (pp. 422-431). Philadelphia: F. A. Davis.

Ray, M. A. (2006). The Theory of Bureaucratic Caring. In M. Parker (Ed.), *Nursing theories and nursing practice* (2nd ed., pp. 360-368). Philadelphia: F. A. Davis.

Ray, M. A., & Turkel, M. C. (2000). Culturally based caring. In L. Dunphy & J. Winland-Brown (Eds.), *Advanced practice nursing: A holistic approach* (pp. 43-55). Philadelphia: F. A. Davis.

Ray, M., Turkel, M., & Marino, F. (2002). The transformative process for nursing in workforce redevelopment. *Nursing Administration Quarterly, 26*(2), 1-14.

Smircich, L. (1985). Is the concept of culture a paradigm for understanding organizations and ourselves? In P. Frost, L. Moore, M. Louis, L. C. Lundberg, & J. Martin (Eds.), *Organizational culture* (pp. 55-72). Beverly Hills, CA: Sage.

Sorbello, B. (2008). The nurse administrator as caring person: A synoptic analysis applying caring philosophy, Ray's ethical theory of existential authenticity, the ethic of justice, and the ethic of care. *International Journal for Human Caring 12*(1), 44-49.

Strauss, A., & Corbin, J. (1990). *Basics of qualitative research: Grounded theory procedures and techniques.* Newbury Park, CA: Sage.

Talbot, M. (1991). *The holographic universe.* New York: Harper Collins.

Turkel, M. (2001). Applicability of bureaucratic caring theory to contemporary nursing practice: The political and economic dimensions. In M. Parker (Ed.), *Nursing theories and nursing practice* (pp. 433-444). Philadelphia: F. A. Davis.

Turkel, M. (2003). A journey into caring as experienced by nurse managers. *International Journal for Human Caring, 7*(1), 20-26.

Turkel, M., & Ray, M. (2000). Relational complexity: A theory of the nurse-patient relationship within an economic context. *Nursing Science Quarterly, 13*(4), 307-313.

Turkel, M., & Ray, M. (2001). Relational complexity: From grounded theory to instrument development and theoretical testing. *Nursing Science Quarterly, 14*(4), 281-287.

Turkel, M., & Ray, M. (2003). A process model for policy analysis within the context of political caring. *International Journal for Human Caring, 7*(3), 17-25.

Vicenzi, A. E., White, K. R., & Begun, J. W. (1997). Chaos in nursing: Make it work for you. *American Journal of Nursing, 97*(10), 26-31.

Watson, J. (1985). *Nursing: Human science and human care.* Norwalk, CT: Appleton-Century-Crofts.

Watson, J. (2008). Assessing and measuring caring in nursing and health science (2nd ed.). New York: Springer Publishing Co.

Wheatley, M. J. (1999). *Leadership and the new science: Discovering order in a chaotic world.* San Francisco: Berrett-Koehler.

BIBLIOGRAPHY

Primary Sources

Books

Davidson, A., & Ray, M. (In process). Complexity for human-environment well being. New York: Springer Publishing Co.

Ray, M. (in press). *Transcultural caring dynamics in nursing and health care.* Philadelphia: F. A. Davis.

Watson, J., & Ray, M. (Eds.). (1988). *The ethics of care and the ethics of cure: Synthesis in chronicity.* New York: National League for Nursing. (Released, 1989. translated into Swedish.)

Book Chapters

Ray, M. A. (1981). A philosophical analysis of caring within nursing. In M. Leininger (Ed.), *Caring: An essential human need* (pp. 25-36). Thorofare, NJ: Charles B. Slack.

Ray, M. A. (1984). The development of a nursing classification system of institutional caring. In M. Leininger (Ed.), *Care: The essence of nursing and health* (pp. 95-112). Thorofare, NJ: Charles B. Slack.

Ray, M. A. (1985). A philosophical method to study nursing phenomena. In M. Leininger (Ed.), *Qualitative research methods in nursing* (pp. 81-92). New York: Grune & Stratton.

Ray, M. A. (1990). Phenomenological method in nursing research. In N. Chaska (Ed.), *The nursing profession: Turning points* (pp. 173-179). New York: McGraw-Hill.

Ray, M. A. (1991). Caring inquiry: The esthetic process in the way of compassion. In D. Gaut & M. Leininger (Eds.), *Caring: The compassionate healer* (pp. 181-189). New York: National League for Nursing Press.

Ray, M. A. (1992). Phenomenological method for nursing research. In J. Poindexter (Ed.), *Nursing theory. Research & Practice Summer Research Conference monograph* (pp. 163-174). Detroit: Wayne State University.

Ray, M. A. (1994). Environmental encountering through interiority. In E. Schuster & C. Brown (Eds.), *Exploring our environmental connections* (pp. 113-118). New York: National League for Nursing Press.

Ray, M. A. (1994). The quality of authentic presence: Transcultural caring inquiry in primary care. In J. Wang & P. Simoni (Eds.), *Proceedings of First International and Interdisciplinary Health Research Symposium* (pp. 69-72). At Peking Union Medical College Hospital, Beijing, China, and Zhejiang Medical University, Hangzhou, China (Chinese translation). Morgantown, WV: West Virginia University.

Ray, M. A. (1994). The richness of phenomenology: Philosophic, theoretic, and methodologic concerns. In J. Morse (Ed.), *Critical issues in qualitative research methods* (pp. 116-135). Newbury Park, CA: Sage. (Translated into Spanish, 2004.)

Ray, M. A. (1995). Transcultural health care ethics: Pathways to progress. In J. Wang (Ed.), *Health care and culture* (pp. 3-9). Morgantown, WV: West Virginia University.

Ray, M. A. (1997). Illuminating the meaning of caring: Unfolding the sacred art of divine love. In M. S. Roach (Ed.), *Caring from the heart: The convergence between caring and spirituality* (pp. 163-178). New York: Paulist Press.

Ray, M. A. (1999). Caring foundations of deacony. In T. Ryokas & K. Keissling (Eds.), *Spiritus-Lux-Caritas* (pp. 225-236). Lahti, Finland: Deaconal Institution of Lahti. (Translated into German, 1999, University of Heidelberg, Germany.)

Ray, M. A. (1999). Critical theory as a framework to enhance nursing science. In E. Polifroni & M. Welch (Eds.), *Perspectives on philosophy of science in nursing* (pp. 382-386). Philadelphia: Lippincott.

Ray, M. A. (2000). Transcultural assessment of older adults. In S. Koch & S. Garratt (Eds.), *Assessing older people: A practical guide for health professionals.* Sydney, Australia: MacLennan & Petty.

Ray, M. A. (2001). Complex culture and technology: Toward a global caring communitarian ethics of nursing. In R. Locsin (Ed.), *Concerning technology and caring* (pp. 41-52). Westport, CT: Greenwood Publishing Group.

Ray, M. A. (2001). The Theory of Bureaucratic Caring. In M. Parker (Ed.), *Nursing theories and nursing practice* (pp. 422-431). Philadelphia: F. A. Davis.

Ray, M. A. (2006). The Theory of Bureaucratic Caring. In M. Parker (Ed.), *Nursing theories and nursing practice* (2nd ed., pp. 360-368). Philadelphia: F. A. Davis.

Ray, M. (2007). Technological caring as a dynamic of complexity in nursing practice. In A. Barnard & R. Locsin (Eds.). *Perspectives on technology and nursing practice.* United Kingdom: Palgrave.

Ray, M. A., & Turkel, M. C. (2000). Culturally based caring. In L. Dunphy & J. Winland-Brown (Eds.), *Advanced practice nursing: A holistic approach* (pp. 43-55). Philadelphia: F. A. Davis.

Journal Articles

Coffman, S., & Ray, M. A. (1999). Mutual intentionality: A theory of support processes in pregnant African American women. *Qualitative Health Research, 9*(4), 479-492.

Coffman, S., & Ray, M. A. (2002). African American women describe support processes during high-risk pregnancy and postpartum. *Journal of Obstetric, Gynecologic, and Neonatal Nursing, 31*(5), 536-544.

Davidson, A., & Ray, M. (1991). Studying the human-environment relationship using the science of complexity. *ANS Advances in Nursing Science, 14*(2), 73-87.

Ray, M. (1999). Transcultural caring in primary care. *National Academies of Practice Forum, 1*(1), 177-182.

Ray, M. A. (1987). Technological caring: A new model in critical care. *Dimensions of Critical Care Nursing, 2*(3), 166-173.

Ray, M. A. (1989). A theory of bureaucratic caring for nursing practice in the organizational culture. *Nursing Administration Quarterly, 13*(2), 31-42. (Also translated and published in Japanese.)

Ray, M. A. (1992). Critical theory as a framework to enhance nursing science. *Nursing Science Quarterly, 5*(3), 98-101.

Ray, M. A. (1993). A study of care processes using Total Quality Management as a framework in a USAF regional hospital emergency service and related services. *Military Medicine, 158*(6), 396-403.

Ray, M. A. (1993). A theory of bureaucratic caring for nursing practice in the organizational culture. *The Japanese Journal of Nursing Research, 1*, 14-24.

Ray, M. A. (1994). Communal moral experience as the research starting point for health care ethics. *Nursing Outlook, 42*(3), 104-109.

Ray, M. A. (1994). Complex caring dynamics: A unifying model for nursing inquiry. *Theoretic and Applied Chaos in Nursing, 1*(1), 23-32. (Journal renamed *Complexity and Chaos in Nursing.*)

Ray, M. A. (1994). Interpretive analysis of Olson's book, *The Life of Illness: One Woman's Journey. Qualitative Health Research, 2*(2), 250-253.

Ray, M. A. (1994). Transcultural nursing ethics: A framework and model for transcultural ethical analysis. *Journal of Holistic Nursing, 12*(3), 251-264.

Ray, M. A. (1997). Consciousness and the moral ideal: Transcultural analysis of Watson's Transpersonal Caring Theory. *Advanced Nursing Practice Journal, 3*(1), 25-31.

Ray, M. A. (1997). The ethical theory of Existential Authenticity: The lived experience of the art of caring in nursing administration. *Canadian Journal of Nursing Research, 22*(1), 111-126. (Abstract also published in French.)

Ray, M. A. (1998). Complexity and nursing science. *Nursing Science Quarterly, 11*(3), 91-93.

Ray, M. A. (1998). The interface of caring and technology: A new reflexive ethics in intermediate care. *Holistic Nursing Practice, 12*(4), 71-79.

Ray, M. A. (1999). The future of caring in the challenging health care environment. *International Journal for Human Caring, 3*(1), 7-11.

Ray, M. A., Didominic, V. A., Dittman, P. W., Hurst, P. A., Seaver, J. B., Sorbello, B. C., et al. (1995). The edge of chaos: Caring and the bottom line. *Nursing Management, 9*, 48-50.

Ray, M., & Turkel, M. (2001). Impact of TRICARE/managed care on total force readiness. *Military Medicine, 166*(4), 281-289.

Ray, M., Turkel, M., & Marino, F. (2002). The transformative process for nursing in workforce redevelopment. *Nursing Administration Quarterly, 26*(2), 1-14.

Turkel, M., & Ray, M. (2000). Relational complexity: A theory of the nurse-patient relationship within an economic context. *Nursing Science Quarterly, 13*(4), 307-313.

Turkel, M., & Ray, M. (2001). Relational complexity: From grounded theory to instrument development and theoretical testing. *Nursing Science Quarterly, 14*(4), 281-287.

Turkel, M., & Ray, M. (2003). A process model for policy analysis within the context of political caring. *International Journal for Human Caring, 7*(3), 17-25.

Turkel, M., & Ray, M. (2004). Creating a caring practice environment through self-renewal. *Nursing Administration Quarterly, 28*(4), 249-254.

Turkel, M., & Ray, M. A. (2005). Models of caring practice. [Editorial.] *International Journal for Human Caring, 9*(3), 7-8.

Dissertation

Ray, M. (1981a). A study of caring within an institutional culture. *Dissertation Abstracts International, 42*(06). (University Microfilm No. 8127787.)

Secondary Sources

Books

Johns, C. (2000). *Becoming a reflective practitioner.* Oxford, England: Blackwell Science.

Nyberg, J. J. (1998). *A caring approach in nursing administration.* Niwot, CO: University Press of Colorado.

Book Chapters

Coffman, S. (2007). Caring, the essence of nursing. In A. Berman, S. Snyder, B. Kozier, & G. Erb (Eds.), *Fundamentals of nursing: Concepts, process, and practice* (8th ed., pp. 444-458). Upper Saddle River, NJ: Prentice Hall.

Tappen, R., Turkel, M., & Hall, R. (1997). Nursing in transition: A response to the changing health care system. In A. Moorehead & P. Huber (Eds.), *Nursing roles: Evolving or recycled?* Thousand Oaks, CA: Sage.

Turkel, M. (2000). Directing and organizing patient care. In M. Tappen (Ed.), *Leadership and management* (4th ed.). Philadelphia: F. A. Davis.

Turkel, M. (2001). Challenging contemporary practices in critical care settings. In N. Locsin (Ed.), *Advancing technology, caring and nursing.* Westport, CT: Auburn House.

Turkel, M. (2006). Applications of Marilyn Ray's Theory of Bureaucratic Caring. In M. Parker (Ed.), *Nursing theories and nursing practice* (2nd ed., pp. 369-379). Philadelphia: F. A. Davis.

Journal Articles

Barry, C. D. (2001). Creating a quilt: An aesthetic expression of caring for nursing students. *International Journal for Human Caring, 6*(1), 25-29.

Cody, W. K. (1998). Critical theory and nursing science: Freedom in theory and practice. *Nursing Science Quarterly, 11*(2), 44-46.

Davidhizar, R. (2002). Management toolbox: Strategies for effective confrontation. *Radiologic Technology, 73*(5), 476-478.

Davis, R. (1997). Community caring: An ethnographic study within an organizational culture. *Public Health Nursing, 14*(2), 92-100.

Davis, R. (2000). Holographic community: Reconceptualizing the meaning of community in an era of health care reform. *Nursing Outlook, 48*(6), 294-301.

DeMarco, R. F. (1998). Caring to confront in the workplace: An ethical perspective for nurses. *Nursing Outlook, 46*(3), 130-135.

Fulbrook, P. (1999). On the receiving end: Experiences of being a relative in critical care. Part 2. *Nursing in Critical Care, 4*(4), 179-185.

Gaydos, H. L. (2001). On calling and character: Caring as archetypal act. *International Journal for Human Caring, 5*(1), 8-13.

Goldberg, B. (1998). Connection: An exploration of spirituality in nursing care. *Journal of Advanced Nursing, 27*(4), 836-842.

Huffman, C. (1997). The nurse-technology relationship: The case of ultrasonography. *Journal of Obstetric, Gynecologic and Neonatal Nursing, 26*(6), 673-682.

Jakobsson, L. (1997). Met and unmet nursing care needs in men with prostate cancer: An explorative study. Part II. *European Journal of Cancer Care, 6*(2), 117-123.

Jones, J. (1997). Your experiences: The guiding light of a good yarn: How stories from the past provide a link to the future of emergency nursing practice. *Australian Emergency Nursing Journal, 1*(2), 42-46.

Käppeli, S. (2001). Compassion—A forgotten tradition of nursing? *Pflege, 14*(5), 293-306.

King, S. J. (2000). Caring for adolescent females with anorexia nervosa: Registered nurses' perspective. *Journal of Advanced Nursing, 32*(1), 139-147.

Pelletier, D. (2000). Australian clinicians and educators identify gaps in specialist cardiac nursing practice. *Australian Journal of Advanced Nursing, 17*(3), 24-30.

Schoenhofer, S. O. (1998). Giving of oneself on another's behalf: The phenomenology of everyday caring. *International Journal for Human Caring, 2*(2), 23-29.

Turkel, M. (2001). Struggling to find a balance: The paradox between caring and economics. *Nursing Administration Quarterly, 26*(1), 67-82.

Turkel, M. (2003). A journey into caring as experienced by nurse managers. *International Journal for Human Caring, 7*(1), 20-26.

Turkel, M. (2007). Dr. Marilyn Ray's Theory of Bureaucratic Caring. *International Journal for Human Caring, 11*(4), 57-70.

Turkel, M., Tappen, R., & Hall, R. (1999). Moments of excellence. *Journal of Gerontological Nursing, 25*(1), 7-12.

Turkel, M. C. (2000). Relational complexity: A theory of the nurse-patient relationship within an economic context. *Nursing Science Quarterly, 13*(4), 307-313.

Turkel, M. J. (1999). Moments of excellence: Nurses' response to role redesign in long-term care. *Journal of Gerontological Nursing, 25*(1), 7-12.

Valentine, K. (1989). Caring is more than kindness: Modeling its complexities. *Journal of Nursing Administration, 19*(11), 28-34.

Walsh, M. (2000). Chaos, complexity and nursing. *Nursing Standard, 14*(32), 39-42.

Wuest, J. (1997). Fraying connections of caring women: An exemplar of including difference in the development of explanatory frameworks. *Canadian Journal of Nursing Research, 29*(2), 99-116.

Wuest, J. (2001). Precarious ordering: Toward a formal theory of women's caring. *Journal of Health Care for Women International, 22*(1/2), 167-193.

Theses and Dissertations

Czerenda, A. J. (2006). "The show must go on": A caring inquiry into the meaning of widowhood and health for older Indian widows. D.N.S. dissertation, Florida Atlantic University, United States—Florida. Retrieved April 4, 2008, from ProQuest Digital Dissertations database. (Publication No. AAT 3222085.)

Hilsenbeck, J. R. (2006). Unveiling the mystery of covenantal trust: The theory of the social process between the nurse manager and the chief nursing officer. D.N.S. dissertation, Florida Atlantic University, United States—Florida. Retrieved April 4, 2008, from ProQuest Digital Dissertations database. (Publication No. AAT 3244888.)

Quinn, C. M. (2000). The lived experience of caring and the nurse executive: A phenomenological study. *Dissertation Abstracts International, 38*(04). (University Microfilms No. 1398084.)

Swinderman, T. D. (1997). Caring in nurse managers as described by staff nurses. *Dissertation Abstracts International, 35*(06). (University Microfilms No. 1385321.)

Swinderman, T. D. (2005). The magnetic appeal of nurse informaticians: Caring attractor for emergence. D.N.S. dissertation, Florida Atlantic University, United States—Florida. Retrieved April 4, 2008, from ProQuest Digital Dissertations database. (Publication No. AAT 3162666.)

Turkel, M. J. (1997). Struggling to find a balance: A grounded theory study of the nurse-patient relationship within an economic context. *Dissertation Abstracts International, 58*(08). (University Microfilms No. 9805958.)

Wright, C. A. (2001). Public health nurse managers' perception of Total Quality Management initiatives. *Dissertation Abstracts International, 39*(02). (University Microfilms No. 1401204.)

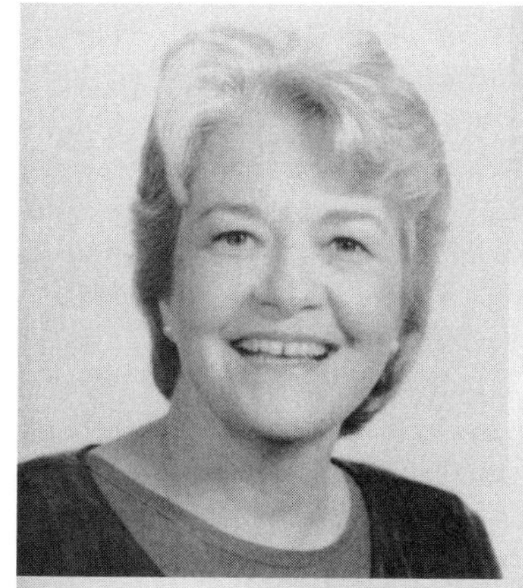

CHAPTER

9

Patricia Benner

Caring, Clinical Wisdom, and Ethics in Nursing Practice

Karen A. Brykczynski

"The nurse-patient relationship is not a uniform, professionalized blueprint but rather a kaleidoscope of intimacy and distance in some of the most dramatic, poignant, and mundane moments of life" (Benner, 1984a).

CREDENTIALS AND BACKGROUND OF THE PHILOSOPHER

Patricia Benner was born in Hampton, Virginia, and spent her childhood in California, where she received her early and professional education. Majoring in nursing, she obtained a baccalaureate of arts degree from Pasadena College in 1964. In 1970, she earned a master's degree in nursing, with major emphasis in medical-surgical nursing, from the University of California, San Francisco (UCSF), School of Nursing. Her PhD in stress, coping, and health was conferred in 1982 at University of California, Berkeley, and her dissertation was published in 1984 (Benner, 1984b). Benner has a wide range of clinical experience, including acute medical-surgical, critical care, and home health care. She has held staff and head nurse positions.

Benner has a rich background in research and began this part of her career in 1970 as a postgraduate nurse researcher in the School of Nursing at UCSF. Upon completion of her doctorate in 1982, Benner achieved the position of associate professor in the Department of Physiological Nursing at UCSF and became a tenured professor in 1989. In 2002, she moved to the Department of Social and Behavioral Sciences at UCSF, where she was professor and first occupant of the Thelma Shobe Cook Endowed Chair

Previous authors: Jullette C. Mitre, Sr., Judith E. Alexander, and Susan L. Keller. The author wishes to express appreciation to Patricia Benner for critiquing this chapter.

in Ethics and Spirituality. She taught at the doctoral and master's levels and served on three to four dissertation committees per year. She retired from full-time teaching in 2008 but continues to be involved in presentations and consultation, as well as writing and research projects.

Benner acknowledges that her thinking in nursing has been influenced greatly by Virginia Henderson. Henderson (1989) commented that Benner's *From Novice to Expert: Excellence and Power in Clinical Nursing Practice* (1984a) had the potential to materially affect the practice and preparation of nurses for practice. The Institute for Nursing Healthcare Leadership commemorated the impact of this landmark book on nursing practice with a celebration 20 years after its publication, at the conference "Charting the Course: The Power of Expert Nurses to Define the Future," which was held in Boston in September of 2003. In the Foreword to Benner's work, *The Primacy of Caring: Stress and Coping in Health and Illness* (Benner & Wrubel, 1989), Henderson made the following comment regarding the publication:

> . . . a wide-ranging and scholarly work that demonstrates familiarity with an impressive body of literature, dating back to ancient Greece, that bears on the argument underlying their central themes of caring, stress and coping (p. ix).

The research described in the book by Benner, Tanner, and Chesla (1996), *Expertise in Nursing Practice: Caring, Clinical Judgment, and Ethics*, is a continuation and expansion of the research described in *From Novice to Expert.* In the Foreword to the 1996 book, Barbara Stevens Barnum wrote the following:

> This work continues to challenge our traditional understanding of what it means to know, to be, and to act skillfully and ethically in nursing practice. Equally important, the book enables the reader to see how we might begin to shape our systems to better accommodate expert caring work. One of the truths of learning made clear by this work is that clinical learning is a dialogue between principles and practice (pp. vii-viii).

Clinical Wisdom in Critical Care: A Thinking-in-Action Approach, by Benner, Hooper-Kyriakidis, and Stannard (1999), constitutes phase two of the articulation research of critical care nursing practice begun in *Expertise in Nursing Practice: Caring, Clinical Judgment, and Ethics.* Articulation refers to "describing, illustrating, and giving language to taken-for-granted areas of practical wisdom, skilled know-how, and notions of good practice" (Benner et al., 1999, p. 5). In the first Foreword to this book, Joan Lynaugh wrote the following:

> Perhaps the most important accomplishment of this text is its insistence on incorporating all the elements of critical care: clinical thinking and thinking ahead, caregiving to patients and families, ethical and moral issues, dealing with breakdown and technological hazard, communication and negotiation among all participants, teaching and coaching, and understanding the linkages between the larger systems and the individual patient (Benner et al., 1999, p. vi).

In the second Foreword, Joyce Clifford wrote the following of the work:

> . . . provides the nurse administrator a wonderful understanding of the way organizational design can facilitate the caregiving process of clinical experts . . . [and] also provides guidance to those entrusted with the development of practice environments that promote the clinical learning and advancement of those just entering the profession (Benner et al., 1999, p. vii).

Benner has published extensively and has been the recipient of numerous honors and awards, including the 1984, 1989, 1996, and 1999 *American Journal of Nursing (AJN)* Book of the Year awards for *From Novice to Expert: Excellence and Power in Clinical Nursing Practice* (1984a), *The Primacy of Caring: Stress and Coping in Health and Illness* (1989, with Wrubel), *Expertise in Nursing Practice: Caring, Clinical Judgment, and Ethics* (1996, with Tanner and Chesla), and *Clinical Wisdom in Critical Care: A Thinking-in-Action Approach* (1999, with

Hooper-Kyriakidis & Stannard), respectively. *The Crisis of Care: Affirming and Restoring Caring Practices in the Helping Professions* (1994), edited by Susan S. Phillips and Patricia Benner, was selected for the CHOICE list of Outstanding Academic Books for 1995. Benner's books have been translated into 10 languages. Several of her articles also have been translated and read worldwide. Benner received the *AJN* media CD-ROM of the year award for *Clinical Wisdom and Interventions in Critical Care: A Thinking-in-Action Approach* (2001, with Hooper-Kyriakidis & Stannard).

In 1985, Benner was inducted into the American Academy of Nurses. She received the National League for Nursing's Linda Richards Award for leadership in education in 1989. In 1990, she received the Excellence in Nursing Research and Excellence in Nursing Education Award from the Organization of Nurse Executives—California. She also received the Alumnus of the Year Award from Point Loma Nazarene College (formerly Pasadena College) in 1993. In 1994, Benner became an Honorary Fellow in the Royal College of Nursing, United Kingdom. In 1995, she received the Helen Nahm Research Lecture Award from the faculty at UCSF in recognition of her contribution to nursing science and research.

Benner received an award for outstanding contributions to the profession from the National Council of State Boards of Nursing in 2002, for her work on developing an instrument to capture the sources and nature of nursing errors. The instrument Taxonomy of Error, Root Cause and Practice (TERCAP) is an electronic data collection tool that can be used to examine practice breakdown (Benner et al., 2002; Benner & Malloch, 2010). In 2003, Benner received an award for 20 years of collecting and extending clinical wisdom, experiential learning, and caring practices from the Institute for Nursing Health Care Leadership. She received the American Association of Colleges of Nursing Pioneering Spirit Award in May 2004 for her work on skill acquisition and articulating nursing knowledge in critical care. In 2007, she was selected for the UCSF School of Nursing's Centennial Wall of Fame. She is invited worldwide to lecture and lead workshops on health, stress and coping, skill acquisition, and ethics. Patricia Benner and her husband and colleague, Richard Benner, consults with nurses in hospitals around the world regarding their approach to clinical practice development models (CPDMs) (Benner & Benner, 1999).

Benner was appointed Nursing Education Study Director for the Carnegie Foundation's Preparation for the Professions Program (PPP) in March 2004. This is a nationwide study that is part of a series of studies on professional education that focus on the shift from technical professionalism to civic professionalism. According to this perspective, teachers are engaged as mentors in apprenticeships with learners to promote learning to see and think like professional practitioners—in this case, nurses (www.nursing.ubc.ca).

PHILOSOPHICAL SOURCES

Benner studies clinical nursing practice in an attempt to discover and describe the knowledge embedded in nursing practice. She maintains that knowledge accrues over time in a practice discipline and is developed through dialogue in relationship and situational contexts. She refers to this work as *articulation research,* as was noted earlier. One of the first philosophical distinctions that Benner made was to differentiate between practical and theoretical knowledge. Benner stated that knowledge development in a practice discipline "consists of extending practical knowledge (know-how) through theory-based scientific investigations and through the charting of the existent 'know-how' developed through clinical experience in the practice of that discipline" (1984a, p. 3). She believes that nurses have been delinquent in documenting their clinical learning, and "this lack of charting of our practices and clinical observations deprives nursing theory of the uniqueness and richness of the knowledge embedded in expert clinical practice" (Benner, 1983, p. 36). Benner has contributed extensively to the description of the know-how of nursing practice.

Citing Kuhn (1970) and Polanyi (1958), philosophers of science, Benner (1984a) emphasizes the difference between "knowing how," a practical knowledge that may elude precise abstract formulations, and "knowing that," which lends itself to theoretical explanations. Knowing that is the way an individual comes to know by establishing causal relationships between events. Knowing how is skill acquisition that may defy knowing that, that is, an individual may know how before a theoretical explanation is developed. Benner (1984a) maintains that practical knowledge may extend theory or may be developed before scientific formulations. Clinical situations are always more varied and complicated than theoretical accounts; therefore, clinical practice is an area of inquiry and a source of knowledge development. Clinical practice embodies the notion of excellence. By studying practice, nurses can uncover new knowledge. Nursing must develop the knowledge base of its practice (know-how), and, through scientific investigation and observation, it must begin to record and develop the know-how of clinical expertise. Ideally, practice and theory set up a dialogue that creates new possibilities. Theory is derived from practice, and practice is altered or extended by theory.

Hubert Dreyfus introduced Benner to phenomenology. Stuart Dreyfus, in operations research, and Hubert Dreyfus, in philosophy, both professors at the University of California at Berkeley, developed the Dreyfus Model of Skill Acquisition (Dreyfus & Dreyfus, 1980; Dreyfus & Dreyfus, 1986), which Benner applied in her work, *From Novice to Expert.* She credits Jane Rubin's (1984) scholarship, teaching, and colleagueship as sources of inspiration and influence, especially in relation to the works of Heidegger (1962) and Kierkegaard (1962). Richard Lazarus (Lazarus & Folkman, 1984; Lazarus, 1985) mentored her in the field of stress and coping. Judith Wrubel has been a participant and co-author with Benner for years, collaborating on the ontology of caring and caring practices (Benner & Wrubel, 1989). Additional philosophical and ethical influences on Benner's work include Joseph Dunne (1993), Knud Løgstrup (1995a, 1995b, 1997), Alistair MacIntyre (1981, 1999), Kari Martinsen (Alvsvåg, 2010), Maurice Merleau-Ponty (1962), Onora O'Neill (1996), and Charles Taylor (1971, 1982, 1989, 1991, 1993, 1994).

Benner (1984a) adapted the Dreyfus model to clinical nursing practice. The Dreyfus brothers developed the skill acquisition model by studying the performance of chess masters and pilots in emergency situations (Dreyfus & Dreyfus, 1980; Dreyfus & Dreyfus, 1986). This model is situational and describes five levels of skill acquisition and development: (1) novice, (2) advanced beginner, (3) competent, (4) proficient, and (5) expert. The model posits that changes in four aspects of performance occur in movement through the levels of skill acquisition as follows: (1) movement from a reliance on abstract principles and rules to the use of past, concrete experience, (2) shift from reliance on analytical, rule-based thinking to intuition, (3) change in the learner's perception of the situation from viewing it as a compilation of equally relevant bits to viewing it as an increasingly complex whole, in which certain parts stand out as more or less relevant, and (4) passage from a detached observer, standing outside the situation, to one of a position of involvement, fully engaged in the situation (Benner, Tanner, & Chesla, 1992).

Because the model is situation based and is not trait based, the level of performance is not an individual characteristic of an individual performer, but instead is a function of a given nurse's familiarity with a particular situation in combination with her or his educational background. The performance level can be determined only by consensual validation of expert judges and by assessment of the outcomes of the situation (Benner, 1984a). In applying the model to nursing, Benner noted that "experience-based skill acquisition is safer and quicker when it rests upon a sound educational base" (1984a, p. xix). Benner (1984a) defines skill and skilled practice to mean implementing skilled nursing interventions and clinical judgment skills in actual clinical situations. In no case does this refer to context-free psychomotor skills or other demonstrable enabling skills outside the context of nursing practice.

In subsequent research undertaken to further explicate the Dreyfus model, Benner identified two interrelated aspects of practice that also distinguish the levels of practice from advanced beginner to expert (Benner et al., 1992, 1996). First, clinicians at different levels of practice live in different clinical worlds, recognizing and responding to different situated needs for action. Second, clinicians develop what Benner terms *agency,* or the sense of responsibility toward the patient, and evolve into fully participating members of the healthcare team.

Benner attempted to highlight the growing edges of clinical knowledge rather than to describe a typical nurse's day. Benner's explanation of nursing practice goes beyond the rigid application of rules and theories and is based on "reasonable behavior that responds to the demands of a given situation" (1984a, p. xx). The skills acquired through nursing experience and the perceptual awareness that expert nurses develop as decision makers from the "gestalt of the situation" lead them to follow their hunches as they search for evidence to confirm the subtle changes they observe in patients (1984a, p. xviii).

The concept that experience is defined as the outcome when preconceived notions are challenged, refined, or refuted in actual situations is based on the works of Heidegger (1962) and Gadamer (1970). As the nurse gains experience, clinical knowledge becomes a blend of practical and theoretical knowledge. Expertise develops as the clinician tests and modifies principle-based expectations in the actual situation. Heidegger's influence is evident in this and in Benner's subsequent writings on the primacy of caring. Benner refutes the dualistic Cartesian descriptions of mind-body person and espouses Heidegger's phenomenological description of person as a self-interpreting being who is defined by concerns, practices, and life experiences. Persons are always situated, that is, they are engaged meaningfully in the context of where they are. Persons come to situations with an understanding of the self in the world. Heidegger (1962) termed *practical knowledge* as the kind of knowing that occurs when an individual is involved in the situation. Persons share background meanings, skills, and habits derived from their cultural practices.

By virtue of being humans, we have embodied intelligence, meaning that we come to know things by being in situations. When a familiar situation is encountered, there is embodied recognition of its meaning. For example, having previously witnessed someone developing a pulmonary embolus, a nurse notices qualitative nuances and has recognition ability for observing it before other nurses who have not seen it before. Benner and Wrubel (1989) stated, "Skilled activity, which is made possible by our embodied intelligence, has been long regarded as 'lower' than intellectual, reflective activity" but argue that intellectual, reflective capacities are dependent on embodied knowing (p. 43). Embodied knowing and the meaning of being are premises for the capacity to care; things matter and "cause us to be involved in and defined by our concerns" (p. 42).

While doing her doctoral studies at Berkeley, Benner was a research assistant to Richard S. Lazarus (Lazarus, 1985; Lazarus & Folkman, 1984), who is known for his development of stress and coping theory. As part of Lazarus' larger study, Benner conducted a study of midcareer males' meaning of work and coping, which was published as *Stress and Satisfaction on the Job: Work Meanings and Coping of Mid-Career Men* (1984b). In this study, *coping* is defined as a form of practical knowledge, and it was determined that work meanings influence what is experienced as stress and what coping options are available to the individual. Lazarus' Theory of Stress and Coping is described as phenomenological, that is, the person is understood to constitute and be constituted by meanings. Stress is described as the disruption of meanings, and coping is what the person does about the disruption. Both doing something and refraining from doing something about the stressful situation are ways of coping. Coping is bound by the meanings inherent in what the person interprets as stressful. The person must be understood as a "participant self" in a situation that is shaped by reflective and nonreflective meanings and concerns (Benner & Wrubel, 1989, p. 63). Different possibilities arise from the way the person is in the situation. Benner uses this key concept to describe clinical nursing practice in terms of nurses making a positive difference by being in the situation in a caring way.

Benner's approach to knowledge development that began with *From Novice to Expert* (1984a) constitutes the commencement of a growing, living tradition for learning from clinical nursing practice through collection and interpretation of exemplars (Benner, 1994; Benner & Benner, 1999; Benner, et al., 1996; Benner, et al., 1999). Benner and Benner stated the following:

> Effective delivery of patient/family care requires collective attentiveness and mutual support of good practice embedded in a moral community of practitioners seeking to create and sustain good practice.... This vision of practice is taken from the Aristotelian tradition in ethics (Aristotle, 1985) and the more recent articulation of this tradition by Alasdair MacIntyre (1981), where practice is defined as a collective endeavor that has notions of good internal to the practice.... However, such collective endeavors must be comprised of individual practitioners who have skilled know how, craft, science, and moral imagination, who continue to create and instantiate good practice (Benner & Benner, 1999, pp. 23-24).

Benner expresses that nursing is a cultural paradox in a highly technical society that is slow to value and articulate caring practices. She feels that the value of extreme individualism makes it difficult to perceive the brilliance of caring in expert nursing practice. Benner (2003) calls for a relational ethic that is based on practice to balance the dominant focus on rights and justice.

Major Concepts & Definitions

NOVICE

In the novice stage of skill acquisition in the Dreyfus model, the person has no background experience of the situation in which he or she is involved. Context-free rules and objective attributes must be given to guide performance. There is difficulty discerning between relevant and irrelevant aspects of a situation. Generally, this level applies to students of nursing, but Benner has suggested that nurses at higher levels of skill in one area of practice could be classified at the novice level if placed in an area or situation unfamiliar to them (Benner, 1984a).

ADVANCED BEGINNER

The advanced beginner stage in the Dreyfus model develops when the person can demonstrate marginally acceptable performance, having coped with enough real situations to note, or to have pointed out by a mentor, the recurring meaningful components of the situation. The advanced beginner has enough experience to grasp aspects of the situation (Benner, 1984a). Unlike attributes and features, aspects cannot be objectified completely because they require experience based on recognition in the context of the situation.

Nurses functioning at this level are guided by rules and are oriented by task completion. They have difficulty grasping the current patient situation in terms of the larger perspective. However, Dreyfus and Dreyfus (1996) state the following:

> Through practical experience in concrete situations with meaningful elements which neither the instructor nor student can define in terms of objective features, the advanced beginner starts intuitively to recognize these elements when they are present. We call these newly recognized elements "situational" to distinguish them from the objective elements of the skill domain that the beginner can recognize prior to seeing concrete examples (p. 38).

Clinical situations are viewed by nurses who are in the advanced beginner stage as a test of their abilities and the demands of the situation placed on them rather than in terms of patient needs and responses (Benner et al., 1992). Advanced

Major Concepts & Definitions—cont'd

beginners feel highly responsible for managing patient care, yet they still rely on the help of those who are more experienced (Benner et al., 1992). Benner places most newly graduated nurses at this level.

COMPETENT

Through learning from actual practice situations and by following the actions of others, the advanced beginner moves to the competent level (Benner et al., 1992). The competent stage of the Dreyfus model is typified by considerable conscious and deliberate planning that determines which aspects of current and future situations are important and which can be ignored (Benner, 1984a).

Consistency, predictability, and time management are important in competent performance. A sense of mastery is acquired through planning and predictability (Benner et al., 1992). The level of efficiency is increased, but "the focus is on time management and the nurse's organization of the task world rather than on timing in relation to the patient's needs" (Benner et al., 1992, p. 20). The competent nurse may display hyperresponsibility for the patient, often more than is realistic, and may exhibit an ever-present and critical view of the self (Benner et al., 1992).

The competent stage is most pivotal in clinical learning, because the learner must begin to recognize patterns and determine which elements of the situation warrant attention and which can be ignored. The competent nurse devises new rules and reasoning procedures for a plan while applying learned rules for action on the basis of relevant facts of that situation. To become proficient, the competent performer must allow the situation to guide responses (Dreyfus & Dreyfus, 1996). Studies point to the importance of active teaching and learning in the competent stage to coach nurses who are making the transition from competency to proficiency (Benner et al., 1996; Benner et al., 1999).

PROFICIENT

At the proficient stage of the Dreyfus model, the performer perceives the situation as a whole (the total picture) rather than in terms of aspects, and the performance is guided by maxims. The proficient level is a qualitative leap beyond the competent. Now the performer recognizes the most salient aspects and has an intuitive grasp of the situation based on background understanding (Benner, 1984a).

Nurses at this level demonstrate a new ability to see changing relevance in a situation, including recognition and implementation of skilled responses to the situation as it evolves. They no longer rely on preset goals for organization, and they demonstrate increased confidence in their knowledge and abilities (Benner et al., 1992). At the proficient stage, there is much more involvement with the patient and family (see the Case Study). The proficient stage is a transition into expertise (Benner et al., 1996).

EXPERT

The fifth stage of the Dreyfus model is achieved when "the expert performer no longer relies on analytical principle (rule, guideline, maxim) to connect her or his understanding of the situation to an appropriate action" (Benner, 1984a, p. 31). Benner described the expert nurse as having an intuitive grasp of the situation and as being able to identify the region of the problem without losing time considering a range of alternative diagnoses and solutions. There is a qualitative change as the expert performer "knows the patient," meaning knowing typical patterns of responses

Continued

MAJOR CONCEPTS & DEFINITIONS—cont'd

and knowing the patient as a person. Key aspects of the expert nurse's practice are as follows (Benner et al., 1996):

- Demonstrating a clinical grasp and resource based practice
- Possessing embodied know-how
- Seeing the big picture
- Seeing the unexpected

The expert nurse has this ability to recognize patterns on the basis of deep experiential background. For the expert nurse, meeting the patient's actual concerns and needs is of utmost importance, even if it means planning and negotiating for a change in the plan of care. There is almost a transparent view of the self (Benner et al., 1992).

ASPECTS OF A SITUATION

The aspects are the recurring meaningful situational components recognized and understood in context because the nurse has previous experience (Benner, 1984a).

ATTRIBUTES OF A SITUATION

The attributes are measurable properties of a situation that can be explained without previous experience in the situation (Benner, 1984a).

COMPETENCY

Competency is "an interpretively defined area of skilled performance identified and described by its intent, functions, and meanings" (Benner, 1984a, p. 292). This term is unrelated to the competent stage of the Dreyfus model.

DOMAIN

This is an area of practice having a number of competencies with similar intents, functions, and meanings (Benner, 1984a).

EXEMPLAR

An exemplar is an example of a clinical situation that conveys one or more intents, meanings, functions, or outcomes easily translated to other clinical situations (Benner, 1984a).

EXPERIENCE

Experience is not a mere passage of time, but an active process of refining and changing preconceived theories, notions, and ideas when confronted with actual situations; it implies there is a dialogue between what is found in practice and what is expected (Benner & Wrubel, 1982).

MAXIM

This is a cryptic description of skilled performance that requires a certain level of experience to recognize the implications of the instructions (Benner, 1984a).

PARADIGM CASE

A paradigm case is a clinical experience that stands out and alters the way the nurse will perceive and understand future clinical situations (Benner, 1984a). Paradigm cases create new clinical understanding and open new clinical perspectives and alternatives.

SALIENCE

Salience describes a perceptual stance or embodied knowledge whereby aspects of a situation stand out as more or less important (Benner, 1984a).

ETHICAL COMPORTMENT

Good conduct born out of an individualized relationship with the patient which involves engagement in a particular situation and entails a sense

Major Concepts & Definitions—cont'd

of membership in the relevant professional group. It is socially embedded, lived and embodied in practices, ways of being, and responding to a clinical situation that promote the well being of the patient (Day & Benner, 2002). "Clinical and ethical judgments are inseparable and must be guided by being with and understanding the human concerns and possibilities in concrete situations" (Benner, 2000, p. 305).

HERMENEUTICS

Hermeneutics means "interpretive." The term derives from biblical and judicial exegesis. As used in research, hermeneutics refers to describing and studying "meaningful human phenomena in a careful and detailed manner as free as possible from prior theoretical assumptions, based instead on practical understanding" (Packer, 1985, pp. 1081-1082).

USE OF EMPIRICAL EVIDENCE

Benner's early work focused on the anticipatory socialization of nurses. Benner and Kramer (1972) studied the differences between nurses who worked in special care units and those who worked in regular hospital units. Benner was a research consultant for a nursing activity study conducted in 1974 and 1975 to determine the use and productivity of nursing personnel. Concurrently, she was a consultant on a study of new nurse-work entry. Benner and Benner (1979) conducted a systematic evaluation of the competencies, the job finding, and the work-entry problems of new graduate nurses. Benner also studied methods of increasing teacher competencies through the use of a mobile microteaching laboratory.

From 1978 to 1981, Benner was the author and project director of a federally funded grant, Achieving Methods of Intraprofessional Consensus, Assessment and Evaluation, known as the AMICAE project. This research led to the publication of *From Novice to Expert* (1984a) and numerous articles. Benner directed the AMICAE project to develop evaluation methods for participating schools of nursing and hospitals in the San Francisco area. It was an interpretive, descriptive study that led to the use of Dreyfus' five levels of competency to describe skill acquisition in clinical nursing practice. In describing the interpretive approach, Benner (1984a) explains that it seeks a rich description of nursing practice from observation and narrative accounts of actual nursing practice to provide the text for interpretation (hermeneutics).

Nurses' descriptions of patient care situations in which they made a positive difference "present the uniqueness of nursing as a discipline and an art" (Benner, 1984a, p. xxvi). More than 1200 nurse participants completed questionnaires and interviews as part of the AMICAE project. Paired interviews with preceptors and preceptees were "aimed at discovering if there were distinguishable, characteristic differences in the novice's and expert's descriptions of the same clinical incident" (Benner, 1984a, p. 14). Additional interviews and participant observations were conducted with 51 nurse-clinicians and other newly graduated nurses and senior nursing students to "describe characteristics of nurse performance at different stages of skill acquisition" (Benner, 1984a, p. 15). The purpose "of the inquiry has been to uncover meanings and knowledge embedded in skilled practice. By bringing these meanings, skills, and knowledge into public discourse, new knowledge and understandings are constituted" (Benner, 1984a, p. 218).

Thirty-one competencies emerged from the analysis of transcripts of interviews about nurses' detailed descriptions of patient care episodes that included their intentions and interpretations of events. From these competencies, which were identified from actual practice situations, the following seven domains were derived inductively on the basis of similarity of function and intent (Benner, 1984a):

1. The helping role
2. The teaching-coaching function
3. The diagnostic and patient monitoring function
4. Effective management of rapidly changing situations
5. Administering and monitoring therapeutic interventions and regimens
6. Monitoring and ensuring the quality of health-care practices
7. Organizational work role competencies

Each domain was developed using the related competencies from actual practice situation descriptions. Benner presented the domains and competencies of nursing practice as an open-ended interpretive framework for enhancing the understanding of the knowledge embedded in nursing practice. As a result of the socially embedded, relational, and dialogical nature of clinical knowledge, domains and competencies should be adapted for use in each institution through the study of clinical practice at each specific locale (Benner & Benner, 1999). Such adaptations have been implemented in many institutions for nursing staff in hospitals around the world (Alberti, 1991; Balasco & Black, 1988; Brykczynski, 1998; Dolan, 1984; Gaston, 1989; Gordon, 1986; Hamric, Whitworth, & Greenfield, 1993; Lock & Gordon, 1989; Nuccio, et al., 1996; Silver, 1986a, 1986b). The domains and competencies have been useful for ongoing articulation of the knowledge embedded in advanced practice nursing (Brykczynski, 1999; Fenton, 1985; Fenton & Brykczynski, 1993; Lindeke, Canedy, & Kay, 1997; Martin, 1996).

Benner and Wrubel (1989) have further explained and developed the background to their ongoing study of the knowledge embedded in nursing practice in *The Primacy of Caring: Stress and Coping in Health and Illness.* They note that the primacy of caring is three-pronged "as the producer of both stress and coping in the lived experience of health and illness . . . as the enabling condition of nursing practice (indeed any practice), and the ways that nursing practice based in such caring can positively affect the outcome of an illness" (1989, p. 7).

Benner extended the research presented in *From Novice to Expert* (1984a) and features this work in *Expertise in Nursing Practice* (1996b). This latter book is based on a 6-year study of 130 hospital nurses, primarily critical care nurses, examining the acquisition of clinical expertise and the nature of clinical knowledge, clinical inquiry, clinical judgment, and expert ethical comportment. The key aims of the extension of this research were as follows:

- Delineate the practical knowledge embedded in expert practice.
- Describe the nature of skill acquisition in critical care nursing practice.
- Identify institutional impediments and resources for the development of expertise in nursing practice.
- Begin to identify educational strategies that encourage the development of expertise.

In the introduction to the 1996 work, Benner stated, "In the study we found that examining the nature of the nurse's agency, by which we mean the sense and possibilities for acting in particular clinical situations, gave new insights about how perception and action are both shaped by a practice community" (Benner et al., 1996, p. xiii). This study resulted in a clearer understanding of the distinctions between engagement with a problem or situation and the requisite nursing skills of interpersonal involvement. It appears that these nursing skills are learned over time experientially. The skill of involvement seems central in gaining nursing expertise. Understanding of the interlinkage of clinical and ethical decision making (i.e., how an individual's notions of good and poor outcomes and visions of excellence shape clinical judgments and actions) was enhanced by this research. This study represents phase one of the articulation project designed to describe the nature of critical care nursing practice.

Phase two took place from 1996 to 1997 and included 76 nurses (32 of them advanced practice nurses) from six different hospitals. This work is presented in the book published in 1999 by Benner and colleagues, *Clinical Wisdom in Critical Care.* The following nine domains of critical care nursing practice were identified as broad themes in this work:

1. Diagnosing and managing life-sustaining physiological functions in unstable patients
2. Using the skilled know-how of managing a crisis
3. Providing comfort measures for the critically ill
4. Caring for patients' families
5. Preventing hazards in a technological environment
6. Facing death: end-of-life care and decision making
7. Communicating and negotiating multiple perspectives
8. Monitoring quality and managing breakdown
9. Using the skilled know-how of clinical leadership and the coaching and mentoring of others

These nine domains of critical care nursing practice were used as broad themes to interpret the data and incorporate descriptions of the following six aspects of clinical judgment and skillful comportment:

1. Reasoning-in-transition
2. Skilled know-how
3. Response-based practice
4. Agency
5. Perceptual acuity and the skill of involvement
6. Links between clinical and ethical reasoning

Identification of clinical grasp and clinical forethought (two pervasive habits of thought linked with action in nursing practice in phase two of this articulation project) enriched the understanding of clinical judgment (Benner et al., 1999). Benner explained that clinical grasp is as follows:

> . . . clinical inquiry in action that includes problem identification and clinical judgment across time about the particular transitions of particular patients and families. It has four components: making qualitative distinctions, engaging in detective work, recognizing changing clinical relevance, and developing clinical knowledge in specific patient populations (Benner et al., 1999, p. 317).

She added that clinical forethought, although it plays a role in clinical grasp, "also plays an essential role in structuring the practical logic of clinicians. Clinical forethought refers to at least four habits of thought and action: future think, clinical forethought about specific diagnoses and injuries, anticipation of risks for particular patients, and seeing the unexpected" (Benner et al., 1999, p. 317).

MAJOR ASSUMPTIONS

Benner incorporates the following assumptions (as delineated in Brykczynski's 1985 dissertation; see also Benner 1984a) in her ongoing articulation research:

- There are no interpretation-free data. This abandons the assumption from natural science that there is an independent reality whose meaning can be represented by abstract terms or concepts (Taylor, 1982).
- There are no nonreactive data. This abandons the false belief from natural science that one can neutrally observe brute data (Taylor, 1982).
- Meanings are embedded in skills, practices, intentions, expectations, and outcomes. They are taken for granted and often are not recognized as knowledge. According to Polanyi (1958), a context possesses existential meaning, and this distinguishes it from "denotative or, more generally, representative meaning" (p. 58). He claims that transposing a significant whole in terms of its constituent parts deprives it of any purpose or meaning.
- People who share a common cultural and language history have a background of common meanings that allows for understanding and interpretation. Heidegger (1962) refers to this as *primordial understanding,* after the writings of Dilthey (1976) in the late 1800s and early 1900s, asserting that cultural organization and meanings precede and influence individual understanding.
- The meanings embedded in skills, practices, intentions, expectations, and outcomes cannot be made completely explicit; however, they can be interpreted by someone who shares a similar language and cultural background and can be validated consensually by participants and relevant practitioners. Humans are self-interpreting beings (Heidegger, 1962). Hermeneutics is the interpretation of cultural contexts and meaningful human action.

- Humans are integrated, holistic beings. The mind-body split is abandoned. Embodied intelligence enables skilled activity that is transformed through experience and mastery (Dreyfus & Dreyfus, 1980; Dreyfus & Dreyfus, 1986). Benner stated, "This model assumes that all practical situations are far more complex than can be described by formal models, theories and textbook descriptions" (1984a, p. 178). The hierarchical elevation of intellectual, reflective activity above embodied skilled activity ignores the point that skilled action is a way of knowing and that the skilled body may be essential for the more highly esteemed levels of human intelligence (Dreyfus, 1979).

Benner and her collaborators explicated the themes of nursing, person, situation, and health in their publications.

Nursing

Nursing is described as a caring relationship, an "enabling condition of connection and concern" (Benner & Wrubel, 1989, p. 4). "Caring is primary because caring sets up the possibility of giving help and receiving help" (Benner & Wrubel, 1989, p. 4). "Nursing is viewed as a caring practice whose science is guided by the moral art and ethics of care and responsibility" (Benner & Wrubel, 1989, p. xi). Benner and Wrubel (1989) understand nursing practice as the care and study of the lived experience of health, illness, and disease and the relationships among these three elements.

Person

Benner and Wrubel (1989) use Heidegger's phenomenological description of person, which they describe as "A person is a self-interpreting being, that is, the person does not come into the world predefined but gets defined in the course of living a life. A person also has . . . an effortless and nonreflective understanding of the self in the world" (p. 41). "The person is viewed as a participant in common meanings" (Benner & Wrubel, 1989, p. 23).

Finally, the person is embodied. Benner and Wrubel (1989) have conceptualized the following four major aspects of understanding that the person must deal with:

1. The role of the situation
2. The role of the body
3. The role of personal concerns
4. The role of temporality

Together, these aspects of the person make up the person in the world. This view of the person is based on the works of Heidegger (1962), Merleau-Ponty (1962), and Dreyfus (1979, 1991). Their goal is to overcome Cartesian dualism, the view that the mind and body are distinct, separate entities (Visintainer, 1988).

Benner and Wrubel (1989) define *embodiment* as the capacity of the body to respond to meaningful situations. On the basis of the work of Merleau-Ponty (1962), Dreyfus (1979, 1991), and Dreyfus and Dreyfus (1986), they outline the following five dimensions of the body (Benner & Wrubel, 1989):

1. The unborn complex, unacculturated body of the fetus and newborn baby
2. The habitual skilled body complete with socially learned postures, gestures, customs, and skills evident in bodily skills such as sense perception and "body language" that are "learned over time through identification, imitation, and trial and error" (Benner & Wrubel, 1989, p. 71)
3. The projective body that is set (predisposed) to act in specific situations (e.g., opening a door or walking)
4. The actual projected body indicating an individual's current bodily orientation or projection in a situation that is flexible and varied to fit the situation, such as when an individual is skillful in using a computer
5. The phenomenal body, the body aware of itself with the ability to imagine and describe kinesthetic sensations

Benner and Wrubel (1989) point out that nurses attend to all of these dimensions of the body and seek to understand the role of embodiment in particular situations of health, illness, and recovery.

Health

On the basis of the work of Heidegger (1962) and Merleau-Ponty (1962), Benner and Wrubel focus "on the lived experience of being healthy and being ill" (1989, p. 7). *Health* is defined as what can be assessed, whereas *well-being* is the human experience of health or wholeness. Well-being and being ill are understood as distinct ways of being in the world. Health is described as not just the absence of disease and illness. Also, on the basis of the work of Kleinman, Eisenberg, and Good (1978), a person may have a disease and not experience illness, because illness is the human experience of loss or dysfunction, whereas disease is what can be assessed at the physical level (Benner & Wrubel, 1989).

Situation

Benner and Wrubel (1989) use the term *situation* rather than *environment,* because *situation* conveys a social environment with social definition and meaningfulness. They use the phenomenological terms *being situated* and *situated meaning,* which are defined by the person's engaged interaction, interpretation, and understanding of the situation. "Personal interpretation of the situation is bounded by the way the individual is in it" (Benner & Wrubel, 1989, p. 84). This means that each person's past, present, and future, which include their own personal meanings, habits, and perspectives, influence the current situation.

THEORETICAL ASSERTIONS

Benner (1984a) stated that there is always more to any situation than theory predicts. The skilled practice of nursing exceeds the bounds of formal theory. Concrete experience facilitates learning about the exceptions and shades of meaning in a situation. The knowledge embedded in practice can lead to discovering and interpreting theory, precedes and extends theory, and synthesizes and adapts theory in caring nursing practice. Some of the relationship statements included in Benner's work follow:

- "Discovering assumptions, expectations, and sets can uncover an unexamined area of practical knowledge that can then be systematically studied and extended or refuted" (Benner, 1984a, p. 8).
- Clinical knowledge is embedded in perceptions rather than precepts.
- "Perceptual awareness is central to good nursing judgment and . . . [for the expert] begins with vague hunches and global assessments that initially bypass critical analysis; conceptual clarity follows more often than it precedes" (Benner, 1984a, p. xviii).
- Formal rules are limited and discretionary judgment is needed in actual clinical situations.
- Clinical knowledge develops over time, and each clinician develops a personal repertoire of practice knowledge that can be shared in dialogue with other clinicians.
- "Expertise develops when the clinician tests and refines propositions, hypotheses, and principle based expectations in actual practice situations" (Benner, 1984a, p. 3).

LOGICAL FORM

Through qualitative descriptive research, Benner applied the Dreyfus Model of Skill Acquisition to clinical nursing practice. By following the model's logical sequence, Benner was able to identify the performance characteristics and teaching-learning needs inherent at each level of skill. In reporting her research, Benner used exemplars taken directly from interviews and observation of expert practice to help the reader form a clear picture of such practice. The goal of Benner's research is to bring meanings and knowledge embedded in skilled practice into public discourse. Benner (1984a) claims that new knowledge and understanding are constituted by articulating meanings, skills, and knowledge that previously were taken for granted and embedded in clinical practice.

ACCEPTANCE BY THE NURSING COMMUNITY

Practice

Benner describes clinical nursing practice by using an interpretive phenomenological approach. *From Novice to Expert* (1984a) includes several examples of the application of her work in practice settings (Dolan, 1984; Huntsman, Lederer, & Peterman, 1984; Ullery, 1984). As noted earlier, Benner's approach has been used to aid in the development of clinical promotion ladders, new graduate orientation programs, and clinical knowledge development seminars. Symposia focusing on excellence in nursing practice have been held for staff development, recognition, and reward, and as a way to demonstrate clinical knowledge development in practice (Dolan, 1984). Fenton (1984) reported the use of Benner's approach in an ethnographic study of the performance of clinical nurse-specialists. Her findings included identification and description of competencies of nurses functioning at an advanced level of preparation. Balasco and Black (1988) and Silver (1986a, 1986b) used Benner's work as a basis for differentiating clinical knowledge development and career progression in nursing.

Neverveld (1990) used Benner's rationale and format in her development of basic and advanced preceptor workshops. Farrell and Bramadat (1990) used Benner's paradigm case analysis in a collaborative educational project between a university school of nursing and a tertiary care teaching hospital to better understand the development of clinical reasoning skills in actual practice situations. Crissman and Jelsma (1990) applied Benner's findings in developing a cross-training program to address staffing imbalances. They delineated specific cross-training performance objectives for novice nurses, but also provided support for the experiential judgment needed to function in unfamiliar settings by designating a preceptor in the clinical area. The aim is for the novice to be able to perform more like an advanced beginner, with an experienced nurse available as a resource.

Benner has been cited extensively in nursing literature regarding nursing practice concerns and the role of caring in such practice. She continues to advance understanding of the knowledge embedded in clinical situations through publications (Benner 1985a, 1985b, 1987; Benner & Tanner, 1987; Benner, et al., 1996; Benner et al., 1999). Benner edited a clinical exemplar series in the *American Journal of Nursing* during the 1980s. (See this chapter in the fifth edition of this book [2002].) In 2001, she began editing a series called "Current Controversies in Critical Care" in the *American Journal of Critical Care.* (See the *Journals* listing in this chapter's bibliography.) As was noted earlier, Benner's work with the National Council of State Boards of Nursing constitutes a major contribution to error recognition and enhancement of the safety of nursing practice (Benner et al., 2002; Benner & Malloch, 2010).

Education

Benner (1982) has critiqued the concept of competency-based testing by contrasting it with the complexity of the proficiency and expert stages described in the Dreyfus Model of Skill Acquisition and the 31 competencies described in the AMICAE project (Benner, 1984a). In summary, she stated, "Competency-based testing seems limited to the less situational, less interactional areas of patient care where the behavior can be well defined and patient and nurse variations do not alter the performance criteria" (1982, p. 309).

Fenton (1984, 1985) applied the domains of clinical nursing practice as the basis for studying the skilled performance of clinical nurse specialists (CNSs). Her analysis validated that the CNSs studied demonstrated competencies in common with those skills of expert nurses reported in the AMICAE project. She also identified additional areas of skilled performance for CNSs, including the consulting role, and she delineated five preliminary categories relevant for curriculum evaluation in the graduate program. Ethical, clinical, and political dilemmas, positions, or stances that promote success or failure, and new knowledge that blends the empirical and the theoretical, were among these categories.

According to Barnum (1990), it was not Benner's development of the seven domains of nursing practice that has had the greatest impact on nursing education, but the "appreciation of the utility of the Dreyfus model in describing learning and thinking in our discipline" (p. 170). As a result of Benner's application of the Dreyfus model, nursing educators have realized that learning needs at the early stages of clinical knowledge development are different from those required at later stages. These differences need to be acknowledged and valued to develop nursing education programs appropriate for the background experience of the students . . . While some nurses have come to appreciate knowledge that is developed in practice, others find extant theories that are taught in academia useful for nursing practice applications.

In *Expertise in Nursing Practice,* Benner and colleagues (1996) emphasized the importance of learning the skills of involvement and caring through practical experience, the articulation of knowledge with practice, and the use of narratives in undergraduate education. This work provides further support for the thesis that it may be better to place a new graduate with a competent nurse preceptor who can explain nursing practice in ways that the beginner comprehends, rather than with the expert, whose intuitive knowledge may elude beginners who do not have the experienced know-how to grasp the situation.

In *Clinical Wisdom in Critical Care,* Benner and colleagues (1999) urged greater attention to experiential learning and presented the work as a guide to teaching. They designed a highly interactive CD-ROM to accompany the book (Benner et al., 2001). The results of the recently completed national study of nursing education are forthcoming by Benner, Sutphen, Leonard, and Day (2008). Benner reported that the study was designed to identity and describe "signature pedagogies" that maximize the nurse's ability to cope with the challenges of nursing that have developed during the 30 years since the last national study of nursing education (Schwartz, 2005).

Research

The preceding example by Fenton (1984, 1985) presented an application of educational research. Lock and Gordon (1989), medical anthropologists who had been research assistants on the AMICAE project, extended the inquiry to study the formal models used in nursing practice and medicine. They concluded that formal models serve as maps that direct care, substitute knowledge, and result in conformity. Gordon (1984) cautions that a misuse of formal models occurs when nurses apply models without using judgment, when they use models to exert control, when they use language from models that may cover up meanings, or when they do not understand the meaning of the models. And finally, "formal models should be used with discretion" as tools and should not eclipse the relational, holistic, intuitive aspects of nursing (p. 242).

FURTHER DEVELOPMENT

Benner's philosophy of nursing practice provides concept definitions and in-depth descriptions from nursing practice. From these situated descriptions, competencies in seven domains have been derived from actual nursing practice (Benner, 1984a). Additionally, nine domains have been described for critical care nursing practice (Benner et al., 1999), and these domains and competencies have been modified to reflect advanced practice nursing (Brykczynski, 1999; Fenton, 1984, 1985; Fenton & Brykczynski, 1993). These descriptions of nursing practice follow Benner's approach to maintaining the context of the clinical situation, so that the descriptions are holistic or synthetic and are not procedural and elemental.

The competencies within each domain are in no way intended as an exhaustive list. Instead, the situation-based interpretive approach to describing nursing practice seeks to overcome some of the problems of reductionism and the problem of global and overly general descriptions based on nursing process categories (Benner, 1984a). In a further description of this approach, Benner (1992) examined the role of narrative accounts for understanding the notion of good or ethical caring in expert clinical nursing practice. "The narrative memory of the actual concrete event is taken up in embodied know-how and comportment, complete with emotional responses to situations. The narrative memory can evoke perceptual or sensory memories that enhance pattern recognition" (p. 16).

Dunlop (1986) explored the nursing literature related to the science of caring. She drew a distinction between a science *for* caring and a science *of* caring. She stated, "A science of caring implies that caring can be operationalized in some way as a set of behaviors, which can be observed, counted or measured" (p. 666). Benner has taken a hermeneutical approach to uncover the knowledge embedded in clinical nursing practice. Dunlop stated, "As she does this, she is also uncovering the nursing-caring with which it is deeply intertwined" (p. 668). Dunlop noted that "it does not provide us with any universal truths about caring in general or about nursing-caring in particular—indeed it does not make any such pretension" (p. 668).

CRITIQUE

Simplicity

Benner has developed interpretive descriptive accounts of clinical nursing practice. The concepts are the levels of skilled practice from the Dreyfus model, including novice, advanced beginner, competent, proficient, and expert. She used these five concepts to describe nursing practice based on interviews, observations, and the analysis of transcripts of exemplars that nurses provided. From these descriptions, competencies were identified, and these were grouped inductively into seven domains of nursing practice on the basis of common intentions and meanings (Benner, 1984a). Benner and colleagues' (1996) study of critical care nursing explored the differentiation of levels of practice in depth and suggested, as noted earlier, that nurses at different levels live in different worlds in the Heideggerian sense. Benner's ongoing articulation research project has produced nine domains of critical care nursing practice (Benner et al., 1999). The model is relatively simple with regard to the five stages of skill acquisition, and it provides a comparative guide for identifying levels of nursing practice from individual nurse descriptions and observations of actual nursing practice. The interpretations are validated by consensus.

A degree of complexity is encountered in the subconcepts for differentiation among the levels of competency and the need to identify meanings and intentions. This interpretive approach is designed to overcome the constraints of the rational-technical approach to the study and description of practice. Although a de-contextualized (object) description of the novice level of performance is possible, such a description of expert performance would be difficult, if not impossible, and is of limited usefulness because of the limits of objectification. In other words, the philosophical problem of infinite regress would be encountered in attempts to specify all the aspects of expert practice. Instead, a holistic understanding of the particular situation is required for expert performance.

Generality

The novice to expert skill acquisition model has universal characteristics, that is, it is not restricted by age, illness, health, or location of nursing practice. However, the characteristics of theoretical universality imply properties of operationalization for prediction that are not a part of this perspective. Indeed, this phenomenological perspective critiques the limits of universality in studies of human practices. The interpretive model of nursing practice has the potential for universal application as a framework, but the descriptions are limited by dependence on the actual clinical nursing situations from which they must be derived. Its use depends on an understanding of the five levels of competency and the ability to identify the characteristic intentions and meanings inherent at each level of practice.

Although clinical knowledge is relational and contextual and involves local, specific, historical issues, it is generalizable in terms of the translation of meanings to similar situations (Guba & Lincoln, 1982).

To capture the contextual and relational aspects of practice, Benner uses narrative accounts of actual clinical situations and maintains that this approach enables the reader to recognize similar intents and meanings, although the objective circumstances may be quite different. An example of generalizability or transferability as used here follows: Upon reading or hearing a narrative about a nurse connecting with a family whose child is dying, other nurses can relate the knowledge and meanings conveyed to experiences that they may have had with families of patients of any age who were dying.

Empirical Precision

The model was tested using qualitative methods; 31 competencies, 7 domains of nursing practice, and 9 domains of critical care nursing practice were derived inductively. Subsequent research suggests that the framework is applicable and useful for continued development of knowledge embedded in nursing practice. This approach to knowledge development honors the primacy of caring and the central ethic of care and responsibility embedded in expert nursing practice, which do not show up if we use only scientific, technical, and organizational strategies for legitimizing expert nursing care (Benner, 1999).

The use of an alternative qualitative process of discovering nursing knowledge makes it difficult to address the body of Benner's work within a rational-empirical framework for critique. Whereas, positivistic science seeks theories to be applied in practice using a quantitative approach, the qualitative interpretive approach describes expert nursing practice with exemplars. Benner's work can be considered as hypothesis generating rather than hypothesis testing. Benner provides no universal "how to" for nursing practice, but instead provides a methodology for uncovering and entering into the situated meaning of expert nursing care. Altmann (2007) pointed out that most of the criticism of Benner's work has developed from misinterpretation of her philosophy as theory and evaluation of her qualitative research with quantitative parameters.

Derivable Consequences

Although clinical nurses around the world enthusiastically received *From Novice to Expert* (1984a), some academicians and administrators initially interpreted it as promoting traditionalism and devaluing education and theory for nursing practice (Christman, 1985). Benner's qualitative interpretive approach to interpretation of the meaning and level of nursing practice creates doubt among objective researchers who seek precision and control. An ongoing debate developed over cognitive interpretations of Benner's concepts of expertise and intuition (Benner, 1996b; Cash, 1995; Darbyshire, 1994; English, 1993; Paley, 1996). Yet it was never intended that these phenomenological concepts be operationalized and objectified.

Benner's perspective is phenomenological, not cognitive. She stated, "Clinical judgment and caring practices require attendance to the particular patient across time, taking into account changes and what has been learned. In this vision of clinical judgment, skilled know-how and action are linked" (Benner, 1999, p. 316). The strength of the Benner model is that data-based research contributes to the science of nursing as a practice discipline (Darbyshire, 1994). The significance of Benner's research findings lies in her conclusion that "a nurse's clinical knowledge is relevant to the extent to which its manifestation in nursing skills makes a difference in patient care and patient outcomes" (Benner & Wrubel, 1982, p. 11).

Generalization is approached through an understanding of common meanings, skills, practices, and embodied capacities rather than through general abstract laws that explain and predict. Such common meanings, skills, and practices are socially embedded in nurse schooling and in the practice and tradition of nursing. The knowledge embedded in clinical nursing practice should be brought forth as public knowledge to further a greater understanding of nursing practice. Benner (1984a) believes that the scope and complexity of nursing practice are too extensive for nurses to rely on idealized, de-contextualized views of practice or experiments. Benner (1992) stated, "The platonic quest to get to the general so that we can get beyond the vagaries of experience was a misguided turn.... We can redeem the turn if we subject our theories to our unedited, concrete, moral experience and acknowledge that skillful ethical comportment calls us not to be beyond experience but tempered and taught by it" (p. 19).

The generalizations possible with the interpretive approach are depicted through exemplars that demonstrate relational and contextually relevant intents and aspects of clinical knowledge. The applicability and relevance of the common approaches used for universality or generalization in physics and the natural sciences are questioned by the interpretive approach, that claims that the basis for generalization in clinical knowledge cannot be structural or mechanistic, but must be based on common meanings and practices. Preferred strategies for generalization in clinical practice are based on the skilled knowledge, intent, content, and notion of good in clinical knowledge depicted by exemplars that illustrate the role of the situation.

Benner claims that nurses need to overcome the limits of subject-object descriptions. Her call is to "increase public storytelling" to validate nursing as an ethical caring practice, and "to extend, alter, and preserve ethical distinctions and concerns" (Benner, 1992, pp. 19-20). Benner (1996a) stated, "We have overlooked practitioner stories that demonstrate that compassion can be wise and, in the long run, less costly than 'defensive' adversarial commodified technocures" (pp. 35-36). Benner's work is useful in that it frames nursing practice in the context of what nursing actually is and does.

SUMMARY

Benner seeks to affirm and restore nurses' caring practices during a time when nurses are rewarded more for efficiency, technical skills, and measurable outcomes. She maintains that caring practices are imbued with knowledge and skill about everyday human needs, and that in order to be experienced as caring, these practices must be attuned to the particular person who is being cared for and to the particular situation as it unfolds. Benner's philosophy of nursing practice is a dynamic, emerging holistic perspective that holds philosophy, practice, research, and theory as interdependent, interrelated, and hermeneutic. Her hope voiced in the preface of *From Novice to Expert* (1984a) saying that domains and competencies would not be deified by system builders seems to have been largely realized, as those who have sought to apply these concepts have honored the contextual background on which they are based.

Benner maintains that there is excellence and power in clinical nursing practice that can be made visible through what she describes as *articulation research.* Intricate nuanced descriptions of situational contexts are the essence of this research approach, which dictates that data are to be collected through situation-based dialogue and observation of actual practice. The situational context guides interpretation of meanings such that there is agreement among interpreters. This is a holistic approach that emphasizes identification and description of meanings embedded in clinical practice. The holistic approach is maintained throughout the research process from beginning to end. The situational context is maintained as narratives are interpreted through dialogue among researchers and clinicians.

Case Study

A case study from the peer-identified nurse expert project that this author (Brykczynski, 1993-1995, 1998) conducted as part of a nursing service clinical ladder enhancement process is selected here to illustrate how Benner's approach can be applied to knowledge development in clinical nursing practice. This project was undertaken to identify and describe expert staff nursing practices at our institution. Exemplars were obtained and participant observations were conducted to yield narrative text that then was interpreted through Benner's multiphase interpretive phenomenological process (Benner, 1984a, 1994). In the final phase of data analysis, Benner's domains and competencies of nursing practice (Benner, 1984a) were incorporated as an interpretive framework. A critical aspect of using Benner's approach is the realization that the domains and competencies form a dynamic evolving interpretive framework that is used in interpreting the narrative and observational data collected. They are not used initially as a prescriptive abstract theoretical framework that might circumscribe the study.

The nurse who described this situation had approximately 8 years of experience in critical care, and she noted that this was significant to her practice because it taught her how to integrate taking care of a family in crisis along with taking care of a critically ill patient. This was a paradigm case for the nurse, who learned many things from it that affected her future practice. Mrs. Walsh is a pseudonym for a woman in her 70s who was in critical condition following repeat coronary artery bypass graft (CABG) surgery. Her family lived nearby when Mrs. Walsh had her first CABG surgery. They had moved out of town but returned to our institution, where the first surgery had been performed successfully. Mrs. Walsh remained critically ill and unstable for several weeks before her death. Her family was very anxious because of Mrs. Walsh's unstable and deteriorating condition, and for the first few weeks, a family member was always with her, 24 hours a day.

The nurse became involved with this family while Mrs. Walsh was still in surgery, because family members were very anxious that the procedure was taking longer than it had the first time and made repeated calls to the critical care unit to ask about the patient. The nurse met with the family and offered to go into the operating room to talk with the cardiac surgeon so as to better inform the family of their mother's status.

One of the helpful things the nurse did to assist this family was to establish a consistent group of nurses to work with Mrs. Walsh, so that family members could establish trust and feel more confident about the care their mother was receiving. This eventually enabled family members to leave the hospital for intervals to get some rest. The nurse related that this was a family whose members were affluent, educated, and well informed, and that they came in prepared with lists of questions. A consistent group of nurses who were familiar with Mrs. Walsh's particular situation helped both family members and nurses to be more satisfied and less anxious. The family developed a close relationship with the three nurses who consistently cared for Mrs. Walsh and shared with them details about Mrs. Walsh and her life.

The nurse related that there was a tradition in this particular critical care unit not to involve family members in care. She broke that tradition when she responded to the son's and the daughter's helpless feelings by teaching them some simple things that they could do for their mother. They learned to give some basic care, such as bathing her. The nurse acknowledged that involving family members in direct patient care with a critically ill patient is complex and requires knowledge and sensitivity. She believes that a developmental process is involved when nurses learn to work with families.

She noted that after a nurse has lots of experience and feels very comfortable with highly technical skills, it becomes okay for family members to be in the room when care is provided. She pointed out that direct observation by anxious family members can be disconcerting to those who are insecure with their skills when family members ask things like, "Why are you doing this? Nurse 'So and So' does it differently." She commented that nurses learn to be flexible and to reset priorities. They should be able to let some things wait that do not need to be done right away to give the family some time with the patient. One of the things that the nurse did to coordinate care was to meet with the family to see what times worked best for them; then she posted family time on the patient's activity schedule outside her cubicle to communicate the plan to others involved in Mrs. Walsh's care.

When Mrs. Walsh died, the son and daughter wanted to participate in preparing her body. This had never been done in this unit, but after checking to see that there was no policy forbidding it, the nurse invited them to participate. They turned down the lights, closed the doors, and put music on; the nurse, the patient's daughter, and the patient's son all cried together while they prepared Mrs. Walsh to be taken to the morgue. The nurse took care of all intravenous lines and tubes while the children bathed her. The nurse provided evidence of how finely tuned her skill of involvement was with this family when she explained that she felt uncomfortable at first because she thought that the son and daughter should be sharing this time alone with their mother. Then she realized that they really wanted her to be there with them. This situation taught her that families of critically ill patients need care as well. The nurse explained that this was a paradigm case that motivated her to move into a CNS role, with expansion of her sphere of influence from her patients during her shift to other shifts, other patients and their families, and other disciplines.

Domain: The Helping Role of the Nurse

This narrative exemplifies the meaning and intent of several competencies in this domain, in particular creating a climate for healing and providing emotional and informational support to patients' families (Benner, 1984a). Incorporating the family as participants in the care of a critically ill patient requires a high level of skill that cannot be developed until the nurse feels competent and confident in technical critical care skills. This nurse had many years of experience in this unit, and she felt that providing care for their mother was so important to these children that she broke tradition in her unit and taught them how to do some basic comfort and hygiene measures. The nurse related that the other nurses in this critical care unit held the belief that active family involvement in care was intrusive and totally out of line. A belief such as this is based on concerns for patient safety and efficiency of care, yet it cuts the family off from being fully involved in the caring relationship. This nurse demonstrated moral courage, commitment to care, and advocacy in going against the tradition in her unit of excluding family members from direct care. She had 8 years of experience in this unit, and her peers respected her, so she was able to change practice by starting with this one patient-family situation and involving the other two nurses who were working with them.

Chesla's (1996) research points to a gap between theory and practice with respect to including families in patient care. Eckle (1996) studied family presence with children in emergency situations and concluded that in times of crisis, the needs of families must be addressed to provide effective and compassionate care. The skilled practice of including the family in care emerged as significantly meaningful in the narrative text from the peer-identified nurse expert study. This was defined as an additional competency in the domain called the *helping role of the nurse* and was named *maximizing the family's role in care* (Brykczynski, 1998). The intent of this competency is to assess each situation as it arises and develops over time, so that family involvement in care can adequately address specific patient-family needs, and so they are not excluded from involvement nor do they have participation thrust upon them.

This narrative illustrates how Benner's approach is dynamic and specific for each institution. The belief that being attuned to family involvement in care is in part a developmental process is supported by Nuccio and colleagues' (1996) description of this aspect of care in the CPDM at their institution. They observed that novice nurses begin by recognizing their feelings associated with family-centered care, while expert nurses develop creative approaches to include patients and families in care. The intricate process of finely tuning the nurse's collaboration with families in critical care is delineated further by Levy (2004) in her interpretive phenomenological study that articulates the practices of nurses with critically burned children and their families.

CRITICAL THINKING *Activities*

1. Describe clinical situations from your own experience or those of colleagues that you have observed that illustrate how nurses at various levels of skill development from

novice to expert involve patients and families in care.

2. Discuss the clinical narrative provided here in terms of the rights and justice approach to ethical decision making, and then describe what the care and responsibility approach to relational ethics would add to this perspective. You may want to refer to Benner's (2003) chapter, "Finding the Good Behind the Right," to assist you in responding to this challenge.
3. Describe and give examples of what is meant by the statement that caring practices, intervention skills, clinical judgment, and collaboration skills articulated with Benner's approach can increase the visibility of nursing practice in the following three senses: (1) to the individual nurse, (2) to nursing colleagues, and (3) to the healthcare system.
4. Obtain a videotape of the movie *At First Sight,* produced by MGM in 1999. View it and identify examples from the movie to illustrate the phenomenology of how the massage therapist, played by Val Kilmer, constructed his world as a blind person; contrast this with how his architect love interest, played by Mira Sorvino, constructed her world as a sighted person. Articulate how the massage therapist was like a novice when his sight was restored, and relate insights gained from this exercise to skill development in nursing practice.

POINTS FOR *Further Study*

- Patricia Benner home page. Accessed March 21, 2008, at: http://www.bennerassociates.com
- Hubert Dreyfus home page. Accessed March 21, 2008, at: http://ist-socrates.berkeley.edul~hdreyfus
- The Carnegie Foundation for the Advancement of Teaching, Professional and Graduate Education. Accessed March 21, 2008, at: http://www.carnegiefoundation.org
- Brykczynski, K. A. (2010). Benner's philosophy in nursing practice. In Alligood, M. Nursing theory: Utilization and Application (4th ed. pp. 137-159). St. Louis: Mosby.
- Benner, P. (2001). *From novice to expert: Commemorative edition.* Upper Saddle River, NJ: Prentice Hall. (Re-published edition of the original 1984 work.)
- Benner, P., Tanner, C., & Chesla, C. (1992). *From beginner to expert: Clinical knowledge in critical care nursing* [Video]. New York: Helene Fuld Trust Fund. Available from FITNE, Inc., at: http://www.fitne.net/
- Benner, P., Stannard, D., & Hooper-Kyriakidis, P. (2001). *Clinical wisdom and interventions in Critical Care: A Thinking-in-Action Approach* (CD-ROM). Philadelphia: W. B. Saunders.

REFERENCES

Alberti, A. M. (1991). Advancing the scope of primary nurses in the NICU. *Journal of Perinatal and Neonatal Nursing, 5*(3), 44-50.

Altmann, T. K. (2007). An evaluation of the seminal work of Patricia Benner: Theory or philosophy? *Contemporary Nurse, 25*(1-2), 114-123.

Alvsvåg, H. (2010). Kari Martinsen: Philosophy of caring. In A. M. Tomey & M. R. Alligood (Eds.), *Nursing theorists and their work* (7th ed.). St. Louis: Mosby, 165-189.

Aristotle (1985). *Nicomachean ethics* [T. Irwin, Trans.]. Indianapolis: Hackett.

Balasco, E. M., & Black, A. S. (1988). Advancing nursing practice: Description, recognition, and reward. *Nursing Administration Quarterly, 12*(2), 52-62.

Barnum, B. (1996). Foreword. In P. Benner, C. Tanner, & C. Chesla (Eds.), *Expertise in nursing practice: Caring clinical judgment, and ethics.* New York: Springer.

Barnum, B. J. (1990). *Nursing theory: Analysis, application, evaluation.* Glenview, IL: Scott, Foresman.

Benner, P. (1982, May). Issues in competency-based training. *Nursing Outlook, 20*(5), 303-309.

Benner, P. (1983). Uncovering the knowledge embedded in clinical practice. *Image: The Journal of Nursing Scholarship, 15*(2), 36-41.

Benner, P. (1984a). *From novice to expert: Excellence and power in clinical nursing practice.* Menlo Park, CA: Addison-Wesley.

Benner, P. (1984b). *Stress and satisfaction on the job: Work meanings and coping of mid-career men.* New York: Praeger.

Benner, P. (1985a). The oncology clinical nurse specialist: An expert coach. *Oncology Nursing Forum, 12*(2), 40-44.

Benner, P. (1985b). Quality of life: A phenomenological perspective on explanation, prediction, and understanding in nursing science. *ANS Advances in Nursing Science, 8*(1), 1-14.

Benner, P. (1987, Sept.). A dialogue with excellence. *American Journal of Nursing, 87*(9), 1170-1172.

Benner, P. (1992). The role of narrative experience and community in ethical comportment. *ANS Advances in Nursing Science, 14*(2), 1-21.

Benner, P. (1994). The tradition and skill of interpretive phenomenology in studying health, illness, and caring practices. In P. Benner (Ed.), *Interpretive phenomenology: Embodiment, caring, and ethics in health and illness* (pp. 99-126). Thousand Oaks, CA: Sage.

Benner, P. (1996a). Embodiment, caring and ethics: A nursing perspective: The 1995 Helen Nahm lecture. *The Science of Caring, 8*(2), 30-36.

Benner, P. (1996b). A response by P. Benner to K. Cash. Benner and expertise in nursing: A critique. *International Journal of Nursing Studies, 33*(6), 669-674.

Benner, P. (1999). Claiming the wisdom and worth of clinical practice. *Nursing and Health Care Perspectives, 20*(6), 312-319.

Benner, P. (2000). The quest for control and the possibilities of care. In M. A. Wrathall & J. Malpas (Eds.), *Heidegger, coping and cognitive science: Essays in honor of Hubert L. Dreyfus* (vol 2, pp. 293-383). Cambridge, MA: M. I. T. Press.

Benner, P. (2003). Finding the good behind the right: A dialogue between nursing and bioethics. In F. G. Miller, J. C. Fletcher, &. J. M. Humber (Eds.), *The nature and prospect of bioethics: Interdisciplinary perspectives* (pp. 113-139). Totowa, NJ: Humana Press.

Benner, P., & Benner, R. V. (1979). *The new nurses' work entry: A troubled sponsorship.* New York: Tiresias.

Benner, P., & Benner, R. V. (1999). The clinical practice development model: Making the clinical judgment, caring and collaborative work of nurses visible. In B. Haag-Heitman (Ed.), *Clinical practice development: Using novice to expert theory* (pp. 17-42). Gaithersburg, MD: Aspen.

Benner, P., Hooper-Kyriakidis, P., & Stannard, D. (1999). *Clinical wisdom in critical care: A thinking-in-action approach.* Philadelphia: W. B. Saunders.

Benner, P., & Kramer, M. (1972, Jan.). Role conceptions and integrative role behavior of nurses in special care and regular hospital nursing units. *Nursing Research, 21*(1), 20-29.

Benner, P., & Malloch, K., with M. Ferrell (Ed.). (2010). *Nursing pathways for patient safety.* Philadelphia: Elsevier International Press.

Benner, P., Sheets, V., Uris, P., Malloch, K., Schwed, K., & Jamison, D. (2002). Individual, practice, and system causes of errors in nursing: A taxonomy. *Journal of Nursing Administration, 32*(10), 509-523.

Benner, P., Stannard, D., & Hooper-Kyriakidis, P. (2001). *Clinical wisdom and interventions in critical care: A thinking-in-action approach* (CD-ROM). Philadelphia: W. B. Saunders.

Benner, P., Sutphen, M., Leonard, V., & Day, L. (2008). *Educating nurses: Teaching and learning in a complex practice of care.* The Carnegie Foundation for the Achievement of Teaching. 2008 Marion Woodward Lecture. University of British Columbia, Vancouver.

Benner, P., & Tanner, C. (1987, Jan.). Clinical judgment: How expert nurses use intuition. *American Journal of Nursing, 87*(1), 23-31.

Benner, P., Tanner, C., & Chesla, C. (1992). From beginner to expert: Gaining a differentiated clinical world in critical care nursing. *ANS Advances in Nursing Science, 14*(3), 13-28.

Benner, P., Tanner, C., & Chesla, C. (1996). *Expertise in nursing practice: Caring, clinical judgment, and ethics.* New York: Springer.

Benner, P., & Wrubel, J. (1982). Skilled clinical knowledge: The value of perceptual awareness. *Nurse Educator, 7*(3), 11-17.

Benner, P., & Wrubel, J. (1989). *The primacy of caring: Stress and coping in health and illness.* Menlo Park, CA: Addison-Wesley.

Brykczynski, K. A. (1985). Exploring the clinical practice of nurse practitioners. [Doctoral dissertation, University of California, San Francisco.] *Dissertation Abstracts International*, 46, 3789B. (University Microfilms No. DA8600592.)

Brykczynski, K. A. (1993-1995). Principal investigator. Developing a profile of expert nursing practice. Project of the UTMB Nursing Service Task Force studying expert nursing practice, supported by UTMB Joint Ventures. Galveston, TX: University of Texas Medical Branch.

Brykczynski, K. A. (1998). Clinical exemplars describing expert staff nursing practice. *Journal of Nursing Management, 6*, 351-359.

Brykczynski, K. A. (1999). An interpretive study describing the clinical judgment of nurse practitioners. *Scholarly Inquiry for Nursing Practice: An International Journal, 13*(2), 141-166.

Cash, K. (1995). Benner and expertise in nursing: A critique. *International Journal of Nursing Studies, 32*(6), 527-534.

Chesla, C. A. (1996). Reconciling technologic and family care in critical-care nursing. *Image: The Journal of Nursing Scholarship, 28*(3), 199-203.

Christman, L. (1985). [Review of *From Novice to Expert* (1984) by Patricia Benner.] *Nursing Administration Quarterly, 9*(4), 87-89.

Clifford, J. (1999). Foreword. In P. Benner, P. Hooper-Kyriakidis, & D. Stannard (Eds.). *Clinical wisdom in critical care: A thinking-in-action approach.* Philadelphia: W. B. Saunders.

Crissman, S., & Jelsma, N. (1990). Cross-training: Practicing effectively on two levels. *Nursing Management, 21*(3), 64a-64h.

Darbyshire, P. (1994). Skilled expert practice: Is it "all in the mind"? A response to English's critique of Benner's novice to expert model. *Journal of Advanced Nursing, 19*, 755-761.

Day, L., & Benner, P. (2002). Ethics, ethical comportment, and etiquette. *American Journal of Critical Care, 11*(1), 76-79.

Dilthey, W. (1976). *Selected writings.* [H. P. Rickman, Trans. & Ed.] London: Cambridge University Press. (Original work published 1833-1911.)

Dolan, K. (1984). Building bridges between education and practice. In P. Benner (Ed.), *From novice to expert: Excellence and power in clinical nursing practice* (pp. 275-284). Menlo Park, CA: Addison-Wesley.

Dreyfus, H. L. (1979). *What computers can't do.* New York: Harper & Row.

Dreyfus, H. L. (1991). *Being-in-the-world: A commentary on being and time dimension. I.* Cambridge, MA: M. I. T. Press.

Dreyfus, H. L., & Dreyfus, S. E. (1986). *Mind over machine.* New York: The Free Press.

Dreyfus, H. L., & Dreyfus, S. E. (1996). The relationship of theory and practice in the acquisition of skill. In P. Benner, C. Tanner, & C. Chesla (Eds.), *Expertise in nursing practice: Caring, clinical judgment, and ethics* (pp. 29-47). New York: Springer.

Dreyfus, S. E., & Dreyfus, H. L. (1980, Feb.). *A five-stage model of the mental activities involved in directed skill acquisition.* Unpublished report supported by the Air Force Office of Scientific Research, USAF (Contract F49620-79-c-0063). Berkeley, CA: University of California, Berkeley.

Dunlop, M. J. (1986). Is a science of caring possible? *Journal of Advanced Nursing, 11*, 661-670.

Dunne, J. (1993). *Back to the rough ground: Practical judgment and the lure of technique.* Notre Dame. IN: Indiana University Press.

Eckle, N. J. (1996). Family presence—Where would you want to be? *Critical Care Nurse, 16*(1), 102.

English, I. (1993). Intuition as a function of the expert nurse: A critique of Benner's novice to expert model. *Journal of Advanced Nursing, 18*, 387-393.

Farrell, P., & Bramadat, I. J. (1990). Paradigm case analysis and stimulated recall: Strategies for developing clinical reasoning skills. *Clinical Nurse Specialist, 4*(3), 153-157.

Fenton, M. V. (1984). Identification of the skilled performance of master's prepared nurses as a method of curriculum planning and evaluation. In P. Benner (Ed.), *From novice to expert: Excellence and power in clinical nursing practice* (pp. 262-274). Menlo Park, CA: Addison-Wesley.

Fenton, M. V. (1985). Identifying competencies of clinical nurse specialists. *Journal of Nursing Administration, 15*(12), 31-37.

Fenton, M. V., & Brykczynski, K. A. (1993). Qualitative distinctions and similarities in the practice of clinical nurse specialists and nurse practitioners. *Journal of Professional Nursing, 9*(6), 313-326.

Gadamer, G. (1970). *Truth and method.* London: Sheer & Ward.

Gaston, C. (1989). Inservice education: Career development for South Australian nurses. *Australian Journal of Advanced Nursing, 6*(4), 5-9.

Gordon, D. R. (1984). Research application: Identifying the use and misuse of formal nursing models in nursing practice. In P. Benner (Ed.), *From novice to expert: Excellence and power in clinical nursing practice* (pp. 225-243). Menlo Park, CA: Addison-Wesley.

Gordon, D. R. (1986). Models of clinical expertise in American nursing practice. *Social Science and Medicine, 22*(9), 953-961.

Guba, E. G., & Lincoln, Y. S. (1982). Epistemological and methodological bases of naturalistic inquiry. *Educational Communications and Technology Journal, 30*, 233-252.

Hamric, A. B., Whitworth, T. R., & Greenfield, A. S. (1993). Implementing a clinically focused advancement system. *Journal of Nursing Administration, 23*(9), 20-28.

Heidegger, M. (1962). *Being and time.* [J. MacQuarrie & E. Robinson, Trans.] New York: Harper & Row.

Henderson, V. (1989). Foreword. In P. Benner & J. Wrubel (Eds.), *The primacy of caring: Stress and coping in health and illness.* Menlo Park, CA: Addison-Wesley.

Huntsman, A., Lederer, J. R., & Peterman, E. M. (1984). Implementation of staff nurse III at El Camino Hospital. In P. Benner (Ed.), *From novice to expert: Excellence and power in clinical nursing practice* (pp. 244-257). Menlo Park, CA: Addison-Wesley.

Kierkegaard, S. (1962). *The present age.* [A. Dur, Trans.] New York: Harper & Row.

Kleinman, A., Eisenberg, L., & Good, B. (1978). Culture, illness, and care: Clinical lessons from anthropologic and cross-cultural research. *Annals of Internal Medicine, 88*, 251-258.

Kuhn, T. S. (1970). *The structure of scientific revolutions* (2nd ed.). Chicago: University of Chicago Press.

Lazarus, R. S. (1985). The trivialization of distress. In J. C. Rosen & L. J. Solomon (Eds.), *Preventing health risk behaviors and promoting coping with illness* (vol 8, pp. 279-298). Hanover, NH: University Press of New England.

Lazarus, R. S., & Folkman, S. (1984). *Stress appraisals and coping.* New York: Springer.

Levy, K. (2004). Practices that facilitate critically burned children's healing. *Qualitative Health Research, 13*(10), 1-21.

Lindeke, L. L., Canedy, B. H., & Kay, M. M. (1997). A comparison of practice domains of clinical nurse specialists and nurse practitioners, *Journal of Professional Nursing, 13*(5), 281-287.

Lock, M., & Gordon, D. R. (Eds.). (1989). *Biomedicine examined.* Boston, MA: Kluwer Academic.

Løgstrup, K. E. (1995a). *Metaphysics* (vol I; R. L. Dees, Trans.). Milwaukee, WI: Marquette University Press.

Løgstrup, K. E. (1995b). *Metaphysics* (vol II; R. L. Dees, Trans.). Milwaukee, WI: Marquette University Press.

Løgstrup, K. E. (1997). *The ethical demand* (with introduction by A. MacIntyre & H. Fink). Notre Dame, IN: University of Notre Dame Press.

Lynaugh, J. (1999). Foreword. In P. Benner, P. Hooper-Kyriakidis, & D. Stannard (Eds.), *Clinical wisdom in critical care: A thinking-in-action approach.* Philadelphia: W. B. Saunders.

MacIntyre, A. (1981). *After virtue: a study in moral theory.* Notre Dame, IN: University of Notre Dame.

MacIntyre, A. (1999). *Dependent rational animals: Why human beings need the virtues.* Chicago: Open Court.

Martin, L. L. (1996). *Factors affecting performance of advanced nursing practice.* [Doctoral dissertation, Virginia Commonwealth University, School of Nursing.] (University Microfilms No. 9627443.)

Merleau-Ponty, M. (1962). *Phenomenology of perception.* [C. Smith, Trans.] London: Routledge and Kegan Paul.

Neverveld, M. E. (1990, July/Aug.). Preceptorship: One step beyond. *Journal of Nursing Staff Development, 6*(4), 186-189, 194.

Nuccio, S. A., Lingen, D., Burke, L. J., Kramer, A., Ladewig, N., Raum, J., et al. (1996). The clinical practice developmental model: The transition process. *Journal of Nursing Administration, 26*, 29-37.

O'Neill, O. (1996). *Towards justice and virtue: A constructive account of practical reasoning.* Cambridge, MA: Cambridge University Press.

Packer, M. J. (1985). Hermeneutic inquiry in the study of human conduct. *American Psychologist, 40*(10), 1081-1093.

Paley, J. (1996). Intuition and expertise: Comments on the Benner debate. *Journal of Advanced Nursing, 23*(4), 665-671.

Phillips, S., & Benner, P. (Eds.). (1994). *The crisis of care: Affirming and restoring caring practices in the helping professions.* Washington, DC: Georgetown University Press.

Polanyi, M. (1958). *Personal knowledge.* Chicago: University of Chicago Press.

Rubin, J. (1984). *Too much of nothing: Modern culture, the self and salvation in Kierkegaard's thought.* [Unpublished doctoral dissertation.] Berkeley, CA: University of California, Berkeley.

Schwartz, A. (2005). State of nursing education. *Science of Caring, 17*(1), 12-15.

Silver, M. (1986a). A program for career structure: A vision becomes a reality. *The Australian Nurse, 16*(2), 44-47.

Silver, M. (1986b). A program for career structure: From neophyte to expert. *The Australian Nurse, 16*(2), 38-41.

Taylor, C. (1971). Interpretation and the sciences of man. *The Review of Metaphysics, 25*, 3-34.

Taylor, C. (1982). Theories of meaning. Dawes Hicks Lecture. Read November 6, 1980. *Proceedings of the British Academy* (pp. 283-327). Oxford, UK: University Press.

Taylor, C. (1989). *Sources of the self: The making of modern identity.* Cambridge, MA: Harvard.

Taylor, C. (1991). *Ethics of authenticity.* Cambridge, MA: Harvard.

Taylor, C. (1993). Explanation and practical reason. In M. Nussbaum & A. Sen (Eds.). *The quality of life* (pp. 208-231). Oxford, UK: Clarendon.

Taylor, C. (1994). Philosophical reflections on caring practices. In S. S. Phillips & P. Benner (Eds.), *The crisis of care: Affirming and restoring caring practices in the helping professions* (pp. 174-187). Washington, DC: Georgetown University Press.

Ullery, J. (1984). Focus on excellence. In P. Benner (Ed.), *From novice to expert: Excellence and power in clinical nursing practice* (pp. 258-261). Menlo Park, CA: Addison-Wesley.

Visintainer, M. (1988). [Review of the book *The Primacy of Caring: Stress and Coping in Health and Illness.] Image: The Journal of Nursing Scholarship, 20*(2), 113-114.

BIBLIOGRAPHY*

Primary Sources

Books

Benner, P. (2001). *From novice to expert.* [Commemorative edition.] Upper Saddle River, NJ: Prentice Hall.

Benner, P. (2004). *The use of nursing narratives for reflecting on ethical and clinical judgment.* Tokyo, Japan: Shorinsha Publishers.

Gordon, S., Benner, P., & Noddings, N. (Eds.). (1996). *Caregiving readings in knowledge, practice, ethics, and politics.* Philadelphia: University of Pennsylvania Press.

Book Chapters

Benner, P. (1997). A dialogue between virtue ethics and care ethics. In D. Thomasma (Ed.), *The moral philosophy of Edmund Pellegrino* (pp. 47-61). Dordrecht, Netherlands: Kluwer.

Benner, P. (1998). When health care becomes a commodity: The need for compassionate strangers. In J. F. Kilner, R. D. Orr, & J. A. Shelly (Eds.), *The changing face of health care* (pp. 119-135). Grand Rapids, MI: William B. Eerdmans.

Benner, P. (1999). Parish nursing in the context of caring practices. In A. Solari-Twaddell (Ed.). *Parish nursing.* Thousand Oaks, CA: Sage.

Benner, P. (2001). The phenomenon of care. In S. K. Tombs (Ed.), *Handbook of phenomenology and medicine* (pp. 351-369). Dordrecht, Netherlands: Kluwer Academic Publishers.

Benner, P. (2002). Learning through experience and expression: Skillful ethical comportment in nursing practice. In E. D. Pellegrino, D. C. Thomasma, & J. L. Kissel (Eds.), *The healthcare professional as friend and healer: Building on the work of Edmund Pellegrino* (pp. 49-64). Washington, DC: Georgetown University Press.

Benner, P. (2003). Clinical reasoning articulating experiential learning in nursing practice. In O. Slevin & L. Basford (Eds.), *Theory and practice of nursing* (2nd ed., pp. 176-186). London, UK: Nelson Thornes Ltd.

Benner, P. (2005). Stigma and personal responsibility: Moral dimensions of a chronic illness. In R. B. Purtillo, G. M. Jensen, & R. C. Brasic (Eds.). *Educating for moral action: A sourcebook in health and rehabilitation ethics.* Philadelphia: F. A. Davis Co.

Benner, P. (2007). Experiential learning, skill acquisition and gaining clinical knowledge. In K. Obsborn, A. Wraa, A. Watson , & C. Wraa (Eds.). *Medical-surgical nursing.* Saddleback, NJ: Prentice-Hall.

Benner, P. (2007). Interpretive phenomenology. In L. M. Given (Ed.). *The Sage encyclopedia of qualitative methods.* Thousand Oaks, CA: Sage.

Benner, P., & Leonard, V. W. (2005). Patient concerns and choices and clinical judgment in EBP. In B. Melnyk & E. Fineout-Overholt (Eds.). *Evidence-based practice in nursing and healthcare: A guide to best practices.* Philadelphia: Lippincott

Benner, P., & Gordon, S. (1996). Caring practice. In S. Gordon, P. Benner, & N. Noddings (Eds.), *Caregiving, readings in knowledge, practice, ethics and politics* (pp. 40-55). Philadelphia: University of Pennsylvania Press.

Benner, P., & Leonard, V. W. (2005). Patient concerns, choices, and clinical judgment in evidence-based practice. In B. M. Mszurek (Ed.). *Evidence-based practice in nursing & healthcare: A guide to best practice* (pp. 163-182).

Benner P., & Sutphen, M. (2007). Clinical reasoning, decision-making in action: Thinking critically and clinically. In R. Hughes (Ed.), *Patient safety and quality for nursing center for primary care, prevention, & clinical partnerships.* Rockville, MD: Agency for Healthcare Research and Quality.

Journal Articles

Benner, P. (1996). A dialogue between virtue ethics and care ethics. *Theoretical Medicine, 23,* 1-15.

Benner, P. (1996). A response by P. Benner to K. Cash, Benner expertise in nursing: A critique. *International Journal of Nursing Studies, 33*(6), 669-674.

Benner, P. (2000). Seeing the person beyond the disease: Current controversies in critical care. *American Journal of Critical Care, 10*(2), 60-62.

Benner, P. (2000). The roles of embodiment, emotion and lifeworld for rationality and agency in nursing practice. *Nursing Philosophy, 1,* 5-19.

Benner, P. (2000). The wisdom of our practice. *AJN, 100*(10), 99-101, 103, 105.

Benner, P. (2001). Breathing new life into practice communities. *American Journal of Critical Care, 10*(3), 188-190.

Benner, P. (2001). Creating a culture of safety and improvement: A key to reducing medical error. *American Journal of Critical Care, 10*(4), 281-284.

Benner, P. (2001). Curing, caring, and healing in medicine: Symbiosis and synergy or syncretism? *Park Ridge Center Bulletin, 23,* 11-12.

Benner, P. (2001). Death as a human passage: Compassionate care for persons dying in critical care units. *American Journal of Critical Care, 10*(5), 355-359.

Benner, P. (2001). Developing clinical expertise in undergraduate education [in Japanese]. *Expert Nurse, 12*(15), 107-113.

Benner, P. (2001). Seeing the person beyond the disease: Current controversies in critical care. *American Journal of Critical Care, 10*(2), 121-124.

Benner, P. (2001). Taking a stand on experiential learning and good practice. *American Journal of Critical Care, 10*(1), 60-62.

Benner, P. (2002). Caring for the silent patient. *American Journal of Critical Care, 11*(5), 480-481.

Benner, P. (2002). Creating compassionate institutions that foster agency and respect. *American Journal of Critical Care, 11*(2), 164-166.

Benner, P. (2002). Living organ donors: Respecting the risks involved in the "gift of life." *American Journal of Critical Care, 11*(3), 266-268.

Benner, P. (2002). One year after September 11: Revisiting our ethical visions of freedom and justice. *American Journal of Critical Care, 11*(6), 572-573.

Benner, P. (2003). Avoiding ethical emergencies. *American Journal of Critical Care, 12*(1), 71-72.

Benner, P. (2003). Beware of technological imperatives and commercial interests that prevent best practices! *American Journal of Critical Care, 12*(5), 469-471.

Benner, P. (2003). [Book review for *From detached concern to empathy: Humanizing medical practice*, J. Halpern, Ed.] *The Cambridge Quarterly for Health Care Ethics, 12*(1), 134-136.

Benner, P. (2003). Creating a more responsible public dialogue about the social, ethical, and legal aspects of genomics. *American Journal of Critical Care, 12*(3), 259-261.

Benner, P. (2003). Enhancing patient advocacy and social ethics: Current controversies in critical care. *American Journal of Critical Care, 12*(4), 374-375.

Benner, P. (2003). Reflecting on what we care about: Current controversies in critical care. *American Journal of Critical Care, 12*(2), 165-166.

Benner, P. (2004). Designing formal classification systems to better articulate knowledge, skills, and meanings in nursing practice. *American Journal of Critical Care, 13*(5), 426-430.

Benner, P. (2004). Listening to past leaders. *American Journal of Critical Care, 13*(6), 510-511.

Benner, P. (2004). Nursing leaders as moral sources: In honor of Dr. Gloria Smith. *American Journal of Critical Care, 13*(3), 242-243.

Benner, P. (2004). Relational ethics of comfort, touch and solace—Endangered arts? *American Journal of Critical Care, 13*(4), 346-349.

Benner, P. (2004). Seeing the person beyond the disease: Current controversies in critical care. *American Journal of Critical Care, 13*(1), 75-78.

Benner, P. (2004). The dangers of geneticism. *Journal of Midwifery and Women's Press,* May-June; *49*(3), 260-262.

Benner, P. (2005). Extending the dialogue about classification systems and the work of professional nurses. *American Journal of Critical Care, 14*(3), 242-272.

Benner P. (2005). Honoring the good behind rights and justice in healthcare when more than justice is needed. *American Journal of Critical Care, 14*(2), 152-156.

Benner, P. (2005). Using the Dreyfus Model of Skill Acquisition to describe and interpret skill acquisition and clinical judgment in nursing practice and education. *The Bulletin of Science, Technology and Society Special Issue: Human Expertise in the Age of the Computer, 24*(3), 188-199.

Benner, P., Brennan, M. R., Sr., Kessenich, C. R., & Letvak, S. A. (1996). Critique of Silva's philosophy, science and theory: Interrelationships and implications for nursing research. *Image: The Journal of Nursing Scholarship, 29*(3), 214-215.

Benner, P., Ekegren, K., Nelson, G., Tsolinas, T., & Ferguson-Dietz, L. (1997). The nurse as a wise, skillful and compassionate stranger. *American Journal of Nursing, 97*(11), 27-34.

Benner, P., Kerchner, S., Corless, I. B., & Davies, B. (2003). Current controversies in critical care: Attending death as a human passage: Core nursing principles for end-of-life care. *American Journal of Critical Care, 12*(6), 558-561.

Benner P., & Sutphen, M. (2007). Learning across the professions: The clergy, a case in point. *Journal of Nursing Education, 46*(3).

Benner, P., Sutphen, M., Leonard, V., & Day, L. (2007). Learning to see and think like a nurse: Clinical reasoning and caring practices. *Journal of Japanese Society of Nursing Research, 30*(1), 20-24.

Benner, P., Stannard, D., & Hooper, P. L. (1996). "Thinking-in-action" approach to teaching clinical judgment: A classroom innovation for acute care advanced practice nurses. *Advanced Practice Nursing Quarterly, 1,* 70-77.

Benner, P., Tanner, C. A., & Chesla, C. A. (1996). Nurse practitioner extra: Becoming an expert nurse. (Adapted with permission from Benner, Tanner, & Chesla [Eds.]. *Expertise in nursing practice: Caring, clinical judgment, and ethics.* New York: Springer Publishing.) *AJN, 97*(6), Contin Care Extra Ed, 16BBB, 16DDD.

Benner, P., Tanner, C. A., & Chesla, C. A. (1996). The social fabric of nursing knowledge. (Adapted with permission from Benner, Tanner, & Chesla [Eds.]. *Expertise in nursing practice: Caring, clinical judgment, and ethics.* New York: Springer Publishing.) *AJN, 97*(7), Nurse Pract Extra Ed, 16BBB.

Benner, P., et al. (1996). Survey reactions of nursing leaders: A grim prognosis for health care? *AJN, 96*(11), 43.

Brant, M., Rosen, L., & Benner, P. (1998, Nov.). Nurses as skilled samaritans: The nurse as wise, skillful, and compassionate stranger. *AJN, 98*(4), Contin Care Extra Ed, 22-23.

Cohen H., & Benner, P. (2002). Errors in nursing: Individual, practice, and system causes of errors in nursing: A taxonomy. *JONA, 32*(10), 509-523.

Dracup, K., Cronenwett, L., Meleis, A., & Benner, P. (2005). Reflections on the doctorate of nursing practice. *Nursing Outlook,* Jul-Aug *53*(4):177-182.

Ekegren, K., Nelson, G., Tsolinas, A., Ferguson-Dietz, L., & Benner, P. (1997). The nurse as wise, skillful, and compassionate stranger. *AJN, 97,* 26-34.

Emami, A., Benner, P., & Ekman, S. L. (2001). A sociocultural health model for late-in-life immigrants. *Journal of Transcultural Nursing, 12*(1), 15-24.

Emami, A., Benner, P., Lipson, J. G., & Ekman, S. L. (2001). Health as continuity and balance in life. *Western Journal of Nursing Research, 22,* 812-825.

Fowler, M., & Benner, P. (2001). The new code of ethics for nurses: A dialogue with Marsha Fowler. *American Journal of Critical Care, 10*(6), 434-437.

Harrington, C., Crider, M. C., Benner, P., & Malone, R. (2005). Advanced nursing training in health policy: Designing and implementing a new program. *Policy, Politics & Nursing Practice, 6*(2), 99-108.

Puntillo, K. A., Benner, P., Drought, T., Drew, B., Stotts, N., Stannard, D., et al. (2001). End-of-life issues in intensive care units: A national random survey of nurses' knowledge and beliefs. *American Journal of Critical Care, 10*(4), 216-229.

Spichiger, E., Wallhagen, M., & Benner, P. (2005). Nursing as a caring practice from a phenomenological perspective. *Scandinavian Journal of Caring Sciences, 19*(4), 303-309.

Sullivan, W., & Benner, P., (2005). Challenges to professionalism: Work integrity and the call to renew and strengthen the social contract of the professions. *American Journal of Critical Care, 14*(1), 78-84.

Weiss, S. M., Malone, R. E., Merighi, J. R., & Benner, P. (2002). Economism, efficiency, and the moral ecology of good nursing practice. *Canadian Journal of Nursing Research, 34*(2), 95-119.

Secondary Sources

Doctoral Dissertations

The following doctoral dissertations were supervised by Patricia Benner:

Boller, J. E. (2001). The ecology of exercise: An interpretive phenomenological account of exercise in the lifeworld of persons on maintenance hemodialysis. [Doctoral dissertation, University of California, San Francisco.] *Dissertation Abstracts International,* B62/12, 5638. (University Microfilms No. 3034743.)

Brykczynski, K. A. (1985). Exploring the clinical practice of nurse practitioners. [Doctoral dissertation, University of California, San Francisco.] *Dissertation Abstracts International, 46,* 3789B. (University Microfilms No. DA8600592.)

Chan, G. K. (2005). E.R.= exit required. A philosophical, theoretical, and phenomenological investigation of care at the end-of-life in the emergency department. [Doctoral dissertation, University of California, San Francisco.] *Dissertation Abstracts International,* B66/06, 3054. (University Microfilms No. 3179943.)

Chesla, C. A. (1988). Parents' caring practices and coping with schizophrenic offspring, an interpretive study. [Doctoral dissertation, University of California, San Francisco.] *Dissertation Abstracts International* 49-B, 2563. (University Microfilms No. AAD88-13331.)

Cho, A. (2001). Understanding the lived experience of heart transplant recipients in North America and South Korea: An interpretive phenomenological cross-cultural study. [Doctoral dissertation, University of California, San Francisco.] *Dissertation Abstracts International,* B62/12, 5639. (University Microfilms No. 3034721.)

Day, L. J. (1999). Nursing care of potential organ donors: An articulation of ethics, etiquette and practice. [Doctoral dissertation, University of California, San Francisco.] *Dissertation Abstracts International, 60-B,* 5431. (University Microfilms No. AADAA-19951464.)

Doolittle, N. (1990). Life after stroke. [Doctoral dissertation, University of California, San Francisco.] *Dissertation Abstracts International, 51-B,* 1742. (University Microfilms No. AAD90-24963.)

Dunlop, M. (1990). Shaping nursing knowledge: An interpretive analysis of curriculum documents from NSW Australia. [Doctoral dissertation, University of California, San Francisco.] *Dissertation Abstracts International, 51-B,* 659. (University Microfilms No. AAD90-16380.)

Gordon, D. (1984). Expertise, formalism, and change in American nursing practice: A case study. Medical anthropology program. [Doctoral dissertation, University of California, San Francisco.] *Dissertation Abstracts International, 46-A,* 738. (University Microfilms No. AAD85-09101.)

Hartfield, M. (1985). Appraisal of anger situations and subsequent coping responses in hypertensive and normotensive adults: A comparison. [Doctoral dissertation, University of California, San Francisco.] *Dissertation Abstracts International, 46-B,* 4452. (University Microfilms No. AAD85-24005.)

Hooper, P. L. (1995). Expert titration of multiple vasoactive drugs in post-cardiac surgical patients: An interpretive study of clinical judgment and perceptual acuity. [Doctoral dissertation, University of California, San Francisco.] *Dissertation Abstracts International, 57-B,* 238. (University Microfilms No. AAD85-19614338.)

Kesselring, A. (1990). The experienced body, when taken-for-grantedness falters: A phenomenological study of living with breast cancer. [Doctoral dissertation, University of California, San Francisco.] *Dissertation Abstracts International, 52-B,* 1955. (University Microfilms No. AAD91-19579.)

Kinavey, C. (2003). Adolescents living with spina bifida: Moving from parental to self-care. [Doctoral dissertation, University of California, San Francisco.] *Dissertation Abstracts International.* (University Microfilms No. 3051044.)

Leonard, V. W. (1993). Stress and coping in the transition to parenthood of first time mothers with career commitments: An interpretive study. [Doctoral dissertation, University of California, San Francisco.] *Dissertation Abstracts International, 54-A,* 3221. (University Microfilms No. AAD94-02354.)

Lionberger, H. (1986). Phenomenological study of therapeutic touch in nursing practice: An interpretive study of nurses' practice of therapeutic touch. [Doctoral dissertation, University of California, San Francisco.] *Dissertation Abstracts International, 46-B,* 2624. (University Microfilms No. AAD85-24008.)

MacIntyre, R. (1993). Sex, drugs, and T-cell counts in the gay community: Symbolic meanings among gay men with asymptomatic HIV infections (immune deficiency). [Doctoral dissertation, University of California, San Francisco.] *Dissertation Abstracts International, 54-B,* 4601. (University Microfilms No. AAD94-06617.)

Mahrer-Imhof, R. (2003). Couples' daily experiences after the onset of cardiac disease: An interpretive phenomenological study. [Doctoral dissertation, University of California, San Francisco.]

Malone, R. (1995). The almshouse revisited: Heavy users of emergency services. [Doctoral dissertation, University of California, San Francisco.] *Dissertation Abstracts International, 56-B,* 6036. (University Microfilms No. AADAA-19606591.)

McKeever, L. C. (1988). Menopause: An uncertain passage. An interpretive study. [Doctoral dissertation, University of California, San Francisco.] *Dissertation Abstracts International, 49-B,* 3677. (University Microfilms No. AAD88-24678.)

Plager, K. A. (1995). Practical well-being in families with school-age children: An interpretive study. [Doctoral dissertation, University of California, San Francisco.] *Dissertation Abstracts International, 56-B,* 6039. (University Microfilms No. AADAA-16906593.)

Popell, C. L. (1983). An interpretive study of stress and coping among parents of school-age developmentally disabled children. [Doctoral dissertation, Wright Institute of Graduate Psychology.] *Dissertation Abstracts International, 44-B,* 1604. (University Microfilms No. AAD83-20854.)

Prakke, H. (2004). Articulating maternal caregivers' concerns, knowledge and needs. [Doctoral dissertation,

University of California, San Francisco.] *Dissertation Abstracts International.* (University Microfilms No. 3149700.)

Raingruber, B. J. (1998). Moving in a climate of care: Styles and patterns of interaction between nurse-therapists and clients: An interpretive study. [Doctoral dissertation, University of California, San Francisco.] *Dissertation Abstracts International, 58-B*, 6482. (University Microfilms No. AAD98-18661.)

Rodriguez, L. (2007). Student and faculty experiences of practice breakdown and error in nursing school. [Doctoral dissertation, University of California, San Francisco.] *Dissertation Abstracts International.* (University Microfilms No. 3289350.)

Schilder, E. (1986). The use of physical restraints in an acute care medical ward (immobilization). [Doctoral dissertation, University of California, San Francisco.] *Dissertation Abstracts International, 47-B*, 4826. (University Microfilms No. AAD87-08453.)

SmithBattle, L. (1992). Caring for teenage mothers and their children: Narratives of self and ethics of intergenerational caregiving. [Doctoral dissertation, University of California, San Francisco.] *Dissertation Abstracts International, 53-B*, 4594. (University Microfilms No. AAD93-03555.)

Spichiger, E. (2004). Dying patients' and their families' experiences of hospital end-of-life care. [Doctoral dissertation, University of California, San Francisco.] *Dissertation Abstracts International.* (University Microfilms No. 3136071.)

Stannard, P. (1997). Reclaiming the house: An interpretive study of nurse-family interactions and activities in critical care. [Doctoral dissertation, University of California, San Francisco.] *Dissertation Abstracts International, 58-B*, 4147. (University Microfilms No. AAD98-06902.)

Stevens, M. (1984). Adolescents coping with hospitalization for surgery. [Doctoral dissertation, University of California, San Francisco.] *Dissertation Abstracts International, 45-B*, 3977. (University Microfilms No. AAD85-03742.)

Stuhlmiller, C. (1991). An interpretive study of appraisal and coping of rescue workers in an earthquake disaster: The Cypress collapse. [Doctoral dissertation, University of California, San Francisco.] *Dissertation Abstracts International, 52-B*, 4671. (University Microfilms No. AAD92-05240.)

Warnian, L. (1987). *A hermeneutical study of group psychotherapy.* [Unpublished doctoral dissertation.] Berkeley, CA: University of California, Berkeley.

Weiss, S. M. (1996). Possibility or despair: Biographies of aging. [Doctoral dissertation, University of California, San Francisco.] *Dissertation Abstracts International, 57-B*, 3662. (University Microfilms No. AAD96-34295.)

Videotape

Moccia, R. (1987). *Nursing theory: A circle of knowledge* (Videotape). New York: National League for Nursing.

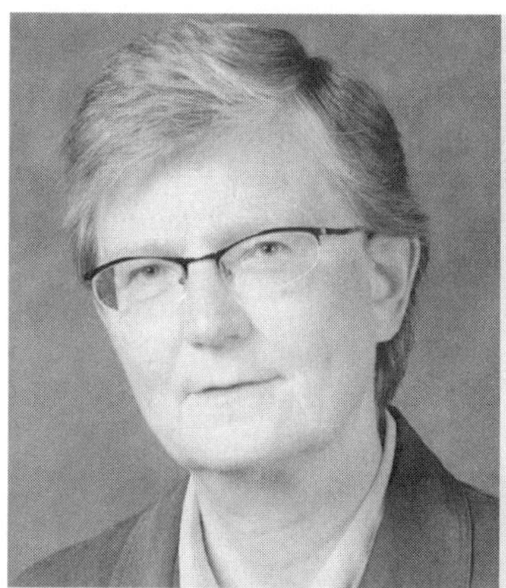

Photo credit: Lars Jakob Løtvedt, Bergen Norway.

CHAPTER 10

Kari Martinsen

1943-present

Philosophy of Caring

Herdis Alvsvåg

"Nursing is founded on caring for life, on neighbourly love, . . . At the same time it is necessary that the nurse is professionally educated" (Martinsen, 2006, p. 78).

CREDENTIALS AND BACKGROUND OF THE THEORIST

Kari Marie Martinsen, a nurse and philosopher, was born in Oslo, the capital of Norway, in 1943, during the WW II German occupation of Norway. Her parents were both engaged in the Resistance Movement. After the war, moral and sociopolitical discussions dominated home life, a home that consisted of three generations: a younger sister, parents, and a grandmother. Both parents were economists who were educated at the University of Oslo. Her mother worked all of her adult life outside the home.

After high school, Martinsen began her studies at Ullevål College of Nursing in Oslo, graduating in 1964. She worked in clinical practice at Ullevål hospital for 1 year, while doing preparatory studies for university entry. Before embarking upon a university degree, she specialized as a psychiatric nurse in 1966 and worked for 2 years at Dikemark Psychiatric Hospital near Oslo, where she also was engaged for several years in psychiatric care of outpatients.

While practicing as a nurse, she became concerned about social inequalities in general and in the health service in particular. Health, illness, care, and treatment were obviously distributed unequally. She also became disturbed over perceived discrepancies between healthcare theories, ideals, and goals on the one hand, and practical results of nursing, medicine, and the health service on the other. She began to pose questions about how a society and a profession must be constituted to support and aid the ill and the unemployed. One particularly poignant question was, How the nursing profession must operate

Translators: Vigdis Elisabeth Brekke, Bjørn Follevåg, and Kirsten Costain Schou.

if it is not to let down its weakest patients and those that need care the most. The obvious follow-up question was how the nurse might be able to care for the patient when medical science first and foremost relates to patient's diseases? In other words, Martinsen wanted to know how we who represent the health services provide adequate nursing for the subjects of our care, when we are so closely allied with a science that objectifies the patient. She posed questions about whether that same objectification will increase with the emphasis on a scientific base for the discipline of nursing.

These fundamental questions urged Martinsen to take up additional studies, this time for a bachelor's degree in psychology at the University of Oslo in 1968, with the goal of obtaining a master's degree in psychology. As a prerequisite, she needed an intermediate examination in physiology and another free credit at the intermediate level; here she chose philosophy. This encounter with philosophy and phenomenology changed her plans drastically. She realized that philosophy rather than psychology might better illuminate the existential questions with which she was concerned. The study of phenomenology attracted her to the University of Bergen, Norway's second largest city.

From 1972 to 1974, she attended the Department of Philosophy at the University of Bergen. In her work for the graduate degree in philosophy (Magister artium), Martinsen grappled philosophically with questions that had disturbed her as a citizen, a professional, and a healthcare worker. The dissertation *Philosophy and Nursing: A Marxist and Phenomenological Contribution* (Martinsen, 1975) created an instant debate and received much critical attention. The dissertation directed a critical gaze toward the nursing profession for its refusal to take up or take seriously the consequences of the nursing discipline uncritically adopting the characteristics of a profession, and uncritically embracing only a scientific basis for nursing. Such a development might contribute to distancing nurses from the patients who need them most. This dissertation, the first written by a nurse in Norway, analyzed the discipline of nursing from a critical philosophical and social perspective.

During the mid-1970s, Norway experienced a marked shortage of nursing teachers. The rectors of three nursing colleges in Bergen took the initiative to establish a temporary nursing teacher–training course to address this problem. The course was established jointly by the University of Bergen, the county authorities, and three nursing colleges. A nurse with university level qualifications was needed to head the program. Martinsen was asked to be Dean of the Faculty of Nursing Teachers' Training in Bergen, which she accepted from 1976 to 1977.

Through her philosophical studies and the sociological issues she encountered in practical nursing and in nursing education, Martinsen developed an interest in nursing history. How did education of nurses in Norway begin, who was responsible for its inception, and what did they wish to achieve? In order to look more closely at some of these issues, Martinsen applied for and received a grant from the Norwegian Nurses' Association in 1976. She was affiliated with the Department of Hygiene and Social Medicine at the University of Bergen, where she lectured not only to her students in the nursing teachers' training program but also to medical students in social medicine.

At that time, an intense debate over nursing education was raging in Norway. A public commission proposed retention of the traditional 3-year degree but eventually agreed to alter this to a system of stage-based qualification. This meant that after completion of 1 year, a student became a qualified care assistant, and after 2 additional years, a qualified nurse. This implied the end of the principle of a comprehensive 3-year degree. Nurses throughout the country, with the Norwegian Nurses' Association at the forefront, marched in protest to save the 3-year nursing degree. Sides in this debate remained rigidly opposed, and the tone of the political discourse on the issue of nursing education was heated. Martinsen threw herself into this debate. She suggested that nursing education be changed to a 4-year program, but she also gave her approval to the principle of stage-based education. She sketched an educational model in which one is qualified as a care assistant after 2 years and as a nurse after 4 years (Martinsen, 1976). With the comprehensive 3-year degree as the stated goal for the nursing association, her suggestion was viewed as a provocation.

In 1978, she received a grant from Norway's General Science Research Council. At this time, she was attached to the History Department at the University of Oslo, where she worked on her new project on the social history of nursing, while lecturing master's degree students in sociopolitical history. From 1981 to 1985, she was a scientific assistant at the History Department at the University of Bergen. In addition to conducting her own research, Martinsen lectured and supervised master's degree students in feminist history and developed a database of Norwegian feminist history.

The period from 1976 to 1986 can be described as a historical phase in Martinsen's work (Kirkevold, 2000). She published several historical articles (Martinsen, 1977, 1978, 1979a, 1979b). Close collaborators during this phase were Anne Lise Seip, professor of social history, Ida Blom, professor of feminist history, and Kari Wærness, professor of sociology. In 1979, Martinsen and Wærness published a "lit torch" of a book with the provocative title, *Caring Without Care?* (Martinsen & Wærness, 1979). In this book, the authors raised important questions about whether nurses were "moving away" from the sickbed, whether caring for the ill and infirm was disappearing with the advent of increasingly technical care and treatment, and whether nurses were becoming administrators and researchers who increasingly relinquished the concrete execution of care to other occupational groups.

Aiding ill and care-dependent people was considered women's work, and this view has long historical roots. However, the existence of the professionally trained nurse is not very old in Norway, originating in the late 1800s. The deaconesses (Christian lay sisters), who were educated at different deaconess houses in Germany, were the first trained health workers in Norway. Martinsen described how these first trained nurses built up a nursing education in Norway, and how they expanded and wrote textbooks and practiced nursing both in institutions and in homes. They were the forerunners of Norway's public health system. This pioneer period was described by Martinsen in her book, *Nursing History: Frank and Engaged Deaconesses: A Caring Profession Emerges 1860-1905* (Martinsen, 1984). Based on this work, Martinsen attained the doctor of philosophy degree from the University of Bergen in 1984.

In defense of her dissertation, Martinsen had to prepare two lectures: "Health Policy Problems and Health Policy Thinking behind the Hospital Law of 1969" (Martinsen, 1989a), and "The Doctors' Interest in Pregnancy—Part of Perinatal Care: The Period ca. 1890-1940" (Martinsen, 1989b). This work emerged from her 10-year historical phase, beginning in the mid-70s, when she wrote about nursing's social history and feminist history, as well as on the social history of medicine.

From 1986, Martinsen worked for 2 years as Associate Professor at the Department of Health and Social Medicine at the University of Bergen. She lectured and supervised master's degree students, in addition to writing a series of philosophical and historical papers, published in 1989 under the title *Caring, Nursing and Medicine: Historical-Philosophical Essays* (Martinsen, 1989c). With this book, the threads of Martinsen's historical phase were drawn together, marking the beginning of a more philosophical period (Kirkevold, 2000). The book has several editions, and the 2003 publication includes a lengthy interview with the author (Karlsson & Martinsen, 2003). Fundamental problems in caring and interpretations of the meaning of discernment are what preoccupied Martinsen from 1985 to 1990. In a Danish anthology published in 1990, she contributed a paper entitled "Moral Practice and Documentation in Practical Nursing." Here she writes:

> Moral practice is based upon *caring.* Caring does not merely form the value foundation of nursing; it is a fundamental precondition of our life . . . Discernment demands emotional involvement and the capacity for situational analysis in order to assess

> alternatives for action . . . To learn moral practice in nursing is to learn how the moral is founded in concrete situations. It is accounted for through experiential objectivity or through discretion, in action or in speech. In both cases learning good nursing is of the essence (Martinsen, 1990, pp. 60, 64-65).

In 1990, Martinsen moved to Denmark for a 5-year period. She was employed at the University of Århus to establish master's degree and PhD programs in nursing. Her philosophical foundation was further developed during these years mainly through encounters with Danish life philosophy (Martinsen, 2002a) and theological tradition. In *Caring, Nursing and Medicine: Historical-Philosophical Essays,* Martinsen (1989c, 2003b) had connected the concept of caring to the German philosopher Martin Heidegger (1889-1976). While she was living in Denmark, Heidegger's role as a Nazi sympathizer during WW II became public knowledge. At that time, a series of academic articles were published, which proved that Heidegger was a member of the national Socialist Party in Germany, and that he had betrayed his Jewish colleagues and friends such as Edmund Husserl (1859-1938) and Hannah Arendt (1906-1975). Heidegger was banned from teaching for several years after the war because of his involvement with the Nazis (Lubcke, 1983).

Martinsen confronted Heidegger and her own thinking about his philosophy in *From Marx to Løgstrup: On Morality, Social Criticism and Sensuousness in Nursing* (Martinsen, 1993b). Precisely because life and learning cannot be separated, it became important for Martinsen to go to sources other than Heidegger to illustrate the fundamental aspects of caring. Knud E. Løgstrup (1905-1981) was the Danish theologian and philosopher who became her alternative source, although the two never met. Martinsen knew him through his books and via his wife Rosemarie Løgstrup, who was originally German. She met her husband in Germany, where both were studying philosophy. She later translated his books into German.

While Martinsen lived and worked in Denmark, she met with Patricia Benner on several occasions for public dialogues in Norway and Denmark, and again in 1996 in California. One of these dialogues was later published with the title, "Ethics and Vocation, Culture and the Body" (Martinsen, 1997b); it took place at a conference at the University of Tromsø.

Martinsen also had important dialogues with Katie Eriksson, the Finnish professor of nursing. They met in Norway, Denmark, Sweden, and Finland. In the beginning, their discussions were tense and strained, but over time, they developed into fruitful and enlightening conversations that later were published as *Phenomenology and Caring: Three Dialogues* (Martinsen, 1996). Martinsen's first chapter in this book is titled "Caring and Metaphysics—Has Nursing Science Got Room for This?" the second, "The Body and Spirit in Practical Nursing," and the third, "The Phenomenology of Creation—Ethics and Power: Løgstrup's Philosophy of Religion Meets Nursing Practice." These headings employ impressive language, similar to that of the dialogues that Martinsen conducted with Benner; in her preface to the book, she elaborates:

> The words about which we speak and write are compassion, hope, suffering, pain, sacrifice, shame, violation, doubt. These are "big words." But they are no bigger than their location in life, our everyday nursing situation. Mercy, writes the Danish theologian and philosopher Løgstrup, is the renewal of life, it is to afford others life . . . . What else is nursing but to release the patient's possibilities for living a meaningful life within the life cycle we inhabit between life and death? We must venture into life amongst our fellow humans in order to experience the actual meaning of these big words (Martinsen, 1996, p. 7).

While Martinsen was teaching in Århus, she became Adjunct Professor at the Department of Nursing Science at the University of Tromsø in 1994. In 1997, she moved north and become a full-time professor. However, needing more time for her research and writings, she left after only 1 year in this position to become a freelancer in 1998.

The period from 1990 is characterized by philosophical research. Fundamental philosophical and ontological questions and their meaning for nursing dominated Martinsen's thought. During this period, in addition to her own books, she worked on a variety of projects and published in several journals and anthologies. Books from this period have already been mentioned (Martinsen, 1993b, 1996). In 2000, *The Eye and the Call* (Martinsen, 2000b) was published. The titles of the chapters in this book ring more poetically than before: "To See with the Eye of the Heart," "Ethics, Culture and the Vulnerability of the Flesh," "The Calling—Can We Be Without It?" and "The Act of Love and the Call."

Martinsen also worked with ideas about space and architecture. According to her, space and architecture can influence human dignity. She first wrote about this idea in an article with the poetic title, "The House and the Song, the Tears and the Shame: Space and Architecture as Caretakers of Human Dignity" (Martinsen, 2001). In 2004, she was working on a book project about space and architecture within the health service. This has been interrupted because of her engagement in discussions about the role of evidence-based medicine in nursing practice (Martinsen 2005, 2008).

Martinsen has held positions at two nursing colleges. From 1989 to 1990, she was employed as researcher at Bergen Deaconess University College, Bergen. From 1999 to 2004, she was adjunct Professor at Lovisenberg Deaconess University College, Oslo. Ideas and academic ventures sprouted and flourished easily around her, and she drew others into academic projects. She edited a collection of articles which several nursing college teachers contributed to, called *The Thoughtful Nurse* (Martinsen, 1993a). Lovisenberg Deaconess University College in Oslo, with Martinsen's assistance, took the initiative to publish a new edition of the first Norwegian nursing textbook, which was originally published in 1877 (Nissen, 2000). In this edition, Martinsen (2000a) wrote an Afterword, placing the text within a context of academic nursing. Together with a colleague in Oslo, Martinsen edited another collection of articles. In addition to the editors, college lecturers again contributed articles to the book, published as *Ethics, Discipline, and Refinement: Elizabeth Hagemann's Ethics Book—New Readings* (Martinsen & Wyller, 2003). This book provides an analysis of a text on ethics for nurses published in 1930 and used as a textbook right up to 1965. When the ethics text was republished in 2003, it was interpreted in the light of two French philosophers, Pierre Bourdieu (1930-2002) and Michel Foucault (1926-1984), as well as the German sociologist Max Weber (1864-1920).

With these last publications, Martinsen returned to her roots in history. Historical and philosophical threads seem to merge. Both are present in different phases of her thought, but they color her work differently during the different periods.

In 2002, Martinsen made her way back to the University of Bergen as professor at the Department of Public Health and Primary Health Care section for nursing science. Teaching master's and doctoral students was central. She arranged doctoral courses and was much in demand in the Nordic countries as supervisor and lecturer. Again, she experienced a lack of time for her research. Therefore, she became a part-time professor at Bergen Deaconess University College in 2006, and from 2007, a full-time professor at Harstad University College, in northern Norway.

THEORETICAL SOURCES

What is Martinsen's *theoretical background*? In her analysis of the profession of nursing in the early 1970s, Martinsen looked to three philosophers in particular: Karl Marx (1818-1883), the German philosopher, politician, and social theorist; Edmund Husserl (1859-1938), the German philosopher and founder of phenomenology; and Merleau-Ponty (1908-1961), the French philosopher and phenomenologist of the body. Later, she broadened her theoretical sources to include other philosophers, theologians, and sociologists.

Karl Marx: Critical Analysis—A Transformative Practice

Marxist philosophy gave Martinsen some analytical tools with which to describe the reality of the discipline of nursing and the social crisis in which it found itself. This crisis consisted of the failure of the discipline to examine and recognize its nature as fragmented, specialized, and technically calculating, as it pretends to hold a holistic perspective on care. She found that the discipline was part of positivism and the capitalist system, without praxis of liberation. A "reversed care–law" rules in such a way that those who need care most receive the least. Marx criticized individualism and the satisfaction of the needs of the rich at the expense of the poor. Martinsen's view is that it is important to expose this phenomenon when it occurs in the health service. Such exposure of this reality can be a force for change. She maintains that we must question the nature of nursing, its content and inner structure, its historical origins, and the genesis of the profession. This can result in a critical nursing practice in which the practitioner views her occupation and profession in a historical and social context. Thus her historical interest has a critical and transformative intention.

Edmund Husserl: Phenomenology as the Natural Attitude

Husserl's phenomenology is important for Martinsen's critiques of science and positivism. Positivism's view of the self lies in its attitude of objectification and its dehumanizing (in the sense of reducing self to the nature of "thing"), calculating attitude toward the person. Husserl viewed phenomenology as a strict science. The strict methodological processes of phenomenology produce an attitude of composed reflection over our scientific reality, so that we may uncover structures and contexts within which we otherwise perform taken-for-granted and unconscious work. This practice is about making the taken-for-granted problematic. By problematizing taken-for-granted self-understanding, we find opportunities to grasp "the thing itself," which will always reveal itself perspectively. Phenomenology works with the prescientific, what we encounter in the natural attitude, when we are directed toward something with the intent to recognize and understand it meaningfully. Phenomenology insists upon context, wholeness, involvement, engagement, the body, and the lived life. We live in contexts, in time and space, and we live historically. The body cannot be divided into body and soul; it is a wholeness that relates to other bodies, to things in the world, and to nature.

Merleau-Ponty: The Body as the Natural Attitude

Merleau-Ponty builds upon Husserl's thought, but focuses more than any other thinker on the human body in the world. Both Husserl and Merleau-Ponty criticized Descartes (1596-1650), who separates the person from the world in which one lives with other persons. The body is representing the natural attitude in the world. The nursing profession relates to the body in all its aspects. We use our own bodies in the performance of caring, and we relate to other bodies who are in need of nursing, treatment, and care. Our bodies and those of our patients express themselves through actions, attitudes, words, tone of voice, and gestures. Phenomenology involves acts of interpretation, description, and recognition of lived life, the everyday life that people live together with others in a mutual natural world, including the professional contexts in which caring is performed.

Martin Heidegger: Existential Being as Caring

Martin Heidegger (1889-1976) was a German phenomenologist and a student of Husserl, among others. He investigated existential being, that is to say, that which is and how it is. Martinsen connects the concept of caring to Heidegger because he "has caring as a central concept in his thought . . . . The point is to try to elicit the fundamental qualities of caring, or what caring is and encompasses" (Martinsen, 1989c, p. 68). She continues: "An analysis of our practical life and an analysis of what caring is, are inseparable. To investigate the one is at the same time to investigate the other. Together, they form an inseparable unit. Caring is a fundamental concept in understanding the person" (Martinsen, 1989c, p. 69). With phenomenology and Heidegger as a backdrop, Martinsen gives content and substance to caring: caring will always have at least two parts as a precondition. One is concerned and anxious for the other. Caring involves how we relate to each other, and how we show concern for each other in our daily life. Caring is the most natural and the most fundamental aspect of human existence.

As was mentioned earlier, Martinsen revised her perspective on Heidegger (Martinsen, 1993b). At the same time, she did not reject "Heidegger's original and acute thought" (Martinsen, 1993b, p. 17). She turns back to Heidegger when she explains what it means to dwell. Heidegger had examined precisely the concept that to dwell is always to live amongst things (Martinsen, 2001). Here we may note that Heidegger reinforces an idea also maintained by Merleau-Ponty: that the things we surround ourselves with are not merely things for us, objectively speaking, but they actually participate in shaping our lives. We leave something of ourselves within these things when we dwell amidst them. It is the body that dwells, surrounded by an environment.

Knud Eiler Løgstrup: Ethics as a Primary Condition of Human Existence

K. E. Løgstrup (1905-1981), the Danish philosopher and theologian, became important for Martinsen in the "void" left by Heidegger. Løgstrup can be summarized through two intellectual strands: phenomenology and creation theology, the latter containing his philosophy of religion (creation theology should not be confused with the more recent "creationism" in the United States). As a phenomenologist, he sought to reveal and analyze the essential phenomena of human existence. Through his phenomenological investigations, Løgstrup arrived at what he termed *sovereign* or *spontaneous life utterances:* trust, hope, compassion, and the openness of speech. That these are essential is to say that they are precultural characteristics of our existence. As characteristics, they provide conditions for our culture, conditions for our existence; they make human community possible (Lubcke, 1983). According to Heidegger, caring is such a characteristic. In Løgstrup's opinion, the sovereign life utterances were the necessary characteristics for human coexistence.

Martinsen maintains that for Løgstrup, metaphysics and ethics are interwoven in the concept of creation:

> They are characteristic phenomena which sustain us in such a way that caring for the other arises out of the condition of our having been created. Caring for the other reveals itself in human relationship through trust, open speech, hope and compassion. These phenomena, which Løgstrup also calls sovereign life utterances, are "born ethical" whish means that they are essentially ethical. Trust, open speech, hope and compassion are fundamentally good in them selves without requiring our justification. If we try to gain dominance over them, they will be destroyed. Metaphysics and ethics, or rather metaphysical ethics, is practical. It is linked to questions of life in which the person is stripped of omnipotence (Martinsen, 1993b, pp. 17-18).

We must care for that which exists, not seek to control it: "Western culture is singular in its need to understand and control. It has moved away from the cradle of our culture and our religion in the narrative of creation from the Old Testament. In The Old Testament 'guarding,' 'watching,' and 'caring' on one side, and cultivating and using on the other, formed a unified opposition" (Martinsen, 1996, p. 79). That these are unified opposites is to say that they singularly and in themselves are opposites that separate and are insurmountable, but when they are adjusted to one another, they enter into an opposition that unifies and creates a sound whole. To care for, guide and guard, cultivate and make use of, that is to say, cultivate and use in a caring manner as a unified opposition, means that we do not become domineering and exploitative, but restrained and considerate in our dealings with one another and with nature.

The ethical question is how a society combats suffering and takes care of those who need help. In a nursing context, Martinsen formulates this very question like this: "How do we as nurses take care of the person's eternal meaning, the individual's unending worth—independent of what the individual is capable of, can be useful for or can achieve? Can I bear to see the other as the other, and yet not as fundamentally different from myself?" (Martinsen, 1993b, p. 18).

Max Weber: Vocation as the Duty to Serve One's Neighbor through One's Work

Max Weber (1864-1920) was a German sociologist who made a major impact on the philosophy of social science. Weber sought to understand the meaning of human action. He was also a critic of the society he saw emerging with the advent of industrialization. In Weber, Martinsen found a new alliance, in addition to Marx, in the criticism of both capitalism and science. While Løgstrup was a philosopher of religion, Weber was a sociologist of religion. Weber also criticized the West for its boundless intervention and its boundless consumption. Science disenchants the created world precisely because it relates to what was created as objects in its objectification of all that exists (Martinsen, 2000b, 2001, 2002b).

To a great extent, Martinsen joins Weber in her explication of vocation (Martinsen, 2000b). Weber looked to Martin Luther (1483-1546), who discussed vocation in the secular sense, as follows:

> Vocation is work in the sense of a life's occupation or a restricted field of work, in which the individual will endow his fellow person . . . The young Luther linked vocation to work, and understood it as an act of neighbourly love. Vocation is understood on the basis of the notion of creation, that we are created in order to care for one another through work (Martinsen 2000b, pp. 94-95).

In other words, vocation is in the service of creation. With reference to the young Luther, Martinsen wrote that vocation "means that we are placed in life contexts which demand something of us. It is a challenge that I, in this my vocation, meet and attend to my neighbour. It lies in Existence as a law of life" (Martinsen, 1996, p. 91).

Michel Foucault: The Effect of His Method Intensifying Phenomenologists' Phenomenology

Phenomenologists underscore the importance of history for our experience. Martinsen (1975) referred to Foucault in her dissertation in philosophy, but was especially concerned with this philosopher in connection with her historical works from 1976 (Martinsen 1978, 1989a, 2001, 2002b, 2003a). Foucault (1926-1984) was a French philosopher and historian of ideas. He was concerned with the notions of fracture and difference, rather than continuity and context. He claimed that within each historical epoch and within the different cultures, there reside some shared common structures, systems of terms and forms of thought that shape societies. In this way, Foucault confronted subjective philosophy, which emphasizes the person as a private and independent individual. For example, Foucault asked which fundamental conditions were present during the historical epoch in which institutions for the insane were created. In later epochs, he defined the insane as mentally ill. Something new had happened; what did it depend on? Why did it happen and what was to be achieved in society? What actions were undertaken; were there alliances of power and did they involve establishing order and discipline? To question in this way is to dig through several layers of understanding, getting beyond the general conception in order to understand the meaning of history in a new and different way. Foucault elicits the basic social distinctions that make it possible to characterize people. They are dug out of tacit preconditions (Lubcke, 1983). In this way Foucault's method intensified the phenomenological process. He asked us to think anew and differently from the existing mode of thinking within the epoch and within the contexts in which we live. The gaze became not only descriptive, but also critical.

Martinsen stated that, in caring for the other, we relate to the other in a different way and look for things different from those that are looked for within natural science and objectify medicine using their "classification gaze" and "examining gaze" (Martinsen, 1989b, pp. 142-168; Martinsen, 2000a). Such gazes require special space; caring requires different types of space in order to develop different types of knowledge. The questions we must bring with us into caring in the health service are these: Which disciplinary characteristics or structures are found in our practice today, in nursing practice and its spatial arrangements? What will it mean to think differently from those of our particular epoch? Is it here we find critical nursing, and if so, what are the implications for today's health service and research?

Paul Ricoeur: The Bridge-Builder

Ricoeur (1913-2005) is a French philosopher. His position is often designated as *critical hermeneutics* or *hermeneutic phenomenology.* He seeks to build a bridge between natural science and human science, between phenomenology and structuralism and other opposing positions. He focuses on topics such as time and narrative, language and history, discernment and science. Ricoeur is concerned with human communication, on what it is to understand one another. He points to everyday language and its many meanings, in contrast to the language of science. Martinsen states:

> The culture of medicine is dominated by an abstract conceptual language in which words are embedded in different classifications, and in which they are not always in accordance with actual practical and concrete situations. . . . In everyday language of the caring tradition on the other hand, words are followed by the manner in which they unfold in different contexts of meaning within concrete caring—in the company of the patient and the professional community. When spoken in everyday language, the words are distinguished by their power of expression. They strike a tone (Martinsen, 1996, p. 103).

Martinsen referred to several parallels in the philosophy of language of Løgstrup and Ricoeur.

Major Concepts & Definitions

Martinsen is reluctant to provide definitions of terms, since definitions have a tendency to close off concepts. Rather, she maintains, the content of concepts should be presented. It is important to circumscribe the meaningful content of a term, explain what the term means, but avoid having terms locked up in definitions.

CARE

Care "forms not only the value base of nursing, but is a fundamental precondition for our lives. Care is the positive development of the person through the Good" (Martinsen, 1990, p. 60). Care is a trinity: relational, practical, and moral simultaneously (Alvsvåg, 2003; Martinsen, 2003b). Caring is directed outward toward the situation of the other. In professional contexts, caring requires education and training. "Without professional knowledge, concern for the patient becomes mere sentimentality" (Martinsen, 1990, p. 63). She is clear that guardianship negligence or sentimentality are not expressions of care.

PROFESSIONAL JUDGMENT AND DISCERNMENT

These qualities are linked to the concrete. It is through the exercise of professional judgment in practical, living contexts that we learn clinical observation. It is "training not only to see, listen and touch clinically, but to see, listen and touch clinically in a good way" (Martinsen, 1993b, p. 147). The patient makes an impression on us, we are moved bodily, and the impression is sensuous. "Because perception has an analogue

Continued

MAJOR CONCEPTS & DEFINITIONS—cont'd

character, it evokes variation and context in the situation" (Martinsen, 1993b, p. 146). One thing is reminiscent of another, and this recollection creates a connection between the impressions in the situation, professional knowledge, and previous experience. Discretion expresses professional knowledge through the natural senses and everyday language (Martinsen, 2005, 2006).

MORAL PRACTICE IS FOUNDED ON CARE

"Moral practice is when empathy and reflection work together in such a way that caring can be expressed in nursing" (Martinsen, 1990, p. 60). Morality is present in concrete situations and must be accounted for. Our actions need to be accounted for; they are learned and justified through the objectivity of empathy, which consists of empathy and reflection. This means in concrete terms to discover how the other will best be helped, and the basic conditions are recognition and empathy. Sincerity and judgment enter into moral practice (Martinsen, 1990).

PERSON-ORIENTED PROFESSIONALISM

Person-oriented professionalism is "to demand professional knowledge which affords the view of the patient as a suffering person, and which protects his integrity. It challenges professional competence and humanity in a benevolent reciprocation, gathered in a communal basic experience of the protection and care for life . . . It demands an engagement in what we do, so that one wants to invest something of oneself in encounters with the other, and so that one is obligated to do one's best for the person one is to care for, watch over or nurse. It is about having an understanding of one's position within a life context that demands something from us, and about placing the other at the centre, about the caring encounter's orientation toward the other" (Martinsen, 2000b, pp. 12, 14).

SOVEREIGN LIFE UTTERANCES

Sovereign life utterances are phenomena that accompany the Creation itself. They exist as precultural phenomena in all societies; they are present as potentials. They are beyond human control and influence, and are therefore sovereign. Sovereign life utterances are openness, mercy, trust, hope, and love. These are phenomena that we are given in the same way that we are given time, space, air, water, and food (Alvsvåg, 2003). Unless we receive them, life disintegrates. Life is self-preservation through reception (Martinsen, 2000b). Sovereign life utterances are preconditions for care, simultaneously as caring actions are necessary conditions for the realization of sovereign life utterances in the concrete life. We can act in such a way that openness, trust, hope, mercy, and love are realized through our interactions, or we can shut them out. Without their presence in our actions, caring cannot be realized. At the same time, caring actions clear the way for the realization of sovereign life utterances in our personal and our professional lives. Care can bring the patient to experience the meaning of love and mercy; caring can light hope or give it sustenance, and caring can be that which makes trust and openness foremost in relations with the nurse. In the same way, lack of care can block the other's experience of mercy; it can create mistrust and an attitude of restraint in relation to the health service.

THE UNTOUCHABLE ZONE

This term refers to a zone that we must not interfere with in encounters with the other and encounters with nature. It refers to boundaries for which we must have respect. The untouchable

MAJOR CONCEPTS & DEFINITIONS—cont'd

zone creates a certain protective distance in the relation; it ensures impartiality and demands argumentation, theory, and professionalism. In caring, the untouchable zone is united with its opposite, which is openness, in which closeness, vulnerability, and motive have their correct place. Openness and the untouchable zone constitute a unifying contradiction in caring (Martinsen, 1990, 2006).

VOCATION

Vocation "is a demand life makes to me in a completely human way to encounter and care for one's fellow person. Vocation is given as a law of life concerning neighborly love which is foundationally human" (Martinsen, 2000b, p. 87). It is an ethical demand to take care of one's neighbor. For this reason, nursing requires a personal refinement, in addition to professional knowledge (Malchau, 2000).

THE EYE OF THE HEART

This concept stems from the parable of the Good Samaritan. The heart says something about the existence of the whole person, about being touched or moved by the suffering of the other and the situation the other experiences. In sensuousness and perception, we are moved before we understand, but we are also challenged by the afterthought of understanding. To see and be seen with the eye of the heart is a form of participatory attention based on a reciprocation that unifies perception and understanding, in which the eye's understanding is led by the senses (Martinsen, 2000b, 2006).

THE REGISTERING EYE

The registering eye is objectifying, and the perspective is that of the observer. It is concerned with finding connections, systematizing, ranking, classifying, and placing in a system. The registering eye represents an alliance between modern natural science, technology, and industrialization. If one as a patient is exposed to, or if one as a professional employs, this gaze in a one-sided manner, compassion is lifted out of the situation, and the will to life is reduced (Martinsen, 2000b).

EMPIRICAL EVIDENCE

In Martinsen's philosophy of caring, language and reflection involved in professional judgment and narrative are ways of accounting convincingly for case conditions, situations, and phenomena (Martinsen, 1997a, 2002c, 2003c, 2004b, 2005). She states that obvious perceptions must be accounted for convincingly. With reference to Husserl, she points to different forms of evidence: the undoubtable (apodictic), the exhaustive, and the partial. Each type represents different evidential requirements. Facts, themes, and situations provide different forms of evidence. For example, we cannot accept mathematical evidence that is undoubtable and transfer this to physical objects and persons. In the field of caring, it is discernment and narrative that can clarify the empirical facts of a case in an evidentiary, enlightening, or convincing manner (Martinsen 2003c, 2004b, 2005, 2008). To exercise discretion is to interpret the impressions we get of the patient. The professional knowledge and experience one has built up give one a horizon of understanding that is flexible in encounters with the patient's situation (Martinsen, 1990, 2002c). The narrative can both describe and prescribe action (Kjær, 2000; Martinsen, 1997a). "A good narrative tells existential morality into being, and makes practical action unavoidable" (Martinsen, 1993b, p. 161).

MAJOR ASSUMPTIONS

Nursing

Although care goes beyond nursing, caring is fundamental to nursing and to other work of a caring nature. Caring involves having consideration for, taking care of, and being concerned about the other. When we speak about caring, three things must be simultaneously present; we could call them the "trinity of caring": caring must be relational, practical, and moral (Alvsvåg, 2003).

- *Relational* means that caring requires at least two people. Martinsen describes it thus:

  The one has concern for the other. When the one suffers, the other will "grieve" (in the sense of suffer with) and *provide for* the alleviation of pain. . . . Caring is the most natural and the most fundamental aspect of the person's existence. In caring, the relationship between people is the most essential element. . . . The essence of the person is that one is created for the sake of others—for one's own sake. . . . The point here is that caring always presupposes others. Further, that I can never understand myself or realise myself alone or independent of others (Martinsen, 1989c, p. 69).
- Caring is *practical.* It is about concrete and practical action. Caring is trained and learned through its practice.
- Caring is also *moral*: "If caring is to be genuine, I must relate to the other from an *attitude* (mood, 'befindlichkeit') which acknowledges the other in light of *his* situation. . . . [We must] neither overestimate nor underestimate his ability to help himself" (Martinsen, 1989c, p. 71).

Caring requires a correct understanding of the situation, which presupposes a good evaluation of the goals inherent in the caring situation: "Performing nursing is essentially directed towards persons not capable of self-help, who are ill and in need of care. To encounter the ill person with caring through nursing involves a set of preconditions such as knowledge, skills, and organization" (Martinsen, 1989c, p. 75). We need training in all types of caring work. We must practice and reflect alone and with others in order to develop professional judgment. Caring and professional judgment are integrated in nursing (Martinsen, 1990, 1997a, 2003c, 2004b, 2005, 2006).

Person

It is the meaning-bearing fellowship of tradition that turns the individual into a person. The person cannot be torn away from the social milieu and the community of persons (Martinsen, 1975). In one way, there is a parallel between the person and the body. It is as bodies that we relate to ourselves, to others, and to the world (Alvsvåg, 2000; Martinsen, 1997a). The body is a unit of soul and flesh, or spirit and flesh. The person is bodily, and as bodies we both perceive and understand.

Health

Health is discussed from a sociohistorical perspective. Two rival historical health ideals, the classical Greek and the modern one of intervention and expansion, form the background when Martinsen writes: "Health does not only reflect the condition of the organism, it is also an expression of the current level of competence in medicine. To put it pointedly, the tendencies of the modern concept of health are such that if one has an unnecessary 'defect' or an organ which 'could' be better, one is not completely healthy" (Martinsen, 1989c, p. 146). The modern reductionist health ideal on which modern medicine is built is both analytical and individualistic; it is oriented toward all that is not "good enough." Combined with medicine's autonomy and resources, it has yielded success in terms of treatment. Martinsen is concerned with the point that this ideology does not withstand critical examination. Medicine's sometimes damaging effects and insufficient service for people with chronic diseases and illnesses bring Martinsen to turn toward the conservative, classical health ideal. What is important is to cure sometimes, help often, and comfort always. This requires society to offer people the opportunity to live the best life possible and the individual to live sensibly; both requirements have environmental implications. We must not change the environment at such a speed and to such an extent that the change exceeds our knowledge base; restraint and caution are required (Martinsen, 1989c, 2003b).

Environment: Space and Situation

The person is always in a particular situation in a particular space. In space are found time, ambience, and power (Martinsen, 2001, 2002b, 2002c). Martinsen asks what time, architecture, and knowledge do to the ambience of a space. Architecture, our interaction with each other, use of objects, words, knowledge, our being-in-the-room—all set the tone and color the situation and the space. The person enters into universal space, natural space, but through dwelling creates cultural space. We build houses with rooms, and the activities of the health service take place in different rooms. "The sick-room is important as a physical, material and constructed place, but it is also a place we share with other people. . . . The room with its interior and objects makes visible the patient's and the nurse's interpretation of it" (Martinsen, 2001, pp. 175-176). Our challenge is to give patients and each other dignity in these spaces. What is needed then is deliberate knowledge gathered in slowed down, deliberate spaces, "space in which to perceive—smell, listen, see and care" (Martinsen, 2001, p. 176).

THEORETICAL ASSERTIONS

People are created dependent and relational. Care is fundamental to human life. As humans, we live not merely in fellowship with one another, but we also enter into relationships with animals and with nature, and we relate to a creative force that sustains the whole. The person is fundamentally dependent upon community and the creation. To the created belong the sovereign life utterances, "These are firstly *given to* us, and secondly they are *sovereign.* That is to say it is impossible for the person to avoid their power. . . . These are phenomena which are present in the service of life. They create life, they release life's possibilities" (Martinsen, 1996, p. 80).

The body is created as a whole, that is to say that need and spirit, or body and spirit, enter into a benevolent interaction, in which sensing cannot be avoided. Martinsen (1996) writes the following:

> Sensing initiates interaction and maintains it. Care of the body becomes central. In this respect, nursing is secular vocational work which through professional care of the body protects and provides space for the life possibilities of the patient. The vocation is seen as a demand life makes on us to care for our neighbour, in this case the patient, through our work. It is work in the service of life processes. Vocation, the body and work are seen as a counterweight to the new (bodiless) spirituality in nursing (p. 72).

Love of one's neighbor is coupled with a concrete, practical, professional, and moral discernment.

Sensuous and experience-based knowledge is the most fundamental and essential for the practice of nursing. Caring is learned through practical experience in concrete situations under the supervision of expert and experienced nurses (Martinsen, 1993b, 2003b).

Metaphysics is not speculation about that of which we cannot know anything. It is an interpretation of phenomena we all recognize through our senses and can experience. These phenomena are prescientific and foundational.

LOGICAL FORM

Martinsen's logical form can be described as inductive and analogous. The inductive aspect of her thought has its source in that experiences in life and in the health service are the starting point for her theoretical works. She turns toward philosophy and history in the hope of gaining greater insight and understanding of the concrete work of nursing and the lived life. In her meeting with the philosophy of life and the phenomenology of creation, she encounters the ontological and metaphysical in a different way than that of traditional philosophy. Life utterances, the creation, time, and space are ontological and metaphysical facts. Analogy would say that we think these facts and recognize them in our concrete experiences in our practical life. They come to expression in meetings between persons, in narratives, and in the exercise of discernment. "In this way, metaphysics pries at the empirical," writes Martinsen with reference to Løgstrup (Martinsen, 1996). Further, she states, "The narrative takes time, it is slow. It provides context through analogous forms of recognition, that is to say, it is relevant to us when we can recognize ourselves in the life phenomena it relates" (Martinsen, 2002b, p. 267).

Kirkevold (1998) writes the following:

> Martinsen does not mean to present a logically constructed theory. On the contrary, she distances herself from that view of knowledge that insists theory have a logical structure of terms, principles and rules. Martinsen's theory is an interpretive analysis of caring, upon which the author tries to shed light from several perspectives. Her treatment of this phenomenon must be said to be both extensive and thorough (p. 180).

APPLICATIONS BY THE NURSING COMMUNITY

Practice

Martinsen herself is reluctant to provide concrete directions for practical nursing. However, she recommends that nurses "think along" and assess what she writes and speaks about in their own lives, their own practice and experience, and, against this background, imagine their own way to alternatives for action. This is how Kirkevold (1998) puts it:

> Martinsen's theory of caring is practically relevant as an overarching/general philosophy of nursing. It is clearly articulated and encompasses a precise formulation of how (one ought) to understand and approach patients and nursing. Its strength is the ability to promote reflection upon nursing practice in different contexts, in that it gives a clear picture of what the author believes must be present so that nursing may be considered caring or moral practice (p. 181).

Many of these texts have, she maintains:

> . . . a normative character, and are intended to mobilize a counter-culture in nursing, which does not only revolutionize the discipline of nursing and its practice, but which also stands as a resisting force against the societal tendency in opposition to the concept of care. . . . In recent years the personal, inspiring and poetic style has become more pronounced. It communicates Martinsen's normatively founded philosophy of caring in a gripping way, and has therefore had great impact on nurses and students (Kirkevold, 1998, p. 204).

Martinsen herself addresses practicing nurses through their professional journal, *Sykepleien.* Kirkevold writes: "In choosing the journal *Nursing* as a main vehicle for communicating her academic work, she has underscored her roots in practical nursing rather than in science" (Kirkevold, 1998, p. 203).

Education

Most nursing colleges in Norway and Denmark make good use of Martinsen's texts, and her works form part of the curriculum at a variety of educational levels. Her books are reprinted regularly and have had considerable impact. Several prescribed texts for nursing education have dealt with her thought (Alvsvåg, 2003; Kirkevold 1998; Kristoffersen, 2002; Mekki & Tollefsen, 2000; Nielsen, 2003). In addition, other books have been written for nursing education in which the aim is to make Martinsen's thinking relevant for both nursing generally and for specific professional issues. For example, several college lecturers in Norway and Denmark produced an article compilation in 2000, which gives an introduction to Martinsen's thought and for which the target group is students (Alvsvåg & Gjengedal, 2000). In 2002, the book *The Philosophy of Caring in Practice: Thinking with Kari Martinsen in Nursing,* was published

(Austgard, 2002). In this book, concrete situations of caring are presented, illustrating how philosophy might influence practical nursing. The book was also translated into Danish in 2004 (Austgard, 2004).

In 2003, a Danish nurse wrote a textbook of spiritual care. Central to the book is Martinsen's thinking, in addition to that of Katie Eriksson and Joyce Travelbee (Overgaard, 2003). In the *Danish Encyclopedia of Nursing,* published in 2008, Kari Martinsen is portrayed in a separate article, while several other articles refer to her thinking on caring and judgment (Jørgensen & Lyngaa, 2008).

Research

In the same way as one in practical nursing can "think along" and assess what she writes, her writings can also be applied in research. Countless dissertations based on practical, concrete, and more theoretical issues discuss the relationship between empirical experience in light of Martinsen's terminology and philosophy. In 1993, as Martinsen turned 50, the book, *Wisdom and Skill,* was published (Kirkevold, Nortvedt, & Alvsvåg, 1993) in which Kirkevold states that Martinsen's thought and works have created a critical and constructive role model for research and professional development (Kirkevold, 1993). Ruth Olsen writes about the reflective practitioner (Olsen, 1993), involving ideas subsequently elaborated in her doctoral dissertation, later published under the title *Wise with Experience? On Sensation and Attention, Knowledge and Reflection in Practical Nursing* (Olsen, 1998). In her 2003 doctoral dissertation, Danish nursing scholar Kirsten Beedholm analyzes, with inspiration from the French philosopher Foucault's archeological method and Martinsen's readings of Løgstrup's texts (Beedholm, 2003). In another doctoral dissertation from 2006, the Norwegian pedagogue Pål Henning Walstad addresses Kari Martinsen's Grundtvig-Løgstrupian influence, calling it *Care for Life,* and discusses this in relation to practical work and professional education (Walstad, 2006). Moreover, nursing teacher Betty-Ann Solvoll has in her 2007 doctoral dissertation done a field study of nursing education and is discussing the data in relation to Martinsen's reflections on care (Solvoll, 2007).

FURTHER DEVELOPMENT

Caring can be understood on several levels: ontological, concrete, and practical, or at the level of system or organization. In nursing, we are encouraged to act in a professional and moral manner, so that caring and life utterances are given the space they need to emerge in nurse-patient encounters. We are continuously challenged to reflect critically over whether this happens or not. It would involve the manifestation of a person-oriented professionalism, the manifestation of loving deeds in the profession, over and over (Martinsen, 1993b, 2000b).

It is important, moreover, to develop a mode of thinking about caring in nursing research. Science in nursing might face certain boundaries. The challenge is to develop a type of research which does not impoverish practice, but which upgrades the available knowledge and wisdom developed through practice, in other words to develop or create a practice-oriented research, a cooperation between researcher and practitioner (Martinsen, 1989c, 1993b). Kirkevold writes as follows:

> Martinsen's theory is especially important because it is one of the few existing Norwegian nursing theories, and because it is one of the first Nordic nursing theories that gives expression to a new understanding of reality and the need for new nursing theories based upon this (Kirkevold, 1998, p. 182).

At the organizational and social levels, the concept of care is also highly relevant. It is important to develop social systems and organizations, such as the health service, so that a person-oriented professionalism can be facilitated. Martinsen writes about both a merciful and a political Samaritan (Martinsen, 1993b, 2000b, 2003b). What is important at both organizational and social levels is how the political

Samaritans facilitate the work of the merciful Samaritans.

CRITIQUE

Clarity

Marinsen's theory clearly states that life has been created and given to us. We have been created in dependence on each other and on nature. Caring for each other and for nature is fundamental. Our challenge as nurses from her perspective is to meet patients and their families with person-oriented professionality, and that is at the heart of person-oriented professionality.

Simplicity

At first glance, Martinsen's theory seems complex. At the same time, the question must be asked whether this is because she turns so many of our familiar assumptions on their heads, for example, that we as human beings are free, independent, and boundless in our capacity for activity and interference with creation. Western societies live in a culture of individualism. Her view of humanity can be described as *collectivist.* She uses a poetic and philosophical rather than a scientific mode of speaking, which might also seem alien in a scientized society. She writes about general phenomena that affect us all, and that we can easily recognize in our personal lives, either occupationally or in daily life. Seen this way, the theory of caring is not hard to understand. Martinsen asks that we read slowly while imagining our own experiences in light of what she writes (Martinsen, 2000b).

Generality

Because Martinsen's nursing theory deals with essential phenomena of life and nursing, phenomena present in all human situations, it can be seen as relevant to patients in general (Martinsen, 2006). Her theory of care "seems to be relevant for all patients who, because of illness or other reasons, need help and assistance" (Kirkevold, 1998, p. 181).

Empirical Precision

The patient's and the nurse's worlds of experience are diverse, nuanced, and multifaceted. A nuanced and varied language is required to deal with a multifaceted reality, one that is on par with what is to be described. This language is close to philosophy and also to everyday language; it is a poetic language. We may say that the poetic language is the most precise in describing manifold phenomena and situations open to interpretation. Reflection on professional judgment and professional narratives creates the contexts of a community of nursing and the tradition of nursing; we recognize situations and thus find professional and moral insight. This enables us to perform situation-dependent, good nursing—a professional moral practice.

Derivable Consequences

Martinsen's theory of caring is a critique of the prevailing system and at the same time an inspiration to individuals in concrete caring situations (Gjengedal, 2000). Gjengedal writes that Martinsen's motivation for theoretical work "has precisely a practical point of departure, a wish to understand and protect against devaluation of the aspect of care in nursing" (Gjengedal, 2000, p. 38). Devaluation of caring might occur if one uncritically accepts "a scientific perspective blind to the lived life and all that gives meaning to being" (Gjengedal, 2000, p. 54).

Lived life is built on basic structures; being has meaning and this meaning exists from the beginning of life. As persons and as nurses, we are challenged to live in a way that allows positive meaning to be expressed in our human relations, for example, in relations between patients and their family members. How we express this in a concrete way in a nursing context is for us as professionals to decide, but the philosophy on which Martinsen bases her thinking can provide ideas for our own reflection in specific situations.

Specific situations present themselves with both possibilities and limitations. Socially created structural arrangements such as lack of personnel, financial resources, and lack of institutional beds present serious limitations on a daily basis. Opportunities for caring become more accessible within a caring community and are shaped by politically aware people:

> A caring community is not dictatorial, nor is it society's passive extended arm. The caring community exists only to the extent that we struggle for its existence. We must form it ourselves: through solidarity, through morally responsible action, through the fight for greater equality and for community and social integration. Caring is an active and radical concept (Martinsen, 1989c, p. 62).

It is important to create conditions for good and equitable health care and living standards for all, but in the fight over limited budgetary resources, to take as our starting point those who are weakest, who most need help, it is about turning the inverted law of care around such that those who have least receive most.

SUMMARY

Martinsen has both personal and sociopolitical interest in the ill and in those who, for other reasons, fall outside of society. Her theoretical stance can be called critical and phenomenological. She takes as her starting point the idea that human beings are created and are beings for whom we have administrative responsibility. We are relational and dependent on each other and on the Creation. Therefore, caring, solidarity, and moral practice are unavoidable realities for us.

In her thought on the subject of caring, Martinsen challenges society, the politics of health care, and healthcare workers themselves to realize the values inherent in caring through concrete policies and practical nursing. She deliberately gives few directives for action. Rather, she asks us to think ourselves into the situations of patients and family members and to arrive at the best choices for action based on a rich situational understanding, professional insight, and a caring attitude.

Martinsen's thought has provoked, engaged, and created debate and professional development in nursing in the Nordic countries over the past 30 years. Her thought challenges us to both think and act well and correctly, critically, and differently in nursing, in education, and in research. Martinsen's "caring thought" contributes to the enlightenment of nursing and nursing research through its perspectives, concepts, and insights based on historical and philosophical scholarship and research.

Case Study

As nurses, we meet patients and their family members in many different life situations. Patients may be of all age groups, acutely or chronically ill, might return to life and health, or are coming to the end of their lives and must face death as a reality. Nurses meet patients and family members in their homes, at the hospital or the nursing home, in the school health service, at the local clinic, and so forth. Some meetings with patients and family members make a greater impression on us than others, and all meetings represent situations of learning in more than one way.

Against this background, write a brief case study from your personal experience, or make one up and discuss how caring is expressed in the situation.

CRITICAL THINKING Activities

Imagine and present as a starting point a concrete situation with which you have personal experience as an active participant, or in an observational role.

1. Discuss how caring and professional judgment and discretion are expressed in the situation.
2. From the starting point of the situation in the first item, discuss what is meant by person-oriented professionalism and moral practice.

POINTS FOR *Further Study*

- Martinsen, K. (2006). *Care and vulnerability*. Oslo: Akribe (English original).
- Martinsen, K. (2008). Modernitet, avtrylling og skam. En måte å lese vestens medisin på i det moderne. In K. A. Petersen & M. Høyen (red.). *At sette spor på en vandring fra Aquinas til Bordieu—æresbog til Staf Callewaert.* Forlag@hexis.dk [Modernity, disenchantment and shame. A way of reading Western medicine in the modern. In K. A. Petersen & M. Høyen (ed.). *Leaving a trail on the way from Aquinas to Bordieu—honorary volume for Staf Callewaert.* Forlag@hexis.dk]

REFERENCES*

Alvsvåg, H. (2000). Menneskesynet—Fra kroppsfenomenologi til skapelsesfenomenologi. I H. Alvsvåg & E. Gjengedal (red.), *Omsorgstenkning. En innføring i Kari Martinsens forfatterskap.* Bergen: Fagbokforlaget. [The view of the person—From the phenomenology of the body to creation phenomenology. In H. Alvsvåg & E. Gjengedal (Eds.), *Caring thought: An introduction to the writings of Kari Martinsen.* Bergen: Fagbokforlaget.]

Alvsvåg, H. (2003). Omsorg—Med utgangspunkt i Kari Martinsens omsorgstenkning. I B. K. Nielsen (red.), *Sygeplejebogen 2, 1. del Teoretisk-metodisk grundlag for klinisk sygepleje.* København: Gads Forlag. [Caring—From the starting point of Kari Martinsen's philosophy. In B. K. Nielsen (Ed.), *Nursing textbook 2, part 1. Theoretical-methodologic basis of clinical nursing.* Copenhagen: Gads Forlag.]

Alvsvåg, H., & Gjengedal, E. (red.) (2000). *Omsorgstenkning. En innføring i Kari Martinsens forfatterskap.* Bergen: Fagbokforlaget. [*Caring thought: An introduction to the writings of Kari Martinsen.* Bergen: Fagbokforlaget.]

Austgard, K. (2002). *Omsorgsfilosofi i praksis. A tenke med Kari Martinsen i sykepleien.* Oslo: Cappelen Akademisk Forlag. [*Philosophy of caring in practice. Thinking with Kari Martinsen in nursing.* Oslo: Cappelen Akademisk Forlag.]

Austgard, K. (2004). *Omsorgsfilosofi i praksis. At tænke med Kari Martinsen i sygeplejen.* København: Akademisk Forlag. [*Philosophy of Caring in Practice: Thinking with Kari Martinsen in Nursing.* Copenhagen: Akademisk Forlag.]

Beedholm, K. (2003). *Forandring og træghed i den sygeplejefaglige diskurs.* Viborg: Forlaget PUC. [*Change and inertia in the discourse of nursing studies.* Viborg: Forlaget PUC.]

Gjengedal, E. (2000). Omsorg og sykepleie. I H. Alvsvåg & E. Gjengedal (red.), *Omsorgstenkning: En innføring i Kari Martinsens forfatterskap.* Bergen: Fagbokforlaget. [Caring and nursing. In H. Alvsvåg & E. Gjengedal (Eds.), *Caring thought: An introduction to the writings of Kari Martinsen.* Bergen: Fagbokforlaget.]

Jørgensen, B. B. & Lyngaa, J. (ed.) (2008). *Sygeplejeleksikon.* København: Munksgaard. [*Encyclopedia of Nursing.* Copenhagen: Munksgaard.]

Karlsson, B., & Martinsen, K. (2003). Prolog. In K. Martinsen, *Omsorg, sykepleie og medisin.* 2. utgave. Oslo: Universitetsforlaget. [Prologue. In K. Martinsen. *Caring, nursing and medicine: Historical-philosophical essays* (2nd ed.). Oslo: Universitetsforlaget.]

Kirkevold, M. (1993). Innledning. I M. Kirkevold, F. Nortvedt, & H. Alvsvåg (red.), *Klokskap og kyndighet. Kari Martinsens innflytelse på norsk og dansk sykepleie.* Oslo: ad Notam Gyldendal. [Introduction. In M. Kirkevold, F. Nortvedt, & H. Alvsvåg (Eds.), *Wisdom and skill: Kari Martinsen's influence on Norwegian and Danish nursing.* Oslo: ad Notam Gyldendal.]

Kirkevold, M. (1998). *Sykepleieteorier—Analyse og evaluering.* Oslo: ad Notam Gyldendal. 2. utgave. [*Nursing theories—Analysis and evaluation* (2nd ed.). Oslo: ad Notam Gyldendal.]

Kirkevold, M. (2000). Utviklingstrekk i Kari Martinsens forfatterskap. I H. Alvsvåg & E. Gjengedal (red.), *Omsorgstenkning—En innføring i Kari Martinsens forfatterskap.* Bergen: Fagbokforlaget. [Developmental characteristics in the writings of Kari Martinsen. In H. Alvsvåg & E. Gjengedal (Eds.), *Caring thought: An introduction to the writings of Kari Martinsen.* Bergen: Fagbokforlaget.]

Kirkevold, M., Nortvedt, F., & Alvsvåg, H. (red.) (1993). *Klokskap og kyndighet. Kari Martinsens innflytelse på norsk og dansk sykepleie.* Oslo: Gyldendal Academisk. [*Wisdom and skill. Kari Martinsen's influence on Norwegian and Danish nursing.* Oslo: Gyldendal Academisk.]

Kjær, T. (2000). Fænomenologi, etikk og fortælling: I H. Alvsvåg & E. Gjengedal (red.), *Omsorgstenkning—En innføring i Kari Martinsens forfatterskap.* Bergen: Fagbokforlaget. [Phenomenology, ethics and narrative. In H. Alvsvåg & E. Gjengedal (Eds.), *Caring thought: An introduction to the writings of Kari Martinsen.* Bergen: Fagbokforlaget.]

Kristoffersen, N. J. (2002). *Generell sykepleie.* Oslo: Universitetsforlaget. [*Fundamental nursing.* Oslo: Universitetsforlaget.]

Lubcke, P. (red.) (1983). *Politikens filosofiske leksikon.* København: Politikens Forlag. [*Politiken's philosophical lexicon.* Copenhagen: Politikens Forlag.]

*Norwegian titles are provided with approximate translation into English.

Malchau, S. (2000). Kaldet. I H. Alvsvåg & E. Gjengedal (red.), *Omsorgstenkning—En innføring i Kari Martinsens forfatterskap.* Bergen: Fagbokforlaget. [The call. In H. Alvsvåg & E. Gjengedal (Eds.), *Caring thought: An introduction to the writings of Kari Martinsen.* Bergen: Fagbokforlaget.]

Martinsen K. (1975). *Filosofi og sykepleie. Et marxistisk og fenomenologisk bidrag.* Filosofisk institutes stensilserie nr. 34. Bergen: Universitetet i Bergen. [*Philosophy and nursing: A Marxist and phenomenological contribution* (Philosophical institute's stencil series no. 34). Bergen: University of Bergen.]

Martinsen, K. (1976). Historie og sykepleie—Momenter til en utdanningsdebatt. *Kontrast, 7*, 430-446. [History and nursing—Elements of an educational debate. *Contrast, 7*, 430-446.]

Martinsen, K. (1977). Nightingale—Ingen opprører bak myten. *Sykepleien 18*(65), 1022-1025. [Nightingale—No rebel behind the myth. *Nursing, 18*(65), 1022-1025.]

Martinsen, K. (1978). Det 'kliniske blikk' i medisinen og i sykepleien. *Sykepleien, 20*(66), 1271-1272. [The 'clinical gaze' in medicine and in nursing. *Nursing, 20*(66), 1271-1272.]

Martinsen, K. (1979a). Den engelske sanitation—Bevegelsen, hygiene og synet på sykdom. I Ø. Larsen (red.), *Synet på sykdom.* Oslo: Seksjon for medisinsk historie, Universitetet i Oslo. [The English sanitation movement, hygiene and the view of illness. In Ø. Larsen (Ed.), *The view of illness.* Oslo: University of Oslo (Section for medical history).]

Martinsen, K. (1979b). Diakonissesykepleiens framvekst. Fra vekkelser og kvinneforeninger til moderhus og fattigomsorg. I NAVF's sekretariat for kvinneforskning (red.), *Lønnet og ulønnet omsorg. En seminarrapport.* Arbeidsnotat nr. 5/79. Oslo: NAVF. [Development of the professional trained Christian nurses. From revival and woman's charitable groups to the mother house and care of the poor. In NAVF's Secretariat for Feminist Research (Ed.), *Paid and unpaid care: A seminar report.* Working paper no. 5/79. Oslo: NAVF.]

Martinsen, K. (1984). *Sykepleiens historie. Freidige og uforsagte diakonisser. Et omsorgsyrke vokser fram 1860-1905.* Oslo: Aschehoug/Tanum-Norli. [*History of nursing: Frank and engaged deaconesses: A caring profession emerges 1860-1905.* Oslo: Aschehoug/Tanum-Norli.]

Martinsen, K. (1989a). Helsepolitiske problemer og helsepolitisk tenkning bak sykehusloven av 1969. I K. Martinsen, *Omsorg, sykepleie og medisin. Historisk-filosofiske essays.* Oslo: Tano Forlag. [Health policy problems and health policy thinking behind the hospital law of 1969. In K. Martinsen, *Caring, nursing and medicine: Historical-philosophical essays.* Oslo: Tano Forlag.]

Martinsen, K. (1989b). Legers interesse for svangerskapet—En del av den perinatale omsorg. Tidsrommet ca. 1890-1940. I K. Martinsen, *Omsorg, sykepleie og medisin. Historisk-filosofiske essays.* Oslo: Tano Forlag. [The doctor's interest in pregnancy—Part of perinatal care: The period ca. 1890-1940. In K. Martinsen, *Caring, nursing and medicine: Historical-philosophical essays.* Oslo: Tano Forlag.]

Martinsen, K. (1989c). *Omsorg, sykepleie og medisin. Historisk-filosofiske essays.* Oslo: Tano Forlag. [*Caring, nursing and medicine: Historical-philosophical essays.* Oslo: Tano Forlag.]

Martinsen, K. (1990). Moralsk praksis og dokumentasjon i praktisk sykepleie. I T. Jensen, L. U. Jensen, & W. C. Kim (red.), *Grundlagsproblemer i sygeplejen. Etik, videnskabsteori, ledelse & samfunn.* Aarhus: Philosophia. [Practice and documentation in practical nursing. In T. Jensen, L. U. Jensen, & W. C. Kim (Eds.), *Foundational problems in nursing: Ethics, theories of science, leadership and society.* Aarhus: Philosophia.]

Martinsen, K. (red.) (1993a). *Den omtenksomme sykepleier.* Oslo: Tano. [*The thoughtful nurse.* Oslo: Tano.]

Martinsen, K. (1993b). *Fra Marx til Løgstrup. Om moral, samfunnskritikk og sanselighet i sykepleien.* Oslo: Tano Forlag. [*From Marx to Løgstrup: On morality, social criticism and sensuousness in nursing.* Oslo: Tano Forlag.]

Martinsen, K. (1996). *Fenomenologi og omsorg. Tre dialoger.* Oslo: Tano-Aschehoug. [*Phenomenology and caring: Three dialogues.* Oslo: Tano-Aschehoug.]

Martinsen, K. (1997a). De etiske fortellinger. *Omsorg, 1*(14), 58-63. [The ethical narratives. *Caring, 1*(14), 58-63.]

Martinsen, K. (1997b). Etikk og kall, kultur og kropp—En dialog med Patricia Benner. I M. Sæther (red.), *Sykepleiekonferanse på Nordkalottens tak.* Tromsø: Universitetet i Tromsø. [Ethics and vocation, culture and the body—A dialogue with Patricia Benner. In M. Sæther (Ed.), *Nursing conference on the roof of Nordkalotten.* Tromsø: University of Tromsø.]

Martinsen, K. (2000a). Kjærlighetsgjerningen og kallet. Betraktninger omkring Rikke Nissens "Lærebog i Sygepleje for diakonisser". I R. Nissen, *Lærebog i Sygepleie. Med etterord av Kari Martinsen.* Oslo: Gyldendal Akademisk. [The loving act and the call. Reflections on Rikke Nissen's *textbook of nursing for deaconesses.* In R. Nissen, *Textbook of nursing. With afterword by Kari Martinsen.* Oslo: Gyldendal Akademisk.]

Martinsen, K. (2000b). *Øyet og kallet.* Bergen: Fagbokforlaget. [*The eye and the call.* Bergen: Fagbokforlaget.]

Martinsen, K. (2001). Huset og sangen, gråten og skammen. Rom og arkitektur som ivaretaker av menneskets verdighet. I T. Wyller (red.), *Skam. Perspektiver på skam, ære og skamløshet i det moderne.* Bergen: Fagbokforlaget. [The house and the song, the tears and the shame: Space and architecture as caretakers of human dignity. In T. Wyller (Ed.), *Shame. Perspectives on shame, honor and shamelessness in modernity.* Bergen: Fagbokforlaget]

Martinsen, K. (2002a). Livsfilosofiske betraktninger. *Diakoninytt, 3*(118), 8-12. [Reflections on the philosophy of life. *Deaconry News, 3*(118), 8-12.]

Martinsen, K. (2002b). Rommets tid, den sykes tid, pleiens tid. I I. T. Bjørk, S. Helseth, & F. Nortvedt (red.), *Møte mellom pasient og sykepleier.* Oslo: Gyldendal Akademisk. [The room's time, the ill person's time, nursing time. In I. T. Bjørk, S. Helseth, & F. Nortvedt (Eds.), *The meeting between patient and nurse.* Oslo: Gyldendal Akademisk.]

Martinsen, K. (2002c). Samtalen, kommunikasjonen og sakligheten i omsorgsyrkene. *Omsorg, 1*(19), 14-22. [Conversation, communication and professionality in the caring professions. *Caring, 1*(19), 14-22.]

Martinsen, K. (2003a). Disiplin og rommelighet I K. Martinsen & T. Wyller (red.), *Etikk, disiplin og dannelse. Elisabeth Hagemanns etikkbok—Nye lesinger.* Oslo: Gyldendal Akademisk. [Discipline and spaciousness. In K. Martinsen & T. Wyller (Eds.), *Ethics, discipline and refinement: Elizabeth Hagemann's ethics book—New readings.* Oslo: Gyldendal Akademisk.]

Martinsen, K. (2003b). *Omsorg, sykepleie og medisin. Historisk-filosofiske essays.* 2. utgave. Oslo: Universitetsforlaget. [*Caring, nursing and medicine: Historical-philosophical essays* (2nd ed.). Oslo: University Press.]

Martinsen, K. (2003c). Talens åpenhet og evidens—Dialog med Jens Bydam. *Klinisk Sygepleje,* 4(17), 36-46. [The openness of speech and evidence—Dialogue with Jens Bydam. *Clinical Nursing, 4*(17), 36-46.]

Martinsen, K. (2004b). Skjønn—Språk og distanse—Dialog med Jens Bydam. *Klinisk Sygepleje, 2*(18), 50-56. [Discernment—Language and distance—Dialogue with Jens Bydam. *Clinical Nursing,* 2(18), 50-56.]

Martinsen, K. (2005). *Samtalen, skjønnet og evidensen.* Oslo: Akribe. [*Dialog, Discernment and the Evidence.* Oslo: Akribe.]

Martinsen, K. (2006). *Care and Vulnerability.* Oslo: Akribe (English original).

Martinsen, K. (2008). *Å se og å innse—om ulike former for evidens.* Oslo: Akribe. [*To see and to realize—on various forms of evidence.* Oslo: Akribe.] (In process with Katie Ericsson).

Martinsen, K., & Wærness, K. (1979). *Pleie uten omsorg?* Oslo: Pax Forlag A/S. [*Caring without care?* Oslo: Pax Forlag.]

Martinsen, K., & Wyller, T. (red.) (2003). *Etikk, disiplin og dannelse. Elisabeth Hagemanns etikkbok—Nye lesinger.* Oslo: Gyldendal Akademisk. [*Ethics, discipline and refinement: Elizabeth Hagemann's ethics book—New readings.* Oslo: Gyldendal Akademisk.]

Mekki, T. E., & Tollefsen, S. (2000). *På terskelen. Introduksjon til sykepleie som fag og yrke.* Oslo: Akribe. [*On the threshold: Introduction to nursing as discipline and profession.* Oslo: Akribe.]

Nielsen, B. K. (ed.) (2003). *Sygeplejenbogen 2, 1. del.* Teoretisk-metodisk grundlag for klinisk sygepleje. København: Gads Forlag. [*Nursing textbook 2, part 1. Theoretical-methodic basis of clinical nursing.* Copenhagen: Gads Forlag.]

Nissen, R. (2000). *Lærebog i Sygepleie. Med etterord av Kari Martinsen.* Oslo: Gyldendal Akademisk. [*Textbook of nursing. With an afterword by Kari Martinsen.* Oslo: Gyldendal Akademisk.]

Olsen, R. (1993). Den reflekterte praktiker—Rapport fra et sykehjem. I Kirkevold, M., Nortvedt, F., & Alvsvåg, H. (red.), *Klokskap og kyndighet. Kari Martinsens innflytelse på norsk og dansk sykepleie.* Oslo: ad Notam Gyldendal (s. 200-208). [The reflective practitioner—Report from a nursing home. In M. Kirkevold, F. Nortvedt, & H. Alvsvåg (Eds.), *Wisdom and skill. Kari Martinsen's influence on Norwegian and Danish nursing* (pp. 200-208). Oslo: ad Notam Gyldendal.]

Olsen, R. H. (1998). *Klok av erfaring? Om sansing og oppmerksomhet, kunnskap og refleksjon i praktisk sykepleie.* Oslo: Tano Aschehoug. [*Wise with experience? On Sensation and Attention, Knowledge and Reflection in practical nursing.* Oslo: Tano Aschehoug.]

Overgaard, A. E. (2003). *Åndelig omsorg—En lærebog.* København: Nytt Nordisk Forlag Arnold Busck. [*Spiritual care—Textbook.* Copenhagen: Nyt Nordisk Forlag Arnold Busck.]

Solvoll, B.A. (2007). *Omsorgsferdigheter som pedagogisk prosjekt—en feltstudie i sykepleieutdanningen.* Oslo: Universitetet i Oslo, Det medisinske fakultet, nr. 540. [*Caring skills as pedagogical project—a field study in nursing education.* Oslo: University of Oslo, Faculty of medicine, Doctoral dissertations no. 540.]

Walstad, P.B. (2006). *Dannelse og Duelighed for livet. Dannelse og yrkesutdanning i den grundtvigske tradisjon.* Trondheim: Norges teknisk-naturvitenskapelige universitet, NTNU Doctoral dissertations 2006:88. [*Education and Capability for life. Education and professional training in the Grundtvigian tradition.* Trondheim: Norges teknisk-naturvitenskapelige universitet, NTNU Doctoral dissertations 2006:88.]

BIBLIOGRAPHY*

Primary Sources

Books

Martinsen K. (1975). Filosofi og sykepleie. Et marxistisk og fenomenologisk bidrag. Filosofisk institutts stensilserie nr. 34. Bergen: Universitetet i Bergen. [Philosophy and nursing: A Marxist and phenomenological contribution.

*Norwegian titles are provided with approximate translation into English.

Philosophical Institute's stencil series no. 34. Bergen: University of Bergen.]

Martinsen, K. (1979). Medisin og sykepleie, historie og samfunn. Oslo: Norsk Sykepleierforbund. [Medicine and nursing, history and society. Oslo: The Norwegian Nursing Association.]

Martinsen, K. (1984). Sykepleiens historie. Freidige og uforsagte diakonisser. Et omsorgsyrke vokser fram 1860-1905. Oslo: Aschehoug/Tanum-Norli. [History of nursing: Frank and engaged deaconesses. A caring profession emerges 1860-1905. Oslo: Aschehoug/Tanum-Norli.]

Martinsen, K. (1989). Omsorg, sykepleie og medisin. Historisk-filosofiske essays. Oslo: Tano Forlag. [Caring, nursing and medicine. Historical-philosophical essays. Oslo: Tano Forlag.]

Martinsen, K. (red.) (1993). Den omtenksomme sykepleier. Oslo: Tano. [The thoughtful nurse. Oslo: Tano.]

Martinsen, K. (1993). Fra Marx til Løgstrup. Om moral, samfunnskritikk og sanselighet i sykepleien. Oslo: Tano Forlag. [From Marx to Løgstrup. On morality, social criticism and sensuousness in nursing. Oslo: Tano Forlag.]

Martinsen, K. (1996). Fenomenologi og omsorg. Tre dialoger. Oslo: Tano-Aschehoug. [Phenomenology and caring. Three dialogues. Oslo: Tano-Aschehoug.]

Martinsen, K. (2000). Øyet og kallet. Bergen: Fagbokforlaget. [The eye and the call. Bergen: Fagbokforlaget.]

Martinsen, K., & Wærness, K. (1979). Pleie uten omsorg? Oslo: Pax Forlag A/S. [Caring without care? Oslo: Pax Forlag.]

Martinsen, K., & Wyller, T. (red.) (2003). Etikk, disiplin og dannelse. Elisabeth Hagemanns etikkbok—Nye lesinger. Oslo: Gyldendal Akademisk. [Ethics, discipline and refinement. Elizabeth Hagemann's ethics book—New readings. Oslo: Gyldendal Akademisk.]

Martinsen, K. (2005). Samtalen, skjønnet og evidensen. Oslo: Akribe. Dialog, discernment and evidence. Oslo: Akribe.

Martinsen, K. (2006). Care and Vulnerability. Oslo: Akribe (English original).

Martinsen, K. (2008). Å se og å innse—om ulike former for evidens. Oslo: Akribe. [To see and to realize—on various forms of evidence. Oslo: Akribe.] (In process with Katie Ericsson).

Book Chapters

Martinsen, K. (1972). Samfunnets krise og sykepleiernes oppgave. I I. K. Haugen, T. Malmin, S. Midtgaard, & K. Nicolaysen (red.), *Pedialogen* (s. 3-14). Oslo: Norsk Sykepleierforbund. [The crises of society and the nursing objectives. In I. K. Haugen, T. Malmin, S. Midtgaard, & K. Nicolaysen (Eds.), *Pedialog* (pp. 3-14). Oslo: Norwegian Nursing Association.]

Martinsen, K. (1972). Sykepleie som sosial-moralsk praksis. I I. K. Haugen, T. Malmin, S. Midtgaard, & K. Nicolaysen (red.), *Pedialogen* (s. 15-36). Oslo: Norsk Sykepleierforbund. [Nursing as social and moral practice. In I. K. Haugen, T. Malmin, S. Midtgaard, & K. Nicolaysen (Eds.), *Pedialog* (pp. 15-36). Oslo: Norwegian Nursing Association.]

Martinsen, K. (1978). Fra ufaglært fattigsykepleie til profesjonelt yrke—Konsekvenser for omsorg. I B. Persson, K. Ravn, & R. Truelsen (red.), *Fokus på sygeplejen-79. Årbok* (s. 128-157). København: Munksgaard. [From unskilled nursing the poor to professional occupation—Consequences for nursing. In B. Persson, K. Ravn, & R. Truelsen (Eds.), *Focus on nursing* (Annual 79, pp. 128-157). Copenhagen: Munksgaard.]

Martinsen, K. (1979). Den engelske sanitation-bevegelsen, hygiene og synet på sykdom. I Ø. Larsen (red.), *Synet på sykdom* (s. 78-87). Oslo: Seksjon for medisinsk historie, Universitetet i Oslo. [The English sanitation movement: Hygiene and the view of illness. In Ø. Larsen (Ed.), *The view of illness* (pp. 78-87). Oslo: University of Oslo, Section for Medical History.]

Martinsen, K. (1979). Diakonissesykepleiens framvekst. Fra vekkelser og kvinneforeninger til moderhus og fattigomsorg. I NAVF's sekretariat for kvinneforskning (red.), *Lønnet og ulønnet omsorg. En seminarrapport* (Arbeidsnotat nr. 5, s. 135-170). Oslo: NAVF. [Development of the professional trained Christian nurses: From revival and woman's charitable groups to the mother house and care of the poor. In NAVF's Secretariat for Feminist Research (Ed.), *Paid and unpaid care: A seminar report* (Working paper no. 5, pp. 135-170). Oslo: NAVE]

Martinsen, K. (1979). Diakonissene. I E. Mehlum (red.), *Bak maskinene, under fanene.* Utgitt i forbindelse med "Kristiania-utstillingen" om arbeidsfolk i byen for 100 år siden (s. 54-56). Oslo: Tiden. [Deconesses. In E. Mehlum (Ed.), *Behind the machines and the banners* (pp. 54-56). Oslo: Tiden.] (Published in connection with "The Christiania (Oslo) exhibition" on the condition of workers 100 years ago.)

Martinsen, K. (1979). Sykepleien, historien og den omvendte omsorgen. I R. Wendt (red.), *Utveckling av omvårdnadsarbete* (s. 90-102). Lund: Studentlitteratur. [Nursing, history and the converse caring. In R. Wendt (Ed.), *Development of health care* (pp. 90-102). Lund: Studentlitteratur.]

Martinsen, K. (1979). Sykepleien i historisk perspektiv: Fra omsorg mot egenomsorg. I M. S. Fagermoen & R. Nord (red.), *Sykepleie: Teori/praksis* (s. 5-23). Oslo: Norwegian Nursing Association. [Nursing in a historical perspective: From care to self caring. In M. S. Fagermoen & R. Nord (Eds.), *Nursing: Theory/practice* (pp. 5-23). Oslo: Norwegian Nursing Association.]

Martinsen, K. (1981). Diakonisser. I H. F. Dahl, J. Elster, I. Iversen, S. Nørve, T. I. Romøren, R. Slagstad, m.fl. (red.), *Pax leksikon.* Oslo: Pax Forlag (s. 89-90). [Deaconessses. In H. F. Dahl, J. Elster, I. Iversen, S. Nørve, T. I. Romøren, R. Slagstad, et al. (Eds.), *Pax lexicon* (pp. 89-90). Oslo: Pax Forlag.]

Martinsen, K. (1981). Guldberg, Cathinka. I H. F. Dahl, J. Elster, I. Iversen, S. Nørve, T. I. Romøren, R. Slagstad, m.fl. (red.), *Pax leksikon* (s. 553-554). Oslo: Pax forlag. [Guldberg, Cathinka. In H. F. Dahl, J. Elster, I. Iversen, S. Nørve, T. I. Romøren, R. Slagstad, et al. (Eds.), *Pax lexicon* (pp. 553-554). Oslo: Pax Forlag.]

Martinsen, K. (1981). Nightingale, Florence. I H. F. Dahl, J. Elster, I. Iversen, S. Nørve, T. I. Romøren, R. Slagstad, m.fl. (red.), *Pax leksikon* (s. 448-449). [Nightingale, Florence. In H. F. Dahl, J. Elster, I. Iversen, S. Nørve, T. I. Romøren, R. Slagstad, et al. (Eds.), *Pax lexicon* (pp. 448-449). Oslo: Pax Forlag.]

Martinsen, K. (1981). Omsorg i sykepleie. I E. Barnes & S. Solbak (red.), *Sykepleielære 1. Lærebok for hjelpepleiere* (Kap. 3). Oslo: Aschehoug. [Care in nursing. In E. Barnes & S. Solbak (Eds.), *Nursing textbook 1. Textbook for licensed practical nurses* (Chapter 3). Oslo: Aschehoug.]

Martinsen, K. (1981). Sykepleier. I H. F. Dahl, J. Elster, I. Iversen, S. Nørve, T. I. Romøren, R. Slagstad, m.fl. (red.), *Pax leksikon* (s. 179-180). [Nurse. In H. F. Dahl, J. Elster, I. Iversen, S. Nørve, T. I. Romøren, R. Slagstad, et al. (Eds.), *Pax lexicon* (pp. 179-180). Oslo: Pax Forlag.]

Martinsen, K. (1981). Sykepleieraksjonen 1972. I H. F. Dahl, J. Elster, I. Iversen, S. Nørve, T. I. Romøren, R. Slagstad, m.fl. (red.), Pax leksikon (s. 180-181). Oslo: Pax forlag. [Nurses on strike 1972. In H. F. Dahl, J. Elster, I. Iversen, S. Nørve, T. I. Romøren, R. Slagstad, et al. (Eds.), *Pax lexicon* (pp. 180-181). Oslo: Pax Forlag.]

Martinsen, K. (1981). Sykepleierforbund, Norsk (NSF). I H. F. Dahl, J. Elster, I. Iversen, S. Nørve, T. I. Romøren, R. Slagstad, m.fl. (red.), *Pax leksikon* (s. 181-183). Oslo: Pax Forlag. [Nursing association. In H. F. Dahl, J. Elster, I. Iversen, S. Nørve, T. I. Romøren, R. Slagstad, et al. (Eds.), *Pax lexicon* (pp. 181-183). Oslo: Pax Forlag.]

Martinsen, K. (1981). Trekk av hjelpepleiernes historie. I E. Barnes & S. Solbak (red.), *Sykepleielære 1. Lærebok for hjelpepleiere.* (Kap. 2). Oslo: Aschehoug. [Aspects of licensed practical nurse history. In E. Barnes & S. Solbak (Eds.), *Nursing textbook 1. Textbook for licensed practical nurses* (Chapter 2). Oslo: Aschehoug.]

Martinsen, K. (1985). Organisering av omsorg: diakonisser i Norge. I J. Bjørgum, K. Gundersen, S. Lie, & K. Vogt (red.), *Kvinnenes kulturhistorie* (s.131-134). Oslo: Universitetsforlaget. [Organization of care: deaconesses in Norway. In J. Bjørgum, K. Gundersen, S. Lie, & K. Vogt (Eds.), *Woman's cultural history* (pp. 131-134). Oslo: Universitetsforlaget.]

Martinsen, K. (1986). Sykepleierne—Helsemisjonerer, oppdragere og profesjonelle yrkeskvinner. I. Fredriksen & H. Rømer (red.), I *Kvinder, Mentalitet og arbejde. Kvindehistorisk forskning i Norden* (s. 151-156). Aarhus: Aarhus universitetsforlag. [Nurses—Health missionaries, educators and professional working woman. In I. Fredriksen & H. Rømer (Eds.), *Woman, mentality and work: Research on feminist history in Nordic countries* (pp. 151-156). Aarhus: Aarhus universitetsforlag.]

Martinsen, K. (1987). Ledelse og omsorgsrasjonalitet—Gir patriarkatbegrepet innsikt? I NAVFs sekretariat for kvinneforskning (red.), *Kjønn og makt: teoretiske perspektiver* (s. 18-26). Arbeidsnotat nr. 2. Oslo: NAVE [Leadership and rationality of care—Does the concept of patriarchy yield insight? In *Gender and power: theoretical perspectives* (Working paper no. 2, pp. 18-26). Oslo: NAVF.]

Martinsen K. (1989). Omsorg i sykepleien—In moralsk utfordring. I B. Persson, J. Petersen, & R. Truelsen (red.), *Fokus på sygeplejen-90* (s. 181-200). København: Munksgaard. [Caring in nursing—A moral challenge. In B. Persson, J. Petersen, & R. Truelsen (Eds.), *Focus on Nursing—90* (pp. 181-200). Copenhagen: Munksgaard.]

Martinsen, K. (1990). Fra resultater til situasjoner: Omsorg, makt og solidaritet. I Samkvind (Center for samfundsvidenskabelig kvindeforskning). *Kvinder og kommuner i Norden* (s. 61-82), København: Samkvind. [From results to situations: Care, power and solidarity. In Samkvind (Center for Feminist Research), *Woman and municipals in Nordic country* (pp. 61-82). Copenhagen: Samkvind.]

Martinsen, K. (1990). Moralsk praksis og dokumentasjon i praktisk sykepleie. I T. Jensen, L. U. Jensen, & W. C. Kim (red.), *Grundlagsproblemer i sygeplejen. Etik, videnskabsteori, ledelse & samfunn* (s. 60-84). Aarhus: Philosophia. [Moral practice and documentation in practical nursing. In T. Jensen, L. U. Jensen, & W. C. Kim, *Foundational problems in nursing: Ethics, theories of science, leadership and society* (pp. 60-84). Aarhus: Philosophia.]

Martinsen, K. (1993). Etikk og diakoni. I P. Frølich, J. Midtbø, & A. Tang, *Bergen Diakonissehjem 75 år* (s. 22-26). Bergen: Bergen Diakonissehjem. [Etichs and Diaconi. In P. Frølich, J. Midtbø, & A. Tang, *Bergen Diakonissehjem 75 years* (pp. 22-26). Bergen: Bergen Diakonissehjem.]

Martinsen, K. (1993). Omsorgens filosofi og dens praksis. I H. M. Dahl (red.), *Omsorg og kjærlighet i velfærdsstaten* (Samfundsvidenskabelig kvindeforskning/Cekvina (s. 7-23). Århus: Universitetet i Århus. [Caring philosophy and its practice. In H. M. Dahl (Ed.), *Care and love in the welfare state* (Social scientifically woman studies, pp. 7-23). Århus: The University of Århus.]

Martinsen, K. (1995). Omsorgsfeltet i den kliniske sygepleje. I I. Andersen & M. G. Erikstrup (red.), *Statens sundhedsvidenskabelige forskningsråds sygeplejeforskningsinitiativ. Betydning for sygeplejepraksis* (s. 31-43). Århus: Århus Universitet. [Area for care in clinical nursing. In I. Andersen & M. G. Erikstrup (Eds.), *The state's initiative in nursing science. The significance for nursing practice* (pp. 31-43). Århus: Århus University.]

Martinsen, K. (1997). Etikk og kall, kultur og kropp—En dialog med Patricia Benner. I M. Sæther (red.), *Sykepleiekonferanse på Nordkalottens tak* (s. 111-157). Tromsø: Universitetet i Tromsø. [Ethics and vocation, culture and the body—A dialogue with Patricia Benner. In M. Sæther (Ed.), *Nursing conference on the roof of Nordkalotten* (pp. 111-157). Tromsø: University of Tromsø.]

Martinsen, K. (1999). Etikken og kulturen, og kroppens sårbarhet. I K. Christensen & L. J. Syltevik (red.), *Omsorgens forvitring? En antologi om utfordringer i velferdsstaten—Tilegnet Kari Wærness* (s. 241-269). Bergen: Fagbokforlaget. [Ethics and culture, and vulnerability of the body. In K. Christensen & L. J. Syltevik (Eds.), *Weathering of caring? An anthology about challenges in the welfare state—Dedicate Kari Wærness* (pp. 241-269). Bergen: Fagbokforlaget.]

Martinsen, K. (2000). Kjærlighetsgjerningen og kallet. Betraktninger omkring Rikke Nissens "Lærebog i Sygepleje for diakonisser". I R. Nissen, *Lærebog i Sygepleie. Med etterord av Kari Martinsen* (s. 245-300). Oslo: Gyldendal Akademisk. [The loving act and the call. Reflections on Rikke Nissen's *Textbook of nursing for deaconesses.* In R. Nissen, *Textbook of nursing. With afterword by Kari Martinsen* (pp. 245-300). Oslo: Gyldendal Akademisk.]

Martinsen, K. (2001). Huset og sangen, gråten og skammen. Rom og arkitektur som ivaretaker av menneskets verdighet. I T. Wyller (red.), *Skam: Perspektiver på skam, ære og skamløshet i det moderne* (s. 167-190). Bergen: Fagbokforlaget. [The house and the song, the tears and the shame: Space and architecture as caretakers of human dignity. In T. Wyller (Ed.), *Shame: Perspectives on shame, honor and shamelessness in modernity* (pp. 167-190). Bergen: Fagbokforlaget.]

Martinsen, K. (2002). Rikke Nissen. Kjærlighetsgjerningen og sykestuen. I R. Birkelund (red.), *Omsorg, kald og kamp. Personer og ideer i sygeplejens historie* (s. 305-328). København: Munksgaard forlag. [The loving act and the room for the sick. In R. Birkelund (Ed.), *Care, vocation and love in action and the sick-room. Persons and ideas in nursing history* (pp. 305-328). Copenhagen: Munksgaard.]

Martinsen, K. (2002). Rommets tid, den sykes tid, pleiens tid. I I. T. Bjørk, S. Helseth, & F. Nortvedt (red.), *Møte mellom pasient og sykepleier* (s. 250-271). Oslo: Gyldendal Akademisk. [The room's time, the ill person's time, nursing time. In I. T. Bjørk, S. Helseth, & F. Nortvedt (Eds.), *The meeting between patient and nurse* (pp. 250-271). Oslo: Gyldendal Akademisk.]

Martinsen, K. (2003). Disiplin og rommelighet. I K. Martinsen & T. Wyller (red.), *Etikk, disiplin og dannelse. Elisabeth Hagemanns etikkbok—Nye lesinger* (s. 51-85). Oslo: Gyldendal Akademisk. [Discipline and spaciousness. In K. Martinsen & T. Wyller (Eds.), *Ethics, discipline and refinement. Elizabeth Hagemann's ethics book—New readings* (pp. 51-85). Oslo: Gyldendal Akademisk.]

Martinsen, K. (2005). Å bo på sykehuset og erfare arkitektur. I K. Larsen (red.), *Arkitektur, kropp og læring.* København: Reitzels forlag. [To dwell in hospitals and experience architecture. In K. Larsen (Ed.), *Architecture, body and learning.* Copenhagen: Reitzels forlag.]

Martinsen, K. (2005). Sårbarheten og omveiene. Løgstrup og sykepleien. I D. Bugge, P. Bøvadt and P. Sørensen (red.). *Løgstrups mange ansikter* (s. 255-270). Fredriksberg: Anis. [Vulnerability and detours. Løgstrup and nursing. In D. Bugge, P. Bøvadt and P. Sørensen (ed.). *Løgstrup's many faces* (pp. 255-270). Fredriksberg: Anis.]

Martinsen, K. (2007). Angår du meg? Etisk fordring og disiplinert godhet. I H. Alvsvåg & O. Førland (red.). *Engasjement og læring* (s. 315-344). Oslo: Akribe. [Do you concern me? Etical demand and disciplined goodness. In H. Alvsvåg & O. Førland (ed.). *Commitment and learning* (pp 315-344) Oslo: Akribe.]

Martinsen, K., K. Beedholm and K. Fredriksen (2007). Metadebatten der forsvandt. I K. Fredriksen, K. Lomborg and U. Zeitler (red.). *Perspektiver på forskning* (s. 43-55). Århus: JCVU udviklingsinitiativet for sygeplejerskeuddannelsen. [The Meta debate that disappeared. In K. Fredriksen, K. Lomborg and U. Zeitler (ed.). *Perspectives on research* (pp 43-55). Århus: JCVU udviklingsinitiativet for sygeplejerskeuddannelsen.

Martinsen, K. (2008). Modernitet, avtrylling og skam. En måte å lese vestens medisin på i det moderne. In K. A. Petersen and M. Høyen (red.). *At sette spor på en vandring fra Aquinas til Bordieu—æresbog til Staf Callewaert.* Forlag@hexis.dk [Modernity, disenchantment and shame. A way of reading Western medicine in the modern. In K. A. Petersen and M. Høyen (ed.). *Leaving a trail on the way from Aquinas to Bordieu—honorary volume for Staf Callewaert.* Forlag@hexis.dk]

Journal Articles

Martinsen, K. (1976). Historie og sykepleie—Momenter til en utdanningsdebatt. *Kontrast, 7*(12), 430-446. [History and nursing—Elements of an educational debate. *Contrast, 7*(12), 430-446.]

Martinsen, K. (1977). Nightingale—Ingen opprører bak myten. *Sykepleien, 18*(65), 1022-1025. [Nightingale—No rebel behind the myth. *Nursing, 18*(65), 1022-1025.]

Martinsen, K. (1978). Det 'kliniske blikk' i medisinen og i sykepleien. *Sykepleien, 20*(66), 1271-1272. [The "clinical gaze" in medicine and in nursing. *Nursing, 20*(66), 1271-1272.]

Martinsen, K. (1981). Omsorgens filosofi og omsorg i praksis. *Sykepleien, 8*(69), 4-10. [The philosophy of caring—And the practice. *Nursing, 8*(69), 4-10.]

Martinsen, K. (1982). Den tvetydige veldedigheten. *Sosiologi i dag,* temanummer *Kvinner og omsorgsarbeid, 1*(12), 29-41. [The ambiguity of charity. *Sociology, 1*(12), 29-41.]

Martinsen, K. (1982). Diakonissene—De første faglærte sykepleiere. *Sykepleien, 7*(70), 6-9. [The deaconesses—The first professionally trained nurses. *Nursing, 7*(70), 6-9.]

Martinsen, K. (1985). Kallsarbeidere og yrkeskvinner: Diakonissene—Våre første sykepleiere. *Forskningsnytt*, temanummer: *Kvinner og arbeid, 1*, 18-23. [Woman with a calling and a profession: The deaconesses—Our first nurses. *News in Science, 1*, 18-23.]

Martinsen, K. (1985). Sykepleiertradisjonen—Et nødvendig korrektiv til dagens sykepleieforskning. *Sykepleien, 15*(73), 6-14. [The nursing tradition—A necessary corrective to today's nursing science. *Nursing, 15*(73), 6-14.]

Martinsen, K. (1986). Omsorg og profesjonalisering—Med fagutviklingen i sykepleien som eksempel. *Nytt om kvinneforskning, 2*(10), 21-32. [Care and professionalism—An example from the development in nursing. *News in Woman Science, 2*(10), 21-32.]

Martinsen, K. (1987). Arbeidsdeling—Kjønn og makt. *Sykepleien, 1*(74), 18-23. [Division of labor—Gender and power. *Nursing, 1*(74), 18-23.]

Martinsen, K. (1987). Endret kunnskapsideal og to pleiegrupper. *Sykepleien, 4*(74), 20-25. [A changing paradigm and two types of nurses. *Nursing, 4*(74), 20-25.]

Martinsen, K. (1987). Helsepolitiske problemer og helsepolitisk tenkning bak sykehusloven av 1969. *Historisk tidsskrift, 3*(66), 357-372. [Health policy problems and health policy thinking underlying the new hospital law. *History, 3*(66), 357-372.]

Martinsen, K. (1987). Ledelse og omsorgsrasjonalitet—Gir patriarkatbegrepet innsikt? *Sykepleien, 1*(74), 18-23. [Management and caring rationality—Does the concept of patriarchate give insight? *Nursing, 1*(74), 18-23.]

Martinsen, K. (1987). Legers interesse for svangerskapet—En del av den perinatale omsorg. Tidsrommet ca. 1890-1940. *Historisk tidsskrift, 3*(66), 373-390. [Doctors' interests in pregnancy—A part of perinatal care. *History, 3*(66), 373-390.]

Martinsen, K. (1987). Norsk Sykepleierskeforbund på barrikadene for utdanning fra første stund. *Sykepleien, 3*(74), 6-12. [The Norwegian Nursing Association on the barricades from day one. *Nursing, 3*(74), 6-12.]

Martinsen, K. (1988). Ansvar og solidaritet. En moralfilosofisk og sosialpolitisk forståelse av omsorg. *Sykepleien, 12*(75), 17-21. [Responsibility and solidarity. A moral-philosophical and sociopolitical understanding of caring. *Nursing, 12*(75) 17-21.]

Martinsen, K. (1988). Etikk og omsorgsmoral. *Sykepleien, 13*(75), 16-20. [Ethics and the moral practice of caring. *Nursing, 13*(75), 16-20.]

Martinsen, K. (1990). Diakoni er fellesskap og samhørighet. *Under Ulriken, 5*(30), 6-10. [Diaconi is community and fellowship. *Under Ulrikken, 5*(30), 6-10.]

Martinsen, K. (1991). Omsorg og makt, ord og kropp i sykepleien. *Sykepleien, 2*(78), 2-11, 29. [Caring and power, word and body in nursing profession. *Nursing, 2*(78), 2-11, 29.]

Martinsen, K. (1991). Under kjærlig forskning. Fenomenologiens åpning for den levde erfaring i sykepleien. *Perspektiv—Sygeplejersken, 36*(91), 4-15. [Compassionate research. Phenomenology opening up for lived experience in nursing. *Perspective—Nursing* (Danish), *36*(91), 4-15.]

Martinsen, K. (1993). Grunnforskning—Trofast og troløs forskning—Noen fenomenologiske overveielser. *Tidsskrift for Sygeplejeforskning, 1*(9), 7-28. [Basic research—Faithful and faithless research—Some phenomenological considerations. *Nursing Research* (Danish), *1*(9), 7-28.]

Martinsen, K. (1997). De etiske fortellinger. *Omsorg, 1*(14), 58-63. [The ethical narratives. *Caring, 1*(14), 58-63.]

Martinsen, K. (1997). Kallet—Kan vi være det foruten? *Tidsskrift for sygeplejeforskning, 2*(13), 9-41. [The vocation—Can we do without it? *Nursing Science, 2*(13), 9-41.]

Martinsen, K. (1998). Det fremmede og vedkommende (I). *Klinisk Sygepleje, 1*(12), 13-19. [Strangeness and relevant (I). *Clinical Nursing, 1*(12), 13-19.]

Martinsen, K. (1998). Det fremmede og vedkommende (II). *Klinisk Sygepleje, 1-2*(12), 78-84. [Strangeness and relevans (II). *Clinical Nursing, 2*(12), 78-84.]

Martinsen, K. (2001). Er det mørketid for filosofien? Et svar til Marit Kirkevold. *Tidsskrift for sygeplejeforskning* (dansk), *1*(17), 19-23. [Is Philosophy in shadow? A replay to Marit Kirkevold. *Nursing Science* (Danish), *1*(17), 19-23.]

Martinsen, K. (2002). Livsfilosonske betraktninger. I *Diakoninytt, 3*(118), 8-12. [Reflections on the philosophy of life. *Deaconry News, 3*(118), 8-12.]

Martinsen, K. (2002). Samtalen, kommunikasjonen og sakligheten i omsorgsyrkene. *Omsorg, 1*(19), 14-22. [Conversation, communication and professionality in the caring professions. *Caring, 1*(19), 14-22.]

Martinsen, K. (2003). Talens åpenhet og evidens—Dialog med Jens Bydam. *Klinisk Sygepleje, 4*(17), 36-46. [The openness of speech and evidence—Dialogue with Jens Bydam. *Clinical Nursing, 4*(17), 36-46.]

Martinsen, K. (2004). Skjønn—Språk og distanse: dialog med Jens Bydam. *Klinisk Sygepleje, 2*(18), 50-56. [Discernment—Language and distance: Dialogue with Jens Bydam. *Clinical Nursing, 2*(18), 50-56.]

Martinsen, K. (2008). Innfallet—og dets betydning i liv og arbeid. Metafysisk inspirerte overveielser over innfallets natur og måter å vise seg på. *Klinisk Sygepleje, 1*(22), . . . [The Innfall (impulse)—and its significance in life and work. Metaphysically inspired reflections on the nature of the Innfall and its ways of showing itself. *Clinical Nursing, 1* (22) . . .]

Martinsen, K., & Wærness, K. (1976). Sykepleierrollen—En undertrykt kvinnerolle i helsesektoren (I). *Sykepleien, 4*(64), 220-224. [The nursing role—An oppressed female role in National Health Service. *Nursing, 4*(64), 220-224.]

Martinsen, K., & Wærness, K. (1976). Sykepleierrollen—En undertrykt kvinnerolle i Helsesektoren (II). *Sykepleien, 5*(64), 274-275, 281-282. [The nursing role—An oppressed female role in National Health Service. *Nursing, 5*(64), 274-275, 281-282.]

Martinsen, K., & Wærness, K. (1980). Klientomsorg og profesjonalisering. *Sykepleien, 4*(68), 12-14. [Client care and the professionalization. *Nursing, 4*(68), 12-14.]

Publications in Press

Martinsen, K. (2008). Å se og å innse—om ulike former for evidens. Oslo: Akribe. [To see and to realize—on various forms of evidence. Oslo: Akribe.] (In process with Katie Eriksson).

Martinsen, K. (2008). Rom og rommelighet. Bergen: Fagbokforlaget. [Room and spaciousness. Bergen: Fagbokforlaget.]

Secondary Sources

Alvsvåg, H., & Gjengedal, E. (red.) (2000). Omsorgstenkning. En innføring i Kari Martinsens forfatterskap. Bergen: Fagbokforlaget. [Caring thought: An introduction to the writings of Kari Martinsen. Bergen: Fagbokforlaget.]

Austgard, K. (2002). Omsorgsfilosofi i praksis. Å tenke med filosofen Kari Martinsen i sykepleien. Oslo: Cappelen Akademisk Forlag. [Philosophy of caring in practice: Thinking with philosopher Kari Martinsen in nursing. Oslo: Cappelen Akademisk Forlag.]

Beedholm,K. (2003). Forandring og træghed i den sygeplejefaglige diskurs. Viborg: Forlaget PUC, Denmark. [Change and inertia in the discourse of nursing studies. Viborg: Forlaget PUC, Denmark.]

Jørgensen, B.B. and Lyngaa, J. (red.) (2008). Sygeplejeleksikon. København: Munksgaard. [Encyclopedia of Nursing. Copenhagen: Munksgaard.]

Kirkevold, M., Nortvedt, F., & Alvsvåg, H. (red.) (1993). Klokskap og kyndighet. Kari Martinsens innflytelse på norsk og dansk sykepleie. Oslo: Gyldendal Academisk. [Wisdom and skill: Kari Martinsen's influence on Norwegian and Danish nursing. Oslo: Gyldendal Academisk.]

Mekki, T. E., & Tollefsen, S. (2000). På terskelen. Introduksjon til sykepleie som fag og yrke. Oslo: Akribe. [On the threshold: An introduction to nursing as discipline and profession. Oslo: Akribe.]

Olsen, R. (1998). Klok av erfaring? Om sansing og oppmerksomhet, kunnskap og refleksjon i praktisk sykepleie. Oslo: Tano Aschehoug. [Wise with experience? On sensation and attention, knowledge and reflection in practical nursing. Oslo: Tano Aschehoug.]

Overgaard, A. E. (2003). Åndelig omsorg—En lœrebog. Kari Martinsen, Katie Eriksson og Joyce Travelbee i nytt lys. København: Nyt Nordisk Forlag Arnold Busck. [Spiritual care—A textbook. Kari Martinsen, Katie Eriksson and Joyce Travelbee in a new light. Copenhagen: Nyt Nordisk Forlag Arnold Busck.]

Solvoll, B.A. (2007). Omsorgsferdigheter som pedagogisk prosjekt—en feltstudie I sykepleieutdanningen. Oslo: Universitetet i Oslo, Det medisinske Fakultet, nr 540. [Caring skills as pedagogical project—a field study in nursing education. Oslo: University of Oslo, Faculty of Medicine, Doctoral dissertations no 540.]

Walstad, P.B. (2006). Dannelse og Duelighed for livet. Dannelse og yrkesutdanning i den grundtvigske tradisjon. Trondheim: Norges teknisk-naturvitenskapelige universitet. Doctoral dissertation 2006:88. [Education and Capability for life. Education and professional training in the Grundtvigian tradition. Trondheim: Norges teknisk-naturvitenskapelige universitet, NTNU Doctoral dissertations 2006:88.]

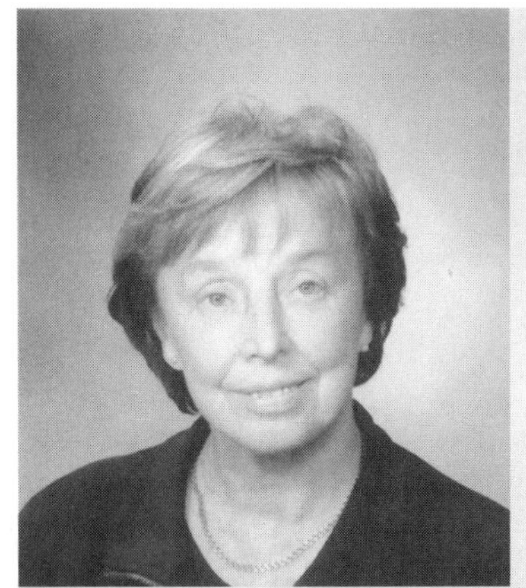

CHAPTER

11

Katie Eriksson

1943-present

Theory of Caritative Caring

Unni Å. Lindström, Lisbet Lindholm, and Joan E. Zetterlund

"Caritative caring means that we take "caritas" into use when caring for the human being in health and suffering...Caritative caring is a manifestation of the love that 'just exists'... Caring communion, true caring, occurs when the one caring in a spirit of caritas alleviates the suffering of the patient" (Eriksson, 1992c, pp. 204, 207).

CREDENTIALS OF THE THEORIST

Katie Eriksson is one of the pioneers of caring science in the Nordic countries. When she started her career 30 years ago, she had to open the way for a new science. We who have followed her work and progress in Finland have noticed her excellent ability from the very beginning to have designed caring science as a discipline, while at the same time with her excellent pedagogical skill bringing to life the abstract substance of caring.

Eriksson was born on November 18, 1943, in Jakobstad, Finland. She belongs to the Finland-Swedish minority in Finland, and her native language is Swedish. She is a 1965 graduate of the Helsinki Swedish School of Nursing, and in 1967, she completed her public health nursing specialty education at the same institution. She graduated in 1970 from the nursing teacher education program at Helsinki Finnish School of Nursing. She continued her academic studies at University of Helsinki, where she received her MA degree in philosophy in 1974 and her licentiate degree in 1976; she defended her doctoral dissertation in pedagogy (*The Patient Care Process—An Approach to Curriculum Construction within Nursing Education: The Development of a Model for the Patient Care Process and an Approach for Curriculum Development Based on the Process of Patient Care*) in 1982 (Eriksson, 1974, 1976, 1981). In 1984, she was appointed Docent of Caring Science (part time) at University of Kuopio, the first docentship in caring science in the Nordic countries. She was appointed Professor of Caring Science at Åbo Akademi University in 1992. Between 1993 and

1999, she also held a professorship in caring science at University of Helsinki, Faculty of Medicine, where she has been a docent since 2001. Since January 1, 1996, she has served as Director of Nursing at Helsinki University Central Hospital, with responsibilities for research and development of caring science in connection with her professorship at Åbo Akademi University.

At the end of the 1960s and beginning of the 1970s, Eriksson worked in various fields of nursing practice, but she continued her studies at the same time. Her main area of work, however, has been in teaching and research. Since the beginning of the 1970s, Eriksson has systematically deepened her thoughts about caring, partly through the development of an ideal model for caring that has formed the basis for the caritative caring theory, and partly through the development of an autonomous, humanistically oriented caring science. Eriksson is one of the few caring science researchers in the Nordic countries who has developed a caring theory, and she has been a forerunner of basic research in caring science.

Eriksson's scientific career and professional experience comprise two periods: the years 1970 to 1986 at Helsinki Swedish School of Nursing, and the period from 1986, when she was invited to found the Department of Caring Science at Åbo Akademi University, which she has directed since 1987.

In 1972, after teaching for 2 years at the nursing education unit at Helsinki Swedish School of Nursing, she was assigned to start and develop an educational program to prepare nurse educators at that institution. Such a program taught in the Swedish language had not existed in Finland. This education program, with initial collaboration with University of Helsinki, was the beginning of caring science didactics. Under Eriksson's leadership, Helsinki Swedish School of Nursing developed one of the leading educational programs in caring science and nursing in the Nordic countries. It became the forerunner of education based on caring science and also of integration of research in the education. Eriksson was in charge of the program for 2 years, until she became dean at Helsinki Swedish School of Nursing in January 1974. She remained the dean until September 1986, when she was nominated to plan and start academic education and research at Åbo Akademi University.

Toward the end of the 1980s, nursing science became a university subject in Finland, and professorial chairs were established at four Finnish universities and at the Finland-Swedish university, Åbo Akademi University. In 1986, Eriksson was called to plan an education and research program within the subject of caring science at Åbo Akademi University's Faculty of Education in Vaasa, Finland. A fully developed education program for health care, with three focus areas or options and a research education program for caring science, was created. The result of her planning was the establishment of the Department of Caring Science in 1987. It became an autonomous department within the Faculty of Education of Åbo Akademi University until 1992, when a new faculty, the Faculty of Social and Caring Sciences, was founded. A result of her work was that the education program for the MA in health and the caring science didactic education program were developed.

In 1987, a doctoral program was started under Eriksson's direction, and 32 doctoral dissertations have been published at the department. At her own department, Eriksson, with her staff and researchers, has further developed the caritative theory of caring and caring science as an academic discipline. The department today has a leading position in the Nordic countries with students and researchers from those countries.

In addition to her work with teaching, research, and supervision, Eriksson is the dean of the Department of Caring Science. One of her central tasks has been to develop Nordic and other international contacts within caring science.

Eriksson has been a very popular guest and keynote speaker, not only in Finland, but in all the Nordic countries and at various international congresses. In 1977, she was a guest speaker at Symposium of Medical and Nursing Education in Istanbul, Turkey; in 1978, she participated in the foundation of medical care teacher education in Reykjavik, Iceland;

in 1982, she presented her nursing care didactic model at the First Open Conference of the Workgroup of European Nurse-Researchers in Uppsala, Sweden; and for several years, she participated in education and advanced education of nurses at the Statens Utdanningscenter for Helsopersonell (Federal Education Center for Nursing Staff) in Oslo, Norway. In 1988, she taught a course titled "Basic Research in Nursing Care Science" at the University in Bergen, Norway, and a course called "Nursing Care Science's Theory of Science and Research" at Umeå University in Sweden. She has worked as consultant at many educational institutions in Sweden; since 1975, she has been a regular lecturer at Nordiska Hälsovårdsskolan (The Nordic School of Public Health) in Gothenburg, Sweden. In 1991, she was a guest speaker at the 13th International Association for Human Caring (IAHC) Conference in Rochester, New York; in 1992, she presented her theory at the 14th IAHC Conference in Melbourne, Australia; and in 1993, she was the keynote speaker at the 15th IAHC Conference, Caring as Healing: Renewal Through Hope, in Portland, Oregon (Eriksson, 1994b).

Since 1985, she has been a yearly keynote speaker at the annual congresses for nurse managers and, since 1996, at the annual caring science symposia in Helsinki, Finland. In many public dialogues with Professor Kari Martinsen from Norway, Eriksson has discussed basic questions about caring and caring science. Some of the dialogues have been published (Martinsen, 1996).

Eriksson has worked as a leader of many symposia: in 1975, for The Nordic Symposium about the Nursing Care Process (the first Nordic Nursing Care Science Symposium in Finland); in 1982, for The Symposium in Basic Research in Nursing Care Science; in 1985, for The Nordic Symposium in Nursing Care Science; in 1989, for the Nordic symposium titled "Humanistic Caring"; in 1991, for the Nordic Caring Science Conference, "Caritas & Passio in Vaasa, Finland"; and in 1993, for the Nordic Caring Science Conference, "To Care or Not to Care—The Key Question" in Nursing in Vaasa, Finland.

Eriksson's caritative theory of caring came into clearer focus internationally in 1997, when the IAHC for the first time arranged its research conference in a European country. The Department of Caring Science had the honor of serving as the host of this conference, which was arranged in Helsinki, Finland, in 1997, with the topic, "Human Caring: The Primacy of Love and Existential Suffering."

Eriksson is a member of several editorial committees for international journals in nursing and caring science. She has been invited to many universities in Finland and other Nordic countries as a faculty opponent for doctoral students and an expert consultant in her field. She is not only an advisor for her own research students but also a supervisor for research students at Kuopio and Helsinki Universities, where she is an associate professor (docent). Eriksson served as chairperson of the Nordic Academy of Caring Science from 1999 to 2002.

Eriksson has produced an extensive list of textbooks, scientific reports, professional journal articles, and short papers. Her publications started at the beginning of the 1970s and include a total of about 400 titles. Some of her publications have been translated into other languages, mainly into Finnish. *Vårdandets Idé [The Idea of Caring]* has been published in Braille. Her first English translation, *The Suffering Human Being [Den Lidande Människan]*, was published in 2006 by Nordic Studies Press in Chicago.

Eriksson has received many awards and honors for her professional and academic accomplishments, of which we want to mention several. In 1975, Eriksson was nominated by Finland to receive the 3M-ICN (International Council of Nurses) Nursing Fellowship award; in 1987, she was awarded the Sophie Mannerheim Medal of the Swedish Nursing Association in Finland; and in 1998, she received the Caring Science Gold Mark for academic nursing care at Helsinki University Central Hospital. Also in 1998, she received an Honorary Doctorate in Public Health from the Nordic School of Public Health, in Gothenburg, Sweden. Other awards include the 2001 Åland Islands medal for caring science activity in the province and the

2003 Topelius Medal, instituted by Åbo Akademi University in acknowledgment of good research. In 2003, she was honored nationally as a Knight, First Class, of the Order of the White Rose of Finland.

THEORETICAL SOURCES

Ever since the middle of the 1970s, Eriksson's leading thoughts have been not only to develop the substance of caring, but also to develop caring science as an independent discipline (Eriksson, 1988). From the beginning, Eriksson wanted to go back to the great Greek classics by Plato, Socrates, and Aristotle, from whom she found her inspiration for the development of both the substance and the discipline of caring science (Eriksson, 1987a). From her basic idea of caring science as a humanistic science, she developed a meta-theory that she refers to as "the theory of science for caring science" (Eriksson, 1988, 2001).

When developing caring science as an academic discipline, her most important sources of inspiration besides Plato and Aristotle were Swedish theologian Anders Nygren (1972) and Hans-Georg Gadamer (1960/1994). Nygren and later Tage Kurtén (1987) have provided her with support for her division of caring science into systematic and clinical caring science. Eriksson introduces Nygren's concepts of motive research, context of meaning, and basic motive, which give the discipline a structure. The aim of motive research is to find the essential context, the leading idea of caring. The idea of motive research applied to caring science is, in an objective way, to show the characteristics of caring (Eriksson, 1992c).

The basic motive in caring science and caring is *caritas,* which constitutes the leading idea and keeps the various elements together. It gives both the substance and the discipline of caring science a distinctive character. In development of the basic motive, St. Augustine (1957) and Søren Kierkegaard (1843/1943) become important sources. In further development of the discipline, Eriksson's thinking has been influenced by sources of theory of science such as Thomas Kuhn (1971) and Karl Popper (1997), and later by the American philosopher Susan Langer (1942) and the Finnish philosophers Eino Kaila (1939) and Georg von Wright (1986), all of whom support the human science idea that science cannot exist without values.

For many years, Eriksson collaborated with Håkan Törnebohm (1978), holder of the first Nordic professorial chair in the theory of science at the University of Gothenburg, Sweden. It is especially Törnebohm's research in and development of paradigms related to the development of various scientific cultures that inspired Eriksson (Eriksson, 1989; Lindström, 1992).

The thought that concepts have both meaning and substance has been prominent in Eriksson's scientific work. This appears through a systematic analysis of fundamental concepts with the help of a semantic method of analysis rooted in the idea of hermeneutics, which professor in education Peep Koort (1975) developed. Koort, who was Eriksson's mentor, was unmistakably her most important source of inspiration in her scientific work. Building on the foundation of his methodology, Eriksson subsequently developed a model for concept development that has been of great importance to many researchers in their scientific work.

In her formulation of the caritative caring ethic, which Eriksson conceives as an ontological ethic, Emmanuel Lévinas' (1988) idea that ethics precedes ontology has been a guiding principle. Eriksson agrees especially with Lévinas' thought that the call to serve precedes dialogue, that ethics is always more important in relations with other human beings. The fundamental substance of ethics—caritas, love, and charity—is supported further by Aristotle's (1993), Nygren's (1972), Kierkegaard's (1843/1943), and St. Augustine's (1957) ideas. In the formulation of caritative ethics, Eriksson has been inspired by Kierkegaard's ideas of the innermost spirit of a human being as a synthesis of the eternal and temporal, and that acting ethically is to will absolutely or to will the eternal (Kierkegaard, 1843/1943). She stresses the importance of the knowledge of history of ideas for the preservation of the whole of spiritual culture and finds support for this in Nikolaj Berdâev (1990), the Russian philosopher and historian. In intensifying the basic conception of the human being as body, soul, and spirit, Eriksson carries on an interesting dialogue with several theologians like Gustaf Wingren (1960/1996), António Barbosa da Silva (1993), and Tage Kurtén (1987), while developing the subdiscipline she refers to as *caring theology.*

Perhaps the most prominent feature of Eriksson's thinking has been her clear formulation of the ontological, epistemological, and ethical basic assumptions with regard to the discipline of caring science. In the field of caring science, historical sources like Plato, Aristotle, and Socrates have served as guides for Eriksson whenever she has been looking for a basis for the substance of caring in its original historical form.

MAJOR CONCEPTS & DEFINITIONS

CARITAS

Caritas means love and charity. In caritas, eros and agapé are united, and caritas is by nature unconditional love. Caritas, which is the fundamental motive of caring science, also constitutes the motive for all caring. It means that caring is an endeavor to mediate faith, hope, and love through tending, playing, and learning.

CARING COMMUNION

Caring communion constitutes the context of the meaning of caring and is the structure that determines caring reality. Caring gets its distinctive character through caring communion (Eriksson, 1990). It is a form of intimate connection that characterizes caring. Caring communion requires meeting in time and space, an absolute, lasting presence (Eriksson, 1992c). Caring communion is characterized by intensity and vitality, and by warmth, closeness, rest, respect, honesty, and tolerance. It cannot be taken for granted but pre-supposes a conscious effort to be with the other. Caring communion is seen as the source of strength and meaning in caring. Eriksson (1990) writes in *Pro Caritate,* referring to Lévinas:

> Entering into communion implies creating opportunities for the other—to be able to step out of the enclosure of his/her own identity, out of that which belongs to one towards that which does not belong to one and is nevertheless one's own—it is one of the deepest forms of communion (pp. 28-29).

Joining in a communion means creating possibilities for the other. Lévinas suggests that considering someone as one's own son implies a relationship "beyond the possible" (1985, p. 71; 1988). In this relationship, the individual perceives the other person's possibilities as if they were his or her own. This requires the ability to move toward that which is no longer one's own but which belongs to oneself. It is one of the deepest forms of communion (Eriksson, 1992b). Caring communion is what unites and ties together and gives caring its significance (Eriksson, 1992a).

THE ACT OF CARING

The act of caring contains the caring elements (faith, hope, love, tending, playing, and learning), involves the categories of infinity and eternity, and invites to deep communion. The act of caring is the art of making something very special out of something less special.

CARITATIVE CARING EFFECTS

Caritative caring ethics comprises the ethics of caring, the core of which is determined by the caritas motive. Eriksson makes a distinction between caring ethics and nursing ethics. She also defines the foundations of ethics in care and its essential substance. Caring ethics deals with the basic relation between the patient and the nurse—the way in which the nurse meets the patient in an ethical sense. It is about the approach we have toward the patient. Nursing ethics deals with the ethical principles and rules that guide

MAJOR CONCEPTS & DEFINITIONS—cont'd

my work or my decisions. Caring ethics is the core of nursing ethics. The foundations of caritative ethics can be found not only in history, but also in the dividing line between theological and human ethics in general. Eriksson has been influenced by Nygren's (1966) human ethics and Lévinas' (1988) "face ethics," among others. Ethical caring is what we actually make explicit through our approach and the things we do for the patient in practice. An approach that is based on ethics in care means that we, without prejudice, see the human being with respect, and that we confirm his or her absolute dignity. It also means that we are willing to sacrifice something of ourselves. The ethical categories that emerge as basic in caritative caring ethics are human dignity, the caring communion, invitation, responsibility, good and evil, and virtue and obligation. In an ethical act, the good is brought out through ethical actions (Eriksson, 1995, 2003).

DIGNITY

Dignity constitutes one of the basic concepts of caritative caring ethics. Human dignity is partly absolute dignity, partly relative dignity. Absolute dignity is granted the human being through creation, while relative dignity is influenced and formed through culture and external contexts. A human being's absolute dignity involves the right to be confirmed as a unique human being (Eriksson, 1988, 1995, 1997a).

INVITATION

Invitation refers to the act that occurs when the carer welcomes the patient to the caring communion. The concept of invitation finds room for a place where the human being is allowed to rest, a place that breathes genuine hospitality, and where the patient's appeal for charity meets with a response (Eriksson, 1995; Eriksson & Lindström, 2000).

SUFFERING

Suffering is an ontological concept described as a human being's struggle between good and evil in a state of becoming. Suffering implies in some sense dying away from something, and through reconciliation, the wholeness of body, soul, and spirit is re-created, when the human being's holiness and dignity appear. Suffering is a unique, isolated total experience and is not synonymous with pain (Eriksson, 1984, 1993).

SUFFERING RELATED TO ILLNESS, TO CARE, AND TO LIFE

These are three different forms of suffering. Suffering related to illness is experienced in connection with illness and treatment. When the patient is exposed to suffering caused by care or absence of caring, the patient experiences suffering related to care, which is always a violation of the patient's dignity. Not to be taken seriously, not to be welcome, being blamed, and being subjected to the exercise of power are various forms of s uffering related to care. In the situation of being a patient, the entire life of a human being may be experienced as suffering related to life (Eriksson, 1993, 1994a; Lindholm & Eriksson, 1993).

THE SUFFERING HUMAN BEING

The suffering human being is the concept that Eriksson uses to describe the patient. The patient refers to the concept of *patiens* (Latin), which means "suffering." The patient is a suffering human being, or a human being who suffers and patiently endures (Eriksson, 1994a; Eriksson & Herberts, 1992).

RECONCILIATION

Reconciliation refers to the drama of suffering. A human being who suffers wants to be confirmed in his or her suffering and be given time and space to suffer and reach reconciliation.

Continued

MAJOR CONCEPTS & DEFINITIONS—cont'd

Reconciliation implies a change through which a new wholeness is formed of the life the human being has lost in suffering. In reconciliation, the importance of sacrifice emerges (Eriksson, 1994a). Having achieved reconciliation implies living with an imperfection with regard to oneself and others but seeing a way forward and a meaning in one's suffering. Reconciliation is a prerequisite of caritas (Eriksson, 1990).

CARING CULTURE

Caring culture is the concept that Eriksson (1987a) uses instead of environment. It characterizes the total caring reality and is based on cultural elements such as traditions, rituals, and basic values. Caring culture transmits an inner order of value preferences or ethos, and the different constructions of culture have their basis in the changes of value that ethos undergoes. If communion arises based on the ethos, the culture becomes inviting. Respect for the human being, his or her dignity and holiness, forms the goal of communion and participation in a caring culture. The origin of the concept of culture is to be found in such dimensions as reverence, tending, cultivating, and caring; these dimensions are central to the basic motive of preserving and developing a caring culture (Eriksson, 1987a; Eriksson & Lindström, 2003).

USE OF EMPIRICAL EVIDENCE

From the beginning development of her theory, Eriksson has firmly established it in empiricism by systematically employing a hermeneutical and hypothetical deductive approach. Eriksson, in conformity with a human science and hermeneutical way of thinking, has developed a caring science concept of evidence (Eriksson, Nordman, & Myllymäki, 1999). As her main argument for this, she points out that the concept of evidence in natural science is too narrow to capture and reach the depth of the complex caring reality. Her concept of evidence is derived from Gadamer's concept of truth (Gadamer, 1960/1994), which encompasses the true, the beautiful, and the good. She points out, in accordance with Gadamer, that evidence cannot be connected solely with a method and empirical data. Evidence in a human science perspective contains two aspects: a conceptual, logical one, which she calls ontological, and an empirical one, each pre-supposing the other. The evidence concept developed by Eriksson has been shown to be empirically evident when tested in two comprehensive empirical studies where the idea was to develop evidence-based caring cultures in seven caring units in the Hospital District of Helsinki and Uusimaa (Eriksson & Nordman, 2004).

During the 1970s, Eriksson initially developed a nursing care process model (Eriksson, 1974), which later, in her doctoral dissertation (1981), was formulated as a theory. Since then, Eriksson, step by step, has deepened her conceptual and logical understanding of the basic concepts and phenomena that have emerged from the theory. She has tested their validity in empirical contexts, where the concepts have assumed contextual and pragmatic attributes. This logical way of working, a constant movement between logical and empirical evidence, has been summarized by Eriksson in her model of concept development (Eriksson, 1997b). The validity of this model has been tested in several doctoral dissertations since 1995 (Kasén, 2002; Lindwall, 2004; Nåden, 1998; Rundqvist, 2004; Sivonen, 2000; von Post, 1999). She started more comprehensive systematic as well as clinical research programs on caring when she was appointed director of the Department of Caring Science at Åbo Akademi University. All 32 doctoral dissertations written at the Department of Caring Science between 1992 and 2008 are in different ways a test and validation of her ideas and theory.

MAJOR ASSUMPTIONS

Eriksson distinguishes between two kinds of major assumptions: axioms and theses. She regards axioms as fundamental truths in relation to the conception of the world; theses are fundamental statements concerning the general nature of caring science, and their validity is tested through basic research. Axioms and theses jointly constitute the ontology of caring science and therefore also are the foundation of its epistemology (Eriksson, 1988, 2001). The caritative theory of caring is based on the following axioms and theses, as modified and clarified from Eriksson's basic assumptions with her approval (Eriksson, 2002). The axioms are as follows:

- The human being is fundamentally an entity of body, soul, and spirit.
- The human being is fundamentally a religious being.
- The human being is fundamentally holy. Human dignity means accepting the human obligation of serving with love, of existing for the sake of others.
- Communion is the basis for all humanity. Human beings are fundamentally interrelated to an abstract and/or concrete other in a communion.
- Caring is something human by nature, a call to serve in love.
- Suffering is an inseparable part of life. Suffering and health are each other's prerequisites.
- Health is more than the absence of illness. Health implies wholeness and holiness.
- The human being lives in a reality that is characterized by mystery, infinity, and eternity.

The theses are as follows:

- Ethos confers ultimate meaning on the caring context.
- The basic motive of caring is the caritas motive.
- The basic category of caring is suffering.
- Caring communion forms the context of meaning of caring and derives its origin from the ethos of love, responsibility, and sacrifice, namely, caritative ethics.
- Health means a movement in becoming, being, and doing while striving for wholeness and holiness, which is compatible with endurable suffering.
- Caring implies alleviation of suffering in charity, love, faith, and hope. Natural basic caring is expressed through tending, playing, and learning in a sustained caring relationship, which is asymmetrical by nature.

The Human Being

The conception of the human being in Eriksson's theory is based on the axiom that the human being is an entity of body, soul, and spirit (Eriksson, 1987a, 1988). She emphasizes that the human being is fundamentally a religious being, but all human beings have not recognized this dimension. The human being is fundamentally holy, and this axiom is related to the idea of human dignity, which means accepting the human obligation of serving with love and existing for the sake of others. Eriksson stresses the necessity of understanding the human being in his ontological context. The human being is seen as in constant becoming; he is constantly in change and therefore never in a state of full completion. He is understood in terms of the dual tendencies that exist within him, engaged in a continued struggle and living in a tension between being and nonbeing. Eriksson sees the human being's conditional freedom as a dimension of becoming. She links her thinking with Kierkegaard's (1843/1943) ideas of free choice and decision in the human being's various stages—aesthetic, ethical, and religious stages—and she thinks that the human being's power of transcendency is the foundation of real freedom. The dual tendency of the human being also emerges in his effort to be unique, while he simultaneously longs for belonging in a larger communion.

The human being is fundamentally dependent on communion; he is dependent on another, and it is in the relationship between a concrete other (human being) and an abstract other (some form of God) that the human being constitutes himself and his being (Eriksson, 1987a). The human being seeks a communion where he can give and receive love, experience faith and hope, and be aware that his existence here and now has meaning. According to Eriksson (1987b), the human being we meet in care is creative and imaginative, has desires and wishes, and is able to experience phenomena; therefore, a description of the human being only in terms of his needs is insufficient. When the human being is entering the caring context, he or she becomes a patient in the original sense of the concept—a suffering human being (Eriksson, 1994a).

Caritas

Love and charity, or caritas, as the basic motive of caring has been found in Eriksson (1987b, 1990, 2001) as a principal idea even in her early works. The caritas motive can be traced through semantics, anthropology, and the history of ideas (Eriksson, 1992c). According to Nygren (1966), *caritas* means human love and charity. Anthropologically, the essence of the human being is love. Giving love is a human characteristic (Lévinas, 1988). The history of ideas indicates that the foundation of the caring professions through the ages has been an inclination to help and minister to those suffering (Lanara, 1981).

Caritas constitutes the motive for caring, and it is through the caritas motive that caring gets its deepest formulation. This motive, according to Eriksson, is also the core of all teaching and fostering growth in all forms of human relations. In caritas, the two basic forms of love—eros and agapé (Nygren, 1966)—are combined. When the two forms of love combine, generosity becomes a human being's attitude toward life, and joy its form of expression. The motive of caritas becomes visible in a special ethical attitude in caring, or what Eriksson calls a *caritative outlook,* which she formulates and specifies in caritative caring ethics (Eriksson, 1995). Caritas constitutes the inner force that is connected with the mission to care. A carer who works in love also beams forth what Eriksson calls *claritas,* or the strength and light of beauty.

Caritas comprises love for one's neighbor and for God, a human being's love for himself, a human being's love for everything created, and God's love for human beings. Eriksson sees expressions of love as a development of the original virtues of mercy and the theological virtues of faith, hope, and love (Eriksson, 1987a, 1990). From the idea of caritas, Eriksson has derived her whole caritative caring theory.

Caring

In accordance with the fundamental assumptions of caring science, Eriksson sees caring as ontological and an expression of caritas (Eriksson, 1988). Caring is something natural and original. Eriksson thinks that the substance of caring can be understood only by a search for its origin. This origin is in the origin of the concept and in the idea of natural caring. The fundamentals of natural care are constituted by the idea of motherliness, which implies cleansing and nourishing, and spontaneous and unconditional love.

Natural basic caring is expressed through tending, playing, and learning in a spirit of love, faith, and hope. The characteristics of tending are warmth, closeness, and touch; playing is an expression of exercise, testing, creativity, and imagination, and desires and wishes; learning is aimed at growth and change. To tend, play, and learn implies sharing, and sharing, Eriksson (1987a) says, is "presence with the human being, life and God" (p. 38). True care therefore is "not a form of behavior, not a feeling or state. It is to be there—it is the way, the spirit in which it is done, and this spirit is caritative" (Eriksson, 1998, p. 4). Eriksson brings out that caring through the ages can be seen as various expressions of love and charity, with a view toward alleviating suffering and serving life and health. In her later texts, she stresses that caring also can be seen as a search for truth, goodness, beauty, and the eternal, and for what is permanent in caring, and making it visible or evident (Eriksson, 2002). Her constant search has been centered on the question of what is care (the caring fundamentals) in caring. Eriksson emphasizes that caritative caring relates to the innermost core of nursing, and she has distinguished between traditions that she calls *caring nursing* and *nursing care.*

She means that nursing care is based on the nursing care process, and that it represents good care only when it is based on the innermost core of caring. Caring nursing represents a kind of caring without prejudice that emphasizes the patient and his or her suffering and desires (Eriksson, 1994a).

Caritative caring arises in the encounter with the suffering human being in a caring relationship that involves caring communion (Eriksson, 1998). The core of the caring relationship, between nurse and patient as described by Eriksson (1993), is an open invitation that contains affirmation that the other is always welcome. The constant open invitation is involved in what Eriksson (2003) today calls the *act of caring.* The act of caring expresses the innermost spirit of caring and re-creates the basic motive of caritas. The caring act expresses the deepest holy element, the safeguarding of the individual patient's dignity. In the caring act, the patient is invited to a genuine sharing, a communion, in order to make the caring fundamentals alive and active (Eriksson, 1987a) (i.e., appropriated to the patient). The appropriation has the consequence of somehow restoring the human being and making him or her more genuinely human. In an ontological sense, the ultimate goal of caring, according to Eriksson, cannot be only health; it reaches further and includes human life in its entirety. Because the mission of the human being is to serve, to exist for the sake of others, the ultimate purpose of caring is to bring the human being back to this mission (Eriksson, 1994a).

Ethos

Eriksson uses the concept of ethos in accordance with Aristotle's (1935, 1997) idea that ethics is derived from ethos. In Eriksson's sense, the ethos of caring science, as well as that of caring, consists of the idea of love and charity and respect and honor of the holiness and dignity of the human being. Ethos is the sounding board of all caring. Ethos is ontology in which there is an "inner ought to," a target of caring "that has its own language and its own key" (Eriksson, 2003, p. 23). Good caring and true knowledge become visible through ethos. Ethos originally refers to home, or to the place where a human being feels at home. It symbolizes a human being's innermost space, where he appears in his nakedness (Lévinas, 1989). Ethos and ethics belong together, and in the caring culture, they become one (Eriksson, 2003). Eriksson thinks that *ethos* means that we feel called to serve a particular task. This ethos she sees as the core of caring culture. Ethos, which forms the basic force in caring culture, reflects the prevailing priority of values through which the basic foundations of ethics and ethical actions appear.

Suffering

At the beginning of the 1990s, when Eriksson reintroduced the idea of suffering as a basic category of caring, she returned to the fundamental historical conditions of all caring, the idea of charity as the basis of alleviating suffering (Eriksson, 1984, 1993, 1994a, 1997a). This meant a change in the view of caring reality to a focus on the suffering human being. In an ontological sense, Eriksson sees all suffering as a fight between evil and good. Her starting point is that suffering is an inseparable part of human life, and that it has no distinct reason or definition. It has many faces and many characteristics, but it lacks an explicit language. Suffering as such has no meaning, but a human being can ascribe meaning to it by becoming reconciled to it. Eriksson makes a distinction between endurable and unendurable suffering and thinks that an unendurable suffering paralyzes the human being, preventing him or her from growing, while endurable suffering is compatible with health. In its deepest meaning, all suffering can be described in some sense as a form of dying, but it also can lead to renewal. Every human being's suffering is enacted in a drama of suffering. Alleviating a human being's suffering implies being a co-actor in the drama and confirming his or her suffering. A human being who suffers wants to have the suffering confirmed and be given time and space to become reconciled to it. The ultimate purpose of caring is to alleviate suffering. Eriksson has described three different forms: suffering related to illness, suffering related to care, and suffering related to life (Eriksson, 1993, 1994a, 1997a).

Health

Eriksson considers health in many of her earlier writings in accordance with an analysis of the concept in which she defines health as soundness, freshness, and well-being. The subjective dimension, or well-being, is emphasized strongly (Eriksson, 1976). In the current axiom of health, she states that it is more than absence of illness; *health* implies being whole in body, soul, and spirit. *Health* means as a pure concept wholeness and holiness (Eriksson, 1984). In accordance with her view of the human being, Eriksson has developed various premises regarding the substance and laws of health, which have been summed up in an ontological health model. She sees health as both movement and integration. Health is a movement between actual and potential in a human being's active becoming, and it is an integrated part of human life. The health premise is a movement comprising various partial premises: health as movement implies a change; a human being is being formed or destroyed, but never completely; health is movement between actual and potential; health is movement in time and space; health as movement is dependent on vital force on vitality of body, soul, and spirit; the direction of this movement is determined by the human being's needs and desires; the will to find meaning, life, and love constitutes the source of energy of the movement; and health as movement strives toward a realization of one's potential (Eriksson, 1984).

In the ontological conception, health is conceived as a becoming, a movement toward a deeper wholeness and holiness. As a human being's inner health potential is touched, a movement occurs that becomes visible in the different dimensions of health as doing, being, and becoming with a wholeness unique to human beings (Eriksson, Bondas-Salonen, Fagerström, Herberts, & Lindholm, 1990). In doing, the person's thoughts concerning health are focused on healthy life habits and avoiding illness; in being, the person strives for balance and harmony; in becoming, the human being becomes whole on a deeper level of integration.

Eriksson (1997a) sees that health and suffering belong together. Health becomes wholeness only through its combination with suffering. Health and suffering are two sides of the same movement, and they are integrated into each other and constantly present in a human being's life. In the health dimension of doing, human beings are unfamiliar with their suffering and want to explain it away. In the health dimension of being, they seek harmony and want to get away from suffering. In becoming, human beings are not unfamiliar with suffering; instead, they strive to reconcile themselves to the circumstances of life. Eriksson (1994a) thinks that suffering can give health meaning by making the human being conscious of the contrasts of health and suffering.

THEORETICAL ASSERTIONS

Eriksson's fundamental idea when formulating theoretical assertions is that they connect four levels of knowledge: the meta-theoretical, the theoretical, the technological, and caring as art. The generation of theory takes place through dialectical movement between these levels, but here deduction constitutes the basic epistemological idea (Eriksson, 1981). The theory of science for caring science, which contains the fundamental epistemological, logical, and ethical standpoints, is formed on the meta-theoretical level. Eriksson (1988), in accordance with Nygren (1972), sees the basic motive as the element that permeates the formation of knowledge at all levels and gives scientific knowledge its unique characteristics. A common, clearly formulated ontology constitutes the foundation of both the caritative caring theory and caring science as a discipline. In accordance with Lévinas' (1988) thinking, Eriksson is of the opinion that ethics precedes ontology. The caritas motive, the ethos of love and charity, and the respect and reverence for human holiness and dignity, which determine the nature of caring, give the caritative caring theory its feature. This ethos, which encircles caring as science and as art, permeates caring culture and creates the preconditions for caring. The ethos is reflected in the process of nursing care, in the documentation, and in various care planning models.

Caring communion constitutes the context of meaning from which the concepts in the theory are to be understood. Human suffering forms the basic category of caring and summons the carer to true caring (i.e., serving in love and charity). In the act of caring, the suffering human being, or patient, is invited and welcomed to the caring communion, where the patient's suffering can be alleviated through the act of caring in the drama of suffering that is unique to every human being. Alleviation of suffering implies that the carer is a co-actor in the drama, confirms the patient's suffering, and gives time and space to suffer until reconciliation is reached. Reconciliation is the ultimate aim of health or being and signifies a reestablishment of wholeness and holiness (Eriksson, 1997a).

The outer structure of caring is constituted by the nursing care process, structured as a hermeneutic course of events in which understanding is a necessary prerequisite of action. It creates a caring culture in which caritative caring is made possible.

LOGICAL FORM

Meta-theory has always had a fundamental place in Eriksson's thinking and thought patterns, and her epistemological work is anchored in Aristotle's theory of knowledge (Aristotle, 1935). Searching for knowledge, which is intrinsically hermeneutic, and which has taken place within the scope of an articulated theoretical perspective, is to be understood as a search for the original text in a historical-hermeneutic tradition, that which in the old hermeneutic sense represents truth (Gadamer, 1960/1994). To achieve the depth in the development of knowledge and theory she has consistently striven for, Eriksson has used various logical models for the hypothetical deductive method and hermeneutics guiding principles.

The logical form is constituted both in Eriksson's caritative theory of caring and in caring science as a discipline (Eriksson & Lindström, 1997). Eriksson stresses the importance of the logical form being created on the basis of the substance of caring (i.e., caritas), not on the basis of method. It is thus deduction combined with abduction that has formed the guiding logic. The language, words, and concepts are the carriers of the content of meaning, and Eriksson stresses the necessity of choosing words, concepts, and language that correspond to the tradition of human science.

In the dynamic change between the natural world and the world of science, there has constantly occurred a striving toward the source of the true, the beautiful, and the good—that which is evident. Eriksson (1999) shapes her theory of scientific thought, in which reflection moves between patterns at different levels, and the repertory of interpretation is subject to the theoretical perspective. The movement takes place distinctly between *dóxa* (empirical-perceptive knowledge) and *episteme* (rational-conceptual knowledge), and "the infinite." Movement thus takes place between the two basic epistemological categories of the theory of knowledge: perception and conception. The infinite reaches beyond rational concept-forming knowledge, in which epistemological categories mainly take the form of symbols and metaphors.

Eriksson has consistently applied three forms of inference—deduction, induction, and abduction or retroduction (Eriksson & Lindström, 1997)—that have given the theory a logical external structure. The substance of her caring theory has moved simultaneously by abductive leaps (Peirce, 1990; Eriksson & Lindström, 1997), which sometimes have created a new chaos but have carried Eriksson's thinking toward new discoveries. Through abduction, the ideal model for caritative caring has been shaped, proceeding from historical and self-evident suppositions (Nygren, 1972). Eriksson in this way has made use of old original texts that testify to caritative caring as her research material. Through induction and deduction, the validity of the theory has been tested continually.

Theory as conceived by Eriksson is in accordance with the Greek concept of theory, *theoria*, in the sense of seeing the beautiful and the good, participating in the common, and dedicating it to others (Gadamer, 2000, p. 49). Theory and practice are different aspects of the same core. The convincing force and potential of the whole theory are found in its innermost core, caritas, around which the generation of theory takes place. The caring substance is formed in a dialectical movement between the potential and the actual, the abstract general and the concrete individual. With the help of logical abstract thinking combined with the logic of the heart (Pascal, 1971), the Theory of Caritative Caring becomes perceptible through the art of caring.

ACCEPTANCE BY THE NURSING COMMUNITY

Practice

A characteristic feature of Eriksson's manner of working is her way of structuring abstract thinking as a natural and obvious precondition of clinical activity and an evidence-based form of caring that opens up a deeper insight. Eriksson uses the concept of caring as art as an expression of a caring practice in which the abstract generality appears in a unique individual caritative act of caring.

Several nursing units in the Nordic countries have based their practice and caring philosophy on Eriksson's ideas and her caritative theory of caring. These include several clinics in the Hospital District of Helsinki and Uusimaa in Finland, Stiftelsen Hemmet in the Åland Islands of Finland, and Stora Sköndal in Sweden. Because Eriksson's thinking and process model of caring are general, the nursing care process model has proved to be applicable in all contexts of caring, from acute clinical caring and psychiatric care to health-promoting and preventive care.

Since the 1970s, Eriksson's nursing care process model has been systematically used, tested, and developed as a basis of nursing care and documentation at Helsinki University Central Hospital. From the beginning of the 1990s, Eriksson has served as director of the clinical research program, "In the World of the Patient." This program comprises a number of empirical studies in various clinics within the whole district of university hospitals. In various studies, Eriksson's theory has been tested, and the results have been presented in doctoral and master's theses and published in professional and scientific journals. The study, "In the Patient's World II: Alleviating the Patient's Suffering—Ethics and Evidence" will lead to recommendations for the care of patients and is an ongoing research project that will become a handbook for clinical caring science.

Theoretical assumptions, assertions, and nursing care process model form the basis of the development of caring, planning and documentation. Eriksson's model has been subjected to more comprehensive academic research (Fagerström, 1999; Kärkkäinen & Eriksson, 2003, 2004; Lukander, 1995; Turtiainen, 1999). Eriksson's thinking has been influential in nursing leadership and nursing administration, where the caritative theory of nursing forms the core of the development of nursing leadership at various levels of the nursing organization. That Eriksson's ideas about caring and her nursing care process model work in practice has been verified by everything from a multiplicity of essays and tests of learning in clinical practice to master's theses, licentiates' theses, and doctoral dissertations produced all over the Nordic countries.

Education

Since the 1970s, Eriksson's theory has been integrated into the education of nurses at various levels, and her books have been included continuously in the examination requirements in various forms of nursing education in the Nordic countries. The education for master's and doctoral degrees that started in 1986 at the Department of Caring Science, Åbo Akademi University, has been based entirely on Eriksson's ideas, and her caritative caring theory forms the core of the development of substance in education and research.

Eriksson started the first Finnish-Swedish education of caring science teachers in 1970. She subsequently for 15 years had the advantage of working with a team of teachers who have integrated her ideas and her caritative caring theory, while at the same time developing caring didactics. Eriksson worked intensively to develop the caring science curriculum. In her book on didactics of caring (Eriksson, 1985), Eriksson further developed her curriculum theory and didactics. Her theory of caring didactics is based on a dialectic between a clearly articulated ontology, epistemology, and ethos, which results in didactics, an art of teaching that is hermeneutical by nature. The caring science concepts and the theory run like a main thread through whole education, independently of the level. Eriksson's buildup of caring science as a humanistic autonomous discipline, with its subdisciplines such as caring ethics, caring theology, and the history of ideas of caring (Eriksson, 1988, 2001), forms the basic structure of the organization of the curriculum and teaching on numerous levels (Eriksson, 1986).

Development of the caring science–centered curriculum and caring didactics continued in the educational and research program in caring science didactics. Development of teachers within the education of nurses forms a part of the master's degree program and has resulted in the first doctoral dissertation in the didactics of caring science (Ekebergh, 2001).

Eriksson realized at an early stage the importance of integrating academic courses in the education of nurses; nowadays, academic courses in caring science based on Eriksson's theory are offered as part of the continuing education of those who work in clinical practice. Approximately 200 nurses take part annually in these academic courses.

Because Eriksson sees caring science not as profession oriented but as a "pure" academic discipline, it has aroused interest among students in other disciplines and other occupational groups, such as teachers, social workers, psychologists, and theologians. Eriksson stresses that it is necessary for doctors as well to study caring science, so that genuine interdisciplinary cooperation is achieved between caring science and medicine.

Research

Eriksson and her teaching and research colleagues at the Department of Caring Science have designed a research program based on her caring science tradition. This program comprises systematic caring science, clinical caring science, the didactics of caring science, caring administration, and interdisciplinary research. Eriksson's caritative caring theory has been tested and further developed in various contexts with different methodological approaches, both within the department's own research projects and in the 32 doctoral dissertations that so far have been published at the department.

Eriksson has always emphasized the importance of basic research as necessary for clinical research, and her main thesis is that substance should direct the choice of research method. In her book, *Pausen (The Pause)* (Eriksson, 1987b), she describes how the research object is structured, starting from the caritative theory of caring. In her book, *Broar (Bridges)* (Eriksson, 1991), she describes the research paradigm and various methodological approaches based on a human science perspective. During the first few years, the emphasis lay on basic research, with the focus on development of the basic concepts and assumptions of the theory and on the fundamentals of history and the history of ideas. An especially strong point in Eriksson's research is the clearly formulated theoretical perspective that confers explicitness and greater depth to the generation of knowledge. The development of the theory and research have always moved hand in hand with the focus on various dimensions of the theory, and in this connection, we wish to illustrate some central results of the research.

Eriksson has always emphasized the necessity of an exhaustive and systematic analysis of basic concepts, and she has developed her own model of concept development (Eriksson, 1991, 1997b), which has proved fruitful and is used by many researchers, including Nåden (1998) in his study of the art of caring, von Post (1999) in her study of the concept of natural care, Sivonen (2000) in studies of the concepts of soul and spirit, and Kasén (2002) in her study of the concept of the caring relationship. Other studies have focused on the concept of dignity (Edlund, 2002), the concepts of power and authority (Rundqvist, 2004), and the concept of the body in a perioperative context (Lindwall, 2004).

Continued development of Eriksson's concept of health took place in the research project Den Mångdimensionella Hälsan (Multidimensional Health), which was in progress during the years 1987 to 1992 and resulted in the ontological health model (Eriksson, 1994a; Eriksson et al., 1990; Eriksson & Herberts, 1992). The project included several studies resulting in a number of master's theses. Of these, Lindholm's study of young people's conception of health (1998; Lindholm & Eriksson, 1998) and Bondas' study of women's health during the perinatal period (2000; Bondas & Eriksson, 2001) led to doctoral dissertations.

The ontological health model subsequently formed the basis for several studies. Wärnå (2002), in her study concerning the worker's health, related Aristotle's theory of virtue to Eriksson's ontological health model. The result of the study opened a new line of thought in preventive health service in working environments; continued research and development are now in progress in a number of factories in the wood-processing industry in Finland.

Since the mid-1980s, when suffering as the basic category in caring was made explicit in Eriksson's theory, examples of research related to suffering have been legion. One is Wiklund's (2000) study of suffering as struggle and drama, among both patients who had undergone coronary bypass surgery and patients addicted to drugs. In several clinical studies, Råholm focused on suffering and alleviation of suffering in patients undergoing coronary bypass surgery (Råholm, Lindholm, & Eriksson, 2002; Råholm, 2003). The manifestation of suffering in a psychiatric context has been studied by Fredriksson, who illustrates the possibilities of the caring conversation in the alleviation of suffering (Fredriksson, 2003; Fredriksson & Eriksson, 2003; Fredriksson & Lindström, 2002). In a Norwegian study, Nilsson (2004) studied suffering in patients in psychiatric noninstitutional care units with a high degree of ill health and found that the experience of loneliness is of basic importance. Caspari (2004) in her study illustrated the importance of aesthetics for health and suffering.

In a cooperative project between researchers in Sweden and Finland, the suffering of women with breast cancer has been studied. This project comprises, among other things, intervention studies, in which the importance of different forms of care for the alleviation of suffering has been illustrated (Arman, Rehnsfeldt, Lindholm, & Hamrin, 2002; Arman-Rehnsfeldt & Rehnsfeldt, 2003; Lindholm, Nieminen, Mäkelä, & Rantanen-Siljamäki, 2004). Arman-Rehnsfeldt, in her dissertation, illustrated how the drama of suffering is formed among these women (Arman, 2003).

Continuous research has been carried out since the 1970s, with a view toward developing caring science as an academic discipline, and a theory of science for caring science has been formulated (Eriksson, 1988, 2001; Eriksson & Lindström, 2000, 2003; Lindström, 1992). Eriksson has developed subdisciplines of caring science, which means that researchers of caring science and other scientific disciplines enter into dialogues with each other, and constitute a research area. An example of this is the development of caritative caring ethics (Andersson, 1994; Eriksson, 1991, 1995; Fredriksson & Eriksson, 2001; Råholm & Lindholm, 1999; Råholm et al., 2002). Another interesting subdiscipline that Eriksson has developed is caring theology, within which she has articulated spiritual and doctrinal questions in caring with a scientific group of themes, and in this respect has cleared the way for new thinking. Caring theology, which has aroused great interest among caregivers in clinical practice, nowadays can be studied in academic courses.

Many researchers at universities, institutes of higher education, and clinics all over the Nordic countries make use of Eriksson's ideas and theory. This is evident in how frequently her literature is referenced. (Further discussion of this is not within the scope of this chapter.)

FURTHER DEVELOPMENT

Eriksson continues developing her thinking and the caritative caring theory with unabated energy and constantly finds new ways, while at the same time recreating and deepening what has been stated before. Systematic research and the development of caritative caring theory, as well as the discipline of caring science, take place chiefly within the scope of the research programs in her own department with her own staff and the postdoctoral group. The dissertation topics of doctoral candidates are connected with the research programs and form an important contribution of knowledge to the ongoing development of Eriksson's thinking. During the last few years, Eriksson has emphasized the necessity of basic research in clinical caring science, where she has especially stressed the understanding of the research object, caring reality. She describes the object of research from three points of view: the experienced world, praxis as activity, and the real reality, which stretches beyond the empirical reality and constitutes the infinite. In the real reality, which carries the attributes of mystery, one finds something of the deepest potential of caring, and it is a reality that can be understood in Gadamer's sense, in the old Greek meaning of praxis, as a way of living, a mode of being, that is, an ontology (Gadamer, 2000). The development of knowledge in caring science becomes fundamentally different depending on what object of knowledge constitutes the focus of research (Eriksson & Lindström, 2003). Another central area of interest for Eriksson (2003) today is formed by the development of caritative caring ethics (i.e., the question of ethos, the basic values of caring, the ethical fundamentals of caring, and appropriation in the act of caring). Continued development of the caritative theory of caring also occurs, as has emerged before, through continued implementation and testing in various clinical contexts.

CRITIQUE

Clarity

The strong point of Eriksson's theory is the overall logical structure of the theory, in which every new concept becomes a part of an ever more comprehensive whole in which an element of internal logic can be seen clearly in the development of substance. Her main thesis has always been that basic conceptual clarity will be needed before it becomes meaningful to develop the contextual features of the theory. Eriksson has used concept analysis and analysis of ideas as central methods, which has led to semantic and structural clarity. It has at the same time meant that the concepts may have assumed dimensions that have been regarded as strange to those who are not familiar with the theoretical perspective in which the development of the theory has taken place. We, who have for many years had the opportunity to follow Eriksson's work, have time and again been able to realize that her way of thinking forms a logical whole, where the abstract scientific reveals the concrete in a new understanding (i.e., provides an experience of evidence and verifies the convincing force of the theory).

Simplicity

The theoretical clarity of Eriksson's theory reflects the simplicity of the theory by showing the general in a clear and logical conceptual entirety. The hermeneutic approach has deepened the understanding of the substance and thus contributed to the simplicity of the theory (Gadamer, 1960/1994). The simplicity also can be understood as an expression of Gadamer's concept of theory by making it comprehensible that theory and practice belong together and reflect two sides of the same reality. Eriksson agrees with Gadamer's thought that understanding includes application, and the theory opens the way to deeper participation and communion. Eriksson (2003) formulates this process by the statement that "ideals reach reality and reality reaches the ideals" (p. 26).

Generality

Eriksson's theory is general in the sense that it aims at creating an ontological and ethical basis of caring, while at the same time it constitutes the core of the discipline and thus involves epistemology as well. Eriksson's theory is also general as a result of the wide convincing force it receives through its theoretical core concepts and its theoretical axioms and theses. There may be a risk that a too-general theory becomes diffuse in relation to different caring contexts. Eriksson, however, has always stressed the importance of describing the core concepts on an optimal level of abstraction in order to include all of the complex caring reality that simultaneously carries a wealth of signification that opens up understanding in various caring contexts.

Empirical Precision

Eriksson's thinking as a whole has reached an understanding that extends to other disciplines and professions. She has developed a language and a rhetoric that can reach researchers as well as practitioners in the human scientific field. The empirical precision of Eriksson's theory is manifested through a combination of the clarity, simplicity, and generality of the theory combined with a rich substance and a clearly formulated ethos.

Derivable Consequences

Eriksson's work on developing her caritative caring theory for 30 years has been successful, and there is evidence that her thinking is of great importance to clinical practice, research, and education, and also to the development of the discipline. By her development of the caritative theory of care, Eriksson has created her own caring science tradition, a tradition that has grown strong, and it is no exaggeration to say that it has set the tone in the Nordic countries.

SUMMARY

Eriksson has been a guide and visionary who has gone before and "ploughed new furrows" in theory development for many years. Eriksson's caritative theory and her whole caring science thinking have developed over the course of 30 years. Characteristic of her thinking is that while she is working at an abstract level developing concepts and theory, the theory is rooted in clinical reality and teaching. The whole caritative theory and the caring that are built up around the theoretical core get their distinctive character and deeper meaning through the ethos of caritas, love, and compassion that permeates the whole. The ultimate goal of caring is to alleviate suffering and serve life and health. The conception of the human being as an entity of body, soul, and spirit, with a core of holiness and dignity, constitutes one of the basic axioms.

Knowledge formation, which Eriksson sees as a hermeneutic spiral, starts from the thought that ethics preceded ontology. In a concrete sense, this implies that the thought of human holiness and dignity is always kept alive in all phases of the search for knowledge. Ethics precedes ontology in theory as well as in practice.

Eriksson's caring science tradition and discipline of caring science form a basis for the activity at the Department of Caring Science at Åbo Akademi University. Eriksson's caritative caring theory and the discipline of caring science have inspired many in the Nordic countries, and they are used as the basis for research, education, and clinical practice. Many of her original textbooks, published mainly in Swedish, have been translated into Finnish, Norwegian, and Danish.

Case Study

The case presented is a philosophy of practice, by Ulf Donner, leader of the Foundation Home at the psychiatric nursing home in Finland that for 15 years has based its practice on Eriksson's caritative theory of caring.

Even at an early stage in our serving in caring science, we caregivers recognized ourselves in the caring science theory, which stresses the healing force of love and compassion in the form of tending, playing, and learning in faith, hope, and charity. The caritative culture is made visible with the help of rituals, symbols, and traditions, for instance, with the stone that burns with the light of the Trinity and the daily common time for spiritual reflection. In every meeting with the suffering human being, the attributes of love and charity are striven for, and the day involves discussions of reconciliation, forgiveness, and how we as caregivers can tend by nourishing and cleansing on the level of becoming, being, and doing. In the struggle in love and compassion to reach a fellow human being who, because of suffering, has withdrawn from the communion to find common horizons, the sacrifice of the caregiver is constantly available.

We work with people who often have the feeling that they do not deserve the love they encounter and who, in various ways, try to convince us caregivers of this. We experience patients' disappointment in their destructive acts, and we constantly have to remember that it may be broken promises that produce such dynamics. Sometimes, it may be difficult to recognize that suffering expressed in this way in an abstract sense seeks an embrace that does not give way but is strong enough to give shelter to this suffering, in a way that makes a becoming movement possible. In recognizing what is bad and what is difficult, horizons in the field of force are expanded, and the possibility of bringing in a ray of light and hope is opened.

As caregivers, we constantly ask ourselves whether the words, the language we use, bring promise, and how we can create linguistic footholds in the void by means of images and symbols. In our effort to nourish and cleanse, that which constitutes the basic movement of tending, we often recognize the importance of teaching the patient to be able to mourn disappointments and affirm the possibilities of forgiveness in the movement of reconciliation.

We also try to bring about the open invitation to the suffering human being to join a communion with the help of myths, legends, and tales concerned with human questions about evil vs. good and about eternity and infinity. Reading aloud with common reflective periods often provides us caregivers a possibility of getting closer to patients without getting too close, and opens the door for the suffering the patient bears.

In the act of caring, we strive for openness with regard to the patient's face and a confirmative attitude that responds to the appeal that we can recognize that the patient directs to us. When we as caregivers respond to the patient's appeal for charity, we are faced with the task of confirming the holiness of the other as a human being. Our constant effort is to make it possible for the patient to reestablish his or her dignity, accomplish his or her human mission, and enter true communion.

CRITICAL THINKING *Activities*

1. Reflect on the meaning of caritas as the ethos of caring.
   a. How is caritas culture formed in a care setting?
   b. How do caritative elements appear in caring?
   c. Try to formulate an ethics based on caritas.
2. Health and suffering are each other's preconditions. Think about what this means for the care of a patient.
3. How have you recognized the elements of caring—faith, hope, love and tending, playing, and learning—in a concrete caring situation? Give examples.
4. The most usual form of suffering related to care, suffering as a consequence of lack of caritative caring, is a violation of a human being's dignity. Think about a situation where this may occur and what can be done in order to prevent suffering related to care.

POINTS FOR *Further Study*

- Eriksson, K. (2007). Becoming through suffering—The path to health and holiness. *International Journal of Human Caring, 11*(2), 8-16.
- Eriksson, K. (2007). The theory of caritative caring: A vision. *Nursing Science Quarterly, 20*(3), 201-202.
- Eriksson, K. (2006). *The suffering human being.* Chicago: Nordic Studies Press. [English translation of *Den Lidande Människan.* Stockholm: Liber Förlag, 1994.]

REFERENCES

Andersson, M. (1994). Integritet som begrepp och princip. En studie av ett vårdetiskt ideal i utveckling. Doktorsavhandling, Turku, Finland, Åbo Akademis Förlag, [Integrity as a concept and as a principle in health care ethics. Doctoral dissertation, Turku, Finland. Åbo Akademi University Press.]

Aristotle (1935). Metaphysics, X-XIV oeconomica magna moralia. (H. Tredennick & G. C. Armstrong, Trans.). Cambridge, MA: Harvard University Press.

Aristotle. (1993). Den nikomachiska etiken. Gothenburg, Sweden: Daidalos. [The nicomachean ethics (M. Ringbom, Trans. & Commentary). Gothenburg, Sweden: Daidalos.]

Aristotle. (1997). Retoriikka. Helsinki, Finland: Gaudeamus. [Rhetoric (P. Hohti, Trans.). Helsinki, Finland: Gaudeamus.]

Arman, M. (2003). Lidande i existens i patientens värld—Kvinnors upplevelser av att leva med bröstcancer. Doktorsavhandling, Turku, Finland, Åbo Akademis Förlag. [Suffering and existence in the patient's world—Women's experiences of living with breast cancer. Doctoral dissertation, Turku, Finland, Åbo Akademi University Press.]

Arman, M., Rehnsfeldt, A., Lindholm, L., & Hamrin, E. (2002). The face of suffering among women with breast cancer—Being in a field of forces. Cancer Nursing, 25(2), 96-103.

Arman-Rehnsfeldt, M., & Rehnsfeldt, A. (2003). Vittnesbördet som etisk grund i vårdandet. I K. Eriksson & U. Å. Lindström (red.), Gryning II. Klinisk vårdvetenskap (s. 109-121), Vaasa, Finland: Institutionen för vårdvetenskap, Åbo Akademi. ["Bearing witness as an ethical base in caring." In K. Eriksson & U. Å. Lindström (Eds.), Dawn II. Clinical caring science (pp. 109-121). Vaasa, Finland: Department of Caring Science, Åbo Akademi.]

Barbosa da Silva, A. (1993). Vetenskap och människosyn i sjukvården: en introduktion till vetenskapsfilosofi och vårdetik. Stockholm: Svenska hälso och sjukvårdens tjänstemannaförbund, (SHSTF). [Science and view of human nature in nursing: an introduction to philosophy of science and caring ethics. Stockholm: Svenska hälso och sjukvårdens tjänstemannaförbund, (SHSTF).]

Berdâev, N. A. (1990). Historiens mening: ett försök till en filosofi om det mänskliga ödet. Skellefteå, Sweden: Artos. [The meaning of history: an attempt at philosophy of human fate. Skellefteå, Sweden: Artos.]

Bondas, T. (2000). Att vara med barn: en vårdvetenskaplig studie av kvinnors upplevelser under perinatal tid. Doktorsavhandling, Turku, Finland, Åbo Akademis Förlag. [To be with child: a study of women's lived experiences during the perinatal period from a caring science perspective. Doctoral dissertation, Turku, Finland, Åbo Akademi University Press.]

Bondas, T., & Eriksson, K. (2001). Women's lived experiences of pregnancy: A tapestry of joy and suffering. Qualitative Health Research, 11(6), 824-840.

Caspari, S. (2004). Det Gyldne snitt. Den estetiske dimensjon et etisk anliggende. Doktorsavhandling, Turku, Finland: Åbo Academis Förlag. [The golden section. The aesthetic dimension—A source of health. Doctoral dissertation. Turku, Finland, Åbo Akademi University Press.]

Edlund, M. (2002). Människans värdighet—Ett grundbegrepp inom vårdvetenskapen. Doktorsavhandling, Turku, Finland, Åbo Akademis Förlag. [Human dignity—A basic caring science concept. Doctoral dissertation, Turku, Finland, Åbo Akademi University Press.]

Ekebergh, M. (2001). Tillägnandet av vårdveteskaplig kunskap. Reflexionens betydelse för lärandet. Doktorsavhandling, Turku, Finland, Åbo Akademis Förlag. [Acquiring caring science knowledge—The importance of reflection for learning. Doctoral dissertation, Turku, Finland, Åbo Akademi University Press.]

Eriksson, K. (1974). Vårdprocessen (kompendium). Helsinki, Finland: Helsingfors svenska sjukvårdsinstitut. [The nursing care process (Compendium). Helsinki, Finland: Helsingfors svenska sjukvårdsinstitut.]

Eriksson, K. (1976). Hälsa. En teoretisk och begreppsanalytisk studie om hälsan och dess natur som mål för hälsovårdsedukation. Licentiatavhandling, Helsinki, Finland: Institutionen för pedagogik, Helsingfors universitet. [Health. A conceptual analysis and theoretical study of health and its nature as a goal for health care education. Unpublished Licentiate thesis, Helsinki, Finland: Department of Education, University of Helsinki.]

Eriksson, K. (1981). Vårdprocessen—En utgångspunkt för läroplanstänkande inom vårdutbildningen. Utvecklande av en vårdprocessmodell samt ett läroplanstänkande utgående från vårdprocessen, n. 94. Helsinki, Finland: Helsingfors universitet, Pedagogiska Institutionen. [The nursing care process—An approach to curriculum construction within nursing education. The development of a model for the nursing care process and an approach for curriculum development based on the process of nursing care (No. 94). Helsinki, Finland: Department of Education, University of Helsinki.]

Eriksson, K. (1984). Hälsans idé. Stockholm: Almqvist & Wiksell. [The idea of health. Stockholm: Almqvist & Wiksell.]

Eriksson, K. (1985). Vårddidaktik. Stockholm: Almqvist & Wiksell, [Caring didactics. Stockholm: Almqvist & Wiksell.]

Eriksson, K. (1986). Annual report. Helsingfors: Svenska Sjukvårdsinstitut.

Eriksson, K. (1987a). Vårdandets idé. Stockholm: Almqvist & Wiksell. [The idea of caring. Stockholm: Almqvist & Wiksell.]

Eriksson, K. (1987b). Pausen. En beskrivning av vårdvetenskapens kunskapsobjekt. Stockholm: Almqvist & Wiksell. [The pause: A description of the knowledge object of caring science. Stockholm: Almqvist & Wiksell.]

Eriksson, K. (1988). Vårdvetenskap som disciplin, forsknings- och tillämpningsområde (Vårdforskningar 1/1988). Vaasa, Finland: Institutionen för vårdvetenskap, Åbo Akademi. [Caring science as a discipline, field of research and application (Caring research 1/1988). Vaasa, Finland: Department of Caring Science, Åbo Akademi.]

Eriksson, K. (1989). Caring paradigms. A study of the origins and the development of caring paradigms among nursing students. Scandinavian Journal of Caring Sciences, 3(4), 169-176.

Eriksson, K. (1990). Pro Caritate. En lägesbestämning av caritativ vård. Vårdforskningar 2/1990. Vaasa, Finland: Institutionen för vårdvetenskap, Åbo Akademi. [Caritative caring—A positional analysis. Vaasa, Finland: Department of Caring Science, Åbo Akademi.]

Eriksson, K. (1991). Broar. Introduktion i vårdvetenskaplig metod. Vaasa, Finland: Institutionen för vårdvetenskap, Åbo Akademi. [Bridges. Introduction to the methods of caring science (test ed.). Vaasa, Finland: Department of Caring Science, Åbo Akademi.]

Eriksson, K. (1992a). The alleviation of suffering—The idea of caring. Scandinavian Journal of Caring Sciences, 6(2), 119-123.

Eriksson, K. (1992b). Different forms of caring communion. Nursing Science Quarterly, 5, 93.

Eriksson, K. (1992c). Nursing: The caring practice "being there." In D. Gaut (Ed.), The practice of caring in nursing (pp. 201-210). New York: National League for Nursing Press.

Eriksson, K. (1993). Lidandets idé. I K. Eriksson (red.), Möten med lidanden. Vårdforskning 4/1993 (s. 1-27). Vaasa, Finland: Institutionen för vårdvetenskap, Åbo Akademi. [The idea of suffering. In K. Eriksson (Ed.), Encounters with suffering (pp. 1-27). Vaasa, Finland: Department of Caring Science, Åbo Akademi.]

Eriksson, K. (1994a). Den lidande människan. Stockholm: Liber Förlag. [The suffering human being. Stockholm: Liber Förlag.] [English translation published in 2006 by Nordic Studies Press, Chicago.]

Eriksson, K. (1994b). Theories of caring as health. In D. Gaut & A. Boykin (Eds.), Caring as healing: Renewal through hope (pp. 3-20). New York: National League for Nursing Press.

Eriksson, K., (Ed.). (1995). Mot en caritativ vårdetik (Vårdforskning 5/1995). Vaasa, Finland: Institutionen för vårdvetenskap, Åbo Akademi. [Toward a caritative caring ethic (Caring research 5/1995). Vaasa, Finland: Department of Caring Science, Åbo Akademi.]

Eriksson, K. (1997a). Caring, spirituality and suffering. In M. S. Roach (Ed.), Caring from the heart: the convergence between caring and spirituality (pp. 68-84). New York: Paulist Press.

Eriksson, K. (1997b). Perustutkimus ja käsiteanalyysi. I M. Paunonen & J. Vehviläinen-Julkunen, Hoitotieteen tutkimusmetodiikka (s. 50-75). Helsinki Porvoo, Finland: WSOY. [Basic research and concept analysis. In M. Paunonen & J. Vehviläinen-Julkunen, The research methodology of caring science (pp. 50-75). Helsinki Porvoo, Finland: WSOY.]

Eriksson, K. (1998). Understanding the world of the patient, the suffering human being: The new clinical paradigm from nursing to caring. In C. E. Guzzetta (Ed.), Essential readings in holistic nursing (pp. 3-9). Gaithersburg, MD: Aspen.

Eriksson, (1999, November). Teoriutveckling inom vårdvetenskapen. Human vetenskaplig angreppspunkt. Stockholm: Nordisk Akademi för Sykepleievitenskap, Kongress i Stockholm. [Theory development in caring science. A humanistic approach. Stockholm: Nordisk Akademi för Sykepleievitenskap, Kongress i Stockholm.]

Eriksson, K. (2001). Vårdvetenskap som akademisk disciplin (Vårdforskning 7/2001). Vaasa, Finland: Institutionen för vårdvetenskap, Åbo Akademi. [Caring science as an academic discipline (Caring research 7/2001). Vaasa, Finland: Department of Caring Science, Åbo Akademi.]

Eriksson, K. (2002). Caring science in a new key. Nursing Science Quarterly, 15(1), 61-65.

Eriksson, K. (2003). Ethos. I K. Eriksson & U. Å. Lindström (red.), Gryning II. Klinisk vårdvetenskap (s. 21-34). Vaasa, Finland: Institutionen för vårdvetenskap, Åbo Akademi. [Ethos, in K. Eriksson & U. Å. Lindström (Eds.), Dawn II. Clinical caring science (pp. 21-34). Vaasa, Finland: Department of Caring Science, Åbo Akademi.]

Eriksson, K., Bondas-Salonen, T., Fagerström, L., Herberts, S., & Lindholm, L. (1990). Den mångdimensionella hälsan—En pilotstudie över uppfattningar bland patienter, skolungdomar och lärare (Projektrapport). Vaasa, Finland: Vasa Sjukvårdsdistrikt kf. och Institutionen för vårdvetenskap, Åbo Akademi. [Multidimensional health—A pilot study of how patients, school students, and teachers experience health (Project Rep. 1). Vaasa, Finland: Vasa Sjukvårdsdistrikt kf. och Institutionen för vårdvetenskap, Åbo Akademi.]

Eriksson, K., & Herberts, S. (1992). Den mångdimensionella hälsan. En studie av hälsobilden hos sjukvårdsledare och sjukvårdspersonal (Projektrapport 2). Vaasa, Finland: Vasa sjukvårdsdistrikt kf. och Institutionen för vårdvetenskap, Åbo Akademi. [The multidimensional health. A study of the view of health among health care leaders and health care personnel (Project Rep. 2). Vaasa, Finland: Vasa sjukvårdsdistrikt kf. och Institutionen för vårdvetenskap, Åbo Akademi.]

Eriksson, K., & Lindström, U. Å. (1997). Abduction—A way to deeper understanding of the world of caring. Scandinavian Journal of Caring Sciences, 11(4), 195-198.

Eriksson, K., & Lindström, U. Å. (2000). Siktet, sökandet, slutandet—Om den vårdvetenskapliga kunskapen. I K. Eriksson & U. Å. Lindström (red.), Gryning—En vårdvetenskaplig antologi (s. 5-18). Vaasa, Finland: Institutionen för vårdvetenskap, Åbo Akademi. [In the prospect of, searching for, and ending of—The caring science knowledge. In K. Eriksson & U. Å. Lindström (Eds.), Dawn. An anthology of caring science (pp. 5-18). Vaasa, Finland: Department of Caring Science, Åbo Akademi.]

Eriksson, K., & Lindström, U. Å. (2003). Klinisk vårdvetenskap. I K. Eriksson & U. Å. Lindström (red.), Gryning II. Klinisk vårdvetenskap (s. 3-20). Vaasa, Finland: Institutionen för vårdvetenskap, Åbo Akademi. [Clinical caring science. In K. Eriksson & U. Å. Lindström (Eds.), Dawn II. Clinical caring science (pp. 3-20). Vaasa, Finland: Department of Caring Science, Åbo Akademi.]

Eriksson, K., & Nordman, T. (2004). Trojanska hästen II. Utvecklande av evidensbaserade vårdande kulturer. Vaasa, Finland: Institutionen för vårdvetenskap, Åbo Akademi. [Trojan Horse II. The development of evidence-based caring cultures. Vaasa, Finland; The Department of Caring Science, Åbo Akademi University.]

Eriksson K., Nordman T., & Myllymäki, I., (1999). Den trojanska hästen. Evidensbaserat vårdande och vårdarbete ur ett vårdvetenskapligt perspektiv (Rapport 1). Institutionen för vårdvetenskap. Vaasa, Finland: Åbo Akademi; Helsingfors universitetscentralsjukhus & Vasa sjukvårdsdistrikt. [The Trojan horse. Evidence-based caring and nursing care in a caring science perspective. (Report). Department of Caring Science. Vaasa, Finland: Åbo Akademi; Helsingfors universitetscentralsjukhus & Vasa sjukvårdsdistrikt.]

Fagerström, L. (1999). The patients' caring needs. To understand and measure the unmeasurable. Doctoral dissertation. (Turku, Finland, Åbo Akademi University Press.)

Fredriksson, L. (2003). Det vårdande samtalet. Doktorsavhandling, Åbo Akademis Förlag, Turku, Finland. [The caring conversation. Doctoral dissertation, Turku, Finland, Åbo Akademi University Press.]

Fredriksson, L., & Eriksson, K. (2001). The patient's narrative of suffering—A path to health? An interpretative research synthesis on narrative understanding. Scandinavian Journal of Caring Sciences, 15(1), 3-11.

Fredriksson, L., & Eriksson, K. (2003). The ethics of the caring conversation. Nursing Ethics, 10(2), 138-148.

Fredriksson, L., & Lindström, U. Å. (2002). Caring conversations—Psychiatric patients' narratives about suffering. Journal of Advanced Nursing, 40(4), 396-404.

Gadamer, H-G. (1994). Truth and method (2nd rev. ed., J. Weinsheimer & D. G. Marshall, Trans.). New York: Continuum. [Original work published 1960.]

Gadamer, H-G. (2000). Teoriens lovprisning, Århus: Systeme. [Praise the theory. New Haven: Yale University Press, 1998.] [German orig: Lob der Theorie, 3. Auflage, 1991.]

Kaila, E. (1939). Den mänskliga kunskapen: vad den är och vad den icke är. Helsinki, Finland: Söderström. [Human knowledge: What it is and what it is not (G. H. von Wright, Trans.). Helsinki, Finland: Söderström.]

Kasén, A. (2002). Den vårdande relationen. Doktorsavhandling, Turku, Finland, Åbo Akademis Förlag. [The caring relationship. Doctoral dissertation Turku, Finland, Åbo Akademi University Press.]

Kierkegaard, S. (1943). Antingen—Eller [Orig. 1843. Enten—Eller.]. Utgiver under pseudonymen Victor Eremita. Köpenhamn: Meyer. [Either/or. Princeton, N. J.: Princeton University Press, 1987. [Original work published 1843.]

Koort, P. (1975). Semantisk analys och konfigurationsanalys. Lund, Sweden: Studentlitteratur. [Semantic analysis and analysis of configuration. Lund, Sweden: Studentlitteratur.]

Kuhn, T. (1971). The structure of scientific revolutions. Chicago: University of Chicago Press.

Kurtén, T. (1987). Grunder för en kontextuell teologi: ett wittgensteinskt sätt att närma sig teologin I diskussion med Anders Jeffner. Turku, Finland: Åbo Akademis Förlag. [Bases for a contextual theology: a Wittgensteinian way of approaching theology in a discussion with Anders Jeffner. Turku, Finland: Åbo Akademi University Press.]

Kärkkäinen, O., & Eriksson, K. (2003). Evaluation of patient records as a part of developing a nursing care classification. Journal of Clinical Nursing, 12(2), 198-205.

Kärkkäinen, O., & Eriksson, K. (2004). Structuring the documentation of nursing care on the basis of a theoretical process model. Scandinavian Journal of Caring Sciences, 18(2), 229-236.

Lanara, V. (1981). Heroism as a nursing value. Athens, Greece: Sisterhood Evniki.

Langer, S. K. (1942). Filosofi i en ny tonart. Stockholm: Geber. [Philosophy in a new key. Stockholm: Geber.]

Lévinas, E. (1985). Ethics and infinity. Pittsburgh: Duquesne University Press.

Lévinas, E. (1988). Etik och oändlighet. Stockholm-Lund: Symposion. [Ethics and infinity. Stockholm-Lund: Symposion.]

Lévinas, E. (1989). The Lévinas reader (S. Hand, Ed.). Oxford: Blackwell.

Lindholm, L. (1998). Den unga människans hälsa och lidande. Doktorsavhandling, Vaasa, Finland. Institutionen för vårdvetenskap, Åbo Akademi. [The young person's health and suffering. Doctoral dissertation, Vaasa, Finland. Åbo Akademi, Department of Caring Science.]

Lindholm, L., & Eriksson, K. (1993). To understand and to alleviate suffering in a caring culture. Journal of Advanced Nursing, 18, 1354-1361.

Lindholm, L., & Eriksson, K. (1998). The dialectic of health and suffering: An ontological perspective on young people's health. Qualitative Health Research, 8(4), 513-525.

Lindholm, L., Nieminen, A-L., Mäkelä, C., & Rantanen-Siljamäki, S. (2004). Significant others—A source of strength in the care of women with breast cancer. Manuscript submitted for publication.

Lindström, U. Å. (1992). De psykiatriska specialsjukskötarnas yrkesparadigm. Doktorsavhandling, Turku, Finland. Åbo Akademis Förlag. [The professional paradigm of the qualified psychiatric nurses. Doctoral dissertation, Turku, Finland, Åbo Akademi University Press.]

Lindwall, L. (2004). Kroppen som bärare av hälsa och lidande. Doktorsavhandling, Turku, Finland, Åbo Akademis Förlag. [The body as a carrier of health and suffering. Doctoral dissertation, Turku, Finland, Åbo Akademi University Press.]

Lukander, E. (1995). Developing and testing a method: Nursing audit, for evaluation of nursing care. Licentiate thesis, Kuopion yliopisto, Kuopio, Finland.

Martinsen, K., (Ed.). (1996). Fenomenologi og omsorg. Oslo, Norway: TANO. [Phenomenology and care. Oslo, Norway: TANO.]

Nilsson, B. (2004). Savnets tone i ensomhetens melodi. Ensomhet hos aleneboende personer med alvorlig psykisk lidelse. Doktorsavhandling, Turku, Finland, Åbo Akademis Förlag. [The tune of want in the loneliness melody. Doctoral dissertation, Turku, Finland, Åbo Akademi University Press.]

Nygren, A. (1966). Eros och agapé. Stockholm: Aldus Bonniers. [Eros and agapé. Stockholm: Aldus Bonniers.]

Nygren, A. (1972). Meaning and method: prolegomena to a scientific philosophy of religion and a scientific theology. London: Epworth Press.

Nåden, D. (1998). Når sykepleie er kunstutøvelse. En undersøkelse av noen nødvendige forutsetninger for sykepleie som kunst. Doktorsavhandling, Vaasa, Finland. Institutionen för vårdvetenskap, Åbo Akademi. [When caring is an exercise of art. An examination of some necessary preconditions of nursing as art. Doctoral dissertation, Department of Caring Science, Åbo Akademi, Vaasa, Finland.]

Pascal, B. (1971). Tankar. Uddevalla, Sweden: Bohusläningens AB. [Thoughts. Uddevalla, Sweden: Bohusläningens AB.]

Peirce, C. S. (1990). Pragmatism och kosmologi. Valda uppsatser. Gothenburg, Sweden: Daidalos. [Pragmatism and cosmology (Chosen essays). Gothenburg, Sweden: Daidalos.]

Popper, K. R. (1997). Popper i urval av Miller. Kunskapsteori, vetenskapsteori. Stockholm: Thales. [Popper in selection of Miller. Theory of knowledge and theory of science. Stockholm: Thales.]

Rundqvist, E. (2004). Makt som fullmakt. Ett vårdvetenskapligt perspektiv. Doktorsavhandling, Åbo Akademis Förlag, Turku, Finland. [Power as authority. A caring science perspective. Doctoral dissertation, Åbo Akademi University Press, Turku, Finland.]

Råholm, M-B. (2003). I kampens och modets dialektik. Doktorsavhandling, Åbo Akademis Förlag, Turku, Finland. [In the dialectic of struggle and courage. Dissertation, Åbo Akademi University Press, Turku, Finland.]

Råholm, M-B., & Lindholm, L. (1999). Being in the world of the suffering patient: A challenge to nursing ethics. Nursing Ethics, 6, 528-539.

Råholm, M-B., Lindholm, L., & Eriksson, K. (2002). Grasping the essence of the spiritual dimension reflected through the horizon of suffering—An interpretative research synthesis. The Australian Journal of Holistic Nursing, 9, 4-12.

Sivonen, K. (2000). Vården och det andliga. En bestämning av begreppet 'andlig' ur ett vårdvetenskapligt perspektiv. Doktorsavhandling, Turku, Finland, Åbo Akademis Förlag. [Care and the spiritual dimension. A definition of the concept of "spiritual" in a caring science perspective. Doctoral dissertation, Turku, Finland, Åbo Akademi University Press.]

St. Augustine, A. (1957). Bekännelser. Stockholm: Söderström. [Confessions. Stockholm: Söderström.]

Turtiainen, A-M. (1999). Hoitotyön käytännön kuvaamisen yhtenäistäminen: Belgialaisen hoitotyön minimitiedoston (BeNMDS) kulttuurinen adaptio Suomeen. Doktorsavhandling, Väitöskirja, Kuopion yliopisto, Kuopio, Finland. [Methods to describe nursing with uniform language: The cross-cultural adaptation process of the Belgium Nursing Minimum Data Set in Finland. Doctoral dissertation, Kuopio University, Kuopio, Finland.]

Törnebohm, H. (1978). Paradigm i vetenskapsteorin (Del 2. Rapport nr. 100). Gothenburg, Sweden: Institutionen för vetenskapsteori, Göteborgs universitet. [Paradigms in the theory of science (Part 2 Report nr. 100). Gothenburg, Sweden: Institutionen för vetenskapsteori, Göteborgs universitet.]

von Post, I. (1999). Professionell naturlig vård ur anestesi och operationassjuksköterskors perspektiv. Doktorsavhandling, Åbo Akademis Förlag, Turku, Finland. [Professional natural care from the perspective of nurse anesthetists and operating room nurses. Doctoral dissertation, Turku, Finland, Åbo Akademi University Press.]

von Wright, G. H. (1986). Vetenskapen och förnuftet. Helsinki, Finland: Söderström. [Science and reason. Helsinki, Finland: Söderström.]

Wiklund, L. (2000). Lidandet som kamp och drama. Doktorsavhandling, Turku, Finland, Åbo Akademis Förlag. [Suffering as struggle and as drama. Doctoral dissertation, Turku, Finland, Åbo Akademi University Press.]

Wingren, G. (1996). Predikan: en principiell studie. Lund, Sweden: Gleerup. [The sermon: a study based on principles. Lund, Sweden: Gleerup.] [Original work published 1960.]

Wärnå, C. (2002). Dygd och hälsa. Doktorsavhandling, Turku, Finland, Åbo Akademis Förlag. [Virtue and health. Doctoral dissertation, Turku, Finland, Åbo Akademi University Press.]

BIBLIOGRAPHY

Primary Sources

Articles in Scientific Journals With Referee Practice

Arman, M., Rehnsfeldt, A., Lindholm, L., Hamrin, E., & Eriksson, K. (2004). Suffering related to health care: A study of breast cancer patients' experiences. *International Journal of Nursing Practice, 10*(6), 248-256.

Bondas, T., & Eriksson, K. (2001). Women's lived experiences of pregnancy: A tapestry of joy and suffering. *Qualitative Health Research, 11*(6), 824-840.

Caspari, S., Nåden, D., & Eriksson, K. (2006). The aesthetic dimension in hospitals—An investigation into strategic plans. *International Journal of Nursing Studies, 43*, 851-859.

Caspari, S., Nåden, D., & Eriksson, K. (2007). Why Not ask The Patient? An Evaluation of the Aesthetic Surroundings in Hospital by Patients. *Quality Management in Health Care, 16*(3), 280-292.

Eriksson, K. (1976). Nursing—Skilled work or a profession. *International Nursing Review, 23*(4), 118-120.

Eriksson, K. (1979). Semantiska och kulturella aspekter på hälsobegreppet. *Finska Läkaresällskapets handlingar*, 74-81. [Semantic and cultural aspects of the concept of health. *Finska Läkaresällskapets handlingar*, 74-81.]

Eriksson, K. (1980). Hoitotieteen loogiset ja tieteenteoreettiset perusteet. *Sosiaalinen aikakauskirja, 14*(5), 6-10. [The theory of science and logical basics of caring science. *Sosiaalinen aikakauskirja, 14*(5), 6-10.

Eriksson, K. (1980). Hoitotieteen teoreettisista malleista, käsitejärjestelmistä ja niiden merkityksestä alan kehittämisessä. *Sosiaalilääketieteellinen aikakauslehti, 17*(2), 66-70. [The importance of caring scientific theoretical models and concept systems for the development of the science. *Sosiaalilääketieteellinen aikakauslehti, 17*(2), 66-70.]

Eriksson, K. (1982). Sjukskötarnas strävan efter högskoleutbildning. *Kasvatus, 13*(3), 192-194. [The nurses strive for a university education. *Kasvatus, 13*(3), 192-194.]

Eriksson, K. (1989). Caring paradigms. A study of the origins and the development of caring paradigms among nursing students. *Scandinavian Journal of Caring Sciences, 3*(4), 169-176.

Eriksson, K. (1989). Det finns en gemensam substans i allt vårdandet. *Vård i Norden, 15*(2), 27-28. [There is a common substance in all caring. *Nordic of Journal Nursing Research and Clinical Studies, 15*(2), 27-28.]

Eriksson, K. (1989). Motivforskning inom vårdvetenskapen. En beskrivning av vårdvetenskapens grundmotiv. *Hoitotiede, 1*(2), 61-67. [Motive research within caring science. A description of the basic motive in caring science. *Journal of Nursing Science, 1*(2), 61-67.]

Eriksson, K. (1990). Nursing science in a Nordic perspective. Systematic and contextual caring science. A study of the basic motive of caring and context. *Scandinavian Journal of Caring Sciences, 4*(1), 3-5.

Eriksson, K. (1992). Different forms of caring communion. *Nursing Science Quarterly, 5*, 93.

Eriksson, K. (1992). The alleviation of suffering—The idea of caring. *Scandinavian Journal of Caring Sciences, 6*(2), 119-123.

Eriksson, K. (1994). Hälsovårdskandidatutbildningen vid Helsingfors universitet—Historisk tillbakablick och visioner. *Hoitotiede, 3*, 122-126. [The bachelor's degree in health care at Helsinki University—A historical retrospect and visions. *Journal of Nursing Science, 3*, 122-126.]

Eriksson, K. (1995). Ars moriendi är ars vivendi. *Finsk tidskrift, 10*, 641-645. [Ars moriendi is ars vivendi. *Finsk tidskrift, 10*, 641-645.]

Eriksson, K. (1995). Teologi og bioetik. *Vård i Norden, 1*, 33. [Theology and bio-ethics. *Nordic Journal of Nursing Research and Clinical Studies, 1*, 33.]

Eriksson, K. (1997). Understanding the world of the patient, the suffering human being—The new clinical paradigm from nursing to caring. *Advanced Practice Nursing Quarterly, 3*(1), 8-13.

Eriksson, K. (1998). Hälsans tragedy. *Finsk tidskrift, 10*, 590-599. [The tragedy of health. *Finsk tidskrift, 10*, 590-599.]

Eriksson, K. (2002). Caring science in a new key. *Nursing Science Quarterly, 15*(1), 61-65.

Eriksson, K. (2007a). Becoming through suffering—The path to health and holiness. *International Journal of Human Caring, 11*(2), 8-16.

Eriksson, K. (2007b). The theory of caritative caring: A vision. *Nursing Science Quarterly, 20*(3), 201-202.

Eriksson, K., Bondas, T., Lindholm, L., Kasén, A., & Matilainen, D. (2002). Den vårdvetenskapliga forskningstraditionen vid Institutionen för vårdvetenskap, Åbo Akademi. *Hoitotiede, 14*(6), 307-315. [The tradition of research at the Department of Caring Science, Åbo Akademi University. *Journal of Nursing Science, 14*(6), 307-315.]

Eriksson, K., Herberts, S., & Lindholm, L. (1994). Bilder av lidande—Lidande i belysning av aktuell vårdvetenskaplig forskning. *Hoitotiede, 4*, 155-162. [Views of suffering—Suffering in the light of current research within caring science. *Journal of Nursing Science, 4*, 155-162.]

Eriksson, K., & Lindström, U. Å. (1997). Abduction—A way to deeper understanding of the world of caring. *Scandinavian Journal of Caring Sciences, 11*(4), 195-198.

Eriksson, K., & Lindström, U. Å. (1999). Abduktion och pragmatism—Två vägar till framsteg inom vårdvetenskapen. *Hoitotiede, 11*(5), 292-299. [Abduction and pragmatism—Two ways to progress within caring science. *Journal of Nursing Science, 11*(5), 292-299.]

Eriksson, K., & Lindström, U. Å. (1999). En vetenskapsteori för vårdvetenskapen. *Hoitotiede, 11*(6), 358-364. [A theory of science for caring science. *Journal of Nursing Science, 11*(6), 358-364.]

Eriksson, K., & Lindström, U. Å. (1999). The fundamental idea of quality assurance. *International Journal for Human Caring, 3*(3), 21-27.

Eriksson, K., & von Post, I. (1999). A hermeneutic textual analysis of suffering and caring in the perioperative context. *Journal of Advanced Nursing, 30*(4), 983-989.

Fagerström, L., Eriksson, K., & Bergbom Engberg, I. (1998). The patient's perceived caring needs as a message of suffering. *Journal of Advanced Nursing, 28*(5), 978-987.

Fagerström, L., Eriksson, K., & Bergbom Engberg, I. (1999). The patient's perceived caring needs—Measuring the unmeasurable. *International Journal of Nursing Practice, 5*(4), 199-208.

Fredriksson, L., & Eriksson, K. (2001). The patient's narrative of suffering—A path to health? An interpretetative research synthesis on narrative understanding. *Scandinavian Journal of Caring Sciences, 15*(1), 3-11.

Fredriksson, L., & Eriksson, K. (2003). The ethics of the caring conversation. *Nursing Ethics, 10*(2), 138-148.

Herberts, S., & Eriksson, K. (1995). Nursing leaders' and nurses' view of health. *Journal of Advanced Nursing, 22*, 868-878.

Kärkkäinen, O., Bondas, T. & Eriksson, K. (2005). Documentation of individualized patient care: a qualitative metasynthesis. *Nursing Ethics, 12*(2), 123-132.

Kärkkäinen, O., & Eriksson, K. (2003). Evaluation of patient records as a part of developing a nursing care classification. *Journal of Clinical Nursing, 12*(2), 198-205.

Kärkkäinen, O., & Eriksson, K. (2004a). A theoretical approach to documentation of care. *Nursing Science Quarterly, 17*(3), 2-6.

Kärkkäinen, O., & Eriksson, K. (2004b). Structuring the documentation on nursing care on the basis of a theoretical caring process model. *Scandinavian Journal of Caring Sciences, 18*(2), 229-236.

Kärkkäinen, O., & Eriksson, K. (2005). Recording the content of the caring process. *Journal of Nursing Management, 13*, 202-208.

Lindholm, L., & Eriksson, K. (1993). To understand and to alleviate suffering in a caring culture. *Journal of Advanced Nursing, 18*, 1354-1361.

Lindholm, L., & Eriksson, K. (1998). The dialectic of health and suffering: An ontological perspective on young people's health. *Qualitative Health Research, 8*(4), 513-525.

Nåden, D., & Eriksson, K. (2000). The phenomenon of confirmation—An aspect of nursing as an art. *International Journal for Human Caring, 4*(3), 23-28.

Nåden, D., & Eriksson, K. (2002). Encounter: A fundamental category of nursing as an art. *International Journal for Human Caring, 6*(1), 34-40.

Nåden, D., & Eriksson, K. (2003). Semantisk begrepsanalyse—Et grunnleggende aspekt i en disiplins teoriutvikling. *Vård i Norden, 23*(1), 21-26. [Semantic concept analysis—A fundamental aspect in the theory development of a discipline. *Nordic Journal of Nursing Research and Clinical Studies, 23*(1), 21-26.]

Nåden, D., & Eriksson, K. (2004a). Understanding the importance of values and moral attitudes in nursing care in preserving human dignity. *Nursing Science Quarterly, 17*(1), 86-91.

Nåden, D., & Eriksson, K. (2004b). Values and moral attitudes in nursing care. Understanding the patient perspective. *Norsk Tidskrift for Sygepleieforskning, 6*(1), 3-17.

Rehnsfeldt, A. & Eriksson, K. (2004). The progression of suffering implies alleviated suffering. *Scandinavian Journal of Caring Sciences, 18*(3), 264-272.

Rudolfsson, G., von Post, I., & Eriksson, K. (2007). The development of caring in the perioperative culture—nurse leaders' perspective on the struggle to retain sight of the patient. *Nursing Administration Quarterly, 31*(4), 312-324.

Rudolfsson, G., von Post, I., & Eriksson, K. (2007). The expression of caring within the perioperative dialogue: a hermeneutic study. *International Journal of Nursing Studies, 44*, 905-915.

Råholm, M-B., & Eriksson, K. (2001). Call to life: Exploring the spiritual dimension as a dialectic between suffering and desire experienced by coronary bypass patients. *International Journal for Human Caring, 5*(1), 14-20.

Råholm, M-B., Lindholm, L., & Eriksson, K. (2002). Grasping the essence of the spiritual dimension reflected through the horizon of suffering: An interpretative research synthesis. *The Australian Journal of Holistic Nursing, 9*(1), 4-13.

von Post, I., & Eriksson, K. (2000). The ideal and practice concepts of 'professional nursing care.' *International Journal for Human Caring, 4*(1), 14-22.

Wikström-Grotell, C., Lindholm, L., & Eriksson, K. (2002). Det mångdimensionella rörelsebegreppet i fysioterapin—En kontextuell analys. *Nordisk Fysioterapi, 6*, 146-184. [The multidimensional concept of movement in physiotherapy—A contextual analysis. *Nordisk Fysioterapi, 6*, 146-184.]

Wärnå, C., Lindholm, L., & Eriksson, K. (2007). Virtue and health—finding meaning and joy in working life. *Scandinavian Journal of Caring Sciences, 21*, 191-198.

Articles in Compilation Works and Proceedings With Referee Practice

Compilation Works

Eriksson, K. (1971). En analys av sjuksköterskeutbildningen utgående från en utbildningsteknologisk model. I *Sairaanhoidon vuosikirja VIII* (s. 54-77). Helsinki, Finland: Sairaanhoitajien Koulutussäätiö. [An analysis of nursing education from an educational-technological model. In *Health care yearbook VIII* (pp. 54-77). Helsinki, Finland: Sairaanhoitajien Koulutussäätiö.]

Eriksson, K. (1974). Sairaanhoidon kehittäminen oppiaineena. I *Sairaanhoidon vuosikirja XI* (s. 9-21). Helsinki, Finland: Sairaanhoitajien Koulutussäätiö. [The development of health care as a subject. In *Health care yearbook XI* (pp. 9-21). Helsinki, Finland: Sairaanhoitajien Koulutussäätiö.]

Eriksson, K. (1977). Hälsa—En teoretisk och begreppsanalytisk studie om hälsa och dess nature. I *Sairaanhoidon vuosikirja XIV* (s. 55-195). [Health—A conceptual analysis and theoretical study of health and its nature. In *Health care yearbook XIV* (pp. 155-195). Helsinki, Finland: Sairaanhoitajien Koulutussäätiö.]

Eriksson, K. (1978). Modellen—Ett sätt att beskriva vårdskeendet. I *Sairaanhoidon vuosikirja XV* (s. 189-225). Helsinki, Finland: Sairaanhoitajien Koulutussäätiö. [The model—A way of describing the act of nursing care. In *Health care yearbook XV* (pp. 189-225). Helsinki, Finland: Sairaanhoitajien Koulutussäätiö.]

Eriksson, K. (1982). Den vårdvetenskapscentrerade läroplanen—Ett alternativ för dagens vårdutbildning. I *Sairaanhoidon vuosikirja XIX* (s. 173-187). Helsinki, Finland: Sairaanhoitajien Koulutussäätiö. [The caring science centered curriculum—An alternative for health education today. In *Health care yearbook XIX* (pp. 173-187). Helsinki, Finland: Sairaanhoitajien Koulutussäätiö.]

Eriksson, K. (1983). Den fullvuxna insulindiabetikern i hälsovårdens vårdprocess. I *Sairaanhoidon vuosikirja XIX* (s. 428-430). Helsinki, Finland: Sairaanhoitajien Koulutussäätiö. [The adult insulin-dependent diabetic in the health care nursing process. In *Health care yearbook XIX* (pp. 428-430). Helsinki, Finland: Sairaanhoitajien Koulutussäätiö.]

Eriksson, K. (1983). Vårdområdet finner sin profil—Den vårdvetenskapliga eran har inlets. I *Epione, Jubileumsskrift 1898-1983* (s. 12-17). [The area of caring finds its profile—The caring science era has begun. In *Epione, Jubilee-script 1898-1983* (pp. 12-17). Helsinki, Finland: SSY-Sjuksköterskeföreningen i Finland.]

Eriksson, K. (1986). Hoito, Caring—Hoitotyön primaari substanssi. Puheenvuoro 2. I T. Martikainen & K. Manninen (red.), *Hoitotyö ja koulutus* (s. 17-41). Hämeenlinna, Finland: Sairaanhoitajien Koulutussäätiö. [Caring—The primary substance of nursing. Speech 2. In T. Martikainen & K. Manninen (Eds.), *Nursing and education* (pp. 17-41). Hämeenlinna, Finland: Sairaanhoitajien Koulutussäätiö.]

Eriksson, K. (1987). Vårdvetenskapen som humanistisk vetenskap. I *Hoitotiede vuosikirja (s. 68-77)* [Caring science as a humanistic science. *Journal of Nursing Science Yearbook* 68-77.]

Eriksson, K. (1988). Vårdandets idé och ursprung. I *Panakeia. Vårdvetenskaplig årsbok* (s. 17-35). Stockholm: Almqvist & Wiksell. [The origin and idea of caring. In *Panakeia. Caring science yearbook* (pp. 17-35). Stockholm: Almqvist & Wiksell.]

Eriksson, K. (1989). Ammatillisuus hoitamisessa. I *Hoitoopin perusteet* (2: 2 yppl., s. 125-129). Vaasa, Finland: Sairaanhoitajien Koulutussäätiö. [Professionalism in caring. In *The basics of nursing science* (2nd ed., pp. 125-129). Vaasa, Finland: Sairaanhoitajien Koulutussäätiö.]

Eriksson, K. (1990). Framtidsvisioner—om utvecklingen av sjukskötarens arbete. I *Epione, Jubileumsskrift 1898-1988* (s. 28-38). Helsinki, Finland: SSY-sjuksköterskeföreningen i Finland r.f. [Future visions of the development of the nurse's work. In *Epione, Jubilee-script 1898-1988* (pp. 28-38). Helsinki, Finland: SSY-sjuksköterskeföreningen i Finland r.f.]

Eriksson, K. (1991). Hälsa är mera än frånvaro av sjukdom. I *Centrum för vårdvetenskap, Vård—Utbildning—Utveckling—Forskning* (s. 1-2, 29-35). Stockholm: Karolinska Institutet. [Health is more than the absence of illness. In *Centrum för vårdvetenskap, Vård—Utbildning—Utveckling—Forskning* (pp. 1-2, 29-35). Stockholm: Karolinska Institutet.]

Eriksson, K. (1992). Nursing: The caring practice "being there." In D. Gaut (Ed.), *The practice of caring in nursing* (pp. 201-210). New York: National League for Nursing Press.

Eriksson, K. (1993). De första åren—Några reflektioner kring den vårdvetenskapliga eran. I *Epione, Jubileumsskrift 1898-1993* (s. 7-15). Helsinki, Finland: SSY-Sjuksköterskeföreningen. [The first years—Reflections upon the era of caring science. In *Epione, Jubilee-script 1898-1993* (pp. 7-15). Helsinki, Finland: SSY-Sjuksköterskeföreningen.]

Eriksson, K. (1994). Theories of caring as health. In D. Gaut & A. Boykin (Eds.), *Caring as healing: Renewal through hope* (pp. 3-20). New York: National League for Nursing Press.

Eriksson, K. (1994). Vårdvetenskapen som autonom discipline. I H. Willman (red.), *Hygieia. Hoitotyön vuosikirja 1994* (s. 87-91).). Helsinki, Finland: Kirjayhtymä. [Caring science as an autonomous discipline. In H. Willman (Ed.), *Hygieia. Nursing yearbook 1994* (pp. 87-91). Helsinki, Finland: Kirjayhtymä.]

Eriksson, K. (1996). Efterskrift—Om vårdvetenskapens möjligheter och gränser. I K. Martinsen (red.),

Fenomenologi og omsorg (s. 140-150). Oslo, Norway: TANO. [Postscript—About the possibilities and boundaries of caring science. In K. Martinsen (Ed.), *Phenomenology and caring* (pp. 140-150). Oslo, Norway: TANO.]

Eriksson, K. (1996). Om dokumentation—Vad den är och inte är. I K. Dahlberg (red.), *Konsten att dokumentera omvårdnad* (s. 9-13). Lund, Sweden: Studentlitteratur. [On documentation—What it is and what it is not. In K. Dahlberg (ed.), *The art of documenting care* (pp. 9-13). Lund, Sweden: Studentlitteratur.]

Eriksson, K. (1996). Om människans värdighet. I T. Bjerkreim, J. Mathinsen, & R. Nord (red.), *Visjon, viten og virke. Festskrift till sykepleieren Kjellaug Lerheim, 70 år* (s. 79-86). Oslo, Norway: Universitetsförlaget. [On human dignity. In T. Bjerkreim, J. Mathinsen, & R. Nord (Eds.), *Vision, knowledge and influence. Jubilee-script for the nurse Kjellaug Lerheim, 70 years* (pp. 79-86). Oslo, Norway: Universitetsförlaget.]

Eriksson, K. (1997). Caring, spirituality and suffering. In M. S. Roach (Ed.), *Caring from the heart: The convergence between caring and spirituality* (pp. 68-84). New York: Paulist Press.

Eriksson, K. (1997). Mot en vårdetisk teori. I *Hoitotyön vuosikirja* 1997. Pro Nursing RY:n vuosikirja, Hygieia (s. 9-23). Helsinki, Finland: Kirjayhtymä. [Toward an ethical caring theory. In *Nursing yearbook* 1997. Pro Nursing RY:s yearbook, Hygieia (pp. 9-23). Helsinki, Finland: Kirjayhtymä.]

Eriksson, K. (1997). Perustutkimus ja käsiteanalyysi. I M. Paunonen & K. Vehviläinen-Julkunen (red.), *Hoitotieteen tutkimusmetodiikka* (s. 50-75). Helsinki, Finland: WSOY. [Basic research and conceptual analysis. In M. Paunonen & K. Vehviläinen-Julkunen (Eds.), *The research methodology of caring science* (pp. 50-75). Helsinki, Finland: WSOY.]

Eriksson, K. (1998). Epione—Vårdandets ethos. I *Epione, Jubileumsskrift 1898-1998* Helsinki, Finland: SSY-Sjuksköterskeföreningen. [Epione—The ethos of caring. In *Epione, Jubilee-script 1898-1998.* Helsinki, Finland: SSY-Sjuksköterskeföreningen.]

Eriksson, K. (1998). Människans värdighet, lidande och lidandets ethos. I *Suomen Mielenterveysseura, Tuhkaa ja linnunrata. Henkisyys mielenterveystyössä* (s. 67-82). Helsinki: Suomen Mielenterveysseura, SMS-julkaisut. [Human dignity, suffering and the ethos of suffering. In *Ashes and the Milky Way: Spirituality in mental health care nursing* (pp. 67-82). Helsinki: Suomen Mielenterveysseura, SMS-julkaisut.]

Eriksson, K. (1998). Understanding the world of the patient, the suffering human being: The new clinical paradigm from nursing to caring. In C. E. Guzzetta (Ed.), *Essential readings in holistic nursing* (pp. 3-9). Gaithersburg, MD: Aspen Publications.

Eriksson, K. (1999). Tillbaka till Popper och Kuhn—En evolutionär epistemologi för vårdvetenskapen. I J. Kinnunen, P. Meriläinen, K. Vehviläinen-Julkunen, & T. Nyberg (red.), *Terveystieteiden monialainen tutkimus ja yliopistokoulutus. Suunnistuspoluilta tiedon valtatielle. Professor Sirkka Sinkkoselle omistettu juhlakirja* (s. 21-35). Kuopio, Finland: Kuopion yliopiston julkaisuja E, Yhteiskuntatieteet 74. [Back to Popper and Kuhn—An evolutionary epistemology for caring science. In J. Kinnunen, P. Meriläinen, K. Vehviläinen-Julkunen, & T. Nyberg (Eds.), *The multiscientific health science university education and research. Paths to the highway of science. A jubilee book dedicated to Professor Sirkka Sikkonen* (pp. 21-35). Kuopio, Finland: Kuopion yliopiston julkaisuja E, Yhteiskuntatieteet 74.]

Eriksson, K. (1999). Vårdvetenskapen—En akademisk disciplin. I S. Janhonen, I. Lepola, M. Nikkonen, & M. Toljamo (red.), *Suomalainen hoitotiede uudelle vuosituhannelle. Professori Maija Hentisen juhlakirja* (s. 59-64). Oulu, Finland: Oulun yliopiston hoitotieteen ja terveyshallinnon laitoksen julkaisuja 2. [Caring science—An academic discipline. In S. Janhonen, I. Lepola, M. Nikkonen, & M. Toljamo (Eds.), *The Finnish caring science in the new millennium. A jubilee-script dedicated to Professor Maija Hentinen* (pp. 59-64). Oulu, Finland: Oulun yliopiston hoitotieteen ja terveyshallinnon laitoksen julkaisuja 2.]

Eriksson, K. (2000). Caritas et passio—Liebe und leiden—Als grundkategorien der pflegewissenschaft. I T. Strom, *Diakonie an der Schwelle zum neuen Jahrtausend.* Heidelberg, Germany: Diakoniewissenschaftlichen Instituts, Universität Heidelberg. [Caritas et passio—Love and suffering as basic categories in caring science. In T. Strom, *The diaconate on the threshold of the new millennium.* Heidelberg, Germany: Diakoniewissenschaftlichen Instituts, Universität Heidelberg.]

Eriksson, K. (2002). Rakkaus—Diakoniatieteen ydin ja ethos? I M. Lahtinen & T. Toikkanen (red.), *Anno Domini. Diakoniatieteen vuosikirja 2002* (s. 155-164). Tampere, Finland: Tammerpaino. [Love—The core and ethos of deacony? In M. Lahtinen & T. Toikkanen (Eds.), *Anno Domini. Diakonic yearbook 2002* (pp. 155-164). Tampere, Finland: Tammerpaino.]

Eriksson, K. (2003). Diakonian erityisyys hoitotyössä. I M. Lahtinen & T. Toikkanen (red.), *Anno domini. Diakoniatieteen vuosikirja 2003* (s. 120-126). Tampere, Finland: Tammerpaino. [The uniqueness of deacony in nursing. In M. Lahtinen & T. Toikkanen (Eds.), *Anno Domini. Diakonic yearbook 2003* (pp. 120-126). Tampere, Finland: Tammerpaino.]

Eriksson, K., & Hamrin, E. (1988). Vårdvetenskapen formas—En tillbakablick och ett framtidsperspektiv. I *Panakeia, vårdvetenskaplig årsbok* (s. 9-16). Stockholm: Almqvist & Wiksell. [Caring science is formed—A historical and futuristic perspective. In *Panakeia, caring science yearbook* (pp. 9-16). Stockholm: Almqvist & Wiksell.]

Eriksson, K., Nordman, T., & Kasén, A. (1998). Reflective practice: A way to the patient's world and caring, the core of nursing. In C. Johns & D. Freshwater (Eds.), *Transforming nursing through reflective practice.* Oxford: Blackwell Science.

Eriksson, K., & Willman, H. (1972). Kohti parempaa ohjausta. I *Sairaanhoidon vuosikirja IX* (s. 131-139). Helsinki, Finland: Sairaanhoitajien Koulutussäätiö. [Toward a better counseling. In *Health care yearbook IX* (pp. 131-139). Helsinki, Finland: Sairaanhoitajien Koulutussäätiö.]

Books and Monographs

Eriksson, K. (1974). *Sjuksköterskeyrket—Hantverk eller profession.* Sjuksköterskors samarbete i Norden. Rapport från SSN:s expertgrupp för klargörande av vårdfunktionsområdet. Helsinki, Finland: SSN. [*The nursing profession—Skill or profession.* Collaboration of nurses in the Nordic countries. Report from SSN's expert group for the clarification of nursing. Helsinki, Finland: SSN.]

Eriksson, K. (1975). *Den teoretiska utgångspunkten för vårdprocessen.* Rapport från SSN:s symposium i Helsingfors. Helsinki, Finland: SSN. [*The theoretical starting point of the nursing care process.* A report from SSN:s symposium in Helsinki. Helsinki, Finland: SSN.]

Eriksson, K. (1976). Hoitotapahtuma. *Hoito-oppi 2.* Helsinki, Finland: Sairaanhoitajien Koulutussäätiö. [The nursing care process. *Nursing science 2.* Helsinki, Finland: Sairaanhoitajien Koulutussäätiö.]

Eriksson, K. (1976). *Hälsa. En teoretisk och begreppsanalytisk studie om hälsan och dess natur som mål för hälsovårdsedukation.* Licentiatavhandling, Helsinki, Finland: Institutionen för pedagogik, Helsingfors universitet. [*Health. A conceptual analysis and theoretical study of health and its nature as a goal for health care education.* Unpublished licentiate thesis, Helsinki, Finland: Department of Education University of Helsinki.]

Eriksson, K. (1979). *Vårdprocessen.* Stockholm: Almqvist & Wiksell. [*The nursing care process.* Stockholm: Almqvist & Wiksell.]

Eriksson, K. (1981). *Vårdprocessen—En utgångspunkt för läroplanstänkande inom vårdutbildningen. Utvecklande av en vårdprocessmodell samt ett läroplanstänkande utgående från vårdprocessen* (Nr. 94). Helsinki, Finland: Helsingfors universitet, Pedagogiska Institutionen. [*The nursing care process—An approach to curriculum construction within nursing education. The development of a model for the nursing care process and an approach for curriculum development based on the process of nursing care* (No. 94). Helsinki, Finland: Department of Education University of Helsinki.]

Eriksson, K. (1982). *Vårdprocessen.* (2:a uppl.). Stockholm: Almqvist & Wiksell. [*The nursing care process* (2nd ed.). Stockholm: Almqvist & Wiksell.]

Eriksson, K. (1983). *Introduktion till vårdvetenskap.* Stockholm: Almqvist & Wiksell. [*An introduction to caring science.* Stockholm: Almqvist & Wiksell.]

Eriksson, K. (1984). *Hälsans idé.* Stockholm: Almqvist & Wiksell. [*The idea of health.* Stockholm: Almqvist & Wiksell.]

Eriksson, K. (1985). *Johdatus hoitotieteeseen.* Helsinki, Finland: Sairaanhoitajien Koulutussäätiö. [*An introduction to caring science.* Helsinki, Finland: Sairaanhoitajien Koulutussäätiö.]

Eriksson, K. (1985). *Vårddidaktik.* Stockholm: Almqvist & Wiksell. [*Caring didactics.* Stockholm: Almqvist & Wiksell.]

Eriksson, K. (1985). *Vårdprocessen* (3: e uppl.). Stockholm: Almqvist & Wiksell. [*The nursing care process* (3rd ed.). Stockholm: Almqvist & Wiksell.]

Eriksson, K. (1986). *Hoito-opin didaktiikka.* Helsinki, Finland: Sairaanhoitajien Koulutussäätiö. [*The didactics of caring science.* Helsinki, Finland: Sairaanhoitajien Koulutussäätiö.]

Eriksson, K. (1986). *Introduktion till vårdvetenskap* (2:a uppl.). Stockholm: Almqvist & Wiksell. [An introduction to caring science (2nd ed.). Stockholm: Almqvist & Wiksell.]

Eriksson, K. (1987). *Hoitamisen idea.* Forssa, Finland: Sairaanhoitajien Koulutussäätiö. [*The idea of caring.* Forssa, Finland: Sairaanhoitajien Koulutussäätiö.]

Eriksson, K. (1987). *Pausen. En beskrivning av vårdvetenskapens kunskapsobjekt.* Stockholm: Almqvist & Wiksell. [*The pause. A description of the knowledge object of caring science.* Stockholm: Almqvist & Wiksell.]

Eriksson, K. (1987). *Vårdandets idé.* Stockholm: Almqvist & Wiksell. [*The idea of caring.* Stockholm: Almqvist & Wiksell.]

Eriksson, K. (1988). *Hoito tieteenä.* Forssa, Sweden: Sairaanhoitajien Koulutussäätiö. [*Caring as a science.* Forssa, Sweden: Sairaanhoitajien Koulutussäätiö.]

Eriksson, K. (1989). *Caritas-idea.* Helsinki, Finland: Sairaanhoitajien Koulutussäätiö. [*The idea of caritas.* Helsinki, Finland: Sairaanhoitajien Koulutussäätiö.]

Eriksson, K. (1989). *Hälsans idé.* (2:a uppl.). Stockholm: Almqvist & Wiksell. [*The idea of health* (2nd ed.). Stockholm: Almqvist & Wiksell.]

Eriksson, K. (1989). *Terveyden idea.* Helsinki, Finland: Sairaanhoitajien Koulutussäätiö. [*The idea of health.* Helsinki, Finland: Sairaanhoitajien Koulutussäätiö.]

Eriksson, K. (1992). *Broar. Introduktion i vårdvetenskaplig metod.* Vaasa, Finland: Institutionen för vårdvetenskap, Åbo Akademi. [*Bridges. Introduction to the methods of caring science.* Vaasa, Finland: Department of Caring Science, Åbo Akademi.]

Eriksson, K. (1994). *Den lidande människan.* Stockholm: Liber Förlag. [*The suffering human being.* Stockholm: Liber Förlag.]

Eriksson, K. (1995). *Det lidende menneske* (Danish translation). Copenhagen: Munksgaard. [*The suffering human being* (Danish translation). Copenhagen: Munksgaard.]

Eriksson, K. (1995). *Den lidende menneske* (Norwegian translation). Oslo: TANO. [*The suffering human being* (Norwegian translation). Oslo: TANO.]

Eriksson, K. (1996). *Omsorgens idé* (Danish translation). Copenhagen: Munksgaard. [*The idea of caring* (Danish translation). Copenhagen: Munksgaard.]

Eriksson, K. (1997). *Vårdandets idé* (Kassettband). Talboksoch punktskriftsbiblioteket. Stockholm: Almqvist & Wiksell. [*The idea of caring* (Audiotape). Talboksoch punktskriftsbiblioteket. Stockholm: Almqvist & Wiksell.]

Eriksson, K. (2001). *Gesundheit. Ein Schlüsselbegriff der Pflegetheorie.* (German translation). Bern, Germany: Verlag Hans Huber. [*The idea of health* (German translation). Bern, Germany: Verlag Hans Huber.]

Eriksson, K. (2006). *The suffering human being.* Chicago: Nordic Studies Press. [English translation of: *Den lidande människan.* Stockholm, Sweden: Liber Förlag. 1994.]

Eriksson, K., & Barbosa da Silva, A. (Eds.). (1994). *Usko ja terveys—johdatus hoitoteologiaan.* (Finnish translation). Helsinki, Finland: Sairaanhoitajien Koulutussäätiö. [*Caring theology* (Finnish translation). Helsinki, Finland: Sairaanhoitajien Koulutussäätiö.]

Eriksson, K., Byfält, H., Leijonqvist, G-B., Nyberg, K., & Uuspää, B. (1986). *Vårdteknologi.* Stockholm: Almqvist & Wiksell. [*Caring technology.* Stockholm: Almqvist & Wiksell.]

University and Department Publications

Eriksson, K. (1988). Vårdvetenskap som disciplin, forsknings- och tillämpningsområde. Vårdforskningar 1/1988. Vaasa, Finland: Institutionen för vårdvetenskap, Åbo Akademi. [Caring science as a discipline, field of research and application. Vaasa, Finland: Department of Caring Science, Åbo Akademi.]

Eriksson, K. (1990). Pro Caritate. En lägesbestämning av caritativ vård. Vårdforskningar 2/1990. Vaasa, Finland: Institutionen för vårdvetenskap, Åbo Akademi. [Pro Caritate. Caritative caring—A positional analysis. Vaasa, Finland: Department of Caring Science, Åbo Akademi.]

Eriksson, K. (1991). Att lindra lidande. I K. Eriksson & A. Barbosa da Silva (red.), Vårdteologi. Vårdforskningar 3/1991 (s. 204-221). Vaasa, Finland: Institutionen för vårdvetenskap, Åbo Akademi. [To alleviate suffering. In K. Eriksson & A. Barbosa da Silva (Eds.), Caring theology (pp. 204-221). Vaasa, Finland: Department of Caring Science, Åbo Akademi.]

Eriksson, K. (1991). Vårdteologins framväxt. I K. Eriksson & A. Barbosa da Silva (red.), Vårdteologi. Vårdforskningar 3/1991 (s. 1-25). [The growth of caring theology. In K. Eriksson & A. Barbosa da Silva (Eds.), Caring theology (pp. 1-25). Vaasa, Finland: Department of Caring Science, Åbo Akademi.]

Eriksson, K. (1993). Lidandets idé. I K. Eriksson (red.), Möten med lidanden. Vårdforskningar 4/1993 (s. 1-27). Vaasa, Finland: Institutionen för vårdvetenskap, Åbo Akademi. [The idea of suffering. In K. Eriksson (Ed.), Encounters with suffering (pp. 1-27). Vaasa, Finland: Department of Caring Science, Åbo Akademi.]

Eriksson, K. (red.). (1993). Möten med lidanden. Vårdforskning 4/1993. Vaasa, Finland: Institutionen för vårdvetenskap, Åbo Akademi. [Encounters with suffering. Vaasa, Finland: Department of Caring Science, Åbo Akademi.]

Eriksson, K. (red.). (1995). Den mångdimensionella hälsan—Verklighet och visioner. Slutrapport. Vaasa, Finland: Vasa sjukvårdsdistrikt kf. och Institutionen för vårdvetenskap, Åbo Akademi. [Multidimensional health—Visions and reality. Final report. Vaasa, Finland: Vasa sjukvårdsdistrikt kf. och Institutionen för vårdvetenskap, Åbo Akademi.]

Eriksson, K. (1995). Mot en caritativ vårdetik. I K. Eriksson (red.), Mot en caritativ vårdetik. Vårdforskning 5/1995 (s. 9-40). Vaasa, Finland: Institutionen för vårdvetenskap, Åbo Akademi. [Toward a caritative caring ethic. In K. Eriksson (Ed.), Toward a caritative caring ethic. Caring research 5/1995. (pp. 9-40). Vaasa, Finland: Department of Caring Science, Åbo Akademi.]

Eriksson, K. (1995). Vad är vårdetik? I K. Eriksson (red.), Mot en caritativ vårdetik. Vårdforskning 5/1995 (s. 1-8). Vaasa, Finland: Institutionen för vårdvetenskap, Åbo Akademi. [What is caring ethic? In K. Eriksson (Ed.), Toward a caritative caring ethic (pp. 1-8). Vaasa, Finland: Department of Caring Science, Åbo Akademi.]. Caring research 5/1995.

Eriksson, K. (1997). Att insjukna i demens—Ett tungt lidande för patient och anhöriga. I B. Beck-Friis & G. Grahn (red.), Leva med demenshandikapp. Lund, Sweden: Lunds universitet: Stiftelsen Silviahemmet. [Becoming ill with dementia—A burdensome suffering for the patient and his/her family. In B. Beck-Friis & G. Grahn (Eds.), Living with the handicap of dementia (Action in favor of people suffering from neurodegenerative diseases). Lund, Sweden: Lunds universitet, Stiftelsen Silviahemmet.]

Eriksson, K. (1998). Vårdvetenskapens framväxt som akademisk disciplin—Ett finlandssvenskt perspektiv. I K. Eriksson (red.), Jubileumsskrift 1987-1997 (s. 1-7). Vaasa, Finland: Institutionen för vårdvetenskap, Åbo Akademi. [The growth of caring science as an academic discipline—A Finland-Swedish perspective. In K. Eriksson (Ed.), Jubilee-script 1987-1997 (pp. 1-7). Vaasa, Finland: Department of Caring Science, Åbo Akademi.]

Eriksson, K. (2001). Vårdvetenskap som akademisk disciplin. Vårdforskning 7/2001. Vaasa, Finland: Institutionen för vårdvetenskap, Åbo Akademi. [Caring science as an academic discipline. Caring research 7/2001. Vaasa, Finland: Department of Caring Science, Åbo Akademi.]

Eriksson, K. (2002). Den trojanske hest. Evidensbasering og sygepleje. (Danish translation). Copenhagen:

Gads Förlag. [The Trojan horse. Evidence-based nursing and caring through a caring science perspective (Danish translation). Copenhagen: Gads Förlag.]

Eriksson, K. (2002). Idéhistoria som deldisciplin inom vårdvetenskapen. I K. Eriksson & D. Matilainen (red.), Vårdandets och vårdvetenskapens idéhistoria. Strövtåg i spårandet av "caritas originalis." Vårdforskning 8/2002 (s. 1-14). Vaasa, Finland: Institutionen för vårdvetenskap, Åbo Akademi. [The history of ideas as a sub-discipline within caring science. In K. Eriksson & D. Matilainen (Eds.), The history of ideas of caring and caring science. Wanderings in search of "caritas originalis." Caring research 8/2002 (pp. 1-14). Vaasa, Finland: Department of Caring Science, Åbo Akademi.]

Eriksson, K. (2002). Vårdandets idéhistoria. I K. Eriksson & D. Matilainen (red.), Vårdandets och vårdvetenskapens idéhistoria. Strövtåg i spårandet av "caritas originalis." Vårdforskning 8/2002 (s. 15-34). Vaasa, Finland: Institutionen för vårdvetenskap, Åbo Akademi. [The history of ideas of caring. In K. Eriksson & D. Matilainen (Eds.), The history of ideas of caring and caring science. Wanderings in search of "caritas originalis." Caring research 8/2002 (pp. 15-34). Vaasa, Finland: Department of Caring Science, Åbo Akademi.]

Eriksson, K. (2003). Ethos. I K. Eriksson & U. Å. Lindström (red.), Gryning II. Klinisk vårdvetenskap (s. 21-34). Vaasa, Finland: Institutionen för vårdvetenskap, Åbo Akademi. [Ethos. In K. Eriksson & U. Å. Lindström (Eds.), Dawn II. Clinical caring science (pp. 21-34). Vaasa, Finland: Department of Caring Science, Åbo Akademi.]

Eriksson, K., & Barbosa da Silva, A. (1991). Vårdteologi som vårdvetenskapens deldisciplin. I K. Eriksson & A. Barbosa da Silva (red.), Vårdteologi. Vårdforskningar 3/1991 (s. 26-64). Vaasa, Finland: Institutionen för vårdvetenskap, Åbo Akademi. [Caring theology as a sub-discipline of caring science. In K. Eriksson & A. Barbosa da Silva (Eds.), Caring theology. Caring research 3/1991 (pp. 26-64). Vaasa, Finland: Department of Caring Science, Åbo Akademi.]

Eriksson, K., Bondas-Salonen, T., Fagerström, L., Herberts, S., & Lindholm, L. (red.). (1990). Den mångdimensionella hälsan. En pilotstudie över uppfattningar bland patienter, skolungdomar och lärare (Projektrapport 1). Vaasa, Finland: Vasa sjukvårdsdistrikt kf. och Institutionen för vårdvetenskap, Åbo Akademi. [Multidimensional health. A pilot study of understanding health among patients, students and teachers (Project Rep. 1). Vaasa, Finland: Vasa sjukvårdsdistrikt kf. och Institutionen för vårdvetenskap, Åbo Akademi.]

Eriksson, K., & Herberts, S. (1991). Tron i hälsans tjänst. I K. Eriksson & A. Barbosa da Silva (red.), Vårdteologi. Vårdforskningar 3/1991 (s. 222-258). Vaasa Finland: Institutionen för vårdvetenskap, Åbo Akademi. [Faith in the service of health. In K. Eriksson & A. Barbosa da Silva (Eds.), Caring theology. Caring research 3/1991 (pp. 222-258). Vaasa Finland: Department of Caring Science, Åbo Akademi.

Eriksson, K., & Herberts, S. (1992). Den mångdimensionella hälsan. En studie av hälsobilden hos sjukvårdsledare och sjukvårdspersonal (Projektrapport 2). Vaasa, Finland: Vasa sjukvårdsdistrikt kf och Institutionen för vårdvetenskap, Åbo Akademi. [Multidimensional health. A study of the views of health among health care leaders and health care personnel (Project Rep. 2). Vaasa, Finland: Vasa sjukvårdsdistrikt kf och Institutionen för vårdvetenskap, Åbo Akademi.]

Eriksson, K., & Herberts, S. (1993). Lidande—En begreppsanalytisk studie. I K. Eriksson (red.), Möten med lidanden. Vårdforskningar 4/1993 (s. 29-54). Vaasa, Finland: Institutionen för vårdvetenskap, Åbo Akademi. [A study of suffering—A concept analysis. In K. Eriksson (Ed.), Encounters with suffering. Caring research 4/1993 (pp. 29-54). Vaasa, Finland: Department of Caring Science, Åbo Akademi.]

Eriksson, K., Herberts, S., & Lindholm, L. (1993). Bilder av lidande—Lidande i belysning av aktuell vårdvetenskaplig forskning. I K. Eriksson (red.), Möten med lidanden. Vårdforskningar 4/1993 suffering (s. 55-78). Vaasa, Finland: Institutionen för vårdvetenskap, Åbo Akademi. [Views of suffering—Suffering in the light of current caring science research. In K. Eriksson (Ed.), Encounters with suffering. Caring research 4/1993 (pp. 55-78). Vaasa, Finland: Department of Caring Science, Åbo Akademi.]

Eriksson, K., & Koort, P. (1973). Sjukvårdspedagogik (Kompendium). Helsinki, Finland: Helsingfors svenska sjukvårdsinstitut. [The pedagogy of nursing care (Compendium). Helsinki, Finland: Helsingfors svenska sjukvårdsinstitut.]

Eriksson, K., & Lindholm, L. (1993). Lidande och kärlek ur ett psykiatriskt vårdperspektiv—En casestudie av mötet mellan mänskligt lidande och kärlek. I K. Eriksson (red.), Möten med lidanden. Vårdforskningar 4/1993 suffering (s. 79-137). Vaasa, Finland: Institutionen för vårdvetenskap, Åbo Akademi. [Love and suffering through a psychiatric caring perspective—A case study of the encounters with human love and suffering. In K. Eriksson (Ed.), Encounters with suffering. Caring research 4/1993 (pp. 79-137). Vaasa, Finland: Department of Caring Science, Åbo Akademi.]

Eriksson, K., & Lindström, U. Å. (2000). Gryning. En vårdvetenskaplig antologi. Vaasa, Finland: Institutionen för vårdvetenskap, Åbo Akademi. [Dawn. An anthology of caring science. Vaasa, Finland: Department of Caring Science, Åbo Akademi.]

Eriksson, K., & Lindström, U. Å. (2000). Siktet, Sökandet, slutandet. I K. Eriksson & U. Å. Lindstöm (red.), Gryning. En vårdvetenskaplig antologi (s. 5-18). Vaasa, Finland:

Institutionen för vårdvetenskap, Åbo Akademi. [Envisioning, seeking and ending. In K. Eriksson & U. Å. Lindström (eds.), Dawn. An anthology of caring science (pp. 5-18). Vaasa, Finland: Department of Caring Science, Åbo Akademi.]

Eriksson, K., & Lindström, U. Å. (2003). Klinisk vårdvetenskap. I K. Eriksson & U. Å. Lindström (red.), Gryning II. Klinisk vårdvetenskap (s. 3-20). Vaasa, Finland: Institutionen för vårdvetenskap, Åbo Akademi. [Clinical caring science. In K. Eriksson & U. Å. Lindström (Eds.), Dawn II. Clinical caring science (pp. 3-20). Vaasa, Finland: Department of Caring Science, Åbo Akademi.

Eriksson, K., & Lindström, U. Å. (2007). Vårdvetenskapens vetenskapsteori på hermeneutisk grund—några grunddrag. I K. Eriksson, U. Å. Lindström, D. Matilainen & L. Lindholm (red.), Gryning III. Vårdvetenskap och hermeneutik (s. 5-20). Vaasa, Finland: Enheten för vårdvetenskap, Åbo Akademi. [The theory of science for caring science on a hermeneutic foundation—some basic features. In K. Eriksson, U. Å. Lindström, D. Matilainen & L. Lindholm (Eds.), Dawn III. Caring science and hermeneutics (pp. 5-20). Vaasa, Finland: Department of Caring Science, Åbo Akademi.]

Eriksson, K., & Matilainen, D. (red.). (2002). Vårdandets och vårdvetenskapens idéhistoria. Strövtåg i spårandet av "caritas originalis". Vårdforskning 8/2002. Vaasa, Finland: Institutionen för vårdvetenskap, Åbo Akademi. [Eriksson, K., & Matilainen, D. (eds.). The history of ideas of caring and caring science. Wanderings in search of "caritas originalis." Caring research 8/2002. Vaasa, Finland: Department of Caring Science, Åbo Akademi.]

Eriksson, K., & Matilainen, D. (red.). (2004). Vårdvetenskapens didaktik. Caritativ didaktik i vårdandets tjänst. Vårdforskningar 9/2004. Vaasa, Finland: Institutionen för vårdvetenskap, Åbo Akademi. [The didactics of caring science. Caritative didactics in the service of caring. Vaasa, Finland: Department of Caring Science, Åbo Akademi.]

Eriksson, K., & Nordman, T. (2004). Den trojanska hästen II—Utvecklande av evidensbaserade vårdande kulturer. Vaasa, Finland: Institutionen för vårdvetenskap, Åbo Akademi. [The Trojan horse II—Development of evidence-based caring cultures. Vaasa, Finland: Department of Caring Science, Åbo Akademi.]

Eriksson K., Nordman T., & Myllymäki I. (1999). Den trojanska hästen. Evidensbaserat vårdande och vårdarbete ur ett vårdvetenskapligt perspektiv cultures (Rap. 1). Vaasa, Finland: Institutionen för vårdvetenskap, Åbo Akademi; Helsingfors universitetscentralsjukhus & Vasa sjukvårdsdistrikt. [The Trojan horse II—Development of evidence-based caring cultures (Rep. 1). Vaasa, Finland: Institutionen för vårdvetenskap, Åbo Akademi; Helsingfors universitetscentralsjukhus & Vasa sjukvårdsdistrikt.

Herberts, S., & Eriksson, K. (1995). Vårdarnas etiska profil. I K. Eriksson (red.), Mot en caritativ vårdetik. Vårdforskning 5/1995 (s. 41-62). Vaasa, Finland: Institutionen för vårdvetenskap, Åbo Akademi. [The ethical profile of the carers. In K. Eriksson (Ed.), Toward a caritative caring ethic. Caring research 5/1995 (pp. 41-62). Vaasa, Finland: Department of Caring Science, Åbo Akademi.]

Secondary Sources

Doctoral Dissertations

Andersson, M. (1994). Integritet som begrepp och princip. En studie av ett vårdetiskt ideal i utveckling. Doktorsavhandling, Turku, Finland, Åbo Akademis Förlag. [Integrity as a concept and as a principle in health care ethics. Doctoral dissertation, Turku, Finland, Åbo Akademi University Press.]

Arman, M. (2003). Lidande och existens i patientens värld. Kvinnors upplevelser av att leva med bröstcancer. Doktorsavhandling, Turku, Finland, Åbo Akademis Förlag. [Suffering and existence in the patient's world. Women's experiences of living with breast cancer. Doctoral dissertation, Turku, Finland, Åbo Akademi University Press.]

Bondas, T. (2000). Att vara med barn: en vårdvetenskaplig studie av kvinnors upplevelser under perinatal tid. Doktorsavhandling, Turku, Finland, Åbo Akademis Förlag. [To be with child: a study of women's lived experiences during the perinatal period from a caring science perspective. Doctoral dissertation, Turku, Finland, Åbo Akademi University Press.]

Caspari, S. (2004). Det gyldne snitt. Den estetiske dimensjon, en kilde til helse og et etisk anliggende. Doktorsavhandling, Turku, Finland, Åbo Akademis Förlag. [The golden section. The aestethic dimension—a source of health. Doctoral dissertation, Turku, Finland, Åbo Akademi University Press.]

Edlund, M. (2002). Människans värdighet-ett grundbegrepp inom vårdvetenskapen. Doktorsavhandling, Turku, Finland, Åbo Akademis Förlag. [Human dignity—A basic caring science concept. Doctoral dissertation, Turku, Finland, Åbo Akademi University Press.]

Ekebergh, M. (2001). Tillägnandet av vårdvetenskaplig kunskap. Reflexionens betydelse för lärandet. Doktorsavhandling, Turku, Finland, Åbo Akademis Förlag. [Acquiring caring science knowledge—The importance of reflection for learning. Doctoral dissertation, Turku, Finland, Åbo Akademi University Press.]

Fagerström, L. (1999). The patient's caring needs. To understand and to measure the unmeasurable. Doctoral dissertation, Turku, Finland, Åbo Akademi University Press.

Fredriksson, L. (2003). Det vårdande samtalet. Doktorsavhandling, Turku, Finland, Åbo Akademis Förlag. [The caring conversation. Doctoral dissertation, Turku, Finland, Åbo Akademi University Press.

Hilli, Y. (2007). Hemmet som ethos. En idéhistorisk studie av hur hemmet som ethos blev evident i hälsosysterns vårdande under 1900-talets första hälft. Doktorsavhandling, Turku, Finland, Åbo Akademis Förlag. [The home as ethos. A history of ideas study of how the home as ethos became evident in public health nurses' caring during the first half of the 20th century. Doctoral dissertation, Turku, Finland, Åbo Akademi University Press.]

Karterud, D. (2006). Den etiske akten—Den caritative etikken når pasientens fordringer er av eksistensiell art. Doktorsavhandling, Turku, Finland, Åbo Akademis Förlag. [The ethical act—caring ethics when the patients' demands are existential. Doctoral dissertation, Turku, Finland, Åbo Akademi University Press.]

Kasén, A. (2002). Den vårdande relationen. Doktorsavhandling, Turku, Finland, Åbo Akademis Förlag. [The caring relationship. Doctoral dissertation, Turku, Finland, Åbo Akademi University Press.]

Kärkkäinen, O. (2005). Documentation of Patient Care as Evidence of Caring Substance. Doctoral dissertation, Vaasa, Finland: Department of Caring Science, Åbo Akademi University.

Lassenius, E. (2005). Rummet i vårdandets värld. Doktorsavhandling, Turku, Finland, Åbo Akademis Förlag. [The space in the world of caring. Doctoral dissertation, Turku, Finland, Åbo Akademi University Press.]

Lindholm, L. (1998). Den unga människans hälsa och lidande. Doktorsavhandling, Vaasa, Finland: Institutionen för vårdvetenskap, Åbo Akademi. [The young person's health and suffering. Doctoral dissertation, Vaasa, Finland: Department of Caring Science, Åbo Akademi University.]

Lindström, U. Å. (1992). De psykiatriska specialsjukskötarnas yrkesparadigm. Doktorsavhandling, Turku, Finland, Åbo Akademis Förlag. [The professional paradigm of the qualified psychiatric nurses. Doctoral dissertation, Turku, Finland, Åbo Akademi University Press.]

Lindwall, L. (2004). Kroppen som bärare av hälsa och lidande. Doktorsavhandling, Turku, Finland, Åbo Akademis Förlag. [The body as a carrier of health and suffering. Doctoral dissertation, Turku, Finland, Åbo Akademi University Press.]

Matilainen, D. (1997). Idémönster i Karin Neuman-Rahns livsgärning och författarskap—En idéhistorisk-biografisk studie i psykiatrisk vård i Finland under 1900-talets första hälft. Doktorsavhandling, Turku, Finland, Åbo Akademis Förlag. [Patterns of ideas in Karin Neuman-Rahns' life-work and writings—A study of psychiatric care in Finland in the former part of the twentieth century, based on biography and the history of ideas. Doctoral dissertation, Turku, Finland, Åbo Akademi University Press.]

Nilsson, B. (2004). Savnets tone i ensomhetens melodi. Ensomhet hos aleneboende personer med alvorlig psykisk lidelse. Doktorsavhandling, Turku, Finland, Åbo Akademis Förlag. [The tune of want in the loneliness melody. Doctoral dissertation, Turku, Finland, Åbo Akademi University Press.]

Nordman, T. (2006). Människan som patient i en vårdande kultur. Doktorsavhandling, Vaasa, Finland: Enheten för vårdvetenskap, Åbo Akademi. [A human being as a patient in a caring culture. Doctoral dissertation, Vaasa, Finland: Department of Caring Science, Åbo Akademi University.]

Nyback, M-H. (2008). Generic and professional caring in a Chinese setting—an ethnographic study. Doctoral dissertation, Turku, Finland, Åbo Akademi University Press.

Nåden, D. (1998). När sykepleie er kunstutøvelse. En undersøkelse av noen nødvendige forutsetninger for sykepleie som kunst. Doktorsavhandling, Vaasa, Finland: Institutionen för vårdvetenskap, Åbo Akademi. [When caring is an exercise of art. An examination of some necessary preconditions of nursing as an art. Doctoral dissertation, Vaasa, Finland: Department of Caring Science, Åbo Akademi University.]

Rehnsfeldt, A. (1999). Mötet med patienten i ett livsavgörande skede. Doktorsavhandling, Turku, Finland, Åbo Akademi. [The encounter with the patient in a life-changing process. Doctoral dissertation, Turku, Finland, Åbo Akademi University Press.]

Roxberg, Å. (2005). Vårdande och icke-vårdande tröst. Doktorsavhandling, Turku, Finland: Åbo Akademis Förlag. [Caring and non-caring consolation. Doctoral dissertation, Turku, Finland, Åbo Akademi University Press.]

Rudolfsson, G. (2007). Den perioperativa dialogen—en gemensam värld. Doktorsavhandling, Vaasa, Finland: Enheten för vårdvetenskap, Åbo Akademi. [The perioperative dialogue—a common world. Doctoral dissertation, Vaasa, Finland: Department of Caring Science, Åbo Akademi University.]

Rundqvist, E. (2004). Makt som fullmakt. Ett vårdvetenskapligt perspektiv. Doktorsavhandling, Turku, Finland, Åbo Akademis Förlag. [Power as authority. A caring science perspective. Doctoral dissertation, Turku, Finland, Åbo Akademi University Press.]

Råholm, M-B. (2003). I kampens och modets dialektik. Doktorsavhandling, Turku, Finland, Åbo Akademis Förlag. [In the dialectic of struggle and courage. Doctoral dissertation, Turku, Finland, Åbo Akademi University Press.]

Sæteren, B. (2006). Kampen for livet i vemodets slør. Å leve i spenningsfeltet mellom livets mulighet og dødens nødvendighet. Doktorsavhandling, Turku, Finland, Åbo Akademis Förlag. [Struggling for life in the veil of pensiveness. A life between the pressure created by the possibility of life and the necessity of death. Doctoral dissertation, Turku, Finland, Åbo Akademi University Press.]

Sivonen, K. (2000). Vården och det andliga. En bestämning av begreppet 'andlig' ur ett vårdvetenskapligt perspektiv. Doktorsavhandling, Turku, Finland, Åbo Akademis Förlag. [Features of spirituality in caring. Doctoral dissertation, Turku, Finland, Åbo Akademi University Press.]

Söderlund, M. (2004). Som drabbad av en orkan. Anhörigas tillvaro när en närstående drabbas av demens. Doktorsavhandling, Turku, Finland, Åbo Akademis Förlag. [As if struck by a hurricane: The situation of the relatives of someone suffering from dementia. Doctoral dissertation, Turku, Finland, Åbo Akademi University Press.]

von Post, I. (1999). Professionell naturlig vård ur anestesoch operationssjuksköterskors perspektiv. Doktorsavhandling, Turku, Finland, Åbo Akademis Förlag. [Professional natural care from the perspective of nurse anesthetists and operating room nurses. Doctoral dissertation, Turku, Finland, Åbo Akademi University Press.]

Wiklund, L. (2000). Lidandet som kamp och drama. Doktorsavhandling, Turku, Finland, Åbo Akademis Förlag. [Suffering as struggle and as drama. Doctoral dissertation, Turku, Finland, Åbo Akademi University Press.]

Wärnå, C. (2002). Dygd och hälsa. Doktorsavhandling, Turku, Finland, Åbo Akademis Förlag. [Virtue and health. Doctoral dissertation, Turku, Finland, Åbo Akademi University Press.]

UNIT

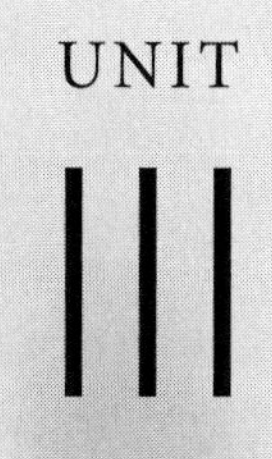

Nursing Models

- *Nursing conceptual models are concepts and their relationships that specify a perspective from which to view phenomena specific to the discipline of nursing.*
- *Different conceptual models provide various perspectives or frameworks for thinking critically and making nursing decisions.*
- *Conceptual models address the broad metaparadigm concepts that are central to their meaning in the context of the particular framework and the discipline of nursing.*

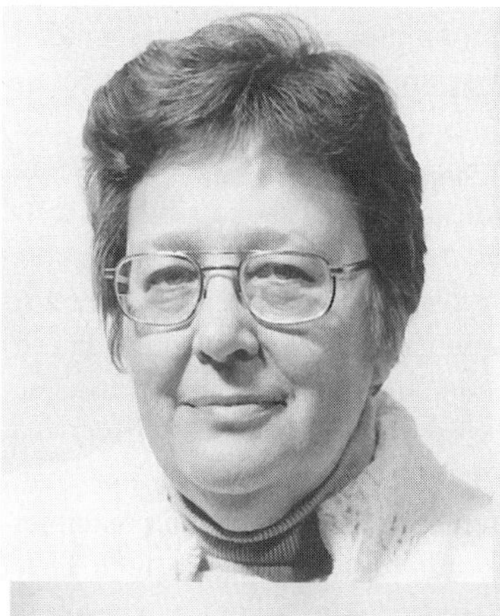

CHAPTER 12

Myra Estrin Levine

1921-1996

The Conservation Model

Karen Moore Schaefer

"Nursing is human interaction" (Levine, 1973, p. 1).

CREDENTIALS AND BACKGROUND OF THE THEORIST*

Levine's mentor during her graduate studies at Wayne State directed her attention to many of the authors who greatly influenced Levine's thinking (1988a).

Levine enjoyed a varied career. She was a private duty nurse (1944), a civilian nurse in the U.S. Army (1945), a preclinical instructor in the physical sciences at Cook County (1947 to 1950), the director of nursing at Drexel Home in Chicago (1950 to 1951), and a surgical supervisor at both the University of Chicago Clinics (1951 to 1952) and Henry Ford Hospital in Detroit (1956 to 1962). Levine worked her way up the academic ranks at Bryan Memorial Hospital in Lincoln, Nebraska (1951), Cook County School of Nursing (1963 to 1967), Loyola University (1967 to 1973), Rush University (1974 to 1977), and the University of Illinois (1962 to 1963, 1977 to 1987). She chaired the Department of Clinical Nursing at Cook County School of Nursing (1963 to 1967) and coordinated the graduate nursing program in oncology at Rush University (1974 to 1977). Levine was the director of the Department of Continuing Education at Evanston Hospital (March to June 1974) and a consultant to the department (July 1974 to 1976). She was an adjunct associate professor of Humanistic Studies at the University of

*The information in this section is informed by Levine's autobiographical chapter (1988a), her curriculum vitae, and the program from the Mid-Year Convocation, Loyola University, Chicago (1992). Previous authors: Karen Moore Schaefer, Gloria S. Artigue, Karen J. Foil, Tamara Johnson, Ann Marriner Tomey, Mary Carolyn Poat, LaDema Poppa, Roberta Woeste, and Susan T. Zoretich.

Illinois (1981 to 1987). In 1987, she became a Professor Emerita, Medical Surgical Nursing, at the University of Illinois at Chicago. In 1974, Levine went to Tel-Aviv University, Israel, as a visiting associate professor and returned as a visiting professor in 1982. She also was a visiting professor at Recanati School of Nursing, Ben Gurion University of the Negev, at Beer Sheva, Israel (March to April, 1982).

Levine received numerous honors, including charter fellow of the American Academy of Nursing (1973), honorary member of the American Mental Health Aid to Israel (1976), and honorary recognition from the Illinois Nurses Association (1977). She was the first recipient of the Elizabeth Russell Belford Award for excellence in teaching from Sigma Theta Tau (1977). Both the first and second editions of her book, *Introduction to Clinical Nursing* (Levine, 1969a; 1973), received *American Journal of Nursing* Book of the Year awards, and her book, *Renewal for Nursing*, was translated into Hebrew (Levine, 1971a). Levine was listed in *Who's Who in American Women* (1977 to 1988) and in *Who's Who in American Nursing* (1987). She was elected fellow of the Institute of Medicine of Chicago (1987 to 1991). The Alpha Lambda Chapter of Sigma Theta Tau recognized Levine for her outstanding contributions to nursing in 1990. In January 1992, she was awarded an honorary doctorate of humane letters from Loyola University, Chicago (Mid-Year Convocation, Loyola University, 1992). Levine was an active leader in the American Nurses Association and the Illinois Nurses Association. After her retirement in 1987, she remained active in theory development and encouraged questions and research about her theory (Levine, 1996).

A dynamic speaker, Levine was a frequent presenter of programs, workshops, seminars, and panels, and a prolific writer regarding nursing and education. She also served as a consultant to hospitals and schools of nursing. Although she never intended to develop theory, she provided an organizational structure for teaching medical-surgical nursing and a stimulus for theory development (Stafford, 1996). "The Four Conservation Principles of Nursing" was the first statement of the conservation principles (Levine, 1967a). Other preliminary work included "Adaptation and Assessment: A Rationale for Nursing Intervention," "For Lack of Love Alone," and "The Pursuit of Wholeness" (Levine, 1966b, 1967b, 1969b). The first edition of her book using the conservation principles, *Introduction to Clinical Nursing*, was published in 1969 (Levine, 1969a). Levine addressed the consequences of the four conservation principles in *Holistic Nursing* (Levine, 1971b). The second edition of *Introduction to Clinical Nursing* was published in 1973 (Levine, 1973). After that, Levine (1984) presented the conservation principles at nurse theory conferences, some of which have been audiotaped, and at the Allentown College of St. Francis de Sales (now DeSales University) Conference.

Levine (1989) published a substantial change and clarification about her theory in "The Four Conservation Principles: Twenty Years Later." She elaborated on how redundancy characterizes availability of adaptive responses when stability is threatened. Adaptation processes establish a body economy to safeguard the individual's stability. The outcome of adaptation is conservation.

She explicitly linked health to the process of conservation to clarify that the Conservation Model views health as one of its essential components (Levine, 1991). Conservation, through treatment, focuses on integrity and the reclamation of oneness of the whole person.

Levine died on March 20, 1996, at the age of 75. She leaves a legacy as an administrator, educator, friend, mother, nurse, scholar, student of humanities, and wife (Pond, 1996). Dr. Baumhart (Mid-Year Convocation, Loyola University, 1992), President of Loyola University, said the following of Levine:

> Mrs. Levine is a renaissance woman . . . who uses knowledge from several disciplines to expand the vision of health needs of persons that can be met by modern nursing. In the Talmudic tradition of her ancestors, [she] has been a forthright spokesperson for social justice and the inherent dignity of [the] human person as a child of God (p. 6).

THEORETICAL SOURCES

From Beland's (1971) presentation of the theory of specific causation and multiple factors, Levine learned historical viewpoints of diseases and learned that the way people think about disease changes over time. Beland directed Levine's attention to numerous authors who became influential in her thinking, including Goldstein (1963), Hall (1966), Sherrington (1906), and Dubos (1961, 1965). Levine uses Gibson's (1966) definition of perceptual systems, Erikson's (1964) differentiation between total and whole, Selye's (1956) stress theory, and Bates' (1967) models of external environment. Levine was proud that Rogers (1970) was her first editor. She acknowledged Nightingale's contribution to her thinking about the "guardian activity" of observation used by nurses to "save lives and increase health and comfort" (Levine, 1992, p. 42).

MAJOR CONCEPTS & DEFINITIONS

The three major concepts of the Conservation Model are (1) wholeness, (2) adaptation, and (3) conservation.

WHOLENESS (HOLISM)

"Whole, health, hale are all derivations of the Anglo-Saxon word *hal*" (Levine, 1973, p. 11). Levine based her use of wholeness on Erikson's (1964, 1968) description of wholeness as an open system. Levine (as cited in 1969a) quotes Erikson, who states, "Wholeness emphasizes a sound, organic, progressive mutuality between diversified functions and parts within an entirety, the boundaries of which are open and fluent" (p. 94). Levine (1996) believed that Erikson's definition set up the option of exploring the parts of the whole to understand the whole. *Integrity* means the oneness of the individuals, emphasizing that they respond in an integrated, singular fashion to environmental challenges.

ADAPTATION

"Adaptation is a process of change whereby the individual retains his integrity within the realities of his internal and external environment" (Levine, 1973, p. 11). Conservation is the outcome. Some adaptations are successful and some are not. Adaptation is a matter of degree, not an all-or-nothing process. There is no such thing as maladaptation.

Levine (1991) speaks of the following three characteristics of adaptation:

1. Historicity
2. Specificity
3. Redundancy

She states, "... every species has fixed patterns of responses uniquely designed to ensure success in essential life activities, demonstrating that adaptation is both historical and specific" (p. 5). In addition, adaptive patterns may be hidden in the individual's genetic code. Redundancy represents the fail-safe options available to individuals to ensure adaptation. Loss of redundant choices through trauma, age, disease, or environmental conditions makes it difficult for the individual to maintain life. Levine (1991) suggests that "the possibility exists that aging itself is a consequence of failed redundancy of physiological and psychological processes" (p. 6).

ENVIRONMENT

Levine (1973) also views each individual as having his or her own environment, both internally and externally. Nurses can relate to the internal environment as the physiological and pathophysiological aspects of the patient. Levine uses Bates' (1967) definition of the

Continued

MAJOR CONCEPTS & DEFINITIONS—cont'd

external environment and suggests the following three levels:

1. Perceptual
2. Operational
3. Conceptual

These levels give dimension to the interactions between individuals and their environments. The perceptual level includes aspects of the world that individuals are able to intercept and interpret with their sense organs. The operational level contains things that affect individuals physically, although they cannot directly perceive them, things such as microorganisms. At the conceptual level, the environment is constructed from cultural patterns, characterized by a spiritual existence and mediated by the symbols of language, thought, and history (Levine, 1973).

ORGANISMIC RESPONSE

The capacity of the individual to adapt to his or her environmental condition is called the organismic response. It can be divided into the following four levels of integration:

1. Fight or flight
2. Inflammatory response
3. Response to stress
4. Perceptual awareness

Treatment focuses on the management of these responses to illness and disease (Levine, 1969a).

Fight or Flight

The most primitive response is the fight or flight syndrome. The individual perceives that he or she is threatened, whether or not a threat actually exists. Hospitalization, illness, and new experiences elicit a response. The individual responds by being on the alert to find more information and to ensure his or her safety and well-being (Levine, 1973).

Inflammatory Response

This defense mechanism protects the self from insult in a hostile environment. It is a way of healing. The response uses available energy to remove or keep out unwanted irritants and pathogens. It is limited in time because it drains the individual's energy reserves. Environmental control is important (Levine, 1973).

Response to Stress

Selye (1956) described the stress response syndrome to predictable, non–specifically induced organismic changes. The wear and tear of life is recorded on the tissues and reflects long-term hormonal responses to life experiences that cause structural change. It is characterized by irreversibility and influences the way patients respond to nursing care.

Perceptual Awareness

This response is based on the individual's perceptual awareness. It occurs only as the individual experiences the world around him or her. The individual uses this response to seek and maintain safety. It is information seeking (Levine, 1967a, 1969b).

Trophicognosis

Levine (1966a) recommended trophicognosis as an alternative to nursing diagnosis. It is a scientific method of reaching a nursing care judgment.

CONSERVATION

Conservation is from the Latin word *conservatio,* which means "to keep together" (Levine, 1973). "Conservation describes the way complex systems are able to continue to function even when severely challenged" (Levine, 1990, p. 192). Through conservation, individuals are able to confront obstacles, adapt accordingly, and maintain their

MAJOR CONCEPTS & DEFINITIONS—cont'd

uniqueness. "The goal of conservation is health and the strength to confront disability" as ". . . the rules of conservation and integrity hold" in all situations in which nursing is required (Levine, 1973, pp. 193-195). The primary focus of conservation is keeping together the wholeness of the individual. Although nursing interventions may deal with one particular conservation principle, nurses also must recognize the influence of the other conservation principles (Levine, 1990).

Levine's (1973) model stresses nursing interactions and interventions that are intended to promote adaptation and maintain wholeness. These interactions are based on the scientific background of the conservation principles. Conservation focuses on achieving a balance of energy supply and demand within the biological realities unique to the individual. Nursing care is based on scientific knowledge and nursing skills. There are four conservation principles.

CONSERVATION PRINCIPLES

The goals of the Conservation Model are achieved through interventions that attend to the conservation principles.

Conservation of Energy

The individual requires a balance of energy and a constant renewal of energy to maintain life activities. Processes such as healing and aging challenge that energy. This second law of thermodynamics applies to everything in the universe, including people.

Conservation of energy has long been used in nursing practice even with the most basic procedures. Nursing interventions "scaled to the individual's ability are dependent upon providing care that makes the least additional demand possible" (Levine, 1990, pp. 197-198).

Conservation of Structural Integrity

Healing is a process of restoring structural and functional integrity through conservation in defense of wholeness (Levine, 1991). The disabled are guided to a new level of adaptation (Levine, 1996). Nurses can limit the amount of tissue involved in disease by early recognition of functional changes and by nursing interventions.

Conservation of Personal Integrity

Self-worth and a sense of identity are important. The most vulnerable become patients. This begins with the erosion of privacy and the creation of anxiety. Nurses can show patients respect by calling them by name, respecting their wishes, valuing personal possessions, providing privacy during procedures, supporting their defenses, and teaching them. "The nurse's goal is always to impart knowledge and strength so that the individual can resume a private life—no longer a patient, no longer dependent" (Levine, 1990, p. 199). The sanctity of life is manifested in all people. "The conservation of personal integrity includes recognition of the holiness of each person" (Levine, 1996, p. 40).

Conservation of Social Integrity

Life gains meaning through social communities, and health is socially determined. Nurses fulfill professional roles, provide for family members, assist with religious needs, and use interpersonal relationships to conserve social integrity (Levine, 1967b, 1969a).

USE OF EMPIRICAL EVIDENCE

Levine (1973) believed that specific nursing activities could be deducted from scientific principles. The scientific theoretical sources have been well researched. She based much of her work on accepted science principles.

MAJOR ASSUMPTIONS

Introduction to Clinical Nursing is a text for beginning nursing students that uses the conservation principles as an organizing framework (Levine, 1969a, 1973). Although she didn't state them specifically as assumptions, Levine (1973) valued "a holistic approach to care of all people, well or sick" (p. 151). Her respect for the individuality of each person is noted in the following statements:

> Ultimately, decisions for nursing interventions must be based on the unique behavior of the individual patient. . . . Patient centered nursing care means individualized nursing care . . . and as such he requires a unique constellation of skills, techniques, and ideas designed specifically for him (1973, p. 6).

Schaefer (1996) identified the following statements as assumptions about the model:

- The person can be understood only in the context of his or her environment (Levine, 1973).
- "Every self-sustaining system monitors its own behavior by conserving the use of the resources required to define its unique identity" (Levine, 1991, p. 4).
- Human beings respond in a singular, yet integrated, fashion (Levine, 1971a).

Nursing

Levine (1973) stated the following about nursing:

> Nursing is a human interaction (p. 1).
>
> Professional nursing should be reserved for those few who can complete a graduate program as demanding as that expected of professionals in any other discipline . . . There will be very few professional nurses (Levine, 1965, p. 214).

Nursing practice is based on nursing's unique knowledge and the scientific knowledge of other disciplines adjunctive to nursing knowledge (Levine, 1988b), as follows:

> It is the nurse's task to bring a body of scientific principles, on which decisions depend, into the precise situation that she shares with the patient. Sensitive observation and the selection of relevant data form the basis for her assessment of his nursing requirements.
>
> The nurse participates actively in every patient's environment and much of what she does supports his adjustments as he struggles in the predicament of illness (Levine, 1966b, p. 2452).

The essence of Levine's theory is as follows:

> . . . when nursing intervention influences adaptation favorably, or toward renewed social well-being, then the nurse is acting in a therapeutic sense; when the response is unfavorable, the nurse provides supportive care (1966b, p. 2450).
>
> The goal of nursing is to promote adaptation and maintain wholeness (1971b, p. 258).

Person

Person is described as a holistic being; wholeness is integrity (Levine, 1991). Integrity means that the person has freedom of choice and movement. The person has a sense of identity and self-worth. Levine also described person as a "system of systems, and in its wholeness expresses the organization of all the contributing parts" (pp. 8-9). Persons experience life as change through adaptation with the goal of conservation. According to Levine (1989), "The life process is the process of change" (p. 326).

Health

Health is socially determined by the ability to function in a reasonably normal manner (Levine, 1969b). Social groups predetermine health. Health is not just an absence of pathological conditions. Health is the return to self; individuals are free and able to pursue their own interests within the context of their own resources. Levine stressed the following:

> It is important to keep in mind that health is also culturally determined—it is not an entity on its own, but rather a definition imparted by the ethos and beliefs of the groups to which individuals belong (M. Levine, personal communication, February 21, 1995).

Even for a single individual, the definition of health will change over time.

Environment

Environment is conceptualized as the context in which individuals live their lives. It is not a passive backdrop. "The individual actively participates in his environment" (Levine, 1973, p. 443). Levine discussed the importance of the internal and external environment to the determinant of nursing interventions to promote adaptation. "All adaptations represent the accommodation that is possible between the internal and external environment" (p. 12).

THEORETICAL ASSERTIONS

Although many theoretical assertions can be generated from Levine's work, the four major assertions follow:

1. "Nursing intervention is based on the conservation of the individual patient's energy" (Levine, 1967a, p. 49).
2. "Nursing intervention is based on the conservation of the individual patient's structural integrity" (Levine, 1967a, p. 56).
3. "Nursing intervention is based on the conservation of the individual patient's personal integrity" (Levine, 1967a, p. 56).
4. "Nursing intervention is based on the conservation of the individual patient's social integrity" (Levine, 1967b, p. 57).

Levine (1991) provided some thoughts about two theories in their early stages of development. The theory of therapeutic intention is intended to provide the basis of nursing interventions that focus on biological realities of the patient. Although not planned as such, the theory naturally flows from the conservation principles. The theory of redundancy expands the redundancy domain of adaptation and offers explanations for redundant options such as those found in aging and the physiological adaptation of a failing heart.

LOGICAL FORM

Levine primarily uses deductive logic. In developing her model, Levine integrates theories and concepts from the humanities and the sciences of nursing, physiology, psychology, and sociology. She uses the information to analyze nursing practice situations and describe nursing skills and activities. With the assistance of many of her students and colleagues, and through her own personal health encounters, Levine has experienced the Conservation Model and its principles operating in practice.

APPLICATIONS TO THE NURSING COMMUNITY

Practice

Levine helps define what nursing is by identifying the activities it encompasses and giving the scientific principles behind them. Conservation principles as a framework are not limited to nursing care in the hospital but can be generalized and used in every environment, hospital, or community (Levine, 1990, 1991). Conservation principles, levels of integration, and other concepts can be used in numerous contexts (Fawcett, 2000). Hirschfeld (1976) has used the principles of conservation in the care of the older adult. Savage and Culbert (1989) used the Conservation Model to establish a plan of care for infants. Dever (1991) based her care of children on the Conservation Model. Roberts, Fleming, and Yeates-Giese (1991) designed interventions for women in labor based on the Conservation Model. Mefford (2000) tested a theory of health promotion for preterm infants derived from Levine's Conservation Model of nursing and found a significant inverse relationship between the consistency of the caregiver and the age at which the infant achieved health, and an inverse relationship between the use of resources by preterm infants during the initial hospital stay and the consistency of caregivers. Cooper (1990) developed a framework for wound care focusing on structural integrity while integrating all the integrities. Leach (2007) published a white paper on use of the Conservation Model to guide wound care practices. Webb (1993) used the Conservation Model to provide care for patients undergoing cancer treatment. Roberts, Brittin, and deClifford (1995) and Roberts, Brittin, Cook, and deClifford (1994) used the Conservation Model to study the boomerang pillow technique effect on respiratory capacity. Taylor (1974) used it to measure the outcomes of nursing care and again in her textbook, *Neurological Dysfunction and Nursing Interventions* (Taylor & Ballenger, 1980). Jost (2000) used the model to develop an assessment of the needs of staff during the experience of change.

Conservation principles have been used as a framework for numerous practice settings in cardiology, obstetrics, gerontology, acute care (neurology), pediatrics, long-term care, emergency care, primary care, neonatology, critical care, and in the homeless community (Savage & Culbert, 1989; Schaefer & Pond, 1991).

Education

Levine (1973) wrote *Introduction to Clinical Nursing* as a textbook for beginning students. It introduced new material into the curricula. She presented an early discussion of death and dying and believed that women should be awakened after a breast biopsy and consulted about the next step.

Introduction to Clinical Nursing provides an organizational structure for teaching medical-surgical nursing to beginning students (Levine, 1969a, 1973). In both the 1969 and 1973 editions, Levine presents a model at the end of each of the first nine chapters. Each model contains objectives, essential science concepts, and nursing process to give nurses a foundation for nursing activities. These models are not part of the Conservation Model. The Conservation Model is addressed in the Introduction and in Chapter 10 of the introductory text. The teachers' manual that accompanies the text remains a timely source of educational principles that may be helpful to both beginning teachers and seasoned teachers (Levine, 1971c).

Critics argue that although the text is labeled introductory, a beginning student would need a fairly extensive background in physical and social sciences to use it (*Canadian Nurse*, 1970). A critic of the second edition suggests that the emphasis of scientific principles is a definite strength, but the text's weakness is that it does not present adequate examples of pathological profiles when disturbances are discussed (*Canadian Nurse*, 1974). For this reason, this one reviewer recommends that the text be used as a supplementary or complementary text, not as a primary text.

Hall (1979) indicates that Levine's model is used as a curriculum model. The model has been integrated successfully into undergraduate and graduate curricula (Grindley & Paradowski, 1991; Schaefer, 1991a).

Research

Fitzpatrick and Whall (1983) state, "All in all, Levine's model served as an excellent beginning. Its contribution has added a great deal to the overall development of nursing knowledge" (p. 115). However, Fawcett (1995) states that to establish credibility, "more systematic evaluations of the use of the model in various clinical situations are needed, as are studies that test conceptual-theoretical-empirical structures directly derived from or linked with the conservation principles" (p. 208). Many research questions can be generated from Levine's model (Radwin & Fawcett, 2002; Schaefer, 1991b). Graduate students and clinical researchers have used the conservation principles as a framework for their research (Ballard, Robley, Barrett, et al., 2006; Cox, 1988; Gagner-Tjellesen, Yurkovich, & Gragert, 2001; Mefford, 2000; Moch, St. Ours, Hall, et al., 2007; Nagley, 1984). Ballard and colleagues used the model to frame their phenomenological study of how participants reconstructed their lives with paraplegia. They found that structural integrity, along with all the other integrities, was used as a basis for defining their new lives.

One of the most important questions to be asked about the model is: What are the human experiences not explained by the model? This question can provide guidance for continued testing of the model's application in nursing practice. For example, as healthcare providers use information from the human genome project, nurse researchers will want to test the ability of the model to explain comprehensive nursing care of the client undergoing genetic counseling. Based on the outcome of testing, hypotheses can be developed and tested to support the prescriptive basis of theories developed from the model.

FURTHER DEVELOPMENT

Levine and others have worked on using the conservation principles as the basis for a nursing diagnosis taxonomy (Stafford, 1996; Taylor, 1989). Additional work has been done on use of Levine's model in administration and with the frail elderly. The model was used to develop a theory of health promotion in preterm infants (Mefford, 2000) and has great potential for studies of sleep disorders and in the development of collaborative and primary care practices as well (Fawcett, 2000). The philosophical, ethical, and spiritual implications of the model are research challenges yet to be realized (Stafford, 1996).

CRITIQUE

Clarity

Levine's model possesses clarity. Fawcett (2000) states, "... Levine's Conservation Model provides nursing with a logically congruent, holistic view of the person" (p. 189). George (2002) affirms, "this theory directs nursing actions that lead to favorable outcomes" (p. 237). The model has numerous terms; however, Levine adequately defines them for clarity.

Simplicity

Although the four conservation principles appear simple initially, they contain subconcepts and multiple variables. Nevertheless, this model is still one of the simpler ones developed.

Generality

The four conservation principles can be used in all nursing contexts.

Empirical Precision

Levine used deductive logic to develop her model, which can be used to generate research questions. As she lived her Conservation Model, she verified the use of inductive reasoning to further develop and inform her model (M. Levine, personal communication, May 17, 1989).

Derivable Consequences

Although some authors question the level of contribution Levine's model provides, the four conservation principles are recognized as one of the earliest nursing models. Furthermore, the model has continued to have utility for nursing practice and research and is receiving increased recognition in this twenty-first century.

SUMMARY

Levine developed her Conservation Model to provide a framework within which to teach beginning nursing students. In the first chapter of her book, she introduced her assumptions about holism, and that the conservation principles support a holistic approach to patient care (Levine, 1969a, 1973). The model is logically congruent, is externally and internally consistent, has breadth as well as depth, and is understood, with few exceptions, by professionals and consumers of health care. Nurses using the Conservation Model can anticipate, explain, predict, and perform patient care. However, its ability to predict outcomes must be tested further. Levine (1990) said, "... everywhere that nursing is essential, the rules of the conservation and the integrity hold" (p. 195).

Case Study*

Yolanda is a 55-year-old married African-American mother of two adult children who has a history of breast cancer. She was diagnosed with fibromyalgia 2 years ago, following years of unexplained muscle aches and what she thought was arthritis. The diagnosis was a relief for her; she was able to read about it and learn how to care for herself. Over the past 2 months, Yolanda stopped taking all of her medicine, because she was seeing a new physician and wanted to start her care at ground zero. In addition to her family responsibilities, she is completing her degree as an English major. At the time of her appointment, she told the nurse practitioner that she was having the worst pain possible.

Using Levine's Conservation Model, the nurse practitioner completed a comprehensive assessment in preparation for developing a plan of care in consultation with the physician. Nursing care is organized according to the conservation principles, with consideration of how the individual adapts to the internal and external environments. Yolanda's diagnosis of fibromyalgia was based on the exclusion of other illnesses with a cluster of symptoms, including pain, fatigue, and sleeplessness (e.g., systemic lupus erythematosus, multiple sclerosis). Laboratory and other diagnostic results all were within normal limits.

The external environment includes perceptual, operational, and conceptual factors. Perceptual factors are those that are perceived through the senses. Yolanda reported a history of unexplained fatigue and pain for years. She recently stopped her medications "to clean my body out." However, she reported that the pain became unbearable and was making it difficult for her to sleep. She noted that when she sleeps at least 6 hours a night, her pain is less intense. With the current insomnia, her pain is very intense.

Operational factors are threats to the environment that the client cannot perceive through the senses. Yolanda reported severe pain in response to both the cold weather and changes in barometric pressure.

The conceptual environment includes cultural and personal values about health care, the meaning of health and illness, knowledge about health care, education, language use, and spiritual beliefs. In response to breast cancer, Yolanda developed her spirituality through prayer and reading the Bible. She believes that this is how she gets through the painful moments of her current illness.

Conservation of energy focuses on the balance of energy input and output to prevent excessive fatigue. Yolanda complains of a fatigue that just "comes over me." She has difficulty doing housework. One day of work usually means one day in bed because of extreme fatigue. Her hemoglobin level and hematocrit are normal; her arterial blood gas results have always been within normal limits. Most diagnostic study values are within normal limits in patients with fibromyalgia, making treatment difficult.

Conservation of structural integrity involves maintaining the structure of the body to promote healing. Because there is no known cause of fibromyalgia, treatment focuses on reducing symptoms. Yolanda's

*This case study is based on raw data from a study in process titled "Fibromyalgia in African American Women: A Phenomenological Investigation," Philadelphia. *Yolanda* is a fictitious name used to protect the privacy and anonymity of the participant.

symptoms could not be traced to any physical or structural alteration, yet she reports severe pain and fatigue. The nurse practitioner knows that it is important to acknowledge the reality of the symptoms and work with the client to determine if activities of daily living result in changes in the pattern of illness. In addition, Yolanda thinks she is going through menopause, and she is having trouble determining if her symptoms are caused by menopause or fibromyalgia.

With continued questioning, the nurse practitioner learns that Yolanda was diagnosed with irritable bowel syndrome several years earlier. She is not worried about constipation but is concerned about sudden diarrhea. She is afraid to go to school; she fears embarrassment because she might have an "accident." Yolanda was taking several medications for her discomfort. One of them made her feel so "hung over" that she stopped taking it after 2 weeks. She was given amitriptyline (Elavil) for sleep. It was the only medicine that helped her get 6 hours of continuous sleep.

Personal integrity involves the maintenance of one's sense of personal worth and self-esteem. Yolanda reported that she lost control when she was diagnosed with breast cancer. A dear friend convinced her to go to church and encouraged her to use prayer. When feeling sorry for herself, she would go into her bedroom and read her Bible, cry by herself, and pray. She believes that prayer and Bible reading helped her heal. She continues to pray and read her Bible to gain the strength she needs to live with her current illness. She also believes that she needs to be able to laugh at herself; humor helps her to feel better. She actively seeks health information, as indicated by her quest to learn about her new diagnosis of fibromyalgia. She is most upset about not being able to walk like she used to walk. One of her favorite pastimes was shopping for shoes at the mall, which now is difficult for her.

Social integrity acknowledges that the patient is a social being. Yolanda is a married mother of three grown children. She keeps a lot of her feelings from her children but does share them with her husband. He is a major source of support for her. He takes her food shopping and makes sure that she gets to her appointments on time. She shared at the time of her visit that she wants to have a picnic for her birthday, but the only way she can do it is to ask her grandchildren to help her husband clean the yard.

Yolanda is a middle-aged woman with a history of severe pain, sleeplessness, and fatigue. Diagnostic studies have been unrevealing, with the exception of multiple tender points. The history of pain and positive tender points supported the diagnosis of fibromyalgia. She has stopped taking all medications and reports that she may be going through menopause. She reports severe pain and fatigue that make it difficult for her to sleep and to do normal housework. Her husband and grandchildren are available to help with chores at home, and she seeks the support of prayer and reading her Bible to ease her discomfort. She also finds that humor helps her to feel better.

The initial plan of care includes (1) validate the illness experience, (2) encourage continued use of prayer, Bible reading, and humor to help her feel better, (3) discuss medication therapy and what might help her achieve restful sleep, (4) refer her for blood work to assess hormone levels, and (5) assist her with determining the meaning of the symptoms (e.g., menopause or fibromyalgia). Yolanda indicated that when she was able to get 6 hours of uninterrupted sleep, her pain was less intense and she felt better. Finding both medication-induced and nonpharmaceutical approaches to improve sleep is a high priority.

The nurse practitioner will assess the outcome of Yolanda's care based on the organismic responses. The following predicted responses suggest adaptation:

- Reports comfort as a result of prayer, Bible reading, and humor
- Distinguishes symptoms of menopause from symptoms of fibromyalgia
- Reports feeling rested after 6 hours of uninterrupted sleep
- Reports a perceived reduction in pain and fatigue
- Collaborates with healthcare providers to manage symptoms of menopause

CRITICAL THINKING Activities

1. Keep a reflective journal about a personal health or illness experience or that of someone very close. Reflect on its consistency with the Conservation Model—how to modify, expand, or delimit to provide a context for explanation.
2. Levine stated, "Health is culturally determined; it is not an entity on its own, but rather a definition imparted by the ethos and beliefs of groups to which the individual belongs" (M. Levine, personal communication, February, 21, 1995).

   Visit a museum and evaluate how artistic expression captures the beliefs of different ethnic groups, and explore how these beliefs shape definitions of health and illness. On the basis of an ethnically derived definition of health, propose ethnically appropriate interventions using Levine's conservation principles.
3. Watch one of the following movies: *City of Joy, Soul Food*, or *The Secret Garden.* Use examples from the movie to support or refute Levine's propositional statements.
4. Apply the Conservation Model to a pathography, such as *Love and Other Infectious Diseases* by Molly Haskell, and explain life with illness. Identify what is unexplained, and suggest how the model might be developed to better encompass the experience.

POINTS FOR Further Study

- Karen Schaefer's chapter, "Levine's Conservation Nursing Model in Nursing Practice" (#10) in a companion Elsevier text, Alligood (2010). *Nursing theory: Utilization & application,* 4th edition.
- Cardinal Stitch University Library; Nursing Theorist: Myra Levine. Accessed September 17, 2007 at: http://library.stitch.edu/research/subjects/nursingtheorists/levine.htm
- Hahn School of Nursing and Health Science, University of San Diego. Accessed December 20, 2004 at: http://www.sandiego.edu/nursing/theory/
- Nursing for Nurses—Levine Conservation Model (Blog). Accessed September 16, 2007 at: http://allnurses.com/forums/f76/levine-conservation-model-48040-print.html
- Mayo Clinic—Nursing Theorist—Myra Levine. Accessed September 17, 2007 at: http://www.mayo.edu/education/nursing-research/levine.html
- *The nursing theorist: Portraits of excellence.* Myra Levine (video, CD, or electronically), by Oakland: Studio III, Oakland, CA. Now available at Fitne, Inc., 5 Depot Street, Athens, Ohio 45701
- Leach, M. J. Using Levine's conservation model to guide practice (white paper). Accessed September 17, 2007 at: http://www.o-m.com/article/6024

REFERENCES

Ballard, N., Robley, L., Barrett, D., Fraser, D., & Mendoza, I. (2006). Patients' recollections of therapeutic paralysis in the intensive care unit. *American Journal of Critical Care, 15*(1), 86-94.

Bates, M. (1967). A naturalist at large. *Natural History, 76*(6), 8-16.

Beland, I. (1971). *Clinical nursing: Pathophysiological and psychosocial implications* (2nd ed.). New York: Macmillan.

Cooper, D. H. (1990). Optimizing wound healing: A practice within nursing domains. *Nursing Clinics of North America, 25*(1), 165-180.

Cox, B. (1988). Pregnancy, anxiety, and time perception (Doctoral dissertation University of Illinois at Chicago, Health Science Center, 1988). *Dissertation Abstracts International, 48,* 2260B. (University Microfilms No. AA18724993)

Dever, M. (1991). Care of children. In K. M. Schaefer & J. B. Pond (Eds.), *The Conservation Model: A framework for nursing practice* (pp. 71-82). Philadelphia: F. A. Davis.

Dubos, R. (1961). *Mirage of health.* Garden City, NY: Doubleday.

Dubos, R. (1965). *Man adapting.* New Haven, CT: Yale University Press.

Erikson, E. H. (1964). *Insight and responsibility.* New York: W. W. Norton.

Erikson, E. H. (1968). *Identity: Youth and crisis.* New York: W. W. Norton.

Fawcett, J. (1995). Levine's Conservation Model. In J. Fawcett (Ed.), *Analysis and evaluation of conceptual models of nursing* (pp. 165-215). Philadelphia: F. A. Davis.

Fawcett J. (2000). Levine's Conservation Model. In J. Fawcett (Ed.), *Analysis and evaluation of contemporary nursing knowledge: Nursing models and theories* (pp. 151-193). Philadelphia: F. A. Davis.

Fitzpatrick, J. J., & Whall, A. L. (1983). *Conceptual models of nursing: Analysis and application.* Bowie, MD: Robert J. Brady.

Gagner-Tjellesen, D., Yurkovich, E. E., & Gragert, M. (2001). Use of music therapy and other ITNIs in acute care. *Journal of Psychosocial Nursing and Mental Health Services, 39*(10), 26-37.

George, J. B. (2002). The Conservation Principles: A model for health. In J. George (Ed.) *Nursing theories: The base for professional nursing practice* (225-240). Upper Saddle River, NJ: Prentice Hall.

Gibson, J. E. (1966). *The senses considered as perceptual systems.* Boston: Houghton Mifflin.

Goldstein, K. (1963). *The organism.* Boston: Beacon Press.

Grindley, J., & Paradowski, M. B. (1991). Developing an undergraduate program using Levine's model. In K. M. Schaefer & J. B. Pond (Eds.), *Levine's Conservation Model: A framework for nursing practice* (pp. 199-208). Philadelphia: F. A. Davis.

Hall, E. T. (1966). *The hidden dimension.* Garden City, NY: Doubleday.

Hall, K. V. (1979). Current trends in the use of conceptual frameworks in nursing education. *Journal of Nursing Education, 18*(4), 26-29.

Hirschfeld, M. J. (1976). The cognitively impaired older adult. *American Journal of Nursing, 76,* 1981-1984.

Jost, S. G. (2000). An assessment and intervention strategy for managing. *Journal of Nursing Administration, 30*(1), 34-40.

Leach, M. J. Using Levine's Conservation Model to Guide Practice (white paper). Accessed September 17, 2007. http://www.o-m.com/article/6024.

Levine, M. E. (1965, June). The professional nurse and graduate education. *Nursing Science, 3,* 206.

Levine, M. E. (1966a). Trophicognosis: An alternative to nursing diagnosis. *American Nurses Association Regional Clinical Conferences, 2,* 55-70.

Levine, M. E. (1966b). Adaptation and assessment: A rationale for nursing intervention. *American Journal of Nursing, 66,* 2450-2454.

Levine, M. E. (1967a). The four conservation principles of nursing. *Nursing Forum, 6,* 45-59.

Levine, M. E. (1967b, Dec.). For lack of love alone. *Minnesota Nursing Accent, 39,* 179.

Levine, M. E. (1969a). *Introduction to clinical nursing.* Philadelphia: F. A. Davis.

Levine, M. E. (1969b). The pursuit of wholeness, *American Journal of Nursing, 69,* 93.

Levine, M. E. (1971a). *Renewal for nursing.* Philadelphia: F. A. Davis.

Levine, M. E. (1971b). Holistic nursing. *Nursing Clinics of North America, 6,* 253-263.

Levine, M. E. (1971c). Instructor's guide to introduction to clinical nursing. Philadelphia: F. A. Davis.

Levine, M. E. (1973). *Introduction to clinical nursing* (2nd ed.). Philadelphia: F. A. Davis.

Levine, M. E. (1984, April). *A conceptual model for nursing: The four conservation principles.* Proceedings from Allentown College of St. Francis Conference, Philadelphia.

Levine, M. E. (1988a). Myra Levine. In T. M. Schoor & A. Zimmerman (Eds.), *Making choices, taking chances: Nurse leaders tell their stories* (pp. 215-228). St. Louis: C. V. Mosby.

Levine, M. E. (1988b). Antecedents from adjunctive disciplines: Creation of nursing theory. *Nursing Science Quarterly, 1*(1), 16-21.

Levine, M. E. (1989). The four conservation principles: Twenty years later. In J. Riehl (Ed.), *Conceptual models for nursing practice* (3rd ed., pp. 325-337). New York: Appleton-Century-Crofts.

Levine, M. E. (1990). Conservation and integrity. In M. Parker (Ed.), *Nursing theories in practice* (pp. 189-201). New York: National League for Nursing.

Levine, M. E. (1991). The conservation principles: A model for health. In K. Schaefer & J. Pond (Eds.), *Levine's Conservation Model: A framework for nursing practice* (pp. 1-11). Philadelphia: F. A. Davis.

Levine, M. E. (1992). Nightingale redux. In B. S. Barnum (Ed.), *Nightingale's notes on nursing* (pp. 39-43). Philadelphia: J. B. Lippincott.

Levine, M. E. (1996). The conservation principles: A retrospective. *Nursing Science Quarterly, 9*(1), 38-41.

Mefford, L. C. (2000). *The relationships of nursing care to health outcomes of preterm infants: Testing a theory of health promotion for preterm infants based on Levine's Conservation Model.* Unpublished doctoral dissertation, University of Tennessee, Knoxville.

Mid-Year Convocation: Loyola University, Chicago. (1992). The Conferring of Honorary Degrees by R. C. Baumhart, Candidate for the degree of Doctor and Humane Letters, p. 6.

Moch, V., St. Ours, C., Hall, S., Bositis, A., Tillery, M., Belcher, A., Krumm, S., & McCorkle, R. (2007). Using a conceptual model in nursing research-mitigating fatigue in cancer patients. Journal *of Advanced Nursing, 58*(5), 503-512.

Nagley, S. J. (1984). Prevention of confusion in hospitalized elderly persons (Doctoral dissertation). *Dissertation Abstracts International, 48,* 1732B. (University Microfilms No. AA18420848) Case Western Reserve University.

Pond, J. B. (1996). Myra Levine, nurse educator and scholar dies. *Nursing Spectrum, 5*(8), 8.

Radwin, L., & Fawcett, J. (2002). A conceptual model based programme of nursing research: Retrospective and prospective applications. *Journal of Advanced Nursing, 40*(3), 355-360.

[Review of the book *Introduction to clinical nursing*]. (1970, Jan.). *Canadian Nurse, 66*, 42.

[Review of the book *Introduction to clinical nursing* (2nd ed.)]. (1974, May). *Canadian Nurse, 70*, 39.

Roberts, J. E., Fleming, N., & Yeates-Giese, D. (1991). Perineal integrity. In K. M. Schaefer & J. B. Pond (Eds.), *The Conservation Model: A framework for nursing practice* (pp. 61-70). Philadelphia: F. A. Davis.

Roberts, K. L., Brittin, M., Cook, M., & deClifford, J. (1994). Boomerang pillows and respiratory capacity. *Clinical Nursing Research, 3*(2), 157-165.

Roberts, K. L., Brittin, M., & deClifford, J. (1995). Boomerang pillows and respiratory capacity in frail elderly women. *Clinical Nursing Research, 4*(4), 465-471.

Rogers, M. E. (1970). *An introduction to the theoretical basis of nursing.* Philadelphia: F. A. Davis.

Savage, T. A., & Culbert, C. (1989). Early intervention: The unique role of nursing. *Journal of Pediatric Nursing, 4*(5), 339-345.

Schaefer, K. M. (1991a). Developing a graduate program in nursing: Integrating Levine's philosophy. In K. M. Schaefer & J. B. Pond (Eds.), *Levine's Conservation Model: A framework for nursing practice* (pp. 209-218). Philadelphia: F. A. Davis.

Schaefer, K. M. (1991b). Levine's conservation principles and research. In K. M. Schaefer & J. B. Pond (Eds.), *Levine's Conservation Model: A framework for nursing practice* (pp. 45-60). Philadelphia: F. A. Davis.

Schaefer, K. M. (1996). Levine's Conservation Model: Caring for women with chronic illness. In P. H. Walker & B. Neuman (Eds.), *Blueprint for use of nursing models: Education, research, practice and administration.* New York: National League for Nursing.

Schaefer, K. M., & Pond, J. B. (Eds.) (1991). *Levine's Conservation Model: A framework for nursing practice.* Philadelphia: F. A. Davis.

Selye, H. (1956). *The stress of life.* New York: McGraw-Hill.

Sherrington, A. (1906). *Integrative function of the nervous system.* New York: Charles Scribner's Sons.

Stafford, M. J. (1996). In tribute: Myra Estrin Levine, Professor Emerita, MSN, RN, FAAN. *Chart, 93*(3), 5-6.

Taylor, J. W. (1974). Measuring the outcomes of nursing care. *Nursing Clinics of North America, 9*, 337-348.

Taylor, J. W. (1989). Levine's conservation principles: Using the model for nursing diagnosis in a neurological setting. In J. P. Riehl-Sisca (Ed.), *Conceptual models for nursing practice* (3rd ed., pp. 349-358). Norwalk, CT: Appleton & Lange.

Taylor, J. W., & Ballenger, S. (1980). *Neurological dysfunction and nursing interventions.* New York: McGraw-Hill.

Webb, H. (1993). Holistic care following a palliative Hartmann's procedure. *British Journal of Nursing, 2*(2), 128-132.

BIBLIOGRAPHY

Primary Sources

Books

Levine, M. E. (1969). *Introduction to clinical nursing.* Philadelphia: F. A. Davis.

Levine, M. E. (1971). *Renewal for nursing.* Philadelphia: F. A. Davis. [Translated into Hebrew, Am Oved, Jerusalem, 1978.]

Levine, M. E. (1973). *Introduction to clinical nursing* (2nd ed.). Philadelphia: F. A. Davis.

Book Chapters

Levine, M. E. (1964). Nursing service. In M. Leeds & H. Shore (Eds.), *Geriatric institutional management.* New York: G. P. Putnam's Sons.

Levine, M. E. (1973). Adaptation and assessment: A rationale for nursing intervention. In M. E. Hardy (Ed.), *Theoretical foundations for nursing.* New York: Irvington.

Levine, M. E. (1988). Myra Levine. In T. M. Schorr & A. Zimmerman (Eds.), *Making choices, taking chances: Nursing leaders tell their stories.* St. Louis: Mosby.

Levine, M. E. (1989). The four conservation principles: Twenty years later. In J. Riehl (Ed.), *Conceptual models for nursing practice* (3rd ed.). New York: Appleton-Century-Crofts.

Levine, M. E. (1990). Conservation and integrity. In M. Parker (Ed.), *Nursing theories in practice* (pp. 189-201). New York: National League for Nursing.

Levine, M. E. (1991). The conservation principles: A model for health. In K. Schaefer & J. Pond (Eds.), *Levine's Conservation Model: A framework for nursing practice* (pp. 1-11). Philadelphia: F. A. Davis.

Levine, M. E. (1992). Nightingale redux. In B. S. Barnum (Ed.), *Nightingale's notes on nursing: Commemorative edition with commentaries by nursing theorists.* Philadelphia: J. B. Lippincott.

Levine, M. E. (1994). Some further thoughts on nursing rhetoric. In J. F. Kikuchi & H. Simmons (Eds.), *Developing a philosophy of nursing* (pp. 104-109). Thousand Oaks, CA: Sage.

Journal Articles

Levine, M. E. (1963). Florence Nightingale: The legend that lives. *Nursing Forum, 2*(4), 24-35.

Levine, M. E. (1964, Feb.). Not to startle, though the way were steep. *Nursing Science, 2*, 58-67.

Levine, M. E. (1964, Dec.). There need be no anonymity. *First, 18*(9), 4.

Levine, M. E. (1965). The professional nurse and graduate education. *Nursing Science, 3*, 206-214.

Levine, M. E. (1965). Trophicognosis: An alternative to nursing diagnosis. *ANA Regional Clinical Conferences, 2*, 55-70.

Levine, M. E. (1966.). Adaptation and assessment: A rationale for nursing intervention. *American Journal of Nursing, 66*(11), 2450-2453.

Levine, M. E. (1967, Dec.). For lack of love alone. Minnesota Nursing *Accent, 39*(7), 179-202.
Levine, M. E. (1967). Medicine-nursing dialogue belongs at patient's bedside. *Chart, 64*(5), 136-137.
Levine, M. E. (1967). The four conservation principles of nursing. *Nursing Forum, 6*, 45-59.
Levine, M. E. (1967). This I believe: About patient-centered care. *Nursing Outlook, 15*, 53-55.
Levine, M. E. (1968, Feb.). Knock before entering personal space bubbles (part 1). *Chart, 65*(2), 58-62.
Levine, M. E. (1968, March). Knock before entering personal space bubbles (part 2). *Chart, 65*(3), 82-84.
Levine, M. E. (1968). The pharmacist in the clinical setting: A nurse's viewpoint. *American Journal of Hospital Pharmacy, 25*(4), 168-171. [Also translated into Japanese and published in *Kyushu National Hospital Magazine* for Western Japan.]
Levine, M. E. (1969, Feb.). Constructive student power. *Chart, 66*(2), 42FF.
Levine, M. E. (1969, Oct.). Small hospital—Big nursing. *Chart, 66*, 265-269.
Levine, M. E. (1969, Nov.). Small hospital—Big nursing. *Chart, 66*, 310-315.
Levine, M. E. (1969). The pursuit of wholeness. *American Journal of Nursing, 69*, 93-98.
Levine, M. E. (1970). Dilemma. *ANA Clinical Conferences*, 338-342.
Levine, M. E. (1970). Breaking through the medications mystique. *American Journal of Hospital Pharmacy, 27*(4), 294-299; *American Journal of Nursing, 70*(4), 799-803.
Levine, M. E. (1970, July/Dec.). Symposium on a drug compendium: View of a nursing educator. *Drug Information Bulletin*, 133-135.
Levine, M. E. (1970). The intransigent patient. *American Journal of Nursing, 70*, 2106-2111.
Levine, M. E. (1971). Consider implications for nursing in the use of physician's assistant. *Hospital Topics, 49*, 60-63.
Levine, M. E. (1971). Holistic nursing. *Nursing Clinics of North America, 6*, 253-264.
Levine, M. E. (1971). The time has come to speak of health care. *AORN Journal, 13*, 37-43.
Levine, M. E. (1972). Benoni. *American Journal of Nursing 72*, (3), 466-468.
Levine, M. E. (1972). Nursing educators—An alienating elite? *Chart, 69*(2), 56-61.
Levine, M. E. (1973). On creativity in nursing. *Image: The Journal of Nursing Scholarship, 3*(3), 15-19.
Levine, M. E. (1974). The pharmacist's clinical role in interdisciplinary care: A nurse's viewpoint. *Hospital Formulary Management, 9*, 47.
Levine, M. E. (1975). On creativity in nursing. *Nursing Digest, 3*, 38-40.
Levine, M. E. (1977). Nursing ethics and the ethical nurse. *American Journal of Nursing, 77*, 845-849.
Levine, M. E. (1978). Cancer chemotherapy: A nursing model. *Nursing Clinics of North America, 13*(2), 271-280.
Levine, M. E. (1978). Does continuing education improve nursing practice? *Hospitals, 52*(21), 138-140.
Levine, M. E. (1978). Kapklavoo and nursing, too (Editorial). *Research in Nursing and Health, 1*(2), 51.
Levine, M. E. (1979). Knowledge base required by generalized and specialized nursing practice. *ANA Publications, (G-127)*, 57-69.
Levine, M. E. (1980). The ethics of computer technology in health care. *Nursing Forum, 19*(2), 193-198.
Levine, M. E. (1982). Bioethics of cancer nursing. *Rehabilitation Nursing, 7*, 27-31, 41.
Levine, M. E. (1982). The bioethics of cancer nursing. *Journal of Enterostomal Therapy, 9*, 11-13.
Levine, M. E. (1988). Antecedents from adjunctive disciplines: Creation of nursing theory. *Nursing Science Quarterly, 1*(1), 16-21.
Levine, M. E. (1988, June). What does the future hold for nursing? 25th Anniversary Address, 18th District. *Illinois Nurses Association Newsletter, XXIV*(6), 1-4.
Levine, M. E. (1989). Beyond dilemma. *Seminars in Oncology Nursing, 5*, 124-128.
Levine, M. E. (1989). Ration or rescue: The elderly in critical care. *Critical Care Nursing, 12*(1), 82-89.
Levine, M. E. (1989). The ethics of nursing rhetoric. *Image: The Journal of Nursing Scholarship, 21*(1), 4-5.
Levine, M. E. (1995). The rhetoric of nursing theory. *Image: The Journal of Nursing Scholarship, 27*(1), 11-14.
Levine, M. E. (1996). On the humanities in nursing. *Canadian Journal of Nursing Research, 27*(2), 19-23.
Levine, M. E. (1996). The conservation principles: A retrospective. *Nursing Science Quarterly, 9*(1), 38-41.
Levine, M. E. (1997). On creativity in nursing. *Image: The Journal of Nursing Scholarship, 29*(3), 216-217.
Levine, M. E., Hallberg, C., Kathrein, M., & Cox, R. (1972). Nursing grand rounds: Congestive failure. *Nursing '72, 2*(10), 18-23.
Levine, M. E., Line, L., Boyle, A., & Kopacewski, E. (1972). Nursing grand rounds: Insulin reactions in a brittle diabetic. *Nursing '72, 2*(5), 6-11.
Levine, M. E., Moschel, P., Taylor, J., & Ferguson, G. (1972). Nursing grand rounds: Complicated case of CVA. *Nursing '72, 2*(3), 3-34.
Levine, M. E., Scanlon, M., Gregor, P., King, R., & Martin, N. (1972). Issues in rehabilitation: The quadriplegic adolescent. *Nursing '72, 2*, 6.
Levine, M. E., Zoellner, J., Ozmon, B., & Simunek, E. (1972). Nursing grand rounds: Severe trauma. *Nursing '72, 2*(9), 33-38.

Secondary Sources

Book Reviews

[Review of the book Introduction to clinical nursing]. (1969, Sept/Oct.). Bedside Nurse, 2, 4.

[Review of the book Introduction to clinical nursing]. (1970, Feb.). Nursing Outlook, 18, 20.

[Review of the book Introduction to clinical nursing]. (1970, Jan.). American Journal of Nursing, 70, 99.

[Review of the book Introduction to clinical nursing]. (1970, Jan.). Canadian Nurse, 66, 42.

[Review of the book Introduction to clinical nursing]. (1970, Oct.). American Journal of Nursing, 70, 2220.

[Review of the book Introduction to clinical nursing]. (1971, April). Nursing Mirror, 132, 43.

[Review of the book Introduction to clinical nursing], (1971, Dec.). Canadian Nurse, 76, 47.

[Review of the book Introduction to clinical nursing], (1971, Dec.). Nursing Mirror, 133, 16.

[Review of the book Introduction to clinical nursing], (1974, Feb.). American Journal of Nursing, 74, 347.

[Review of the book Introduction to clinical nursing]. (1974, May). Canadian Nurse, 70, 39.

[Review of the book Introduction to clinical nursing]. (1974, May). Nursing Outlook, 22, 301.

[Review of the book Introduction to clinical nursing]. (1971, Nov.). Bedside Nurse, 4, 2.

[Review of the book Renewal for nursing]. (1971, Aug.). Supervisor Nurse, 2, 68.

[Review of the book Renewal for nursing]. (1971, Dec.). AANA Journal, 49, 495.

[Review of the book Renewal for nursing]. (1971, Dec.). Canadian Nurse, 67, 47.

[Review of the book Renewal for nursing]. (1971, Dec.). Nursing Mirror, 133, 16.

Book Chapters

Leonard, M. K. (1990). Myra Estrin Levine. In J. B. George (Ed.), *Nursing theories: The base for professional nursing practice* (pp. 181-192). Englewood Cliffs, NJ: Prentice Hall.

MacLean, S. L. (1989). Activity intolerance: Cues for diagnosis. In R. M. Carroll-Johnson (Ed.), *Classification proceedings of the eighth annual conference of North American Nursing Diagnosis Association* (pp. 320-327). Philadelphia: J. B. Lippincott.

McLane, A. (1987). Taxonomy and nursing diagnosis, a critical view. In A. McLane (Ed.), *Classification proceedings of the seventh annual conference of Nursing of North America.* St. Louis: Mosby.

Meleis, A. I. (1985). Myra Levine. In A. I. Meleis (Ed.), *Theoretical nursing: Development and progress* (pp. 275-283). Philadelphia: J. B. Lippincott.

Peiper, B. A. (1983). Levine's nursing model. In J. J. Fitzpatrick & A. L. Whall (Eds.), *Conceptual models of nursing: Analysis and application* (pp. 101-115). Bowie, MD: Robert J. Brady.

Pond, J. B. (1990). Application of Levine's Conservation Model to nursing the homeless community. In M. E. Parker (Ed.), *Nursing theories in practice* (pp. 203-215). New York: National League for Nursing.

Schaefer, K. M. (1990). A description of fatigue associated with congestive heart failure: Use of Levine's Conservation Model. In M. E. Parker (Ed.), *Nursing theories in practice* (pp. 217-237). New York: National League for Nursing.

Schaefer, K. M. (1996). Levine's Conservation Model: Caring for women with chronic illness. In P. H. Walker & B. Neuman (Eds.), *Blueprint for use of nursing models: Education, research, practice and administration* (pp. 187-228). New York: National League for Nursing Press.

Schaefer, K. M. (2001). Levine's Conservation Model: A model for the future of nursing. In Parker, M. E. (Ed.), *Nursing theories and nursing practice* (pp. 103-124). Philadelphia: F. A. Davis.

Schaefer, K. M. (2001). Levine's Conservation Model: Use of the model in nursing practice. In M. R. Alligood & A. Marriner-Tomey (Eds.), *Nursing theory: Utilization & application* (pp. 89-108; Taiwanese ed.). St. Louis: Mosby.

Schaefer, K. M. (2002). Levine's Conservation Model in nursing practice. In M. R. Alligood & A. M. Tomey (Eds.), *Nursing theory: Utilization & application* (2nd ed., pp. 197-217). St. Louis: Mosby.

Taylor, J. W. (1989). Levine's conservation principles: Using the model for nursing diagnosis in a neurological setting. In J. P. Riehl-Sisca (Ed.), *Conceptual models for nursing practice* (3rd ed., pp. 349-358). Norwalk, CT: Appleton & Lange.

Books

Barnum, B. J. S. (1994). *Nursing theory: Analysis application evaluation* (4th ed.). Philadelphia: J. B. Lippincott.

Chinn, P. L., & Kramer, M. K. (1995). *Theory and nursing: A systematic approach* (4th ed.). St. Louis: Mosby.

Clark, M. J. (1992). *Nursing in the community.* Norwalk, CT: Appleton & Lange.

Griffith-Kenney, J. W., & Christensen, P. (1986). *Nursing process: Application of theories, frameworks, and models* (pp. 6, 24-25), St. Louis: Mosby.

Rogers, M. E. (1970). An introduction to the theoretical basis of nursing. Philadelphia: F. A. Davis.

Journal Articles

Ballard, N., Robley, L., Barrett, D., Fraser, D., & Mendoza, I. (2006). Patients' recollections of therapeutic paralysis in the intensive care unit. *American Journal of Critical Care, 15*(1), 86-94.

Brunner, M. (1985). A conceptual approach to critical care nursing using Levine's model. *Focus on Critical Care, 12*(2), 39-40.

Bunting, S. M. (1988, Nov.). The concept of perception in selected nursing theories. *Nursing Science Quarterly, 1*(4), 168-174.

Cooper, D. M. (1990, March). Optimizing wound healing: A practice within nursing's domain. *Nursing Clinics of North America, 25*(1), 165-180.

Crawford-Gamble, P. E. (1986). An application of Levine's conceptual model. *Perioperative Nursing Quarterly, 2*(1), 64-70.

Fawcett, J., Brophy, S. F., Rather, M. L., & Roos, J. (1997). Commentary about Levine's on creativity in nursing. *Image: The Journal of Nursing Scholarship, 29*(3), 218-219.

Fawcett, J., Tulman, L., & Samarel, N. (1995). Enhancing function in life transitions and serious illness. *Advance Practice Nursing Quarterly, 1*, 50-57.

Flaskerud, J. H., & Halloran, E. J. (1980). Areas of agreement in nursing theory development. *ANS Advances in Nursing Science, 3*(1), 1-7.

Falk, K., Swedberg, K., Gaston-Johansson, F., & Ekman, I. (2007). Fatigue is a prevalent and severe symptom associated with uncertainty and sense of coherence in patients with chronic heart failure. *European Journal of Cardiovascular Nursing, 6*, 99-104.

Foreman, M. D. (1989, Feb.). Confusion in the hospitalized elderly: Incidence, onset, and associated factors. *Research in Nursing and Health, 12*(1), 21-29.

Gagner-Tjellesen, D., Yurkovich, E. E., & Gragert, M. (2001). Use of music therapy and other ITNIs in acute care. *Journal of Psychosocial Nursing and Mental Health Services, 39*(10), 26-37.

Hall, K. V. (1979). Current trends in the use of conceptual frameworks in nursing education. *Journal of Nursing Education, 18*(4), 26-29.

Happ, M. B., Williams, C. C., Strumpf, N. E., & Burger, S. G. (1996). Individualized care for frail elderly: Theory and practice. *Journal of Gerontological Nursing, 22*(3), 6-14.

Hirschfeld, M. J. (1976). The cognitively impaired older adult. *American Journal of Nursing, 76*, 1981-1984.

Jost, S. G. (2000). An assessment and intervention strategy for managing staff needs during change. *Journal of Nursing Administration, 30*(1), 34-40.

Langer, V. S. (1990). Minimal handling protocol for the intensive care nursery. *Neonatal Network-Journal of Neonatal Nursing, 9*(3), 23-27.

Lynn-McHale, D. J., & Smith, A. (1991). Comprehensive assessment of families of the critically ill. *AACN Clinical Issues in Critical Care Nursing, 2*(2), 195-209.

Moch, V., St. Ours, C., Hall, S., Bositis, A., Tillery, M., Belcher, A., Krumm, S., & McCorkle, R. (2007). Using a conceptual model in nursing research-mitigating fatigue in cancer patients. Journal *of Advanced Nursing, 58*(5), 503-512.

Molchany, C. B. (1992). Ventricular septal and free wall rupture complicating acute MI. *Journal of Cardiovascular Nursing, 6*(4), 38-45.

Newport, M. A. (1984). Conserving thermal energy and social integrity in the newborn. *Western Journal of Nursing Research, 6*(2), 175-197.

O'Laughlin, K. M. (1986). Change in bladder function in the woman undergoing radical hysterectomy for cervical cancer. *Journal of Obstetrical, Gynecological and Neonatal Nursing, 15*(5), 380-385.

Piccoli, M., & Galvao, C. M. (2001). Perioperative nursing: Identification of the nursing diagnosis infection risk based on Levine's conceptual model (English abstract). *Revista Latino-Americana de Enfermagem, 9*(4), 37-43.

Roberts, K. L., Brittin, M., Cook, M., & deClifford, J. (1994). Boomerang pillows and respiratory capacity. *Clinical Nursing Research, 3*(2), 157-165.

Roberts, K. L., Brittin, M., & deClifford, J. (1995). Boomerang pillows and respiratory capacity in frail elderly women. *Clinical Nursing Research, 4*(4), 465-471.

Savage, T. V., & Culbert, C. (1989). Early intervention: The unique role of nursing. *Journal of Pediatric Nursing, 4*(5), 339-345.

Schaefer, K. M. (1997). Levine's Conservation Model in nursing practice. In M. R. Alligood & A. Marriner Tomey (Eds.), *Nursing theory: Utilization & application* (pp. 89-107). St. Louis: Mosby.

Schaefer, K. M., & Pond, J. (1994). Levine's Conservation Model as a guide to nursing practice. *Nursing Science Quarterly, 7*(2), 53-54.

Schaefer, K. M., & Shober-Potylycki, M. J. (1993). Fatigue in congestive heart failure: Use of Levine's Conservation Model. *Journal of Advanced Nursing, 18*, 260-268.

Schaefer, K. M., Swavely, D., Rothenberger, C., Hess, S., & Willistin, D. (1996). Sleep disturbances post coronary artery bypass surgery. *Progress in Cardiovascular Nursing, 11*(1), 5-14.

Stafford, M. J. (1996). In tribute: Myra Estrin Levine, Professor Emerita, MSN, RN, FAAN. *Chart, 93*(3), 5-6.

Taylor, J. W. (1974). Measuring the outcomes of nursing care. *Nursing Clinics of North America, 9*, 337-348.

Tompkins, E. S. (1980). Effect of restricted mobility and dominance on perceived duration. *Nursing Research, 29*(6), 333-338.

Tribotti, S. (1990). Admission to the neonatal intensive care unit: Reducing the risks. *Neonatal Network, 8*(4), 17-22.

Webb, H. (1993). Holistic care following a palliative Hartmann's procedure. *British Journal of Nursing, 2*(2), 128-132.

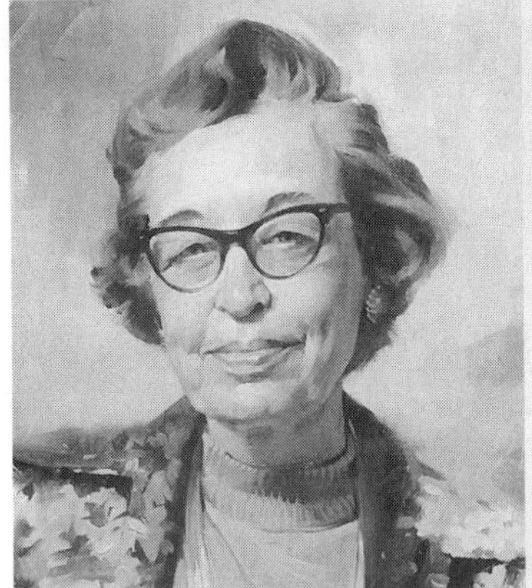

Photo credit: Kathleen Lininger, Austin, TX

CHAPTER

13

Martha E. Rogers

1914-1994

Unitary Human Beings

Mary E. Gunther

"Professional practice in nursing seeks to promote symphonic interaction between man and environment, to strengthen the coherence and integrity of the human field, and to direct and redirect patterning of the human and environmental fields for realization of maximum health potential" (Rogers, 1970, p. 122).

CREDENTIALS AND BACKGROUND OF THE THEORIST

Martha Elizabeth Rogers, eldest of four children of Bruce Taylor Rogers and Lucy Mulholland Keener Rogers, was born May 12, 1914, in Dallas, Texas. Soon after her birth, her family returned to Knoxville, Tennessee. She began her college education (1931 to 1933) studying science at the University of Tennessee. Receiving her nursing diploma from Knoxville General Hospital School of Nursing (1936), she quickly obtained a BS degree from George Peabody College in Nashville, Tennessee (1937). Her other degrees included an MA degree in public health nursing supervision from Teachers College, Columbia University, New York (1945), and an MPH (1952) and an ScD (1954) from Johns Hopkins University in Baltimore.

Rogers' early nursing practice was in rural public health nursing in Michigan and in visiting nurse supervision, education, and practice, in Connecticut. Rogers subsequently established the Visiting Nurse Service of Phoenix, Arizona. For 21 years (from 1954 to 1975), she was professor and head of the Division of Nursing at New York University. After 1975, she continued her duties as professor until she became Professor Emerita in 1979. She held this title until her death on March 13, 1994, at the age of 79.

Rogers' publications include three books and more than 200 articles. She lectured in 46 states, the District of Columbia, Puerto Rico, Mexico, the Netherlands, China, Newfoundland, Columbia, Brazil, and other

Previous authors: Kaye Bultemeier, Mary Gunther, Joann Sebastian Daily, Judy Sporleder Maupin, Cathy A. Murray, Martha Carole Satterly, Denise L. Schnell, and Therese L. Wallace. Earlier editions of this chapter were critiqued by Dr. Lois Meier and Dr. Martha Rogers.

countries (M. Rogers, personal communication, March 1988). Rogers received honorary doctorates from such renowned institutions as Duquesne University, University of San Diego, Iona College, Fairfield University, Emory University, Adelphi University, Mercy College, and Washburn University of Topeka. The numerous awards for her contributions and leadership in nursing include citations for Inspiring Leadership in the Field of Intergroup Relations by Chi Eta Phi Sorority, In Recognition of Your Outstanding Contribution to Nursing by New York University, and For Distinguished Service to Nursing by Teachers College. In addition, New York University houses the Martha E. Rogers Center for the Study of Nursing Science. In 1996, Rogers was inducted posthumously into the American Nurses Association Hall of Fame.

In 1988, colleagues and students joined her in forming the Society of Rogerian Scholars (SRS) and immediately began to publish *Rogerian Nursing Science News,* a members' newsletter, to disseminate theory developments and research studies (Malinski & Barrett, 1994). In 1993, SRS began to publish a refereed journal, *Visions: The Journal of Rogerian Nursing Science.* The society includes a foundation that maintains and administers the Martha E. Rogers Fund. To keep pace with the Society of Rogerian Scholars, see www.societyofregerianscholars.org/biography_mer.html. In 1995, New York University established the Martha E. Rogers Center to provide a structure for continuation of Rogerian research and practice.

A verbal portrait of Rogers includes such descriptive terms as *stimulating, challenging, controversial, idealistic, visionary, prophetic, philosophical, academic, outspoken, humorous, blunt,* and *ethical.* Rogers remains a widely recognized scholar honored for her contributions and leadership in nursing. Butcher (1999) noted, "Rogers, like Nightingale, was extremely independent, a determined, perfectionist individual who trusted her vision despite skepticism" (p. 114). Colleagues consider her one of the most original thinkers in nursing as she synthesized and resynthesized knowledge into "an entirely new system of thought" (Butcher, 1999, p. 111). Today she is thought of as "ahead of her time, in and out of this world" (Ireland, 2000, p. 59).

THEORETICAL SOURCES

Rogers' grounding in the liberal arts and sciences is apparent in both the origin and the development of her conceptual model, published in 1970 as *An Introduction to the Theoretical Basis of Nursing* (Rogers, 1970). Aware of the interrelatedness of knowledge, Rogers credited scientists from multiple disciplines with influencing the development of the Science of Unitary Human Beings. Rogerian science emerged from the knowledge bases of anthropology, psychology, sociology, astronomy, religion, philosophy, history, biology, physics, mathematics, and literature to create a model of unitary human beings and the environment as energy fields integral to the life process. Within nursing, the origins of Rogerian science can be traced to Nightingale's proposals and statistical data, placing the human being within the framework of the natural world. This "foundation for the scope of modern nursing" began nursing's investigation of the relationship between human beings and the environment (Rogers, 1970, p. 30). Newman (1997) describes the Science of Unitary Human Beings as "the study of the moving, intuitive experience of nurses in mutual process with those they serve" (p. 9).

MAJOR CONCEPTS & DEFINITIONS

In 1970, Rogers' conceptual model of nursing rested on a set of basic assumptions that described the life process in human beings. Wholeness, openness, unidirectionality, pattern

Continued

MAJOR CONCEPTS & DEFINITIONS—cont'd

and organization, sentience, and thought characterized the life process (Rogers, 1970).

Rogers postulates that human beings are dynamic energy fields integral with environmental fields. Both human and environmental fields are identified by pattern and characterized by a universe of open systems. In her 1983 paradigm, Rogers postulated four building blocks for her model: energy field, a universe of open systems, pattern, and four dimensionality.

Rogers consistently updated the conceptual model through revision of the homeodynamic principles. Such changes corresponded with scientific and technological advances. In 1983, Rogers changed her wording from that of unitary man to unitary human being, to remove the concept of gender. Additional clarification of unitary human beings as separate and different from the term *holistic* stressed the unique contribution of nursing to health care. In 1992, four dimensionality evolved into pandimensionality. Rogers' fundamental postulates have remained consistent since their introduction; her subsequent writings served to clarify her original ideas.

ENERGY FIELD

An energy field constitutes the fundamental unit of both the living and the nonliving. *Field* is a unifying concept, and *energy* signifies the dynamic nature of the field. Energy fields are infinite and pandimensional. Two fields are identified: the human field and the environmental field. "Specifically human beings and environment are energy fields" (Rogers, 1986b, p. 2). The unitary human being (human field) is defined as an irreducible, indivisible, pandimensional energy field identified by pattern and manifesting characteristics that are specific to the whole and that cannot be predicted from knowledge of the parts. The environmental field is defined as an irreducible, pandimensional energy field identified by pattern and integral with the human field. Each environmental field is specific to its given human field. Both change continuously, creatively, and integrally (Rogers, 1994a).

UNIVERSE OF OPEN SYSTEMS

The concept of the universe of open systems holds that energy fields are infinite, open, and integral with one another (Rogers, 1983). The human and environmental fields are in continuous process and are open systems.

PATTERN

Pattern identifies energy fields. It is the distinguishing characteristic of an energy field and is perceived as a single wave. The nature of the pattern changes continuously and innovatively, and these changes give identity to the energy field. Each human field pattern is unique and is integral with the environmental field (Rogers, 1983). Manifestations emerge as a human-environmental mutual process. Pattern is an abstraction; it reveals itself through manifestation. "Manifestations of pattern have been described as unique and refer to behaviors, qualities, and characteristics of the field" (Clarke, 1986, p. 30). A sense of self is a field manifestation, the nature of which is unique to each individual. Some variations in pattern manifestations have been described in phrases such as "longer vs. shorter rhythms," "pragmatic vs. imaginative," and time experienced as "fast" or "slow." Pattern is changing continually and may manifest disease, illness, or well-being. Pattern change is continuous, innovative, and relative.

PANDIMENSIONALITY

Rogers defines *pandimensionality* as a nonlinear domain without spatial or temporal attributes. The term *pandimensional* provides for an infinite domain without limit. It best expresses the idea of a unitary whole.

USE OF EMPIRICAL EVIDENCE

Being an abstract conceptual system, the Science of Unitary Human Beings does not directly identify testable empirical indicators. Rather, it specifies a worldview and philosophy used to identify the phenomena of concern to the discipline of nursing. As was mentioned previously, Rogers' model emerged from multiple knowledge sources; the most readily apparent of these are the nonlinear dynamics of quantum physics and general system theory.

Evident in her model are the influence of Einstein's (1961) theory of relativity in relation to space-time and Burr and Northrop's (1935) electrodynamic theory relating to electrical fields. By the time von Bertalanffy (1960) introduced general system theory, theories regarding a universe of open systems were beginning to affect the development of knowledge within all disciplines. With general system theory, the term *negentropy* was brought into use to signify increasing order, complexity, and heterogeneity in direct contrast to the previously held belief that the universe was winding down. Rogers, however, refined and purified general system theory by denying hierarchical subsystems, the concept of single causation, and the predictability of a system's behavior through investigations of its parts.

Introducing quantum theory and the theories of relativity and of probability fundamentally challenged the prevailing absolutism. As new knowledge escalated, the traditional meanings of *homeostasis, steady state, adaptation,* and *equilibrium* were questioned seriously. The closed-system, entropic model of the universe was no longer adequate to explain phenomena, and evidence accumulated in support of a universe of open systems (Rogers, 1994b). Continuing development within other disciplines of the acausal, nonlinear dynamics of life validated Rogers' model. Most notable of this development is that of chaos theory, quantum physics' contribution to the science of complexity (or wholeness), that blurs the boundaries between the disciplines, allowing exploration and deepening of the understanding of the totality of human experience.

MAJOR ASSUMPTIONS

Nursing

Nursing is a learned profession and is both a science and an art. It is an empirical science and, like other sciences, that lies in the phenomenon central to its focus. Rogerian nursing focuses on concern with people and the world in which they live—a natural fit for nursing care, as it encompasses people and their environments. The integrality of people and their environments, operating from a pandimensional universe of open systems, points to a new paradigm and initiates the identity of nursing as a science. The purpose of nursing is to promote health and well-being for all persons. The art of nursing is the creative use of the science of nursing for human betterment (Rogers, 1994b). "Professional practice in nursing seeks to promote symphonic interaction between human and environmental fields, to strengthen the integrity of the human field, and to direct and redirect patterning of the human and environmental fields for realization of maximum health potential" (Rogers, 1970, p. 122). Nursing exists for the care of people and the life process of humans.

Person

Rogers defines *person* as an open system in continuous process with the open system that is the environment (integrality). She defines *unitary human being* as an "irreducible, indivisible, pandimensional energy field identified by pattern and manifesting characteristics that are specific to the whole" (Rogers, 1992, p. 29). Human beings "are not disembodied entities, nor are they mechanical aggregates. . . . Man is a unified whole possessing his own integrity and manifesting characteristics that are more than and different from the sum of his parts" (Rogers, 1970, pp. 46-47). Within a conceptual model specific to nursing's concern, people and their environment are perceived as irreducible energy fields integral with one another and continuously creative in their evolution.

Health

Rogers uses health in many of her earlier writings without clearly defining the term. She uses the term *passive health* to symbolize wellness and the absence of disease and major illness (Rogers, 1970). Her promotion of positive health connotes direction in helping people with opportunities for rhythmic consistency (Rogers, 1970). Later, she wrote that wellness "is a much better term . . . because the term *health* is very ambiguous" (Rogers, 1994b, p. 34).

Rogers uses *health* as a value term defined by the culture or the individual. Health and illness are manifestations of pattern and are considered "to denote behaviors that are of high value and low value" (Rogers, 1980). Events manifested in the life process indicate the extent to which a human being achieves maximum health according to some value system. In Rogerian science, the phenomenon central to nursing's conceptual system is the human life process. The life process has its own dynamic and creative unity, inseparable from the environment, and is characterized by the whole (Rogers, 1970).

In "Dimensions of Health: A View from Space," Rogers (1986b) reaffirms the original theoretical assertions, adding philosophical challenges to the prevailing perception of health. Stressing a new worldview that focuses on people and their environment, she lists iatrogenesis, nosocomial conditions, and hypochrondriasis as the major health problems in the United States. Rogers (1986b) writes, "A new world view compatible with the most progressive knowledge available is a necessary prelude to studying human health and to determining modalities for its promotion whether on this planet or in the outer reaches of space" (p. 2).

Environment

Rogers (1994a) defines environment as "an irreducible, pandimensional energy field identified by pattern and manifesting characteristics different from those of the parts. Each environmental field is specific to its given human field. Both change continuously and creatively" (p. 2). Environmental fields are infinite, and change is continuously innovative, unpredictable, and characterized by increasing diversity. Environmental and human fields are identified by wave patterns manifesting continuous mutual change.

THEORETICAL ASSERTIONS

The principles of homeodynamics postulate a way of perceiving unitary human beings. The evolution of these principles from 1970 to 1994 is depicted in Table 13-1. Rogers (1970) wrote, "The life process is homeodynamic. . . . These principles postulate the way the life process is and predict the nature of its evolving" (p. 96). Rogers identified the principles of change as helicy, resonancy, and integrality. The helicy principle describes spiral development in continuous, nonrepeating, and innovative patterning. Rogers' articulation of the principle of helicy describing the nature of change evolved from probabilistic to unpredictable, while remaining continuous and innovative. According to the principle of resonancy, patterning changes with development from lower to higher frequency, that is, with varying degrees of intensity. Resonancy embodies wave frequency and energy field pattern evolution. Integrality, the third principle of homeodynamics, stresses the continuous mutual process of person and environment. The principles of homeodynamics evolved into a concise and clear description of the nature, process, and context of change within human and environmental energy fields (Hills & Hanchett, 2001).

In 1970, Rogers identified the following five assumptions that are also theoretical assertions supporting her model derived from literature on human beings, physics, mathematics, and behavioral science:

1. "Man is a unified whole possessing his own integrity and manifesting characteristics more than and different from the sum of his parts" (energy field) (p. 47).
2. "Man and environment are continuously exchanging matter and energy with one another" (openness) (p. 54).

Table 13-1 *Evolution of Principles of Homeodynamics: 1970, 1983, 1986, and 1992*

An Introduction to the Theoretical Basis of Nursing, 1970	Nursing: A Science of Unitary Man, 1980	Science of Unitary Human Beings: A Paradigm for Nursing, 1983	Dimensions of Health: A View From Space, 1986	Nursing Science and the Space Age, 1992
RESONANCY				
Continuously propagating series of waves between man and environment	Continuous change from lower- to higher-frequency wave patterns in the human and environmental fields	Continuous change from lower- to higher-frequency wave patterns in the human and environmental fields	Continuous change from lower- to higher-frequency wave patterns in the human and environmental fields	Continuous change from lower- to higher-frequency wave patterns in the human and environmental fields
HELICY				
Continuous, innovative change growing out of mutual interaction of man and environment along a spiraling longitudinal axis bound in space-time	Nature of change between human and environmental fields is continuously innovative, probabilistic, and increasingly diverse, manifesting nonrepeating rhythmicities	Continuous innovative, probabilistic, increasing diversity of human and environmental field patterns, characterized by nonrepeating rhythmicities	Continuous, innovative, probabilistic, increasing, and environmental diversity characterized by nonrepeating rhythmicities	Continuous, innovative, unpredictable, increasing diversity of human and environmental field patterns
RECIPROCY				
Continuous mutual interaction between the human field and the environmental field	—	—	—	—
SYNCHRONY				
Change in the human field and simultaneous state of environmental field at any given point in space-time	Continuous, mutual, simultaneous interaction between human and environmental fields	Continuous, mutual human field and environmental field process	Continuous, mutual human field and environmental field process	Continuous, mutual human field and environmental field process

Conceptualized by Joann Daily from the following sources:

Riehl, J. P., & Roy, C. (Eds.). (1980). *Conceptual models for nursing practice* (2nd ed.). New York: Appleton-Century-Crofts.

Rogers, M. E. (1970). *An introduction to the theoretical basis of nursing.* Philadelphia: F. A. Davis.

Rogers, M. E. (1983). Science of unitary human beings: A paradigm for nursing. In I. W. Clements & F. B. Roberts (Eds.), *Family health: A theoretical approach to nursing care.* New York: John Wiley & Sons.

Table revised by Denise Schnell and Therese Wallace in 1988 to include the following source:

Rogers, M. E. (1986b). *Dimensions of health: A view from space* (obtained through personal correspondence with Martha Rogers, March 1988).

Table updated by Cathy Murray from the following source:

Rogers, M. E. (1992). Nursing science and the space age. *Nursing Science Quarterly, 5*(1), 27-34.

3. "The life process evolves irreversibly and unidirectionally along the space-time continuum" (helicy) (p. 59).
4. "Pattern and organization identify man and reflect his innovative wholeness" (pattern and organization) (p. 65).
5. "Man is characterized by the capacity for abstraction and imagery, language and thought, sensation, and emotion" (sentient, thinking being) (p. 73).

LOGICAL FORM

Rogers uses a dialectic method as opposed to a logistical, problematic, or operational method, that is, Rogers explains nursing by referring to broader principles that explain human beings. She explains human beings through principles that characterize the universe, based on the perspective of a whole that organizes the parts.

Rogers' model of unitary human beings is deductive and logical. The theory of relativity, the general system theory, the electrodynamic theory of life, and many other theories contributed ideas for Rogers' model. Unitary human beings and environment, the central components of the model, are integral with one another. The basic building blocks of her model are energy field, openness, pattern, and pandimensionality providing a new worldview. These concepts form the basis of an abstract conceptual system defining nursing and health. From the abstract conceptual system, Rogers derived the principles of homeodynamics, which postulate the nature and direction of human beings' evolution. Although Rogers invented the words *homeodynamics* (similar state of change and growth), *helicy* (evolution), *resonancy* (intensity of change), and *integrality* (wholeness), all definitions are etymologically consistent and logical.

ACCEPTANCE BY THE NURSING COMMUNITY

Practice

The Rogerian model is an abstract system of ideas from which to approach the practice of nursing. Rogers' model, stressing the totality of experience and existence, is relevant in today's healthcare system, where continuum of care is more important than episodic illness and hospitalization. This model provides the abstract philosophical framework from which to view the unitary human-environmental field phenomenon. Within the Rogerian framework, nursing is based on theoretical knowledge that guides nursing practice. The professional practice of nursing is creative and imaginative and exists to serve people. It is rooted in intellectual judgment, abstract knowledge, and human compassion.

Historically, nursing has equated practice with the practical and theory with the impractical. More appropriately, theory and practice are two related components in a unified nursing practice. Alligood (1994) articulates how theory and practice direct and guide each other as they expand and increase unitary nursing knowledge. Nursing knowledge provides the framework for the emergent artistic application of nursing care (Rogers, 1970).

Within Rogers' model, the critical thinking process directing practice can be divided into three components: pattern appraisal, mutual patterning, and evaluation. Cowling (2000) states that pattern appraisal is meant to avoid, if not transcend, reductionistic categories of physical, mental, spiritual, emotional, cultural, and social assessment frameworks. Through observation and participation, the nurse focuses on human expressions of reflection, experience, and perception to form a profile of the patient. Mutual exploration of emergent patterns allows identification of unitary themes predominant in the pandimensional human-environmental field process. Mutual understanding implies knowing participation but does not lead to the nurse's prescribing change or predicting outcomes. As Cowling (2000) explains, "A critical feature of the unitary pattern appreciation process, and also of healing through appreciating wholeness, is a willingness on the part of the scientist or practitioner to let go of expectations about change" (p. 31). Evaluation centers on the perceptions emerging during mutual patterning.

Noninvasive patterning modalities used within Rogerian practice include, but are not limited to, acupuncture, aromatherapy, therapeutic touch, massage, guided imagery, meditation, self-reflection, guided reminiscence, journal keeping, humor, hypnosis, sleep, hygiene, dietary manipulation, music, and physical exercise (Alligood, 1991a; Bultemeier, 1997; Kim, Park, & Kim, 2008; Larkin, 2007; Levin, 2006; Lewandowski, et al., 2005; MacNeil, 2006; Siedliecki & Good, 2006; Smith, Kemp, Hemphill, & Vojir, 2002; Smith & Kyle, 2008; Walling, 2006). Barrett (1998) notes that integral to these modalities are "meaningful dialogue, centering, and pandimensional authenticity (genuineness, trustworthiness, acceptance, and knowledgeable caring)" (p. 138). Nurses participate in the lived experience of health in a multitude of roles, including "facilitators and educators, advocates, assessors, planners, coordinators, and collaborators," by accepting diversity, recognizing patterns, viewing change as positive, and accepting the connectedness of life (Malinski, 1986, p. 27) These roles may require the nurse to "let go of traditional ideas of time, space, and outcome" (Malinski, 1997, p. 115).

The Rogerian model provides a challenging and innovative framework from which to plan and implement nursing practice, which Barrett (1998) defines as the "continuous process (of voluntary mutual patterning) whereby the nurse assists clients to freely choose with awareness ways to participate in their well-being" (p. 136).

Education

Rogers clearly articulated guidelines for the education of nurses within the Science of Unitary Human Beings. Rogers discusses structuring nursing education programs to teach nursing as a science and as a learned profession. Barrett (1990b) calls Rogers a "consistent voice crying out against antieducationalism and dependency" (p. 306). Rogers' model clearly articulates values and beliefs about human beings, health, nursing, and the educational process. As such, it has been used to guide curriculum development in all levels of nursing education (Barrett, 1990b; DeSimone, 2006; Hellwig & Ferrante, 1993; Mathwig, Young, & Pepper, 1990). Rogers (1990) stated that nurses must commit to lifelong learning and noted, "The nature of the practice of nursing (is) the use of knowledge for human betterment" (p. 111).

Rogers advocated separate licensure for nurses prepared with an associate's degree and those with a baccalaureate degree, recognizing that there is a difference between the technically oriented and the professional nurse. In her view, the professional nurse must be well rounded and educated in the humanities, sciences, and nursing. Such a program would include a basic education in language, mathematics, logic, philosophy, psychology, sociology, music, art, biology, microbiology, physics, and chemistry; elective courses could include economics, ethics, political science, anthropology, and computer science (Barrett, 1990b). With regard to the research component of the curriculum, Rogers (1994b) stated the following:

> Undergraduate students need to be able to identify problems, to have tools of investigation and to do studies that will allow them to use knowledge for the improvement of practice, and they should be able to read the literature intelligently. People with master's degrees ought to be able to do applied research.... The theoretical research, the fundamental basic research is going to come out of doctoral programs of stature that focus on nursing as a learned field of endeavor (p. 34).

Barrett (1990b) notes that with increasing use of technology and increasing severity of illness of hospitalized patients, students may be limited to observational experiences in these institutions. Therefore, the acquisition of manipulative technical skills must be accomplished in practice laboratories and at alternative sites, such as clinics and home health agencies. Other sites for education include health promotion programs, managed care programs, homeless shelters, and senior centers.

Research

Rogers' conceptual model provides a stimulus and direction for research and theory development in nursing science. Fawcett (2000), who insists that the level of abstraction affects direct empirical observation and testing, endorses the designation of the Science of Unitary Human Beings as a conceptual model rather than a grand theory. She states clearly that the purpose of the work determines its category. Conceptual models "identify the purpose and scope of nursing and provide frameworks for objective records of the effects of nursing" (Fawcett, 2005, p. 18).

Emerging from Rogers' model are theories that explain human phenomena and direct nursing practice. The Rogerian model, with its implicit assumptions, provides broad principles that conceptually direct theory development. The conceptual model provides a stimulus and direction for scientific activity. Relationships among identified phenomena generate both grand (further development of one aspect of the model) and middle range (description, explanation, or prediction of concrete aspects) theories (Fawcett, 1995).

Two prominent grand nursing theories grounded in Rogers' model are Newman's health as expanding consciousness and Parse's human becoming (Fawcett, 2005). Numerous middle range theories have emerged from Rogers' three homeodynamic principles as follows: (1) helicy, (2) resonancy, and (3) integrality (Figure 13-1). Exemplars of middle

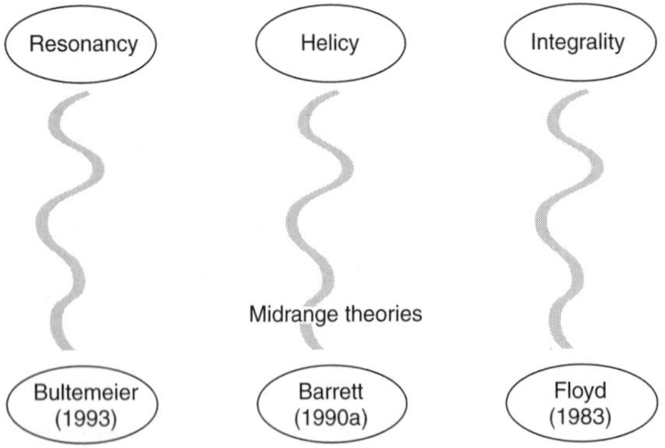

Figure 13-1 Theory development within the Science of Unitary Human Beings.

range theories derived from homeodynamic principles include power-as-knowing-participation-in-change (helicy) (Barrett, 1990a), the theory of perceived dissonance (resonancy) (Bultemeier, 1997), and the theory of interactive rhythms (integrality) (Floyd, 1983). In her overview of Rogerian science–based theories, Malinski (2006) identifies work within specific concepts: (1) self-transcendence (Reed, 1991, 2003), enlightenment (Hills & Hanchett, 2001), and spirituality (Malinski, 1994; Smith, 1994); (2) turbulence (Butcher, 1993) and dissonance (Bultemeier, 1997); (3) aging (Alligood & McGuire, 2000; Butcher, 2003); (4) intentionality (Zahourek, 2005); and (5) caring (Smith, 1999). Other middle range theories encompass the phenomena of human field motion (Ference, 1986), as well as creativity, actualization, and empathy (Alligood, 1991b).

Rogers (1986a) maintains that research in nursing must examine unitary human beings as integral with their environment. Therefore, the intent of nursing research is to examine and understand a phenomenon and, from this understanding, design patterning activities that promote healing. To obtain a clearer understanding of lived experiences, the person's perception and sentient awareness of what is occurring are imperative. The variety of events associated with human phenomena provides the experiential data for research that is directed toward capturing the dynamic, ever-changing life experiences of human beings. Selecting the correct method for examining the person and the environment as health-related phenomena is the challenge of the Rogerian researcher. Both quantitative and qualitative approaches have been used in the Science of Unitary Human Beings research, although not all researchers agree that both are appropriate. Researchers do agree that ontological and epistemological congruence between the model and the approach must be considered and reflected by the research question (Barrett, Cowling, Carboni, & Butcher, 1997). Quantitative experimental and quasi-experimental designs are not appropriate, because their purpose is to reveal causal relationships. Descriptive, explanatory, and correlational designs are more appropriate, because they recognize "the unitary nature of the phenomenon of interest" and may "propose evidence of patterned mutual change among variables" (Sherman, 1997, p. 132).

Specific research methods emerging from middle range theories based on the Rogerian model capture the human-environmental phenomena. As a means of capturing the unitary human being, Cowling (1998) describes the process of pattern appreciation using the combined research and practice case study method. Case study attends to the whole person (irreducibility), aims at comprehending the essence (pattern), and respects the inherent interconnectedness of phenomena. A pattern profile is composed through a synopsis and synthesis of the data (Barrett, et al., 1997). Other innovative methods of recording and entering the human-environmental field phenomenon include photo-disclosure (Bultemeier, 1997), hermeneutic text interpretation (Alligood, 2002; Alligood & Fawcett, 1999), and measurement of the effect of dialogue combined with noninvasive modalities (Leddy & Fawcett, 1997).

Rogerian instrument development is extensive and ever-evolving. A wide range of instruments for measuring human-environmental field phenomena have emerged (Table 13-2). The continual emergence of middle range theories, research approaches, and instruments demonstrates recognition of the importance of Rogerian science to nursing.

FURTHER DEVELOPMENT

Rogers (1986a) believed that knowledge development within her model was a "never-ending process" using "a multiplicity of knowledge from many sources . . . to create a kaleidoscope of possibilities" (p. 4). Recent explorations by Rogerian scholars into Buddhist, Hindu, and aboriginal philosophies exemplify this belief in an essential unity (Madrid, 1997).

Fawcett (2005) identified the following three rudimentary theories developed by Rogers from the Science of Unitary Human Beings:

1. Theory of accelerating evolution
2. Theory of rhythmical correlates of change
3. Theory of paranormal phenomena

Further explication and testing of these theories and the homeodynamic principles will contribute to nursing science knowledge.

CRITIQUE

Simplicity

Ongoing studies and work within the model have served to simplify and clarify some of the concepts and relationships. However, when the model is examined in total perspective, some still classify it as complex. With its continued use in practice, research, and education, nurses will come to appreciate the model's elegant simplicity. As Whall (1987) notes, "With only three principles, a few major concepts, and five assumptions, Rogers has explained the nature of man and the life process" (p. 154).

Generality

Rogers' conceptual model is abstract and therefore generalizable and powerful. It is broad in scope, providing a framework for the development of nursing knowledge through the generation of grand and middle range theories.

Empirical Precision

Early criticisms of the model identified its major limitations as difficult-to-understand principles, lack of operational definitions, and inadequate tools for measurement (Butterfield, 1983). Drawing on knowledge from a multitude of scientific fields, Rogers' conceptual model is deductive in logic with an inherent lack of immediate empirical support (Barrett, 1990b). As Fawcett (1995) points out, failure to properly categorize the work as a conceptual model rather than as a theory leads to "considerable misunderstandings and inappropriate expectations" (p. 29), which can result in the work being labeled inadequate.

As noted earlier, the development of the model by Rogerian scientists has resulted in the generation of testable theories accompanied by tools of measurement.

Table 13-2 Research Instruments and Practice Tools Derived From the Science of Unitary Human Beings

Instrument	Description
Human Field Motion Test (HFMT) (Ference, 1980, 1986; Young et al., 2001)	Measures human field motion by means of semantic differential ratings of the concepts My Motor Is Running and My Field Expansion.
Perceived Field Motion Scale (PFM) (Yarcheski & Mahon, 1991; Young et al., 2001)	Measures the perceived experience of motion by means of semantic differential ratings of the concept My Field Motion.
Human Field Rhythms (HFR) (Yarcheski & Mahon, 1991; Young et al., 2001)	Measures the frequency of rhythms in the human-environmental energy field mutual process by means of a one-item visual analogue scale.
Index of Field Energy (IFE) (Gueldner, as cited in Watson et al., 1997; Young et al., 2001)	Measures human field dynamics by means of semantic differential ratings of 18 pairs of simple black-and-white line drawings.
The Well-being Picture Scale (Gueldner et al., 2005)	Revision of the Index of Field Energy. A 10-item non–language-based pictorial scale that measures general well-being.
Power as Knowing Participation in Change Tool (PKPCT) (Barrett, 1984, 1986, 1990a; Watson et al., 1997; Young et al., 2001)	Measures the person's capacity to participate knowingly in change by means of semantic differential ratings of the concepts Awareness, Choices, Freedom to Act Intentionally, and Involvement in Creating Changes.
Diversity of Human Field Pattern Scale (DHFPS) (Hastings-Tolsma, 1993; Watson et al., 1997; Young et al., 2001)	Measures diversity of human field pattern, or degree of change in the evolution of human potential throughout the life process, by means of Likert scale ratings of 16 items.
Human Field Image Metaphor Scale (HFIMS) (Johnston, 1993a, 1993b, 1994; Young et al., 2001)	Measures the individual's awareness of the infinite wholeness of the human field by means of Likert scale ratings of 14 metaphors that represent perceived potential and 11 metaphors that represent perceived field integrality.
Temporal Experience Scale (TES) (Paletta, 1988, 1990; Young et al., 2001)	Measures subjective experience of temporal awareness by means of Likert scale ratings of 24 metaphors representing the factors of time dragging, time racing, and timelessness.
Assessment of Dream Experience (ADE) (Watson, 1994, 1999; Watson et al., 1997; Young et al., 2001)	Measures dreaming as a beyond waking experience by means of Likert scale ratings of the extent to which 20 items describe what the individual's dreams have been like during the past 2 weeks.
Person-Environment Participation Scale (PEPS) (Leddy, 1995, 1999; Young et al., 2001)	Measures the person's experience of continuous human-environment mutual process by means of semantic differential ratings of 15 bipolar adjectives representing the content areas of comfort, influence, continuity, ease, and energy.
Leddy Heartiness Scale (LHS) (Leddy, 1996; Young et al., 2001)	Measures the person's perceived purpose and power to achieve goals by means of Likert scale ratings of 26 items representing meaningfulness, ends, choice, challenge, confidence, control, capability to function, and connections.
McCanse Readiness for Death Instrument (MRDI) (McCanse, 1988; 1995)	Measures physiological, psychological, sociological, and spiritual aspects of healthy field pattern, as death is developmentally approached by means of a 26-item structured interview questionnaire.

Table 13-2 ***Research Instruments and Practice Tools Derived From the Science of Unitary Human Beings—cont'd***

Mutual Exploration of the Healing Human-Environmental Field Relationship (Carboni, 1992; Young et al., 2001)	Measures nurses' and clients' experiences and expressions of changing configurations of energy field patterns of the healing human-environmental field relationship using semi-structured and open-ended items. Forms for a nurse and a single client and for a nurse and two or more clients are available.
Practice Tool and Citation	**Description**
Nursing Process Format (Falco & Lobo, 1995)	Guides use of a Rogerian nursing process, including nursing assessment, nursing diagnosis, nursing planning for implementation, and nursing evaluation, according to the homeodynamic principles of integrality, resonancy, and helicy.
Assessment Tool (Smith et al., 1991)	Guides use of a Rogerian nursing process, including assessment, diagnosis, implementation, and evaluation, according to the homeodynamic principles of complementarity (i.e., integrality), resonancy, and helicy, for patients hospitalized in a critical care unit and their family members, using open-ended questions.
Critical Thinking for Pattern Appraisal, Mutual Patterning, and Evaluation Tool (Bultemeier, 2002)	Provides guidance for the nurse's application of pattern appraisal, mutual patterning, and evaluation, as well as areas for the client's self-reflection, patterning activities, and personal appraisal.
Nursing Assessment of Patterns Indicative of Health (Madrid & Winstead-Fry, 1986)	Guides assessment of patterns, including relative present, communication, sense of rhythm, connection to environment, personal myth, and system integrity.
Assessment Tool for Postpartum Mothers (Tettero et al., 1993)	Guides assessment of mothers experiencing the challenges of their first child during the postpartum period.
Assessment Criteria for Nursing Evaluation of the Older Adult (Decker, 1989)	Guides assessment of the functional status of older adults living in their own homes, including demographic data, client prioritization of problems, sequential patterning (e.g., family of origin culture, past illnesses), rhythmical patterning (e.g., healthcare usage, medication usage, social contacts, acute illnesses), and cross-sectional patterning (e.g., current living arrangements and health concerns, cognitive and emotional status).
Holistic Assessment of the Chronic Pain Client (Garon, 1991)	Guides holistic assessment of clients living in their own homes and experiencing chronic pain, including the environmental field, the community, and all systems in contact with the client; the home environment; client needs and expectations; client and family strengths; the client's pain experience—location, intensity, cause, meaning, effects on activities, life, and relationships, relief measures, and goals; and client and family feelings about illness and pain.

Continued

Table 13-2 Research Instruments and Practice Tools Derived From the Science of Unitary Human Beings—cont'd

Human Energy Field Assessment Form (Wright, 1989, 1991)	Used to record findings related to human energy field assessment as practiced in therapeutic touch, including location of field disturbance on a body diagram and strength of the overall field and intensity of the field disturbance on visual analogue scales.
Family Assessment Tool (Whall, 1981)	Guides assessment of families in terms of individual subsystem considerations, interactional patterns, unique characteristics of the whole family system, and environmental interface synchrony.
An Assessment Guideline for Work with Families (Johnston, 1986)	Guides assessment of the family unit, in terms of definition of family, family organization, belief system, family developmental needs, economic factors, family field and environmental field complementarity, communication patterns, and supplemental data, including health assessment of individual family members, developmental factors, member interactions, and relationships.
Nursing Process Format for Families (Reed, 1986)	Guides the use of a developmentally oriented nursing process for families.
A Conceptual Tool Kit for Community Health Assessment (Hanchett, 1979)	Tools used to guide assessment of the energy, individuality, and pattern and organization of a community.
Community Health Assessment (Hanchett, 1988)	Guides assessment of a community in areas of diversity; rhythms, including frequencies of colors, rhythms of light, and patterns of sound; motion; experience of time; pragmatic-imaginative-visionary worldviews; and sleep-wake beyond waking rhythms.

From Fawcett, J. (2005). *Contemporary nursing knowledge: Analysis and evaluation of nursing models and theories* (pp. 337-339). Philadelphia: F. A. Davis. Used with permission.

Derivable Consequences

Rogers' science has the fundamental intent of understanding human evolution and its potential. It "coordinates a universe of open systems to identify the focus of a new paradigm and initiate nursing's identity as a science" (Rogers, 1989, p. 182).

Although all the metaparadigm concepts are explored, the emphasis is on the integrality of human-environmental field phenomena. Rogers suggested many ideas for future studies; on the basis of this and the research of others, it can be said that the conceptual model is useful. Such utility has been proven in the arenas of practice, education, and research.

SUMMARY

The Rogerian model emerged from a broad historical base and has moved to the forefront as scientific knowledge has evolved. Understanding the concepts and principles of the Science of Unitary Human Beings requires a foundation in general education, a willingness to let go of the traditional, and an ability to perceive the world in a new and creative way. Emerging from a strong educational base, this model provides a challenging framework from which to provide nursing care. The abstract ideas expounded in the Rogerian model and their congruence with modern scientific knowledge spur new and challenging theories that further the understanding of the unitary human being. Nursing scholars and practitioners are carrying Rogers' ideas into the next century.

Case Study

Charlie Dee is a 56-year-old male with a 30-year history of smoking two packs of cigarettes a day. He is seeing nurse practitioner, Sandra Gee, for the first time after being diagnosed with chronic obstructive pulmonary disease. Pattern appraisal begins with eliciting the client's description of his experience with this disease, his perceptions of his health, and how the disease is expressed (symptoms). Mr. Dee states that he has a productive cough that is worse in the morning, gets short of breath whenever he is physically active, and always feels tired. Through specific questions, the nurse practitioner discovers that Mr. Dee has experienced a change in his sleep patterns and nutritional intake. He is sleeping for shorter periods and eating less. She also learns that Mr. Dee's wife smokes, and that they have indoor cats for pets. He does not think that his wife will be amenable to changing her habits or getting rid of the cats. During this appraisal, the nurse seeks to discover what is important to Mr. Dee and how he defines *healthy*.

Mutual patterning involves sharing knowledge and offering choices. Upon completion of the appraisal, the nurse summarizes what she has been told and how she understands it. In this way, the nurse and the client can reach consensus about what activities would be acceptable to Mr. Dee. Ms. Gee provides information about the disease and suggestions that will increase his comfort. Noninvasive interventions include breathing retraining, recommendations for a high protein-high calorie diet, eating smaller meals more frequently, sleeping with the head elevated, and using progressive relaxation exercises at bedtime. The nurse recommends that the Dee's buy a HEPA filter and humidifier to assist in removing environmental pollutants and maintaining proper humidity in the home.

Because Mr. Gee has expressed a desire to quit smoking, the nurse suggests that he use forms of centering, such as guided imagery and meditation, to supplement the nicotine patches prescribed by his physician. She also provides him with written material about the disease that he can share with his wife. At the end of the visit, Mr. Dee states that he feels better knowing that he has the power to change some things about his life.

CRITICAL THINKING Activities

1. Review two research articles that use Rogerian science as the framework to guide the research process.
2. Identify the middle range theory that was developed or guided the research process.
3. What philosophical tenets from Nightingale contributed to the basis for development of the Rogerian model?
4. Locate three publications, and discuss how the authors used Rogerian science in nursing education.
5. Analyze your clinical practice, and identify areas in which practice based on Rogerian science would improve nursing care. Enumerate the changes and the anticipated positive outcomes.

POINTS FOR Further Study

- Society of Rogerian Scholars (SRS), supporting the development of Unitary Health Care and the Science of Unitary Human Beings. New York University College of Nursing, 246 Greene Street, New York, NY 10003-6677, available at: http://medweb.uwcm.ac.uk/martha/society/htm

Publications

- *Visions: The Journal of Rogerian Nursing Science*
- *Rogerian Nursing Science News SRS Newsletter*

Websites

- Martha E. Rogers Home Page and Listserv at: http://medweb.uwcm.uk/martha (Maintained by Francis C. Biley, PhD, RN, Cardiff University, Wales, UK.)
- Rogerian Nursing Science Wiki at: http://rogeriannursingscience.wikispaces.com/ (Created by H. K. Butcher, RN, PhD, University of Iowa College of Nursing. The intended purpose is twofold: [1] to bring together a collaborative participative community to co-create a definitive comprehensive explication of the SUHB; [2] to create an on-line resource that anyone can access for all those who want to learn how Rogerian nursing science serves as a foundation for nursing research, practice, education, and administration.)
- New York University, Martha E. Rogers Center at: http://www.nyu.edu/nursing/bulletin/centers
- American Nurses Association Hall of Fame Inductee Page at: http://nursingworld.org/Functional/MenuCategoAboutANA
- Martha E. Rogers Gravesite at: http://www.aahn.org/gravesites/rogers.html

REFERENCES

Alligood, M. R. (1991a). Guided reminiscence: A Rogerian based intervention. *Rogerian Nursing Science News, 3*(3), 1-3.

Alligood, M. R. (1991b). Testing Rogers' theory of accelerating change: The relationship among creativity, actualization, and empathy in persons 18 to 92 years of age. *Western Journal of Nursing Research, 13*, 84-96.

Alligood, M. R. (1994). Toward a unitary view of nursing practice. In M. Madrid & E. A. M. Barrett (Eds.), *Rogers' scientific art of nursing practice* (pp. 223-240). New York: National League for Nursing.

Alligood, M. R. (2002). A theory of the art of nursing discovered in Rogers' Science of Unitary Human Beings. *International Journal for Human Caring, 6*(2), 55-60.

Alligood, M. R., & Fawcett, J. (1999). Acceptance of an invitation to dialogue: Examination of an interpretive approach for the science of unitary human beings. *Visions: Journal of Rogerian Nursing Science, 7*(1), 5-13.

Alligood, M. R. & McGuire, S. L. (2000). Perception of time, sleep patterns and activity in senior citizens: A test of the Rogerian theory of aging. *Visions: The Journal of Rogerian Nursing Science, 8*, 6-14.

Barrett, E. A. M. (1984). An empirical investigation of Martha E. Rogers' principle of helicy: The relationship of human field motion and power. Dissertation Abstracts International, 45, 615A.

Barrett, E. A. M. (1986). Investigation of the principle of helicy: The relationship of human field motion and power. In V. M. Malinski (Ed.), *Explorations on Martha Rogers' science of unitary human beings* (pp. 173-188). Norwalk, CT: Appleton-Century-Crofts.

Barrett, E. A. M. (1990a). An instrument to measure power-as-knowing-participation-in-change. In O. Strickland & C. Waltz (Eds.), *The measurement of nursing outcomes: Measuring clients self-care and coping skills* (Vol. 4, pp. 159-180). New York: Springer.

Barrett, E. A. M. (1990b). *Visions of Rogers' science-based nursing.* New York: National League for Nursing.

Barrett, E. A. M. (1998). A Rogerian practice methodology for health patterning. *Nursing Science Quarterly, 11*(4), 136-138.

Barrett, E. A. M., Cowling, W. R., Carboni, J. T., & Butcher, H. K. (1997). Unitary perspectives on methodological practices. In M. Madrid (Ed.), *Patterns of Rogerian knowing* (pp. 47-62). New York: National League for Nursing.

Bultemeier, K. (1997). Photo-disclosure: A research methodology for investigating the unitary human being. In M. Madrid (Ed.), *Patterns of Rogerian knowing.* New York National League for Nursing Press.

Bultemeier, K. (2002). Rogers' science of unitary human beings in nursing practice. In M. R. Alligood & A. Marriner Tomey (Eds.), *Nursing theory: Utilization and application* (2nd ed., pp. 267-288). St. Louis: Mosby.

Burr, H. S., & Northrup, F. S. C. (1935). The electrodynamic theory of life. *Quarterly Review of Biology, 10*, 322-323.

Butcher, H. K. (1993). Kaleidoscoping in life's turbulence: From Seurat's art to Rogers' nursing science. In M. E. Parker (Ed.), *Patterns of nursing theories in practice* (pp. 183-198). New York: National League for Nursing.

Butcher, H. K. (1999). Rogerian ethics: An ethical inquiry into Rogers' life and science. *Nursing Science Quarterly, 5*, 111-118.

Butcher, H. K. (2003). Aging as emerging brilliance: Advancing Rogers' unitary theory of aging. *Visions: The Journal of Rogerian Nursing Science, 11*, 55-66.

Butterfield, S. E. (1983). In search of commonalties: Analysis of two theoretical frameworks. *International Journal of Nursing Studies, 20*(1), 15-22.

Carboni, J. T. (1992). Instrument development and the measurement of unitary constructs. *Nursing Science Quarterly, 5*, 134-142.

Clarke, P. N. (1986). Theoretical and measurement issues in the study of field phenomena. *ANS Advances in Nursing Science, 9*(1), 29-39.

Cowling, W. R. (1998). Unitary case inquiry. *Nursing Science Quarterly, 11*(4), 139-141.

Cowling, W. R. (2000). Healing as appreciating wholeness. *ANS Advances in Nursing Science, 22*(3), 16-32.

Decker, K. (1989). Theory in action: The geriatric assessment team. *Journal of Gerontological Nursing, 15*(10), 25-28.

DeSimone, B. B. (2006). Curriculum design to promote the critical thinking of accelerated bachelor's degree nursing students. *Nurse Educator, 31*(5), 213-217.

Einstein, A. (1961). *Relativity.* New York: Crown.

Falco, S. M., & Lobo, M. L. (1995). Martha E. Rogers. In J. B. George (Ed.), *Nursing theories. The base for professional nursing practice* (4th ed., pp. 229-248). Norwalk, CT: Appleton & Lange.

Fawcett, J. (1995). *Analysis and evaluation of conceptual models of nursing* (3rd ed.). Philadelphia: F. A. Davis.

Fawcett, J. (2000). *Analysis and evaluation of contemporary nursing knowledge: Nursing models and theories.* Philadelphia: F. A. Davis.

Fawcett, J. (2005). *Contemporary nursing knowledge: Analysis and evaluation of nursing models and theories.* Philadelphia: F. A. Davis.

Ference, H. M. (1980). *The relationship of time experience, creativity traits, differentiation and human field motion. An empirical investigation of Rogers' correlates of synergistic human development.* Dissertation Abstracts International, 40, 5206B.

Ference, H. M. (1986). The relationship of time experience, creativity traits, differentiation, and human field motion. In V. M. Malinski (Ed.), *Explorations in Martha Rogers' science of unitary human beings* (pp. 95-106). Norwalk, CT: Appleton-Century-Crofts.

Floyd, J. A. (1983). Research using Rogers' conceptual system: Development of a testable theorem. *ANS Advances in Nursing Science, 5*(2), 37-48.

Garon, M. (1991). Assessment and management of pain in the home care setting: Application of Rogers' science of unitary human beings. *Holistic Nursing Practice, 6*(1), 47-57.

Gueldner, S. H., Michel, Y., Bramlett, M. H., Liu, C., Johnston, L. W., Endo, E., Minegishi, H., & Carlyle, M. S. (2005). The Well-Being Picture Scale: A revision of the Index of Field Energy. *Nursing Science Quarterly, 18*(1), 42-50.

Hanchett, E. S. (1979). *Community health assessment: A conceptual tool kit.* New York: Wiley.

Hanchett, E. S. (1988). *Nursing frameworks and community as client: Bridging the gap.* Norwalk, CT: Appleton & Lange.

Hastings-Tolsma, M. T. (1993). The relationship of diversity of human field pattern to risk-taking and time experience: An investigation of Rogers' principles of homeodynamics (Doctoral dissertation, New York University, 1992). *Dissertation Abstracts International, 53*, 4029B.

Hellwig, S. D., & Ferrante, S. (1993). Martha Rogers' model in associate degree education. *Nurse Educator, 18*(5), 25-27.

Hills, R. G. S., & Hanchett, E. (2001). Human change and individuation in pivotal life situations: Development and testing the theory of enlightenment *Visions: The Journal of Rogerian Nursing Science, 9*(1), 6-19.

Ireland, M. (2000). Martha Rogers' odyssey. *American Journal of Nursing*, 100(10), 59.

Johnston, L. W. (1993a). *The development of the human field image metaphor scale.* Dissertation Abstracts International, 54, 1890B.

Johnston, L. W. (1993b). The development of the human field image metaphor scale. *Visions: Journal of Rogerian Nursing Science, 1*, 55-56.

Johnston, L. W. (1994). Psychometric analysis of Johnston's human field image metaphor scale. *Visions: The Journal of Rogerian Nursing Science, 2*(1), 7-11.

Johnston, R. L. (1986). Approaching family intervention through Rogers' conceptual model. In A. L. Whall (Ed.), *Family therapy theory for nursing. Four approaches* (pp. 11-32). Norwalk, CT: Appleton-Century-Crofts.

Kim, T. S., Park, J. S., & Kim, M. A. (2008). The relation of meditation to power and well-being. *Nursing Science Quarterly, 21*(1), 49-58.

Larkin, D. M. (2007). Ericksonian hypnosis in chronic care support groups: A Rogerian exploration of power and self-defined health-promoting goals. *Nursing Science Quarterly, 20*(4), 357-369.

Leddy, S. K. (1995). Measuring mutual process: Development and psychometric testing of the person-environment participation scale. *Visions: The Journal of Rogerian Nursing Science, 3*(1), 20-31.

Leddy, S. K. (1996). Development and psychometric testing of the Leddy healthiness scale. *Research in Nursing and Health, 19*(5), 431-440.

Leddy, S. K. (1999). Further exploration of the psychometric properties of the Person-Environment Participation Scale: Differentiating instrument reliability and construct validity. *Visions: The Journal of Rogerian Nursing Science, 7*, 55-57.

Leddy, S. K., & Fawcett, J. (1997). Testing the theory of healthiness: Conceptual and methodological issues. In M. Madrid (Ed), *Patterns of Rogerian knowing* (pp. 75-86). New York: National League for Nursing.

Levin, J. D. (2006). Unitary transformative practice: Using metaphor and imagery for self-reflection and theory informed practice. *Visions: The Journal of Rogerian Nursing Science, 14*(1), 27-35.

Lewandowski, W., Good, M., & Drauker, C. B. (2005). Changes in the meaning of pain with the use of guided imagery. *Pain Management Nursing, 6*(2), 58-67.

MacNeil, M. S. (2006). Therapeutic touch, pain, and caring: Implications for nursing practice. *International Journal for Human Caring, 10*(1), 40-48.

Madrid, M. (Ed.). (1997). *Patterns of Rogerian knowing.* New York: National League for Nursing.

Madrid, M. & Winstead-Fry, P. (1986). Rogers' conceptual model. In P. Winstead-Fry (Ed.), *Case studies in nursing theory* (pp. 73-102). New York: National League for Nursing.

Malinski, V. M. (Ed.) (1986). *Explorations on Martha Rogers' science of unitary human beings.* New York: Appleton-Century-Crofts.

Malinski, V. M. (1994). Spirituality: A pattern manifestation of the human/environment mutual process. *Visions: The Journal of Rogerian Nursing Science, 2*, 12-18.

Malinski, V. M. (1997). Rogerian health patterning: Evolving into the 21st century. *Nursing Science Quarterly, 10*(3), 115-116.

Malinski, V. M. (2006). Rogerian science-based nursing theories. *Nursing Science Quarterly, 19*(1), 7-12.

Malinski, V. M., & Barrett, E. A. M. (1994). *Martha E. Rogers: Her life and her work.* Philadelphia: F. A. Davis.

Mathwig, G. M., Young, A. A., & Pepper, J. M. (1990). Using Rogerian science in undergraduate and graduate nursing education. In E. A. M. Barrett (Ed.), *Visions of Rogers' science-based nursing* (pp. 319-334). New York: National League for Nursing.

McCanse, R. L. (1988). *Healthy death readiness: Development of a measurement instrument.* Dissertation Abstracts International, 48, 2606B.

McCanse, R. L. (1995). The McCanse Readiness for Death Instrument (MRDI): A reliable and valid measure for hospice care. *Hospice Journal: Physical, Psychosocial, and Pastoral Care of the Dying, 10*(1), 15-26.

Newman, M. A. (1997). A dialogue with Martha Rogers and David Bohm about the science of unitary human beings. In M. Madrid (Ed.), *Patterns of Rogerian knowing* (pp. 3-10). New York: National League for Nursing.

Paletta, J. L. (1988). *The relationship of temporal experience to human time.* Dissertations Abstracts International, 49, 1621B-1622B.

Paletta, J. L. (1990). The relationship of temporal experience to human time. In E. A. M. Barrett (Ed.), *Visions of Rogers' science-based nursing* (pp. 239-254). New York: National League for Nursing.

Reed, P. G. (1986). The developmental conceptual framework: Nursing reformulations and applications for family therapy. In A. L. Whall (Ed.), *Family therapy for nursing. Four approaches* (pp. 69-91). Norwalk, CT: Appleton-Century-Crofts.

Reed, P. G. (1991). Toward a nursing theory of self-transcendence: Deductive reformulation using developmental theories. *ANS Advances in Nursing Science, 13*(4), 64-77.

Reed, P. G. (2003). The theory of self-transcendence. In M. J. Smith & P. R. Liehr (Eds.), *Middle range theory for nursing* (pp. 145-166). New York: Springer.

Riehl, J. P., & Roy, C. (Eds.). (1980). *Conceptual models for nursing practice* (2nd ed.). New York: Appleton-Century-Crofts.

Rogers, M. E. (1970). *An introduction to the theoretical basis of nursing.* Philadelphia: F. A. Davis.

Rogers, M. E. (1980). *The science of unitary man. Tape V: Health and illness* (Audiotape). New York: Media for Nursing.

Rogers, M. E. (1983). Science of unitary human beings: A paradigm for nursing. In I. W. Clements & F. B. Roberts, *Family health: A theoretical approach to nursing care* (pp. 219-227). New York: John Wiley & Sons.

Rogers, M. E. (1986a). Science of unitary human beings. In V. M. Malinski (Ed.), *Explorations in Martha Rogers' science of unitary human beings* (pp. 3-8). Norwalk, CT: Appleton-Century-Crofts.

Rogers, M. E. (1986b). *Dimensions of health: A view from space.* Paper presented at the conference on "Law and Life in Space," September 12, 1986. Center for Aerospace Sciences, University of North Dakota.

Rogers, M. E. (1989). Nursing: A science of unitary human beings. In J. P. Riehl-Sisca (Ed.), *Conceptual models for nursing practice* (3rd ed., pp. 181-188). Norwalk, CT: Appleton-Century-Crofts.

Rogers, M. E. (1990). Space-age paradigm for new frontiers in nursing. In M. E. Parker (Ed.), *Nursing theories in practice* (pp. 105-114). New York: National League for Nursing.

Rogers, M. E. (1992). Nursing science and the space age. *Nursing Science Quarterly, 5*(1), 27-34.

Rogers, M. E. (1994a). Nursing science evolves. In M. Madrid & E. A. M. Barrett (Eds.), *Rogers' scientific art of nursing practice* (pp. 3-9). New York: National League for Nursing.

Rogers, M. E. (1994b). The science of unitary human beings: Current perspectives. *Nursing Science Quarterly, 7*(1), 33-35.

Sherman, D. W. (1997). Rogerian science: Opening new frontiers of nursing knowledge through its application in quantitative research. *Nursing Science Quarterly, 10*(3), 131-135.

Siedliecki, S. L. & Good, M. (2006). Effect of music on power, pain, depression and disability. *Journal of Advanced Nursing, 54*(5), 553-562.

Smith, D. W. (1994). Toward developing a theory of spirituality. *Visions: The Journal of Rogerian Nursing Science, 2*, 35-43.

Smith, K., Kupferschmid, B. J., Dawson, C., & Briones, T. L. (1991). A family-centered critical care unit. *AACN Clinical Issues, 2*, 258-268.

Smith, M. C. (1999). Caring and the science of unitary human beings. *Advances in Nursing Science, 21*(4), 14-28.

Smith, M. C., Kemp, J., Hemphill, L., & Vojir, C. P. (2002). Outcomes of therapeutic massage for hospitalized cancer patients. *Journal of Nursing Scholarship, 34*(3), 257-262.

Smith, M. C. & Kyle, L. (2008). Holistic foundations of aromatherapy for nursing. *Holistic Nursing Practice, 22*(1), 3-11.

Tettero, I., Jackson, S., & Wilson, S. (1993). Theory to practice: Developing a Rogerian-based assessment tool. *Journal of Advanced Nursing, 18*, 776-782.

von Bertalanffy, L. (1960). *General system theory: Foundations, developments, application.* New York: George Braziller.

Walling, A. (2006). Therapeutic modulation of the psychoneuroimmune system by medical acupuncture creates enhanced feelings of well-being. *Journal of the American Academy of Nurse Practitioners, 18*(4), 135-143.

Watson, J. (1994). Relationship of sleep-wake rhythm, dream experience, human field motion, and time experience in older women. (Doctoral dissertation, New York University, 1993). *Dissertation Abstracts International, 54(12)*, 6137B.

Watson, J. (1999). Measuring dreaming as a beyond waking experience in Rogers' conceptual model. *Nursing Science Quarterly, 12*, 245-250.

Watson, J., Barrett, E. A. M., Hastings-Tolsma, M., Johnston, L., & Gueldner, S. (1997). Measurement in Rogerian science: A review of selected instruments. In M. Madrid (Ed.), *Patterns of Rogerian knowing* (pp 87-99). New York: National League for Nursing.

Whall, A. L. (1981). Nursing theory and the assessment of families. *Journal of Psychiatric Nursing and Mental Health Services, 19*(1), 30-36.

Whall, A. L. (1987). A critique of Rogers' framework. In R. R. Parse (Ed.), *Nursing science: Major paradigms, theories, and critiques* (pp. 147-158). Philadelphia: W. B. Saunders.

Wright, S. M. (1989). *Development and construct validity of the energy field assessment form.* Dissertation Abstracts International, 49, 3113B.

Wright, S.M. (1991). Validity of the human energy field assessment form. *Western Journal of Nursing Research, 13*, 635-647.

Yarcheski, A., & Mahon, N. E. (1991). An empirical test of Rogers' original and revised theory of correlates in adolescents. *Research in Nursing and Health, 14*, 447-455.

Young, A., Taylor, S. G., & McLaughlin-Renpenning, K. (2001). *Connections: Nursing research, theory, and practice.* St. Louis: Mosby.

Zahourek, R. P. (2005). Intentionality: Evolutionary development in healing: A grounded theory study for holistic nursing. *Journal of Holistic Nursing, 23*, 89-109.

BIBLIOGRAPHY

Primary Sources

Books

Rogers, M. E. (1961). *Educational revolution in nursing.* New York: Macmillan.

Rogers, M. E. (1964). *Reveille in nursing.* Philadelphia: F. A. Davis.

Rogers, M. E. (1970). *An introduction to the theoretical basis of nursing.* Philadelphia: F. A. Davis.

Book Chapters

Rogers, M. E. (1977). Nursing: To be or not to be. In B. Bullough & V. Bullough (Eds.), *Expanding horizons for nursing.* New York: Springer.

Rogers, M. E. (1978). Emerging patterns in nursing education. In *Current perspectives in nursing education* (Vol. II, pp. 1-8). St. Louis: Mosby.

Rogers, M. E. (1980). Nursing: A science of unitary man. In J. P. Riehl & C. Roy, *Conceptual models for nursing practice* (2nd ed., pp. 329-337). New York: Appleton-Century-Crofts.

Rogers, M. E. (1981). Science of unitary man: A paradigm for nursing. In G. E. Laskar, *Applied systems and cybernetics* (Vol. IV, pp. 1719-1722). New York: Pergamon.

Rogers, M. E. (1983). Beyond the horizon. In N. L. Chaska, *The nursing profession: A time to speak.* New York: McGraw-Hill.

Rogers, M. E. (1983). The family coping with a surgical crisis: Analysis and application of Rogers' theory to nursing care. (Rogers' response). In I. W. Clements & F. B. Roberts, *Family health: A theoretical approach to nursing care.* New York: John Wiley & Sons.

Rogers, M. E. (1985). High touch in a high-tech future. In National League for Nursing, *Perspectives in nursing—1985-1987* (pp. 25-31). New York: National League for Nursing.

Rogers, M. E. (1985). Nursing education: Preparing for the future. In National League for Nursing, *Patterns of education: The unfolding of nursing* (pp. 11-14). New York: National League for Nursing.

Rogers, M. E. (1985). Science of unitary human beings: A paradigm for nursing. In R. Wood & J. Kekhababh, *Examining the cultural implications of Martha E. Rogers' science of unitary human beings* (pp. 13-23). Lecompton, KS: Wood-Kekhababh Associates.

Rogers, M. E. (1986). Science of unitary human beings. In V. M. Malinski, *Explorations on Martha Rogers: Science of unitary human beings* (pp. 3-8). Norwalk, CT: Apple-ton-Century-Crofts.

Rogers, M. E. (1987). Nursing research in the future. In J. Roode (Ed.), *Changing patterns in nursing education* (pp. 121-123). New York: National League for Nursing.

Rogers, M. E. (1987). Rogers' science of unitary human beings. In R. R. Parse, *Nursing science: Major paradigms, theories, and critiques* (pp. 139-146). Philadelphia: W. B. Saunders.

Rogers, M. E. (1989). Nursing: A science of unitary human beings. In J. P. Riehl-Sisca (Ed.), *Conceptual models for nursing practice* (3rd ed., pp. 181-188). Norwalk, CT: Appleton & Lange.

Rogers, M. E. (1990). Nursing: Science of unitary, irreducible, human beings: Update 1990. In E. A. M. Barrett, *Visions of Rogers' science-based nursing.* New York: National League for Nursing.

Rogers, M. E. (1992). Nightingale's notes on nursing: Prelude to the 21st century. In F. Nightingale, *Notes on nursing; What it is and what it is not* (Commemorative edition, pp. 58-62). Philadelphia: J. B. Lippincott.

Rogers, M. E., Doyle, M. B., Racolin, A., & Walsh, P. C. (1990). A conversation with Martha Rogers on nursing in space. In E. A. M. Barrett (Ed.), *Visions of Rogers' science-based nursing* (pp. 375-386). New York: National League for Nursing.

Journal Articles

Rogers, M. E. (1963). Building a strong educational foundation. *American Journal of Nursing, 63,* 94-95.

Rogers, M. E. (1963). Some comments on the theoretical basis of nursing practice. *Nursing Science, 1,* 11-13, 60-61.

Rogers, M. E. (1963). The clarion call. *Nursing Science, 1,* 134-135.

Rogers, M. E. (1964). Professional standards: Whose responsibility? *Nursing Science, 2,* 71-73.

Rogers, M. E. (1965). Collegiate education in nursing (Editorial). *Nursing Science, 3*(5), 362-365.

Rogers, M. E. (1965). Higher education in nursing (Editorial). *Nursing Science, 3*(6), 443-445.

Rogers, M. E. (1965). Legislative and licensing problems in health care. *Nursing Administration Quarterly, 2,* 71-78.

Rogers, M. E. (1965). What the public demands of nursing today. *RN, 28,* 80.

Rogers, M. E. (1966). Doctoral education in nursing. *Nursing Forum, 5*(2), 75-82.

Rogers, M. E. (1968). Nursing science: Research and researchers. *Teachers College Record, 69,* 469.

Rogers, M. E. (1969). Nursing education for professional practice. *Catholic Nurse, 18*(1), 28-37, 63-64.

Rogers, M. E. (1969). Preparation of the baccalaureate degree graduate. *New Jersey State Nurses Association Newsletter, 25*(5), 32-37.

Rogers, M. E. (1970). Yesterday a nurse, tomorrow a manager: What now? *Journal of New York State Nurses Association, 1*(1), 15-21.

Rogers, M. E. (1972). Nursing's expanded role . . . and other euphemisms. *Journal of New York State Nurses Association,* 3(4), 5-10.

Rogers, M. E. (1972). Nursing: To be or not to be? *Nursing Outlook,* 20(1), 42-46.

Rogers, M. E. (1975). Euphemisms and nursing's future. *Image: The Journal of Nursing Scholarship,* 7(2), 3-9.

Rogers, M. E. (1975). Forum: Professional commitment in nursing. *Image: The Journal of Nursing Scholarship, 2,* 12-13.

Rogers, M. E. (1975). Nursing is coming of age. *American Journal of Nursing, 75*(10), 1834-1843, 1859.

Rogers, M. E. (1975). Reactions to the two foregoing presentations. *Nursing Outlook, 20,* 436.

Rogers, M. E. (1975). Research is a growing word. *Nursing Science, 31,* 283-294.

Rogers, M. E. (1975). Yesterday a nurse, today a manager: What now? *Image; The Journal of Nursing Scholarship 2,* 12-13.

Rogers, M. E. (1977). Legislative and licensing problems in health care. *Nursing Administration Quarterly,* 2(3), 71-78.

Rogers, M. E. (1978). A 1985 dissent (Peer review). *Health/PAC Bulletin, 80,* 32-35.

Rogers, M. E. (1979). Contemporary American leaders in nursing: An oral history. An interview with Martha E. Rogers. *Kango Tenbo, 4*(12), 1126-1138.

Rogers, M. E. (1985). The nature and characteristics of professional education for nursing. *Journal of Professional Nursing, 1*(6), 381-383.

Rogers, M. E. (1985). The need for legislation for licensure to practice professional nursing. *Journal of Professional Nursing, 1*(6), 384.

Rogers, M. E. (1988). Nursing science and art A prospective. *Nursing Science Quarterly, 1*(3), 99-102.

Rogers, M. E. (1989). Creating a climate for the implementation of a nursing conceptual framework. *Journal of Continuing Education in Nursing,* 20(3), 112-116.

Rogers, M. E. (1990). AIDS: Reason for optimism. *Philippine Journal of Nursing, 60(2),* 2-3.

Rogers, M. E. (1994). The science of unitary human beings: Current perspectives. *Nursing Science Quarterly, 7*(1), 33-35.

Rogers, M. E., & Malinski, V. (1989). Vital signs in the science of unitary human beings. *Rogerian Nursing Science News, 1*(3), 6.

Audiotapes

Rogers, M. E. (1980). The science of unitary man. Tape I: Unitary man and his world: A paradigm for nursing (Audiotape). New York: Media for Nursing.

Rogers, M. E. (1980). The science of unitary man. Tape II: Developing an organized abstract system (Audiotape). New York: Media for Nursing.

Rogers, M. E. (1980). The science of unitary man. Tape III: Principles and theories (Audiotape). New York: Media for Nursing.

Rogers, M. E. (1980). The science of unitary man. Tape IV: Theories of accelerating change, paranormal phenomenon, and other events (Audiotape). New York: Media for Nursing.

Rogers, M. E. (1980). The science of unitary man. Tape V: Health and illness (Audiotape). New York: Media for Nursing.

Rogers, M. E. (1980). The science of unitary man. Tape VI: Interventive modalities: Translating theories into practice (Audiotape). New York: Media for Nursing.

Rogers, M. E. (1984). Paper presented at Nurses Theorist Conference, Edmonton, Alberta, Canada (Audiotape). Available through Kennedy Recordings, R. R. 5, Edmonton, Alberta, Canada TSP 4B7 (Tel: 403-470-0013).

Rogers, M. E. (1987). Rogers' framework (Audiotape). Nurse Theorist Conference held in Pittsburgh, PA. Available through Meetings International, 1200 Delor Avenue, Louisville, KY 40217.

Videotapes

Distinguished leaders in nursing—Martha Rogers (Videotape). (1982). Capitol Heights, MD: The National Audiovisual Center. Available through National Institutes of Health, National Library of Medicine, Bethesda, MD 20894, and from Sigma Theta Tau International, 550 West North Street, Indianapolis, IN 46202.

The nurse theorist: Portraits of excellence—Martha Rogers (Video/DVD). (1988). Produced by Fuld Video Project, Oakland, CA: Studio III, available from Fitne, Inc., Athens, Ohio.

Dissertation

Rogers, M. E. (1954). The association of maternal and fetal factors with the development of behavior problems among elementary school children. (Doctoral dissertation, Baltimore: Johns Hopkins University, 1954).

Secondary Sources

Books

Barrett, E. A. M. (1990). *Visions of Rogers' science-based nursing.* New York: National League for Nursing.

Barrett, E. A. M. & Malinski, V. M. (1994). *Martha E. Rogers: 80 years of excellence.* New York: Society of Rogerian Scholars.

Madrid, M. (1997). *Patterns of Rogerian knowing.* New York: National League for Nursing.

Madrid, M., & Barrett, E. A. M. (1994). *Rogers' scientific art of nursing practice.* New York: National League for Nursing.

Malinski, V. M. (Ed.). (1986). *Explorations on Martha Rogers' science of unitary human beings.* Norwalk, CT: Appleton-Century-Crofts.

Sarter, B. (1988). *The stream of becoming: A study of Martha Rogers' theory.* New York: National League for Nursing.

Book Chapters

Garon, M. (2002). Science of Unitary Human Beings: Martha E. Rogers. In J. B. George (ed.), *Nursing theories: The base for professional practice* (5th ed., pp. 269-294). Upper Saddle River, NJ: Prentice Hall.

Gunther, M. (2006a). Martha E. Rogers: Unitary Human Beings. In A. Marriner Tomey & M. R. Alligood (Eds.) *Nursing theorists and their work* (6th ed., pp. 244-266). St. Louis: Mosby Elsevier.

Gunther, M. (2006b). Rogers' Science of Unitary Human Beings in nursing practice. In M. R. Alligood & A. Marriner Tomey (Eds.), *Nursing theory: Utilization and application* (3rd ed., pp. 283-305). St. Louis: Mosby Elsevier.

Hemphill, J. C. & Quillen, S. I. (2005). Martha Rogers' model: Science of unitary beings. In J. J. Fitzpatrick & A. L. Whall (Eds.), *Conceptual models of nursing: Analysis and application* (4th ed.). Upper Saddle River, NJ: Pearson Prentice Hall.

Lutjens, L. R. (1995). Martha Rogers: The Science of Unitary Human Beings. In C. M. McQuiston & A. A. Webb (Eds.), *Foundations of nursing theory: Contributions of 12 key theorist* (pp. 3-28). Thousand Oaks, CA: Sage.

Wills, E. (2007). Grand nursing theories based on unitary process. In M. McEwen & E. M. Wills (Eds.), *Theoretical basis for nursing* (2nd ed., pp. 201-223). Philadelphia: Lippincott Williams & Wilkins.

Sitzman, K. & Eichenberger, L. W. (2004). Martha Rogers' Unitary Human Beings. In K. Sitzman & L. W. Eichenberger, *Understanding the work of nurse theorists: A creative beginning* (pp. 143-148). Boston: Jones & Bartlett.

Journal Articles

Alligood, M. R. (2002). A theory of the art of nursing discovered in Rogers' science of unitary human beings. *International Journal of Human Caring, 6*(2), 55-60.

Alligood, M. R. & Fawcett, J. (2004). An interpretive study of Martha Rogers' conception of pattern. *Visions: The Journal of Rogerian Science, 12*(1), 8-13.

Barnes, S. J., & Adair, B. (2002). The cognitive-sensitive approach to dementia parallels with the science of unitary human beings. *Journal of Psychosocial Nursing and Mental Health Services*, 40(11), 30-37, 44-45.

Barrett, E. A. M. (2000). Speculations on the unpredictable future of the science of unitary human beings. *Visions: The Journal of Rogerian Science, 8*(1), 15-25.

Barrett, E. A. M. (2006). The theoretical matrix for a Rogerian nursing practice. *Theoria Journal of Nursing Theory, 15*(4), 11-15.

Biley, F. C. (2000). Nursing for the new millennium: Martha Rogers and the science of unitary human beings. *Theoria: Journal of Nursing Theory, 9*(3), 19-22.

Biley, A. & Biley, F. C. (2006). Nursing models and theories: More than just passing fads. *Theoria Journal of Nursing Theory, 15*(4), 16-22.

Butcher, H. K. (2000). Critical theory and Rogerian science: Incommensurable or reconcilable. *Visions: The Journal of Rogerian Science, 8*(1), 50-57.

Butcher, H. K. (2000). Rogerian-praxis: A synthesis of Rogerian practice models and theories. *Rogerian Nursing Science News, 12*(1), 2.

Butcher, H. K. (2002). Living in the heart of helicy: An inquiry into the meaning of compassion and unpredictability within Rogers' nursing science. *Visions: The Journal of Rogerian Science, 10*(1), 6-22.

Butcher, H. K. (2004). Written expression and the potential to enhance knowing participation in change. *Visions: The Journal of Rogerian Science, 12*(1), 37-50.

Butcher, H. K. (2005). The unitary field pattern portrait research method: facets, processes, and findings. *Nursing Science Quarterly, 18*(4), 293-297.

Butcher, H. K. (2006). Unitary pattern-based praxis: A nexus of Rogerian cosmology, philosophy, and science. *Visions: The Journal of Rogerian Science, 14*(2), 8-33.

Cowling, W. R. (2001). Unitary appreciative inquiry. *ANS Advances in Nursing Science, 23*(4), 32-48.

Cowling, W. R. (2004). Despair: A unitary appreciative inquiry. *Advances in Nursing Science, 27*(4), 287-300.

Cowling, W. R. (2004). Pattern, participation, praxis, and power in unitary appreciative inquiry. *Advances in Nursing Science, 27*(3), 202-214.

Cowling, W. R. (2005). Despairing women and healing outcomes: A unitary appreciative nursing perspective. *Advances in Nursing Science, 28*(2), 94-106.

Cowling, W. R. (2006). A unitary healing praxis model for women in despair. *Nursing Science Quarterly, 19*(2), 123-132.

Cowling, W. R. (2007). A unitary participatory vision of nursing knowledge. *Advances in Nursing Science, 30*(1), 61-70.

Cowling, W. R. & Taliaferro, D. (2004). Emergence of a healing-caring perspective: Contemporary conceptual and theoretical directions. *Journal of Theory Construction & Testing, 8*(2), 54-59.

Cox, T. (2003). Theory and exemplars of advanced practice spiritual intervention. *Complementary Therapies in Nursing & Midwifery, 9*, 30-34.

Davis, L. A. (2006). The experience of time and nursing practice. *Visions: The Journal of Rogerian Science, 14*(1), 36-44.

DiJoseph, J. & Cavendish, R. (2005). Expanding the dialogue on prayer relevant to holistic care. *Holistic Nursing Practice, 19*(4), 147-155.

Eschiti, V. S. (2006). Journey into chaos: Quantifying the human energy field. *Visions: The Journal of Rogerian Science, 14*(1), 50-57.

Fawcett, J. (2003). The nurse theorists: 21st century updates—Martha E. Rogers. *Nursing Science Quarterly, 16*(1), 44-51.

Fawcett, J. (2003). The science of unitary human beings: Analysis of qualitative research approaches. *Visions: The Journal of Rogerian Science, 11*(1), 7-20.

Fawcett, J., & Alligood, M. R. (2001). SUHB instruments: An overview of research instruments and clinical tools derived from the science of unitary human beings. *Theoria: Journal of Nursing Theory, 10*(3), 5-12.

France, N., Fields, A., & Garth, K. (2004). "You're just shoved to the corner:" The lived experience of Black nursing students being isolated and discounted: A pilot study. *Visions: The Journal of Rogerian Science, 12*(1), 28-36.

Frimel, T. J. (2001). Holistic modalities. Florence Nightingale, Martha Rogers and the art of feng shui. *Beginnings, 21*(1), 10.

Green, A. (2006). A person-centered approach to palliative care nursing. *Journal of Hospice and Palliative Nursing, 8*(5), 294-301.

Hanley, M. A. & Fenton, M. V. (2007). Exploring improvisation in nursing. *Journal of Holistic Nursing, 25*(2), 126-133.

Hardin, S. R. (2003). Spirituality as integrality among chronic heart failure patients: A pilot study. *Visions: The Journal of Rogerian Science, 11*(1), 43-53.

Hastings-Tolsma, M. (2006). Toward a theory of diversity of human field pattern. *Visions: The Journal of Rogerian Science, 14*(2), 34-47.

Hikosaka, A., Hiramatsu, N., Oikawa, M., Shibata, M., & Hanchett, E. (2001). Martha Rogers and the polar bears: A cross-cultural study, session on the principles of homeodynamics. *Visions: The Journal of Rogerian Nursing Science, 9*(1), 58-60.

Hurley, M. (2005). A Rogerian exploration of nurse managers' experience of job satisfaction, stress, and power. *Visions: The Journal of Rogerian Science, 13*(1), 12-26.

Johnston, L. W. (2001). An exploration of individual preferences for audio enhancement of the dying environment. *Visions: The Journal of Rogerian Nursing Science, 9*(1), 20-26.

Kao, H. S., Hsu, M., & Cheng, S. (2006). A Chinese view of the Western nursing metaparadigm. *Journal of Holistic Nursing, 24*(2), 92-101.

Kelly, A. E., Sullivan, P., Fawcett, J., & Samarel, N. (2004). Therapeutic touch, quiet time, and dialogue: Perceptions of women with breast cancer. *Oncology Nursing Forum, 31*(3), 625-631.

Kim, T. S. (2001). Relation of magnetic field therapy to pain and power over time in persons with chronic primary headache: A pilot study. *Visions: The Journal of Rogerian Nursing Science, 9*(1), 27-42.

Kim, T. S. (2004). The concept of magnetism from a Rogerian perspective. *Theoria Journal of Nursing Theory, 13*(4), 4-9.

Leddy, S. K. (2003). A unitary-based nursing practice theory: Theory and application. *Visions: The Journal of Rogerian Science, 11*(1), 21-28.

Leddy, S. K. (2004). Human energy: A conceptual model of unitary nursing practice. *Visions: The Journal of Rogerian Science, 12*(1), 14-27.

Lucero, R. J. & Sousa, K. H. (2006). Participation and change in the nurse work environment. *Visions: The Journal of Rogerian Science, 14*(2), 48-59.

Mahoney, J. (2006). Do you feel like you belong? An on-line versus face-to-face pilot study. *Visions: The Journal of Rogerian Science, 14*(1), 16-26.

Malinski, V. M. (2002). Developing a nursing perspective on spirituality and healing. *Nursing Science Quarterly, 15*(4), 281-287.

Malinski, V. M. (2006). Rogerian science-based nursing theories. *Nursing Science Quarterly, 19*(1), 7-12.

O'Mathuna, D. P., Pryjmachuk, S., Spencer, W., & Matthiesen, S. (2002). A critical evaluation of the theory and practice of therapeutic touch. *Nursing Philosophy, 3*(2), 163-176.

Parse, R. R. (2000). Enjoy your flight: Health in the new millennium. *Visions: The Journal of Rogerian Science, 8*(1), 26-31.

Perkins, J. B. (2003). Healing through spirit: The experience of the eternal in the everyday. *Visions: The Journal of Rogerian Science, 11*(1), 29-42.

Phillips, J. R. (2000). Rogerian nursing science and research: A healing process for nursing. *Nursing Science Quarterly, 13*(3), 196-201.

Salerno, E. M. (2002). Hope, power, and perception of self in individuals recovering from schizophrenia: A Rogerian perspective. *Visions: The Journal of Rogerian Science, 10*(1), 23-36.

Schaefer, P., Vaughn, G., Kenner, C., Donohue, F., & Longo, A. (2000). Revision of a parent satisfaction survey based on the parent perspective. *Journal of Pediatric Nursing: Nursing Care of Children and Families, 15*(6), 373-377.

Shearer, N. B. C., Cisar, N., & Greenburg, E. A. (2007). A telephone-delivered empowerment intervention with patients diagnosed with heart failure. *Heart & Lung, 36*(3), 159-169.

Siedliecki, S. L. (2006). Predictors of self-rated health in patients with chronic nonmalignant pain. *Pain Management Nursing, 7*(3), 109-116.

Smith, D. W. & Broida, J. P. (2007). Pandimensional field pattern changes in healers and healees: Experiencing therapeutic touch. *Journal of Holistic Nursing, 25*(4), 217-225.

Smith, L. H. & Guthrie, B. J. (2005). Testing a model: A developmental perspective of adolescent male sexuality. *Journal for Specialists in Pediatric Nursing, 10*(3), 124-138.

Smith, M. C., Reeder, F., Daniel, L., Baramee, J., & Hagman, J. (2003). Outcomes of touch therapies during bone marrow transplant. *Alternative Therapies in Health & Medicine, 9*(1), 40-49.

Talley, B., Rushing, A., Gee, R. M. (2005). Community assessment using Cowling's unitary appreciative inquiry: A beginning exploration. *Visions: The Journal of Rogerian Science, 13*(1), 27-40.

Todaro-Franceschi, V. (2001). Energy: A bridging concept for nursing science. *Nursing Science Quarterly, 14*(2), 132-140.

Todaro-Franceschi, V. (2001). Pandimensional awareness, purposeful change and the kaleidoscopic cosmos. *Visions: The Journal of Rogerian Nursing Science, 9*(1), 52-57.

Ugarizza, D. N. (2002). Intentionality: Applications within selected theories of nursing. *Holistic Nursing Practice, 16*(4), 41-50.

Vitale, A. (2006). The use of selected energy touch modalities as supportive nursing interventions: Are we there yet? *Holistic Nursing Practice, 20*(4), 191-196.

Vitale, A. T. & O'Connor, P. C. (2006). The effect of Reiki on pain and anxiety in women with abdominal hysterectomies: A quasi-experimental pilot study. *Holistic Nursing Practice, 20*(6), 263-274.

Wall, L. M. (2000). Changes in hope and power in lung cancer patients who exercise. *Nursing Science Quarterly, 13*(3), 234-242.

Watson, J. (2002). Changing paradigms in epidemiology: Catching up with Martha Rogers. *Visions: The Journal of Rogerian Science, 10*(1), 37-50.

Watson, J., Sloyan, C. M., & Robalino, J. E. (2000). The time metaphor test re-visited: Implications for Rogerian research. *Visions: The Journal of Rogerian Science, 8*(1), 32-45.

Watson, J., & Smith, M. C. (2002). Caring science and the science of unitary human beings: A trans-theoretical discourse for nursing knowledge development. *Journal of Advanced Nursing, 37*(5), 452-461.

West, M. M. (2002). Early risk indicators of substance abuse among nurses. *Journal of Nursing Scholarship, 34*(2), 187-193.

Winstead-Fry, P. (2000). Rogers' conceptual system and family nursing. *Nursing Science Quarterly, 13*(4), 278-280.

Wright, B. W. (2004). Trust and power in adults: An investigation using Rogers' Science of Unitary Human Beings. *Nursing Science Quarterly, 17*(2), 139-146.

Wright, B. W. (2007). The evolution of Rogers' science of unitary human beings: 21st century reflections. *Nursing Science Quarterly, 20*(1), 64-67.

Yarcheski, A., Mahon, N. E., & Yarcheski, T. J. (2002). Humor and health in early adolescents: Perceived field motion as a mediating variable. *Nursing Science Quarterly, 15*(2), 150-155.

Yarcheski, A., Mahon, N. E., & Yarcheski, T. J. (2004). Health and well-being in early adolescents using Rogers' science of unitary human beings. *Nursing Science Quarterly, 17*(1), 72-77.

Doctoral Dissertations

Alligood, R. R. (2007). *The life pattern of people with spinal cord injury.* Unpublished doctoral dissertation, Virginia Commonwealth University, Richmond, VA.

Brady, N. R. (2004). *A portrait of families with a member labeled schizophrenic.* Unpublished doctoral dissertation, Case Western Reserve University, Cleveland, OH.

Cox, T. (2004). *Risk induced professional caregiver despair: A unitary appreciative inquiry.* Virginia Commonwealth University, Richmond, VA.

Dye, M. K. (2000). *"Getting back into the swing of things:" A Rogerian portrait of living with traumatic brain injury.* Unpublished doctoral dissertation, University of South Carolina, Columbia, SC.

Grantham, C. A. (2005). *Individual and maternal factors influential with male adolescent physical sexual intimacy.* Unpublished doctoral dissertation, University of Michigan, Ann Arbor, MI.

Hegeman, G. B. (2004). *What is the experience of illness as a change agent: A phenomenological and hermeneutical study.* Unpublished doctoral dissertation, Union Institute and University, Cincinnati, OH.

Hurley, M. (2002). *The relations of stress, power, and job satisfaction in female nurse managers within Rogers' Science of Unitary Human Beings (M. E. Rogers, E. A. M. Barrett).* Unpublished doctoral dissertation, New York University, New York.

Jones, R. (2002). *The relations of dyadic trust, sensation-seeking, and sexual imposition with sexual risk behaviors in young, urban women with primary and non-primary male partners.* Unpublished doctoral dissertation, New York University, New York.

Kemp, J. E. (2004). *Women deployed: Pattern profiles of women who served during the Persian Gulf War.* Unpublished doctoral dissertation, University of Colorado Health Sciences Center, Denver, CO.

Kim, T. S. (2000). *Magnetic field therapy: An exploration of its relation to pain and power in adults with chronic primary headache from a Rogerian perspective.* Unpublished doctoral dissertation, New York University, New York.

Larkin, D. M. (2001). *Ericksonian hypnotherapeutic approaches in chronic care support groups: A Rogerian exploration of power and self-defined health promoting goals.* Unpublished doctoral dissertation, New York University, New York.

Lewandowski, W. A. (2002). *Patterning of pain and power with guided imagery: An experimental study of persons experiencing chronic pain.* Unpublished doctoral dissertation, Case Western Reserve University, Cleveland, OH.

Liu, C. F. (2004). *A profile of field energy following a sudden episode of physical disablement: A Rogerian perspective.* Unpublished doctoral dissertation, Pennsylvania State University, University Park, PA.

Massari-Novak, F. (2004). *The relationship between power as knowing participation and transformational leadership in baccalaureate nursing students.* Unpublished doctoral dissertation, Widener University, Chester, PA.

McGee, E. M. (2004). *I'm better for having known you: An exploration of self-transcendence in nurses.* Unpublished doctoral dissertation, Boston College, Boston, MA.

Musker, K. M. (2005). *Life patterns of women transitioning through menopause.* Unpublished doctoral dissertation, Loyola University, Chicago, IL.

Noyes, L. E. (2001). *Stories of the oldest-old as they come to face death.* Unpublished doctoral dissertation, George Mason University, Fairfax, VA.

Pisarek, S. C. (2001). *Cross-cultural comparison of medical ethical decision making.* Unpublished doctoral dissertation, Walden University, Minneapolis, MN.

Quinn-Griffin, M. T. (2001). *Quality of life of patients with mucosal ulcerative colitis following ileal pouch anal anastomosis surgery.* Unpublished doctoral dissertation, Case Western Reserve University, Cleveland, OH.

Ring, M. E. (2006). *Reiki and changes in pattern manifestations: A Unitary Field Pattern Portrait research study.* Unpublished doctoral dissertation, The Catholic University of America, Washington, D.C.

Rushing, A. M. (2005). *The unitary life pattern of a group of people experiencing serenity in recovery from addiction to alcohol/drugs in 12-step programs.* Unpublished doctoral dissertation, Virginia Commonwealth University, Richmond, VA.

Salerno, E. M. (2000). *Hope, power, and perception of self in individuals recovering from schizophrenia: A Rogerian science perspective (Martha Rogers).* Unpublished doctoral dissertation, New York University, New York.

Shearer, N. B. C. (2000). *Facilitators of health empowerment in women.* Unpublished doctoral dissertation, University of Arizona, Tucson, AZ.

Siedlecki, S. L. (2005). *The effect of music on power, pain, depression, and disability: A clinical trial.* Unpublished doctoral dissertation, Case Western Reserve University, Cleveland, OH.

Stiles, K. A. (2007). *Complex holism: New worldview for nursing as lived in nursing practice.* Unpublished doctoral dissertation, California Institute of Integral Studies, San Francisco, CA.

Varela, T. (2001). *The mirror behind the mask: Experiences of five people living with HIV/AIDS (immune deficiency) who practice Santeria.* Unpublished doctoral dissertation, New York University, New York.

Walker, M. J. (2004). *The effects of nurses practicing the HeartTouch technique on hardiness, spiritual well-being, and perceived stress.* Unpublished doctoral dissertation, University of Texas at Austin.

West, M. M. (2000). *An investigation of pattern manifestations in substance abuse-impaired nurses.* Unpublished doctoral dissertation, Widener University School of Nursing, Chester, PA.

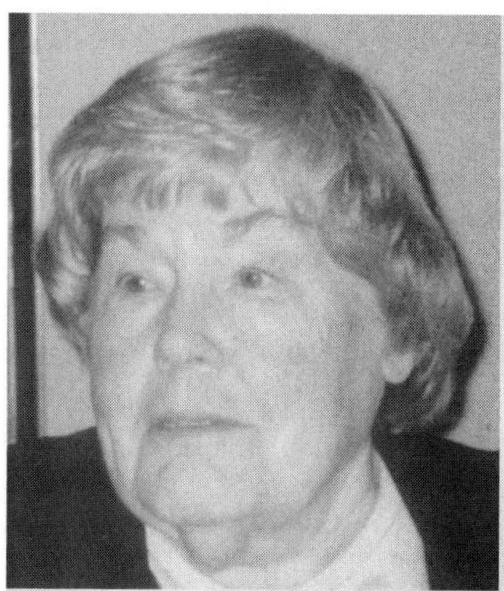

Photo credit: Gerd Bekel Archives, Cloppenburg, Germany.

CHAPTER 14

Dorothea E. Orem

1914-2007

Self-Care Deficit Theory of Nursing

Violeta A. Berbiglia and Barbara Banfield

"Nursing is practical endeavor, but it is practical endeavor engaged in by persons who have specialized theoretic nursing knowledge with developed capabilities to put this knowledge to work in concrete situations of nursing practice" (Orem, 2001, p. 161).

CREDENTIALS AND BACKGROUND OF THE THEORIST

Dorothea Elizabeth Orem, one of America's foremost nursing theorists, was born in Baltimore, Maryland, in 1914. She began her nursing career at Providence Hospital School of Nursing in Washington, DC, where she received a diploma of nursing in the early 1930s. Orem received a BS in Nursing Education from The Catholic University of America (CUA) in 1939, and in 1946, she received an MS in Nursing Education from the same university.

Orem's early nursing experiences included operating room nursing, private duty nursing (home and hospital), hospital staff nursing on pediatric and adult medical and surgical units, evening supervisor in the emergency room, and biological science teaching. Orem held the directorship of both the nursing school and the Department of Nursing at Providence Hospital, Detroit, from 1940 to 1949. After leaving Detroit, she spent 8 years (1949 to 1957) in Indiana working in the Division of Hospital and Institutional Services of the Indiana State Board of Health. Her goal was to upgrade the quality of nursing in general hospitals throughout the state. During this time, Orem developed her definition of nursing practice (Orem, 1956).

In 1957, Orem moved to Washington, DC, to take a position at the Office of Education, U.S. Department of Health, Education, and Welfare, as a curriculum

---

Previous authors: Susan G. Taylor, Angela Compton, Jeanne Donohue Eben, Sarah Emerson, Nergess N. Gashti, Ann Marriner Tomey, Margaret J. Nation, and Sherry B. Nordmeyer. Sang-arun Isaramalai is acknowledged for research and editorial assistance in a previous edition.

consultant. From 1958 to 1960, she worked on a project to upgrade practical nurse training. That project stimulated a need to address the question: What is the subject matter of nursing? As a result, *Guides for Developing Curricula for the Education of Practical Nurses* was developed (Orem, 1959). Later that year, Orem became an assistant professor of nursing education at CUA. She subsequently served as acting dean of the School of Nursing and as associate professor of nursing education. She continued to develop her concepts of nursing and self-care at CUA. Formalization of concepts sometimes was accomplished alone and sometimes with others. Members of the Nursing Models Committee at CUA and the Improvement in Nursing Group, which later became the Nursing Development Conference Group (NDCG), all contributed to the development of the theory. Orem provided intellectual leadership throughout these collaborative endeavors.

In 1970, Orem left CUA and began her own consulting firm. Orem's first published book was *Nursing: Concepts of Practice* (Orem, 1971). She was editor for the NDCG as they prepared and later revised *Concept Formalization in Nursing: Process and Product* (NDCG, 1973, 1979). In 2004, a reprint of the Second Edition was produced and distributed by the International Orem Society for Nursing Science and Scholarship (IOS). Subsequent editions of *Nursing: Concepts of Practice* were published in 1980, 1985, 1991, 1995, and 2001. Orem retired in 1984 and continued working, alone and with colleagues, on the development of Self-Care Deficit Nursing Theory (SCDNT).

Georgetown University conferred on Orem the honorary degree of Doctor of Science in 1976. She received the CUA Alumni Association Award for Nursing Theory in 1980. Other honors received included Honorary Doctor of Science, Incarnate Word College, 1980; Doctor of Humane Letters, Illinois Wesleyan University, 1988; Linda Richards Award, National League for Nursing, 1991; and Honorary Fellow of the American Academy of Nursing, 1992. She was awarded the Doctor of Nursing Honoris Causae from the University of Missouri in 1998.

At age 92, Dorothea Orem's life ended after a period of being bedridden. She died Friday, June 22, 2007, at her residence on Skidaway Island, Georgia. Survivors were her lifelong friend, Walene Shields of Savannah, and her cousin Martin Conover of Minneapolis, Minnesota. Tributes by Dorothea's close colleagues were featured in the IOS official journal, *Self-Care, Dependent-Care & Nursing (SCDCN)*.

Orem's many papers and presentations provide insight into her views on nursing practice, nursing education, and nursing science. Some of these papers are now available to nursing scholars in a compilation edited by Renpenning and Taylor (2003). Other papers of Orem and scholars who worked with her in the development of the theory are archived in Johns Hopkins University.

THEORETICAL SOURCES

Orem (2001) stated, "Nursing belongs to the family of health services that are organized to provide direct care to persons who have legitimate needs for different forms of direct care because of their health states or the nature of their health care requirements" (p. 3). Like other direct health services, nursing has social features and interpersonal features that characterize the helping relations between those who need care and those who provide the required care. What distinguishes these health services from one another is the helping service that each provides. Orem's Self-Care Deficit Nursing Theory provides a conceptualization of the distinct helping service that nursing provides.

Early on, Orem recognized that if nursing was to advance as a field of knowledge and as a field of practice, a structured, organized body of nursing knowledge was needed. From the mid-1950s, when she first put forth a definition of nursing, until shortly before her death in 2007, Orem pursued the development of a theoretical structure that would serve as an organizing framework for such a body of knowledge.

The primary source for Orem's ideas about nursing was her experiences in nursing. Through reflection on nursing practice situations, she was able to identify the proper object, or focus, of nursing. The question that directed Orem's (2001) thinking was, "What condition exists in a person when judgments are made that a nurse(s) should be brought into the situation?"(p. 20). The condition that indicates the need for nursing assistance is "the inability of persons to provide continuously for themselves the amount and quality of required self-care because of situations of personal health" (Orem, 2001, p. 20). It is the proper object or focus that determines the domain and boundaries of nursing, both as a field of knowledge and as a field of practice. The specification of the proper object of nursing marks the beginning of Orem's theoretical work. The efforts of Orem, working independently as well as with colleagues, resulted in the development and refinement of the Self-Care Deficit Nursing Theory (SCDNT). Consisting of a number of conceptual elements and three theories that specify the relationships among these concepts, the SCDNT is a general theory, "one that is descriptively explanatory of nursing in all types of practice situations" (Orem, 2001, p. 22)

In addition to her experiences in nursing practice situations, Orem was well versed in contemporary nursing literature and thought. Her association with nurses over the years provided many learning experiences, and she viewed her work with graduate students and her collaborative work with colleagues as valuable endeavors. Orem cited many other nurses' work in terms of their contributions to nursing, including, but not limited to, Abdellah, Henderson, Johnson, King, Levine, Nightingale, Orlando, Peplau, Riehl, Rogers, Roy, Travelbee, and Wiedenbach.

Orem's familiarity with literature was not limited to nursing literature. In her discussion of various topics related to nursing, Orem cited authors from a number of other disciplines. The influence of scholars such as Allport (1955), Arnold (1960a, 1960b), Barnard (1962), Fromm (1962), Harre (1970), Macmurray (1957, 1961), Maritain (1959), Parsons (1949, 1951), Plattel (1965), and Wallace (1979, 1996) can be seen in Orem's ideas and positions. Familiarity with these sources helps to promote a comprehensive understanding of Orem's work.

Foundational to Orem's SCDNT is the philosophical system of moderate realism. Banfield (1997) conducted a philosophical inquiry to explicate the metaphysical and epistemological underpinnings of Orem's work. This inquiry revealed consistency between Orem's views regarding the nature of reality, the nature of human beings, and the nature of nursing as a science and the ideas and positions associated with the philosophy of moderate realism. Taylor, Geden, Isaramalai, and Wongvatunyu (2000) also explored the philosophical foundations of the SCDNT.

According to the moderate realist position, there is a world that exists independent of the thoughts of the knower. Although the nature of the world is not determined by the thoughts of the knower, it is possible to obtain knowledge about the world.

Orem did not specifically address the nature of reality; however, statements and phrases that she uses reflect a moderate realist position. Four categories of postulated entities are identified as establishing the ontology of the SCDNT (Orem, 2001, p. 141). These four categories are (1) persons in space-time localizations, (2) attributes or properties of these persons, (3) motion or change, and (4) products brought into being.

With regard to the nature of human beings, "the view of human beings as dynamic, unitary beings who exist in their environments, who are in the process of becoming, and who possess free-will as well as other essential human qualities" is foundational to SCDNT (Banfield, 1997, p. 204). This position, which reflects the philosophy of moderate realism, can be seen throughout Orem's work.

Orem (1997) identified "five broad views of human beings that are necessary for developing understanding of the conceptual constructs of self-care deficit nursing theory and for understanding the interpersonal and societal aspects of nursing systems" (p. 28). These are the view of (1) person, (2) agent, (3) user of symbols, (4) organism, and (5) object. The view of human beings as person reflects the philosophical position of moderate realism; it is this position regarding the nature of human beings that is foundational to Orem's work. She made the point that taking a particular view for some practical purpose does not negate the position that human beings are unitary beings (Orem, 1997, p. 31).

The view of person-as-agent is central to the SCDNT. Self-care, which refers to those actions in which a person engages for the purpose of promoting and maintaining life, health, and well-being, is conceptualized as a form of deliberate action. "Deliberate action refers to actions performed by individual human beings who have intentions and are conscious of their intentions to bring about, through their actions, conditions or states of affairs that do not at present exist" (Orem, 2001, pp. 62-63). When engaging in deliberate action, the person acts as an agent. The view of person-as-agent also is reflected in other conceptual elements of the SCDNT. In relation to the view of person-as-agent and the idea of deliberate action, Orem cited a number of scholars, including Arnold, Parsons, and Wallace. She identified seven assumptions regarding human beings that pertain to deliberate action (Orem, 2001, p. 65). These explicit assumptions, while addressing deliberate action, rest upon the implicit assumption that human beings have free will.

The SCDNT represents Orem's work regarding the substance of nursing as a field of knowledge and as a field of practice. She also put forth a position regarding the form of nursing as a science, identifying it as a practical science. The work of Maritain (1959) and Wallace (1979), philosophers associated with the moderate realist tradition, are cited in relation to her ideas about the form of nursing science. In practical sciences, knowledge is developed for the sake of the work to be done. In the case of nursing, knowledge is developed for the sake of nursing practice. Two components make up the practical science: the speculative and the practical. The speculatively practical component is theoretical in nature, while the practically practical component is directive of action. The SCDNT represents speculatively practical knowledge. Practically practical nursing science is made up of models of practice, standards of practice, and technologies.

Orem (2001) identified two sets of speculatively practical nursing science: nursing practice sciences and foundational nursing sciences. The set of nursing practice sciences includes (1) wholly compensatory nursing science, (2) partly compensatory nursing science, and (3) supportive developmental nursing science. The foundational nursing sciences are (1) the science of self-care, (2) the science of the development and exercise of the self-care agency in the absence or presence of limitations for deliberate action, and (3) the science of human assistance for persons with health-associated self-care deficits. In relation to this proposed structure of nursing sciences, Orem stated, "the isolation, naming, and description of the two sets of sciences are based on my understanding of the nature of the practical sciences, on my knowledge of the organization of subject matter in other practice fields, and on my understanding of components of curricula for education for the professions" (pp. 174-175).

In addition to the two components or types of practical science, scientific knowledge necessary for nursing practice includes sets of applied sciences and basic non-nursing sciences. In the development of applied sciences, theories from other fields are used to solve problems in the practice field. These applied nursing sciences have yet to be identified and developed. Box 14-1 depicts the structure of nursing science.

Box 14-1 *Speculatively Practical Nursing Science*

NURSING PRACTICE SCIENCES

Wholly Compensatory Nursing

Partly Compensatory Nursing

Supportive-Developmental Nursing

FOUNDATIONAL NURSING SCIENCES

The Science of Self-Care

The Science of the Development and Exercise of Self-Care Agency in the Absence or Presence of Limitations for Deliberate Action

The Science of Human Assistance for Persons with Health-Associated Self-Care Deficits

APPLIED NURSING SCIENCES

BASIC NON-NURSING SCIENCES

Biological

Medical

Human

Environmental

From Orem, D. E. (2001). *Nursing: Concepts of practice* (6th ed.). St. Louis: Mosby.

Orem's articulation of the form of nursing science provided the framework for the development of a body of knowledge for the education of nurses and for the provision of nursing care in concrete situations of nursing practice. The SCDNT with its conceptual elements and three theories identifies the substance or content of nursing science.

MAJOR CONCEPTS & DEFINITIONS

Orem labeled her self-care deficit nursing theory as a general theory composed of the following three related theories:

1. The theory of self-care, which describes why and how people care for themselves
2. The theory of self-care deficit, which describes and explains why people can be helped through nursing
3. The theory of nursing systems, which describes and explains relationships that must be brought about and maintained for nursing to be produced

The major concepts of Orem's theories are identified here and discussed more fully in Orem (2001), *Nursing: Concepts of Practice* (see Figure 14-1).

SELF-CARE

Self-care comprises the practice of activities that maturing and mature persons initiate and perform, within time frames, on their own behalf in the interest of maintaining life, healthful functioning, continuing personal development, and well-being by meeting known requisites for functional and developmental regulations (Orem, 2001, p. 522).

DEPENDENT CARE

Dependent care refers to the care that is provided to a person who, because of age or related factors, is unable to perform the self-care needed to maintain life, healthful functioning, continuing personal development, and well-being.

SELF-CARE REQUISITES

A self-care requisite is a formulated and expressed insight about actions to be performed that are known or hypothesized to be necessary in the regulation of an aspect(s) of human functioning and development, continuously or under specified conditions and circumstances. A formulated self-care requisite names the following two elements:

1. The factor to be controlled or managed to keep an aspect(s) of human functioning and development within the norms compatible with life, health, and personal well-being
2. The nature of the required action

> Formulated and expressed self-care requisites constitute the formalized purposes of self-care. They are the reasons for which self-care is undertaken; they express the intended or desired result—the goal of self-care (Orem, 2001, p. 522).

UNIVERSAL SELF-CARE REQUISITES

Universally required goals are to be met through self-care or dependent care, and they have their origins in what is known and what is validated, or what is in the process of being validated, about human structural and functional integrity at various stages of the life cycle. The following eight self-care requisites common to men, women, and children are suggested:

1. Maintenance of a sufficient intake of air
2. Maintenance of a sufficient intake of food
3. Maintenance of a sufficient intake of water

Continued

MAJOR CONCEPTS & DEFINITIONS—cont'd

4. Provision of care associated with elimination processes and excrements
5. Maintenance of balance between activity and rest
6. Maintenance of balance between solitude and social interaction
7. Prevention of hazards to human life, human functioning, and human well-being
8. Promotion of human functioning and development within social groups in accordance with human potential, known human limitations, and the human desire to be normal. Normalcy is used in the sense of that which is essentially human and that which is in accordance with the genetic and constitutional characteristics and talents of individuals (Orem, 2001, p. 225).

DEVELOPMENTAL SELF-CARE REQUISITES

Developmental self-care requisites (DSCRs) were separated from universal self-care requisites in the second edition of *Nursing: Concepts of Practice* (Orem, 1980). Three sets of DSCRs have been identified, as follows:

1. Provision of conditions that promote development
2. Engagement in self-development
3. Prevention of or overcoming effects of human conditions and life situations that can adversely affect human development (Orem, 1980, p. 231)

HEALTH DEVIATION SELF-CARE REQUISITES

These self-care requisites exist for persons who are ill or injured, who have specific forms of pathological conditions or disorders, including defects and disabilities, and who are under medical diagnosis and treatment. The characteristics of health deviation as conditions extending over time determine the types of care demands that individuals experience as they live with the effects of pathological conditions and live through their durations.

Disease or injury affects not only specific structures and physiological or psychological mechanisms, but also integrated human functioning. When integrated functioning is affected seriously (severe mental retardation and comatose states), the individual's developing or developed powers of agency are seriously impaired, either permanently or temporarily. In abnormal states of health, self-care requisites arise from both the disease state and the measures used in its diagnosis or treatment.

Care measures to meet existent health deviation self-care requisites must be made action components of individuals' systems of self-care or dependent care. The complexity of self-care or dependent care systems is increased by the number of health deviation requisites that must be met within specific time frames.

THERAPEUTIC SELF-CARE DEMAND

Therapeutic self-care demand consists of the summation of care measures necessary at specific times or over a duration of time to meet all of an individual's known self-care requisites, particularized for existent conditions and circumstances by methods appropriate for the following:

- Controlling or managing factors identified in the requisites, the values of which are regulatory of human functioning (sufficiency of air, water, and food)
- Fulfilling the activity element of the requisite (maintenance, promotion, prevention, and provision) (Orem, 2001, p. 523)

Therapeutic self-care demand at any time (1) describes factors in the patient or the environment that must be held steady within a range of values or brought within and held within such a range for the sake of the patient's life, health, or well-being,

MAJOR CONCEPTS & DEFINITIONS—cont'd

and (2) has a known degree of instrumental effectiveness derived from the choice of technologies and specific techniques for using, changing, or in some way controlling patient or environmental factors.

SELF-CARE AGENCY

The self-care agency is a complex acquired ability of mature and maturing persons to know and meet their continuing requirements for deliberate, purposive action to regulate their own human functioning and development (Orem, 2001, p. 522).

DEPENDENT-CARE AGENCY

Dependent-care agency refers to the acquired ability of a person to know and meet the therapeutic self-care demand of the dependent person and/or regulate the development and exercise of the dependent's self-care agency.

SELF-CARE DEFICIT

Self-care deficit is a relation between persons' therapeutic self-care demands and their powers of self-care agency in which the constituent-developed self-care capabilities within self-care agency are not operable or are not adequate for knowing and meeting some or all components of the existent or projected therapeutic self-care demand (Orem, 2001, p. 522).

NURSING AGENCY

Nursing agency comprises developed capabilities of persons educated as nurses that empower them to represent themselves as nurses and within the frame of a legitimate interpersonal relationship to act, to know, and to help persons in such relationships to meet their therapeutic self-care demands and to regulate the development or exercise of their self-care agency (Orem, 2001, p. 518).

NURSING DESIGN

Nursing design, a professional function performed both before and after nursing diagnosis and prescription, allows nurses, on the basis of reflective practical judgments about existent conditions, to synthesize concrete situational elements into orderly relations to structure operational units. The purpose of nursing design is to provide guides for achieving needed and foreseen results in the production of nursing toward the achievement of nursing goals; these units taken together constitute the pattern that guides the production of nursing (Orem, 2001, p. 519).

NURSING SYSTEMS

Nursing systems are series and sequences of deliberate practical actions of nurses performed at times in coordination with the actions of their patients to know and meet components of patients' therapeutic self-care demands and to protect and regulate the exercise or development of patients' self-care agency (Orem, 2001, p. 519).

HELPING METHODS

A helping method from a nursing perspective is a sequential series of actions that, if performed, will overcome or compensate for the health-associated limitations of persons to engage in actions to regulate their own functioning and development or that of their dependents. Nurses use all methods, selecting and combining them in relation to the action demands on persons under nursing care and their health-associated action limitations, as follows:

- Acting for or doing for another
- Guiding and directing
- Providing physical or psychological support
- Providing and maintaining an environment that supports personal development
- Teaching (Orem, 2001, pp. 55-56)

Continued

MAJOR CONCEPTS & DEFINITIONS—cont'd

BASIC CONDITIONING FACTORS

Basic conditioning factors refer to those factors that condition or affect the value of the therapeutic self-care demand and/or the self-care agency of an individual at particular times and under specific circumstances. Ten factors have been identified:

- Age
- Gender
- Developmental state
- Health state
- Pattern of living
- Healthcare system factors
- Family system factors
- Sociocultural factors
- Availability of resources
- External environmental factors

USE OF EMPIRICAL EVIDENCE

As a practical science, nursing knowledge is developed to inform nursing practice. Orem (2001) stated, "nursing is practical endeavor, but it is practical endeavor engaged in by persons who have specialized theoretic nursing knowledge with developed capabilities to put this knowledge to work in concrete situations of nursing practice" (p. 161). The provision of nursing care occurs in concrete situations. As nurses enter into nursing practice situations, they use their knowledge of nursing science to assign meaning to the features of the situation, to made judgments about what can and should be done, and to design and implement systems of nursing care. From the perspective of the SCDNT, desired nursing outcomes include meeting the patient's therapeutic self-care demand and/or regulating and developing the patient's self-care agency.

The conceptual elements and the three specific theories of the SCDNT are abstractions about the features common to all nursing practice situations. The SCDNT was developed and refined through the use of intellectual processes that focused on nursing practice situations. For example, Orem reflected on her nursing practice experiences to identify the proper object of nursing. In their work related to the SCDNT, the Nursing Development Conference Group (1979) engaged in analysis of nursing cases and in processes of analogical reasoning. In a tribute to Orem, Allison (2008) talks about the Nursing Development Conference Group, saying that "these nurses came together because they were interested in and willing to commit themselves to examining nursing situations in order to formalize ways of thinking about nursing that they felt were descriptive of nursing and would contribute to nursing knowledge" (p. 50). Since the SCDNT was first published, extensive empirical evidence has contributed to the development of theoretical knowledge. Much of this is incorporated into continuing refinement of the theory; however, the basics of the theory remain unchanged.

MAJOR ASSUMPTIONS

Assumptions basic to the general theory were formalized during the early 1970s and were first presented at Marquette University School of Nursing in 1973. Orem (2001) identifies the following five premises underlying the general theory of nursing:

1. Human beings require continuous, deliberate inputs to themselves and their environments to remain alive and function in accordance with natural human endowments.
2. Human agency, the power to act deliberately, is exercised in the form of care for self and others in identifying needs and making needed inputs.

3. Mature human beings experience privations in the form of limitations for action in care for self and others involving making of life-sustaining and function-regulating inputs.
4. Human agency is exercised in discovering, developing, and transmitting ways and means to identify needs and make inputs to self and others.
5. Groups of human beings with structured relationships cluster tasks and allocate responsibilities for providing care to group members who experience privations for making required, deliberate input to self and others (p. 140).

Orem stated pre-suppositions and propositions for the theory of self-care, the theory of self-care deficit, and the theory of nursing systems. These constitute the expression of the theories and are summarized below.

THEORETICAL ASSERTIONS

Presented as a general theory of nursing, one that represents a complete picture of nursing, the SCDNT is expressed in the following three theories:

1. Theory of nursing systems
2. Theory of self-care deficit
3. Theory of self-care

The three constituent theories, taken together in relationship, constitute the SCDNT. The theory of nursing systems is the unifying theory and includes all the essential elements. It subsumes the theory of self-care deficit and the theory of self-care. The theory of self-care deficit develops the reason why a person may benefit from nursing. The theory of self-care, foundational to the others, expresses the purpose, method, and outcome of taking care of self.

Theory of Nursing Systems

The theory of nursing systems proposes that nursing is human action; nursing systems are action systems formed (designed and produced) by nurses through the exercise of their nursing agency for persons with health-derived or health-associated limitations in self-care or dependent care. Nursing agency includes concepts of deliberate action, including intentionality, and the operations of diagnosis, prescription, and regulation. Figure 14-1 shows the basic nursing systems categorized according to the relationship between patient and nurse actions. Nursing systems may be produced for individuals, for persons who constitute a dependent-care unit, for groups whose members have therapeutic self-care demands with similar components or who have similar limitations for

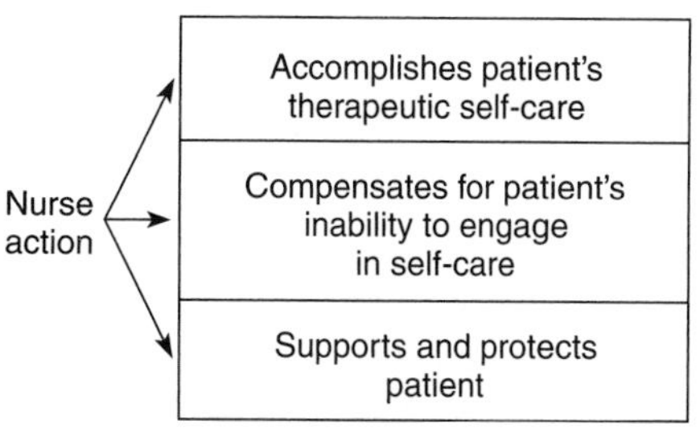

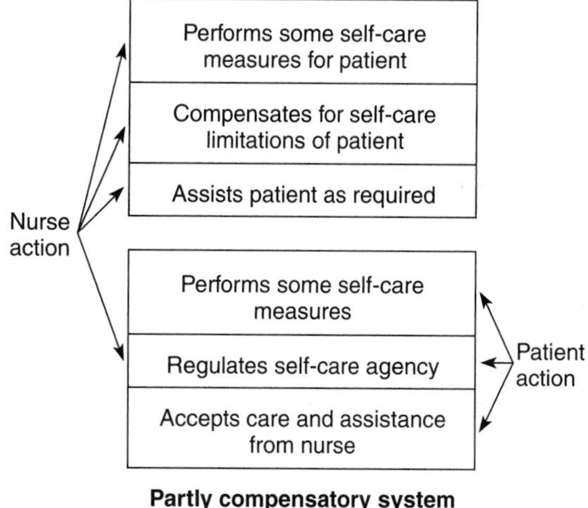

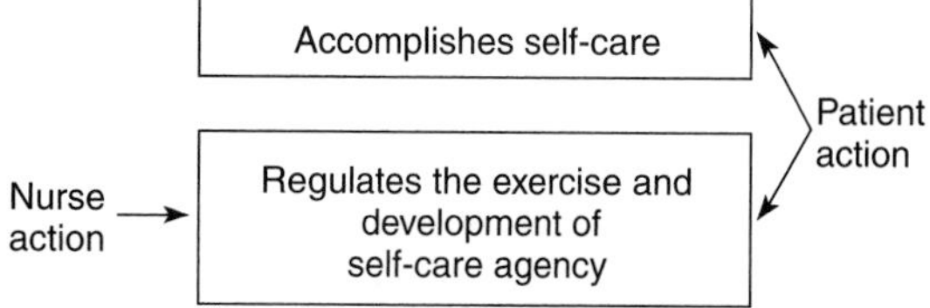

Figure 14-1 Basic nursing systems. (From Orem, D. E. [2001]. *Nursing: Concepts of practice* [6th ed., p. 351]. St. Louis: Mosby.)

engagement in self-care or dependent care, and for families or other multiperson units.

Theory of Self-Care Deficit

The central idea of the theory of self-care deficit is that the requirements of persons for nursing are associated with the subjectivity of mature and maturing persons to health-related or health care–related action limitations. These limitations render them completely or partially unable to know existent and emerging requisites for regulatory care for themselves or their dependents. They also limit the ability to engage in the continuing performance of care measures to control or in some way manage factors that are regulatory of their own or their dependent's functioning and development.

Self-care deficit is a term that expresses the relationship between the action capabilities of individuals and their demands for care. Self-care deficit is an abstract concept that, when expressed in terms of action limitations, provides guides for the selection of methods for helping and understanding patient roles in self-care.

Theory of Self-Care

Self-care is a human regulatory function that individuals must, with deliberation, perform themselves or must have performed for them to maintain life, health, development, and well-being. Self-care is an action system. Elaboration of the concepts of self-care, self-care demand, and self-care agency provides the foundation for understanding the action requirements and action limitations of persons who may benefit from nursing. Self-care, as a human regulatory function, is distinct from other types of regulation of human functioning and development, such as neuroendocrine regulation. Self-care must be learned, and it must be performed deliberately and continuously in time and in conformity with the regulatory requirements of individuals. These requirements are associated with their stages of growth and development, states of health, specific features of health or developmental states, levels of energy expenditure, and environmental factors. The theory of self-care is also extended to a theory of dependent care, wherein the purpose, methods, and outcomes of care of others are expressed (Taylor, Renpenning, Geden, Neuman, & Hart, 2001).

LOGICAL FORM

Orem's insight led to her initial formalization and subsequent expression of a general concept of nursing. This generalization then made possible inductive and deductive thinking about nursing. The form of the theory is shown in the many models that Orem and others have developed, such as those shown in Figure 14-1 and Figure 14-2. Orem described the models and their importance to the development and understanding of the reality of the entities. These models are ". . . directed toward knowing the structure of the processes that are operational or become operational in the production of nursing systems, systems of care for individuals or for dependent-care units or multiperson units served by nurses" (Orem, 1997, p. 31). The overall theory is logically congruent.

ACCEPTANCE BY THE NURSING COMMUNITY

Orem's SCDNT has achieved a significant level of acceptance by the international nursing community, as evidenced by the magnitude of published material. In research, using SCDNT or components, more than 800 references were found (Taylor, 2000). Biggs (2008) updated Taylor's research and found the SCDNT literature to be ever increasing. Berbiglia identified selected practice settings and SCDNT conceptual foci from a review of 3 decades of use of SCDNT in practice and research (1997, 2002, 2006). She publicized selected international SCDNT practice models for the twenty-first century (2006). Allison and McLaughlin-Renpenning (1999) developed a self-care theory approach for nursing administration. SCDNT was introduced as the basic structure for nursing management in German hospital DRG (diagnosis-related group) implementation. The movement toward SCDNT-based nursing management in Germany is credited to Bekel (2002). Although it is difficult to fully assess the international application of the

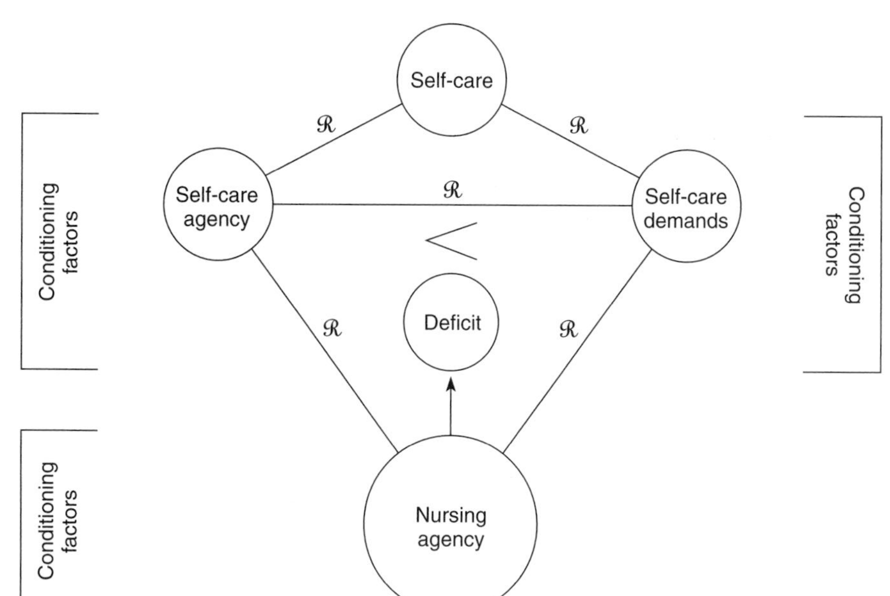

Figure 14-2 A conceptual framework for nursing. *R*, Relationship; <, deficit relationship, current or projected. (From Orem, D. E. [2001]. *Nursing: Concepts of practice* [6th ed., p. 491]. St. Louis: Mosby.)

SCDNT, it is clear that, over time, Germany and Thailand (Harnucharunkul, 2004) have been landmark examples of the successful implementation of the SCDNT.

In 2008, the following U.S. schools (see references for school websites) were among those with SCDNT curriculum frameworks:

- Illinois Wesleyan University School of Nursing (2008)
- University of Tennessee in Chattanooga
- College of Saint Benedict (2008)
- Anderson College
- University of Toledo College of Nursing (2008)
- Alcorn State University Cora S. Balmat School of Nursing (2008)
- Southern University Baton Rouge School of Nursing (2007)

The 10th World Congress for Self-Care and Nursing highlighted SCDNT-based curricula at Illinois Wesleyan University and The University of Tennessee Chattanooga (2008). The influence of Orem's SCDNT continues on the international level through the translation of *Nursing Concepts of Practice* into many languages and the proliferation of SCDNT-based practice, education, and research worldwide.

FURTHER DEVELOPMENT

From the time of publication of the first edition of *Nursing: Concepts of Practice* in 1971, Orem was engaged in continual development of her conceptualizations. She worked by herself and with colleagues. The sixth, and final, edition was completed and published in 2001. Her work with a group of scholars, known as the Orem Study Group, further developed the various conceptualizations and structured nursing knowledge using elements of the theory. This work led to the expression of a theory of dependent care (Taylor et al., 2001) and the foundational science of self-care (Denyes, Orem, & Bekel, 2001). Other scholars have developed models that explain aspects of SCDNT. Philosophical and ethical considerations relative to SCDNT also are available (Banfield, 1997, 2008; Bekel, 1999; Taylor, 1998; Taylor et al., 2000; Taylor & Godfrey, 1999).

Nursing: Concepts of Practice (Orem, 2001) is organized with two foci: nursing as a unique field of knowledge and nursing as practical science. The text includes an expansion, from earlier editions, of content on nursing science and the theory of nursing systems. Important work has been done on the nature of person and interpersonal features of nursing. Orem identified many areas for further development in her descriptions of the stages of theory development. She also described the development of the science of self-care, which could include concepts such as elaboration of operational functions of self-care agency with the elements of sensation and perception, appraisal, and motivation, and determining the relevance of foundational capabilities and dispositions to discreet acts. There is a need to focus on the person in the situation and on capabilities for action and self-management. This content has been expanded in the description of the foundational nursing science of self-care (Denyes et al., 2001).

The International Orem Society for Nursing Science and Scholarship (IOS) was established in 1993. The purpose of the IOS is to advance nursing science and scholarship through the use of Dorothea E. Orem's nursing conceptualizations in nursing education, practice, and research. The IOS publishes *Self-Care, Dependent-Care and Nursing*, an open access online journal on the IOS website (http://www.scdnt.com). Since its inception, the IOS has sponsored international conferences. Gerd Bekel maintains a record of the content of these conferences (gerd.bekel@gbconcept.de).

CRITIQUE

Clarity

The terms Orem used are defined precisely. The language of the theory is consistent with the twenty-first century language used in action theory and philosophy. The terminology of the theory is congruent throughout. The term *self-care* has multiple meanings across disciplines; Orem defined the term and elaborated the substantive structure of the concept in a way that is unique while also congruent with other interpretations. Reference has been made to the difficulty of Orem's language; however, the limitation generally resides in the reader's lack of familiarity with practical science and with the field of action science. Once a basic familiarity with the terminology of the SCDNT is achieved, further reading and studying of Orem's work fosters a comprehensive understanding of her view of nursing as a field of knowledge and as a field of practice.

Simplicity

Orem's theory is expressed in a limited number of terms. These terms are defined and used consistently in the expression of the theory. Orem's general theory, SCDNT, comprises the following three constituent theories: (1) self-care, (2) self-care deficit, and (3) nursing systems. The self-care deficit theory of nursing is a synthesis of knowledge about eight entities, which include self-care (and dependent care), self-care agency (and dependent-care agency), therapeutic self-care demand, self-care deficit, nursing agency, and nursing system. Development of the theory using these entities is parsimonious. The relationship between and among these entities can be presented in a simple diagram. The substantive structure of the theory is seen in the development of these entities. The depth of development of the concepts gives the theory the complexity necessary to describe and understand a human practice discipline.

Generality

Orem (1995) commented on the generality or universality of the theory, as follows:

> The self-care deficit theory of nursing is not an explanation of the individuality of a particular concrete nursing practice situation, but rather the expression of a singular combination of conceptualized properties or features common to all instances of nursing. As a general theory, it serves nurses engaged in nursing practice, in development and validation of nursing knowledge, and in teaching and learning nursing (pp. 166-167).

A review of the research and other literature attests to the generality of the theory.

Empirical Precision

As a general theory, the SCDNT provides a descriptive explanation of why persons require nursing and what processes are needed for production of required nursing care. The concepts of the theory are abstractions of the entities that represent the proper object of nurses in concrete nursing practice situations. Self-care, dependent care, and nursing care all are forms of deliberation action engaged in to achieve a particular purpose. The concepts of therapeutic self-care demand, self-care agency, dependent-care agency, and nursing agency refer to properties of persons. Self-care deficit and dependent-care deficit refer to relationships between properties of persons. Self-care system, dependent-care system, and nursing system are systems of care that are designed and implemented to achieve desired outcomes. Basic conditioning factors refer to factors that condition or influence the variables of persons. These factors may be internal to the person, such as developmental level, or external, such as available resources. In nursing practice situations, the data collected by nurses can be categorized readily according to the concepts of the SCDNT.

For research purposes, both quantitative and qualitative research methods are appropriate for the development of knowledge related to the SCDNT. Specific research methods to be used in any investigation are selected on the basis of the questions being asked. Examples of various approaches can be found in this publication's companion text summary of recent SCDNT-based research (Berbiglia, 2006). Although the concepts of the SCDNT refer to real entities, they are complex in nature. Operationalization of these concepts requires a comprehensive understanding of Orem's work. Instruments to measure some of these concepts have been developed.

In several studies conducted for the purpose of theory testing, instruments designed to measure concepts of the SCDNT have been utilized. According to Orem, the basic conditioning factors condition or influence the therapeutic self-care demand and the self-care agency of persons at particular points in time. General measures of self-care agency, such as the American Society of Anesthesiologists (ASA) scale (Evers, Isenberg, Philipsen, Senten, & Brouns, 1993), have been used to investigate relationships between various basic conditioning factors and self-care agency. These studies usually use correlational designs and statistical techniques and have had mixed findings. Moore and Pichler (2000) reviewed research on basic conditioning factors and concluded that there has been no consensus on the operationalization of these factors. They suggest strategies to address this lack of consensus. The explanation for the lack of expected findings could rest with issues related to measurement and study samples. However, it could well be that the relationships between some of the basic conditioning factors and the variables of therapeutic self-care demand and self-care agency are not captured readily through the use of correlational designs and statistics for aggregates of people.

The current emphasis in SCDNT is on building a body of knowledge based on nursing practice, rather than engaging in theory testing. Instrument development has an important role to play in building nursing knowledge, as well as other types of scholarly work. . . . A great deal of work is needed with regard to the structuring of existent knowledge around the practice sciences and the foundational nursing sciences identified by Orem. Therefore, comprehensive descriptive studies of various populations in terms of their self-care requisites and self-care practices are needed. The structuring of existent knowledge and the findings from descriptive studies will provide a solid base for the development of instruments to measure the concepts of the SCDNT.

Derivable Consequences

The SCDNT differentiates the focus of nursing from other disciplines. Although other disciplines find the theory of self-care helpful and contribute to its development, the theory of nursing systems provides a unique focus for nursing. The significance of Orem's work extends far beyond the development of the SCDNT. In her works, she provided expression of the form of nursing science as practical science, along with a structure for ongoing development of nursing knowledge in the stages of theory development. She presented a visionary view of contemporary nursing practice, education, and knowledge development expressed through the general theory.

SUMMARY

The critical question—What is the condition that indicates that a person needs nursing care?—was the starting point for the development of the SCDNT. Orem noted that it was the inability of persons to maintain on a continuous basis their own care or the care of dependents. From this observation, she began the process of formalizing knowledge about what persons need to do or have done for themselves to maintain health and well-being. When a person needs assistance, what are the appropriate nursing assistive actions? The theory of self-care describes what a person requires and what actions need to be taken to meet those requirements. The theory of self-care deficits describes the limitations involved in meeting requirements for ongoing care and the effects they have on the health and well-being of the person or dependent. The theory of nursing systems provides the structure for examining the actions and antecedent knowledge required to assist the person. These theories also are descriptive of situations involving families and communities.

Orem's work related to nursing as a practical science and the identification of three practice sciences and three foundational nursing sciences provides direction for the development of nursing science. This work offers a structure for the organization of existing nursing knowledge, as well as for the generation of new knowledge.

In an interview with Jacqueline Fawcett (2001), Orem identified factors essential for the development of nursing science. They included the following: (1) a model of practice science, (2) a valid, reliable, general theory of nursing, (3) models of the operations of nursing practice, (4) development of the conceptual structure of the general theory, and (5) integration of the conceptual elements of the theory with the practice operations (p. 36). Orem's work related to the SCDNT and the form of nursing science as a practical science provides a foundation for the development of a body of knowledge. The efforts of nurse scholars and nurse researchers to build on this foundation will result in a body of knowledge that serves nurses in their provision of care to persons requiring nursing.

Case Study

This case study documents an initial interaction between a nurse practitioner and clients, a married couple, in a primary care situation. The constituent units of design for the production of nursing (Orem, 2001, p. 296) provide the outline for the narrative.

Contract for Nursing

Betty is the wife and caregiver of George, who has had Parkinson's disease for 15 years. She is requesting information regarding the possibility of help with long-term care.

An initial assessment leads to the conclusion that no evidence suggests the need for immediate regulatory action. This is always the first step and is based on information about universal self-care requisites focused particularly on maintaining adequate intake of oxygen, safety, or critical health states.

The husband indicates that he is managing well but is frustrated by his inability to do things that he used to be able to do (e.g., going out when or where he wished, using hands for fine motor activities such as photography). George is a 71-year-old man of German origin, who formerly was an engineer. His wife expresses distress with high-risk behavior exhibited by her husband and frustration with her inability to help him recognize and accept the danger of his actions and the limitations caused by the disease and its treatment.

Legitimate Functional Unity of Care Providers

Until the last few years, George was a competent self-carer. He regularly sought medical help and followed physician instructions. Betty has been instrumental in helping him manage his illness. They have frequent contact with the neurologist and the nurse practitioner. George has been hospitalized several times for trauma related to falls. They are a well-groomed couple, well spoken, pleasant, cooperative, communicative, agreeable, responsive to questions, and able to answer questions.

George has stage 3 Parkinson's disease with postural instability (difficulty sitting, standing from sitting position, walking) and lymphedema, especially in his right leg. He has limited sensation and control of his fingers. He is a tall man, which makes it difficult for his wife to assist him.

Betty reports that her husband has stayed out late into early morning hours several times. She didn't know how to locate him. He didn't have needed medications along and required stranger assistance to return home; similar high-risk behavior is repeated regularly. Betty expresses difficulty dealing with these situations.

When out of the house, George behaves as if the environment is safe and his physical limitations don't put him at risk. His disease forced him into early retirement, with a drastic reduction in personal financial resources. He has cognitive limitations associated with the disease and the treatment, among them an inability to process new information, and he does not anticipate potential consequences of his behaviors. The couple lives in an apartment that is handicapped accessible.

Components of the Care System

The couple has an established collaborative care system (Geden & Taylor, 1999). George sees his self-care system as fine—what he can't do, his wife does, and if she is away, she arranges for somebody to help. If he needs help, he can and does get it. This perception is congruent with many collaborative care situations. However, Betty expresses the need for changes in their care system. Frustration with the current situation is evident. The current self-care system in place is by the dependent-care agent; George engages in some actions and makes some judgments within the system. No nursing system is in place. George says he manages well with the assistance of his wife, his physicians, and others who help out.

Therapeutic Self-Care Demand

Components Universal Self-Care Requisites

I. Maintain general good nutrition.
   A. Because of the medications, increased fluids and decreased protein are required.
   B. Because of difficulty swallowing, attention to avoiding foods with high potential for choking is required.
   C. Because of loss of fine motor control, adapted silverware is required.
II. Maintain intake of air using normal care measures.
III. Maintain elimination.
   A. Adaptive devices and personal assistance for getting to bathroom and managing clothing are required because of pathology and mobility limitations.
   B. Constipation is associated with the mobility limitations of parkinsonism and medication side effects, so measures such as increased fluid intake and laxatives may be required.
IV. Maintain a balance between solitude and social interaction.
   A. Neither solitude nor excessive social interaction is appropriate.
V. Maintain a balance between rest and activity.
   A. Neither excessive activity nor rest is appropriate.
   B. A lift chair may be required.
   C. A hospital bed may be needed in the home.
   D. Sleep is disturbed often.
VI. Maintain protection from hazards.
   A. Careful evaluation of potential hazards and means to address them is needed.

VII. Promote normalcy.
   A. Create an environment that allows George to function as normally as possible (e.g., use of adaptive devices, lift chair).

Betty's requisites are those to be expected of a 65-year-old woman. In addition, she needs to make adjustments to her self-care in order to accommodate her husband's demands.

Developmental Self-Care Requisites

Because of progressive chronic disease and unresolved issues, George is unable to progress developmentally; actions to date are unsuccessful in moving him forward with his developmental tasks. The progressive nature of the disease has led to changes in the collaborative care system such that the relationship is becoming more of a dependent-care system. This creates difficulties for both Betty and George. Although he accepts himself as having parkinsonism, he is not realistic about the effect it has on him.

Health Deviation Self-Care Requisites

They need to continue to seek medical attention regularly. Reliance on pharmacological management of pathology, to the exclusion of other management approaches, results in medication side effects that cause more problems to arise.

George accepts himself as a person with Parkinson's disease in need of health care but is frustrated with the disease progression and with its effects on his ability to participate in activities. Both George and Betty are struggling to live with the effects of pathology that will not enable developmental progression. Additional needs were not identified.

Self-Care and Dependent-Care Capabilities

George has severely limited abilities for decision making and self-care. George is unable to manage many activities of daily living, including both physical and decision-making activities; those he can manage require increasingly long periods. This will get progressively worse. Betty expresses the need for assistance in living with her husband in his current health state and with associated care needs. Betty is well informed about the disease process, treatment modalities, and overall self-care requirements associated with the disease, and she is a skilled caregiver. She will continue to manage and control the care system but will find it more and more difficult to do the physical work of taking care of George.

Features of the Nursing System

The nursing system for George and Betty is periodic. It articulates with a dependent-care system, as well as with the self-care systems of both persons. As the disease progresses, assistance will be needed in accessing resources for care and, in some instances, in providing care for George and support for Betty. As noted, Betty wishes to maintain management and control of the care system. She seeks a collaborative role with the nurse practitioner and others. As a first step, the nurse will assist the couple in getting appropriate adaptive equipment, such as a hospital bed and a powered wheelchair. Over time, when a need is identified, home care assistance will be initiated. The nurse and others will help Betty and George determine levels of assistance required. When it is not reasonable for Betty to continue to care for George at home, the physician, the nurse, and others will aid them in relocating George to a residential facility.

The progressive nature of parkinsonism requires a long-term anticipatory approach to care. It requires the involvement of many different persons as the problems change and new demands arise. Attention will have to be paid to Betty's self-care system while she increases her role as dependent caregiver.

CRITICAL THINKING *Activities*

1. Select a nursing situation in which you were involved. Compare the information from that nursing situation with the process of SCDNT. Categorize the data according to the conceptual elements of the SCDNT. Does SCDNT provide a basis for interpreting the data and designing a nursing system to meet the needs for nursing care?

2. Review the case study included in this chapter. Based on your review, design a nursing system that addresses Betty's self-care system while she increases her role as dependent caregiver.
3. Select a research article that references use of SCDNT as the conceptual framework. Is the link to the theory clear? Identify the SCDNT concepts used in the study.
4. Review several definitions of nursing put forth by theorists other than Orem. Compare Orem's description of the proper object of nursing with the others. How are they related?

POINTS FOR *Further Study*

- The official IOS website is available at: http://scdnt.com/
- Selected papers and abstracts from the *10th World Congress Self-care and Nursing* can be found in the IOS journal, *Self-Care, Dependent-Care & Nursing,* on the website at: http://scdnt.com/ja/jarchive.html
- Johns Hopkins Orem Archives at: http://www.medicalarchives.jhmi.edu
- Berbiglia, V. A. (2006,). Orem's self-care deficit nursing theory in practice. In M. R. Alligood & A. M. Tomey (Eds.). *Nursing theory: Utilization & application* (3rd ed., pp. 255-281). St. Louis: Mosby Elsevier.
- Fawcett, J. (1988). *The nurse theorists. Portraits of excellence: Dorothea Orem* (Video/DVD). Athens, OH: Fitne, Inc.
- Fawcett, J. (1992). *Excellence in Action: Dorothea Orem* (Video/DVD). Athens, OH: FITNE, Inc.

REFERENCES

Alcorn State University Cora S. Balmat School of Nursing Academics. Retrieved May 28, 2008 from Alcorn State University Website: http://www.alcorn.edu/Academic/SON/INDEX.HTM

Allison, S. E. (2008). Some early efforts to conceptualize nursing: A tribute to Dorothea E. Orem (Electronic version). *Self-care, Dependent-Care & Nursing*, 16(1), 49-50.

Allison, S. E., & McLaughlin-Renpenning, K. (1999). *Nursing administration in the 21st century.* Thousand Oaks, CA: Sage.

Allport, G. W. (1955). *Becoming.* New Haven: Yale University Press.

Anderson College Academics. Retrieved May 28, 2008 from http://www.anderson.edu/academics/nurs/handbook.pdf

Arnold, M. B. (1960a). *Emotion and personality* (Vol. 1). New York: Columbia University Press.

Arnold, M. B. (1960b). *Emotion and personality* (Vol. 2). New York: Columbia University Press.

Banfield, B. E. (1997). A philosophical inquiry of Orem's self-care deficit nursing theory. *Dissertation Abstracts International, 58*, 5885B.

Banfield, B. E. (2008). Philosophic position on nature of human beings foundational to Orem's self-care deficit nursing theory. *Self-Care, Dependent-Care, & Nursing*, 16(1), 33-40.

Barnard, C. I. (1962). *The functions of the executive.* Cambridge: Harvard University Press.

Bekel, G. (1999). Statements on the object of science: A discussion paper. *International Orem Society Newsletter, 7*(1), 1-3.

Bekel, G. (2002). Development of therapeutic self-care demand for nursing practice situations (Abstract). 7th International Self-Care Deficit Nursing Theory Conference (Abstract 18). MU Sinclair School of Nursing.

Berbiglia, V. A. (1997). Orem's self-care deficit theory in nursing practice. In M. R. Alligood & A. M. Tomey (Eds.), *Nursing theory: Utilization & application* (pp. 129-152). St. Louis: Mosby.

Berbiglia, V. A. (2002). Orem's self-care deficit theory in nursing practice. In M. R. Alligood & A. M. Tomey (Eds.), *Nursing theory: Utilization & application* (2nd ed.) (pp. 239-266). St. Louis: Mosby.

Berbiglia, V. A. (2006). Orem's self-care deficit theory in nursing practice. In M. R. Alligood & A. M. Tomey (Eds.), *Nursing theory: Utilization & application* (3rd ed.) (pp. 255-282). St. Louis: Mosby.

Biggs, A. (2008). Orem's Self-Care Deficit Nursing theory: Update on the state of the art and science. *Nursing Science Quarterly, 21, 200-206*

College of Saint Benedict. Retrieved May 28, 2008 from College of Saint Benedict catalog Website: http://www.csbsju.edu/catalog/1998-2000/programsofstudy/nursing.htm

Denyes, M. J., Orem, D. E., & Bekel, G. (2001). Self-care: A foundational science. *Nursing Science Quarterly, 14*(1), 48-54.

Evers, G. C. M., Isenberg, M. A., Philipsen, H., Senten, M., & Brouns, G. (1993). Validity testing of the Dutch translation of the appraisal of the self-care agency A.S.A. scale. *International Journal of Nursing Studies, 30*(4), 331-342.

Fawcett, J. (2001). The nurse theorists: 21st-century updates—Dorothea E. Orem 2001. *Nursing Science Quarterly,* 14(1):34-38.

Fromm, E. (1962). *The art of loving*. New York: Harper Colophon Books.

Geden, E., & Taylor, S.G. (1999). Theoretical and empirical description of adult couples' collaborative care systems. *Nursing Science Quarterly*, 12(4), 329-334.

Harnucharunkul, Somchit. (2004). Experience of integrating SCDNT in teaching, research and practice in Thailand (Abstract). 8th World Congress SCDNT (p. 23). MU Sinclair.

Harre, R. (1970). *The principles of scientific thinking*. Chicago: University of Chicago Press. Illinois Wesleyan University School of Nursing Curriculum. Retrieved May 28, 2008. From Illinois Wesleyan University School of Nursing site: http://www2.iwu.edu/nursing/curriculum/index.shtml

Macmurray, J. (1957). *The self as agent. London*: Faber and Faber.

Macmurray, J. (1961). *Persons in relation*. New York: Harper and Brothers.

Maratian, J. (1959). *The degrees of knowledge*. New York: Charles Scribner's Sons.

Moore, J. B., & Pichler, V. H. (2000). Measurement of Orem's basic conditioning factors: A review of published research. *Nursing Science Quarterly, 13*(2), 137-142.

Nursing Development Conference Group (NDCG), Orem, D. E. (Ed,). (1973). *Concept formalization in nursing: Process and product.* Boston: Little, Brown & Co.

Nursing Development Conference Group (NDCG), Orem, D. E. (Ed.). (1979). *Concept formalization in nursing: Process and product* (2nd ed.). Boston: Little, Brown & Co

Orem, D. E. (1956). *Hospital nursing service: An analysis.* Report to the Division of Hospital and Institutional Services of the Indiana State Board of Health. Indianapolis: Division of Hospital and Institutional Services.

Orem, D. E. (1959). *Guides for developing curriculum for the education of practical nurses.* Washington, DC: U.S. Department of Health, Education, and Welfare.

Orem, D. E. (1971). *Nursing: Concepts of practice.* New York: McGraw-Hill.

Orem, D. E. (1980). *Nursing: Concepts of practice* (2nd ed.). New York: McGraw-Hill.

Orem, D. E. (1985). *Nursing: Concepts of practice* (3rd ed.). New York: McGraw-Hill.

Orem, D. E. (1991). *Nursing: Concepts of practice* (4th ed.). St. Louis: Mosby.

Orem, D. E. (1995). *Nursing: Concepts of practice* (5th ed.). St. Louis: Mosby.

Orem, D. E. (1997). Views of human beings specific to nursing. *Nursing Science Quarterly, 10*(1), 26-31.

Orem, D. E. (2001). *Nursing: Concepts of practice* (6th ed.). St. Louis: Mosby.

Parson, T. (1949). *Essays in sociological theory*. New York: Free Press.

Parsons, T. (1951. *The social system*. New York: Free Press.

Plattel, M.G. (1965). *Social philosophy*. Pittsburgh: Duquesne University Press. 13(3), 158-163.

Renpenning, K., & Taylor, S. G. (Eds.). (2003). *Self-care theory in nursing: Selected papers of Dorothea Orem.* New York: Springer.

Southern University Baton Rouge School of Nursing (2007, Spring). *Nursing Student Handbook.* (Southern University Baton Rouge School of Nursing Southern University System, Baton Rouge, LA.)

Taylor, S. G. (1998). The development of self-care deficit nursing theory: An historical analysis. *International Orem Society Newsletter, 6*(2), 7-10.

Taylor, S., Geden, E., Isaramalai, S., & Wongvatunyu, S. (2000). Orem's self-care deficit nursing theory: Its philosophical foundation and the state of the science. *Nursing Science Quarterly, 13*(2), 104-109.

Taylor, S. G., & Godfrey, N. S. (1999). Ethical issues. The ethics of Orem's theory—third in a series of articles. *Nursing Science Quarterly, 12*(3), 202-207.

Taylor, S. G., Renpenning, K., Geden, E., Neuman, B., & Hart, M. (2001). A theory of dependent care. *Nursing Science Quarterly*. 14(3), 39-47.

University of Tennessee in Chattanooga Academic, Retrieved May 28, 2008 from University of Tennessee in Chattanooga Website: http://www.utc.edu/Academic/Nursing/philosophy.php

University of Toledo College of Nursing, Retrieved May 28, 2008 from University of Toledo College of Nursing website: http://www.bgsu.edu/colleges/hhs/advising/page30505.html

Wallace, W. A. (1979). *From a realist point of view.* Washington, DC: University Press of America.

Wallace, W. A. (1996). *The modeling of nature, philosophy of science and philosophy of nature in synthesis.* Washington, DC: Catholic University of America Press.

BIBLIOGRAPHY

Primary Sources

Books

Nursing Development Conference Group (NDCG), Orem, D. E. (Ed.). (1972). *Concept formalization in nursing: Process and product.* Boston: Little, Brown & Co.

Nursing Development Conference Group (NDCG), Orem, D. E. (Ed.). (1979). *Concept formalization in nursing: Process and product* (2nd ed.). Boston: Little, Brown & Co.

Orem, D. E. (Ed.). (1959). *Guides for developing curriculum for the education of practical nurses.* Vocational Division #274. Trade and Industrial Education #68. Washington, DC: U.S. Department of Health, Education, and Welfare.

Orem, D. E. (1971). *Nursing: Concepts of practice.* New York: McGraw-Hill.

Orem, D. E. (1980). *Nursing: Concepts of practice* (2nd ed.). New York: McGraw-Hill.

Orem, D. E. (1985). *Nursing: Concepts of practice* (3rd ed.). New York: McGraw-Hill.

Orem, D. E. (1991). *Nursing: Concepts of practice* (4th ed.). St. Louis: Mosby.

Orem, D. E. (1995). *Nursing: Concepts of practice* (5th ed.). St. Louis: Mosby.

Orem, D. E. (2001). *Nursing: Concepts of practice* (6th ed.). St. Louis: Mosby.

Orem, D. E., & Parker, K. S. (Eds.). (1963). *Nurse practice education workshop proceedings.* Washington, DC: The Catholic University of America.

Orem, D. E., & Parker, K. S. (Eds.). (1964). *Nursing content in preservice nursing curriculum.* Washington, DC: The Catholic University of America Press.

Renpenning, K., & Taylor, S. G. (Eds.). (2003). *Self care theory in nursing: Selected papers of Dorothea Orem.* New York: Springer Publishing.

Book Chapters

Orem, D. E. (1966). Discussion of paper—Another view of nursing care and quality. In K. M. Straub & K. S. Parker (Eds.), *Continuity of patient care: The role of nursing.* Washington, DC: The Catholic University of America Press.

Orem, D. E. (1969). Inservice education and nursing practice forces effecting nursing practice. In D. K. Petrowski & K. M. Staub (Eds.), *School of nursing education.* Washington, DC: The Catholic University of America Press.

Orem, D. E. (1981). Nursing: A triad of action systems. In G. E. Lasker (Ed.), *Applied systems and cybernetics. Systems research in health care, biocybernetics, and ecology* (Vol. IV). New York: Pergamon Press.

Orem, D. E. (1982). Nursing: A dilemma for higher education. In Sr. A. Power (Ed.), *Words commemorated: Essays celebrating the centennial of Incarnate Word College.* San Antonio, TX: Incarnate Word College.

Orem, D. E. (1983). The self-care deficit theory of nursing: A general theory. In I. Clements & F. Roberts (Eds.), *Family health: A theoretical approach to nursing care.* New York: Wiley Medical Publications.

Orem, D. E. (1984). Orem's conceptual model and community health nursing. In M. K. Asay & C. C. Ossler (Eds.), *Proceedings of the Eighth Annual Community Health Nursing Conference: Conceptual models of nursing applications in community health nursing.* Chapel Hill, NC: University of North Carolina, Department of Public Health Nursing, School of Public Health.

Orem, D. E. (1988). Nursing administration: A theoretical approach. In B. Henry, C. Arndt, M. DiVincenti, & A. M. Tomey (Eds.), *Dimensions of nursing administration.* Boston: Blackwell Scientific.

Orem, D. E. (1990). A nursing practice theory in three parts, 1956-1989. In M. E. Parker (Ed.), *Nursing theories in practice.* New York: National League for Nursing.

Orem, D. E., & Taylor, S. (1986). Orem's general theory of nursing. In P. Winstead-Fry (Ed.), *Case studies in nursing theory* (pp. 37-71; Pub. No. 15-2152). New York: National League for Nursing.

Journal Articles

Denyes, M. J., Orem, D. E., & Bekel, G. (2001). Self-care: A foundational science. *Nursing Science Quarterly, 14*(1), 48-54.

Orem, D. E. (1962, Jan.). The hope of nursing. *Journal of Nursing Education, 1*, 5.

Orem, D. E. (1979, March). Levels of nursing education and practice. *Alumnae Magazine, 68*, 2-6.

Orem, D. E. (1985, May/June). Concepts of self-care for the rehabilitation client. *Rehabilitation Nursing, 10*(3), 33-36.

Orem, D. E. (1988, May). The form of nursing science. *Nursing Science Quarterly, 1*(2), 75-79.

Orem, D. E. (1997). Views of human beings specific to nursing. *Nursing Science Quarterly, 10*(1), 26-31.

Orem, D. E., & O'Malley, M. (1952, Aug.). Diagnosis of hospital nursing problems. *Hospitals, 26*, 63.

Orem, D. E., & Vardiman, E. (1995, Winter). Orem's nursing theory and positive mental health: Practical considerations. *Nursing Science Quarterly, 8*(4), 165-173.

Secondary Sources

Dissertations

Ahrens, S. L. G. (2001). The development and testing of the Heart Failure Self-Care Inventory: An instrument for measuring heart failure self-care. *Dissertation Abstracts International, 62*, 5636B.

Anderson, J. A. M. (1996). Basic conditioning factors, self-care agency, self-care, and well-being in homeless adults. *Dissertation Abstracts International, 57*, 2473B.

Asdornwised, U. P. (2000). Self-care and dependent-care experiences of Thai patients recovering from coronary artery bypass graft surgery: An ethnographic study. *Dissertation Abstracts International, 61*, 1318B.

Baiardi, J. M. (1997). The influence of health status, burden, and degree of cognitive impairment on the self-care agency and dependent-care agency of caregivers of elders. *Dissertation Abstracts International, 58*, 5885B.

Banfield, B. E. (1997). A philosophical inquiry of Orem's self-care deficit nursing theory. *Dissertation Abstracts International, 58*, 5885B.

Bess, C. J. (1995). Abilities and limitation of adult type II diabetic patients with integrating of self-care practices into their daily lives. *Dissertation Abstracts International, 56*, 3688B.

Brown, K. L. G. (1996). Grief as a basic conditioning factor affecting the self-care agency and self-care of family caregivers of persons with neurotrauma. *Dissertation Abstracts International, 57*, 7447B.

Callaghan, D. M. (2000). The relationships among health-promoting self-care behaviors, self-care, self-efficacy, and self-care agency. *Dissertation Abstracts International, 61*, 3504B.

Canty, J. L. (1993). An investigation of life change events, hope, and self-care agency in inner city adolescents. *Dissertation Abstracts International, 54*, 2992B.

Chen, Y. M. (1996). Relationships among health control orientation, self-efficacy, self-care, and subjective well-being in the elderly with hypertension. *Dissertation Abstracts International, 57*, 3652B.

Cooksey-James, T. J. (1999). Utilization of prenatal care by women of St. Thomas, United States Virgin Islands: A descriptive study. *Dissertation Abstracts International, 61*, 2470B.

Cull, V. V. (1995). Exposure to violence and self-care practices of adolescents. *Dissertation Abstracts International, 56*, 3690B.

Cutler, C. G. (1998). The relationship of self-care agency, self-efficacy, and social support to post-hospitalization adjustment of patients with a mood disorder. *Dissertation Abstracts International, 59*, 0600B.

Dato, C. (2002). A. The relationship of perceived social support, positive symptoms, negative symptoms, and self-care actions in adults with schizophrenia living in the community. *Dissertation Abstracts International, 63*, 1266B.

Demasters, J. J. (1999). Women and the hormone replacement therapy decision: A study of concerns, values, and behaviors using a multiattribute utility model. *Dissertation Abstracts International, 59*, 5784B.

Dennis, C. (1998). Self-care agency, learned helplessness, and health status in elderly adults. *Dissertation Abstracts International, 59*, 1582B.

Dreher, H. M. (2000). The effect of caffeine reduction on sleep and well-being in persons with HIV (immune deficiency). *Dissertation Abstracts International, 61*, 4649B.

Gallegos, E. C. (1997). The effect of social, family and individual conditioning factors on self-care agency and self-care of adult Mexican women. *Dissertation Abstracts International, 58*, 5889B.

Good, M. P. L. (1992). Comparison of the effects of relaxation and music on post-operative pain. *Dissertation Abstracts International, 53*, 1783B.

Haas, D. L. (1991). The relationship between coping dispositions and power components of dependent-care agency in parents of children with special health care needs. *Dissertation Abstracts International, 52*, 1351B.

Hoffart, M. B. (1995). Weaving the fabric of life: A phenomenological inquiry of solitude experienced by school age children (emotional control). *Dissertation Abstracts International, 56*, 5417B.

Isaramalai, S. (2002). Developing a cross-cultural measure of the Self-As-Carer Inventory questionnaire for the Thai population. *Dissertation Abstracts International, 63*, 2307B.

Keatley, V. M. (1998). Critical incident stress in generic baccalaureate students. *Dissertation Abstracts International, 59*, 2124B.

Kleinbeck, S. V. M. (1996). Postdischarge surgical recovery of adult laparoscope outpatients. *Dissertation Abstracts International, 57*, 989B.

Koster, M. K. (1995). A comparison of the relationship among self-care agency, self-determinism, and absenteeism in two groups of school-age children. *Dissertation Abstracts International, 56*, 541B.

Lee, M. B. (1996). Power, self-care, and health in women living in urban squatter settlements in Karachi, Pakistan: A test of Orem's theory. *Dissertation Abstracts International, 57*, 7451B.

Macmurray, J. (1957). *The self as agent*. New York: Harper & Brothers.

Macmurray, J. (1961). *Persons in relation*. New York: Harper & Brothers.

Magnan, M. A. (2001). Self-care and health in persons with cancer-related fatigue: Refinement and evaluation of Orem's self-care framework. *Dissertation Abstracts International, 62*, 5644B.

Malathum, P. (2001). A model of factors contributing to perceived abilities for health-promoting self-care of community-dwelling Thai older adults. *Dissertation Abstracts International, 62*, 5034B.

Maritain, J. (1959). The *degrees of knowledge*. New York: Charles Scribner's Sons.

McKinney, M. L. (2000). Hardiness, threat appraisal, self-care capability, and caregiving characteristics as predictors of emotions and perceived health in family caregivers of cancer patients. *Dissertation Abstracts International, 61*, 2992B.

Metcalfe, S. A. (1997). Self-care actions as a function of the therapeutic self-care demand and self-care agency in individuals with chronic obstructive pulmonary disease. *Dissertation Abstracts International, 57*, 7453B.

Meyer, G. L. (2000). The art of watching out: Vigilance in women who have migraine headaches. *Dissertation Abstracts International, 61*, 0781B.

Morgan, M. J. (1998). Self-care agency in people with end-stage renal disease. *Dissertation Abstracts International, 59*, 1048B.

Neuman, B. (1996). Relationship between children's descriptions of pain, self-care, and dependent-care and basic conditioning factors of development, gender, and ethnicity: "Bears in my throat." *Dissertation Abstracts International, 57*, 2482B.

Nicholson, L. L. (2002). Self-care activities and quality of life in ovarian cancer survivors. *Dissertation Abstracts International, 63*, 1272B.

O'Connor, N. A. (1995). Maieutic dimensions of self-care agency: Instrument development. *Dissertation Abstracts International, 56*, 2563B.

Parsons, T. (1949). *The structure of social action*. Glencoe, Illinois: The Free Press.

Parsons, T. (1951). *The social system*. New York: Free Press.

Pettine, A. (1995). Development of self-care: A problem for elementary-age children? *Dissertation Abstracts International, 56*, 3479B.

Plattel, M. G. (1965). *Social philosophy*. Pittsburgh: Duquesne: University Press.

Raithel, J. A. (2000). Maintaining normalcy when managing the chronic physical illness of asthma. *Dissertation Abstracts International, 61*, 0782B.

Renker, P. R. (1998). Physical abuse, social support, self-care agency, self-care practices, and late adolescent pregnancy outcomes. *Dissertation Abstracts International, 58*, 5891B.

Rieg, L. C. (2000). Information retrieval of self-care and dependent-care agents using NetWellnessRTM, a consumer health information network. *Dissertation Abstracts International, 61*, 5801B.

Robinson, M. K. (1996). Determinants of functional status in chronically ill adults. *Dissertation Abstracts International, 56*, 5424B.

Schmidt, C. A. (1997). Mothers' views concerning the development of self-care agency in school-age children with diabetes. *Dissertation Abstracts International, 59*, 0162B.

Sonninen, A. L. (1997). Testing reliability and validity of the Finnish version of the Appraisal of Self-care Agency (ASA) scale with elderly Finns. *Dissertation Abstracts International, 60*, 0604C.

Surit, P. (2002). Health beliefs, social support, and self-care behaviors of older Thai persons with non-insulin-dependent diabetes mellitus (NIDDM). *Dissertation Abstracts International, 63*, 1276B.

Taggert, H. M. (2000). Tai Chi, balance, functional mobility, fear of falling, and health perception among older women. *Dissertation Abstracts International, 61*, 2994B.

Tiansawad, S. (1995). Self-care abilities and practices for prevention of HIV infection among rural Thai women who attended mobile family planning clinic. *Dissertation Abstracts International, 55*, 3241B.

Vogt, C. A. (1995). A comparison of educational models in determining patients' knowledge and behaviors concerning advance directives. *Dissertation Abstracts International, 55*, 3843B.

Wang, H. H. (1998). A model of self-care and well-being of rural elderly women in Taiwan. *Dissertation Abstracts International, 59*, 2689B.

Weber, N. A. (2000). Explication of the structure of the secondary concept of women's self-care developed within Orem's self-care deficit theory: Instrumentation, psychometric evaluation and theory-testing. *Dissertation Abstracts International, 61*, 1331B.

White, M. M. (2000). Predictors of self-care agency among community-dwelling older adults. *Dissertation Abstracts International, 61*, 1332B.

Zehnder, N. R. (1996). The influence of basic conditioning factors on menopausal self-care agency and menopausal self-care in midlife women. *Dissertation Abstracts International, 57*, 7460B.

CHAPTER

15

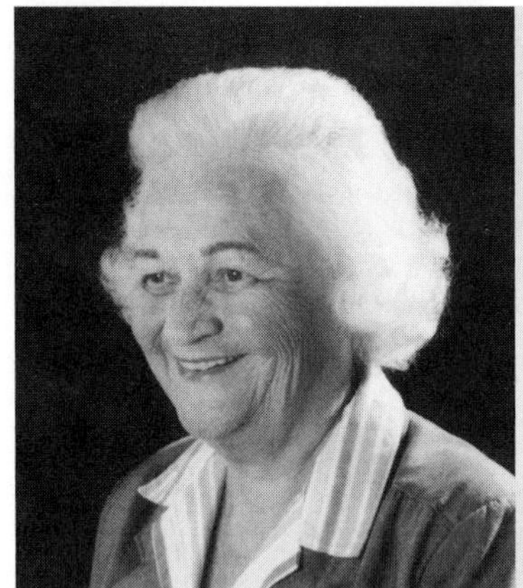

Photo courtesy of Patricia Messmer, PhD, RN-BC, FAAN

Imogene M. King, EdD, RN, FAAN

1923-2007

Conceptual System and Middle Range Theory of Goal Attainment

Christina L. Sieloff and Patricia R. Messmer

"Theory is an abstraction that implies prediction based in research. Theory without research and research without some theoretical basis will not build scientific knowledge for a discipline" (King, 1977, p. 23).

CREDENTIALS AND BACKGROUND OF THE THEORIST

The Nightingale Tribute to Imogene King

Imogene M. King was born on January 30, 1923, in West Point, Iowa; died December 24, 2007, in St. Petersburg, Florida; and is buried in Fort Madison, Iowa. Imogene received a diploma in Nursing from St. John's Hospital School of Nursing, St. Louis, Missouri, in 1945. While working in a variety of staff nurse roles, Imogene began course work toward a Bachelor of Science in Nursing Education, which she received from St. Louis University in 1948; she received a Master of Science in Nursing from St. Louis University in 1957. From 1947 to 1958, King worked as an instructor in medical-surgical nursing and was an assistant director at St. John's Hospital School of Nursing. King went on to study with Mildred Montag as her dissertation chair at Teachers College, Columbia University, New York, receiving a Doctor of Education (EdD) in 1961.

From 1968 to 1972, King was the director of the School of Nursing at Ohio State University in Columbus. While at Ohio State, her book, *Toward a Theory for Nursing: General Concepts of Human Behavior* (1971), was published. In this early work,

---

Previous authors: C. L. Sieloff, M. L. Ackermann, S. A. Brink, J. A. Clanton, C. G. Jones, A. Marriner Tomey, S. L. Moody, G. L. Perlich, D. L. Price, & B. B. Prusinski.

The authors encourage all readers to read Dr. King's original materials in conjunction with this chapter.

King concluded, "a systematic representation of nursing is required ultimately for developing a science to accompany a century or more of art in the everyday world of nursing" (1971, p. 129). Her book subsequently was awarded the *American Journal of Nursing* Book of the Year Award in 1973 (King, 1995a).

From 1961 to 1966, King was an assistant and associate professor of nursing at Loyola University in Chicago, where she developed a master's degree program in nursing based on a nursing conceptual framework. Her first theory article appeared in 1964 in the *Nursing Science* journal with the nurse theorist, Dr. Martha Rogers, from New York University as the editor.

Between 1966 and 1968, King served as Assistant Chief of Research Grants Branch, Division of Nursing, in the U.S. Department of Health, Education, and Welfare, under Jessie Scott. While Imogene was in Washington, D.C., her article "A Conceptual Frame of Reference for Nursing" was published in *Nursing Research* (1968).

From 1968 to 1972, Imogene served as Director of the Nursing Department at Ohio State University. In 1980, King was awarded an honorary PhD from Southern Illinois University (Messmer, 2000).

King then returned to Chicago in 1972 as a professor in the Loyola University graduate program. She also served as the Coordinator of Research in Clinical Nursing at the Loyola Medical Center, Department of Nursing, from 1978 to 1980. In May 1998, King received an honorary doctorate from Loyola University, where her "Nursing Collection" is housed.

From 1972 to 1975, King was a member of the Defense Advisory Committee on Women in the Services for the U.S. Department of Defense. She also was elected alderman for a 4-year term (1975-1979) in Ward 2, Wood Dale, Illinois, in 1975.

In 1980, King was appointed professor at the University of South Florida, College of Nursing, in Tampa, Florida (Houser & Player, 2007). In 1981, the manuscript for her second book, *A Theory for Nursing: Systems, Concepts, Process,* was published. In addition to her first two books, she authored multiple book chapters and articles in professional journals, and a third book, *Curriculum and Instruction in Nursing: Concepts and Process,* was published in 1986. King retired in 1990 and was named professor emeritus at the University of South Florida and continued to guest lecture.

King continued to provide community service and to help plan care through her conceptual system and theory at various healthcare organizations, including Tampa General Hospital (Messmer, 1995). King never really retired, as she was always there for students, faculty, and colleagues who were using her theory, and even went "round the clock" to implement her theory at Tampa General Hospital. King also served on the nursing advisory board, and guest lectured at the University of Tampa.

In 1948, King joined the American Nurses Association (ANA) as a member of the Missouri Nurses Association and was active in Illinois and Ohio as well. Upon her move to Tampa, Florida, she became very active member in the Florida Nurses' Association (FNA) and FNA District 4, Tampa. King held offices in various organizations, including President of the Florida Nurses Foundation, served on the FNA and the FNA District IV boards, and frequently was a delegate from the FNA to the ANA House of Delegates. In 1997, King received a gold medallion from Governor Chiles for advancing the nursing profession in the State of Florida. King was inducted into the FNA Hall of Fame and the ANA Hall of Fame in 2004. In 1994, King also was inducted into the American Academy of Nursing (AAN), served on the AAN Theory Expert Panel, and in 2005, was inducted as an AAN Living Legend. In 1996, King received the Jessie M. Scott Award at the ANA Convention. King was thrilled when Jessie Scott was there for the presentation, and she was on the floor of the ANA House of Delegates to hear President Clinton's congratulations on ANA's 100th anniversary and his admiration of his mother as a nurse anesthetist.

King was the keynote speaker for the 37th Annual Isabel Maitland Stewart Conference in Research in Nursing at Teachers College, Columbia University, in 2000 (Messmer & Fawcett, 2008; Messmer, 2008) and was very pleased when Mildred Montag came for her presentation. King was inducted into the Teachers College, Columbia University of Hall of Fame, in 1999.

The King International Nursing Group (KING) was created to facilitate the dissemination and utilization of King's conceptual system, the Theory of Goal Attainment, and related theories. Even after the organization became inactive, King consulted with members of the organization on an individual basis regarding her theory.

King was one of the original Sigma Theta Tau International (STTI) Virginia Henderson Fellows, and she received the STTI Elizabeth Russell Belford Founders Award for Excellence in Education in 1989 (Messmer, 2007). King was keynote speaker at two STTI theory conferences in 1992, and presented at multiple regional, national, and international STTI conferences on application of her theory.

King communicated regularly with undergraduate, graduate, and doctoral students who were learning about theories within her conceptual system. King served as advisor for Sieloff's (1996) development of an instrument to measure the power of a nursing group within an organization, Killeen's (1996) instrument to measure patient satisfaction with professional nursing care and Frey's (1995) seminal work on adolescent patients diagnosed with type 1 diabetes.

King also was recognized as one of the early nurse theorists through her publications, *Toward a Theory for Nursing* (1971) and *A Theory for Nursing: Systems, Concepts and Process* (1981), which were translated into Japanese, Spanish, and German. In addition, Imogene authored numerous articles on her theory and served on the editorial board of *Nursing Science Quarterly.* King authored several chapters in various books, for example, Frey & Sieloff's *Advancing King's Systems Framework and Theory of Nursing* (1995), and Sieloff and Frey's *Middle Range Theories for Nursing Practice Using King's Conceptual System* (2007).

King (1971) describes the purpose of her first book as follows:

> . . . propos[ing] a conceptual frame of reference for nursing. . .intended to be utilized specifically by students and teachers, and also by researchers and practitioners, to identify and analyze events in specific nursing situations. The conceptual system suggests that the essential characteristics of nursing are those properties that have persisted in spite of environmental changes (p. ix). It is a way of thinking about the real world of nursing; . . . an approach for selecting concepts perceived to be fundamental for the practice of professional nursing; [and] shows a process for developing concepts that symbolize experiences within the physical, psychological, and social environment in nursing (p. 125).

King's (1981) concepts are presented in the Major Concepts & Definitions box.

MAJOR CONCEPTS & DEFINITIONS

"Concepts give meaning to our sense perceptions and permit generalizations about persons, objects, and things" (King, 1995a, p. 16). A limited number of definitions based on the systems framework are listed below. The remainder of King's definitions can be found in her 1981 book.

HEALTH

"Health is defined as dynamic life experiences of a human being, which implies continuous adjustment to stressors in the internal and external environment through optimum use of one's resources to achieve maximum potential for daily living" (King, 1981, p. 5).

NURSING

"Nursing is defined as a process of action, reaction, and interaction whereby nurse and client share information about their perceptions in the nursing situation" (King, 1981, p. 2).

SELF

"The self is a composite of thoughts and feelings which constitute a person's awareness of his [/her]

MAJOR CONCEPTS & DEFINITIONS—cont'd

individual existence, his [/her] conception of who and what he [/she] is. A person's self is the sum total of all he [/she] can call his [/hers]. The self includes, among other things, a system of ideas, attitudes, values, and commitments. The self is a person's total subjective environment. It is a distinctive center of experience and significance. The self constitutes a person's inner world as distinguished from the outer world consisting of all other people and things. The self is the individual as known to the individual. It is that to which we refer when we say, 'I'" (Jersild, 1952, p. 10).

USE OF EMPIRICAL EVIDENCE

King (1971) spoke of concepts as "abstract ideas that give meaning to our sense perceptions, permit generalizations, and tend to be stored in our memory for recall and use at a later time in new and different situations" (pp. 11-12). King (1984) defined *theory* as "a set of concepts, which, when defined, are interrelated and observable in the world of nursing practice" (p. 11). Theory serves to build "scientific knowledge for nursing" (King, 1995b, p. 24). King (1971) provided the criteria to evaluate a theory focusing on "What research findings have been reported to verify the concepts or test the theoretical basis presented and is it useful in adding one's understanding of the world and of the nursing discipline?" (p. 18).

King (1975a) identified at least two methods for developing theory as follows: (1) a theory can be developed and then tested in research, and (2) research can provide data from which a theory may be developed. King's opinion (1978) was that, "in today's world of building knowledge for a complex profession such as nursing, one must consider these two strategies."

King cited many research studies in her 1981 book, especially regarding the development of her concepts. Within the personal system, King examined studies related to perception by Allport (1955), Kelley and Hammond (1964), Ittleson and Cantril (1954), and others. In developing her definition of space, King used studies from Sommer (1969) and Ardrey (1966) and noted Minckley's (1968) research. For the concept of time, she acknowledged Orme's (1969) work.

Within the interpersonal system, King presented communication theories and models, citing the studies of Watzlawick, Beavin, and Jackson (1967) and Krieger (1975). King examined studies by Whiting (1955), Orlando (1961), and Diers and Schmidt (1977) for information on interaction. King also noted Dewey and Bentley's (1949) theory of knowledge, which addressed self-action, interaction, and transaction in *Knowing and the Known,* and Kuhn's (1975) work on transactions.

Commenting on research existing at that time, particularly operations research regarding patient care, King (1975b) noted that "...most studies have centered on technical aspects of patient care and of the healthcare systems rather than on patient aspects directly.... Few problems have been stated that begin with what the patient's condition demands or what the patient wants" (p. 9).

In her 1981 book, King further discussed that "several theoretical formulations about interpersonal relations and nursing process have been described in nursing situations" (pp. 151-152), citing studies by Peplau (1952), Orlando (1961), Paterson and Zderad (1976), and Yura and Walsh (1978) to support her ideas on the transactional process in her theory of goal attainment.

Developing the Conceptual System

In preparation of her 1971 book, King posed the following questions:

- What is the goal of nursing?
- What are the functions of nurses?
- How can nurses continue to expand their knowledge to provide quality care? (pp. 30, 39)

As a result of a review of 20 years of nursing literature (before 1971), King identified multiple concepts used by nurses to describe nursing. Figure 15-1 demonstrates the conceptual system that provided "one approach to studying systems as a whole rather than as isolated parts of a system" (King, 1995a, p. 18), and was "designed to explain (the) organized wholes within which nurses are expected to function" (1995b, p. 23).

King (1981) used a systems approach in the development of her conceptual systems and the middle range Theory of Goal Attainment. King noted that, "some scientists who have been studying systems have noted that the only way to study human beings interacting with the environment is to design a conceptual framework of interdependent variables and interrelated concepts" (King, 1981, p. 10). King (1995a) believed that her "framework differs from other conceptual schema in that it is concerned not with fragmenting human beings and the environment but with human transactions in different kinds of environments" (p. 21).

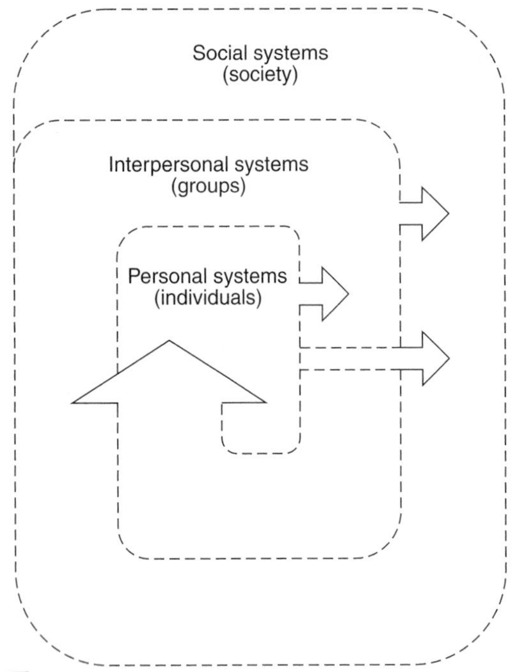

Figure 15-1 Dynamic conceptual systems. (From King, I. [1981]. *A theory for nursing: Systems, concepts, process* [p. 11]. New York: Delmar. Used with permission from I. King.)

"An awareness of the complex dynamics of human behavior in nursing situations prompted [King's] formulation of a conceptual framework that represents personal, interpersonal, and social systems as the domain of nursing" (King, 1981, p. 130). Each of the three systems identified human beings as the basic element in the system, thus "the unit of analysis in [the] framework [was] human behavior in a variety of social environments" (King, 1995a, p. 18). Individuals exist within personal systems, and King provided an example of a total system as being a patient or a nurse. King believed that it is necessary to understand the concepts of body image, growth and development, perception, self, space, and time to comprehend human beings as persons.

Interpersonal systems are formed when two or more individuals interact, forming dyads (two people) or triads (three people). The dyad of a nurse and a patient is one type of interpersonal system. Families, when acting as small groups, also can be considered interpersonal systems. Comprehension of the interpersonal system requires an understanding of the concepts of communication, interaction, role, stress, and transaction.

A comprehensive interacting system consists of groups that make up society, and is referred to as a *social system.* Religious, educational, and healthcare systems are examples of social systems. The influential behavior of an extended family on an individual's growth and development in society is another example of the influence of a social system. Within a social system, the concepts of authority, decision making, organization, power, and status are essential for system understanding.

"The concepts in the framework are the organizing dimensions and represent knowledge essential for understanding the interactions between the three systems" (King, 1995a, p. 18). Concepts were placed in the personal system because they primarily related to individuals, whereas concepts were placed in the interpersonal system because they "emphasized interactions between two or more persons" (King, 1995a, p. 18). Concepts were placed in the social system because they "provided knowledge for nurses to function in larger systems" (King, 1995a, p. 18). However, King (1995a) clearly identified that "the concepts in the framework are not limited to only one of the dynamic interacting systems but cut across all three systems" (p. 19).

King's Middle Range Theory of Goal Attainment

In 1981, King derived the middle range Theory of Goal Attainment from her conceptual system. The question that motivated King to develop a theory was, "What is the nature of nursing?" (King, 1995b, p. 25). She answered, "the way in which nurses, in their role, do with and for individuals that differentiates nursing from other health professionals" (King, 1995b, p. 26). This question and answer guided her development of the Theory of Goal Attainment.

King (1995b) used the following criteria to develop the theory:

- "What are the philosophical assumptions?"
- "Are the concepts clearly identified and defined?"
- "Are the concepts related in propositional statements or models?"
- "Does the theory generate questions to be answered, or hypotheses to be tested in research, to generate knowledge and affirm the theory?"

"The human process of interactions formed the basis for designing a model of transactions that depicts theoretical knowledge used by nurses to help individuals and groups attain goals" (1995a, p. 27) (Figure 15-2).

King (1995b) stated the following:

> "Mutual goal setting [between a nurse and a client] is based on (a) nurses' assessment of a client's concerns, problems, and disturbances in health; (b) nurses' and clients' perceptions of the interference; and (c) their sharing of information whereby each functions to help the client attain the goals identified. In addition, nurses interact with family members when clients cannot verbally participate in the goal setting" (p. 28).

To test her theory, King (1981) conducted research, identifying that her study varied from previous studies in that it "described the nurse-patient interaction process that leads to goal attainment" (p. 153). King's research described a process that led to goal attainment and studied nurse-patient interactions to determine whether nurses made transactions. King used a method of nonparticipant observation to collect information about nurse-patient interactions on a patient care unit in a hospital setting. Patients and nurses volunteered to participate in the study. King then trained graduate students in the nonparticipant observation technique before collecting data. She examined multiple interactions and recorded verbal and nonverbal behaviors as raw data. King also developed a goal-oriented nursing record that nurses could use to determine if they were making transactions leading to goal attainment (King, 1981, pp. 163-177).

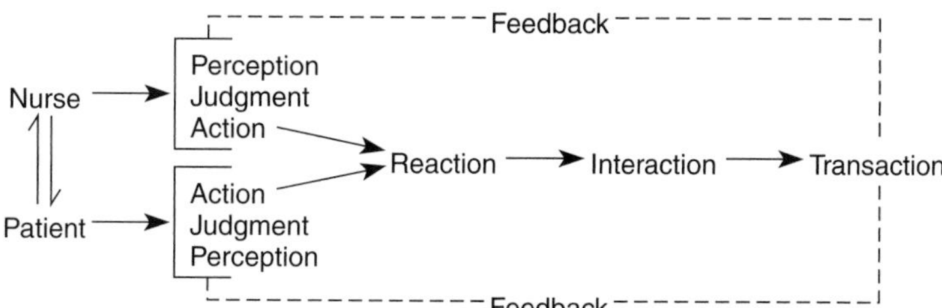

Figure 15-2 A process of human interactions that lead to transactions: A model of transaction. (From King, I. [1981]. *A theory for nursing: Systems, concepts, process* [p. 61]. New York: Delmar. Used with permission from I. King.)

MAJOR ASSUMPTIONS

King's personal philosophy about human beings and life influenced her assumptions, including those related to the environment, health, nursing, individuals, and nurse-patient interactions. King's conceptual system and Theory of Goal Attainment are "based on an overall assumption that the focus of nursing is human beings interacting with their environment, leading to a state of health for individuals, which is an ability to function in social roles" (King, 1981, p. 143).

Nursing

"Nursing is an observable behavior found in the healthcare systems in society" (King, 1971, p. 125). The goal of nursing "is to help individuals maintain their health so they can function in their roles" (King, 1981, pp. 3-4). Nursing is an interpersonal process of action, reaction, interaction, and transaction. Perceptions of a nurse and a patient also influence the interpersonal process.

Person

Specific assumptions related to persons, or individuals, are detailed in *A Theory for Nursing: Systems, Concepts, Process* (King, 1981). In addition, the following assumptions were detailed in King's subsequent works:

- Individuals are spiritual beings (I. King, personal communication, July 11, 1996).
- Individuals have the capacity to think, know, make choices, and select alternative courses of action (King, 1981).
- Individuals have the ability through their language and other symbols to record their history and preserve their culture (King, 1986).
- Individuals are open systems in transaction with the environment. Transaction connotes that no separateness exists between human beings and the environment (King, 1981).
- Individuals are unique and holistic, are of intrinsic worth, and are capable of rational thinking and decision making in most situations (King, 1995b).
- Individuals differ in their needs, wants, and goals (King, 1995b).

Health

Health is a dynamic state in the life cycle; illness interferences with that process. Health "implies continuous adjustment to stress in the internal and external environment through optimum use of one's resources to achieve maximum potential for daily living" (King, 1981, p. 5).

Environment

King (1981) believed that "an understanding of the ways that human beings interact with their environment to maintain health was essential for nurses" (p. 2). Open systems imply that interactions occur between the system and the system's environment, inferring that the environment is changing constantly. "Adjustments to life and health are influenced by [an] individual's interaction with environment . . . Each human being perceives the world as a total person in making transactions with individuals and things in the environment" (King, 1981, p. 141).

THEORETICAL ASSERTIONS

King's Theory of Goal Attainment (1981) focuses on the interpersonal system and the interactions that take place between individuals, specifically in the nurse-patient relationship. In the nursing process, each member of the dyad perceives the other, makes judgments, and takes actions. Together, these activities culminate in reaction. Interaction results and, if perceptual congruence exists and disturbances are conquered, transactions occur. The system is open to permit feedback because each phase of the activity potentially influences perception.

King (1981) developed eight propositions in her Theory of Goal Attainment. These propositions are detailed in Box 15-1 and describe the relationships between concepts. Diagrams follow each proposition. When the propositions were analyzed, 23 relationships were not specified; 22 relationships were positive, and no relationship was negative (Austin & Champion, 1983) (Figure 15-3). In addition, King (1981) derived seven hypotheses from the Theory of

Box 15-1 *Propositions Within King's Theory of Goal Attainment*

1. If perceptual congruence (PC) is present in nurse-client interactions (I), transactions (T) will occur.
   $PC(I) \xrightarrow{+} T$
2. If nurse and client make transactions (T), goals will be attained (GA).
   $T \xrightarrow{+} GA$
3. If goals are attained (GA), satisfactions (S) will occur.
   $GA \xrightarrow{+} S$
4. If goals are attained (GA), effective nursing care (NC_e) will occur.
   $GA \xrightarrow{+} NC_e$
5. If transactions (T) are made in nurse-client interactions (I), growth and development (GD) will be enhanced.
   $(I)T \xrightarrow{+} GD$
6. If role expectations and role performance as perceived by nurse and client are congruent (RCN), transactions (T) will occur.
   $RCN \xrightarrow{+} T$
7. If role conflict (RC) is experienced by nurse and client or both, stress (ST) in nurse-client interactions (I) will occur.
   $RC(I) \xrightarrow{+} ST$
8. If nurses with special knowledge and skills communicate (CM) appropriate information to clients, mutual goal setting (T) and goal attainment (GA) will occur. [Mutual goal setting is a step in transaction and thus has been diagrammed as transaction.]
   $CM \xrightarrow{+} T \xrightarrow{+} GA$

From Austin, J. K., & Champion, V. L. (1983). King's theory of nursing: Explication and evaluation. In P. L. Chinn (Ed.), *Advances in nursing theory development* (p. 55). Rockville, MD: Aspen.

	PA	T	GA	S	NC_e	GD	RCN	RC	ST	CM
PA		+	+	+	+	+	?	?	?	?
T			+	+	+	+	+	?	?	?
GA				+	+	+	+	?	?	+
S					?	?	+	?	?	+
NC_e						?	+	?	?	+
GD							+	?	?	+
RCN								?	?	?
RC									+	?
ST										?
CM										

Figure 15-3 Relationship table. CM, Communicate; GA, goals attained; GD, growth and development; NC_e effective nursing care; PC, Perceptional Congruence; RC, role conflict; RCN, role congruency; S, satisfactions; ST, stress; T, transactions. (Note to editors: restore the proper order—this Figure has not been changed from 6e) thanks (From Austin, J. K., & Champion, V. L. [1983]. King's theory for nursing: Explication and evaluation. In P. L. Chinn [Ed.], *Advances in theory development* [p. 58]. Rockville, MD: Aspen.)

Goal Attainment, which are found in *A Theory for Nursing: Systems, Concepts, Process.*

LOGICAL FORM

In the initial framework suggested in her 1968 article, King identified the following four comprehensive concepts that center on human beings:

1. Health
2. Interpersonal relationships
3. Perceptions
4. Social systems

King viewed individuals as open systems with energy exchange taking place within, and external to, human beings. Although King's original framework was abstract and dealt with "only a few elements of concrete situations" (King, 1981, p. 128), King believed that her four "universal ideas (social systems, health, perception, and interpersonal relations) were relevant in every nursing situation" (King, 1981, p. 128).

Later, King (1975a) identified that her "personal approach to synthesizing knowledge for nursing was to use data and information available from (1) research in nursing and related fields, and (2) 25 years in active practice, teaching, and research. From all the knowledge available, a theoretical framework, relevant for nursing, was formulated" (p. 36). In 1978, King indicated that theory development is composed of inductive and deductive reasoning, with theory's primary purpose being the generation of knowledge through research.

King (1981) then began further development of her conceptual system and proposed the middle range Theory of Goal Attainment to describe "the nature of nurse-client interactions that lead to achievement of goals" (p. 142) as follows:

> Nurses purposely interact with clients to mutually establish goals, and to explore and agree on means to achieve goals. Mutual goal setting is based on nurses' assessment of clients' concerns, problems, and disturbances in health, their perceptions of problems, and their sharing information to move toward goal attainment (pp. 142-143).

In her 1981 publication, King spoke of fewer dichotomies between health and illness, referring to illness as interference in the life cycle. Through reformulation, King provided a more open system relationship between person and environment. King also revised her terminology, using *adjustment* instead of *adaptation,* and *person, human being,* and *individual* rather than *man.*

A logical progression of development existed in the conceptual system from 1971 to 1981, with King deriving her middle range Theory of Goal Attainment from her conceptual system. The Theory of Goal Attainment "organize[s] elements in the process of nurse-client interactions that result in outcomes, that is, goals attained" (King, 1981, p. 143).

King (1971) initially had stated the following:

> . . . [I]f nurses are to assume the roles and responsibilities expected of them, . . . the discovery of knowledge must be disseminated in such a way that they are able to use it in their practice. . . . Descriptive data collected systematically provide cues for generating hypotheses for research in human behavior in nursing situations (p. 128).

During a 1978 nursing theorist conference, King indicated that if nurses were taught this process, they could begin to predict outcomes in nursing. Later, in 1981, King added, "this theory should serve as a standard of practice related to nurse-patient interactions and is, in this sense, a normative theory" (p. 145). Clements and Roberts (1983) expanded on these ideas to show the process of the Theory of Goal Attainment in relation to various nursing situations, including the health of families.

ACCEPTANCE BY THE NURSING COMMUNITY

Practice

King's (1971) early publication led to nursing curriculum development and practice application at Ohio State and other universities. In her 1981 book, King identified that "theory, because it is abstract, cannot be immediately applied to nursing practice or to concrete nursing education programs. When empirical referents are identified, defined and described, . . . theory is useful and can be applied in concrete situations" (p. 157). However, "knowledge of the concepts can be applied in concrete situations" (p. 41).

Professionals in most nursing specialty areas have used the concepts of King's (1981) Theory of Goal Attainment in nursing practice. Its relationship to practice is obvious because the nurse functions primarily through interactions with individuals and groups within the environment. Even before King's conceptual system was published, Brown and Lee (1980) stated "this proposed intrasystems model provides an approach for stimulating continued learning, for establishing innovative foundations for nursing practice, and for generating inquiry through research" (p. 469). King (1984) believes that "nurses, who have knowledge of the concepts of this Theory of Goal Attainment, are able to perceive what is happening to patients and family members and are able to suggest approaches for coping with the situations" (p. 12).

King also developed a documentation system, the goal-oriented nursing record (GONR), to accompany the middle range Theory of Goal Attainment, and to record goals and outcomes. The GONR is a method of collecting data, identifying problems, and implementing and evaluating care that has been used effectively in patient settings. The theory and the GONR are useful in practice, because nurses have the ability to provide individualized plans of care while encouraging active participation from patients in the decision-making phase (King, 1984). Nurses also can use the GONR approach to document the effectiveness of nursing care. "The major elements in this record system are: (a) data base, (b) nursing diagnosis, (c) goal list, (d) nursing orders, (e) flow sheets, (f) progress notes, and (g) discharge summary" (King, 1995b, pp. 30-31).

Healthcare professionals have implemented King's (1981) conceptual system and middle range Theory of Goal Attainment in various national and international practice settings (King, 2006, 2007). The following briefly identifies some of these settings, and the references detail additional settings. Jolly and Winker (1995) described the application of the Theory of Goal Attainment within the context of nursing administration. Alligood (1995) applied the Theory of Goal Attainment to adult patients within orthopedic nursing settings. Laben, Sneed, and Seidel (1995) used goal attainment in short-term group psychotherapy. Coker and colleagues (1995) used the conceptual system to implement nursing diagnoses in a Canadian community hospital, and Fawcett, Vaillancourt, and Watson (1995) used the conceptual system within a large Canadian tertiary care hospital. Viera and Rossi (2000) used King's conceptual system to study nursing diagnoses with puerperal women. Williams (2001) applied King's work in emergency and rural nursing. The Theory of Goal Attainment provided the framework for Daniel's (2002) descriptive study of the perceptions of young adults with chronic inflammatory bowel disease.

In addition to application of the Theory of Goal Attainment with individual or groups of patients or clients, King's conceptual system has been applied to nursing practice. In 1989, Elberson described how King's conceptual system could be applied to nursing administrative practice. Sieloff (1995b) defined the health of a social system. Sieloff began to develop a middle range theory of group power within organizations in 1989. King's theory was further refined and revised (1995a, 2007). Olsson and Forsdahl (1996) examined the role of the new nurse in a Norwegian hospital. King (2007) further clarified the application of her conceptual system within a healthcare organization.

Previous publications have obviously supported the acceptance of King's work in the nursing community. Frey, Sieloff, and Norris (2002) provided an overview of the impact of King's work in the past, present, and future. The acceptance of King's work in the future was further supported by several other publications. King (2007) described her theory of goal attainment and the transaction process as viewed in the twenty-first century. Lane-Tillerson (2007) emphasized that "the idea of continuous advancement is central to Imogene King's (1981) conceptual framework" (p. 141), and imagined nursing practice in 2050, using King's conceptual system, providing support that King's work will be accepted by the nursing community in the years to come. Khowaja (2006) described the use of King's conceptual system and Theory of Goal Attainment (1981) in the development of a clinical pathway. Killeen and King (2007) provided additional support and addressed the use of King's conceptual system with nursing informatics and nursing classification systems for global communications.

Education

Nursing faculty at several universities, such as King and Daubenmire (1973) at Ohio State University; Gold, Haas, and King (2000) at Loyola University in Chicago; and Gulitz and King (1988) at the University of South Florida used King's concepts to design curricula in nursing programs. In 1980, Brown and Lee reported that King's concepts were useful in developing a framework for "use in nursing education, nursing practice, and for generating hypotheses for research . . . [They] provide a systematic means of viewing the nursing profession, organizing a body of knowledge for nursing, and clarifying nursing as a discipline" (p. 468). King's conceptual system and theory also have application for nursing education internationally as described by Rooke (1995b) for a Swedish educational setting and Bello (2000) for Portuguese undergraduate students.

The literature also includes the application of King's work to patient education. Palmer (2006) identified patient education implications for nurses working with older adults.

Research

Many research studies have used King's work as a theoretical basis. Several studies are mentioned here as examples, and others are listed in the bibliography.

Many researchers have used concepts from King's conceptual system. Winker (1995) developed a systems view of health. Rooke (1995a) identified the implications of space for nursing. Sieloff (1995a) defined the health of a social system.

Other researchers have used King's (1981) conceptual system as a theoretical base. This group includes the following:

- McKinney and Dean (2000) applied the conceptual system to "study child abuse and the development of alcohol use/dependence in adult females" (p. 73).
- Gerstle (2001) explored relationships among nurses' moral judgments, their perceptions and judgments of pain, and selected nurse factors, using the conceptual system.
- Lane-Tillerson, Davis, Killion, and Baker (2005) evaluated nursing outcomes when working with African American adolescent girls in relation to a weight loss and weight management program.
- Khowaja (2006) utilized King's conceptual system and theory of goal attainment to develop a clinical pathway.
- Frey, Ellis, and Naar-King (2007) examined the congruency between King's conceptual system and multisystemic therapy.

Researchers also have developed many middle range theories using King's conceptual system (King, 1978). Some of these theories include Frey's theory of families, children, and chronic illness (Frey, 1995), Killeen's theory of patient satisfaction with professional nursing care (1996, 2007), Sieloff's theory of group power within organizations (Sieloff, 1995b, 2003, 2007), Wicks' theory of family health (Wicks, 1995; Wicks, Rice, & Talley, 2007), Doornbos' (2000, 2007) theory related to family health, and the advance directive decision-making model of Goodwin, Kiehl, and Peterson (2002). Fairfax (2007) derived a theory of quality of life of stroke survivors. In addition, other middle range theories have been identified (Sieloff & Frey, 2007).

Research also has been conducted using the concepts of the Theory of Goal Attainment (King, 1981). Hanucharurnkui and Vinya-nguag (1991) used goal attainment to study the outcomes of self-care on postoperative patients' recovery and satisfaction. Froman (1995) studied the perceptual congruency between nurses and patients experiencing medical-surgical conditions. Hanna's (1995) use of the Theory of Goal Attainment promoted the health behavior of adolescents, and Kameoka (1995) analyzed nurse-patient interactions. Anderson (2000) studied parental perceptions of family-centered care provided to children with cleft lip or palate, and Mahon (2001) studied the congruency of patient and nurse expectations and perceptions on postsurgical units.

FURTHER DEVELOPMENT

Over the years, King demonstrated consistently her belief in the need for further testing of the Theory of Goal Attainment. "Any profession that has as its primary mission the delivery of social services requires continuous research to discover new knowledge that can be applied to improve practice" (King, 1971, p. 112). "Because the conceptual systems framework has been synthesized from basic elements in nursing, it will persist into the Twenty one century despite professional and social changes" (King, 1995a, p. 15).

In 1995, Fawcett and Whall identified the following five major areas in which further development of King's work would be helpful:

1. The concept of environment would benefit from additional definition and clarification.
2. King's views of illness, health, and wellness will benefit from additional clarification and discussion.
3. Middle range theories that are implied rather than explicit, such as those of Rooke (1995b), will benefit from development into formal theories. Sieloff & Frey (2007) examined the status of middle range theory development from within King's conceptual system. In 2007, Fawcett examined the development of middle range theory, from within King's conceptual system, and made the following recommendations:
   a) The credibility of King's conceptual system could be further supported through "a meta-analysis or other integrative review of the results obtained from empirical tests of . . . the middle range theory propositions" (Fawcett, 2007, p. 301).
   b) "Additional metatheoretical research is needed to specify the relations between the concepts within the personal, interpersonal, and social systems" (Fawcett, 2007, p. 301).
   c) Continued empirical testing of all middle range theories is also needed.
   d) Additional research instruments need to be developed to measure middle range theory concepts. The utility of those instruments then needs to be evaluated in terms of their utility for practice (Fawcett, 2007).
4. Future linkages between King's (1981) conceptual system and other existing middle range theories should continue in a manner that ensures congruency between the conceptual system and the specific middle range theory.
5. Empirical testing should continue for the Theory of Goal Attainment (King, 1981) and other middle range theories developed within King's conceptual system (Fawcett & Whall, 1995).

CRITIQUE

Simplicity

King's definitions are clear and are conceptually derived from research literature that existed at the time the definitions were published. King's (1978) Theory of Goal Attainment presents ten major concepts, making the theory complex. However, these concepts are easily understood and, with the exception of the concept of self, they have been derived from the research literature.

Generality

King's (1981) Theory of Goal Attainment has been criticized for having limited application in areas of nursing in which patients are unable to interact competently with the nurse. King has responded that 70% of communication is nonverbal and describes the following:

> Try observing a good nurse interact with a baby or a child who has not yet learned the language. If you systematically recorded your observations, you would be able to analyze the behaviors and find many transactions at a nonverbal level. I have a beautiful example of that when I was working side by side with a graduate student in a neuro unit

> with a comatose patient. I was talking to the patient, explaining everything that was happening and showing the graduate student what I believe to be important in nursing care. When the patient regained consciousness a few days later, she asked the nurse in the unit to find that wonderful nurse who was the only one who explained what was happening to her. She wanted to thank her. I made transactions. I could observe her muscle movement. She was trying to help us communicate with her as the resident was poking a tube down her throat.

A nurse-midwife reports observing transactions between mothers and newborns. Psychiatric nurses have reported to me the value of my theory in their practice. So the need in nursing is to broaden nurses' knowledge of communication, and that is what my theory is all about (I. King, personal communication, 1985).

Healthcare professionals have documented additional examples of the application of the Theory of Goal Attainment with psychiatric patients (Kemppainen, 1990; Laben et al., 1995; Ng & Tsang, 2002), patients with acute and chronic orthopedic problems (Alligood, 1995), and developmentally disabled patients (Messmer, 1995). Kameoka, Funashima, and Sugimori (2007) tested a proposition of the theory and explored "the characteristics of nurses whose degree of goal attainment and satisfactions in interactions with patients were both high" (p. 261). King believed that critics assume that a theory will address every person, event, and situation, which is clearly impossible. King reminded critics that even Einstein's theory of relativity could not be tested completely until space travel made testing possible (I. King, personal communication, 1985).

Empirical Precision

King gathered empirical data on the nurse-patient interaction process that leads to goal attainment. A descriptive study was conducted to identify the characteristics of transaction and whether nurses made transactions with patients. From a sample of seventeen patients, goals were attained in twelve cases (70% of the sample). King (1981) believed that, if nursing students were taught the transactual process in the Theory of Goal Attainment and it is used in nursing practice, goal attainment can be measured and the effectiveness of nursing care can be demonstrated.

King continued to serve as a consultant to researchers who tested hypotheses derived from her theory. Since the publication of her theory in 1981, multiple research studies provide additional and ongoing evidence of the empirical precision of the Theory of Goal Attainment.

Froman (1995) tested perceptual congruency between nurses and patients who were experiencing medical-surgical problems. Hanna (1995) tested the Theory of Goal Attainment in promoting health behaviors of adolescents. Using the Theory of Goal Attainment, Kameoka (1995) analyzed interactions between nurses and patients. Additional research projects are currently ongoing, and others are listed in this chapter's bibliography.

Derivable Consequences

King's (1981) middle range Theory of Goal Attainment focuses on all aspects of the nursing process: assessment, planning, implementation, and evaluation. King believed that nurses must assess to set mutual goals, plan to provide alternative means to achieve goals, and evaluate to determine whether goals are attained. King, a renowned nurse theorist, "provided a theory that deals with choice, alternatives, the participation of all individuals in decision making and, specifically, deals with outcomes of nursing care" (I. King, personal communication, 1985).

Healthcare professionals have used, and continue to use, King's conceptual system and middle range Theory of Goal Attainment to implement theory-based practice in various nursing practice settings in Asia (Chugh, 2005), Australia (Khowaja, 2006), Canada, China (Cheng, 2006), Japan (Kameoka, Funashima, & Sugimori, 2007), Portugal (Chaves & de Araujo, 2006), Sweden (Rooke, 1995a, 1995b) and the United States (Frey, Rooke, Sieloff, Messmer & Kameoka, 1995).

King's work has demonstrated over time to be a structured framework for curriculum development at various educational levels. King and other nurse scientists and researchers have used her conceptual system for theory testing and theory development at the middle range level.

SUMMARY

Imogene King contributed to the advancement of nursing knowledge through the development of her conceptual system and middle range Theory of Goal Attainment. By focusing on the attainment of goals, or outcomes, by nurse-patient partnerships, King provided a conceptual system and middle range theory that has demonstrated its usefulness to nurses both in the present and in the future. Nurses from a variety of settings, working with different patient populations from around the world, continue to use King's work to improve the quality of patient care.

Case Study

Upon receiving an assignment at the start of the shift, Colin Jennings, RN, makes initial rounds of the patients. One patient, Amed Kyzeel, as reported by nurses on the previous shift, has been difficult to work with, demanding the attention of staff throughout the shift.

Mr. Jennings visits Mr. Kyzeel last during rounds so that additional time is available for an assessment. Upon entering Mr. Kyzeel's room, Mr. Jennings asks how he is feeling. Mr. Kyzeel complains about a variety of minor concerns. Accepting that Mr. Kyzeel's perceptions are unique and valid to him, Mr. Jennings spends a few minutes just listening.

Because he knows that Mr. Kyzeel is to be discharged today, he asks what the patient knows about his pending discharge and his goals for the day. Mr. Kyzeel admits that he is concerned about leaving the hospital, because he does not know what he can expect during the first 24 hours at home. Mr. Jennings talks with the patient about his concerns, asking him what goals he might want to achieve while in the hospital and upon returning home. Mr. Kyzeel identifies two to three goals that he would like to achieve in the hospital and says that he would like to have someone to stay with him at his home for the first night.

Of the goals identified, Mr. Jennings and Mr. Kyzeel identify which are the most important and the order in which Mr. Kyzeel would like to achieve them. Once this is done, Mr. Jennings and Mr. Kyzeel identify activities that can be done by the patient and the staff to achieve these goals. Before leaving the room, Mr. Jennings and Mr. Kyzeel agree on the goals, their priority, and the specific activities that are to be done.

Having established times when Mr. Jennings and Mr. Kyzeel would briefly talk to evaluate achievement of the goals, Mr. Jennings leaves the room and Mr. Kyzeel begins to work on the activities he needs to accomplish.

CRITICAL THINKING *Activities*

1. Develop your personal definitions of *environment, health, nursing,* and *person,* and compare your definitions with King's. Identify the similarities and differences. Develop a plan to use King's conceptual system and Goal Attainment Theory in your practice.
2. Analyze an interaction you have had with a patient. Were you able to achieve a transaction? If so, think about why you were successful; if not, reflect to identify why.
3. Does the healthcare agency's philosophy encourage involvement of the patients in their care? If so, does mutual goal setting occur? If not, what changes would you suggest to more actively involve patients in their care?
4. Analyze the goal-setting process that occurs between the direct care staff and the nursing administration in a healthcare agency. Does

mutual goal setting occur? Discuss possible changes in the organizational culture to facilitate mutual goal setting.

5. Develop a quality improvement plan to review patient outcomes based on application of mutual goal setting. Encourage documentation of the improvement in effectiveness and efficiency of the care provided based on the use of King's Theory of Goal Attainment.

POINTS FOR *Further Study*

Publications

- King, I. M. (2006). A system approach in nursing administration: Structure, process, and outcome. *JONA 30*(2), 100-104.
- King, I. M. (2007). King's conceptual system, theory of goal attainment, and transaction process in the 21st century. *Nursing Science Quarterly 20*(2), 109-116.
- King, I. (2007). King's structure, process, and outcomes in the 21st century. In C. L. Sieloff, & M. A. Frey (Eds.), *Middle range theory development using King's conceptual system* (pp. 3-11). New York: Springer Publishing Company.
- Sieloff, C. L., & Frey, M. A. (Eds.). (2007). *Middle range theory development using King's conceptual system.* New York: Springer Publishing Company.

Websites

- Mayo Clinic. Accessed February 1, 2008: http://www.mayo.edu/education/nursing-research/king.html
- Nurses.info. Accessed February 1, 2008: http://www.nurses.info/nursing_theory_person_king_imogene.htm
- Nursing Inquiry. Accessed February 1, 2008: http://www.geocities.com/nursinginquiry2002/anabelle/imogeneking3.html
- NurseScribe. Accessed February 1, 2008: http://www.enursescribe.com/imogene_king.htm
- Nursingtheory.net. Accessed February 1, 2008: http://www.nursingtheory.net/models_generalsystems.html

REFERENCES

Alligood, M. R. (1995). Theory of goal attainment: Application to adult orthopedic nursing. In M. A. Frey & C. L. Sieloff (Eds.), *Advancing King's systems framework and theory of nursing* (pp. 209-222). Thousand Oaks, CA: Sage.

Allport, F. H. (1955). *Theories of perception and the concept of structure.* New York: John Wiley & Sons.

Anderson, K. G. (2000). Perceptions of family centered care of parents of children with cleft lip and/or palate. *Masters Abstracts International, 38-06*, 1580.

Ardrey, R. (1966). *The territorial imperative.* New York: Atheneum.

Austin, J. K., & Champion, V. L. (1983). King's theory for nursing: Explication and evaluation. In P. Chinn (Ed.), *Advances in nursing theory development* (pp. 49-61). Rockville, MD: Aspen.

Bello, I. T. R. (2000). Imogene King's theory as the foundation for the set of a teaching-learning process with undergraduation [sic] students [Portuguese]. *Texto & Contexto Enfermagem, 9*(2 Part 2), 646-657.

Brown, S. T., & Lee, B. T. (1980). Imogene King's conceptual framework: A proposed model for continuing nursing education. *Journal of Advanced Nursing, 5*(5), 467-473.

Chaves, E. S., & de Araujo, T. L. (2006). Nursing care for an adolescent with cardiovascular risk [Portuguese]. *Ciencia, Cuidado e Saude, 5*(1), 82-87.

Cheng, M. (2006). Using King's goal attainment theory to facilitate drug compliance in a psychiatric patient [Chinese]. *Journal of Nursing, 53*(3), 90-97.

Chugh, D. (2005). Care analysis using goal attainment model. *Asian Journal of Cardiovascular Nursing, 13*(2), 2-6.

Clements, I. W., & Roberts, F. B. (1983). *Family health: A theoretical approach to nursing care.* New York: John Wiley & Sons.

Coker, E., Fridley, T., Harris, J., Tomarchio, D., Chan, V., & Caron, C. (1995). Implementing nursing diagnoses within the context of King's conceptual framework. In M. A. Frey & C. L. Sieloff (Eds.), *Advancing King's systems framework and theory of nursing* (pp. 161-175). Thousand Oaks, CA: Sage.

Daniel, J. M. (2002). Young adults' perceptions of living with chronic inflammatory bowel disease. *Gastroenterology Nursing, 25*(3), 83-94.

Dewey, J., & Bentley, A. (1949). *Knowing and the known.* Boston: Beacon Press.

Diers, D., & Schmidt, R. (1977). Interaction analysis in nursing research. In P. Verhonick (Ed.), *Nursing research II* (pp. 77-132). Boston: Little, Brown.

Doornbos, M. M. (2000). King's systems framework and family health: The derivation and testing of a theory. *Journal of Theory Construction & Testing, 4*(1), 20-26.

Doornbos, M. M. (2007). King's conceptual system and family health theory in the families of adults with persistent mental illness—An evolving conceptualization. In C. L. Sieloff & M. A. Frey (Eds). *Middle range theory development using King's conceptual system* (pp. 31-49). New York: Springer Publishing Company.

Elberson, K. (1989). Applying King's model to nursing administration. In Henry, B., DiVicenti, M., Arndt, C., & Marriner, A. (Eds.), *Dimensions of nursing administration: Theory, research, education and practice* (pp. 47-53). Boston: Blackwell Scientific Publications.

Fairfax, J. (2007). Development of a middle range theory of quality of life of stroke survivors derived from King's conceptual system. In C. L. Sieloff & M. A. Frey (Eds). *Middle range theory development using King's conceptual system* (pp. 124-137). New York: Springer Publishing Company.

Fawcett, J. (2007). Development of middle range theories based on King's conceptual system: A commentary on progress and future directions. In C. L. Sieloff & M. A. Frey (Eds). *Middle range theory development using King's conceptual system* (pp. 297-307). New York: Springer Publishing Company.

Fawcett, J. M., Vaillancourt, V. M., & Watson, C. A. (1995). Integration of King's framework into nursing practice. In M. A. Frey & C. L. Sieloff (Eds.), *Advancing King's systems framework and theory of nursing* (pp. 176-191). Thousand Oaks, CA: Sage.

Fawcett, J. M., & Whall, A. L. (1995). State of the science and future directions. In M. A. Frey & C. L. Sieloff (Eds.), *Advancing King's systems framework and theory of nursing* (pp. 327-334). Thousand Oaks, CA: Sage.

Frey, M. A. (1995). Toward a theory of families, children, and chronic illness. In M. A. Frey & C. L. Sieloff (Eds.), *Advancing King's systems framework and theory of nursing* (pp. 109-125). Thousand Oaks, CA: Sage.

Frey, M. A., Ellis, D. A., & Naar-King, S. (2007). Testing nursing theory with intervention research: The congruency between King's conceptual system and multisystemic therapy. In C. L. Sieloff & M. A. Frey (Eds). *Middle range theory development using King's conceptual system* (pp. 273-286). New York: Springer Publishing Company.

Frey, M., Rooke. L. Sieloff, C, Messmer, P., Kameoka, T. (1995). Implementing King's conceptual framework and theory of goal attainment in Japan, Sweden and United States. *Image 27*(2), 127-130.

Frey, M. A., & Sieloff, C. L. (Eds). (1995). *Advancing King's framework and theory for nursing*. Thousand Oaks, CA: Sage.

Frey, M. A., Sieloff, C. L., & Norris, D. M. (2002). King's conceptual system and theory of goal attainment: Past, present, and future. *Nursing Science Quarterly, 15*

Froman, D. (1995). Perceptual congruency between clients and nurses: Testing King's theory of goal attainment. In M. A. Frey & C. L. Sieloff (Eds.), *Advancing King's systems framework and theory of nursing* (pp. 223-238). Thousand Oaks, CA: Sage.

Gerstle, D. S. (2001). Relationships among registered nurses' moral judgment and their perception and judgment of pain, and selected nurse factors (Imogene King). *Dissertation Abstracts International, 62-04B*, 1803.

Gold, C., Haas, S., & King, I. (2000). Conceptual frameworks: Putting the nursing focus into core curricula. *Nurse Educator, 25*(2), 95-98.

Goodwin, Z., Kiehl, E. M., & Peterson, J. Z. (2002). King's theory as foundation for an advance directive decision-making model. *Nursing Science Quarterly, 15*(3), 237-241.

Gulitz, E., & King, I. (1988). King's general system model: Application to curriculum development. Nursing Science Quarterly 3(2), 128-132.

Hanna, K. M. (1995). Use of King's theory of goal attainment to promote adolescents' health behavior. In M. A. Frey & C. L. Sieloff (Eds.), *Advancing King's systems framework and theory of nursing* (pp. 239-250). Thousand Oaks, CA: Sage.

Hanucharurnkui, S., & Vinya-nguag, P. (1991). Effects of promoting patients' participation in self-care on postoperative recovery and satisfaction with care. *Nursing Science Quarterly, 4*(1), 14-20.

Houser, B. P., & Player, K. N. (2007). Imogene King. In *Pivotal Moments in Nursing* (Vol. 2). Sigma Theta Tau International Honor Society of Nursing. Indianapolis, IN, 106-131,

Ittleson, W., & Cantril, H. (1954). *Perception: A transactional approach.* Garden City, NY: Doubleday.

Jersild, A. T. (1952). *In search of self.* New York: Teachers College Press.

Jolly, M. L., & Winker, C. K. (1995). Theory of goal attainment in the context of organizational structure. In M. A. Frey & C. L. Sieloff (Eds.), *Advancing King's systems framework and theory of nursing* (pp. 305-316). Thousand Oaks, CA: Sage.

Kameoka, T. (1995). Analyzing nurse-patient interactions in Japan. In M. A. Frey & C. L. Sieloff (Eds.), *Advancing King's systems framework and theory of nursing* (pp. 251-260). Thousand Oaks, CA: Sage.

Kameoka, T., Funashima, N., & Sugimori, M. (2007). If goals are attained, satisfaction will occur in nurse-patient interaction: An empirical test. In C. L. Sieloff & M. A. Frey (Eds). *Middle range theory development using King's conceptual system* (pp. 261-272). New York: Springer Publishing Company.

Kelley, K. J., & Hammond, K. R. (1964). An approach to the study of clinical inference. *Nursing Research, 13*(4), 314-322.

Kemppainen, J. K. (1990). Imogene King's theory: A nursing case study of a psychotic client with human immunodeficiency virus infection. *Archives of Psychiatric Nursing, 4*(6), 384-388.

Khowaja, D. (2006). Utilization of King's interacting systems framework and theory of goal attainment with new multidisciplinary model: Clinical pathway. *Australian Journal of Advanced Nursing, 24*(2), 44-50.

Killeen, M. B. (1996). *Patient-consumer perceptions and responses to professional nursing care: Instrument development.* Unpublished doctoral dissertation, Wayne State University, Detroit.

Killeen, M. B. (2007). Development and initial testing of a theory of patient satisfaction with nursing care. In C. L. Sieloff & M. A. Frey (Eds). *Middle range theory development using King's conceptual system* (pp. 138-163). New York: Springer Publishing Company.

Killeen, M. B., & King, I. M. (2007). Use of King's conceptual system, nursing informatics, and nursing classification systems for global communication. *International Journal of Nursing Terminologies and Classifications, 18*(2), 51-57.

King, I. M. (1964). Nursing theory: Problems and prospects. *Nursing Science, 1*(3), 394-403.

King, I. M. (1968). A conceptual frame of reference for nursing. *Nursing Research, 17*(1), 27-31.

King, I. M. (1971). *Toward a theory for nursing: General concepts of human behavior.* New York: John Wiley & Sons.

King, I. M. (1975a). A process for developing concepts for nursing through research. In P. Verhonick (Ed.), *Nursing research.* Boston: Little, Brown.

King, I. M. (1975b). Patient aspects. In L. J. Schumann, R. D. Spears, Jr., & J. P. Young (Eds.), *Operations research in health care: A critical analysis.* Baltimore: Johns Hopkins University Press.

King, I. M. (1977). Knowledge development in nursing: A process. In I. M. King, & J. Fawcett (Eds.). *The language of nursing theory and metatheory.* (pp. 19-25). Indianapolis: Sigma Theta Tau International Center Nursing Press.

King, I. M. (Speaker). (1978). *Speech presented at 2nd Annual Nurse Educators' Conference.* Chicago: Teach 'Em.

King, I. M. (1981). *A theory for nursing: Systems, concepts, process.* New York: John Wiley & Sons.

King, I. M. (1984). Effectiveness of nursing care: Use of a goal oriented nursing record in end stage renal disease. *American Association of Nephrology Nurses and Technicians Journal, 11*(2), 11-17, 60.

King, I. M. (1986). *Curriculum and instruction in nursing: Concepts and process.* Norwalk, CT: Appleton-Century-Crofts.

King, I. M. (1995a). A systems framework for nursing. In M. A. Frey & C. L. Sieloff (Eds.), *Advancing King's systems framework and theory of nursing* (pp. 14-22). Thousand Oaks, CA: Sage.

King, I. M. (1995b). The theory of goal attainment. In M. A. Frey & C. L. Sieloff (Eds.), *Advancing King's systems framework and theory of nursing* (pp. 23-32). Thousand Oaks, CA: Sage.

King, I. M. (2006). A system approach in nursing administration: structure, process and outcome. *JONA, 30*(2), 100-104.

King, I. M. (2007). King's conceptual system, theory of goal attainment, and transaction process in the 21st century. *Nursing Science Quarterly, 20*(2), 109-116.

King, I., & Daubenmire, J. (1973). Nursing process models: A systems approach. *Nursing Outlook, 13*(19), 50-51.

Krieger, D. (1975). Therapeutic touch: The imprimatur of nursing. *American Journal of Nursing, 75*(5), 784-787.

Kuhh, A. (1975). *Unified social science.* Homewood, IL: Dorsey.

Laben, J. K., Sneed, L. D., & Seidel, S. L. (1995). Goal attainment in short-term group psychotherapy settings: Clinical implications for practice. In M. A. Frey & C. L. Sieloff (Eds.), *Advancing King's systems framework and theory of nursing* (pp. 261-277). Thousand Oaks, CA: Sage.

Lane-Tillerson, C. (2007). Imaging practice in 2050. King's conceptual framework. *Nursing Science Quarterly, 20*(2), 140-143.

Lane-Tillerson, C., Davis, B. L., Killion, C. M., & Baker, S. (2005). Evaluating nursing outcomes: A mixed-methods approach. *Journal of National Black Nurses Association, 16*(2), 20-26.

Mahon, P. Y. (2001). Bridging the gap in patient satisfaction: Congruency of patient-nurse expectation and perception. *Dissertation Abstracts International, 61-10B*, 5237.

McKinney, N. L., & Dean, P. R. (2000). Application of King's theory of dynamic interacting systems to the study of child abuse and the development of alcohol use/dependence in adult females. *Journal of Addictions Nursing, 12*(2), 73-82.

Messmer, P. R. (1995). Implementation of theory-based nursing practice. In M. A. Frey & C. L. Sieloff (Eds.), *Advancing King's systems framework and theory of nursing* (pp. 294-304). Thousand Oaks, CA: Sage.

Messmer, P. R. (2000). Imogene M. King. In V. L. Bullough & L. Sentz (Eds.), *American nursing: A biographical dictionary* (Vol. 3; pp. 164-166). New York: Springer Publishing Company.

Messmer, P. R. (2007). Tribute to the Theorists: Imogene M. King Over the Years. *Nursing Science Quarterly, 20*(3), 198.

Messmer, P. R., & Fawcett, J. (2008). In memoriam: Imogene M. King 1923-2007 *Nursing Science Quarterly, 21*(2).

Messmer, P (2008). Worldview 2008. A Global nursing perspective In honor of Imogene M. King. *Reflections* 1st quarter.

Minckley, B. B. (1968). Space and place in patient care. *American Journal of Nursing, 68*(3), 510-516.

Ng, B. F. L., & Tsang, H. W. H. (2002). A program to assist people with severe mental illness in formulating realistic life goals. *Journal of Rehabilitation, 68*(4), 59-66.

Olsson, H., & Forsdahl, T. (1996). Expectations and opportunities of newly employed nurses at the University Hospital, Tromso, Norway. *Social Sciences in Health: International Journal of Research and Practice, 2*(1), 14-22.

Orlando, I. J. (1961). *The dynamic nurse-patient relationship: Functions, process, principles.* New York: G. P. Putnam's Sons.

Orme, J. E. (1969). *Time, experience and behavior.* New York: American Elsevier.

Palmer, J. A. (2006). Nursing implications for older adult patient education. *Plastic Surgical Nursing, 26*(4), 189-194.

Paterson, J., & Zderad, L. (1976). *Humanistic nursing.* New York: John Wiley & Sons.

Peplau, H. E. (1952). *Interpersonal relations in nursing.* New York: G. P. Putnam's Sons.

Rooke, L. (1995a). The concept of space in King's systems framework: Its implications for nursing. In M. A. Frey & C. L. Sieloff (Eds.), *Advancing King's systems framework and theory of nursing* (pp. 79-96). Thousand Oaks, CA: Sage.

Rooke, L. (1995b). Focusing on King's theory and systems framework in education by using an experiential learning model: A challenge to improve the quality of nursing care. In M. A. Frey & C. L. Sieloff (Eds.), *Advancing King's systems framework and theory of nursing* (pp. 278-293). Thousand Oaks, CA: Sage.

Sieloff, C. L. (1995a). Defining the health of a social system within Imogene King's framework. In M. A. Frey & C. L. Sieloff (Eds.), *Advancing King's systems framework and theory of nursing* (pp. 137-146). Thousand Oaks, CA: Sage.

Sieloff, C. L. (1995b). Development of a theory of departmental power. In M. A. Frey & C. L. Sieloff (Eds.), *Advancing King's systems framework and theory of nursing* (pp. 46-65). Thousand Oaks, CA: Sage.

Sieloff, C. L. (1996). *Development of an instrument to estimate the actualized power of a nursing department.* Unpublished doctoral dissertation, Wayne State University, Detroit.

Sieloff, C. L. (2003). Measuring nursing power within organizations. *Journal of Nursing Scholarship, 35*(2), 183-187.

Sieloff, C. L. (2007). The theory of group power within organizations—Evolving conceptualization within King's conceptual system. In C. L. Sieloff & M. A. Frey (Eds). *Middle range theory development using King's conceptual system* (pp. 196-214). New York: Springer Publishing Company.

Sieloff, C. L., & Frey, M. (2007). *Middle range theories for nursing practice using King's interacting systems framework.* New York: Springer.

Sommer, R. (1969). *Personal space.* Englewood Cliffs, NJ: Prentice-Hall.

Viera, C. S., & Rossi, L. (2000). Nursing diagnoses from NANDA's taxonomy in women with a hospitalized preterm child and King's Conceptual System [Portuguese]. *Revista Latin-Americana de Enfermagem, 8*(6), 110-116.

Watzlawick, P., Beavin, J. W., & Jackson, D. D. (1967). *Pragmatics of human communication.* New York: Norton.

Whiting, J. F. (1955). Q-sort technique for evaluating perceptions of interpersonal relationship. *Nursing Research, 4*, 71-73.

Wicks, M. N. (1995). Family health as derived from King's framework. In M. A. Frey & C. L. Sieloff (Eds.), *Advancing King's systems framework and theory of nursing* (pp. 97-108). Thousand Oaks, CA: Sage.

Wicks, M. N., Rice, M. C., & Talley, C. H. (2007). Further exploration of family health within the context of chronic obstructive pulmonary disease. In C. L. Sieloff & M. A. Frey (Eds). *Middle range theory development using King's conceptual system* (pp. 215-236). New York: Springer Publishing Company.

Williams, L. A. (2001). Imogene King's interacting systems theory—Application in emergency and rural nursing. *Online Journal of Rural Nursing and Health Care, 2*(1). Retrieved January 8, 2004, from CINAHL.

Winker, C. K. (1995). A systems view of health. In M. A. Frey & C. L. Sieloff (Eds.), *Advancing King's systems framework and theory of nursing* (pp. 35-45). Thousand Oaks, CA: Sage.

Yura, H., & Walsh, M. (1978). *The nursing process.* New York: Appleton-Century-Crofts.

BIBLIOGRAPHY

Additional Primary Sources

Books

Fawcett, J., & King, I. (Eds.). (1997). *The language of nursing theory and metatheory.* Indianapolis: Sigma Theta Tau International Center Press.

King, I. M. (1976). *Toward a theory of nursing: General concepts of human behavior* (Sugimori, M., Trans.). Tokyo: Igaku-Shoin.

King, I. M. (1985). *A theory for nursing: Systems, concepts, process* (Sugimori, M., Trans.). Tokyo: Igaku-Shoin.

King, I. M., & Fawcett, J. (1997). *The language of nursing theory and metatheory.* Indianapolis: Sigma Theta Tau International.

Additional Book Chapters

King, I. M. (2007). King's structure, process and outcomes in the 21st century. In C. L. Sieloff & M. A. Frey (Eds). *Middle range theory development using King's conceptual system* (pp. 12-28). New York: Springer Publishing Company.

Journal Articles

Daubenmire, M. J., & King, I. M. (1973). Nursing process models: A systems approach. *Nursing Outlook, 21*(8), 512-517.

King, I. M. (1964). Nursing theory—Problems and prospect. *Nursing Science, 2*(5), 394-403.

King, I. M. (1970). A conceptual frame of reference for nursing. *Japanese Journal of Nursing Research, 3*, 199-204.

King, I. M. (1987). Translating nursing research into practice. *Journal of Neuroscience Nursing, 19*(1), 44-48.

King, I. M. (1990, Fall). Health as the goal for nursing. *Nursing Science Quarterly, 3*(3), 123-128.

King, I. M. (1992). King's theory of goal attainment. *Nursing Science Quarterly, 5*(1), 19-26.

King, I. M. (1994). Quality of life and goal attainment. *Nursing Science Quarterly, 7*(1), 29-32.

King, I. M. (1996). The theory of goal attainment in research and practice. *Nursing Science Quarterly, 9*(2), 61-66.

King, I. M. (1997). King's theory of goal attainment in practice. *Nursing Science Quarterly, 70*(4), 180-185.

King, I. M. (1997). Reflections on the past and a vision for the future. *Nursing Science Quarterly, 10*(1), 15-17.

King, I. M. (1998). Nursing informatics: A universal nursing language. *Florida Nurse, 46*(1), 1-3, 5, 9.

King, I. M. (1998). The Bioethics Focus Group Report. *Florida Nurse, 46*(8), 24.

King, I. M. (1999). A theory of goal attainment: Philosophical and ethical implications. *Nursing Science Quarterly, 12*(4), 292-296.

King, I. M. (2000). Evidence-based nursing practice. *Theoria: Journal of Nursing Theory, 9*(2), 4-9.

Quigley, P., Janzen, S. K., King, I, M., & Goucher, E. (1999). Nurse staffing patient outcomes from one acute care setting within the Department of Veteran's Affairs. *Florida Nurse, 47*(2), 34.

Letter to the Editor

King, I. M., & Whelton, B. J. B. (2001). Reaction to "A nursing theory of person system empathy: Interpreting a conceptualization of empathy in King's Interacting Systems" by M. R. Alligood & B. A. May (Letter to the Editor). *Nursing Science Quarterly, 14*(1), 80-82.

Secondary Sources

Books

Chinn, P. L., & Kramer, M. K. (1995). *Theory and nursing: A systematic approach* (3rd ed.). St. Louis: Mosby.

Fitzpatrick, J. J., & Whall, A. L. (1995). *Conceptual models of nursing: Analysis and application.* Bowie, MD: Robert J. Brady.

George, J. B. (1995). *Nursing theories: The base for professional nursing practice. Englewood* Cliffs, NJ: Prentice-Hall.

Polit, D., & Hungler, B. (1995). *Nursing research: Principles and methods* (5th ed.). Philadelphia: J. B. Lippincott.

Walker, L. O., & Avant, K. C. (1995). *Strategies for theory construction in nursing.* Norwalk, CT: Appleton-Century-Crofts.

Book Chapters

Alligood, M. R. (2007). Rethinking empathy in nursing education: Shifting to a developmental view. In C. L. Sieloff & M. A. Frey (Eds). *Middle range theory development using King's conceptual system* (pp. 287-296). New York: Springer Publishing Company.

Alligood, M. R., Evans, G. W., & Wilt, D. L. (1995). King's interacting system and empathy. In M. A. Frey & C. L. Sieloff (Eds.), *Advancing King's systems framework and theory of nursing* (pp. 66-78). Thousand Oaks, CA: Sage.

Benedict, M., & Frey, M. A. (1995). Theory-based practice in the emergency department. In M. A. Frey & C. L. Sieloff (Eds.), *Advancing King's systems framework and theory of nursing* (pp. 317-324). Thousand Oaks, CA: Sage.

Doornbos, M. M. (1995). Using King's systems framework to explore family health in the families of the young chronically mentally ill. In M. A. Frey & C. L. Sieloff (Eds.), *Advancing King's systems framework and theory of nursing* (pp. 192-205). Thousand Oaks, CA: Sage.

duMont, P. (2007). A theory of asynchronous development: A midlevel theory derived from a synthesis of King and Peplau. In C. L. Sieloff & M. A. Frey (Eds). *Middle range theory development using King's conceptual system* (pp. 50-74). New York: Springer Publishing Company.

Ehrenberger, H. E., Alligood, M. R., Thomas, S. P., Wallace, D. C., & Licavoli, C. M. (2007). Testing a theory of decision making derived from King's systems framework in women eligible for a cancer clinical trial. In C. L. Sieloff & M. A. Frey (Eds). *Middle range theory development using King's conceptual system* (pp. 75-91). New York: Springer Publishing Company.

Fawcett, J. (1995). King's open systems model. In *Analysis and evaluation of conceptual models of nursing* (3rd ed., pp. 109-163). Philadelphia: F. A. Davis.

Frey, M. A. (1995). From conceptual framework to nursing knowledge. In M. A. Frey & C. L. Sieloff (Eds.), *Advancing King's framework and theory for nursing* (pp. 3-13). Thousand Oaks, CA: Sage.

Frey, M. A., & Norris, D. (1997). King's systems framework and theory in nursing practice. In M. R. Alligood & A. Marriner Tomey (Eds.), *Nursing theory: Utilization & application* (pp. 71-88). St. Louis: Mosby.

Hernandez, C. A. (2007). The theory of integration: Congruency with King's conceptual system. In C. L. Sieloff & M. A. Frey (Eds). *Middle range theory development using King's conceptual system* (pp. 105-124). New York: Springer Publishing Company.

Hobdell, E. F. (1995). Using King's interacting systems framework for research on parents of children with neural tube defects. In M. A. Frey & C. L. Sieloff (Eds.), *Advancing King's systems framework and theory of nursing* (pp. 126-136). Thousand Oaks, CA: Sage.

May, B. A. (2007). Relationships among basic empathy, self-awareness, and learning styles of baccalaureate prenursing students within King's personal system. Killeen, M. B. (2007). Development and initial testing of a theory of patient satisfaction with nursing care. In C. L. Sieloff & M. A. Frey (Eds). *Middle range theory development using King's conceptual system* (pp. 164-177). New York: Springer Publishing Company.

Reed, J. E. F. (2007). Social support and health of older adults. In C. L. Sieloff & M. A. Frey (Eds). *Middle range theory development using King's conceptual system* (pp. 92-104). New York: Springer Publishing Company.

Sharts-Hopko, N. C. (1995). Using health, personal, and interpersonal system concepts within the King's systems framework to explore perceived health status during the menopause transition. In M. A. Frey & C. L. Sieloff (Eds.), *Advancing King's systems framework and theory of nursing* (pp. 147-160). Thousand Oaks, CA: Sage.

Sharts-Hopko, N. C. (2007). A theory of health perception: Understanding the menopause transition. In C. L. Sieloff & M. A. Frey (Eds). *Middle range theory development using King's conceptual system* (pp. 178-195). New York: Springer Publishing Company.

Sieloff, C. L. (1995). Imogene King: A conceptual framework for nursing. In C. Metzger McQuiston & A. Webb (Eds.), *Foundations of nursing theory: Contributions of 12 key theorists* (pp. 37-87). Thousand Oaks, California: SAGE Publications.

Sieloff, C. L. (1998). Imogene King: Systems framework and theory of goal attainment. In A. Marriner-Tomey and M. R. Alligood (Eds.), *Nursing theorists and their work* (4th ed.) (pp. 300-319). St. Louis: Mosby-Yearbook, Inc.

Sieloff, C. L., (2002). Imogene King: Systems framework and theory of goal attainment. In A. Marriner-Tomey and M. R. Alligood (Eds.), *Nursing theorists and their work* (5th ed.) (pp. 336-360). St. Louis: Mosby-Yearbook, Inc.

Sieloff, C. L., (2006). Imogene King: Systems framework and theory of goal attainment. In A. Marriner-Tomey and M. R. Alligood (Eds.), *Nursing theorists and their work* (6th ed.) (pp. 336-360). St. Louis: Mosby-Yearbook, Inc.

Sieloff, C. L., Frey, M., & Killeen, M. (2001). Application of King's interacting systems framework. In M. Parker (Ed.), *Nursing theorists and their application in practice.* Philadelphia: F. A. Davis.

Sieloff, C. L., Frey, M., & Killeen, M. (2006). Application of King's Interacting Systems Framework. In M. Parker (Ed.), *Nursing theorists and their application in practice* (2nd ed., pp. 244-267). Philadelphia: F. A. Davis.

Whelton, B. J. B. (2007). The nursing act is an excellent human act: A philosophical analysis derived from classical philosophy and the conceptual system and theory of Imogene King. In C. L. Sieloff & M. A. Frey (Eds). *Middle range theory development using King's conceptual system* (pp. 12-28). New York: Springer Publishing Company.

Zurakowski, T. L. (2007). Theory of social and interpersonal influences on health. In C. L. Sieloff & M. A. Frey (Eds). *Middle range theory development using King's conceptual system* (pp. 237-257). New York: Springer Publishing Company.

Journal Articles

Alligood, M. R., & May, B. A. (2000). A nursing theory of personal system empathy: Interpreting a conceptualization of empathy in King's interacting systems. *Nursing Science Quarterly, 13*(3), 243-247.

Baumann, S. L. (2000). Research issues: Family nursing: Theory-anemic, nursing theory-deprived. *Nursing Science Quarterly, 13*(4), 285-290.

Brooks, E. M., & Thomas, S. (1997). The perception and judgment of senior baccalaureate student nurses in clinical decision making. *ANS Advances in Nursing Science, 19*(3), 50-69.

Calladine, M. L. (1996). Nursing process for health promotion using King's theory. *Journal of Community Health Nursing, 13*(1), 51-57.

Campbell-Begg, T. (2000). A case study using animal-assisted therapy to promote abstinence in a group of individuals who are recovering from chemical addictions. *Journal of Addictions Nursing, 12*(1), 31-35.

Caris-Verhallen, W. M. C. M., Kerkstra, A., van der Heijden, P. G. M., & Bensing, J. M. (1998). Nurse-elderly patient communication in home care and institutional care: An explorative study. *International Journal of Nursing Studies, 35*(1/2), 95-108.

Carter, K. F., & Dufour, L. T. (1994). King's theory: A critique of the critiques. *Nursing Science Quarterly, 7*(3), 128-133.

Crossan, F., & Robb, A. (1998). Role of the nurse: Introducing theories and concepts. *British Journal of Nursing, 7*(10), 608-612.

David, G. L. B. (2000). Ethics in the relationship between nursing and AIDS-afflicted families [Portuguese]. *Texto & Contexto Enfermagem, 9*(2), 590-599.

Doornbos, M. M. (2002). Predicting family health in families with young adults with severe mental illness. *Journal of Family Nursing, 8*(3), 241-263.

Fawcett, J. (2001). Scholarly dialogue. The nurse theorists: 21st-century updates—Imogene M. King. *Nursing Science Quarterly, 14*(4), 311-315.

Frey, M. A. (1996). Behavioral correlates of health and illness in youths with chronic illness. *Advanced Nursing Research, 9*(4), 167-176.

Frey, M. A. (1997). Health promotion in youth with chronic illness: Are we on the right track? *Quality Nursing, 3*(5), 13-18.

Gill, J., Hopwood-Jones, L., Tyndall, J., Gregoroff, S., LeBlanc, P., Lovett, C., et al. (1995). Incorporating nursing diagnosis and King's theory in the O. R. documentation. *Canadian Operating Room Nursing Journal, 13*(1), 10-14.

Husting, P. M. (1997). A transcultural critique of Imogene King's theory of goal attainment. *The Journal of Multicultural Nursing & Health, 3*(3), 15-20.

Jones, S., Clark, V. B., Merker, A., & Palau, D. (1995). Changing behaviors: Nurse educators and clinical nurse specialists design a discharge planning program. *Journal of Nursing Staff Development, 11*(6), 291-295.

Kemppainen, J. K. (1990). Imogene King's theory: A nursing case study of a psychotic client with human immunodeficiency virus infection. *Archives of Psychiatric Nursing, 4*(6), 384-388.

Kline, K. S., Scott, L. D., & Britton, A. S. (2007). The use of supportive-educative and mutual goal setting strategies *to improve self*-management for patients with heart failure. *Home Healthcare News*, 25(8), 502-510.

Kobayashi, F. T. (1970). A conceptual frame of reference for nursing. *Japanese Journal of Nursing Research, 3*(3), 199-204.

Kusaka, T. (1991). Application to the King's goal attainment theory in Japanese clinical setting. *Journal of the Japanese Academy of Nursing Education, 1*(1), 30-31.

Laramee, A. (1999). The building blocks of successful relationships. *Journal of Care Management, 5*(4), 40, 42, 44-45.

Lawler, J., Dowswell, G., Hearn, J., Forster, A., & Young, J. (1999). Recovering from stroke: A qualitative investigation of the role of goal setting in late stroke recovery. *Journal of Advanced Nursing, 30*(2), 401-409.

Lewinson, S. B. (2000). Professionally speaking: Interview with Imogene King. *Nursing Leadership Forum, 4*(3), 91-95.

Lockhart, J. S. (2000). Nurses' perceptions of head and neck oncology patients after surgery: Severity of facial disfigurement and patient gender. *Plastic Surgical Nursing, 20*(2), 68-80.

Long, J. M., Kee, C. C., Graham, M. V., Saethan, T. B., & Dames, F. D. (1998). Medication compliance and the older hemodialysis patient. *American Nephrology Nurses Association Journal, 25*(1), 43-49.

Mayer, B. W. (2000). Female domestic violence victims: Perspectives on emergency care. *Nursing Science Quarterly, 13*(4), 340-346.

McKinney, N., & Frank, D. I. (1998). Nursing assessment of adult females who are alcohol dependent and victims of sexual abuse. *Clinical Excellence for Nurse Practitioners, 2*(3), 152-158.

Messmer, P. R. (2006). Professional model of care: Using King's theory of goal attainment. *Nursing Science Quarterly, 19*(3), 227-228.

Milne, J. (2000). The impact of information on health behaviors of older adults with urinary incontinence. *Clinical Nursing Research, 9*(2), 161-176.

Moreira, T. M. M., & Arajo, T. L. (2002). The conceptual model of interactive open systems and the theory of goal attainment by Imogene King [Portuguese]. *Revista Latino-Americana deEnfermagem, 10*(1), 97-103.

Murray, R. L. E., & Baier, M. (1996). King's conceptual framework applied to a transitional living program. *Perspectives in Psychiatric Care, 32*(1), 15-19.

Nagano, M., & Funashima, N. (1995). Analysis of nursing situations in Japan: Using King's goal attainment theory. *Quality Nursing, 1*(1), 74-78.

Norgan, G. H., Ettipio, A. M., & Lasome, C. E. M. (1995). A program plan addressing carpal tunnel syndrome: The utility of King's goal attainment theory. *American Association of Occupational Health Nurses Journal, 43*(8), 407-411.

Petrich, B. (2000). Medical and nursing students' perceptions of obesity. *Journal of Addictions Nursing, 12*(10), 3-16.

Richard-Hughes, S. (1997). Attitudes and beliefs of Afro-Americans related to organ and tissue donation. *International Journal of Trauma Nursing, 3*(4), 119-123.

Riggs, C. J. (2001). A model of staff support to improve retention in long-term care. *Nursing Administration Quarterly, 25*(2), 43-54.

Scott, L. D. (1998). Perceived needs of parents of critically ill children. *Journal of the Society of Pediatric Nurses, 3*(1), 4-12.

Secrest, J., Iorio, D. H., & Martz, W. (2005). The meaning of work for nursing assistants who stay in long-term care. *International Journal of Older People Nursing, 14*(8b), 90-97.

Sredl, D. (2006). The triangle technique: A new evidence-based educational tool for pediatric medication calculations. *Nursing Education Perspectives, 27*(2), 84-88.

Suslick, D., Secrest, J., Holweger, J., & Myhan, G. (2007). The perianesthesia experience from the patient's perspective. *Journal of PeriAnesthesia Nursing, 22*(1), 10-20.

Tripp-Reimer, T., Woodworth, G., McCloskey, J. C., & Bulechek, G. (1996). The dimensional structure of nursing interventions. *Nursing Research, 45*(1), 10-17.

Tritsch, J. M. (1996). Application of King's theory of goal attainment and the Carondelet St. Mary's case management model. *Nursing Science Quarterly, 11*(2), 69-73.

Ugarriza, D. N. (2002). Intentionality: Applications within selected theories of nursing. *Holistic Nursing Practice, 16*(4), 41-50.

Wadensten, B., & Carlsson, M. (2003). Nursing theory views on how to support the process of aging. *Journal of Advanced Nursing, 42*(2), 118-124.

Walker, K. M., & Alligood, M. R. (2001). Empathy from a nursing perspective: Moving beyond borrowed theory. *Archives of Psychiatric Nursing, 15*(3), 140-147.

Wilkinson, C. R., & Williams, M. (2002). Strengthening patient-provider relationships. *Lippincott's Case Management, 7*(3), 86-102.

Zurakowski, T. L. (2000). The social environment of nursing homes and the health of older residents. *Holistic Nursing Practice, 14*(4), 12-23.

Master's Theses

Allan, N. J. (1995). Goal attainment and life satisfaction among frail elderly. *Masters Abstracts International, 35-05*, 1486.

Aramburu-Drury, C. M. (1996). Exploring the association between body weight and health care avoidance. *Masters Abstracts International, 35-03*, 0725.

Arbeiter, N. A. (1998). The effect of a formal class on advance directives on nurses' perceptions. *Masters Abstracts International, 36-04*, 1059.

Bailey, A. A. (2005). Public health nurses' perceptions of role change. *Masters Abstracts International, 43-04*, 1698.

Bowman, A. M. (2004). Parents' perceptions of quality family-centered nursing care in pediatrics. *Masters Abstracts International, 42-05*, 1679.

Brennan, K. M. (2000). Parents' perceptions of their roles during the treatment of their child's thermal injury. *Masters Abstracts International, 38-06*, 1581.

Dawson, B. W. (1996). The relationship between functional social support, social network and the adequacy of prenatal care. *Masters Abstracts International, 35-01*, 0361.

Federowicz, M. L. (2002). An investigation of clients' perceptions of what constitutes quality nursing care: A phenomenological approach. *Masters Abstracts International, 40-06*, 1501.

Genzel, M. C. (1998). Job satisfaction of the nursing staff development educator. *Masters Abstracts International, 36-04*, 1063.

Johnson, T. (2005). Job satisfaction recruitment and retention of public health nurses. *Masters Abstracts International, 43-05*, 1701.

Kahn, R. (1997). The number and types of interventions developed and employed for a population of ADHD students by an advanced nurse practitioner in a middle-sized urban school district in Michigan Title I Health Program during the 1995-1996 school year. *Masters Abstracts International, 36-01*, 0158.

Kaminski, L. A. (1999). Perceptions of home care nurses as facilitators of discussions and advance directives. *Masters Abstracts International, 37-04*, 1179.

King-Jones, M. J. (2004). Horizontal violence experienced by nursing students. *Masters Abstracts International, 43-05*, 1702.

Leonard, B. M. (1996). Team building using group and peer initiating processes within Imogene King's systems to facilitate CQI (Continuous Quality Improvement). *Masters Abstracts International, 34-06*, 2346.

Luke, J. (2005). Registered nurses' perceptions towards individuals experiencing pain during sickle cell crisis. *Masters Abstracts International, 43-06*, 2196.

McCartan, D. P. (2000). Measurement of the quality of life perceptions of in-home hospice patients: A descriptive/exploratory study. *Masters Abstracts International, 38-06*, 1586.

McGonigle, S. M. (1998). Evaluating outcomes: Client satisfaction with primary nursing in tertiary care. *Masters Abstracts International, 36-04*, 1066.

Mang, A. M. (2001). Parish nursing. *Masters Abstracts International, 40-03*, 674.

Peladeau, N. M. (2006). An empirical study of the stress-coping responses of nurses during the several acute respiratory syndrome (SARS) outbreak. *Masters Abstract International, 44-05*, 2278.

Phillips, E. L. (1995). Diploma nursing students' attitudes toward poverty. *Masters Abstracts International, 33-06*, 1846.

Pinnock-Philp, B. E. (1998). Attitudes toward restricting food in labor: Differences between caregivers in a tertiary care perinatal center and a birthing center. *Masters Abstracts International, 36-06*, 1600.

Prince, S. G. (2005). Comparing two different teaching strategies within a practical nursing diploma program. *Masters Abstracts International, 43-06*, 2199.

Ranta, M. (2000). The effect of mutual goal setting on the self-efficacy to manage heart failure in adults. *Masters Abstracts International, 39-01*, 196.

Rexford, D. S. (2001). Quality of life in a heart failure population. *Masters Abstracts International, 40-01*, 152.

Russo-Meck, P. A. (2004). Career preferences of undergraduate nursing students. *Masters Abstracts International, 43-05*, 1703.

Six, D. M. (1998). Patient satisfaction with prenatal care services in a rural setting: Time. *Masters Abstracts International, 36-06*, 1591.

Skariah, R. A. (1999). Analysis of first nation children's drawings of their perceptions of health. *Masters Abstracts International, 37-04*, 1184.

Sperry, E. J. (1999). Physician perceptions of behaviors associated with the nurse practitioner role. *Masters Abstracts International, 37-06*, 1821.

Stanley, J. M. (2000). Nurses' perceptions of hypnosis. *Masters Abstracts International, 38-03*, 685.

Stover, D. C. (1999). A change in patient satisfaction in the endoscopy laboratory. *Masters Abstracts International, 38-02*, 416.

Tinglin, S. A. (2006). The perceptions of stress in mature female nurses returning to school for graduate studies. *Masters Abstracts International, 44-06*, 2765.

Villanueva-Noble, N. S. (1998). Cross-cultural analysis of perceptions of health in children's drawings: A replicate study (Philippines, Canada). *Masters Abstracts International, 36-04*, 1070.

Doctoral Dissertations

Bigony, M. D. (2007). Perceptions of the nurse-caregiver relationship ands its influence on the utilization of respite care services by spousal caregivers of patients diagnosed with dementia. *Dissertation Abstracts International, 68-04B*, 2243.

Brooks, E. (1995). Exploring the perception and judgment of senior baccalaureate student nurses in clinical decision-making from a nursing theoretical perspective. *Dissertation Abstracts International*, 56-12B, 6667.

duMont, P. (1998). The effects of early menarche on health risk behaviors. *Dissertation Abstracts International*, 60-07B, 3200.

Ehrenberger, H. E. (1998). Testing a theory of decision making derived from King's systems framework in women eligible for a cancer clinical trial. Dissertation *Abstracts International, 60-07B*, 3201.

Gerstle, D. S. (2001). Relationships among registered nurses' moral judgment and their perception and judgment of pain, and selected nurse factors (Imogene King). *Dissertation Abstracts International, 62-04B*, 1803.

Gunther, M. E. (2001). The meaning of high quality nursing care derived from King's interacting systems (Imogene King). *Dissertation Abstracts International, 62-04B*, 1804.

Killeen, M. (1996). Patient-consumer perceptions and responses to professional nursing care: Instrument development. *Dissertation Abstracts International, 57-04B*, 2479.

Maloni, H. W. (2007). An intervention to effect hypertension, glycemic control, diabetes self-management, self-efficacy, and satisfaction with care in type 2 diabetic VA health care users with inadequate functional health literacy skills. *Dissertation Abstracts International, 68-04B*, 2253.

May, B. A. (2000). Relationships among basic empathy, self-awareness, and learning styles of baccalaureate prenursing students within King's personal system. *Dissertation Abstracts International, 61-06b*, 2991.

McKay, T. (1999). An examination of case management nurses' role strain, participative decision making, and their relationships to patient satisfaction: Utilization of King's theory of goal attainment in a managed care environment. *Dissertation Abstracts International, 60-09B*, 4522.

Sieloff, C. L. (1996). Development of an instrument to estimate the actualized power of a nursing department. *Dissertation Abstracts International, 57-04B*, 2484.

Sink, K. K. (2001). Perceptions, informational needs, and feelings of competency of new parents. *Dissertation Abstracts International, 62-01B*, 166.

Whelton, B. T. B. (1996). A philosophy of nursing practice: An application of the Thomistic-Aristotelian concept of nature to the science of nursing. *Dissertation Abstracts International, 57-03A*, 1176.

Winker, C. (1996). A descriptive study of the relationship of interaction disturbance to the organizational health of a metropolitan general hospital. *Dissertation Abstracts International, 57-07B*, 4306.

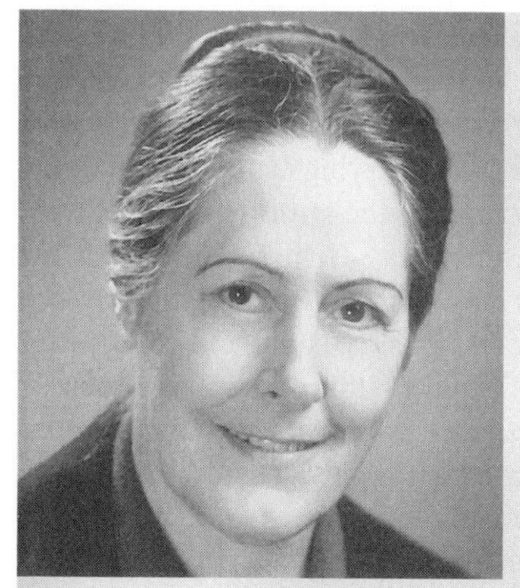

CHAPTER

16

Betty Neuman

1924-present

Systems Model

Barbara T. Freese and Theresa G. Lawson

"The Neuman Systems Model is well positioned as a directive for a truly wholistic perspective for nursing. Its concepts and processes are relevant for the twenty-first century and beyond. Its universal and timeless nature has long proven its value in being utilized effectively by health care professionals in any cultural setting" (B. Neuman, personal communication, December 28, 2007).

CREDENTIALS AND BACKGROUND OF THE THEORIST

Betty Neuman was born in 1924 and grew up on a farm in Ohio. Her rural background helped her develop a compassion for people in need, which has been evident throughout her career. She completed her initial nursing education with double honors at Peoples Hospital School of Nursing (now General Hospital), Akron, Ohio, in 1947. As a young nurse, she moved to California and worked in a variety of roles that included hospital nurse, school nurse, industrial nurse, and clinical instructor at the University of Southern California Medical Center. She earned a baccalaureate degree in public health and psychology with honors (1957) and a master's degree in mental health, public health consultation (1966), from the University of California, Los Angeles (UCLA). She completed a doctoral degree in clinical psychology at Pacific Western University in 1985 (B. Neuman, personal communication, June 3, 1984).

Neuman was a pioneer of nursing involvement in mental health. She and Donna Aquilina were the first two nurses to develop the nurse counselor role within community crisis centers in Los Angeles (B. Neuman, personal communication, June 21, 1992). She developed, taught, and refined a community mental health program for post–master's level nurses at UCLA. She developed and published her first explicit teaching and practice model

Previous authors: Barbara T. Freese, Sarah J. Beckman, Sanna Boxley-Harges, Cheryl Bruick-Sorge, Susan Matthews Harris, Mary E. Hermiz, Mary Meininger, and Sandra E. Steinkeler.

for mental health consultation in the late 1960s, before the creation of her systems model (Neuman, Deloughery, & Gebbie, 1971). Neuman designed a nursing conceptual model for students at UCLA in 1970 to expand their understanding of client variables beyond the medical model (Neuman & Young, 1972). Neuman first published her model during the early 1970s (Neuman & Young, 1972; Neuman, 1974). The first edition of *The Neuman Systems Model: Application to Nursing Education and Practice* was published in 1982; further development and revisions of the model are illustrated in the subsequent editions (Neuman, 1989, 1995, 2002b).

Since developing the Neuman Systems Model, Neuman has been involved in numerous publications, paper presentations, consultations, lectures, and conferences on application and use of the model. She is a Fellow of the American Association of Marriage and Family Therapy, and of the American Academy of Nursing. She taught nurse continuing education at UCLA and in community agencies for 14 years, and was in private practice as a licensed clinical marriage and family therapist, with an emphasis on pastoral counseling. Although retired, she continues to do occasional pastoral and nutritional counseling (B. Neuman, personal communication, December 9, 2007). Neuman lives in Ohio and maintains a leadership role in the Neuman Systems Model Trustees Group. She serves as a consultant nationally and internationally regarding implementation of the model for nursing education programs and for clinical practice agencies (B. Neuman, personal communications, July 18, 2000; February 9, 2004; December 9, 2007).

THEORETICAL SOURCES

The Neuman Systems Model is based on general system theory and reflects the nature of living organisms as open systems (von Bertalanffy, 1968) in interaction with each other and with the environment (Neuman, 1982). Within this model, Neuman synthesizes knowledge from several disciplines and incorporates her own philosophical beliefs and clinical nursing expertise, particularly in mental health nursing.

The model draws from Gestalt theory (Perls, 1973), which describes homeostasis as the process by which an organism maintains its equilibrium, and consequently its health, under varying conditions. Neuman describes adjustment as the process by which the organism satisfies its needs. Many needs exist, and each may disrupt client balance or stability; therefore, the adjustment process is dynamic and continuous. All life is characterized by this ongoing interplay of balance and imbalance within the organism. When the stabilizing process fails to some degree, or when the organism remains in a state of disharmony for too long, illness may develop. If the organism is unable to compensate through illness, death may result (Neuman & Young, 1972).

The model is also derived from the philosophical views of de Chardin and Marx (Neuman, 1982). Marxist philosophy suggests that the properties of parts are determined partly by the larger wholes within dynamically organized systems. With this view, Neuman (1982) confirms that the patterns of the whole influence awareness of the part, which is drawn from de Chardin's philosophy of the wholeness of life.

Neuman used Selye's definition of stress, which is the nonspecific response of the body to any demand made on it. Stress increases the demand for readjustment. This demand is nonspecific; it requires adaptation to a problem, irrespective of the nature of the problem. Therefore, the essence of stress is the nonspecific demand for activity (Selye, 1974). Stressors are the tension-producing stimuli that result in stress; they may be positive or negative.

Neuman adapts the concept of levels of prevention from Caplan's conceptual model (1964) and relates these prevention levels to nursing. Primary prevention is used to protect the organism before it encounters a harmful stressor. Primary prevention involves reducing the possibility of encountering the stressor or strengthening the client's normal line of defense to decrease the reaction to the stressor. Secondary and tertiary prevention are used after the client's encounter with a harmful stressor. Secondary prevention attempts to reduce the effect or possible effect of stressors through early diagnosis and effective treatment of illness symptoms; Neuman describes this as strengthening the internal lines of resistance. Tertiary prevention attempts to reduce the residual stressor effects and return the client to wellness after treatment (Capers, 1996; Neuman, 2002b).

MAJOR CONCEPTS & DEFINITIONS

Betty Neuman (2001) describes the Neuman systems model by stating the following:

> The Neuman systems model reflects nursing's interest in well and ill people as holistic systems and in environmental influences on health. Clients' and nurses' perceptions of stressors and resources are emphasized, and clients act in partnership with nurses to set goals and identify relevant prevention interventions. The individual, family or other group, community, or social issues all are client systems, which are viewed as composites of interacting physiological, psychological, sociocultural, developmental, and spiritual variables (p. 322).

Major concepts identified in the model (see Figure 16-1) are wholistic approach, open system (including function, input and output, feedback, negentropy, and stability), environment (including created environment), client system (including five client variables, basic structure, lines of resistance, normal line of defense, and flexible line of defense), health (wellness to illness), stressors, degree of reaction, prevention as intervention (three levels), and reconstitution (Neuman, 2002b, pp. 12-30; see also Neuman, 1982, 1989, 1995).

WHOLISTIC APPROACH

The Neuman Systems Model is a dynamic, open, systems approach to client care originally developed to provide a unifying focus for defining nursing problems and for understanding the client in interaction with the environment. The client as a system may be defined as a person, family, group, community, or social issue (Neuman, 2002b, p. 15).

Clients are viewed as wholes whose parts are in dynamic interaction. The model considers all variables simultaneously affecting the client system: physiological, psychological, sociocultural, developmental, and spiritual. Neuman included the spiritual variable in the second edition (1989). She changed the spelling of the term *holistic* to *wholistic* in the second edition to enhance understanding of the term as referring to the whole person (B. Neuman, personal communication, June 20, 1988).

OPEN SYSTEM

A system is open when its elements are continuously exchanging information and energy within its complex organization. Stress and reaction to stress are basic components of an open system (Neuman, 2002c, p. 323; see also Neuman, 1982, 1989, 1995).

Function or Process

The client as a system exchanges energy, information, and matter with the environment as it uses available energy resources to move toward stability and wholeness (Neuman, 2002c, p. 323; see also Neuman, 1982, 1989, 1995).

Input and Output

For the client as a system, input and output are the matter, energy, and information that are exchanged between the client and the environment (Neuman, 2002c, p. 323).

Continued

MAJOR CONCEPTS & DEFINITIONS—cont'd

Feedback

System output in the form of matter, energy, and information serves as feedback for future input for corrective action to change, enhance, or stabilize the system (Neuman, 2002c, p. 323).

Negentropy

Neuman defines negentropy as "... a process of energy conservation utilization that assists system progression toward stability or wellness" (Neuman, 2002c, p. 323; see also Neuman, 1982, 1989, 1995).

Stability

Stability is a dynamic and desired state of balance in which the system copes with stressors to maintain an optimal level of health and integrity (Neuman, 2002c, p. 324; see also Neuman, 1982, 1989, 1995).

ENVIRONMENT

As defined by Neuman, "... internal and external forces surrounding and affecting the client at any time comprise the environment" (Neuman, 2002c, p. 322; see also Neuman, 1982, 1989, 1995).

Created Environment

The created environment is developed unconsciously by the client to express system wholeness symbolically. Its purpose is to provide a safe arena for client system functioning, and to insulate the client from stressors (Neuman, 2002b, pp. 19-20; see also Neuman, 1982, 1989, 1995).

CLIENT SYSTEM

The client system is a composite of five variables (physiological, psychological, sociocultural, developmental, and spiritual) in interaction with the environment. The physiological variable refers to body structure and function. The psychological variable refers to mental processes in interaction with the environment. The sociocultural variable refers to the effects and influences of social and cultural conditions. The developmental variable refers to age-related processes and activities. The spiritual variable refers to spiritual beliefs and influences (Neuman, 2002c, p. 322; see also Neuman, 1982, 1989, 1995, 2002b).

Basic Client Structure

The client as a system is composed of a central core surrounded by concentric rings. The inner circle of the diagram (see Figure 16-1) represents the basic survival factors or energy resources of the client. This core structure "... consists of basic survival factors common to all members of the species," such as innate or genetic features (Neuman, 2002c, p. 322; see also Neuman, 1982, 1989, 1995).

Lines of Resistance

A series of broken rings surrounding the basic core structure are called the lines of resistance. These rings represent resource factors that help the client defend against a stressor. An example is the body's immune response system (Neuman, 2002c, p. 323; see also Neuman, 1982, 1989, 1995).

When the lines of resistance are effective, the client system can reconstitute; if they are ineffective, death may ensue. The amount of resistance to a stressor is determined by the interrelationship of the five variables of the client system (Neuman, 2001, p. 322).

Normal Line of Defense

The normal line of defense is the model's outer solid circle. It represents a stability state for the individual or system. It is maintained over time and serves as a standard to assess deviations from the client's usual wellness. It includes system

MAJOR CONCEPTS & DEFINITIONS—cont'd

variables and behaviors such as the individual's usual coping patterns, lifestyle, and developmental stage (Neuman, 2002c, p. 323; see also Neuman, 1982, 1989, 1995). Expansion of the normal line of defense reflects an enhanced wellness state; contraction, a diminished state of wellness (Neuman, 2001, p. 322).

Flexible Line of Defense

The model's outer broken ring is called the flexible line of defense. It is dynamic and can be altered rapidly over a short time. It is perceived as a protective buffer for preventing stressors from breaking through the usual wellness state as represented by the normal line of defense. The relationships of the variables (physiological, psychological, sociocultural, developmental, and spiritual) can affect the degree to which individuals are able to use their flexible line of defense against possible reaction to a stressor or stressors, such as loss of sleep (Neuman, 2002c, p. 323; see also Neuman, 1982, 1989, 1995).

Neuman describes the flexible line of defense as the client system's first protective mechanism. "When the flexible line of defense expands, it provides greater short-term protection against stressor invasion; when it contracts, it provides less protection" (Neuman, 2001, p. 322).

HEALTH

Health includes the full continuum of wellness to illness. It is dynamic and constantly changing. Optimal wellness exists when all system needs are fully met (Neuman, 2002c, p. 323).

Wellness

Wellness exists when the parts of the client system interact in harmony with the whole system. System needs are being met (Neuman, 2002c, p. 324; see also Neuman, 1982, 1989, 1995).

Illness

Illness exists at the opposite end of the continuum from wellness. It occurs when needs are not satisfied, resulting in a state of instability and energy depletion (Neuman, 2002c, p. 324; see also Neuman, 1982, 1989, 1995).

STRESSORS

Stressors are tension-producing stimuli that have the potential to disrupt system stability, leading to an outcome that may be positive or negative. They may arise from the following:

- Intrapersonal forces occurring within the individual, such as conditioned responses
- Interpersonal forces occurring between one or more individuals, such as role expectations
- Extrapersonal forces occurring outside the individual, such as financial circumstances (Neuman, 2002c, p. 324; see also Neuman, 1982, 1989, 1995).

DEGREE OF REACTION

The degree of reaction represents system instability that occurs when stressors invade the normal line of defense (Neuman, 2002c, p. 322; see also Neuman, 1982, 1989, 1995).

PREVENTION AS INTERVENTION

Interventions are purposeful actions to help the client retain, attain, or maintain system stability. They can occur before or after protective lines of defense and resistance are penetrated. Neuman supports beginning intervention when a stressor is suspected or identified. Interventions are based on possible or actual degree of reaction, resources, goals, and anticipated outcomes. Neuman identifies three levels of intervention: (1) primary, (2) secondary, and (3) tertiary (Neuman, 2002c, p. 323; see also Neuman, 1982, 1989, 1995).

Continued

MAJOR CONCEPTS & DEFINITIONS—cont'd

Primary Prevention

Primary prevention is used when a stressor is suspected or identified. A reaction has not yet occurred, but the degree of risk is known. The purpose is to reduce the possibility of encounter with the stressor or to decrease the possibility of a reaction (Neuman, 1982, p. 15; 2002c, p. 323)

Secondary Prevention

Secondary prevention involves interventions or treatment initiated after symptoms from stress have occurred. The client's internal and external resources are used to strengthen internal lines of resistance, reduce the reaction, and increase resistance factors (Neuman, 1982, p. 15; see also Neuman, 2002c, p. 323).

Tertiary Prevention

Tertiary prevention occurs after the active treatment or secondary prevention stage. It focuses on readjustment toward optimal client system stability. The goal is to maintain optimal wellness by preventing recurrence of reaction or regression. Tertiary prevention leads back in a circular fashion toward primary prevention. An example would be avoidance of stressors known to be hazardous to the client (Neuman, 2002c, p. 323; see also Neuman, 1982, 2002b).

RECONSTITUTION

Reconstitution occurs after treatment for stressor reactions. It represents return of the system to stability, which may be at a higher or lower level of wellness than before stressor invasion (Neuman, 2002c, p. 324).

USE OF EMPIRICAL EVIDENCE

Neuman conceptualized the model from sound theories before nursing research was begun on the model. She initially evaluated the utility of the model by submitting a tool to her graduate nursing students at UCLA and published the outcome data in *Nursing Research* (Neuman & Young, 1972). Subsequent nursing research has produced sound empirical evidence in support of the Neuman Systems Model (Figure 16-1).

MAJOR ASSUMPTIONS

Nursing

Neuman (1982) believes that nursing is concerned with the whole person. She views nursing as a "unique profession in that it is concerned with all of the variables affecting an individual's response to stress" (p. 14). The nurse's perception influences the care given; therefore, Neuman (1995) states that the perceptual field of the caregiver and the client must be assessed.

Person

Neuman presents the concept of person as an open client system in reciprocal interaction with the environment. The client may be an individual, family, group, community, or social issue. The client system is a dynamic composite of interrelationships among physiological, psychological, sociocultural, developmental, and spiritual factors (Neuman, 2002c, p. 322).

Health

Neuman considers her work a wellness model. She views health as a continuum of wellness to illness that is dynamic in nature and is constantly changing. Neuman states that "Optimal wellness or stability indicates that total system needs are being met.

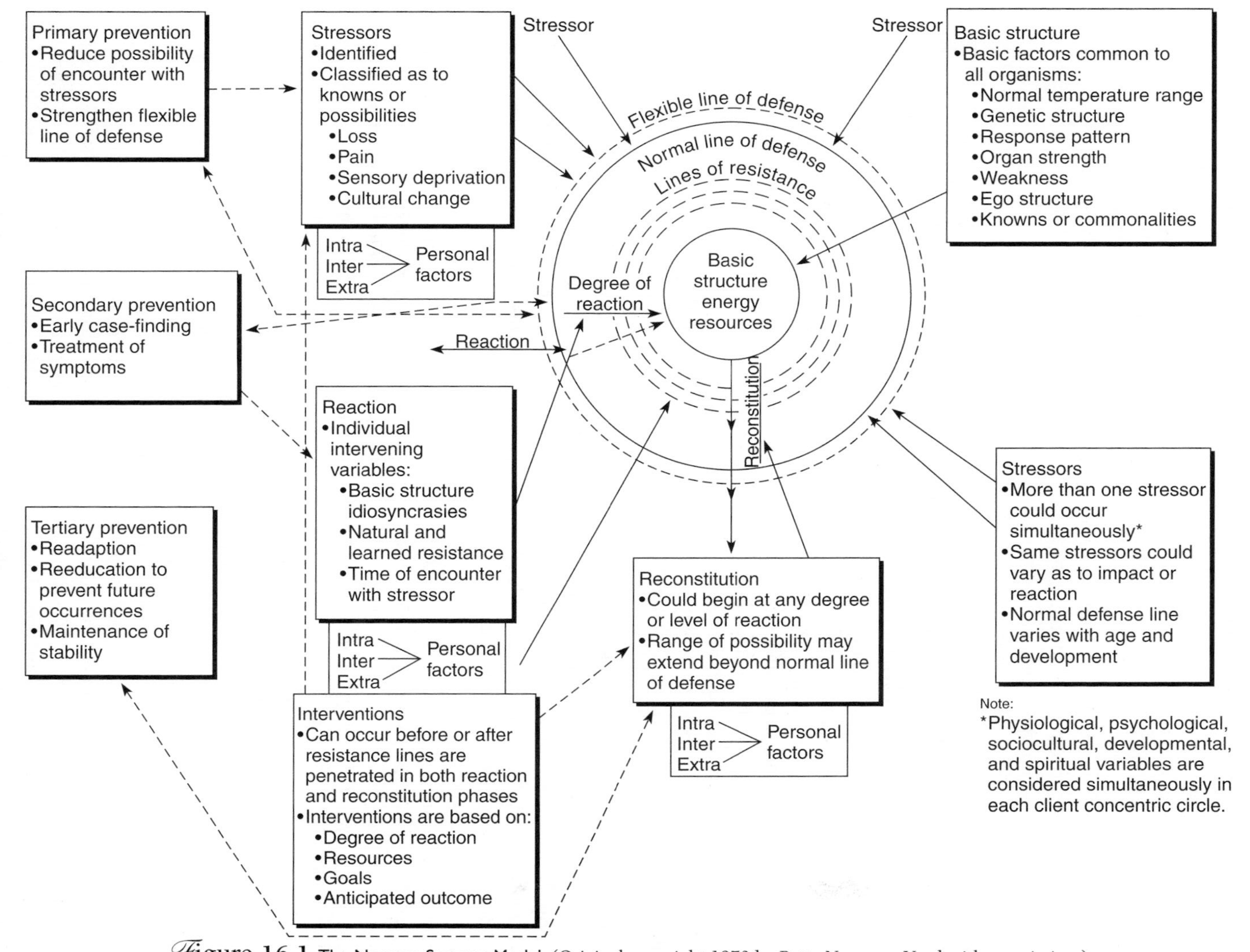

Figure 16-1 The Neuman Systems Model. (Original copyright 1970 by Betty Neuman. Used with permission.)

A reduced state of wellness is the result of unmet systemic needs" (2002c, p. 323).

Environment

Neuman defines *environment* as all the internal and external factors that surround and influence the client system. Stressors (intrapersonal, interpersonal, and extrapersonal) are significant to the concept of environment and are described as environmental forces that interact with and potentially alter system stability (2002c, pp. 322, 324).

Neuman (1995) identifies three relevant environments: (1) internal, (2) external, and (3) created. The internal environment is intrapersonal, with all interaction contained within the client. The external environment is interpersonal or extrapersonal, with all factors arising from outside the client. The created environment is unconsciously developed and is used by the client to support protective coping. It is primarily intrapersonal. The created environment is dynamic in nature and mobilizes all system variables to create an insulating effect that helps the client cope with the threat of environmental stressors by changing the self or the situation. Examples are the use of denial (psychological variable) and life cycle continuation of survival patterns (developmental variable). The created environment perpetually influences and is influenced by changes in the client's perceived state of wellness (Neuman, 1995, 2002c).

THEORETICAL ASSERTIONS

Theoretical assertions are the relationships among the essential concepts of a model (Torres, 1986). The Neuman model depicts the nurse as an active participant with the client and as "concerned with all the variables affecting an individual's response to stressors" (Neuman, 1982, p. 14). The client is in a reciprocal relationship with the environment in that "he interacts with this environment by adjusting himself to it or adjusting it to himself" (Neuman, 1982, p. 14). Neuman links the four essential concepts of person, environment, health, and nursing in her statements regarding primary, secondary, and tertiary prevention. Earlier publications by Neuman stated basic assumptions that linked essential concepts of the model. These statements have been recognized as propositions and serve to define, describe, and link the concepts of the model. Numerous theoretical assertions have been proposed, tested, and published, as noted throughout Neuman and Fawcett (2002).

LOGICAL FORM

Neuman used deductive and inductive logic in developing her model. As was previously discussed, Neuman derived her model from other theories and disciplines. The model is also a product of her philosophy and of observations made in teaching mental health nursing and clinical counseling (Fawcett, Carpenito, et al., 1982).

APPLICATIONS BY THE NURSING COMMUNITY

Alligood (2006) clarifies that a conceptual model provides a frame of reference, while a grand theory proposes direction or action that is testable. The Neuman Systems Model is both a model and a grand nursing theory. As a model, it provides a conceptual framework for nursing practice, research, and education (Freese, Neuman, & Fawcett, 2002; Louis, Neuman, & Fawcett, 2002; Newman, Neuman, & Fawcett, 2002). As a grand theory, it proposes ways of viewing nursing phenomena and nursing actions that are assumed to be true but may form propositions for testing (Neuman, 2002b).

The model serves equally well for all levels of nursing education and for a wide variety of practice areas. It adapts well transculturally and is used frequently for public health nursing in other countries. The model is used extensively in the United States, Canada, and Holland. It has been used throughout the world (Australia, Brazil, Costa Rica, Denmark, Egypt, England, Finland, Ghana, Holland, Hong Kong, Iceland, Japan, Korea, Kuwait, New Zealand, Portugal, Puerto Rico, the Republic of China, Spain, Sweden, Taiwan, Wales, and Yugoslavia).

The ongoing development and universal appeal of the model are reflected in the international Biennial Neuman Systems Model Symposia, which provide a forum across cultures for practitioners, educators, researchers, and students to share information about their use of the model. The first symposium was held in 1986 at Neumann College in Aston, Pennsylvania. Subsequent symposia have been held in Kansas City, Missouri (1988), Dayton, Ohio (1990), Rochester, New York (1993), Orlando, Florida (1995), Boston, Massachusetts (1997), Vancouver, British Columbia (1999), Salt Lake City, Utah (2001), Willow Grove, Pennsylvania (2003), Akron, Ohio (2005), and Ft. Lauderdale, Florida (2007). Each symposium attracts participation from countries throughout the world and from disciplines beyond nursing.

Practice

Use of the Neuman Systems Model for nursing practice facilitates goal-directed, unified, wholistic approaches to client care, yet the model is also appropriate for multidisciplinary use to prevent fragmentation of client care. The model delineates a client system and classification of stressors that can be understood and used by all members of the healthcare team (Mirenda, 1986). Guidelines have been published for use of the model in clinical nursing practice (Freese, et al., 2002) and for the administration of healthcare services (Shambaugh, Neuman, & Fawcett, 2002).

Several instruments have been published to facilitate use of the model. These instruments include an assessment and intervention tool to assist nurses in collecting and synthesizing client data, a format for prevention as intervention, and a format for application of the nursing process within the framework of the Neuman Systems Model (Neuman, 2002a; Russell, 2002).

The Neuman Nursing Process Format consists of three steps: (1) nursing diagnosis, (2) nursing goals, and (3) nursing outcomes. (When used by other disciplines, the term *nursing* is changed accordingly.) Diagnosis involves obtaining a broad, comprehensive data base from which variances from wellness can be determined. Goals are established by negotiation between client and caregiver for desired prescriptive changes to correct variances from wellness. Outcomes are established in relation to the goal for one or more of the three prevention-as-intervention modes. Evaluation then is used to confirm that the desired outcomes have been achieved or to reformulate the goals or outcomes.

Neuman (2002a) outlines her nursing process format clarifying the steps of the process for use of her model in Appendix C (Neuman & Fawcett, 2002, pp. 348-349). Russell (2002) provides a review of clinical tools using the model to guide nursing practice with individuals, families, communities, and organizations.

The breadth of the Neuman model has resulted in its application and adaptation in a variety of nursing practice settings, including hospitals, nursing homes, rehabilitation centers, hospices, mental health units, childbirth centers, and community-based services such as congregational nurse practices. Numerous examples are cited in Neuman's books (1982, 1989, 1995, 2002b). The model's wholistic approach makes it particularly applicable for clients who are experiencing complex stressors that affect multiple client variables such as end-stage kidney disease (Graham, 2006).

The model is used to guide nursing practice in countries throughout the world. As an example, it is used in Holland to guide Emergis, a comprehensive program of mental health that provides psychiatric care for children, adolescents, adults, and elderly, and addiction care and social services (Munck & Merks, 2002). This model has been modified for nursing practice in Malaysia by strengthening the role of the family in caring for patients (Shamsudin, 2002).

Neuman's model provides a systems perspective for use with individuals and families, for community-based practice with groups, and in public health nursing, as its wholistic principles can assist nurses to achieve high-quality care through evidence-based practices (Ume-Nwagbo, Dewan, & Lowry, 2006). Anderson, McFarland, and Helton (1986) used the model for a community health needs assessment in which they identified violence toward women as a major community health concern. This model has been used to promote health for senior citizens at a community nursing center in Pennsylvania (Newman, 2005), to guide a public school nurse clinical practice (Vito, 2005), and as the framework for a parish nurse practice (Kathleen Vito, personal communication, April 21, 2005).

Likewise, the model is functional in the acute care setting. For example, the Children's Hospital of Michigan in Detroit adopted the Neuman Systems Model as the nursing conceptual model to be implemented at their institution. As part of the implementation process, various documents were revised or created to reflect nursing care using concepts of the model, such as the Pediatric Admission Database and the Neuman Process Summary (Torakis & Smigielski, 2000). It is used to guide nursing practice in the Foote Health System in Michigan (Johnson-Crisanti et al., 2005).

The Neuman Systems Model is used effectively to enhance advanced practice nursing (Fawcett, Newman, & McAllister, 2004; Geib, 2006; Gigliotti, 2002). For example, clinical nurse specialists have used the model to identify major health concerns for elderly adults living in the community (Imamura, 2002). The model has also been used to direct the development of guidelines for a community-based Sexual Assault Nurse Examiner program (Melton, Secrest, Chien, & Andersen, 2001).

The model works well for multidisciplinary use. As an example, it is used to guide a team approach to holistic care for older adults after hip fracture (Kain, 2000). It also has proved useful in hospital-based case management in several Kansas hospitals, with the development of case management teams involving social workers and nursing staff (Wetta-Hall, Berry, Ablah, Gillispie, & Stepp-Cornelius, 2004). Further research continues to validate its applicability beyond nursing.

Education

The model is well accepted in academe and is used widely as a curriculum guide. It has been used throughout the United States and in other countries, including Australia, Canada, Denmark, England, Holland, Japan, Korea, Kuwait, Portugal, and Taiwan (Beckman et al., 1994; Lowry, 2002). In an integrative review of use of the model in educational programs at all levels, Lowry (2002) reports that "although the trend is toward eclecticism in nursing education today, the Neuman Systems Model has served many programs well . . ." and frequently is selected in other countries to facilitate student learning (p. 231). Guidelines have been published for use of the model in education for the health professions (Newman et al., 2002).

The model's wholistic perspective provides an effective framework for nursing education at all levels. Lowry and Newsome (1995) reported on a study of 12 associate degree programs that use the model as a conceptual framework for curriculum development. Results indicate that graduates use the model most often in the roles of teacher and care provider, and that they tend to continue practice from a Neuman Systems Model–based perspective following graduation. Neuman's model has been selected for baccalaureate programs on the basis of its theoretical and comprehensive perspectives for a wholistic curriculum, and because of its potential for use with individuals, families, small groups, and the community. Neumann College Division of Nursing was the first school to select the Neuman Systems Model as its conceptual base for its curriculum and approach to client care in 1976.

The model has been used at Lander University in Greenwood, South Carolina, as the framework for baccalaureate nursing education since 1987 (Freese & Lander University Nursing Faculty, 1995). This model provides the framework for nursing education programs at Palm Beach Atlantic University (Alligood, 2004), East Tennessee State University (Lois Lowry, personal communication, April 22, 2005), Purdue University at Fort Wayne (Boxley-Harges, Beckman, & Bruick-Sorge, 2007), and Newberry College (Betsy McDowell, personal communication, January 3, 2007).

The model works equally well to guide clinical learning. For example, it is used with nursing students at a community nursing center (Newman, 2005), and to teach nursing students to promote the health of communities (Falk-Rafael et al., 2004). It is used as a comprehensive framework to organize data collected from maternity patients by undergraduate nursing students at the University of South Florida (Lowry, 2002). Bruick-Sorge (2007) reported using the model in the clinical simulation setting to improve critical thinking skills by using model concepts.

The model's effectiveness as a framework for patient education has been demonstrated. Salvador (2006) reported its use by a group of nurses to develop an oral care guide for patients who have autologous stem cell transplantation. The model's inclusion of both client perception and nurse perception makes it particularly relevant for teaching across cultures. Neuman (2001) stated that several faculty experts are facilitating use of the model in diverse cultures in countries that include Guatemala, Kuwait, Thailand, and Taiwan, and it is used to guide nursing curricula in Jordan, Taiwan, Guam, and Iceland.

The Neuman Systems Model is used to guide learning in classroom and clinical settings for multiple levels of nursing and health-related curricula around the world. Acceptance by the nursing education community is clearly evident. As online nursing education increases, it will be imperative that nurse educators find novel approaches for presenting this information to all levels of students.

Research

A significant amount of research has been conducted over the past decade on the components of the model to generate nursing theory and using the model as a conceptual framework to advance nursing as a scientific discipline. Rules for Neuman Systems Model–Based Nursing Research as specified by Fawcett, a Neuman model trustee, are based on the content of the model and related literature (Fawcett & Gigliotti, 2001). Other guidelines have been published to guide use of the model for nursing research (Louis et al., 2002).

In the third edition of *The Neuman Systems Model,* Louis (1995) discussed its use in nursing research and identified nearly 100 studies, conducted between 1989 and 1993, for which the model provided the organizing framework. The third edition also contains an annotated bibliography of selected studies conducted from 1989 to 1993, with an appendix listing research studies published in journals, dissertations, and master's theses. In the fourth edition of *The Neuman Systems Model*, Fawcett and Giangrande (2002) present an integrated review of 200 research reports of model use that were published through 1997. Skalski, DiGerolamo, and Gigliotti (2006) reported a literature review of 87 Neuman Systems Model–based studies to identify and categorize client system stressors. The Neuman Systems Model is used frequently by nurse researchers as a conceptual framework, as it lends itself to both quantitative and qualitative methods. Recent examples of qualitative studies include studies of raising consciousness in critical care nurses (Moola, 2006), of decision making in asynchronous online education (Molinari, 2001), of the effects of chronic arthritis (Potter & Zauszniewski, 2000), and of the meaning of spirituality among aging adults (Lowry, 2005). Examples of quantitative studies include investigations of problems experienced by infants exposed to tobacco smoke in the environment (Stepans & Knight, 2002; Stepans, Wilhelm, & Dolence, 2006), of coping behaviors of women with family history of breast cancer (Lancaster, 2005), of maternal-student role stress (Gigliotti, 2004, 2007), of physical activity and health-related quality of life in the elderly (Binhosen et al., 2003), of elder abuse (Kottwitz & Bowling, 2003), and of needs of cancer survivors (Narsavage & Romeo, 2003). Jones-Cannon and Davis (2005) implemented a mixed method to examine coping strategies among African American women who care for their aging parents.

This model works well for studying areas of interest across cultures. It was used recently in Malaysia to study patients' spiritual needs and the role of nurses in meeting them (Shamsudin, 2002), to study physical activity and health among elderly persons in Thailand (Binhosen et al., 2003), to compare child health risk factors in Korea and the United States (McDowell, Chang, & Choi, 2003), and to study the effectiveness of a community-based pulmonary rehabilitation program for Thai individuals with chronic obstructive pulmonary disease (Noonhill, Sindhu, Hanucharunkul, & Suwonnaroop, 2007).

Graduate students frequently use the model for dissertations and theses. Recent examples include studies on the relationship among stress, role and job strain, and sleep in middle-aged nurse shift workers (Brown, 2004), on the childhood experiences of women who experience intimate partner violence (Reeves, 2005a, 2005b), on the created environment as a coping strength for homeless abused women (Hemphill, 2006), on the relationship between comfort, spirituality, and quality of life among residents of a long-term care facility in Taiwan (Lee, 2005), and on the relationship between alcohol use and unintentional death in older adults (Rohr, 2006).

Earlier research studies using the Neuman Systems Model are reported in previous editions of this chapter. Additional studies using this model are listed in the bibliography at the end of this chapter.

The Biennial Neuman Systems Model Symposium provides a rich forum for presentation of research (completed and in progress). At the tenth (2005) and eleventh (2007) symposia, nurses from the United States, Canada, and Holland reported on numerous studies that used the model. Studies were reported on the experiences of women related to intimate partner violence (Reeves, 2005b), on perceived health status changes in criminally victimized older adults (Burnett, 2005), on the influence of each variable on perceived health in older adults (Buck, 2005), and on Asian American child-rearing beliefs and practices (McDowell, 2005). Research presented at the eleventh symposium included studies on the lived experience of the chemically dependent nurse (Dittman, 2007), faculty development prior to facilitating online coursework (Greer & Clay, 2007), interventions to reduce nurse burnout (Gunesen, 2007), the discovered strengths of homeless abused women (Hemphill & Quillen, 2007), sleep quality in cardiothoracic surgery patients (Nelson, 2007), and Chinese parent' understanding of child vehicle restraints (Ren, Snowdon, & Thrasher, 2007).

Research projects that were reported at previous symposia (1993 through 2003) are cited in previous editions of this chapter.

The Neuman Systems Model is used extensively to provide the conceptual framework for research projects in the United States and in other countries. Acceptance by the nursing research community is clearly evident.

FURTHER DEVELOPMENT

When published initially, the Neuman Systems Model was described as being at a very early stage of theory development (Walker & Avant, 1983). Although the diagram itself has remained unchanged, the model has been refined based on its use and further developed in subsequent publications (Fawcett, 2001). At least two components have been supported and further developed since 2000. Major developments include spirituality (Beckman et al., 2007; DiJoseph & Cavendish, 2005; Lee, 2005; Lowry, 2005) and the concept of created environment (Hemphill, 2006; Skillen, 2001).

The process of establishing full validity through research continues as with most nursing models. The Neuman Systems Model has demonstrated that it works well pragmatically. Further research on the circular lines surrounding the central core (lines of resistance, normal line of defense, flexible line of defense) will contribute to validity (B. Neuman, personal communication, January 6, 2008).

Establishing full credibility of the model depends on extending the development and testing of middle range theory from it. Neuman and Koertvelyessy identified two theories generated from the model: (1) the theory of optimal client system stability, and (2) the theory of prevention as intervention (Fawcett, 1995b). Breckenridge (1995) described the use of the model to develop middle range theory through research based on practice with nephrology patients. However, Gigliotti (2003) has stated that "... to date, no explicit NSM-derived middle range theories have been developed" (p. 202). Further research based on the Neuman Systems Model is needed to validate the relationship between model concepts and research outcomes (Fawcett & Giangrande, 2002).

The Neuman Systems Model Trustee Group was established in 1988 to preserve, protect, and perpetuate the integrity of the model for the future of nursing (Neuman, 2002d). Its international members, personally selected by Neuman, are dedicated professionals.

The Neuman Systems Model Institute has been organized to generate and test middle range theories derived from the model. Preliminary work that has been completed includes assembling resources, identifying concepts and the relationships among them, and synthesizing existing research based on Neuman Systems Model concepts (Gigliotti, 2003).

CRITIQUE

Neuman developed a comprehensive conceptual model that operationalizes systems concepts that are relevant to the breadth of nursing phenomena. The model's wholistic perspective allows for a wide range of creativity in its use. It remains relevant for use by nursing and by other healthcare professions in the future.

Clarity

Neuman presents abstract concepts that are familiar to nurses. The model's essential concepts of client, environment, health, and nursing are congruent with traditional understanding of the nursing metaparadigm. Concepts defined by Neuman and those borrowed from other disciplines are used consistently throughout the model. However, the model's clarity has been criticized in that concepts need to be defined more completely (August-Brady, 2000; Heyman & Wolfe, 2000).

Simplicity

The model consists of concepts that are organized in a complex, yet logical manner. Multiple interrelationships exist among concepts, and variables tend to overlap to some degree. Distinctions between concepts tend to blur at several points, but loss of theoretical meaning would occur if they were separated completely. Neuman states that the concepts can be separated for analysis, specific goal setting, and interventions (B. Neuman, personal communication, June 21, 1992). This model can be used to explain the client's dynamic state of equilibrium and the reaction or possible reaction to stressors. The concept of prevention as intervention can be used to describe or predict nursing phenomena. The model is complex in nature; therefore, it cannot be described as a simple framework, yet nurses using the model describe it as easy to understand and use across cultures and in a wide variety of practice settings.

Generality

The Neuman Systems Model has been used in a wide variety of nursing situations; it is both comprehensive and adaptable. Some concepts are broad and represent the phenomenon of "client," which may be one person or a larger system. Other concepts are more definitive and identify specific modes of action, such as primary prevention. The model's broad scope allows it to be useful to nurses and to other healthcare professionals in working with individuals, families, groups, or communities in all healthcare settings.

Health professionals beyond nursing can use the model as a framework for care because its wholistic perspective can accommodate varied approaches to client assessment and care. Its systems approach and its emphasis on involving the client as an active participant fit well with contemporary healthcare values such as prevention and interdisciplinary care management.

Empirical Precision

Although the model has not been tested completely, it is used extensively to guide nursing research. Early work (Hoffman, 1982; Louis and Koertvelyessy, 1989) provided initial documentation of empirical support. Continued testing and refinement through the work of the Research Institute and independent nurse researchers will increase the model's empirical precision as research continues and findings from multiple studies are synthesized (Gigliotti, 1999, 2003; Skalski, DiGerolamo, & Gigliotti, 2006).

Derivable Consequences

The derivable consequences of Neuman's conceptual model include guidelines for the professional nurse for assessment of the client system, utilization of the nursing process, and implementation of preventive interventions. The focus on primary prevention and interdisciplinary care is futuristic and serves to improve quality of care. The Neuman nursing process fulfills current health mandates by involving the client actively in negotiating the goals of nursing care (Neuman, 2002a).

Another derivable consequence of the model is its potential to generate nursing theory, for example, the theories of optimal client stability and prevention as intervention (Fawcett, 1995a). The model concepts are relevant for use by health professionals in the twenty-first century. Through continued theory development and research with the model, the nursing profession can expand its scientific knowledge base. According to Fawcett (1989, 1995b), the model meets social considerations of congruence, significance, and utility. The model is broad and systems based. It lends itself well to a comprehensive approach for nurses to respond to the world's rapidly changing healthcare needs.

Application in Practice

Within the three-component Neuman nursing process format, the steps of assessment, intervention, and evaluation are assumed rather than being stated explicitly. Clarifying how the Neuman components of diagnosis, goals, and outcomes fit best with the traditional approach to care planning and delivery would reduce ambiguity for nurses who practice from the traditional perspective.

SUMMARY

The Neuman Systems Model is derived from general systems theory. Its focus is on the client as a system (which may be an individual, family, group, or community) and on the client's responses to stressors. The client system includes five variables (physiological, psychological, sociocultural, developmental, spiritual) and is conceptualized as an inner core (basic energy resources) surrounded by concentric circles that include lines of resistance, a normal line of defense, and a flexible line of defense. Each of the five variables is considered part of each of the concentric circles. Stressors are tension-producing stimuli which may be intrapersonal, interpersonal, or extrapersonal in nature.

The model suggests three levels for nursing interventions (primary prevention, secondary prevention, tertiary prevention), which are based on Caplan's concept of levels of prevention (1964). The purpose of prevention as intervention is to achieve the maximum possible level of client system stability. Neuman suggests a format for the nursing process in which the client as the recipient of care participates actively with the nurse as caregiver to set goals and select interventions.

This model has been well accepted by the nursing community and is used in administration, practice, education, and research. The Neuman Systems Model Trustees Group is actively involved in protecting the integrity of the model and advancing its development. The Neuman Systems Model Research Institute has been established and is working to generate and test middle range theories based on the model.

Case Study

Family as Client

Maria Castillo is a 29-year-old Hispanic American woman who is approximately 38 weeks pregnant and has insulin-dependent gestational diabetes. She and her husband, Juan, have been married for 5 years and have two children—Emilio, age 4, and Dalia, age 2. Juan lost his manufacturing job 4 months ago and has been unable to find work until last week. Maria has been admitted to the maternal unit for uncontrolled diabetes and dehydration. The Castillo's have no family in the area, and young children are not allowed to visit the maternal unit. Juan is concerned about missing time from his new job.

Use the Neuman Systems Model as a conceptual framework to respond to the following:

- Describe the Castillo family as a client system using each of the five variables.
- What stressors, actual and potential, now threaten the family? Which of these stressors are positive and which are negative?
- What additional nursing assessment data are needed considering Maria's medical diagnoses?
- What levels of prevention intervention(s) are appropriate for the Castillo family?
- Describe interventions for each stressor.

CRITICAL THINKING *Activity*

Community as Client

Select one organization with which you are familiar that would be considered a community, based on it having face-to-face interaction and a shared set of interests or values. This could be a church, an employing organization, or a civic group. Use the Neuman Systems Model as a conceptual framework to analyze the organization as a community-client and to support organizational planning, as follows:

- What is the basic structure (core)? What factors in the lines of resistance support the status quo? What factors in the lines of defense support healthy organizational functioning?
- What stressors, actual or potential, that are impacting the organization may disrupt it as a system and result in change?
- What perception of goals by members of the organization would be appropriate for this change?
- What perception of goals by leaders of the organization would be appropriate for this change?
- If these perceptions differ, how can the differences be resolved for mutual goal setting that will be beneficial for the organization?
- What prevention as intervention strategies will support the organization in making changes successfully?

POINTS FOR *Further Study*

- Neuman, B. & Fawcett, J. (2002). *The Neuman systems model* (4th ed.). Upper Saddle River, NJ: Prentice-Hall.
- Neuman, B., & Reed, K. S. (2007). A Neuman systems model perspective on nursing in 2050. *Nursing Science Quarterly, 20*(2), 111-113.
- Geib, K. (2006). Neuman System's Model in nursing practice. In M. R. Alligood, & A. M. Tomey (Eds.), *Nursing theory utilization and application* (3rd ed., pp. 229-254). St. Louis: Mosby-Elsevier. Available at: www.neumansystemsmodel.org
- Lists of Neuman research publications available at: www.neumann.edu/academics/undergrad/nursing/model
- The Neuman Archives that preserve and protect works related to the model are housed in the Neumann College Library in Aston, Pennsylvania.

REFERENCES

Alligood, M. R. (2004). *Welcome: Palm Beach Atlantic University School of Nursing*. West Palm Beach, FL: Palm Beach Atlantic University. Retrieved January 30, 2004, from *http://www.pba.edu/Academic/Nursing.*

Alligood, M. R. (2006). Introduction to nursing theory: History, terminology and analysis. In A. M. Tomey & M. R. Alligood (Eds.), *Nursing theorists and their work* (6th ed., pp. 3-15). St. Louis: Mosby.

Anderson, E., McFarland, J., & Helton, A. (1986). Community-as-client: A model for practice. *Nursing Outlook*, 34(5), 220-224.

August-Brady, M. (2000). Prevention as intervention. *Journal of Advanced Nursing,* 31(6), 1304-1308.

Beckman, S. J., Boxley-Harges, S., Bruick-Sorge, C., Harris, S. M., Hermiz, M. E., Meininger, M., et al. (1994). Betty Neuman systems model. In A. Marriner Tomey (Ed.), *Nursing theorists and their work* (3rd ed., pp. 269-304). St. Louis: Mosby.

Beckman, S., Boxley-Harges, S., Bruick-Sorge, C., & Salmon, B. (2007). Five strategies that heighten nurses' awareness of spirituality to impact client care. *Holistic Nursing Practice,* 21(3), 135-139.

Bertalanffy, L. (1968). *General system theory*. New York: George Braziller.

Binhosen, V., Panuthai, S., Srisuphun, W., Chang, E., Sucamvang, K., & Cioffi, J. (2003). Physical activity and health related quality of life among the urban Thai elderly. *Thai Journal of Nursing Research*, 7(4), 231-243.

Boxley-Harges, S., Beckman, S., & Bruick-Sorge, C. (2007, February). *The NSM lessens the struggles in transitioning to a new curriculum.* Paper presented at the Eleventh Biennial Neuman Systems Model Symposium, Ft. Lauderdale, FL.

Breckenridge, D. M. (1995). Nephrology practice and directions for nursing research. In B. Neuman (Ed.). *The Neuman systems model (3rd* ed. pp. 499-507). Norwalk, CT: Appleton & Lange.

Brown, P.S. (2004). Relationships among life event stress, role and job strain, and sleep in middle-aged female shift workers. *Dissertation Abstracts International, 65*(4), 1774B. (UMI No. 3130329)

Bruick-Sorge, C. (2007, February). *Using simulations to improve students' critical thinking skills in a Neuman-based undergraduate program.* Paper presented at the Eleventh Biennial Neuman Systems Model Symposium, Ft. Lauderdale, FL.

Buck, G. L. (2005). *Wellness: relative importance of variables.* Paper presented at the Tenth Biennial Neuman Systems Model Symposium, Akron, Ohio.

Burnett, H. (2005). *Criminally victimized older adults.* Paper presented at the Tenth Biennial Neuman Systems Model Symposium, Akron, Ohio.

Capers, C. F. (1996). The Neuman systems model: A culturally relevant perspective. *ABNF Journal,* 7(5), 113-117.

Caplan, G. (1964). *Principles of preventive psychiatry.* New York: Basic Books.

DiJoseph, J., & Cavendish, R. (2005). Expanding the dialog on prayer relevant to holistic care. *Holistic Nursing Practice,* 19(4), 147-154.

Dittman, P. W. (2007, February). *"Mountains to climb": The lived experience of chemically dependent nurses pilot study using the Neuman Systems Model.* Paper presented at the Eleventh Biennial Neuman Systems Model Symposium, Ft. Lauderdale, FL.

Falk-Rafael, A. R., Ward-Griffin, C., Laforet-Fliesser, Y., & Beynon, C. (2004). Teaching nursing students to promote the health of communities; a partnership approach. *Nurse Educator,* 29(2), 63-67.

Fawcett, J. (1989). *Analysis and evaluation of conceptual models of nursing* (2nd ed., pp. 172-177). Philadelphia: F. A. Davis.

Fawcett, J. (1995a). Constructing conceptual-theoretical-empirical structures for research. In B. Neuman (Ed.), *The Neuman systems model* (3rd ed., pp. 459-471). Norwalk, CT: Appleton & Lange.

Fawcett, J. (1995b). *Neuman's systems model: Analysis and evaluation of conceptual models of nursing* (3rd ed., pp. 217-275). Philadelphia: F. A. Davis.

Fawcett, J. (2001). Scholarly dialogue. The nurse theorists: 21st-century updates—Betty Neuman. *Nursing Science Quarterly,* 14(3), 211-214.

Fawcett, J., Carpenito, L. J., Efinger, J., Goldblum-Graff, D., Groesbeck, M., Lowry, L. W., et al. (1982). A framework for analysis and evaluation of conceptual models of nursing with an analysis of the Neuman systems model. In B. Neuman (Ed.), *The Neuman systems model: Application to nursing education and practice* (pp. 30-43). Norwalk, CT: Appleton-Century-Crofts.

Fawcett, J., & Giangrande, S. (2002). The Neuman systems model and research: An integrative review. In B. Neuman & J. Fawcett, (Eds.), *The Neuman systems model* (4th ed., pp. 120-149). Upper Saddle River, NJ: Pearson Education.

Fawcett, J., & Gigliotti, E. (2001). Using conceptual models to guide nursing research: The case of the Neuman systems' model. *Nursing Science Quarterly,* 14, 339-345.

Fawcett, J., Newman, D. M. L., & McAllister, M. (2004). Advanced practice nursing and conceptual models of nursing. *Nursing Science Quarterly,* 17(2), 135-138.

Freese, B. T., & Lander University Faculty (1995, Feb.). *Application of the Neuman systems model to education: Baccalaureate workshop.* Paper presented at the Fifth International Neuman Systems Model Symposium, Orlando, FL.

Freese, B. T., Neuman, B., & Fawcett, J. (2002). Guidelines for Neuman systems model-based clinical practice. In B. Neuman & J. Fawcett (Eds.), *The Neuman systems model* (4th ed., pp. 37-42). Upper Saddle River, NJ: Pearson Education.

Geib, K. (2006). Neuman System's Model in nursing practice. In M. R. Alligood & A. M. Tomey (Eds.), *Nursing Theory Utilization and Application, 3rd* edition (pp. 229-254). St. Louis: Mosby-Elsevier

Gigliotti, E. (1999). Women's multiple role stress: Testing Neuman's flexible line of defense. *Nursing Science Quarterly,* 12(1), 36-44.

Gigliotti, E. (2002). A theory-based clinical nurse specialist practice exemplar using Neuman's Systems Model and nursing taxonomies. *Clinical Nurse Specialist: The Journal for Advanced Nursing Practice,* 16(1), 10-16.

Gigliotti, E. (2003). The Neuman systems model institute: Testing middle-range theories. *Nursing Science Quarterly,* 16(3), 201-206.

Gigliotti, E. (2004). Etiology of maternal-student role stress. *Nursing Science Quarterly,* 17(2), 156-164.

Gigliotti, E. (2007). Improving external and internal validity of a model of midlife women's maternal-student role stress. *Nursing Science Quarterly,* 20(2), 161-170.

Graham, J. (2006). Nursing theory and clinical practice: how three nursing models can be incorporated into the care of patients with end stage kidney disease. *Canadian Journal of Nephrology Nurses and Technologists Journal,* 16(4), 28-31.

Greer, A. G., & Clay, M. (2007, February). *Neuman Systems Model: A theoretical perspective for researching the meaning of faculty preparation for online education.* Paper presented at the Eleventh Biennial Neuman Systems Model Symposium, Ft. Lauderdale, FL.

Gunesen, N. (2007, February). *An intervention study to reduce nurse burnout.* Paper presented at the Eleventh Biennial Neuman Systems Model Symposium, Ft. Lauderdale, FL.

Hemphill, J. C. (2006). Discovering strengths of homeless abused women. *Dissertation Abstracts International, 66*(7), 3635B. (UMI No. 3180908)

Hemphill, J. C. & Quillen, J. H. (2007). *Discovering the strengths of homeless and abused women.* Paper presented at the Eleventh Biennial Neuman Systems Model Symposium, Ft. Lauderdale, FL.

Heyman, P. & Wolfe, S. (2000). Neuman systems model. University of Florida. Retrieved January 7, 2008 from http://www.patheyman.com/essays/neuman.

Hoffman, M. K. (1982). From model to theory construction: An analysis of the Neuman health-care system model. In B. Neuman (Ed.), *The Neuman systems model: Application to nursing education and practice* (pp. 44-54). Norwalk, CT: Appleton-Century-Crofts.

Imamura, E. (2002). Amy's chat room: health promotion programmes for community dwelling elderly adults. *International Journal of Nursing Practice* 2002, 8, 61-64.

Johnson-Crisanti, K. J., Burnett, H., Leibowitz, J., Sturtevant, J. R., & Rowley, B. (2005). *Nurses get the third degree—Implementing the Neuman Systems Model.* Paper presented at the Tenth Biennial Neuman Systems Model Symposium, Akron, Ohio.

Jones-Cannon, S. & Davis, B. L. (2005). Coping among African-American daughters caring for aging parents. *Association of Black Nursing Faculty Journal,* 16(6), 118-123.

Kain, H. B. (2000). Care of the older adult following hip fracture. *Holistic Nursing Practice,* 14(4), 24-39.

Kottwitz, D., & Bowling, S. (2003). A pilot study of the Elder Abuse Questionnaire. *Kansas Nurse,* 78(7), 4-6.

Lancaster, D. R. (2005). Coping with appraised breast cancer risk among women with family histories of breast cancer. *Research in Nursing and Health,* 28(2), 144-158.

Lee, F-P. (2005). The relationship of comfort and spirituality to quality of life among long-term care facility residents in southern Taiwan. *Dissertation Abstracts International, 66*(2), 815B. (UMI No. 3163392)

Louis, M. (1995). The Neuman model in nursing research: An update. In B. Neuman (Ed.), *The Neuman systems model* (3rd ed., pp. 473-495). Norwalk, CT: Appleton & Lange.

Louis, M., & Koertvelyessy, A. (1989). Neuman model: Use in research. In B. Neuman (Ed.), *The Neuman systems model* (2nd ed., pp. 93-114). Norwalk, CT: Appleton & Lange.

Louis, M., Neuman, B., & Fawcett, J. (2002). Guidelines for Neuman systems model-based nursing research. In B. Neuman & J. Fawcett (Eds.), *The Neuman systems model* (4th ed., pp. 113-119). Upper Saddle River, NJ: Pearson Education.

Lowry, L.W. (2005, July). *Exploring the meaning of spirituality with aging adults in Appalachia.* Paper presented at the 16th International Nursing Research Congress of Sigma Theta Tau International Nursing Honor Society, Kona, HI.

Lowry, L. W. (2002). The Neuman systems model and education: An integrative review. In B. Neuman & J. Fawcett (Eds.), *The Neuman systems model* (4th ed., pp. 216-237). Upper Saddle River, NJ: Pearson Education.

Lowry, L W., & Newsome, G. G. (1995). Neuman-based associate degree programs: Past, present, and future. In B. Neuman (Ed.), *The Neuman systems model* (3rd ed., pp. 197-214). Norwalk, CT: Appleton & Lange.

McDowell, B. (2005). *Asian-American views on childrearing: assessing the Neuman Systems Model.* Paper presented at the Tenth Biennial Neuman Systems Model Symposium, Akron, Ohio.

McDowell, B. M., Chang, N. J., & Choi, S. S. (2003). Children's health retention in South Korea and the United States: a cross-cultural comparison. *Journal of Pediatric Nursing,* 18(6), 409-415.

Melton, L., Secrest, J., Chien, A., & Andersen, B. (2001). Resources for practice. A community needs assessment for a SANE program using Neuman's model. *Journal of the American Academy of Nurse Practitioners,* 13(4), 178-186.

Mirenda, R. M. (1986). The Neuman systems model: Description and application. In P. Winstead-Fry (Ed.), *Case studies in nursing theory* (pp. 127-167). New York: National League for Nursing.

Molinari, D. (2001). Bridging time and distance: continuing education needs for rural health care providers. *Home Health Care Management & Practice,* 14(1), 54-58.

Moola, S. (2006). Facilitating conscious awareness among critical care nurses. *Dissertation Abstracts International, 66*(8). (UMI No. 0808408)

Munck, C. K., & Merks, A. (2002). Using the Neuman systems model to guide administration of nursing services in Holland: The case of Emergis, institute for mental health care. In B. Neuman & J. Fawcett (Eds.), *The Neuman systems model* (4th ed., pp. 300-316). Upper Saddle River, NJ: Prentice-Hall.

Narsavage, G., & Romeo, E. (2003). Education and support needs of young and older cancer survivors. *Applied Nursing Research,* 16(2), 103-109.

Nelson, K. (2007, February). *Sleep quality in the cardiothoracic surgery patient.* Paper presented at the Eleventh Biennial Neuman Systems Model Symposium, Ft. Lauderdale, FL.

Neuman, B. (1974). The Betty Neuman health care systems model: A total person approach to patient problems. In J. P. Riehl & C. Roy (Eds.), *Conceptual models for nursing practice* (2nd ed., pp. 119-134). NY: Appleton-Century-Crofts.

Neuman, B. (1982). *The Neuman systems model: Application to nursing education and practice.* Norwalk, CT: Appleton-Century-Crofts.

Neuman, B. (1989). *The Neuman systems model* (2nd ed.). Norwalk, CT: Appleton & Lange.

Neuman, B. (1995). *The Neuman systems model* (3rd ed.). Norwalk, CT: Appleton & Lange.

Neuman, B. (2001). The Neuman systems model: A futuristic care perspective. In N. L. Chaska (Ed.), *The nursing profession: Tomorrow and beyond* (pp. 321-329). Thousand Oaks, CA: Sage Publications.

Neuman, B. (2002a). Assessment and intervention based on the Neuman systems model. In B. Neuman & J. Fawcett (Eds.), *The Neuman systems model* (4th ed., pp. 347-359). Upper Saddle River, NJ: Prentice-Hall.

Neuman, B. (2002b). The Neuman systems model. In B. Neuman & J. Fawcett (Eds.), *The Neuman systems model* (4th ed., pp. 3-34). Upper Saddle River, NJ: Prentice-Hall.

Neuman, B. (2002c). The Neuman systems model definitions. In B. Neuman & J. Fawcett (Eds.), *The Neuman systems model* (4th ed., pp. 322-324). Upper Saddle River, NJ: Prentice-Hall.

Neuman, B. (2002d). The Neuman systems model definitions. In B. Neuman & J. Fawcett (Eds.), *The Neuman systems model* (4th ed., pp. 360-363). Upper Saddle River, NJ: Prentice-Hall.

Neuman, B. & Fawcett, J. (2002). *The Neuman Systems Model, (4th* ed.). Upper Saddle River, NJ: Prentice Hall.

Neuman, B., Deloughery, G. W., & Gebbie, M. (1971). *Consultation and community organization in community mental health nursing*. Baltimore: Williams & Wilkins.

Neuman, B., & Young, R. J. (1972, May/June). A model for teaching total person approach to patient problems. *Nursing Research*, 21, 264-269.

Newman, D. M. L. (2005). A community nursing center for the health promotion of senior citizens based on the Neuman Systems Model. *Nursing Education Perspectives*, 26(4), 221-223.

Newman, D. M. L., Neuman, B., & Fawcett, J. (2002). Guidelines for Neuman systems model-based education for the health professions. In B. Neuman & J. Fawcett (Eds.), *The Neuman systems model* (4th ed., pp. 193-215). Upper Saddle River, NJ: Pearson Education.

Noonhill, N., Sindhu, S., Hanucharunkul, S., & Suwonnaroop, N. (2007). An integrated approach to coordination of community resources improves health outcomes and satisfaction in care of Thai patients with COPD. *Thai Journal of Nursing Research*, 11(2), 118-131.

Perls, F. (1973). *The gestalt approach: Eye witness to therapy*. Palo Alto, CA: Science and Behavior Books.

Potter, M. L., & Zauszniewski, J. A. (2000). Spirituality, resourcefulness, and arthritis impact on health perception of elders with rheumatoid arthritis. *Journal of Holistic Nursing*, 18(4), 311-331.

Reeves, A. L. (2005a). Childhood experiences of Appalachian women who have experienced intimate partner violence during adulthood. *Dissertation Abstracts International, 65*(10), 5076B. (UMI No. 3152148)

Reeves, A. L. (2005b). *Childhood experiences of Appalachian women who have experienced intimate partner violence.* Paper presented at the Tenth Biennial Neuman Systems Model Symposium, Akron, Ohio.

Ren, J., Snowdon, A. W., & Thrasher, C. (2007, February). *Chinese parents' knowledge and understanding of vehicle restraint use for their children.* Paper presented at the Eleventh Biennial Neuman Systems Model Symposium, Ft. Lauderdale, FL.

Rohr, K. M. (2006). *Alcohol use and injury-related outcomes in older rural trauma patients.* Unpublished doctoral dissertation, University of North Dakota.

Russell, J. (2002). The Neuman systems model and clinical tools. In B. Neuman & J. Fawcett (Eds.), The Neuman systems model (4th ed., pp. 61-73). Upper Saddle River, NJ: Prentice-Hall.

Salvador, P. T. (2006). Development of an oral care guide for patients undergoing autologous stem cell transplantation. *Canadian Oncology Nursing Journal*, 16(1), 18-20.

Selye, H. (1974). *Stress without distress.* Philadelphia: J. B. Lippincott

Shambaugh, B. F., Neuman, B., & Fawcett, J. (2002). Guidelines for Neuman systems model-based administration of health care services. In B. Neuman & J. Fawcett (Eds.), *The Neuman systems model* (4th ed., pp. 265-270). Upper Saddle River, NJ: Pearson Education.

Shamsudin, N. (2002). Can the Neuman systems model by adapted to the Malaysian nursing context? *International Journal of Nursing Practice*, 8(2), 99-105.

Skalski, C. A., DiGerolamo, L, Gigliotti, E. (2006). Stressors in five client populations: Neuman systems model-based literature review. *Journal of Advanced Nursing*, 56(1), 69-78.

Skillen, D. L. (2001). The created environment for physical assessment by case managers. *Western Journal of Nursing Research*, 23(1), 72-89.

Stepans, M. B. F., & Knight, J. R. (2002). Application of Neuman's framework: infant exposure to environmental tobacco smoke. *Nursing Science Quarterly*, 15(4), 327-334.

Stepans, M. B. F., Wilhelm, S. L., & Dolence, K. (2006). Smoking hygiene: reducing infant exposure to tobacco. *Biological Research for Nursing*, 8(2), 104-114.

Torakis, M. L. & Smigielski, C. M. (2000). Documentation of model-based practice: One hospital's experience. *Pediatric Nursing,* 26(4), 394-399, 428.

Torres, G. (1986). *Theoretical foundations of nursing.* Norwalk, CT: Appleton-Century-Crofts.

Ume-Nwagbo, P. N., Dewan, S. A., & Lowry, L.W. (2006). Using the Neuman systems model for best practices. *Nursing Science Quarterly,* 19(1), 31-35.

Vito, K. (2005). *Application of the Neuman Systems Model in a School Nurse Practice.* Paper presented at the Tenth Biennial Neuman Systems Model Symposium, Akron, Ohio.

Walker, L. O., & Avant, K. (1983). *Strategies for theory construction in nursing.* Norwalk, CT: Appleton-Century-Crofts.

Wetta-Hall, R., Berry, M., Ablah, E., Gillispie, J. M., Stepp-Cornelius, L. K. (2004). Community case management: a strategy to improve access to medical care in uninsured populations. *Care Management Journals,* 5(2), 87-93.

BIBLIOGRAPHY

Primary Sources

Books

Hinton Walker, P., & Neuman, B. (Eds.). (1996). *Blueprint for use of nursing models.* New York: National League for Nursing Press.

Neuman, B. (1982). *The Neuman systems model: Application to nursing education and practice.* Norwalk, CT: Appleton-Century-Crofts.

Neuman, B. (1989). *The Neuman systems model* (2nd ed.). Norwalk, CT: Appleton & Lange.

Neuman, B. (1995). *The Neuman systems model* (3rd ed.). Norwalk, CT: Appleton & Lange.

Neuman, B., Deloughery, G. W., & Gebbie, M. (1971). *Consultation and community organization in community mental health nursing.* Baltimore: Williams & Wilkins.

Neuman, B., & Fawcett, J. (2002). *The Neuman systems model* (4th ed.). Upper Saddle River, NJ: Pearson Education.

Neuman, B. M., & Walker, P. H. (1996). *Blueprint for use of nursing models: Education, research, practice, and administration.* New York: National League for Nursing Press.

Book Chapters

Freese, B. T., Neuman, B., & Fawcett, J. (2002). Guidelines for Neuman systems model-based clinical practice. In B. Neuman & J. Fawcett (Eds.), *The Neuman systems model* (4th ed., pp. 37-42). Upper Saddle River, NJ: Pearson Education.

Louis, M., Neuman, B., & Fawcett, J. (2002). Guidelines for Neuman systems model-based nursing research. In B. Neuman & J. Fawcett (Eds.), *The Neuman systems model* (4th ed., pp. 113-119). Upper Saddle River, NJ: Pearson Education.

Neuman, B. (1974). The Betty Neuman health care systems model: A total person approach to patient problems. In J. P. Riehl & C. Roy (Eds.), *Conceptual models for nursing practice* (pp. 94-104). New York: Appleton-Century-Crofts.

Neuman, B. (1980). The Betty Neuman health care systems model: A total person approach to patient problems. In J. P. Riehl & C. Roy (Eds.), *Conceptual models for nursing practice* (2nd ed., pp. 119-134). New York: Appleton-Century-Crofts.

Neuman, B. (1983). Analysis and application of Neuman's health care model. In I. W. Clements & F. B. Roberts (Eds.), *Family health: A theoretical approach to nursing care* (pp. 239-254, 353-367). New York: John Wiley & Sons.

Neuman, B. (1986). The Neuman systems model explanation: Its relevance to emerging trends toward wholism in nursing. In I. B. Engberg & K. Kuld (Eds.), *Omvårdnad 1986* [Nursing care book]. Mullsjö: Sweden: Omvårdnad's Forum HB.

Neuman, B. (1989). The Neuman nursing process format Adapted to a family case study. In J. P. Riehl & C. Roy (Eds.), *Conceptual models for nursing practice* (pp. 49-62). Norwalk, CT: Appleton & Lange.

Neuman, B. (1990). The Neuman systems model: A theory for practice. In M. E. Parker (Ed.), *Nursing theories in practice* (pp. 24-26). New York: National League for Nursing.

Neuman, B. (1995). In conclusion—Toward new beginnings. In B. Neuman (Ed.), *The Neuman systems model* (3rd ed., pp. 671-703). Norwalk, CT: Appleton & Lange.

Neuman, B. (1995). The Neuman systems model. In B. Neuman (Ed.), *The Neuman systems model* (3rd ed., pp. 3-62). Norwalk, CT: Appleton & Lange.

Neuman, B. (2001). The Neuman systems model: A futuristic care perspective. In N. L Chaska, (Ed.), *The nursing profession: Tomorrow and beyond* (pp. 321-329). Thousand Oaks, CA: Sage Publications.

Neuman, B. (2002). Assessment and intervention based on the Neuman systems model. In B. Neuman & J. Fawcett (Eds.), *The Neuman systems model* (4th ed., pp. 347-359). Upper Saddle River, NJ: Pearson Education.

Neuman, B. (2002). Betty Neuman's autobiography and chronology of the development and utilization of the Neuman systems model. In B. Neuman & J. Fawcett (Eds.), *The Neuman systems model* (4th ed., pp. 325-346). Upper Saddle River, NJ: Pearson Education.

Neuman, B. (2002). The future and the Neuman systems model. In B. Neuman & J. Fawcett (Eds.), *The Neuman systems model* (4th ed., pp. 319-321). Upper Saddle River, NJ: Pearson Education.

Neuman, B. (2002). The Neuman systems model definitions. In B. Neuman & J. Fawcett (Eds.), *The Neuman systems model* (4th ed., pp. 322-324). Upper Saddle River, NJ: Pearson Education.

Neuman, B. (2002). The Neuman systems model. In B. Neuman & J. Fawcett (Eds.), *The Neuman systems model* (4th ed., pp. 3-33). Upper Saddle River, NJ: Pearson Education.

Neuman, B. (2002). The Neuman Systems Model Trustees Group. In B. Neuman & J. Fawcett (Eds.), *The Neuman systems model* (4th ed., pp. 360-363). Upper Saddle River, NJ: Pearson Education.

Neuman, B., & Wyatt, M. (1980). The Neuman stress/adaptation systems approach to education for nurse administrators. In J. P. Riehl & C. Roy (Eds.), *Conceptual models for nursing practice* (2nd ed., pp. 142-150). New York: Appleton-Century-Crofts.

Newman, D. M. L., Neuman, B., & Fawcett, J. (2002). Guidelines for Neuman systems model-based education for the health professions. In B. Neuman & J. Fawcett (Eds.), *The Neuman systems model* (4th ed., pp. 193-215). Upper Saddle River, NJ: Pearson Education.

Shambaugh, B. F., Neuman, B., & Fawcett, J. (2002). Guidelines for Neuman systems model-based administration of health care services. In B. Neuman & J. Fawcett (Eds.), *The Neuman systems model* (4th ed., pp. 265-270). Upper Saddle River, NJ: Pearson Education.

Journal Articles

Deloughery, G. W., Neuman, B. M., & Gebbie, K. M. (1971, Oct). Nurses in community mental health: An informative interpretation for employees of professional nurses. *Public Personnel Review, 32*(4), 215-218.

Neuman, B. (1985, Sept). The Neuman systems model: Its importance for nursing. *Senior Nurse, 3*, 3.

Neuman, B. (1990). Health: A continuum based on the Neuman systems model. *Nursing Science Quarterly, 3*, 129-135.

Neuman, B. (1996). The Neuman systems model in research and practice. *Nursing Science Quarterly, 9*(2), 67-70.

Neuman, B. (1998). NDs should be future coordinators of health care (Letter to the Editor). *Image: The Journal of Nursing Scholarship, 30*, 106.

Neuman, B. (2000). Leadership-scholarship integration: Using the Neuman systems model for 21st century professional nursing practice. *Nursing Science Quarterly, 13*(1), 60-63.

Neuman, B., Chadwick, P. L., Beynon, C. E., Craig, D. M., Fawcett, J., Chang, N. J., et al. (1997). The Neuman systems model: Reflections and projections. *Nursing Science Quarterly, 10*(1), 18-21.

Neuman, B., Deloughery, G. W., & Gebbie, K. M. (1974, Jan.). Teaching organizational concepts to nurses in community mental health. *Journal of Nursing Education, 13*, 1.

Neuman, B. M., Deloughery, G. W., & Gebbie, K. M. (1970). Changes in problem solving ability among nurses receiving mental health consultation: A pilot study. *Communicating Nursing Research, 3*, 41-52.

Neuman, B. M., Deloughery, G. W., & Gebbie, K. M. (1970, Jan./Feb.). Levels of utilization: Nursing specialists in community mental health. *Journal of Psychiatric Nursing and Mental Health Services, 8*(1), 37-39.

Neuman, B. M., Deloughery, G. W., & Gebbie, K. M. (1972, Feb.). Mental health consultation as a means of improving problem solving ability in work groups: A pilot study. *Comparative Group Studies, 3*(1), 81-97.

Neuman, B. M., & Martin, K. S. (1998). Neuman systems model and the Omaha system. *Image: The Journal of Nursing Scholarship, 30*(1), 8.

Neuman, B. M., & Young, R. J. (1972, May/June). A model for teaching total person approach to patient problems. *Nursing Research, 21*, 264-269.

Neuman, B., Newman, D. M. L., & Holder, P. (2000). Leadership-scholarship integration: Using the Neuman systems model for 21st-century professional nursing practice. *Nursing Science Quarterly, 13*(1), 60-63.

Neuman, B., & Reed, K. S. (2007). A Neuman systems model perspective on nursing in 2050. *Nursing Science Quarterly, 20*(2), 111-113.

Neuman, B., & Wyatt, M. A. (1981). Prospects for change: Some evaluative reflections by faculty members from one articulated baccalaureate program. *Journal of Nursing Education, 20*, 40-46.

Secondary Sources

Books

Bertalanffy, L. (1968). *General system theory*. New York: George Braziller.

Caplan, G. (1964). *Principles of preventive psychiatry*. New York: Basic Books.

Fawcett, J. (1989). *Analysis and evaluation of conceptual models of nursing*. Philadelphia: F. A. Davis.

Fawcett, J. (1999). *The relationship of theory and research* (3rd ed.). Philadelphia: Davis.

Fawcett, J. (2000). *Analysis and evaluation of contemporary nursing knowledge: Nursing models and theories*. Philadelphia: Davis.

Lowry, Lois W. (1998). *The Neuman systems model and nursing education: Teaching strategies and outcomes*. Indianapolis: Sigma Theta Tau International: Center Nursing Press.

Meleis, A. I. (1997). *Theoretical nursing: Development and progress* (3rd ed.). Philadelphia: Lippincott.

Perls, F. (1973). *The gestalt approach: Eye witness to therapy*. Palo Alto, CA: Science and Behavior Books.

Reed, K. S. (1993). *Betty Neuman: The Neuman systems model*. Newbury Park, CA: Sage.

Selye, H. (1974). *Stress without distress*. Philadelphia: J. B. Lippincott.

Torres, G. (1986). *Theoretical foundations of nursing*. Norwalk, CT: Appleton-Century-Crofts.

Walker, L. O., & Avant, K. (1983). *Strategies for theory construction in nursing*. Norwalk, CT: Appleton-Century-Crofts.

Book Chapters

Alligood, M. R., & Tomey, A. M. (2002). Introduction to nursing theory: History, terminology and analysis. In A. M. Tomey & M. R. Alligood (Eds.), *Nursing theorists and their works* (5th ed., pp. 3-13). St. Louis: Mosby.

Amaya, M. A. (2002). The Neuman systems model and clinical practice: An integrative review 1974-2000. In B. Neuman & J. Fawcett (Eds.), *The Neuman systems model* (4th ed., pp. 43-60). Upper Saddle River, NJ: Pearson Education.

Beckman, S. J., Boxley-Harges, S., Bruick-Sorge, C., & Eichenaur, J. (1998). Critical thinking, the Neuman systems model, and associate degree education. In L. Lowry (Ed.), *The Neuman systems model and nursing education: Teaching strategies and outcomes* (pp. 53-58). Indianapolis: Center Nursing Press.

Beckman, S. J., Boxley-Harges, S., Bruick-Sorge, C, & Eichenaur, J. (1998). Evaluation modalities for assessing student and program outcomes. In L. Lowry (Ed.), *The Neuman systems model and nursing education: Teaching strategies and outcomes* (pp. 149-160). Indianapolis: Center Nursing Press.

Breckenridge, D. M. (2002). Using the Neuman systems model to guide nursing research in the United States. In B. Neuman & J. Fawcett (Eds.), *the Neuman systems model* (4th ed., pp. 176-182). Upper Saddle River, NJ: Pearson Education.

Busch, P., & Lynch, M. (1998). Creative teaching strategies in a Neuman-based baccalaureate curriculum. In L. Lowry (Ed.), *The Neuman systems model and nursing education: Teaching strategies and outcomes* (pp. 59-70). Indianapolis: Center Nursing Press.

Cammuso, B. S., & Wallen, A. J. (2002). Using the Neuman systems model to guide nursing education in the United States. In B. Neuman & J. Fawcett (Eds.), *The Neuman systems model* (4th ed., pp. 244-253). Upper Saddle River, NJ: Pearson Education.

Chang, N. J., & Freese, B. T. (1998). Teaching culturally competent care: A Korean-American experience. In L. Lowry (Ed.), *The Neuman systems model and nursing education: Teaching strategies and outcomes* (pp. 85-90). Indianapolis: Center Nursing Press.

Crawford, J. A., & Tarko, M. (2002). Using the Neuman systems model to guide nursing practice in Canada. In B. Neuman & J. Fawcett (Eds.), *The Neuman systems model* (4th ed., pp. 90-110). Upper Saddle River, NJ: Pearson Education.

de Kuiper, M. (2002). Using the Neuman systems model to guide nursing education in Holland. In B. Neuman & J. Fawcett (Eds.), *The Neuman systems model* (4th ed., pp. 254-262). Upper Saddle River, NJ: Pearson Education.

Evans, B. (1998). Fourth-generation evaluation and the Neuman systems model. In L. Lowry (Ed.), *The Neuman systems model and nursing education: Teaching strategies and outcomes* (pp. 117-128). Indianapolis: Center Nursing Press.

Fashinpaur, D. (2002). Using the Neuman systems model to guide nursing practice in the United States: Nursing prevention interventions for postpartum mood disorders. In B. Neuman & J. Fawcett (Eds.), *The Neuman systems model* (4th ed., pp. 74-89). Upper Saddle River, NJ: Pearson Education.

Fawcett, J. (1998). Conceptual models and therapeutic modalities in advanced psychiatric nursing practice. In A. W. Burgess (Ed.), *Advanced practice psychiatric nursing* (pp. 41-48). Stamford, CT: Appleton & Lange.

Fawcett, J. (2002). Neuman systems model bibliography. In B. Neuman & J. Fawcett (Eds.), *The Neuman systems model* (4th ed., pp. 364-400). Upper Saddle River, NJ: Pearson Education.

Fawcett, J., & Giangrande, S. K. (2002). The Neuman systems model and research: An integrative review. In B. Neuman & J. Fawcett (Eds.), *The Neuman systems model* (4th ed., pp. 120-149). Upper Saddle River, NJ: Pearson Education.

Freese, B., Beckman, S. J., Boxley-Harges, S., Bruick-Sorge, C, Harris, S. M., Hermiz, et al. (1998). Betty Neuman: Systems model. In A. M. Tomey & M. R. Alligood (Eds.), *Nursing theorists and their work* (4th ed., pp. 267-299). St. Louis: Mosby.

Freese, B. T. (2002). Betty Neuman: Systems model In A. M. Tomey & M. R. Alligood (Eds.), *Nursing theorists and their work* (5th ed., pp. 299-335). St. Louis: Mosby.

Freese, B. T., & Scales, C. J. (1998). NSM-based care as an NLN program evaluation outcome. In L. Lowry (Ed.), *The Neuman systems model and nursing education: Teaching strategies and outcomes* (pp. 135-139). Indianapolis: Center Nursing Press.

Frieburger, O. A. (1998). Overview of strategies that integrate the Neuman systems model, critical thinking, and cooperative learning. In L. Lowry (Ed.), *The Neuman systems model and nursing education: teaching strategies and outcomes* (pp. 79-84). Indianapolis: Center Nursing Press.

Frieburger, O. A. (1998). The Neuman systems model, critical thinking, and cooperative learning in a nursing issues course. In L. Lowry (Ed.), *The Neuman systems model and nursing education: Teaching strategies and outcomes* (pp. 79-84). Indianapolis: Center Nursing Press.

Geib, K. (2006). Neuman System's Model in nursing practice. In M. R. Alligood & A. M. Tomey (Eds.), *Nursing Theory Utilization and Application, 3rd* edition (pp. 229-254). St. Louis: Mosby-Elsevier

Gigliotti, E., & Fawcett, J. (2002). The Neuman systems model and research instruments. In B. Neuman & J. Fawcett

(Eds.), *The Neuman systems model* (4th ed., pp. 150-175). Upper Saddle River, NJ: Pearson Education.

Hassell, J. S. (1998). Critical thinking strategies for family and community client systems. In L. Lowry (Ed.), *The Neuman systems model and nursing education: Teaching strategies and outcomes* (pp. 71-78). Indianapolis: Center Nursing Press.

Lowry, L. W. (1998). Creative teaching and effective evaluation. In L. Lowry (Ed.), *The Neuman systems model and nursing education: Teaching strategies and outcomes* (pp. 17-30). Indianapolis: Center Nursing Press.

Lowry, L. W. (1998). Efficacy of the Neuman systems model as a curriculum framework: A longitudinal study. In L. Lowry (Ed.), *The Neuman systems model and nursing education: Teaching strategies and outcomes* (pp. 139-148). Indianapolis: Center Nursing Press.

Lowry, L. W. (1998). Vision, values, and verities. In L. Lowry (Ed.), *The Neuman systems model and nursing education: Teaching strategies and outcomes* (pp. 167-174). Indianapolis: Center Nursing Press.

Lowry, L. W. (2002). The Neuman systems model and education: An integrative review. In B. Neuman & J. Fawcett (Eds.), *The Neuman systems model* (4th ed., pp. 216-237). Upper Saddle River, NJ: Pearson Education.

Lowry, L. W., Bruick-Sorge, C, Freese, B. T., & Sutherland, R. (1998). Development and renewal of faculty for Neuman-based teaching. In L. Lowry (Ed.), *The Neuman systems model and nursing education: Teaching strategies and outcomes* (pp. 161-166). Indianapolis: Center Nursing Press.

Munck, C. K., & Merks, A. (2002). Using the Neuman systems model to guide administration of nursing services in Holland: The case of Emergis, institute for mental health care. In B. Neuman & J. Fawcett (Eds.), *The Neuman systems model* (4th ed., pp. 300-316). Upper Saddle River, NJ: Pearson Education.

Newsome, G. G., & Lowry, L. W. (1998). Evaluation in nursing: History, models, and Neuman's framework. In L. Lowry (Ed.), *The Neuman systems model and nursing education: Teaching strategies and outcomes* (pp. 37-52). Indianapolis: Center Nursing Press.

Nuttall, P. R., Stittich, E. M., & Flores, F. C. (1998). The Neuman systems model in advanced practice nursing. In L. Lowry (Ed.), *The Neuman systems model and nursing education: Teaching strategies and outcomes* (pp. 109-116). Indianapolis: Center Nursing Press.

Pothiban, L. (2002). Using the Neuman systems model to guide nursing research in Thailand. In B. Neuman & J. Fawcett (Eds.), *The Neuman systems model* (4th ed., pp. 183-190). Upper Saddle River, NJ: Pearson Education.

Reed, K. S. (2002). The Neuman systems model and educational tools. In B. Neuman & J. Fawcett (Eds.), *The Neuman systems model* (4th ed., pp. 238-243). Upper Saddle River, NJ: Pearson Education.

Russell, J. (2002). The Neuman systems model and clinical tools. In B. Neuman & J. Fawcett (Eds.), *The Neuman systems model* (4th ed., pp. 61-73). Upper Saddle River, NJ: Pearson Education.

Sanders, N. F., & Kelley, J. A. (2002). The Neuman systems model and administration of nursing services: An integrative review. In B. Neuman & J. Fawcett (Eds.), *The Neuman systems model* (4th ed., pp. 271-287). Upper Saddle River, NJ: Pearson Education.

Seng, V. S. (1998). Clinical evaluation: The heart of clinical performance. In L. Lowry (Ed.), *The Neuman systems model and nursing education: Teaching strategies and outcomes* (pp. 129-134). Indianapolis: Center Nursing Press.

Strickland-Seng, V. (1998). Clinical evaluation: The heart of clinical performance. In L. Lowry (Ed.), *The Neuman systems model and nursing education: Teaching strategies and outcomes* (pp. 129-134). Indianapolis: Sigma Theta Tau International Center Nursing Press.

Sutherland, R., & Forrest, D. L. (1998). Primary prevention in an associate of science curriculum. In L. Lowry (Ed.), *The Neuman systems model and nursing education: Teaching strategies and outcomes* (pp. 99-108). Indianapolis: Center Nursing Press.

Torakis, M. L. (2002). Using the Neuman systems model to guide administration of nursing services in the United States: Redirecting nursing practice in a freestanding pediatric hospital. In B. Neuman & J. Fawcett (Eds.), *The Neuman systems model* (4th ed., pp. 288-299). Upper Saddle River, NJ: Pearson Education.

Weitzel, A. R., & Wood, K. C. (1998). Community health nursing: Keystone of baccalaureate education. In L. Lowry (Ed.), *The Neuman systems model and nursing education: Teaching strategies and outcomes* (pp. 91-98). Indianapolis: Center Nursing Press.

Journal Articles

August-Brady, M. (2000). Prevention as intervention. *Journal of Advanced Nursing, 31*(6), 1304-1308.

Beckman, S., Boxley-Harges, S., Bruick-Sorge, C., & Salmon, B. (2007). Five strategies that heighten nurses' awareness of spirituality to impact client care. *Holistic Nursing Practice, 21*(3), 135-139.

Beryl-Pilkington, F. (2007). Envisioning nursing in 2050 through the eyes of nurse theorists: King, Neuman, and Roy. *Nursing Science Quarterly, 20*(2):108.

Binhosen, V., Panuthai, S., Srisuphun, W., Chang, E., Sucamvang, K., & Cioffi, J. (2003). Physical activity and health related quality of life among the urban Thai elderly. *Thai Journal of Nursing Research, 7*(4), 231-243.

Dunn, K. S. (2007). Predictors of self-reported health among older African-American central city adults. *Holistic Nursing Practice, 21*(5), 237-243.

Edelman, M., Lunney, M. (2000). You make the diagnosis. Case study: A diabetic educator's use of the Neuman Systems Model. *Nursing Diagnosis, 11*(4), 148, 179-182.

Eilert-Petersson, E., & Olsson, H. Humour and slimming related to the Neuman Systems Model: A study of slimming women in Sweden. *Theoria Journal of Nursing Theory, 12*(3), 4-18.

Falk-Rafael, A. R., Ward-Griffin, C., Laforet-Fliesser, Y., & Beynon, C. (2004). Teaching nursing students to promote the health of communities: a partnership approach. *Nurse Educator, 29*(2), 63-67.

Fawcett, J. (2001). Scholarly dialogue. The nurse theorists: 21st-century updates-Betty Neuman. *Nursing Science Quarterly, 14*(3), 211-214.

Fawcett, J. (2004). Scholarly dialogue. Conceptual models of nursing: international in scope and substance? The case of the Neuman Systems model. *Nursing Science Quarterly. 17*(1), 50-54.

Fawcett, J., & Giangrande, S. K. (2001). Neuman Systems Model-based research: An integrative review project. *Nursing Science Quarterly, 14*(3), 231-238.

Fawcett, J., & Gigliotti, E. (2001). Using conceptual models of nursing to guide nursing research: The case of the Neuman Systems Model. *Nursing Science Quarterly, 14*(4), 339-345.

Fawcett, J., Newman, D. M. L., McAllister, M. (2004). Advanced practice nursing and conceptual models of nursing. *Nursing Science Quarterly, 17*(2), 135-138.

Fuller, C. C., & Hartley, B. (2000). Linear scleroderma: A Neuman nursing perspective. *Journal of Pediatric Nursing: Nursing Care of Children and Families, 15*(3), 168-174.

Gerstle, D. S., All, A. C., & Wallace, D. C. (2001). Quality of life and chronic nonmalignant pain. *Pain Management Nursing, 2*(3), 98-109.

Gigliotti, E. (2001). Empirical tests of the Neuman Systems Model: Relational statement analysis. *Nursing Science Quarterly, 14*(2), 149-157.

Gigliotti, E. (2002). A theory-based clinical nurse specialist practice exemplar using Neuman's Systems Model and nursing's taxonomies. *Clinical Nurse Specialist, 16*(1), 10-16

Gigliotti, E. (2003). Research issues. The Neuman Systems Model Institute: testing middle-range theories. *Nursing Science Quarterly, 16*(3), 201-206.

Gigliotti, E. (2004). Etiology of maternal-student role stress. *Nursing Science Quarterly, 17*(2), 156-164.

Gigliotti, E. (2007). Improving external and internal validity of a model of midlife women's maternal-student role stress. *Nursing Science Quarterly, 20*(2), 161-170.

Graham, J. (2006). Nursing theory and clinical practice: how three nursing models can be incorporated into the care of patients with end stage kidney disease. *CANNT Journal. 16*(4), 28-31.

Jones-Cannon, S., & Davis, B. L. (2005). Coping among African-American daughters caring for aging parents. *ABNF Journal, 16*(6), 118-123.

Kain, H. B. (2000). Care of the older adult following hip fracture. *Holistic Nursing Practice, 14*(4), 24-39.

Kinservik, M. A., & Friedhoff, M. M. (2000). Control issues in toilet training. *Pediatric Nursing, 26*(3), 267-274.

Kottwitz, D., Bowling, S. (2003). A pilot study of the Elder Abuse Questionnaire. *Kansas Nurse, 78*(7), 4-6.

Lancaster, D. R. (2005). Coping with appraised breast cancer risk among women with family histories of breast cancer. *Research in Nursing & Health, 28*(2), 144-158.

Leophonte, P., Delon, S., Dalbies, S., Fontes-Carrere, M., Goncalves de Carvalho, E., & Lepage, S. (2000). Effects of the preparation on anxiety before bronchial fibrescopy. *Recherche En Soins Infirmiers,* (60), 50-66.

Lowry, L., Beckman, S., Gehrling K. R., & Fawcett, J. (2007). Imagining nursing practice: The Neuman Systems Model in 2050. *Nursing Science Quarterly, 20*(3), 226-229.

Lowry, L. W., Burns, C. M., Smith, A. A., & Jacobson, H. (2000). Compete or complement? An interdisciplinary approach to training health professionals. *Nursing and Health Care Perspectives, 21*(2), 76-80.

Malinski, V. M. (2002). Research issues: Developing a nursing perspective on spirituality and healing. *Nursing Science Quarterly, 15*(4), 281-287.

Malinski, V. M. (2003). Research issues. Nursing research and nursing conceptual models: Betty Neuman's Systems Model. *Nursing Science Quarterly, 16*(3), 201.

May, K. M., & Hu, J. (2000). Caregiving and help seeking by mothers of low birthweight infants and mothers of normal birthweight infants. *Public Health Nursing, 17*(4), 273-279.

Melton, L., Secrest, J., Chien, A., & Andersen B. (2000). Resources for practice: A community needs assessment for a SANE program using Neuman's model. *Journal of the American Academy of Nurse Practitioners, 13*(4), 178-186.

Memmott, R. J., Marett, K. M., Bott, R. L., & Duke, L. (2000). Use of the Neuman Systems Model for interdisciplinary teams. *Online Journal of Rural Nursing and Health Care, 1*(2), 9p.

Meyer, T. & Xu, Y. (2005). Academic and clinical dissonance in nursing education: Are we guilty of failure to rescue? *Nurse Educator, 30*(2), 76-79.

Narsavage, G., & Romeo, E. (2003). Education and support needs of young and older cancer survivors. *Applied Nursing Research, 16*(2), 103-109.

Newman, D. M. L. (2005). A community nursing center for the health promotion of senior citizens: Based on the Neuman Systems Model. *Nursing Education Perspectives, 26*(4), 221-223.

Norrish, M. E., Jooste, K. (2001). Nursing care of the patient undergoing alcohol detoxification. *Curationis: South African Journal of Nursing, 24*(3), 36-48.

Olson, R. S. (2001). Community re-entry after critical illness. *Critical Care Nursing Clinics of North America, 13*(3), 449-461.

Potter, M. L., Zauszniewski, J. A. (2000). Spirituality, resourcefulness, and arthritis impact on health perception of elders with rheumatoid arthritis. *Journal of Holistic Nursing, 18*(4), 311-336.

Reed, K. S. (2003). Grief is more than tears. *Nursing Science Quarterly, 16*(1), 77-81.

Shamsudin, N. (2002). Can the Neuman Systems Model be adapted to the Malaysian nursing context? *International Journal of Nursing Practice, 8*(2), 99-105.

Silveira, D. T. (2000). Process of work-health-disease intervention based on Betty Neuman Systems Model. *Revista Gaucha de Enfermagem, 21*(1), 31-43.

Skalski, C. A., DiGerolamo, L., & Gigliotti E. (2006). Stressors in five client populations: Neuman systems model-based literature review. *Journal of Advanced Nursing, 56*(1), 69-78.

Skillen, D. L., Anderson, M. C., Knight, C. L. (2001). The created environment for physical assessment by case managers. *Western Journal of Nursing Research, 23*(1), 72-89.

Spencer, P. (2002). Support system. *Learning Disability Practice, 5*(7), 16-20.

Stepans, M. B. F., & Knight, J. R. (2002). Application of Neuman's framework: Infant exposure to environmental tobacco smoke. *Nursing Science Quarterly, 15*(4), 327-334.

Torakis M. L., & Smigielski, C. M. (2000). Documentation of model-based practice: one hospital's experience. *Pediatric Nursing, 26*(4), 394-399, 428.

Ume-Nwagbo, P. N., DeWan, S. A., & Lowry, L. W. (2006). Using the Neuman systems model for best practices. *Nursing Science Quarterly, 19*(1), 31-35.

Villarruel, A. M., Bishop, T. L., Simpson, E. M., Jemmott, L. S., & Fawcett, J. (2001). Borrowed theories, shared theories, and the advancement of nursing knowledge. *Nursing Science Quarterly, 14*(2), 158-163.

Wetta-Hall, R., Berry, M., Ablah, E., Gillispie, J. M., & Stepp-Cornelius, L. K. (2004). Community case management: a strategy to improve access to medical care in uninsured populations. *Care Management Journals: Journal of Case Management, The Journal of Long Term Home Health Care, 5*(2), 87-93.

Wilson, L. C. (2000). Implementation and evaluation of church-based health fairs. *Journal of Community Health Nursing, 17*(1), 39-48.

Dissertation and Thesis

Alliston, S. A. (2003). Neonatal nurses' attitudes, practices and knowledge of skin care in the extremely low birth weight infant. *Masters Abstracts International, 41*(6), 1704. (UMI No. 1414358)

Annamunthodo Allen, M. (2005). The effects of a prenatal health teaching program. *Masters Abstracts International, 43*(5), 1698. (UMI No. 1425604)

Bagaoisian, C. (2005). Expanding the role of perioperative nursing: An aid to retention and recruitment strategy. *Masters Abstracts International, 43*(3), 820. (UMI No. 1423680)

Bishop, B. D. (2002). Increasing parental knowledge in treatment of childhood fever. *Masters Abstracts International, 40*(6), 1500. (UMI No. 1409021)

Britt, L. (2006). Investigating differences in management of Hyperlipidemia: A comparison of nurse practitioners and physicians. *Masters Abstracts International, 44*(6), 2760. (UMI No. 1435991)

Brown, P. S. (2004). Relationships among life event stress, role and job strain, and sleep in middle-aged female shift workers. *Dissertation Abstracts International, 65*(4), 1774B. (UMI No. 3130329)

Burnett, A. K. (2006). Stress and coping mechanisms of first year university students. *Masters Abstracts International, 44*(1), 312. (UMI No. 1427502)

Casalenuovo, G. A. (2002). Fatigue in diabetes mellitus: Testing a middle range theory of well-being derived from Neuman's theory of optimal client system stability and the Neuman Systems Model. *Dissertation Abstracts International, 63*(5), 2301B. (UMI No. 3054100)

Chun, A. U. (2006). Issues and concerns of transition from a pediatric healthcare facility to an adult healthcare facility for thalassemia patients. *Masters Abstracts International, 44*(5). (UMI No. 1433257)

Collins, T. J. (2000). Adherence *to hypertension management recommendations for patient follow-up care and lifestyle modifications made by military healthcare providers.* Unpublished master's thesis, Uniformed Services University of the Health Sciences.

Curl, E. D. (2005). A comparison of spirituality in vocational nursing students. *Masters Abstracts International, 43*(1), 183. (UMI No. 1421905)

Dash-Martyr, J. M. (2005). Perceptions of the stressors influencing medication compliance of individuals recovering from a mental illness while living in supportive housing. *Masters Abstracts International, 43*(3), 821. (UMI No. 1423679)

Epps, C. D. (2003). Predictors of length of stay, discharge disposition, and hospital charges in elders following hip and knee arthroplasty. *Dissertation Abstracts International, 63*(7), 3229B. (UMI No. 3031152)

Frederick, A. C. (2004). Violence in the dating experiences of college women. *Dissertation Abstracts International, 64*(10), 4863B. (UMI No. 3109275)

Fruehauf, S. L. (2003). Registered nurse first assistants' perceptions of stress when practicing in operating room settings. *Masters Abstracts International, 41*(6), 1705. (UMI No. 1414355)

Geib, K. M. (2004). The relationships among nursing vigilance by nurses, patient satisfaction with nursing vigilance, and patient length of stay in a surgical cardiac care unit. *Dissertation Abstracts International, 64*(11), 5448B. (UMI No. 3114029)

Hansen, C. S. (2001). Is there a relationship between hardiness and burnout in full-time staff nurses versus per diem nurses? *Masters Abstracts International, 30*(1), 193.

Hemphill, J. C. (2006). Discovering strengths of homeless abused women. *Dissertation Abstracts International, 66*(7), 3635B. (UMI No. 3180908)

Huth, M. M. (2003). Imagery to reduce children's postoperative pain. *Dissertation Abstracts International, 63*(7), 3230B. (UMI No. 3058835)

James, B. R. (2002). Wellness program influence on health risk factors and medical costs among Seventh Day Adventists workers. *Dissertation Abstracts International, 62*(8), 3566B. (UMI No. 3023991)

Jones, A. M. (2003). The effect of education on adherence with oral iron supplementation among hemodialysis patients. *Masters Abstracts International, 41*(1), 191. (UMI No. 1410120)

Karr, C. D. (2007). Recognition of stress in emergency room nurses. *Masters Abstracts International, 45*(4). (UMI No. 1441480)

Kimaid, S. W. (2000). The effects of local anesthetics on postoperative pain. *Masters Abstracts International, 38*(6), 1585. (UMI No. 1399703)

Klainin, P. (2003). Occupational stress, dissatisfaction with family relationships, learned resourcefulness, and women's health. *Dissertation Abstracts International, 63*(7), 3231B. (UMI No. 3058838)

Krajewski, L. L. (2004). Legislators' perceptions of respite care for children with special health needs having tracheotomies with or without ventilator assistance. *Masters Abstracts International, 42*(5), 1682. (UMI No. 1418572)

Kristofersdottir, G. (2001). Oncology nurses' perceived knowledge, assessment, and recommendation of alternative therapies. *Masters Abstracts International, 39*(4), 1127. (UMI No. 1403084)

Ladd, K. J. (2000). The effect of social support on the physiological adaptation of an individual receiving an alternate form of nutrition therapy. *Masters Abstracts International, 38*(2), 420. (UMI No. 1397438)

Lapvongwatana P. (2000). Perinatal risk assessment for low birthweight in Thai mothers: Using the Neuman systems model. *Dissertation Abstracts International, 61*(3), 1325B. (UMI No. 9965512)

Lehman, K. L. (2007). Resilience and depressive symptoms in midlife women. *Masters Abstracts International, 45*(4). (UMI No. 1440665)

Lee, F-P. (2005). The relationship of comfort and spirituality to quality of life among long-term care facility residents in southern Taiwan. *Dissertation Abstracts International, 66*(2), 815B. (UMI No. 3163392)

Levi, C. (2001). School nurses' asthma knowledge and management, roles and functions. *Masters Abstracts International, 39*(6), 1558. (UMI No. 1404338)

Lunario, R. A. (2004). The relationship between frequent suctioning and the risk of VAP. *Masters Abstracts International, 42*(5), 1682. (UMI No. 1419228)

MacRae, E. R. (2001). Workplace health promotion and wellness programs: Their nature and scope. *Masters Abstracts International, 39*(4), 1128. (UMI No. 1403161)

Mahon, J. F. (2002). The effect of a dental health education program on the dental health knowledge of inner-city and non-inner-city elementary age children. *Dissertation Abstracts International, 62*(8), 3556B. (UMI No. 3023358)

Manicat-Emo, A. D. (2000). Stress among maternal caregivers of children with acquired brain injury. *Masters Abstracts International, 38*(6), 1586. (UMI No. 1399701)

Mason, S. (2000). The effect of magnetic therapy on the skin oxygenation of individuals with diabetic foot ulcers. *Masters Abstracts International, 38*(5), 1586. (UMI No. 1398939)

McCarthy, S. P. (2004). Prevalence of stressors related to substance use and abuse in a gay male sample. *Masters Abstracts International, 42*(5), 1683. (UMI No. 1419227)

Meisberger, R. J. (2007). Assessment of early goal directed treatment in the adult septic patient. *Masters Abstracts International, 45*(3), 1459. (UMI No. 1441005)

Metzger, M. E. (2007). The use of two peripheral intravenous sites in patients undergoing cardiac catheterization with possible percutaneous coronary intervention. *Masters Abstracts International, 45*(1). (UMI No. 1428486)

Moola, S. (2006). Facilitating conscious awareness among critical care nurses. *Dissertation Abstracts International, 66*(8). (UMI No. 0808408)

Musgrave, C. F. (2001). Religiosity, spiritual well-being, and attitudes toward spiritual care of Israeli oncology nurses. *Dissertation Abstracts International, v*(n), p. (UMI No. 9995617)

Nichols, P. R. (2001). The effects of music on pain and anxiety during intravenous insertion in the emergency department. *Masters Abstracts International, 39*(1), 196. (UMI No. 1400570)

Noorish, M. E. (2004). A holistic nursing care approach in an alcohol detoxification unit. *Masters Abstracts International, 42*(4), 1243. (UMI No. 0666942)

Parkes, V. C. (2005). Young adult males' perceptions of stressors which influence their use of nicotine. *Masters Abstracts International, 43*(1), 191. (UMI No. 1421750)

Poe, M. A. H. (2002). Predictors of spontaneous lacerations in primigravidae. *Dissertation Abstracts International, 61*(11), 5799B. (UMI No. 3066337)

Poppe, C. A. (2006). A survey of senior level baccalaureate students' beliefs about spirituality and spiritual care. *Masters Abstracts International, 44*(4), 1814. (UMI No. 1432264)

Reeves, A. L. (2005). Childhood experiences of Appalachian women who have experienced intimate partner violence during adulthood. *Dissertation Abstracts International, 65*(10), 5076B. (UMI No. 3152148)

Riley-Lawless, K. (2000). The relationship among characteristics of the family environment and behavioral and physiologic cardiovascular risk factors in parents and their adolescent twins. *Dissertation Abstracts International, 61*(3), 1328B. (UMI No. 9965555)

Roberts, M. C. (2003). The relationships among hospital staff nurses' occupational stress, caring behaviors, and spiritual well-being. *Dissertation Abstracts International, 63*(10), 4598B. (UMI No. 3066340)

Robinson-Lewis, P. E. (2005). Middle to older West Indian Canadian adults diagnosed with type two diabetes: Perceptions of stressors related to complying with treatment regimen. *Masters Abstracts International, 43*(3), 823. (UMI No. 1423678)

Rohr, K. M. (2007). Alcohol use and injury-related outcomes in older rural trauma patients. *Dissertation Abstracts International, 67*(9). (UMI No. 3233967)

Ross, J. R. L. (2004). The lived experiences of retired black women who gamble. *Masters Abstracts International, 42*(5), 1683. (UMI No. 1419233)

Sabatini, C. L. (2003). The meaning of the lived experience of adolescent pregnancy to women who gave birth during their teens: a phenomenological study. *Dissertation Abstracts International, 64*(2), 987B. (UMI No. 3080984)

Samuels-Dennis, J. A. (2004). Assessing stressful life events, psychological well-being and coping styles in sole-support parents. *Masters Abstracts International, 42*(5), 1685. (UMI No. 1418930)

Sheridan, M. N. (2005). Students perceptions of their learning experiences in a newly developed diploma program for practical nurses. *Masters Abstracts International, 43*(5), 1704. (UMI No. 1425596)

Simpson, E. M. (2001). Condom use among Black women: A theoretical basis for HIV prevention guided by Neuman Systems Model and Theory of Planned Behavior. *Dissertation Abstracts International, 61*(10), 5240B. (UMI No. 9989654)

Switek, J. A. (2003). The effect of supportive education, as tertiary nursing intervention, on the quality of life of patients with heart failure. *Masters Abstracts International, 41*(3), 765. (UMI No. 1411254)

Swope, E. M. (2001). A study of the quality and intensity of pain and coping strategies in orthopedic patients. *Masters Abstracts International, 39*(2), 487. (UMI No. 1401208)

Utley, C. A. (2003). The lived experience of individuals within the family when one member has migraine headaches. *Masters Abstracts International, 41*(5), 1422. (UMI No. 1413732)

Van Camp, K. L. (2003). Eating disordered behavior among female marathon runners. *Masters Abstracts International, 41*(5), 1423. (UMI No. 1413524)

Wallom, B. L. L. (2001). Coping behaviors and drug use among fifth- and sixth-grade students. *Dissertation Abstracts International, 61*(8), 3076B. (UMI No. 9982666)

Williams, M. K. (2001). The effects of music therapy on anxiety in surgical patients. *Masters Abstracts International, 39*(1), 198. (UMI No. 1400573)

Wojciechowski, C. E. (2005). The living experience of nurses who were participants in malpractice litigation. *Masters Abstracts International, 43*(6), 2204. (UMI No. 1426667)

Young, L. M. (2000). The effects of guided mental imagery on the blood pressure of clients experiencing mild to moderate essential hypertension. *Dissertation Abstracts International, 61*(2), 787B. (UMI No. 9961229)

Zavala-Onyett, N. D. (2001). The impact of a school-based health clinic on school absence. *Masters Abstracts International, 39*(4), 1134. (UMI No. 1403035)

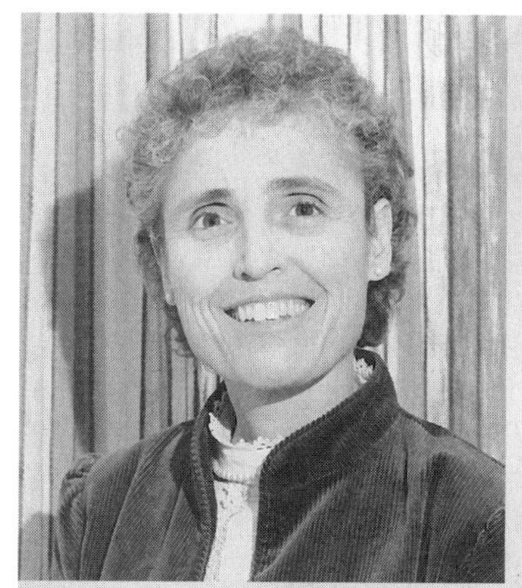

CHAPTER

17

Sister Callista Roy

1939-present

Adaptation Model

Kenneth D. Phillips

"God is intimately revealed in the diversity of creation and is the common destiny of creation; persons use human creative abilities of awareness, enlightenment, and faith; and persons are accountable for the process of deriving, sustaining, and transforming the universe" (Roy, 2000, p. 127).

CREDENTIALS AND BACKGROUND OF THE THEORIST

Sister Callista Roy, a member of the Sisters of Saint Joseph of Carondelet, was born on October 14, 1939, in Los Angeles, California. She received a bachelor's degree in nursing in 1963 from Mount Saint Mary's College in Los Angeles and a master's degree in nursing from the University of California, Los Angeles, in 1966. After earning her nursing degrees, Roy began her education in sociology, receiving both a master's degree in sociology in 1973 and a doctorate in sociology in 1977 from the University of California.

Previous authors: Kenneth D. Phillips, Carolyn L. Blue, Karen M. Brubaker, Julia M. B. Fine, Martha J. Kirsch, Katherine R. Papazian, Cynthia M. Riester, and Mary Ann Sobiech. The author wishes to express appreciation to Sister Callista Roy for critiquing the chapter.

While working toward her master's degree, Roy was challenged in a seminar with Dorothy E. Johnson to develop a conceptual model for nursing. While working as a pediatric staff nurse, Roy had noticed the great resiliency of children and their ability to adapt in response to major physical and psychological changes. Roy was impressed by adaptation as an appropriate conceptual framework for nursing. Roy developed the basic concepts of the model while she was a graduate student at the University of California, Los Angeles, from 1964 to 1966. Roy began operationalizing her model in 1968 when Mount Saint Mary's College adopted the adaptation framework as the philosophical foundation of the nursing curriculum. The Roy Adaptation Model was first presented in the literature in an article published in *Nursing Outlook* in 1970 entitled "Adaptation: A Conceptual Framework for Nursing" (Roy, 1970).

Roy was an associate professor and chairperson of the Department of Nursing at Mount Saint Mary's College until 1982. She was promoted to the rank of professor in 1983 at both Mount Saint Mary's College and the University of Portland. She helped initiate and taught in a summer master's program at the University of Portland. From 1983 to 1985, she was a Robert Wood Johnson postdoctoral fellow at the University of California, San Francisco, as a clinical nurse scholar in neuroscience. During this time, she conducted research on nursing interventions for cognitive recovery in head injuries and on the influence of nursing models on clinical decision making. In 1987, Roy began the newly created position of nurse theorist at Boston College School of Nursing.

Roy has published many books, chapters, and periodical articles and has presented numerous lectures and workshops focusing on her nursing adaptation theory (Roy & Andrews, 1991). The refinement and restatement of the Roy Adaptation Model is published in her 1999 book, *The Roy Adaptation Model* (Roy & Andrews, 1999).

Roy is a member of Sigma Theta Tau, and she received the National Founder's Award for Excellence in Fostering Professional Nursing Standards in 1981. Her achievements include an Honorary Doctorate of Humane Letters by Alverno College (1984), honorary doctorates from Eastern Michigan University (1985) and St. Joseph's College in Maine (1999), and an *American Journal of Nursing* Book of the Year Award for *Essentials of the Roy Adaptation Model* (Andrews & Roy, 1986). Roy has been recognized in the World Who's Who of Women (1979), Personalities of America (1978); as a fellow of the American Academy of Nursing (1978); recipient of a Fulbright Senior Scholar Award from the Australian-American Educational Foundation (1989), and the Martha Rogers Award for Advancing Nursing Science from the National League for Nurses (1991). Roy received the Outstanding Alumna award and the prestigious Carondelet Medal from her alma mater, Mount Saint Mary's. The American Academy of Nursing honored Roy for her extraordinary life achievements by recognizing her as a Living Legend (2007).

THEORETICAL SOURCES

Derivation of the Roy Adaptation Model for nursing included a citation of Harry Helson's work in psychophysics that extended to social and behavioral sciences (Roy, 1984). In Helson's adaptation theory, adaptive responses are a function of the incoming stimulus and the adaptive level (Roy, 1984). A stimulus is any factor that provokes a response. Stimuli may arise from the internal or the external environment (Roy, 1984). The adaptation level is made up of the pooled effect of the following three classes of stimuli:

1. Focal stimuli, which immediately confront the individual
2. Contextual stimuli, which are all other stimuli present that contribute to the effect of the focal stimulus
3. Residual stimuli, environmental factors of which the effects are unclear in a given situation

Helson's work developed the concept of the adaptation level zone, which determines whether a stimulus will elicit a positive or a negative response. According to Helson's theory, adaptation is the process of responding positively to environmental changes (Roy & Roberts, 1981).

Roy (Roy & Roberts, 1981) combined Helson's work with Rapoport's definition of system to view the person as an adaptive system. With Helson's adaptation theory as a foundation, Roy (1970) developed and further refined the model with concepts and theory from Dohrenwend, Lazarus, Mechanic, and Selye. Roy gave special credit to co-authors Driever, for outlining subdivisions of self-integrity, and Martinez and Sato, for identifying common and primary stimuli affecting the modes. Other co-workers also elaborated the concepts. Poush-Tedrow and Van Landingham made contributions to the interdependence mode, and Randell made contributions to the role function mode.

After the development of her model, Roy presented it as a framework for nursing practice, research, and education. Roy (1971) acknowledged that more than 1500 faculty and students contributed to the theoretical development of the adaptation model. She presented the model as a curriculum framework to a large audience at the 1977 Nurse Educator Conference in Chicago (Roy, 1979). And, by 1987, it was estimated that more than 100,000 nurses in the United States and Canada had been prepared to practice using the Roy model.

In *Introduction to Nursing: An Adaptation Model*, Roy (1976a) discussed self-concept and group identity mode. She and her collaborators cited the work of Coombs and Snygg regarding self-consistency and major influencing factors of self-concept (Roy, 1984). Social interaction theories are cited to provide a theoretical basis. For example, Roy (1984) notes that Cooley (1902) theorizes that self-perception is influenced by perceptions of others' responses, termed the "looking glass self." She points out that Mead expands the idea by hypothesizing that self-appraisal uses the generalized other. Roy builds on Sullivan's suggestion that self arises from social interaction (Roy, 1984). Gardner and Erickson support Roy's developmental approaches (Roy, 1984). The other modes—physiological-physical, role function, and interdependence—were drawn similarly from biological and behavioral sciences for an understanding of the person.

Additional development of the model occurred during the later 1900s and into the twenty-first century. These developments included updated scientific and philosophical assumptions; a redefinition of adaptation and adaptation levels; extension of the adaptive modes to group level knowledge development; and analysis, critique, and synthesis of the first 25 years of research based on the Roy Adaptation Model. Roy agrees with other theorists who believe that changes in the person-environment systems of the earth are so extensive that a major epoch is ending (Davies, 1988; De Chardin, 1966). During the 67 million years of the Cenozoic era, the Age of Mammals and an era of great creativity, human life appeared on Earth. During this era, humankind has had little or no influence on the universe (Roy, 1997). "As the era closes, humankind has taken extensive control of the life systems of the earth. Roy claims that we are now in the position of deciding what kind of universe we will inhabit" (Roy, 1997, p. 42). Roy "has made the foci of assumptions of the twenty-first century mutual complex person and environment self-organization and a meaningful destiny of convergence of the universe, persons, and environment in what can be considered a supreme being or God" (Roy & Andrews, 1999, p. 395). According to Roy (1997), "persons are coextensive with their physical and social environments" (p. 34), and they "share a destiny with the universe and are responsible for mutual transformations" (Roy & Andrews, 1999, p. 395). Developments of the model that were related to the integral relationship between person and environment have been influenced by Pierre Teilhard De Chardin's law of progressive complexity and increasing consciousness (De Chardin, 1959, 1965, 1966, 1969) and the work of Swimme and Berry (1992).

MAJOR CONCEPTS & DEFINITIONS

SYSTEM

A system is "a set of parts connected to function as a whole for some purpose and that does so by virtue of the interdependence of its parts" (Roy & Andrews, 1999, p. 32). In addition to having wholeness and related parts, "systems also have inputs, outputs, and control and feedback processes" (Andrews & Roy, 1991, p. 7).

ADAPTATION LEVEL

"Adaptation level represents the condition of the life processes described on three levels as integrated, compensatory, and compromised" (Roy & Andrews, 1999, p. 30). A person's adaptation level is "a constantly changing point, made up of focal, contextual, and residual stimuli, which represent the person's own standard of the range of stimuli

Continued

MAJOR CONCEPTS & DEFINITIONS—cont'd

to which one can respond with ordinary adaptive responses" (Roy, 1984, pp. 27-28).

ADAPTATION PROBLEMS

Adaptation problems are "broad areas of concern related to adaptation. These describe the difficulties related to the indicators of positive adaptation" (Roy & Andrews, 1999, p. 65). Roy (1984) states the following:

> It can be noted at this point that the distinction being made between adaptation problems and nursing diagnoses is based on the developing work in both of these fields. At this point, adaptation problems are seen not as nursing diagnoses, but as areas of concern for the nurse related to adapting person or group (within each adaptive mode) (pp. 89-90).

FOCAL STIMULUS

The focal stimulus is "the internal or external stimulus most immediately confronting the human system" (Roy & Andrews, 1999, p. 31).

CONTEXTUAL STIMULI

Contextual stimuli "are all other stimuli present in the situation that contribute to the effect of the focal stimulus" (Roy & Andrews, 1999, p. 31), that is, "contextual stimuli are all the environmental factors that present to the person from within or without but which are not the center of the person's attention and/or energy" (Andrews & Roy, 1991, p. 9).

RESIDUAL STIMULI

Residual stimuli "are environmental factors within or without the human system with effects in the current situation that are unclear" (Roy & Andrews, 1999, p. 32).

COPING PROCESSES

Coping processes "are innate or acquired ways of interacting with the changing environment" (Roy & Andrews, 1999, p. 31).

INNATE COPING MECHANISMS

Innate coping mechanisms "are genetically determined or common to the species and are generally viewed as automatic processes; humans do not have to think about them" (Roy & Andrews, 1999, p. 46).

ACQUIRED COPING MECHANISMS

Acquired coping mechanisms "are developed through strategies such as learning. The experiences encountered throughout life contribute to customary responses to particular stimuli" (Roy & Andrews, 1999, p. 46).

REGULATOR SUBSYSTEM

Regulator is "a major coping process involving the neural, chemical, and endocrine systems" (Roy & Andrews, 1999, p. 32).

COGNATOR SUBSYSTEM

Cognator is "a major coping process involving four cognitive-emotive channels: perceptual and information processing, learning, judgment, and emotion" (Roy & Andrews, 1999, p. 31).

ADAPTIVE RESPONSES

Adaptive responses are those "that promote integrity in terms of the goals of human systems" (Roy & Andrews, 1999, p. 31).

INEFFECTIVE RESPONSES

Ineffective responses are those "that do not contribute to integrity in terms of the goals of the human system" (Roy & Andrews, 1999, p. 31).

MAJOR CONCEPTS & DEFINITIONS—cont'd

INTEGRATED LIFE PROCESS

Integrated life process refers to the "adaptation level at which the structures and functions of a life process are working as a whole to meet human needs" (Roy & Andrews, 1999, p. 31).

PHYSIOLOGICAL-PHYSICAL MODE

The physiological mode "is associated with the physical and chemical processes involved in the function and activities of living organisms" (Roy & Andrews, 1999, p. 102). Five needs are identified in the physiological-physical mode relative to the basic need of physiological integrity as follows: (1) oxygenation, (2) nutrition, (3) elimination, (4) activity and rest, and (5) protection. Complex processes that include the senses; fluid, electrolyte, and acid-base balance; neurological function; and endocrine function contribute to physiological adaptation. The basic need of the physiological mode is physiological integrity (Roy & Andrews, 1999). The physical mode is "the manner in which the collective human adaptive system manifests adaptation relative to basic operating resources, participants, physical facilities, and fiscal resources" (Roy & Andrews, 1999, p. 104). The basic need of the physical mode is operating integrity.

SELF-CONCEPT-GROUP IDENTITY MODE

The self-concept-group identity mode is one of the three psychosocial modes; "it focuses specifically on the psychological and spiritual aspects of the human system. The basic need underlying the individual self-concept mode has been identified as psychic and spiritual integrity, or the need to know who one is so that one can be or exist with a sense of unity, meaning, and purposefulness in the universe" (Roy & Andrews, 1999, p. 107). "Self-concept is defined as the composite of beliefs and feelings about oneself at a given time and is formed from internal perceptions and perceptions of others' reactions" (Roy & Andrews, 1999, p. 107). Its components include the following: (1) the physical self, which involves sensation and body image, and (2) the personal self, which is made up of self-consistency, self-ideal or expectancy, and the moral-ethical-spiritual self. The group identity mode "reflects how people in groups perceive themselves based on environmental feedback. The group identity mode [is comprised] of interpersonal relationships, group self-image, social milieu, and culture" (Roy & Andrews, 1999, p. 108). The basic need of the group identity mode is identity integrity (Roy & Andrews, 1999).

ROLE FUNCTION MODE

The role function mode "is one of two social modes and focuses on the roles the person occupies in society. A role, as the functioning unit of society, is defined as a set of expectations about how a person occupying one position behaves toward a person occupying another position. The basic need underlying the role function mode has been identified as social integrity—the need to know who one is in relation to others so that one can act" (Hill & Roberts, 1981, pp. 109-110). Persons perform primary, secondary, and tertiary roles. These roles are carried out with both instrumental and expressive behaviors. Instrumental behavior is "the actual physical performance of a behavior" (Andrews, 1991, p. 348). Expressive behaviors are "the feelings, attitudes, likes or dislikes that a person has about a role or about the performance of a role" (Andrews, 1991, p. 348).

Continued

MAJOR CONCEPTS & DEFINITIONS—cont'd

The primary role determines the majority of behavior engaged in by the person during a particular period of life. It is determined by age, sex, and developmental stage (Andrews, 1991, p. 349).

Secondary roles are those that a person assumes to complete the task associated with a developmental stage and primary role (Andrews, 1991, p. 349).

Tertiary roles are related primarily to secondary roles and represent ways in which individuals meet their role associated obligations . . . Tertiary roles are normally temporary in nature, freely chosen by the individual, and may include activities such as clubs or hobbies (Andrews, 1991, p. 349).

The major roles that one plays can be analyzed by imagining a tree formation. The trunk of the tree is one's primary role, or developmental level, such as a generative adult female. Secondary roles branch off from this—for example, wife, mother, and teacher. Finally, tertiary roles branch off from secondary roles—for example, the mother role might involve the role of parent-teacher association president for a given period. Each of these roles is seen as occurring in a dyadic relationship, that is, with a reciprocal role (Roy & Andrews, 1999).

INTERDEPENDENCE MODE

"The interdependence mode focuses on close relationships of people (individually and collectively) and their purpose, structure, and development . . . Interdependent relationships involve the willingness and ability to give to others and accept from them aspects of all that one has to offer such as love, respect, value, nurturing, knowledge, skills, commitments, material possessions, time, and talents" (Roy & Andrews, 1999, p. 111).

The basic need of this mode is termed *relational integrity* (Roy & Andrews, 1999).

Two specific relationships are the focus of the interdependence mode as it applies to individuals. The first is with significant others, persons who are the most important to the individual. The second is with support systems, that is, others contributing to meeting interdependence needs (Roy & Andrews, 1999, p. 112).

Two major areas of interdependence behaviors have been identified: receptive behavior and contributive behavior. These behaviors apply respectively to the "receiving and giving of love, respect and value in interdependent relationships" (Roy & Andrews, 1999, p. 112).

PERCEPTION

"Perception is the interpretation of a stimulus and the conscious appreciation of it" (Pollock, 1993, p. 169). Perception links the regulator with the cognator and connects the adaptive modes (Rambo, 1983).

USE OF EMPIRICAL EVIDENCE

From this beginning, the Roy Adaptation Model has been supported through research in practice and in education (Brower & Baker, 1976; Farkas, 1981; Mastal & Hammond, 1980; Meleis, 1985, 2007; Roy, 1980; Roy & Obloy, 1978; Wagner, 1976). In 1999 (Roy & Andrews, 1999), a group of seven scholars working with Roy conducted a meta-analysis, critique, and synthesis of 163 studies based on the Roy Adaptation Model that had been published in 44 English language journals on five continents and dissertations and theses from the United States. Of these 163 studies, 116 met the criteria established for testing propositions from the model. Twelve generic propositions based on Roy's earlier work were derived. To synthesize the research, findings of each study were used to state ancillary and practice propositions, and support for the propositions was examined. Of 265 propositions tested, 216 (82%) were supported.

MAJOR ASSUMPTIONS

Assumptions from systems theory and assumptions from adaptation level theory have been combined into a single set of scientific assumptions. From systems theory, human adaptive systems are viewed as interactive parts that act in unity for some purpose. Human adaptive systems are complex and multifaceted and respond to a myriad of environmental stimuli to achieve adaptation. With their ability to adapt to environmental stimuli, humans have the capacity to create changes in the environment (Roy & Andrews, 1999). Drawing on characteristics of creation spirituality by Swimme and Berry (1992), Roy combined the assumptions of humanism and veritivity into a single set of philosophical assumptions. Humanism asserts that the person and human experiences are essential to knowing and valuing, and that they share in creative power. Veritivity affirms the belief in the purpose, value, and meaning of all human life. These scientific and philosophical assumptions have been refined for use of the model in the twenty-first century (Box 17-1).

Box 17-1 Vision Basic to Concepts for the Twenty-First Century

SCIENTIFIC ASSUMPTIONS

- Systems of matter and energy progress to higher levels of complex self-organization.
- Consciousness and meaning are constitutive of person and environment integration.
- Awareness of self and environment is rooted in thinking and feeling.
- Humans, by their decisions, are accountable for the integration of creative processes.
- Thinking and feeling mediate human action.
- System relationships include acceptance, protection, and fostering of interdependence.
- Persons and the earth have common patterns and integral relationships.
- Persons and environment transformations are created in human consciousness.
- Integration of human and environment meanings results in adaptation.

PHILOSOPHICAL ASSUMPTIONS

- Persons have mutual relationships with the world and God.
- Human meaning is rooted in an omega point convergence of the universe.
- God is ultimately revealed in the diversity of creation and is the common destiny of creation.
- Persons use human creative abilities of awareness, enlightenment, and faith.
- Persons are accountable for the processes of deriving, sustaining, and transforming the universe.

From Roy, C., & Andrews, H. (1999). *The Roy adaptation model* (2nd ed., p. 35). Upper Saddle River, NJ: Pearson Education, Inc.

Adaptation

Roy has further defined adaptation for use in the twenty-first century (Roy & Andrews, 1999). According to Roy, *adaptation* refers to "the process and outcome whereby thinking and feeling persons, as individuals or in groups, use conscious awareness and choice to create human and environmental integration" (Roy & Andrews, 1999, p. 30). Rather than being a human system that simply strives to respond to environmental stimuli to maintain integrity, every human life is purposeful in a universe that is creative, and persons are inseparable from their environment.

Nursing

Roy defines *nursing* broadly as a "health care profession that focuses on human life processes and patterns and emphasizes promotion of health for individuals, families, groups, and society as a whole" (Roy & Andrews, 1999, p. 4). Specifically, Roy defines nursing according to her model as the science and practice that expands adaptive abilities and enhances person and environmental transformation. She identifies nursing activities as the assessment of behavior and the stimuli that influence adaptation. Nursing judgments are based on this assessment, and interventions are planned to manage the stimuli (Roy & Andrews, 1999). Roy differentiates nursing as a science from nursing as a practice discipline. Nursing science is "a developing system of knowledge about persons that observes, classifies, and relates the processes by which persons positively affect their health status" (Roy, 1984, pp. 3-4). Nursing as a practice discipline is "nursing's scientific body of knowledge used for the purpose of providing an essential service to people, that is, promoting ability to affect health positively" (Roy, 1984, pp. 3-4). "Nursing acts to enhance the interaction of the person with the environment—to promote adaptation" (Andrews & Roy, 1991, p. 20).

Roy's goal of nursing is "the promotion of adaptation for individuals and groups in each of the four adaptive modes, thus contributing to health, quality of life, and dying with dignity" (Roy & Andrews, 1999, p. 19). Nursing fills a unique role as a facilitator of adaptation by assessing behavior in each of these four adaptive modes and factors influencing adaptation and by intervening to promote adaptive abilities and to enhance environment interactions (Roy & Andrews, 1999).

Person

According to Roy, humans are holistic, adaptive systems. "As an adaptive system, the human system is described as a whole with parts that function as unity for some purpose. Human systems include people as individuals or in groups, including families, organizations, communities, and society as a whole" (Roy & Andrews, 1999, p. 31). Despite their great diversity, all persons are united in a common destiny (Roy & Andrews, 1999). "Human systems have thinking and feeling capacities, rooted in consciousness and meaning, by which they adjust effectively to changes in the environment and, in turn, affect the environment" (Roy & Andrews, 1999, p. 36). Persons and the earth have common patterns and mutuality of relations and meaning (Roy & Andrews, 1999). Roy (Roy & Andrews, 1999) defined the person as the main focus of nursing, the recipient of nursing care, a living, complex, adaptive system with internal processes (cognator and regulator) acting to maintain adaptation in the four adaptive modes (physiological, self-concept, role function, and interdependence).

Health

"Health is a state and a process of being and becoming integrated and a whole person. It is a reflection of adaptation, that is, the interaction of the person and the environment" (Andrews & Roy, 1991, p. 21). Roy (1984) derived this definition from the thought that adaptation is a process of promoting physiological, psychological, and social integrity, and that integrity implies an unimpaired condition leading to completeness or unity. In her earlier work, Roy viewed health along a continuum flowing from death and extreme poor health to high-level and peak wellness (Brower & Baker, 1976). During the late 1990s, Roy's writings focused more on health as a process in which health and illness can coexist (Roy & Andrews, 1999). Drawing on the writings of Illich (1974, 1976), Roy wrote, "health is not freedom from the inevitability of death, disease, unhappiness, and stress, but the ability to cope with them in a competent way" (Roy & Andrews, 1999, p. 52).

Health and illness is one inevitable, coexistent dimension of the person's total life experience (Riehl & Roy, 1980). Nursing is concerned with this dimension. When mechanisms for coping are ineffective, illness results. Health ensues when humans continually adapt. As people adapt to stimuli, they are free to respond to other stimuli. The freeing of energy from ineffective coping attempts can promote healing and enhance health (Roy, 1984).

Environment

According to Roy, environment is "all the conditions, circumstances, and influences surrounding and affecting the development and behavior of persons or groups, with particular consideration of the mutuality of person and earth resources that includes focal, contextual, and residual stimuli" (Roy & Andrews, 1999, p. 81). "It is the changing environment [that] stimulates the person to make adaptive responses" (Andrews & Roy, 1991, p. 18). Environment is the input into the person as an adaptive system involving both internal and external factors. These factors may be slight or large, negative or positive. However, any environmental change demands increasing energy to adapt to the situation. Factors in the environment that affect the person are categorized as focal, contextual, and residual stimuli.

THEORETICAL ASSERTIONS

Roy's model focuses on the concept of adaptation of the person. Her concepts of nursing, person, health, and environment are all interrelated to this central concept. The person continually experiences environmental stimuli. Ultimately, a response is made and adaptation occurs. That response may be either an adaptive or an ineffective response. Adaptive responses promote integrity and help the person to achieve the goals of adaptation, that is, they achieve survival, growth, reproduction, mastery, and person and environmental transformations. Ineffective responses fail to achieve or threaten the goals of adaptation. Nursing has a unique goal to assist the person's adaptation effort by managing the environment. The result is attainment of an optimal level of wellness by the person (Andrews & Roy, 1986; Randell, Tedrow, & Van Landingham, 1982; Roy, 1970, 1971, 1980, 1984; Roy & Roberts, 1981).

As an open living system, the person receives inputs or stimuli from both the environment and the self. The adaptation level is determined by the combined effect of focal, contextual, and residual stimuli. Adaptation occurs when the person responds positively to environmental changes. This adaptive response promotes the integrity of the person, which leads to health. Ineffective responses to stimuli lead to disruption of the integrity of the person (Andrews & Roy, 1986; Randell et al., 1982; Roy, 1970, 1971, 1980; Roy & McLeod, 1981).

There are two interrelated subsystems in Roy's model (Figure 17-1). The primary, functional, or control processes subsystem consists of the regulator and the cognator. The secondary, effector subsystem consists of the following four adaptive modes: (1) physiological needs, (2) self-concept, (3) role function, and (4) interdependence (Andrews & Roy, 1986; Limandri, 1986; Mastal, Hammond, & Roberts, 1982; Meleis, 1985, 2007; Riehl & Roy, 1980; Roy, 1971, 1975).

Roy views the regulator and the cognator as methods of coping. The regulator coping subsystem, by way of the physiological adaptive mode, "responds automatically through neural, chemical, and endocrine coping processes" (Andrews & Roy, 1991, p. 14). The cognator coping subsystem, by way of the self-concept, interdependence, and role function adaptive modes, "responds through four cognitive-emotive channels: perceptual information processing, learning, judgment, and emotion" (Andrews & Roy, 1991,

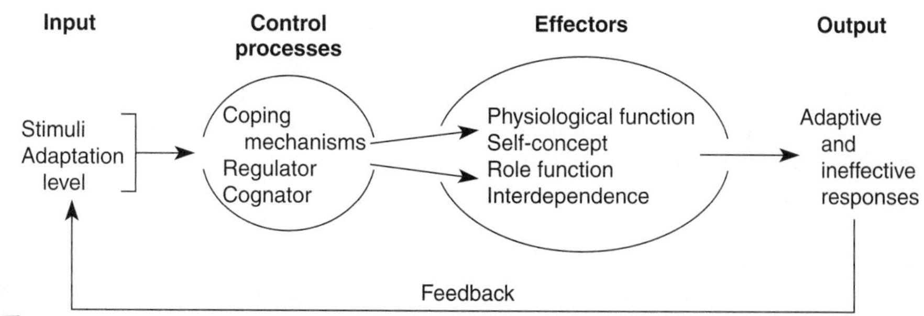

Figure 17-1 Person as an adaptive system. (From Roy, C. [1984]. *Introduction to nursing: An adaptation model* [2nd ed., p. 30]. Englewood Cliffs, NJ: Prentice Hall.)

p. 14). Perception is the interpretation of a stimulus, and perception links the regulator with the cognator in that "input into the regulator is transformed into perceptions. Perception is a process of the cognator. The responses following perception are feedback into both the cognator and the regulator" (Galligan, 1979, p. 67).

The four adaptive modes of the two subsystems in Roy's model provide form or manifestations of cognator and regulator activity. Responses to stimuli are carried out through four adaptive modes. The physiological-physical adaptive mode is concerned with the way humans interact with the environment through physiological processes to meet the basic needs of oxygenation, nutrition, elimination, activity and rest, and protection. The self-concept group identity adaptive mode is concerned with the need to know who one is and how to act in society. An individual's self-concept is defined by Roy as "the composite of beliefs or feelings that an individual holds about him- or herself at any given time" (Roy & Andrews, 1999, p. 49). An individual's self-concept is comprised of the physical self (body sensation and body image) and the personal self (self-consistency, self-ideal, and moral-ethical-spiritual self). The role function adaptive mode describes the primary, secondary, and tertiary roles that an individual performs in society. A role describes the expectations about how one person behaves toward another person. The interdependence adaptive mode describes the interactions of people in society. The major task of the interdependence adaptive mode is for persons to give and receive love, respect, and value. The most important components of the interdependence adaptive mode are a person's significant other (spouse, child, friend, or God) and his or her social support system. The purpose of the four adaptive modes is to achieve physiological, psychological, and social integrity. The four adaptive modes are interrelated through perception (Roy & Andrews, 1999) (Figure 17-2).

The person as a whole is made up of six subsystems. These subsystems (the regulator, the cognator, and the four adaptive modes) are interrelated to form a complex system for the purpose of adaptation.

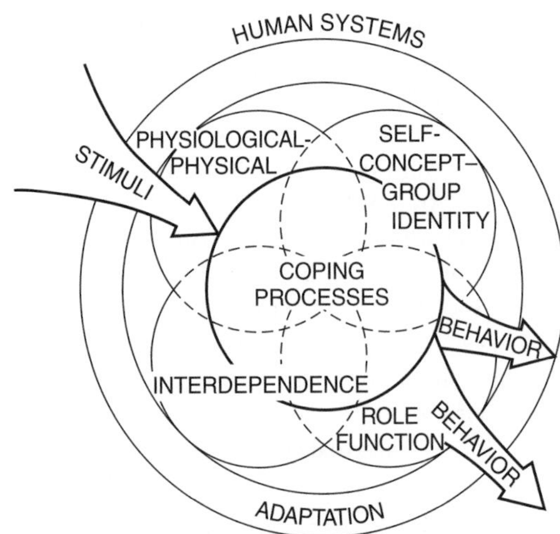

Figure 17-2 Diagrammatic representation of human adaptive systems. (From Roy, C., & Andrews, H. [1999]. *The Roy adaptation model* [2nd ed.]. Upper River Saddle, NJ: Pearson Education, Inc.)

Relationships among the four adaptive modes occur when internal and external stimuli affect more than one mode, when disruptive behavior occurs in more than one mode, or when one mode becomes the focal, contextual, or residual stimulus for another mode (Brower & Baker, 1976; Chinn & Kramer, 2008; Mastal & Hammond, 1980).

With regard to human social systems, Roy broadly categorizes the control processes into the stabilizer and innovator subsystems. The stabilizer subsystem is analogous to the regulator subsystem of the individual and is concerned with stability. To maintain the system, the stabilizer subsystem involves organizational structure, cultural values, and regulation of daily activities of the system. The innovator subsystem is associated with the cognator subsystem of the individual and is concerned with creativity, change, and growth (Roy & Andrews, 1999).

LOGICAL FORM

The Roy Adaptation Model of nursing is both deductive and inductive. It is deductive in that much of Roy's theory is derived from Helson's psychophysics theory. Helson developed the concepts of focal, contextual, and residual stimuli, which Roy (1971) redefined within nursing to form a typology of factors related to adaptation levels of persons. Roy also uses other concepts and theory outside the discipline of nursing and synthesizes these within her adaptation theory.

Roy's adaptation theory is inductive in that she developed the four adaptive modes from research and nursing practice experiences of herself, her colleagues, and her students. Roy built on the conceptual framework of adaptation and developed a step-by-step model by which nurses use the nursing process to administer nursing care to promote adaptation in situations of health and illness (Roy, 1976a, 1980, 1984).

ACCEPTANCE BY THE NURSING COMMUNITY

Practice

The Roy Adaptation Model is deeply rooted in nursing practice, and this, in part, contributes to its continued success (Fawcett, 2002). It remains one of the most frequently used conceptual frameworks to guide nursing practice, and it is used nationally and internationally (Roy & Andrews, 1999; Fawcett, 2005).

Roy's model is useful for nursing practice, because it outlines the features of the discipline and provides direction for practice, education, and research. The model considers goals, values, the patient, and practitioner interventions. Roy's nursing process is well developed. The two-level assessment assists in identification of nursing goals and diagnoses (Brower & Baker, 1976).

Early on, it was recognized as a valuable theory for nursing practice because of the goal that specified its aim for activity and a prescription for activities to realize the goal (Dickoff, James, & Wiedenbach, 1968a, 1968b). The goal of nursing and of the model is adaptation in four adaptive modes in a person's health and illness. The prescriptive interventions are when the nurse manages stimuli by removing, increasing, decreasing, or altering them. These prescriptions may be found in the list of practice-related hypotheses generated by the model (Roy, 1984).

When using Roy's six-step nursing process, the nurse performs the following six functions:

1. Assesses the behaviors manifested from the four adaptive modes
2. Assesses the stimuli for those behaviors and categorizes them as focal, contextual, or residual stimuli
3. Makes a statement or nursing diagnosis of the person's adaptive state
4. Sets goals to promote adaptation
5. Implements interventions aimed at managing the stimuli to promote adaptation
6. Evaluates whether the adaptive goals have been met

By manipulating the stimuli and not the patient, the nurse enhances "the interaction of the person with their environment, thereby promoting health" (Andrews & Roy, 1986, p. 51). The nursing process is well suited for use in a practice setting. The two-level assessment is unique to this model and leads to the identification of adaptation problems or nursing diagnoses.

Roy and colleagues have developed a typology of nursing diagnoses from the perspective of the Roy Adaptation Model (Roy, 1984; Roy & Roberts, 1981). In this typology, commonly recurring problems have been related to the basic needs of the four adaptive modes (Andrews & Roy, 1991).

Intervention is based specifically on the model, but there is a need to develop an organization of categories of nursing interventions (Roy & Roberts, 1981). Nurses provide interventions that alter, increase, decrease, remove, or maintain stimuli (Roy & Andrews, 1999). The nursing judgment model outlined by McDonald and Harms (1966) is recommended by Roy to guide selection of the best intervention for modifying a particular stimulus. According to this model, a number of alternative interventions are generated that may be appropriate for modifying the stimulus. Each possible intervention is judged for the expected consequences of modifying a stimulus, the probability that a consequence will occur (high, moderate, or low), and the value of the change (desirable or undesirable).

Senesac (2003) reviewed the literature for evidence that the Roy Adaptation Model is being implemented in nursing practice. She reported that the

Roy Adaptation Model has been used to the greatest extent by individual nurses to understand, plan, and direct nursing practice in the care of individual patients. Although fewer examples of implementation of the adaptation model are found in institutional practice settings, such examples do exist. She concluded that if the model is to be implemented successfully as a practice philosophy, it should be reflected in the mission and vision statements of the institution, recruitment tools, assessment tools, nursing care plans, and other documents related to patient care.

The Roy Adaptation Model is useful in guiding nursing practice in institutional settings. It has been implemented in a neonatal intensive care unit, an acute surgical ward, a rehabilitation unit, two general hospital units, an orthopedic hospital, a neurosurgical unit, and a 145-bed hospital, among others (Roy & Andrews, 1999).

DeVillers (1998) demonstrated the way in which clinical nurse specialists could use the Roy Adaptation Model to help delineate their roles as expert practitioners in the obstetrical and gynecological setting. She applied Roy's steps of the nursing process and gave specific examples of expert care from each of the adaptive modes.

The Roy Adaptation Model has been applied to the nursing care of individual groups of patients. Examples of the wide range of applications of the Roy Adaptation Model are found in the literature. Villareal (2003) applied the Roy Adaptation Model to the care of young women who were contemplating smoking cessation. The author provides a comprehensive discussion of the use of Roy's six-step nursing process to guide nursing care for young women in their mid-20s who smoked and were members of a closed support group. The researcher performed a two-level assessment. In the first level, stimuli were identified for each of the four adaptive modes. In the second level, the nurse made a judgment about the focal (nicotine addiction), contextual (belief that smoking is enjoyable, makes them feel good, relaxes them, brings them a sense of comfort, and is part of their routine), and residual stimuli (beliefs and attitudes about their body image and that smoking cessation causes weight gain). The nurse made the nursing diagnosis that for this group, a lack of motivation to quit smoking was related to dependency. The women in the support group and the nurse mutually established short-term goals to change behaviors, rather than the long-term goal of smoking cessation. The intervention focused on discussion of the effects of smoking on the body, reasons and beliefs about smoking and smoking cessation, stress management, nutrition, physical activity, and self-esteem. During the evaluation phase, it was determined that the women had moved from pre-contemplation to the contemplation phase of smoking cessation. The author concluded that the Roy Adaptation Model provided a useful framework for providing care to women who smoke.

Samarel, Tulman, and Fawcett (2002) examined the effects of two types of social support (telephone and group social support) and education on adaptation to early-stage breast cancer in a sample of 125 women. Women in the experimental group received both types of social support and education ($n = 34$), while women in the first control group received only telephone support and education, and women in the second control group received only education. Mood disturbance and loneliness were reduced significantly for the experimental group and for the first control group but were not reduced for the second control group. No differences were observed among the groups in terms of cancer-related worry or well-being. This study provides an excellent example of how the Roy Adaptation Model can be used to guide the conceptualization, literature review, theory construction, and development of an intervention.

Samarel and colleagues (1999) developed a resource kit for women with breast cancer. The contents of this kit were derived from the Roy Adaptation Model. The kit contains *The Resource Manual for Women with Breast Cancer,* which collects pertinent information into one source. The manual is divided into eight chapters that are theoretically based on the four adaptive modes. It contains a variety of practice activities to reinforce the information contained in the chapters. The kit contains pamphlets, audiotapes, and videotapes that supplement the narrative in the manual.

Newman (1997a) applied the Roy Adaptation Model to caregivers of chronically ill family members.

With a thorough review of the literature, Newman demonstrated how the Roy Adaptation Model was used to provide care for this population. Newman views the chronically ill family member as the focal stimulus. Contextual stimuli include the caregiver's age, gender, and relationship to the chronically ill family member. The caregiver's physical health status is a manifestation of the physiological adaptive mode. The caregiver's emotional responses to caregiving (shock, fear, anger, guilt, increased anxiety) are effective or ineffective responses of the self-concept mode. Relationships with significant others and support indicate adaptive responses in the interdependence mode. Caregivers' primary, secondary, and tertiary roles are strained by the addition of the caregiving role. Practice and research implications illuminate the applicability of the Roy Adaptation Model for providing care to caregivers of chronically ill family members.

The Roy Adaptation Model has been applied to the care of persons with chronic renal failure who require hemodialysis (Keen et al., 1998), women in menopause (Cunningham, 2002), and to the assessment of an elderly man undergoing a right, below-the-knee amputation. The Roy Adaptation Model has been applied to the care of adolescents with asthma (Hennessy-Harstad, 1999) and inflammatory bowel disease (Decker, 2000) and a 10-month-old child with tracheomalacia (Lankester & Sheldon, 1999). Cook (1999) delineates nursing assessment related to the self-concept of patients with cancer and provides specific interventions to promote adaptation in this group of patients.

Araich (2001) uses a case study to illustrate how theory can be integrated into a cardiac care unit. In this effort, Araich conducts a two-level assessment and describes possible nursing interventions to promote adaptation of persons in cardiac care. Dixon (1999) demonstrates how the Roy Adaptation Model guides community health nursing practice.

Education

The Roy Adaptation Model defines the distinct purpose of nursing for students, which is to promote the adaptation of persons in each of the adaptive modes in situations of health and illness. This model distinguishes nursing science from medical science by having the content of these areas taught in separate courses. She stresses collaboration but delineates separate goals for nurses and physicians. According to Roy (1971), it is the nurse's goal to help the patient put his or her energy into getting well, whereas the medical student focuses on the patient's position on the health-illness continuum with the goal of causing movement along the continuum. She views the model as a valuable tool for analyzing the distinctions between the two professions of nursing and medicine. Roy (1979) believes that curricula based on this model support understanding of theory development by students as they learn about testing theories and experience theoretical insights. Roy (1971, 1979) noted early on that the model clarified objectives, identified content, and specified patterns for teaching and learning.

The adaptation model has been useful in the educational setting and has guided nursing education at Mount Saint Mary's College Department of Nursing in Los Angeles since 1970. As early as 1987, more than 100,000 student nurses had been educated in nursing programs based on the Roy Adaptation Model in the United States and abroad. The Roy Adaptation Model provides educators with a systematic way of teaching students to assess and care for patients within the context of their lives rather than just as victims of illness.

Dobratz (2003) evaluated the learning outcomes of a nursing research course designed from the perspective of the Roy Adaptation Model and described in detail how to teach the theoretical content to students in a senior nursing research course. The evaluation tool was a Likert-type scale that contained seven statements. Students were asked to disagree, agree, or strongly agree with seven statements. Four open-ended questions were included to elicit information from students about the most helpful learning activity, the least helpful learning activity, methods used by the instructor that enhanced learning and grasp of research, and what the instructor could have done to increase learning. The researcher concluded that a research course based on the Roy Adaptation Model helped students put the pieces of the research puzzle together.

Research

If research is to affect practitioners' behaviors, it must be directed toward testing and retesting theories derived from conceptual models for nursing practice. Roy (1984) has stated that theory development and the testing of developed theories are the highest priorities for nursing. The model continues to generate many testable hypotheses to be researched.

Roy's theory has generated a number of general propositions. From these general propositions, specific hypotheses can be developed and tested. Hill and Roberts (1981) have demonstrated the development of testable hypotheses from the model, as has Roy. Data to validate or support the model are created by the testing of such hypotheses; the model continues to generate more of this type of research. The Roy Adaptation Model has been used extensively to guide knowledge development through nursing research (Frederickson, 2000).

Roy (1970) has identified a set of concepts that form a model from which the process of observation and classification of facts would lead to postulates. These postulates concern the occurrence of adaptation problems, coping mechanisms, and interventions based on laws derived from factors that make up the response potential of focal, contextual, and residual stimuli. Roy and colleagues have outlined a typology of adaptation problems or nursing diagnoses (Roy, 1973, 1975, 1976b). Research and testing continue in the areas of typology and categories of interventions that have been derived from the model. General propositions also have been developed and tested (Roy & McLeod, 1981).

Practice-Based Research

DiMattio and Tulman (2003) described changes in functional status and correlates of functional status of 61 women during the 6-week postoperative period following a coronary artery bypass graft. Functional status was measured at 2, 4, and 6 weeks after surgery, using the Inventory of Functional Status in the Elderly and the Sickness Impact Profile. Significant increases were found in all dimensions of functional status except personal at the three measurement points. The greatest increases in functional status occurred at between 2 and 4 weeks after surgery. However, none of the dimensions of functional status had returned to baseline values at the 6-week point. This information will help women who have undergone coronary artery bypass graft surgery to better understand the recovery period and to set more realistic goals.

Young-McCaughan and colleagues (2003) studied the effects of a structured aerobic exercise program on exercise tolerance, sleep patterns, and quality of life in patients with cancer from the perspective of the Roy Adaptation Model. Subjects exercised for 20 minutes, twice a week, for 12 weeks. Significant improvements in exercise tolerance, subjective sleep quality, and psychological and physiological quality of life were demonstrated.

Yeh (2002) tested the Roy Adaptation Model in a sample of 116 Taiwanese boys and girls with cancer (7 to 18 years of age at the time of diagnosis). Two Roy propositions were tested. The first proposition is that environmental stimuli (severity of illness, age, gender, understanding of illness, and communication with others) influence biopsychosocial responses (health-related quality of life [HRQOL]). The second proposition is that the four adaptive modes are interrelated. Using structural equation modeling, the researcher found that severity of illness provided an excellent fit with stage of illness, laboratory values (white blood cell count, hemoglobin, platelets, absolute neutrophil count), and the total number of hospitalizations. Although it is not altogether clear how the focal and contextual stimuli were defined, this study showed that environmental stimuli (severity of illness, age, gender, understanding of illness, and communication with others) influence the biopsychosocial adaptive responses of children to cancer. Finally, this study demonstrated the interrelatedness of the physiological (physical HRQOL), self-concept (disease and symptoms HRQOL), interdependence (social HRQOL), and role function (cognitive HRQOL) adaptive modes.

Woods and Isenberg (2001) provide an example of theory synthesis. In their study of intimate abuse and traumatic stress in battered women, they developed a middle range theory by synthesizing the Roy Adaptation Model with the current literature reporting on intimate abuse and post-traumatic stress disorder. A predictive correlational model was used to examine adaptation as a mediator of intimate abuse and post-traumatic stress disorder. The focal stimulus of this study was the severity of intimate abuse, emotional abuse, and risk of homicide by an intimate partner. Adaptation was operationalized within the four adaptive modes and was tested as a mediator between intimate abuse and post-traumatic stress disorder. Direct relationships were reported between the focal stimulus and intimate abuse, and adaptation in each of the four modes mediated relationships between the focal stimulus and traumatic stress.

Chiou (2000) conducted a meta-analysis of the interrelationships among Roy's four adaptive modes. Using well-defined inclusion and exclusion criteria, a literature search of the *Cumulative Index to Nursing and Allied Health Literature* yielded eight research reports with diverse samples. One in-press report was included. Convenience samples for the nine studies included only adults, and some were elderly. The meta-analysis revealed small to medium correlations between each two mode set and a nonsignificant association between the interdependence and physiological modes. Zhan (2000) found support for Roy's proposition about cognitive adaptive processes in relation to maintaining self-consistency. Using Roy's Cognitive Adaptation Processing Scale (Roy & Zhan, 2001) to measure cognitive adaptation and the Self-Consistency Scale (Zhan & Shen, 1994), Zhan found that cognitive adaptation plays an important role in helping older adults maintain self-consistency in the face of hearing loss. Self-consistency was higher for hearing impaired men than for hearing impaired women, but it did not vary for age, educational level, race, marital status, or income.

Nuamah, Cooley, Fawcett, and McCorkle (1999) studied quality of life in 515 patients with cancer. These researchers clearly established theoretical linkages among the concepts of the Roy Adaptation Model, middle range theory concepts, and empirical indicators. Focal and contextual stimuli were identified. Variables in each of the adaptive modes were operationalized. Using structural equation modeling, the researchers found that two of the environmental stimuli (adjuvant cancer treatment and severity of the disease) explained 59% of the variance in biopsychosocial indicators of the latent variable health-related quality of life. Their findings supported the proposition of the Roy Adaptation Model that environmental stimuli influence biopsychosocial responses.

Samarel and colleagues (1999) used the Roy Adaptation Model to study women's perceptions of adaptation to breast cancer in a sample of 70 women who were participating in an experimental support and education group. The experimental group received coaching; the control group received no coaching. Using quantitative content analysis of structured telephone interviews, the researchers found that 51 of 70 women (72.9%) experienced a positive change toward their breast cancer over the study period, which was indicative of adaptation to the breast cancer. The researchers report qualitative indicators of adaptation for each of Roy's four adaptive modes.

Modrcin-Talbott and colleagues studied self-esteem from the perspective of the Roy Adaptation Model in 140 well adolescents (Modrcin-Talbott, Pullen, Ehrenberger, Zandstra, & Muenchen, 1998b) and 77 adolescents in an outpatient mental health setting (Modrcin-Talbott, Pullen, Zandstra, Ehrenberger, & Muenchen, 1998a). Well adolescents were grouped in terms of early (12 to 14 years), middle (15 to 16 years), or late adolescence (17 to 19 years). Well adolescents were recruited conveniently from a large, southeastern church. Self-esteem in well adolescents did not differ by age group, gender, or whether or not they smoked tobacco. Well adolescents who exercised regularly did score higher on self-esteem. Significant negative relationships were found between self-esteem and depression, state anger, trait anger, anger-in, anger-out, anger control, and anger expression. In the second study, adolescents were sampled from participants of regularly scheduled group sessions as part of an outpatient psychiatric treatment program. Self-esteem significantly differed by age group, with older adolescents scoring lowest on self-esteem. Self-esteem did not differ by gender or whether or not they smoked tobacco. A significant negative relationship was observed between self-esteem and depression. Unlike their study in well adolescents, no statistically significant relationship was found between self-esteem and the dimensions of anger. Self-esteem was not significantly related to parental alcohol use in either group.

Modrcin-Talbott, Harrison, Groer, and Younger (2003) tested the effects of gentle human touch on the biobehavioral adaptation of preterm infants based on the Roy Adaptation Model. According to Roy, infants are born with two adaptive modes: the physiological and interdependence modes. Premature infants often are deprived of human touch, and an environment filled with machines, noxious stimuli, and invasive procedures surrounds them. These researchers found that gentle human touch (focal stimulus) promotes physiological adaptation for premature infants. Heart rate, oxygen saturation stability, increased quiet sleep, less active sleep and drowsiness, decreased motor activity, increased time not moving, and decreased behavioral distress cues were identified as effective responses in the physiological adaptive mode. This study supports Roy's conceptualization of adaptation in infants.

Gallagher (1998) conducted a pilot study to discern if a relationship exists between urogenital distress and the psychosocial impact of urinary incontinence in 17 elderly women. The researcher found significant relationships between urogenital distress and physical activity, social relationships, and travel, which are dimensions of the psychosocial impact of urinary incontinence. Although findings are inconclusive because of a small sample size, the study was framed well in the Roy Adaptation Model and provided important information for future studies.

The University of Montreal Research Team in Nursing Science (Ducharme, Ricard, Duquette, Levesque, & Lachance, 1998; Levesque, Ricard, Ducharme, Duquette, & Bonin, 1998) is studying adaptation to a variety of environmental stimuli. Four groups of individuals were included in their studies as follows: (1) informal family caregivers of a demented relative at home, (2) informal family caregivers of a psychiatrically ill relative at home, (3) nurses as professional caregivers in geriatric institutions, and (4) aged spouses in the community. Using linear structural relations (LISREL), perceived stress (focal stimulus), social support (contextual stimulus), and passive and avoidance coping (coping mechanism) were directly or indirectly linked to psychological distress. This finding supports Roy's proposition that coping promotes adaptation.

Bournaki (1997) studied pain-related responses to venipuncture in school-age children from the perspective of the Roy Adaptation Model. Based on Roy's assumption that "adaptive behavior is a function of the stimulus and adaptation level, that is, the pooled effects of the focal, contextual, and residual stimuli" (Roy & Corliss, 1993, p. 217), Bournaki tested the hypothesis that age, gender, past painful experiences, temperament, medical fears, general fears, and childrearing practices are related to pain location, pain intensity, pain quality, observed behaviors, and heart rate. Findings of this study provided partial support for Roy's proposition that focal and contextual stimuli influence adaptive responses. In this study, pain related to venipuncture was the focal stimulus, and age, gender, past painful experiences, temperament, medical fears, general fears, and childrearing practices were contextual stimuli. Canonical correlation revealed that age (developmental stage), medical fears (self-concept), and two dimensions of temperament—distractibility and threshold (parent-child interdependence)—were related to pain quality, behavioral responses, and heart rate responses. Gender was related to behavioral responses, in that girls cried more often than boys.

Development of Adaptation Research Instruments

The Roy Adaptation Model has provided the theoretical basis for the development of a number of research instruments. Newman (1997b) developed the Inventory of Functional Status–Caregiver of a Child in a Body Cast to measure the extent to which parental caregivers continue their usual activities while a child is in a body cast. Reliability testing indicates that the subscales for household, social, and community childcare of the child in a body cast, childcare of other children, and personal care (rather than the total score) are reliable measures of these constructs. Modrcin-McCarthy, McCue, and Walker (1997) used the Roy Adaptation Model to develop a clinical tool that may be used to identify actual and potential stressors of fragile premature infants and to implement care for them. This tool measures signs of stress, touch interventions, reduction of pain, environmental considerations, state, and stability (STRESS).

Development of Middle Range Theories of Adaptation

Silva (1986) pointed out early on that merely using a conceptual framework to structure a research study is not theory testing. Many researchers have used Roy's model but did not actually test propositions or hypotheses of her model. They have provided face validity of its usefulness as a framework to guide their studies. How theory derives from a conceptual framework must be made explicit; therefore, development and testing of middle range theories derived from the Roy Adaptation Model are needed. Some research of this nature has been conducted with the model, but more is needed for further validation and development of new areas. The model does generate many testable hypotheses related to both practice and nursing theory. The success of a conceptual framework is evaluated, in part, by the number and quality of middle range theories it generates. The Roy Adaptation Model has been the theoretical source of a number of middle range theories. The utility of those theories in practice sustains the life of the model.

Dunn (2004) reports the use of theoretical substruction to derive a middle range theory of adaptation for chronic pain from the Roy Adaptation Model. In Dunn's model of adaptation to chronic pain, pain intensity is specified as the focal stimulus. Contextual stimuli include age, race, and gender. Religious and nonreligious coping are functions of the cognator subsystem. Manifestations of adaptation to chronic pain are its effects on functional ability and psychological and spiritual well-being.

Frame, Kelly, and Bayley (2003) developed the Frame theory of adolescent empowerment by synthesizing the Roy Adaptation Model, Murrell-Armstrong's empowerment matrix, and Harter's developmental perspective. The theory of adolescent empowerment was tested using a quasi-experimental design in which children diagnosed with attention deficit-hyperactivity disorder (ADHD) were randomly assigned to a treatment or a control group. Ninety-two fifth and sixth grade students were assigned to the treatment or the control group. Children in the treatment group attended an eight-session, school nurse–led support group intervention (twice weekly for 4 weeks). The treatment was designed to teach the children about ADHD, the gifts of having ADHD, powerlessness versus empowerment, empowerment with one's feelings, teachers, family, and classmates, and how to learn to relax. Children in the control group received no intervention. Using analysis of covariance, children in the treatment group reported significantly higher perceived social acceptance, perceived athletic competence, perceived physical appearance, and perceived global self-worth.

Jirovec, Jenkins, Isenberg, and Baiardi (1999) have proposed a middle range urine control theory derived from the Roy Adaptation Model, intended to explicate the phenomenon of urine control and to decrease urinary incontinence. According to the theory of urine control, the focal stimulus for urine control is bladder distention. Contextual stimuli include accessible facilities and mobility skills. A residual stimulus is the intense socialization about bladder and sanitary habits that begin in childhood. This theory takes into account physiological coping mechanisms, regulator (spinal reflex mediated by S2 to S4, and coordinated detrusor muscle contraction and sphincter relaxation) and cognator (perception, learning judgment, and awareness of urgency or dribbling). Adaptive responses to prevent urinary incontinence are described for the four adaptive modes. Effective adaptation is defined as continence, and ineffective adaptation is defined as incontinence. The authors provide limited support for the theory of urine control through case studies. The theory of urine control illuminates the complexity, multidimensionality, and holistic nature of adaptation.

Researchers at the University of Montreal have proposed a middle range theory of adaptation to caregiving that is based on the Roy Adaptation Model. This middle range theory has been tested in a number of published studies of informal caregivers of demented relatives at home, informal caregivers of psychiatrically ill relatives at home, professional caregivers of elderly institutionalized patients, and aged spouses in the community. Perceived stress is conceptualized as the focal stimulus. Contextual stimuli include gender, conflicts, and social support. Coping mechanisms include active, passive, and avoidant coping strategies. In this middle range theory, the adaptive (nonadaptive) response (psychological distress) is manifested in the self-concept mode. LISREL analyses have provided support for many of the propositions of this middle range theory of adaptation to caregiving and for the Roy Adaptation Model (Ducharme et al., 1998; Levesque et al., 1998).

Tsai, Tak, Moore, and Palencia (2003) derived a middle range theory of pain from the Roy Adaptation Model. In the theory of chronic pain, chronic pain is the focal stimulus, disability and social support are contextual stimuli, and age and gender are residual stimuli. Perceived daily stress is a coping process. Depression is an outcome variable manifested in all four adaptive modes. Path analysis provided partial support for the theory of chronic pain. Greater chronic pain and disability were associated with greater daily stress, and greater social support was associated with less daily stress. These three variables accounted for 35% of the variance in daily stress. Greater daily stress explained 35% of the variance in depression.

Other middle range theories derived from the Roy Adaptation Model have been proposed, but research reports testing these theories were not found at the time of this literature review. Tsai (2003) has proposed a middle range theory of caregiver stress. Whittemore and Roy (2002) developed a middle range theory of adapting to diabetes mellitus using theory synthesis. Based on an analysis of Pollock's (1993) middle range theory of chronic illness and a thorough review of the literature, reconceptualization of the chronic illness model and the addition of concepts such as self-management, integration, and health-within-illness more specifically extend the Roy Adaptation Model to adapting to diabetes mellitus.

FURTHER DEVELOPMENT

The Roy Adaptation Model is an approach to nursing that has made and continues to make a significant contribution to the body of nursing knowledge, but a few areas remain for development of the model. A more thoroughly defined typology of nursing diagnoses and an organization of categories of interventions would facilitate its use in nursing practice. Overlap in the psychosocial categories of self-concept, role function, and interdependence continues to be noted by scientists who do research from the perspective of the Roy Adaptation Model. Roy recently has redefined health, deemphasizing the concept of a health-illness continuum and conceptualizing health as integration and wholeness of the person. This approach more clearly incorporates the adaptive mechanisms of the comatose patient in response to tactile and verbal stimuli. However, because health was not conceptualized in this manner in the earlier work, this opens up a new area for research. Based on her integrative review of the literature, Frederickson (2000) concluded that there is good empirical support for Roy's conceptualization of person and health. She made the following recommendations for future research. First, there is a need to design studies to test propositions related to environment and nursing. Second, interventions based on the concepts and propositions that have been supported previously should be tested.

CRITIQUE

Clarity

The metaparadigm concepts (person, environment, nursing, and health) of the Roy Adaptation Model are clearly defined and consistent. Roy clearly defines the four adaptive modes (physiological, self-concept, interdependence, and role function). A challenge of the model that was identified is Roy's espousal of a holistic view of the person and environment, while the model views adaptation as occurring in four adaptive modes, and person and environment are conceptualized as two separate entities, with one affecting the other (Malinski, 2000). An answer to this challenge is that Roy's adaptation model is holistic, since change in the internal or external environment (stimulus) leads to response (adapts) as a whole. In fact, Roy's perspective is consistent with other holistic theories, such as psychoneuroimmunology and psychoneuroendocrinology. As one example, psychoneuroimmunology is a theory that proposes a bidirectional relationship between the mind and the immune system. Roy's model is broader than psychoneuroimmunology and provides a theoretical foundation for research about, and nursing care of, the person as a whole.

In more recent writings, Roy has acknowledged the holistic nature of persons who live in a universe that is "progressing in structure, organization, and complexity. Rather than a system acting to maintain itself, the emphasis shifts to the purposefulness of human existence in a universe that is creative" (Roy & Andrews, 1999, p. 35).

Roy has written that other disciplines focus on an aspect of the person, and that nursing views the person as a whole (Roy & Andrews, 1999). "Based on the philosophic assumptions of the nursing model, persons are seen as coextensive with their physical and social environments. The nurse takes a values-based stance, focusing on awareness, enlightenment and faith" (Roy & Andrews, 1999, p. 539). Roy contends that persons have mutual, integral, and simultaneous relationships with the universe and God, and that as humans they "use their creative abilities of awareness, enlightenment, and faith in the processes of deriving, sustaining, and transforming the universe" (Roy & Andrews, 1999, p. 35). Using these creative abilities, persons (sick or well) are active participants in their care and are able to achieve a higher level of adaptation (health).

Mastal and Hammond (1980) discussed difficulties with Roy's model in classifying certain behaviors because concept definitions overlapped. The problem dealt with theory conceptualization and the need for mutually exclusive categories to classify human behavior. Conceptualizing a person's position on the health-illness continuum is no longer a problem because Roy redefined health as personal integration. Other researchers have referred to difficulty in classifying behavior exclusively in one adaptive mode (Bradley & Williams, 1990; Limandri, 1986; Nyqvist & Sjoden, 1993; Silva, 1987). However, this observation supports Roy's proposition that behavior in one adaptive mode affects and is affected by the other modes.

Simplicity

The Roy model includes the concepts of nursing, person, health-illness, environment, adaptation, and nursing activities. It also includes two subconcepts (regulator and cognator) and four modes (physiological, self-concept, role function, and interdependence). This model has several major concepts and subconcepts, so the relational statements are complex until the model is learned.

Generality

The Roy Adaptation Model's broad scope is an advantage, because it may be used for theory building and for deriving middle range theories for testing in studies of smaller ranges of phenomena (Reynolds, 1971). Roy's model (Roy & Corliss, 1993) is generalizable to all settings in nursing practice but is limited in scope, as it primarily addresses the person-environment adaptation of the patient, and information about the nurse is implied.

Empirical Precision

Roy's broad concepts stem from theory in physiological psychology, psychology, sociology, and nursing; empirical data indicate that this general theory base has substance. Roy's model offers direction for researchers who want to incorporate physiological phenomena in their studies. Roy (1980) studied and analyzed 500 samples of patient behaviors collected by nursing students. From this analysis, Roy proposed her four adaptive modes in humans.

Roy (Roy & McLeod, 1981; Roy & Roberts, 1981) has identified many propositions in relation to the regulator and cognator mechanisms and the self-concept, role function, and interdependence modes. These propositions have received varying degrees of support from general theory and empirical data. Most of the propositions are relational statements and can be tested (Tiedeman, 1983). Over the years, many testable hypotheses have been derived from the model (Hill & Roberts, 1981).

The greatest need to increase the empirical precision of the Roy Adaptation Model is for researchers to develop middle range theory based on the Roy Adaptation Model with empirical referents specifically designed to measure concepts proposed in the derived theory. Roy has explicated a significant number of propositions, theorems, and axioms to serve in the development of middle range theory. The holistic nature of the model serves nurse researchers who are interested in the complex nature of physiological and psychosocial adaptive processes.

Derivable Consequences

The Roy Adaptation Model has a clearly defined nursing process and can be useful in guiding clinical practice. This model provides direction for providing nursing care that addresses the holistic needs of the patient. The model is also capable of generating new information through the testing of hypotheses that have been derived from it (Roy & Corliss, 1993; Smith, Garvis, & Martinson, 1983).

SUMMARY

The Roy Adaptation Model has greatly influenced the profession of nursing. It is one of the most frequently used models to guide nursing research, education, and practice. The model is taught as part of the curriculum of most baccalaureate, master's, and doctoral programs of nursing. The influence of the Roy Adaptation Model on nursing research is evidenced by the vast number of qualitative and quantitative research studies it has guided. The Roy Adaptation Model has inspired the development of many middle range nursing theories and the development of adaptation instruments. Sister Callista Roy continues to refine the adaptation model for nursing research, education, and practice.

According to Roy, persons are holistic adaptive systems and the focus of nursing. The internal and external environment consists of all phenomena that surround the human adaptive system and affect their development and behavior. Persons are in constant interaction with the environment and exchange information, matter, and energy, that is, persons affect and are affected by the environment. The environment is the source of stimuli that either threaten or promote a person's existence. For survival, the human adaptive system must respond positively to environmental stimuli. Humans make effective or ineffective adaptive responses to environmental stimuli. Adaptation promotes survival, growth, reproduction, mastery, and transformation of persons and the environment. Roy defines health as a state of becoming an integrated and whole human being.

Three types of environmental stimuli are described in the Roy Adaptation Model. The focal stimulus is that which most immediately confronts the individual and demands the most attention and adaptive energy. Contextual are all other stimuli present in the situation that contribute positively or negatively to the strength of the focal stimulus. Residual stimuli affect the focal stimulus, but their effects are not readily known. These three types of stimuli together form the adaptation level. A person's adaptation level may be integrated, compensatory, or compromised.

Coping mechanisms refer to innate or acquired processes that a person uses to deal with environmental stimuli. Coping mechanisms may be categorized broadly as the regulator or cognator subsystem. The regulator subsystem responds automatically through innate neural, chemical, and endocrine coping processes. The cognator subsystem responds through innate and acquired cognitive-emotive processes that include perceptual and information processing, learning, judgment, and emotion.

Behaviors that manifest adaptation can be observed in four adaptive modes. The physiological mode refers to the person's physical responses to the environment, and the underlying need is physiological integrity. The self-concept mode refers to a person's thoughts, beliefs, or feelings about himself or herself at any given time. The basic need of the self-concept mode is psychic or spiritual integrity. The self-concept is a composite belief about self that is formed from internal perceptions and the perceptions of others. The self-concept mode is comprised of the physical self (body sensation and body image) and the personal self (self-consistency, self-ideal, and the moral-ethical-spiritual self). The role function mode refers to the primary, secondary, and tertiary roles a person performs in society.

The basic need of the role function adaptive mode is social integrity or for one to know how to behave and what is expected of him or her in society. The interdependence adaptive mode refers to relationships among people. The basic need of the interdependence adaptive mode is social integrity or to give and receive love, respect, and value from significant others and social support systems (Table 17-1).

Table 17-1 *Overview of the Adaptive Modes*

Subsystem	Adaptive Mode	Coping Need
REGULATOR Neural Chemical Endocrine	PHYSIOLOGICAL The physiological adaptive mode refers to the way a person, as a physical being, responds to and interacts with the internal and external environment **Basic need:** Physiological integrity	**Oxygenation:** To maintain appropriate oxygenation through ventilation, gas exchange, and gas transport **Nutrition:** To maintain function, to promote growth, and to replace tissue through ingestion and assimilation of food **Elimination:** To excrete metabolic wastes primarily through the intestines and kidney **Activity and rest:** To maintain a balance between physical activity and rest **Protection:** To defend the body against infection, trauma, and temperature changes primarily by way of integumentary structures and innate and acquired immunity **Senses:** To enable persons to interact with their environment by sight, hearing, touch, taste, and smell **Fluid and electrolyte and acid-base balance:** To maintain homeostatic fluid, electrolyte, and acid-base balance to promote cellular, extracellular, and systemic function **Neurological function:** To coordinate and control body movements, consciousness, and cognitive-emotional processes **Endocrine function:** To integrate and coordinate body functions

Continued

Table 17-1 Overview of the Adaptive Modes—cont'd

Subsystem	Adaptive Mode	Coping Need
COGNATOR	SELF-CONCEPT The self-concept adaptive mode refers to the psychological and spiritual characteristics of a person The self-concept consists of the composite of a person's feelings about himself or herself at any given time The self-concept is formed from internal perceptions and the perceptions of others' reactions The self-concept has two major dimensions: the physical self and the personal self **Basic need:** Psychic and spiritual integrity	PHYSICAL SELF **Body sensation:** To maintain a positive feeling about one's physical being (i.e., physical functioning, sexuality, or health) **Body image:** To maintain a positive view of one's physical body and physical appearance PERSONAL SELF **Self-consistency:** To maintain consistent self-organization and to avoid dysequilibrium **Self-ideal or self-expectancy:** To maintain a positive or hopeful view of what one is, what one expects to be, and what one hopes to do **Moral-spiritual-ethical self:** To maintain a positive evaluation of who one is
	INTERDEPENDENCE **Basic need:** Relational integrity or security in nuturing relationships	To maintain close, nurturing relationships with people who are willing to give and receive love, respect, and value
	ROLE FUNCTION **Basic need:** Social integrity	To know who one is and what society's expectations are so that one can act appropriately within society

The goal of nursing is to promote adaptive responses. This is accomplished through a six-step nursing process: assessment of behavior, assessment of stimuli, nursing diagnosis, goal setting, intervention, and evaluation. Nursing interventions focus on managing environmental stimuli by "altering, increasing, decreasing, removing, or maintaining them" (Roy & Andrews, 1999, p. 86).

Meleis (1985) proposed that the focus of nursing theorist works as three types:

1. Those who focus on needs
2. Those who focus on interaction
3. Those who focus on outcome

The Roy Adaptation Model is classified as an outcome theory by Meleis (1985, 2007). Roy, in applying the concepts of system and adaptation to person as the patient of nursing, has presented her articulation of the person for nurses to use as a tool in practice, education, and research. Her conceptions of person and of the nursing process contribute to the science and the art of nursing. The Roy Adaptation Model deserves further study and development by nurse educators, researchers, and practitioners.

Case Study

A 23-year-old male patient is admitted with a fracture of C6 and C7 that has resulted in quadriplegia. He was injured during a football game at the university where he is currently a senior. His career as a quarterback had been very promising. At the time of the injury, contract negotiations were in progress with a leading professional football team.

1. Use Roy's criteria to identify focal and contextual stimuli for each of the four adaptive modes.
2. Consider what adaptations would be necessary in each of the following four adaptive modes: (1) physiological, (2) self-concept, (3) interdependence, and (4) role function.
3. Create an intervention for each of the adaptive modes that will promote adaptation.

CRITICAL THINKING Activities

1. Karen, a recent graduate from a nursing program based on the Roy Adaptation Model, is performing her morning assessments. She enters Mr. Shadeed's room. Mr. Shadeed is awaiting preoperative preparation for a laparotomy to explore an unknown mass. Mr. Shadeed is very irritable this morning. He says that he is thirsty. Karen continues her assessment of Mr. Shadeed. What additional data will she need from each of the four adaptive modes before implementing nursing interventions? What are the focal stimuli, contextual stimuli, and residual stimuli? What is the nursing diagnosis? What are possible interventions? What process can Karen use to select the best nursing intervention?
2. Although it would be easy to assume that Mr. Shadeed's nursing care needs stem from anxiety during the preoperative period, this assumption may or may not be true. Assessment of stimuli in each of the four adaptive modes will enable Karen to assess focal, contextual, and residual stimuli and come to the correct diagnosis. Identify the additional assessment data that Karen will need to collect for each of the following adaptive modes.
   - Physiological adaptive mode
   - Self-concept adaptive mode
   - Role function adaptive mode
   - Interdependence adaptive mode

POINTS FOR Further Study Box

- Roy, C., & Jones, D. (Editors). (2007). *Nursing knowledge development and clinical practice.* New York: Springer.
- Roy, C. (2007). Update from the future: Thinking of theorist Sr. Callista Roy. *Nursing Science Quarterly,* 20(2), 113-116.
- Phillips, K. D. (2006). Roy's adaptation model in nursing practice. In M. R. Alligood, & A. M. Tomey (Eds.), *Nursing theory: Utilization & application* (3rd ed., pp. 307-333). St. Louis: Mosby-Elsevier.
- Sr. Callista Roy. *Portraits of excellence: The nurse theorists video/DVD series,* vol 1. Athens, Ohio: Fitne, Inc.
- Sr. Callista Roy. *Adaptation: Excellence in action video/DVD.* Athens, Ohio: Fitne, Inc.

REFERENCES

Andrews, H. (1991). Overview of the role function mode. In C. Roy & H. Andrews (Eds.), *The Roy adaptation model: The definitive statement* (pp. 347-361). Norwalk, CT: Appleton & Lange.

Andrews, H., & Roy, C. (1986). *Essentials of the Roy adaptation model.* Norwalk, CT: Appleton-Century-Crofts.

Andrews, H., & Roy, C. (1991). Essentials of the Roy adaptation model. In C. Roy & H. Andrews (Eds.), *The Roy adaptation model: The definitive statement* (pp. 3-25). Norwalk, CT: Appleton & Lange.

Araich, M. (2001). Roy's adaptation model: Demonstration of theory integration into process of care in coronary care unit. *ICUs and Nursing Web Journal, 7,* 1-12.

Bournaki, M. C. (1997). Correlates of pain-related responses to venipunctures in school-age children. *Nursing Research, 46,* 147-154.

Bradley, K. M., & Williams, D. M. (1990). A comparison of the preoperative concerns of open heart surgery patients and their significant others. *Journal of Cardiovascular Nursing,* 5, 43-53.

Brower, H. T., & Baker, B. J. (1976). The Roy adaptation model. Using the adaptation model in a practitioner curriculum. *Nursing Outlook, 24,* 686-689.

Chinn, P., & Kramer, M. (2008). *Integrated theory and knowledge development in nursing.* St. Louis: Mosby-Elsevier.

Chiou, C. P. (2000). A meta-analysis of the interrelationships between the modes in Roy's adaptation model. *Nursing Science Quarterly, 13,* 252-258.

Cooley, C. H. (1902). *Human nature and the social order.* New York: Scribner's.

Cook, N. F. (1999). Self-concept and cancer: Understanding the nursing role. *British Journal of Nursing, 8*, 318-324.

Cunningham, D. A. (2002). Application of Roy's adaptation model when caring for a group of women coping with menopause. *Journal of Community Health Nursing, 19*, 49-60.

Davies, P. (1988). *The cosmic blueprint.* New York: Simon & Schuster.

De Chardin, P. T. (1959). *The phenomenon of man.* New York: Harper & Row.

De Chardin, P. T. (1965). *Hymn of the universe.* New York: Harper & Row.

De Chardin, P. T. (1966). *Man's place in nature.* New York: Harper & Row.

De Chardin, P. T. (1969). *Human energy.* New York-Harper & Row.

Decker, J. W. (2000). The effects of inflammatory bowel disease on adolescents. *Gastroenterology Nursing, 23*, 63-66.

DeVillers, M. J. (1998). The clinical nurse specialist as expert practitioner in the obstetrical/gynecological setting. *Clinical Nurse Specialist, 12*, 193-199.

Dickoff, J., James, P., & Wiedenbach, E. (1968a). Theory in a practice discipline. I. Practice oriented discipline. *Nursing Research, 17*, 415-435.

Dickoff, J., James, P., & Wiedenbach, E. (1968b). Theory in a practice discipline. II. Practice oriented research. *Nursing Research, 17*, 545-554.

DiMattio, M. J., & Tulman, L. (2003). A longitudinal study of functional status and correlates following coronary artery bypass graft surgery in women. *Nursing Research, 52*, 98-107.

Dixon, E. L. (1999). Community health nursing practice and the Roy adaptation model. *Public Health Nursing, 16*, 290-300.

Dobratz, M. C. (2003). Putting the pieces together: Teaching undergraduate research from a theoretical perspective. *Journal of Advanced Nursing, 41*, 383-392.

Ducharme, E., Ricard, N., Duquette, A., Levesque, L., & Lachance, L. (1998). Empirical testing of a longitudinal model derived from the Roy adaptation model. *Nursing Science Quarterly, 11*, 149-159.

Dunn, K. S. (2004). Toward a middle-range theory of adaptation to chronic pain. *Nursing Science Quarterly, 77*, 78-84.

Farkas, L. (1981). Adaptation problems with nursing home application for elderly persons: An application of the Roy adaptation nursing model. *Journal of Advanced Nursing, 6*, 363-368.

Fawcett, J. (2002). The nurse theorists: 21st-century updates—Callista Roy. *Nursing Science Quarterly, 15*, 308-310.

Fawcett, J. (2005). Roy's adaptation model. In J. Fawcett (Ed.), *Analysis and evaluation of contemporary nursing knowledge: Nursing models and theories* (2nd ed.) (pp. 364-437). Philadelphia: F. A. Davis.

Frame, K., Kelly, L., & Bayley, E. (2003). Increasing perceptions of self-worth in preadolescents diagnosed with ADHD. *Journal of Nursing Scholarship, 35*, 225-229.

Frederickson, K. (2000). Nursing knowledge development through research: Using the Roy adaptation model. *Nursing Science Quarterly, 13*, 12-16.

Gallagher, M. S. (1998). Urogenital distress and the psychosocial impact of urinary incontinence on elderly women. *Rehabilitation Nursing, 23*, 192-197.

Galligan, A. C. (1979). Addressing small children. Using Roy's concept of adaptation to care for young children. *MCN: American Journal of Maternal Child Nursing, 4*, 24-28.

Hennessy-Harstad, E. B. (1999). Empowering adolescents with asthma to take control through adaptation. *Journal of Pediatric Health Care, 13*, 273-277.

Hill, B. J., & Roberts, C. S. (1981). Formal theory construction: An example of the process. In C. Roy & S. L. Roberts (Eds.), *Theory construction in nursing: An adaptation model.* Englewood Cliffs, NJ: Prentice-Hall.

Illich, I. (1974). Medical nemesis. *Lancet, 1*, 918-921.

Illich, I. (1976). *Limits to medicine: Medical nemesis, the expropriation of health.* London: Boyars.

Jirovec, M. M., Jenkins, J., Isenberg, M., & Baiardi, J. (1999). Urine control theory derived from Roy's conceptual framework. *Nursing Science Quarterly, 12*, 251-255.

Keen, M., Breckenridge, D., Frauman, A. C, Hartigan, M. F., Smith, L., & Butera, E. (1998). Nursing assessment and intervention for adult hemodialysis patients: Application of Roy's adaptation model. *American Nephrology Nurses' Association Journal, 25*, 311-319.

Lankester, K., & Sheldon, L. M. (1999). Health visiting with Roy's model: A case study. *Journal of Child Health Care, 3*, 28-34.

Levesque, L., Ricard, N., Ducharme, F., Duquette, A., & Bonin, J. P. (1998). Empirical verification of a theoretical model derived from the Roy adaptation model: Findings from five studies. *Nursing Science Quarterly, 11*, 31-39.

Limandri, B. J. (1986). Research and practice with abused women—Use of the Roy adaptation model as an explanatory framework. *ANS Advances in Nursing Science, 8*, 52-61.

Malinski, V. M. (2000). Commentary. *Nursing Science Quarterly*, 13, 16-17.

Mastal, M. F., & Hammond, H. (1980). Analysis and expansion of the Roy adaptation model: A contribution to holistic nursing. *ANS Advances in Nursing Science, 2*, 71-81.

Mastal, M. F., Hammond, H., & Roberts, M. P. (1982). Theory into hospital practice: A pilot implementation. *Journal of Nursing Administration, 12*, 9-15.

McDonald, F. J., & Harms, M. (1966). Theoretical model for an experimental curriculum. *Nursing Outlook, 14*, 48-51.

Meleis, A. I. (1985). *Theoretical nursing development and progress.* Philadelphia: J. B. Lippincott.

Meleis, A. I. (2007). *Theoretical nursing development and progress, 4th edition.* Philadelphia: Lippincott Williams & Wilkins.

Modrcin-McCarthy, M. A., McCue, S., & Walker, J. (1997). Preterm infants and STRESS: A tool for the neonatal nurse. *Journal of Perinatal & Neonatal Nursing, 10,* 62-71.

Modrcin-Talbott, M. A., Harrison, L. L., Groer, M. W., & Younger, M. S. (2003). The biobehavioral effects of gentle human touch on preterm infants. *Nursing Science Quarterly, 16,* 60-67.

Modrcin-Talbott, M. A., Pullen, L., Ehrenberger, H., Zandstra, K., & Muenchen, B. (1998a). Self esteem in adolescents treated in an outpatient mental health setting. *Issues in Comprehensive Pediatric Nursing, 21,* 159-171.

Modrcin-Talbott, M. A., Pullen, L., Zandstra, K., Ehrenberger, H., & Muenchen, B. (1998b). A study of self-esteem among well adolescents: Seeking a new direction. *Issues in Comprehensive Pediatric Nursing, 21,* 229-241.

Newman, D. M. (1997a). Responses to caregiving: A reconceptualization using the Roy adaptation model. *Holistic Nursing Practice, 12,* 80-88.

Newman, D. M. (1997b). The Inventory of Functional Status—Caregiver of a Child in a Body Cast. *Journal of Pediatric Nursing, 12,* 142-147.

Nuamah, I. F., Cooley, M. E., Fawcett, J., & McCorkle, R. (1999). Testing a theory for health-related quality of life in cancer patients: A structural equation approach. *Research in Nursing & Health, 22,* 231-242.

Nyqvist, K. H., & Sjoden, P. O. (1993). Advice concerning breast-feeding from mothers of infants admitted to a neonatal intensive-care unit—The Roy adaptation model as a conceptual structure. *Journal of Advanced Nursing, 18,* 54-63.

Pollock, S. E. (1993). Adaptation to chronic illness: A program of research for testing nursing theory. *Nursing Science Quarterly, 6,* 86-92.

Rambo, B. (1983). *Adaptation nursing: Assessment and intervention,* Philadelphia: W. B. Saunders.

Randell, B., Tedrow, M. P., & Van Landingham, J, (1982). *Adaptation nursing: The Roy conceptual model applied.* St. Louis: Mosby.

Reynolds, P. D. (1971). *A primer in theory construction.* Indianapolis: Bobbs-Merrill.

Riehl, J. P., & Roy, C. (1980). *Conceptual models for nursing practice* (2nd ed.) New York: Appleton-Century-Crofts.

Roy, C. (1970). Adaptation: A conceptual framework for nursing. *Nursing Outlook, 18,* 42-45.

Roy, C. (1971). Adaptation: A basis for nursing practice. *Nursing Outlook, 19,* 254-257.

Roy, C. (1973). Adaptation: Implications for curriculum change. *Nursing Outlook, 21,* 163-168.

Roy, C. (1975). A diagnostic classification system for nursing. *Nursing Outlook, 23,* 90-94.

Roy, C. (1976a). *Introduction to nursing: An adaptation model.* Englewood Cliffs, NJ: Prentice-Hall.

Roy, C. (1976b). The impact of nursing diagnosis. *Nursing Digest, 4,* 67-69.

Roy, C. (1979). Relating nursing theory to nursing education: A new era. *Nurse Educator, 4,* 16-21.

Roy, C. (1980). The Roy adaptation model. In J. P. Riehl & C. Roy (Eds.), *Conceptual models for nursing practice* (2nd ed., pp. 179-188). New York: Appleton-Century-Crofts.

Roy, C. (1984). *Introduction to nursing: An adaptation model* (2nd ed.). Englewood Cliffs, NJ: Prentice-Hall.

Roy, C. (1997). Future of the Roy model: Challenge to redefine adaptation. *Nursing Science Quarterly, 10,* 42-48.

Roy, C. (2000). The visible and invisible fields that shape the future of the nursing care system. *Nursing Administration Quarterly, 25*(1), 119-131.

Roy, C., & Andrews, H. (1991). *The Roy adaptation model: The definitive statement.* Norwalk, CT: Appleton & Lange.

Roy, C, & Andrews, H. (1999). *The Roy adaptation model* (2nd ed.). Upper Saddle River, NJ: Pearson Education, Inc.

Roy, C., & McLeod, D. (1981). Theory of the person as an adaptive system. In C. Roy & S. Roberts (Eds.), *Theory construction in nursing: Art adaptation model* (pp. 49-69). Englewood Cliffs, NJ: Prentice-Hall.

Roy, C., & Obloy, M. (1978). The practitioner movement *American Journal of Nursing, 78,* 1698-1702.

Roy, C., & Roberts, S. (1981). *Theory construction in nursing: An adaptation model.* Englewood Cliffs, NJ: Prentice-Hall.

Roy, C., & Zhan, L. (2001). The Roy adaptation model: Theoretical update and knowledge for practice. In M. E. Parker (Ed.), *Nursing theories and nursing practice* (pp. 315-342). Philadelphia: F. A. Davis.

Roy, S. C., & Corliss, C. P. (1993). The Roy adaptation model: Theoretical update and knowledge for practice. In M. E. Parker (Ed.), Patterns of nursing theories in practice. (NLN Pub. 15-2548). New York: National League for Nursing Press.

Samarel, N., Fawcett, J., Tulman, L., Rothman, H., Spector, L., Spillane, P. A., et al. (1999). A resource kit for women with breast cancer: Development and evaluation. *Oncology Nursing Forum, 26,* 611-618.

Samarel, N., Tulman, L., & Fawcett, J. (2002). Effects of two types of social support and education on adaptation to early-stage breast cancer. *Research in Nursing & Health, 25,* 459-470.

Senesac, P. (2003, Spring). Implementing the Roy adaptation model: From, theory to practice. *Roy Adaptation Review,* v4, No 2, Chestnut Hill, MA.

Silva, M. C. (1986). Research testing nursing theory: State of the art *ANS Advances in Nursing Science, 9,* 1-11.

Silva, M. C. (1987). Needs of spouses of surgical patients: A conceptualization within the Roy adaptation model. *Scholarly Inquiry for Nursing Practice, 1,* 29-44.

Smith, C. E., Garvis, M. S., & Martinson, I. M. (1983). Content analysis of interviews using a nursing model: A look at parents adapting to the impact of childhood cancer. *Cancer Nursing, 6,* 269-275.

Swimme, B., & Berry, T. (1992). *The universe story.* San Francisco: Harper.

Tiedeman, M. E. (1983). The Roy adaptation model. In J. Fitzpatrick & A. Whall (Eds.), *The Roy adaptation model* (pp. 157-180). Bowie, MD: Brady.

Tsai, P. F. (2003). Middle-range theory of caregiver stress. *Nursing Science Quarterly, 16,* 137-145.

Tsai, P. F., Tak, S., Moore, C., & Palencia, I. (2003). Testing a theory of chronic pain. *Journal of Advanced Nursing, 43,* 158-169.

Villareal, E. (2003). Using Roy's adaptation model when caring for a group of young women contemplating quitting smoking. *Public Health Nursing, 20,* 377-384.

Wagner, P. (1976). The Roy adaptation model. Testing the adaptation model in practice. *Nursing Outlook, 24,* 682-685.

Whittemore, R., & Roy, C. (2002). Adapting to diabetes mellitus: A theory synthesis. *Nursing Science Quarterly, 15,* 311-317.

Woods, S. J., & Isenberg, M. A. (2001). Adaptation as a mediator of intimate abuse and traumatic stress in battered women. *Nursing Science Quarterly, 14,* 215-221.

Yeh, C. H. (2002). Health-related quality of life in pediatric patients with cancer—A structural equation approach with the Roy adaptation model. *Cancer Nursing, 25,* 74-80.

Young-McCaughan, S., Mays, M. Z., Arzola, S. M., Yoder, L. H., Dramiga, S. A., Leclerc, K. M., et al. (2003). Research and commentary: Change in exercise tolerance, activity and sleep patterns, and quality of life in patients with cancer participating in a structured exercise program. *Oncology Nursing Forum, 30,* 441-454.

Zhan, L. (2000). Cognitive adaptation and self-consistency in hearing-impaired older persons: testing Roy's adaptation model. *Nursing Science Quarterly, 13,* 158-165.

Zhan, L., & Shen, C. (1994). The development of an instrument to measure self-consistency. *Journal of Advanced Nursing, 20,* 509-516.

BIBLIOGRAPHY

Primary Sources

Books

Andrews, H., & Roy, C. (1986). *Essentials of the Roy adaptation model.* Norwalk, CT: Appleton-Century-Crofts.

Boston-Based Adaptation Research in Nursing Society. (1999). *Roy adaptation model-based research: 25 years of contributions to nursing science.* Indianapolis: Sigma Theta Tau International Center Nursing Press.

Riehl, J. P., & Roy, C. (Eds.). (1974). *Conceptual models for nursing practice.* Englewood Cliffs, NJ: Prentice-Hall.

Riehl, J. P., & Roy, C. (Eds.). (1980). *Conceptual models for nursing practice* (2nd ed.). New York: Appleton-Century-Crofts.

Roy, C. (1976). *Introduction to nursing: An adaptation model.* Englewood Cliffs, NJ: Prentice-Hall.

Roy, C. (1982). *Introduction to nursing: An adaptation model* (Japanese translation by Yuriko Kanematsu). Tokyo, Japan: UNI Agency.

Roy, C. (1984). *Introduction to nursing: An adaptation model* (2nd ed.). Englewood Cliffs, NJ: Prentice-Hall.

Roy, C., & Andrews, H. A. (1991). *The Roy adaptation model: The definitive statement.* Norwalk, CT: Appleton & Lange.

Roy, C., & Andrews, H. A. (1999). *The Roy adaptation model* (2nd ed.). Stamford, CT: Appleton & Lange.

Roy, C., & Roberts, S. (1981). *Theory construction in nursing: An adaptation model.* Englewood Cliffs, NJ: Prentice-Hall.

Roy, C., & Jones, D. (Editors). (2007). *Nursing knowledge development and clinical practice.* New York: Springer.

Book Chapters

Barone, S. H., & Roy, C. (1996). The Roy adaptation model in research: Rehabilitation nursing. In P. H. Walker & B. Neuman (Eds.), *Blueprint for use of nursing models: Education, research, practice, and administration* (pp. 64-87). New York: National League for Nursing.

Morgillo-Freeman, S. & Roy, C. (2005). Cognitive behavior therapy and the Roy Adaptation Model: A discussion of theoretical integration. In S. M. Freeman & A. Freeman (Eds.), *Cognitive behavior therapy in nursing practice* (pp. 3-27). New York: Springer

Roy, C. (1974). The Roy adaptation model. In J. P. Riehl & C. Roy (Eds.), *Conceptual models for nursing practice* (pp. 135-144). New York: Appleton-Century-Crofts.

Roy, C. (1980). The Roy adaptation model. In J. P. Riehl & C. Roy (Eds.), *Conceptual models for nursing practice* (2nd ed., pp. 179-188). New York: Appleton-Century-Crofts.

Roy, C. (1981). A systems model of nursing care and its effect on the quality of human life. In G. E. Lasker (Ed.), *Applied systems and cybernetics. Vol. 4. Systems research in health care, biocybernetics, and ecology* (pp. 1705-1714). New York: Pergamon.

Roy, C. (1983). A conceptual framework for clinical specialist practice. In A. B. Hamrick & J. Spross (Eds.), *The clinical nurse specialist in theory and practice* (pp. 3-20). New York: Grune & Stratton.

Roy, C. (1983). Roy adaptation model. In I. Clements & F. Roberts (Eds.), *Family health: A theoretical approach to family health* (pp. 255-278). New York: Wiley.

Roy, C. (1983). Theory development in nursing: A proposal for direction. In N. Chaska (Ed.), *The nursing profession: A time to speak* (pp. 453-467). New York: McGraw-Hill.

Roy, C. (1983). The expectant family: Analysis and application of the Roy adaptation model, and the family in primary care—Analysis and application of the Roy adaptation model. In I. W. Clements & F. B. Roberts (Eds.), *Family health: A theoretical approach to nursing care* (pp. 298-303). New York: John Wiley & Sons.

Roy, C. (1987). Roy's adaptation model. In R. R. Parse (Ed.), *Nursing science: Major paradigms, theories, and critiques* (pp. 35-45). Philadelphia: Saunders.

Roy, C. (1987). The influence of nursing models on clinical decision making II. In K. J. Hannah, M. Reimer, W. C. Mills, & S. Letourneau *(Eds.), Clinical judgment and decision making. The future of nursing diagnosis* (pp. 42-47). New York: Wiley.

Roy, C. (1988). Sister Callista Roy. In T. M. Schorr & A. Zimmerman (Eds.). *Making choices: Taking chances* (pp. 291-298). St. Louis: Mosby.

Roy, C. (1989). The Roy adaptation model. In J. P. Riehl (Ed.), *Conceptual models for nursing practice* (3rd ed., pp. 105-114). Norwalk, CT: Appleton & Lange.

Roy, C. (1991). Altered cognition: An information processing approach. In P. H. Mitchell, L. C. Hodges, M. Muwaswes, & C. A. Walleck (Eds.), *AANN's neuro-science nursing: Phenomenon and practice—Human responses to neurological health problems* (pp. 185-211). Norwalk, CT: Appleton & Lange.

Roy, C. (1991). Structure of knowledge: Paradigm, model, and research specifications for differentiated practice. In I. E. Goertzen (Ed.), *Differentiating nursing practice: Into the twenty-first century* (pp. 31-39). Kansas City, MO: American Academy of Nursing.

Roy, C. (1992). Vigor, variables, and vision: Commentary of Florence Nightingale. In F. Nightingale (Ed.), *Notes on nursing: What it is, and what it is not* (Commemorative edition, pp. 63-71). Philadelphia: Lippincott.

Roy, C. (2000). Alteration in cognitive processing. In C. Stewart-Amidei, J. Kunkel, & K. Bronstein (Eds.), *AANN's neuroscience nursing: Human responses to neurologic dysfunction* (2nd ed., pp. 275-323). Philadelphia: Saunders.

Roy, C. (2000). NANDA and the nurse theorists: The truth of nursing theory. In North American Nursing Diagnosis Association, *Classification of nursing diagnoses* (pp. 59-57). St. Louis: Mosby.

Roy, C. (2001). Alterations in cognitive processing. In C. Stewart-Amidei & J. A. Kunkel (Eds.), AANN's neuroscience nursing: Human responses to neurologic dysfunction (2nd ed., pp. ***-***). Philadelphia: Saunders.

Roy, C. (2007). The Roy Adaptation Model: Historical and philosophical foundations. In Maria Elisa Moreno et al. (Eds.). *Application del model adaptacion en el ciclo vital humano* (2nd ed.). Chia, Columbia: Universidad de La Sabana.

Roy, C., & Anway, J. (1989). Roy's adaptation model: Theories and hypotheses for nursing administration. In B. Henry, M. DiVincenti, C. Arndt, & A. Marriner Tomey (Eds.), *Dimensions of nursing administration: 'Theory, research, education, and practice* (pp. 75-88). Boston: Blackwell Scientific.

Roy, C., & Corliss, C. P. (1993). The Roy adaptation model. Theoretical update and knowledge for practice. In M. E. Parker (Ed.), *Patterns of nursing theories in practice* (pp. 215-229). New York: National League for Nursing Press.

Roy, C., & McLeod, D. (1981). Theory of the person as an adaptive system. In C. Roy & S. L. Roberts (Eds.), *Theory construction in nursing: An adaptation model* (pp. 49-69). Englewood Cliffs, NJ: Prentice-Hall.

Roy, C., & Zhan, L. (2001). The Roy adaptation model: A basis for developing knowledge for practice with the elderly. In M. Parker, (Ed.), *Nursing theories and nursing practice* (pp. 315-342). Philadelphia: F. A. Davis.

Journal Articles

Artinian, N. T., & Roy, C. (1990). Strengthening the Roy adaptation model through conceptual clarification. Commentary (Artinian) and response (Roy). *Nursing Science Quarterly, 3*, 60-66.

Hanna, D. R., & Roy C. (2001). Roy adaptation model perspectives on family. *Nursing Science Quarterly, 14*(1), 9-13.

Pollock, S. E., Frederickson, K., Carson, M. A., Massey, V. H., & Roy, C. (1994). Contributions to nursing science: Synthesis of findings from adaptation model research. *Scholarly Inquiry for Nursing Practice, 8*(4), 361-374.

Roy, C. (1970). Adaptation: A conceptual framework in nursing. *Nursing Outlook, 18*, 42-45.

Roy, C. (1971). Adaptation: A basis for nursing practice. *Nursing Outlook, 19*, 254-257.

Roy, C. (1973). Adaptation: Implications for curriculum change. *Nursing Outlook, 21*, 163-168.

Roy, C. (1975). A diagnostic classification system for nursing. *Nursing Outlook, 23*, 90-94.

Roy, C. (1975). The impact of nursing diagnosis. *AORN Journal, 21*, 1023-1030.

Roy, C. (1976). The Roy adaptation model: Comment *Nursing Outlook, 24*, 690-691.

Roy, C. (1979). Nursing diagnosis from the perspective of a nursing model. *Nursing Diagnosis Newsletter, 6*(3), 1-3.

Roy, C. (1979). Relating nursing theory to nursing education: A new era. *Nurse Educator, 4*(2), 16-21.

Roy, C. (1980). Exposé de Callista Roy sur theories. Exposé de Callista Roy sur l'utilisation de sa theories au nouveau de la recherche. *Acta Nursologica, 3.* [Essay by Castilla Roy on theories. Essay by Castilla Roy on utilization of her theories in new research. *Acta Nursologica*, 3]

Roy, C. (1987). Response to "Needs of spouses of surgical patients, a conceptualization within the Roy adaptation model." *Scholarly Journal for Nursing Practice, 1* (1), 45-50.

Roy, C. (1988). An explication of the philosophical assumptions of the Roy adaptation model. *Nursing Science Quarterly, 1*, 26-34.

Roy, C. (1988). Human information processing and nursing research. *Annual Review of Nursing Research, 6*, 237-262.

Roy, C. (1990). Case reports can provide a standard for care in nursing practice. *Journal of Professional Nursing*, 6(3), 179-180.

Roy, C. (1990). Strengthening the Roy adaptation model through conceptual clarification. *Nursing Science Quarterly, 3*(2), 64-66.

Roy, C. (1991). Theory and research for clinical knowledge development. *Journal of Japanese Nursing Research, 14*(1), 21-29.

Roy, C. (1995). Developing nursing knowledge: Practice issues raised from four philosophical perspectives. *Nursing Science Quarterly, 8*(2), 79-85.

Roy, C. (1997). Future of the Roy model: Challenge to redefine adaptation. *Nursing Science Quarterly, 10*(1), 42-48.

Roy, C. (2000). A theorist envisions the future and speaks to nursing administrators. *Nursing Administration Quarterly, 24*(2), 1-12.

Roy, C. (2000). Critique: Research on cognitive consequences of treatment for childhood acute lymphoblastic leukemia. *Seminars in Oncology Nursing, 16*(4), 291.

Roy, C. (2000). The visible and invisible fields that shape the future of the nursing care system. *Nursing Administration Quarterly, 25*(1), 119-131.

Roy, C. (2003). Reflections on nursing research and the Roy adaptation model. *Japanese Journal of Nursing Research, 36*(1), 7-11.

Roy, C. (2007). Update from the future: Thinking of theorist Sr. Callista Roy. *Nursing Science Quarterly, 20*(2), 113-116.

Whittemore, R., & Roy, C. (2002). Adapting to diabetes mellitus: A theory synthesis. *Nursing Science Quarterly, 15*(4), 311-317.

Dissertation

Roy, C. (1977). *Decision-making by the physically ill and adaptation during illness.* Unpublished doctoral dissertation, University of California, Los Angeles.

Secondary Sources

Book Chapters

Fawcett, J. (2005). Roy's adaptation model. In J. Fawcett (Ed.), *Analysis and evaluation of contemporary nursing knowledge: Nursing models and theories* (pp. 364-437). Philadelphia: F. A. Davis.

Galbreath, J. (2002). Roy adaptation model: Sister Callista Roy. In J. B. George (Ed.), *Nursing theories: The base for professional nursing practice* (pp. 295-338). Upper Saddle River, NJ: Prentice Hall.

Lutjens, L. R. J. (1995). Callista Roy: An adaptation model. In C. M. McQuiston & A. A. Webb (Eds.), *Foundations of nursing theory: Contributions of twelve key theorists* (pp. 91-138). Thousand Oaks, CA: Sage Publications.

Pearson, A., Vaughan, B., & Fitzgerald, M. (1996). An adaptation model for nursing. In *Nursing models for practice* (pp. 110-129). Oxford: Reed Educational and Professional Publishing.

Phillips, K. D. (2002). Roy's adaptation model in nursing practice. In M. R. Alligood & A. M. Tomey (Eds.), *Nursing theory: Utilization & application* (pp. 289-314). St. Louis: Mosby.

Tiedeman, M. E. (2005). Roy's adaptation model. In J. J. Fitzpatrick & A. L. Whall (Eds.), *Conceptual models of nursing: Analysis and application* (4th ed., pp. 146-176). Englewood Cliffs, NJ: Prentice Hall.

Dissertations

Ahern, E. (2006). Elaboration d'un modele theorique de l'agression en milieu psychiatrique et developpement d'instruments de mesure. (Doctoral dissertation. Universite de Montreal, 2006). *Dissertation Abstracts International, 68*, 3698.

Arcamone, A. A. (2005). The effect of prenatal education on adaptation to motherhood after vaginal childbirth in primiparous women as assessed by Roy's four adaptive modes. (Doctoral dissertation. Widener University, 2005). *Dissertation Abstracts International, 66*, 4722.

Beck-Little, R. (2000). Sleep enhancement interventions and the sleep of institutionalized older adults (Doctoral dissertation, University of South Carolina, 2000). *Dissertation Abstracts International, 61*, 3503.

Black, K. D. (2004). Physiologic responses, sense of well-being, self-efficacy for self-monitoring role, perceived availability of social support, and perceived stress in women with pregnancy-induced hypertension. (Doctoral dissertation, Widener University, 2004). *Dissertation Abstracts International, 65*, 1773.

Burns, D. P. (1997). Coping with hemodialysis: A midrange theory deduced from the Roy adaptation model (Doctoral dissertation, Wayne State University, 1997). *Dissertation Abstracts International, 58*, 1206.

Cacchione, P. Z. (1998). Assessment of acute confusion in elderly persons who reside in long-term care facilities (Doctoral dissertation, St. Louis University, 1998). *Dissertation Abstracts International, 59*, 156.

Chayaput, P. (2004). Development and psychometric evaluation of the Thai version of the Coping and Adaptation Processing Scale. (Doctoral dissertation,

Boston College, 2004). *Dissertation Abstracts International, 65*, 2864.

Cheng, S. (2002). A multi-method study of Taiwanese children's pain experience (Doctoral dissertation, University of Colorado Health Sciences Center, 2002). *Dissertation Abstracts International, 63*, 1265.

Chung, C. (1999). Sense of coherence, self-care, and self-actualizing behaviors of Korean menopausal women (Doctoral dissertation, Case Western Reserve University Health Sciences, 1999). *Dissertation Abstracts International, 61*, 776.

Dunn, K. S. (2001). Adaptation to chronic pain: Religious and non-religious coping in Judeo-Christian elders (Doctoral dissertation, Wayne State University, 2001). *Dissertation Abstracts International, 62*, 5640.

Frame, K. R. (2002). The effect of a support group on perceptions of scholastic competence, social acceptance and behavioral conduct in preadolescents diagnosed with attention deficit hyperactivity disorder (Doctoral dissertation, Widener University, 2002). *Dissertation Abstracts International, 63*, 737.

Giedt, J. F. (1999). The psychoneuroimmunological effects of guided imagery in patients on hemodialysis for end-stage renal disease (Doctoral dissertation, Wayne State University, 1999). *Dissertation Abstracts International, 61*, 192.

Gipson-Jones, T. L. (2005). The relationship between work-family conflict, job satisfaction and psychological well-being among African American nurses. (Doctoral dissertation, Hampton University, 2005). *Dissertation Abstracts International, 66*, 2512.

Harner, H. M. (2001). Obstetrical outcomes of teenagers with adult and peer age partners (Doctoral dissertation, University of Pennsylvania, 2001). *Dissertation Abstracts International, 62*, 2256.

Henderson, P. D. (2002). African-American women coping with breast cancer (Doctoral dissertation, Hampton University, 2002). *Dissertation Abstracts International, 63*, 5764.

Hinkle, J. L. (1999). A descriptive study of variables explaining functional recovery following stroke (Doctoral dissertation, University of Pennsylvania, 1999). *Dissertation Abstracts International, 60*, 6021.

Huang, C. M. (2002). Sleep and daytime sleepiness in first-time mothers during early postpartum in Taiwan (Doctoral dissertation, University of Texas at Austin, 2002). *Dissertation Abstracts International*, 64, 3189.

Jenkins, B. E. (2006). Emotional intelligence of faculty members, the learning environment, and empowerment of baccalaureate students. (Doctoral dissertation, Columbia University, 2006). *Dissertation Abstracts International, 67*, 3701.

Kan, E. Z. (2007). Adaptive behaviors and perceptions of recovery following coronary artery bypass graft surgery (Doctoral dissertation, Widener University, 2007). *Dissertation Abstracts International*, 68, 4390.

Kittiwatanapaisan, W. (2002). Measurement of fatigue in myasthenia gravis patients (Doctoral dissertation, University of Alabama at Birmingham, 2002). *Dissertation Abstracts International, 63*, 4595.

Klein, G. J. M. (2000). The relationships among anxiety, self-concept, the impostor phenomenon, and generic senior baccalaureate nursing students' perceptions of clinical competency (Doctoral dissertation, Widener University, 2000). *Dissertation Abstracts International, 61*, 5236.

Kline, N. E. (1999). Sleep disturbances in children receiving short-term, high dose glucocorticoid therapy for acute lymphoblastic leukemia (Doctoral dissertation, Texas Women's University, 1999). *Dissertation Abstracts International, 61*, 194.

Kochniuk, L. (2004). We never buy green bananas: The oldest old. A phenomenological study. (Doctoral dissertation, University of Idaho, 2004). *Dissertation Abstracts International, 65*, 2318.

Kruszewski, A. Z. (1999). Psychosocial adaptation to termination of pregnancy for fetal anomaly (Doctoral dissertation, Wayne State University, 1999). *Dissertation Abstracts International, 61*, 194.

Lefaiver, C. A. (2006). Quality of life: The dyad of caregivers and lung transplant candidates (Doctoral dissertation, Loyola University, 2006). *Dissertation Abstracts International, 67*, 4978.

Lu, Y. (2001). Caregiving stress effects on functional capability and self-care behavior for elderly caregivers of persons with Alzheimer's disease (Doctoral dissertation, Case Western Reserve University, Health Sciences, 2001). *Dissertation Abstracts International, 62*, 1807.

Mahoney, E. T. (2000). The relationships among social support, coping, self-concept, and stage of recovery in alcoholic women (Doctoral dissertation, Catholic University of America, 2000). *Dissertation Abstracts International, 61*, 1872.

Malinski, V. M. (2000). Commentary. *Nursing Science Quarterly*, 13, 16-17.

Otten, R. (2005). History of associate degree nursing at Mount St. Mary's College: 1970-2005 (California). (Doctoral dissertation, Pepperdine University, 2005). *Dissertation Abstracts International, 67*, 492.

Phahuwatanakorn, W. (2004). The relationships between social support, maternal employment, postpartum anxiety, and maternal role competencies in Thai primiparous mothers (Doctoral dissertation, Catholic University of America, 2004). *Dissertation Abstracts International, 64*, 5451.

Sabatini, M. (2003). Exercise and adaptation to aging in older women (Doctoral dissertation, Widener University, 2003). *Dissertation Abstracts International, 64*, 3748.

Saint-Pierre, C. (2003). Elaboration et verification d'un modele predictif de l'adaptation aux roles associes de mere et de travailleuse a statut precaire (Doctoral dissertation. Universite de Montreal, 2003). *Dissertation Abstracts International, 65*, 1252.

Sander, R. A. (2004). Measurement of functional status in the spinal cord injured patient. (Doctoral dissertation, Saint Louis University, 2004). *Dissertation Abstracts International, 65*, 1783.

Salazar-Gonzalez, B. C. (1999). Responses to exercise in elderly Mexican women (Doctoral dissertation, Wayne State University, 1999). *Dissertation Abstracts International, 61*, 197.

Senesac, P. M. (2004). The Roy Adaptation Model: An action research approach to the implementation of a pain management organizational change project. (Doctoral dissertation, Boston College, 2004). *Dissertation Abstracts International, 65*, 2872.

Stephens, K. A. (2005). Preoxygenation practices prior to tracheal suctioning by nurses caring for individuals with spinal cord injury. (Doctoral dissertation, Loyola University, 2005). *Dissertation Abstracts International, 66*, 2518.

Taival, A. S. (1998). The older person's adaptation and the promotion of adaptation in home nursing care: Action research of intervention through training based on the Roy adaptation model (Doctoral dissertation, Tampereen Teknillinen Korkeakoulu, 1998). *Dissertation Abstracts International, 60*, 113.

Thomas-Hawkins, C. (1998). Correlates of changes in functional status in chronic in-center hemodialysis patients (Doctoral dissertation, University of Pennsylvania, 1998). *Dissertation Abstracts International, 59*, 5792.

Toughill, E. H. (2001). Quality of life: The impact of age, severity of urinary incontinence and adaptation (Doctoral dissertation, New York University, 2001). *Dissertation Abstracts International, 61*, 5240.

Tsai, P. F. (1998). Development of a middle-range theory of caregiver stress from the Roy adaptation model (Doctoral dissertation, Wayne State University, 1998). *Dissertation Abstracts International, 60*, 133.

Velos Weiss, J. C. (1998). Lifestyle and angina in the elderly following elective coronary artery bypass graft surgery (Doctoral dissertation, University of Pennsylvania, 1998). *Dissertation Abstracts International, 59*, 1589.

Wood, A. E. (1998). An investigation of stimuli related to baccalaureate nursing students' transition toward role mastery (Doctoral dissertation, University of Tennessee, Knoxville, 1998). *Dissertation Abstracts International, 59*, 4023.

Woods, S. J. (1997). Predictors of traumatic stress in battered women: A test and explication of the Roy adaptation model (Doctoral dissertation, Wayne State University, 1997). *Dissertation Abstracts International, 58*, 1220.

Wright, R. R. (2007). Experiences of emergency nurses: What has been learned from traumatic and violent events? (Doctoral Dissertation, Columbia University, 2007). *Dissertation Abstracts International, 68*, 3698.

Wunderlich, R. J. (2003). An exploratory study of physiological and psychological variables that predict weaning from mechanical ventilation (Doctoral dissertation, Saint Louis University, 2003). *Dissertation Abstracts International, 64*, 3750.

Zbegner, D. K. (2003). An exploratory retrospective study using the Roy Adaptation Model: The adaptive mode variables of physical energy level, self-esteem, marital satisfaction, and parenthood motivation as predictors of coping behaviors in infertile women (Doctoral dissertation, Widener University, 2003). *Dissertation Abstracts International, 64*, 3751.

Journal Articles

Chiou, C. (2000). A meta-analysis of the interrelationships between the modes in Roy's adaptation model. *Nursing Science Quarterly, 13*(3), 252-258.

Dawson, S. (1998). Adult/elderly care nursing: Preamputation assessment using Roy's adaptation model. *British Journal of Nursing, 7* (9), 536, 538-542.

Decker, J. W. (2000). The effects of inflammatory bowel disease on adolescents. *Gastroenterology Nursing, 23(2)*, 63-66.

Dixon, E. L. (1999). Community health nursing practice and the Roy adaptation model. *Public Health Nursing, 16*, 290-300.

Dunn, H. C., & Dunn D. G. (1997). The Roy adaptation model and its application to clinical nursing practice. *Journal of Ophthalmic Nursing and Technology, 6(2)*, 74-78.

Harding-Okimoto, M. B. (1997). Pressure ulcers, self-concept, and body image in spinal cord injury patients. *SCI Nursing, 14(4)*, 111-117.

Hennessy-Harstad, E. B. (1999). Empowering adolescents with asthma to take control through adaptation. *Journal of Pediatric Health Care, 13* (6 Part 1), 273-277.

Ingram, L. (1995). Roy's adaptation model and accident and emergency nursing. *Accident and Emergency Nursing, 3*, 150-153.

LeMone, P. (1995). Assessing psychosexual concerns in adults with diabetes: Pilot project using Roy's modes of adaptation. *Issues in Mental Health Nursing, 16(1)*, 67-78.

Modrcin-McCarthy, M. A., McCue, S., & Walker, J. (1997). Preterm infants and STRESS: A tool for the neonatal nurse. *Journal of Perinatal & Neonatal Nursing, 10*, 62-71.

Modrcin-Talbott, M. A., Pullen, L, Ehrenberger, H., Zandstra, K., & Muenchen, B. (1998). Self-esteem in adolescents treated in an outpatient mental health setting. *Issues in Comprehensive Pediatric Nursing, 21*, 159-171.

Modrcin-Talbott, M. A., Pullen, L., Zandstra, K., Ehrenberger, H., & Muenchen, B. (1998). A study of self-esteem among well adolescents: Seeking a new direction. *Issues in Comprehensive Pediatric Nursing, 21*, 229-241.

Newman, D. M. L., & Fawcett, J. (1995). Caring for a young child in a body cast: Impact on the care giver. *Orthopedic Nursing, 14(1)*, 41-46.

Niska, K. J. (1999). Family nursing interventions: Mexican American early family formation: Third part of a three-part study. *Nursing Science Quarterly, 12(4)*, 335-340.

Niska, K. J. (2001). Mexican American family survival, continuity, and growth: The parental perspective. *Nursing Science Quarterly, 14(4)*, 322-329.

Orsi, A. J., Grandy, C., Tax, A., & McCorkle, R. (1997). Nutritional adaptation of women living with HIV: A pilot study. *Holistic Nursing Practice, 12(1)*, 71-79.

Robinson, J. H. (1995). Grief responses, coping processes, and social support of widows: Research with Roy's model. *Nursing Science Quarterly, 8(4)*, 158-164.

Samarel, N., Fawcett, J., Krippendorf, K., Piacentino, J. C., Eliasof, B., Hughes, P., et al. (1998). Women's perception of group support and adaptation to breast cancer. *Journal of Advanced Nursing, 28(6)*, 1259-1268.

Samarel, N., Fawcett, J., Tulman, L., Rothman, H., Spector, L., Spillane, P. A., et al. (1999). A resource kit for women with breast cancer Development and evaluation. *Oncology Nursing Forum, 26*, 611-618.

Sheppard, V. A., & Cunnie, K. L. (1996). Incidence of diuresis following hysterectomy. *Journal of Post Anesthesia Nursing, 11*, 20-28.

Woods, S. J., & Isenberg, M. A. (2001). Adaptation as a mediator of intimate abuse and traumatic stress in battered women. *Nursing Science Quarterly, 14(3)*, 215-221.

Yeh, C. H. (2001). Adaptation in children with cancer: Research with Roy's model. *Nursing Science Quarterly, 14*, 141-148.

Zhan, L. (2000). Cognitive adaptation and self-consistency in hearing-impaired older persons: Testing Roy's adaptation model. *Nursing Science Quarterly, 13(2)*, 158-165.

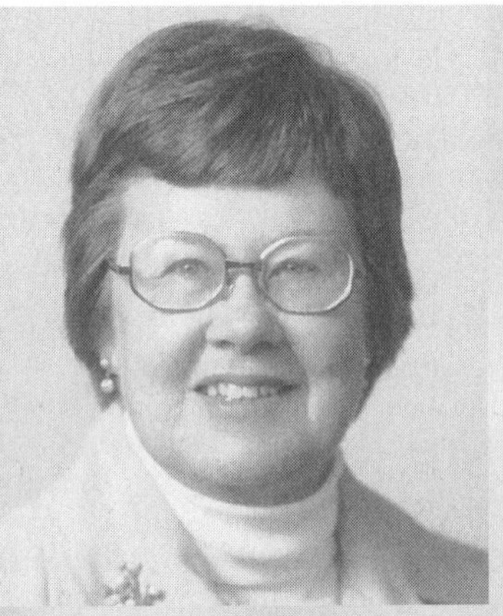

CHAPTER 18

Dorothy Johnson

1919-1999

Behavioral System Model

Bonnie Holaday

"All of us, scientists and practicing professionals, must turn our attention to practice and ask questions of that practice. We must be inquisitive and inquiring, seeking the fullest and truest possible understanding of the theoretical and practical problems we encounter" (Johnson, 1976).

CREDENTIALS AND BACKGROUND OF THE THEORIST

Dorothy E. Johnson was born on August 21, 1919, in Savannah, Georgia. She received her A.A. from Armstrong Junior College in Savannah, Georgia (1938), her B.S.N. from Vanderbilt University in Nashville, Tennessee (1942), and her M.P.H. from Harvard University in Boston (1948).

Johnson's professional experiences involved mostly teaching, although she was a staff nurse at the Chatham-Savannah Health Council from 1943 to 1944. She was an instructor and an assistant professor in pediatric nursing at Vanderbilt University School of Nursing. From 1949 until her retirement in 1978 and her subsequent move to Key Largo, Florida, Johnson was an assistant professor of pediatric nursing, an associate professor of nursing, and a professor of nursing at the University of California in Los Angeles.

In 1955 and 1956, Johnson was a pediatric nursing advisor assigned to the Christian Medical College School of Nursing in Vellore, South India. From 1965 to 1967, she served as chairperson on the committee of the California Nurses Association that developed a position statement on specifications for the clinical specialist. Johnson's publications include four books, more than 30 articles in periodicals, and many papers, reports, proceedings, and monographs (Johnson, 1980).

Of the many honors she received, Johnson (personal correspondence, 1984) was proudest of the 1975 Faculty Award from graduate students, the 1977

Previous authors: Victoria M. Brown, Sharon S. Conner, Linda S. Harbour, Jude A Magers, and Judith K. Watt.

Lulu Hassenplug Distinguished Achievement Award from the California Nurses Association, and the 1981 Vanderbilt University School of Nursing Award for Excellence in Nursing. She died in February 1999 at the age of 80. She was pleased that her Behavioral System Model had been found useful in furthering the development of a theoretical basis for nursing and was being used as a model for nursing practice on an institution-wide basis, but she reported that her greatest satisfaction came from following the productive careers of her students (D. Johnson, personal communication, 1996).

THEORETICAL SOURCES

Johnson's Behavioral System Model (JBSM) was heavily influenced by Florence Nightingale's book, *Notes on Nursing* (Johnson, 1992). Johnson began her work on the model with the premise that nursing was a profession that made a distinctive contribution to the welfare of society. Thus, nursing had an explicit goal of action in patient welfare. Her task was to clarify the social mission of nursing from the "perspective of a theoretically sound view of the person we serve" (Johnson, 1977). She accepted Nightingale's belief that the first concern of nursing is with the "relationship between the person who is ill and their environment, not with the illness" (Johnson, 1977). Johnson (1977) also noted that the "transition from this approach to the more sophisticated and theoretically sounder behavioral system orientation took only a few years and was supported by both my own, and that of many colleagues, growing knowledge about man's action systems and by the rapidly increasing knowledge about behavioral systems." Johnson (1977) came to conceive of nursing's specific contribution to patient welfare as fostering "efficient and effective behavioral functioning in the person, both to prevent illness and during and following illness."

Johnson used the work of behavioral scientists in psychology, sociology, and ethnology to develop her theory. The interdisciplinary literature that Johnson cited focused on observable behaviors that were of adaptive significance. This body of literature influenced the identification and the content of her seven subsystems. Talcott Parsons is acknowledged specifically in early developmental writings presenting concepts of the Johnson Behavioral System Model (Johnson, 1961b). Parsons' (1951, 1964) social action theory stressed a structural-functional approach. One of his major contributions was to reconcile functionalism (the idea that every observable social behavior has a function to perform) with structuralism (the idea that social behaviors, rather than being directly functional, are expressions of deep underlying structures in social systems). Thus, structures (social systems) and all behaviors have a function in maintaining the system. The components of the structure of a social system—goal, set, choice, and behavior—are the same in Parsons' and Johnson's theories.

Johnson also relied heavily on system theory and used concepts and definitions from Rapoport, Chin, von Bertalanffy, and Buckley (Johnson, 1980). In system theory, as in Johnson's theory, one of the basic assumptions embraces the concept of order. Another is that a system is a set of interacting units that form a whole intended to perform some function. Johnson conceptualized the person as a behavioral system, in which the behavior of the individual as a whole is the focus. It is the focus on what the individual does and why. One of the strengths of the Johnson's Behavioral System (JBS) Theory is the consistent integration of concepts defining behavioral systems drawn from general system theory. Some of these concepts include holism, goal seeking, interrelationship/interdependency, stability, instability, subsystems, regularity, structure, function, energy, feedback, and adaptation.

Johnson noted that, although the literature indicates that others support the idea that a person is a behavioral system, and that a person's specific response patterns form an organized and integrated whole, as far as she knew, the idea was original with her. Just as the development of knowledge of the whole biological system was preceded by knowledge of its parts, the development of knowledge of behavioral systems was focused on specific behavioral responses. Empirical literature supporting the notion of the behavioral system as a whole and its usefulness as a framework for nursing decisions in research, education, and nursing practice has accumulated since it was introduced (Benson, 1997; Bhaduri & Jain, 2004; Derdiarian, 1991; Grice, 1997; Holaday, 1981, 1982; Lachicotte & Alexander, 1990; Poster, Dee, & Randell, 1997; Turner-Henson, 1992; Wilkie, 1990; Wilmoth & Ross, 1997; Wilmoth, 2007.)

Developing the Behavioral System Model from a philosophical perspective, Johnson (1980) wrote that nursing contributes by facilitating effective behavioral functioning in the patient before, during, and after illness. She used concepts from other disciplines, such as social learning, motivation, sensory stimulation, adaptation, behavioral modification, change process, tension, and stress, to expand her theory for the practice of nursing.

Major Concepts & Definitions*

BEHAVIOR

Johnson accepted the definition of behavior as expressed by the behavioral and biological scientists, that is, the output of intra-organismic structures and processes as they are coordinated and articulated by and responsive to changes in sensory stimulation. Johnson (1980) focused on behavior affected by the actual or implied presence of other social beings that has been shown to have major adaptive significance.

SYSTEM

Using Rapoport's 1968 definition of *system*, Johnson (1980) stated, "A system is a whole that functions as a whole by virtue of the interdependence of its parts" (p. 208). She accepted Chin's statement that there is "organization, interaction, interdependency, and integration of the parts and elements" (Johnson, 1980, p. 208). In addition, a person strives to maintain a balance in these parts through adjustments and adaptations to the impinging forces.

BEHAVIORAL SYSTEM

A behavioral system encompasses the patterned, repetitive, and purposeful ways of behaving. These ways of behaving form an organized and integrated functional unit that determines and limits the interaction between the person and his or her environment and establishes the relationship of the person to the objects, events, and situations within his or her environment. Usually the behavior can be described and explained. A person as a behavioral system tries to achieve stability and balance through adjustments and adaptations that are successful to some degree for efficient and effective functioning. The system is usually flexible enough to accommodate the influences affecting it (Johnson, 1980).

SUBSYSTEMS

The behavioral system has many tasks to perform; therefore, parts of the system evolve into subsystems with specialized tasks. A subsystem is "a minisystem with its own particular goal and function that can be maintained as long as its relationship to the other subsystems or the environment is not disturbed" (Johnson, 1980, p. 221). The seven subsystems identified by Johnson are open, linked, and interrelated. Input and output are components of all seven subsystems (Grubbs, 1980).

Motivational drives direct the activities of these subsystems, which are continually changing through maturation, experience, and learning. The systems described appear to exist cross culturally and are controlled by biological, psychological, and sociological factors. The seven identified subsystems are attachment-affiliative, dependency, ingestive, eliminative, sexual, achievement, and aggressive-protective (Johnson, 1980).

MAJOR CONCEPTS & DEFINITIONS*—cont'd

Attachment-Affiliative Subsystem

The attachment-affiliative subsystem is probably the most critical, because it forms the basis for all social organization. On a general level, it provides survival and security. Its consequences are social inclusion, intimacy, and formation and maintenance of a strong social bond (Johnson, 1980).

Dependency Subsystem

In the broadest sense, the dependency subsystem promotes helping behavior that calls for a nurturing response. Its consequences are approval, attention or recognition, and physical assistance. Developmentally, dependency behavior evolves from almost total dependence on others to a greater degree of dependence on self. A certain amount of interdependence is essential for the survival of social groups (Johnson, 1980).

Ingestive Subsystem

The ingestive and eliminative subsystems should not be seen as the input and output mechanisms of the system. All subsystems are distinct subsystems with their own input and output mechanisms. The ingestive subsystem "has to do with when, how, what, how much, and under what conditions we eat" (Johnson, 1980, p. 213). "It serves the broad function of appetitive satisfaction" (Johnson, 1980, p. 213). This behavior is associated with social, psychological, and biological considerations (Johnson, 1980).

Eliminative Subsystem

The eliminative subsystem addresses "when, how, and under what conditions we eliminate" (Johnson, 1980, p. 213). As with the ingestive subsystem, the social and psychological factors are viewed as influencing the biological aspects of this subsystem and may be, at times, in conflict with the eliminative subsystem (Loveland-Cherry & Wilkerson, 1983).

Sexual Subsystem

The sexual subsystem has the dual functions of procreation and gratification. Including, but not limited to, courting and mating, this response system begins with the development of gender role identity and includes the broad range of sex-role behaviors (Johnson, 1980).

Achievement Subsystem

The achievement subsystem attempts to manipulate the environment. Its function is control or mastery of an aspect of self or environment to some standard of excellence. Areas of achievement behavior include intellectual, physical, creative, mechanical, and social skills (Johnson, 1980).

Aggressive-Protective Subsystem

The aggressive-protective subsystem's function is protection and preservation. This follows the line of thinking of ethologists such as Lorenz (1966) and Feshbach (1970) rather than the behavioral reinforcement school of thought, which contends that aggressive behavior not only is learned, but has a primary intent to harm others. Society demands that limits be placed on modes of self-protection, and that people and their property be respected and protected (Johnson, 1980).

EQUILIBRIUM

Johnson (1961a) stated that equilibrium is a key concept in nursing's specific goal. It is defined as "a stabilized but more or less transitory, resting state in which the individual is in harmony with himself and with his environment" (p. 65). "It implies that biological and psychological forces are in balance with each other and with impinging social forces" (Johnson, 1961b, p. 11). It is "not synonymous with a state of health, since it may be found either in health or illness" (Johnson, 1961b, p. 11).

Continued

MAJOR CONCEPTS & DEFINITIONS*—cont'd

FUNCTIONAL REQUIREMENTS/ SUSTENAL IMPERATIVES

For the subsystems to develop and maintain stability, each must have a constant supply of function requirements. The environment supplies sustenal imperatives such as protection, nurturance and stimulation. Johnson notes that the biological system and all other living systems have the same requirements.

REGULATION/CONTROL

The interrelated behavioral subsystems must be regulated in some fashion so that their goals can be realized. Regulation implies that deviations will be detected and corrected. Feedback is, therefore, a requirement of effective control. There is self-regulation by the client. The nurse can act as a temporary external regulatory force to preserve the organization and integration of the client's behavior at an optimal level in situations where illness, or under conditions where behavior, constitutes a threat to health.

TENSION

"The concept of tension is defined as a state of being stretched or strained and can be viewed as an end-product of a disturbance in equilibrium" (Johnson, 1961a, p. 10). Tension can be constructive in adaptive change or destructive in inefficient use of energy, hindering adaptation and causing potential structural damage (Johnson, 1961a). Tension is the cue to disturbance in equilibrium (Johnson, 1961b).

STRESSOR

Internal or external stimuli that produce tension and result in a degree of instability are called *stressors*. "Stimuli may be positive in that they are present; or negative in that something desired or required is absent. [Stimuli] . . . may be either endogenous or exogenous in origin [and] may play upon one or more of our linked open systems" (Johnson, 1961b, p. 13). The open-linked systems are in constant interchange. The open-linked systems include the physiological, personality, and meaningful small group (the family) systems and the larger social system (Johnson, 1961b).

*The author acknowledges the contribution of Brown (2006) to this Box.

USE OF EMPIRICAL EVIDENCE

The empirical origins of this theory begin with Johnson's use of systems thinking (synthesis). This process concentrates on the function and behavior of the whole and is focused on an understanding and an explanation of the behavioral system. Johnson's work on the Behavioral System Model corresponded with the "systems age." Buckley's (1968) seminal text was published the same year that Johnson formally presented her theory at Vanderbilt University.

Systems theory, as a basic science, deals on an abstract level with the general properties of systems, regardless of physical form or domain of application. General Systems Theory was founded on the assumption that all kinds of systems had characteristics in common, regardless of their internal nature. Johnson used General System Theory and systems thinking to bring together a body of theoretical constructs, as well as to explain their interrelationships, to identify and describe the mission of nursing. The JBSM provides a framework that is based on her synthesis of the component parts of this system and on a description of the context of relationships with each other (subsystems) and with other systems (environment). Standing in contrast to scientific reductionism, Johnson proposed to view nursing in a holistic manner—a behavioral system. Consistent with systems theory, the JBSM provides an understanding of a system by examining the linkages and interactions between elements that compose the entirety of the system. The paragraphs that follow describe how Johnson incorporated empirical knowledge from other disciplines into the JBSM.

Concepts that Johnson identified and defined in her theory are supported in the literature. She noted that Leitch and Escolona agree that tension produces behavioral changes, and that the manifestation of tension by an individual depends on both internal and external factors (Johnson, 1980). Johnson (1959b) used the work of Selye, Grinker, Simmons, and Wolff to support the idea that specific patterns of behavior are reactions to stressors from biological, psychological, and sociological sources, respectively. Johnson (1961a) suggested a difference in her model from Selye's conception of stress. Johnson's concept of stress "follows rather closely Caudill's conceptualization; that is, that stress is a process in which there is interplay between various stimuli and the defenses erected against them. Stimuli may be positive in that they are present, or negative in that something desired or required is absent" (Johnson, 1961a, pp. 7-8). Selye "conceives stress as 'a state manifested by the specific syndrome which consists of all the nonspecifically induced changes within a biologic system'" (Johnson, 1961a, p. 8).

In *Conceptual Models for Nursing Practice*, Johnson (1980) described seven subsystems that make up her behavioral system. To support the attachment-affiliative subsystem, she cited the work of Ainsworth and Robson. Heathers, Gerwitz, and Rosenthal have described and explained dependency behavior, another subsystem defined by Johnson. The response systems of ingestion and elimination, as described by Walike, Mead, and Sears, are also parts of Johnson's Behavioral System. The works of Kagan and Resnik were used to support the sexual subsystem. The aggressive-protective subsystem, which functions to protect and preserve, is supported by Lorenz and Feshbach (Feshbach, 1970; Johnson, 1980; Lorenz, 1966). According to Atkinson, Feather, and Crandell, physical, creative, mechanical, and social skills are manifested by achievement behavior, another subsystem identified by Johnson (1980).

The restorative subsystem was developed by faculty and clinicians in order to include behaviors such as sleep, play, and relaxation (Grubbs, 1980). Although Johnson (personal communication, 1996) agreed that "there may be more or fewer subsystems" than were originally identified, she did not support restorative as a subsystem of the Behavioral System Model. She believed that sleep is primarily a biological force, not a motivational behavior. She suggested that many of the behaviors identified in infants during their first years of life, such as play, are actually achievement behaviors. Johnson (personal communication, 1996) stated that there was a need to examine the possibility of an eighth subsystem that addresses explorative behaviors; further investigation may delineate it as a subsystem separate from the achievement subsystem.

MAJOR ASSUMPTIONS

Nursing

Nursing's goal is to maintain and restore the person's behavioral system balance and stability or to help the person achieve a more optimum level of balance and functioning. Thus, nursing, as perceived by Johnson, is an external force that acts to preserve the organization and integration of the patient's behavior to an optimal level by means of imposing temporary regulatory or control mechanisms or by providing resources while the patient is experiencing stress or behavioral system imbalance (Brown, 2006). An art and a science, nursing supplies external assistance both before and during system balance disturbance and therefore requires knowledge of order, disorder, and control (Herbert, 1989; Johnson, 1980). Nursing activities do not depend on medical authority, but they are complementary to medicine.

Person

Johnson (1980) viewed the person as a behavioral system with patterned, repetitive, and purposeful ways of behaving that link the person with the environment.

The conception of the person is basically a motivational one. This view leans heavily on Johnson's acceptance of ethology theories, which suggest that innate, biological factors influence the patterning and motivation of behavior. She also acknowledged that prior experience, learning, and physical and social stimuli also influence behavior. She noted that to look at a person as a behavioral system, as well as to be able to see a collection of behavioral subsystems and be knowledgeable about the physiological, psychological, and sociocultural factors operating outside them, was a prerequisite to using this model (author's class notes, 1971).

Johnson identified several assumptions that are critical to understanding the nature and operation of the person as a behavioral system. We assume that there is organization, interaction and interdependency, and integration of the parts of behavior that make up the system. An individual's specific response patterns form an organized and integrated whole. The interrelated and interdependent parts are called *subsystems.* Johnson (1977) further assumed that the behavioral system tends to achieve balance among the various forces operating within and upon it. People strive continually to maintain a behavioral system balance and steady states by more or less automatic adjustments and adaptations to the natural forces impinging upon them. Johnson also recognized that people actively seek new experiences that may temporarily disturb balance.

Johnson further (1977, 1980) assumed that a behavioral system, which both requires and results in some degree of regularity and constancy in behavior, is essential to human beings. Finally, Johnson (1977) assumed that behavioral system balance reflected adjustments and adaptations by the person that are successful in some way and to some degree. This will be true even though the observed behavior may not always match cultural norms for acceptable or health behavior.

Balance is essential for effective and efficient functioning of the person. Balance is developed and maintained within the subsystems(s) or the system as a whole. Changes in the structure or function of a system are related to problems with drive, lack of functional requirements/sustenal imperatives, or a change in the environment. A person's attempt to reestablish balance may require an extraordinary expenditure of energy that leaves a shortage of energy to assist biological processes and recovery.

Health

Johnson perceived health as an elusive, dynamic state influenced by biological, psychological, and social factors. Health is reflected by the organization, interaction, interdependence, and integration of the subsystems of the behavioral system (Johnson, 1980). An individual attempts to achieve a balance in this system, which will lead to functional behavior. A lack of balance in the structural or functional requirements of the subsystems leads to poor health. Thus, when evaluating "health," one focuses on the behavioral system and system balance and stability, effective and efficient functioning, and behavioral system imbalance and instability. The outcomes of behavior system balance are as follows: (1) a minimum expenditure of energy is required (implying that more energy is available to maintain health, or, in the case of illness, that energy is available for the biological processes needed for recovery); (2) continued biological and social survival are ensured; and (3) some degree of personal satisfaction accrues (Grubbs, 1980; Johnson 1980).

Environment

In Johnson's theory, the environment consists of all the factors that are not part of the individual's behavioral system, but that influence the system. The nurse may manipulate some aspects of the environment so that the goal of health or behavioral system balance can be achieved for the patient (Brown, 2006).

The behavioral system "determines and limits the interaction between the person and their environment and establishes the relationship of the person to the objects, events and situations in the environment" (Johnson, 1978). Such behavior is orderly and predictable. It is maintained because it has been functionally efficient and effective most of the time in managing the person's relationship to the environment. It changes when this is no longer the case, or when the person desires a more optimum level of functioning. The behavioral system has many tasks and missions to perform in maintaining its own integrity and in managing the system's relationship to its environment.

The behavioral system attempts to maintain equilibrium in response to environmental factors by adjusting and adapting to the forces that impinge on it. Excessively strong environmental forces disturb the behavioral system balance and threaten the person's stability. An unusual amount of energy is required for the system to reestablish equilibrium in the face of continuing forces (Loveland-Cherry & Wilkerson, 1983).

The environment is also the source of the sustenal imperatives of protection, nurturance, and stimulation that are necessary prerequisites to maintaining health (behavioral system balance) (Grubbs, 1980). When behavioral system imbalance (disequilibrium) occurs, the nurse may need to become the temporary regulator of the environment and provide the person's supply of functional requirements, so the person can adapt to stressors. The type of functional requirements and the amount needed will vary by such variables as age, gender, culture coping ability, and type and severity of illness.

THEORETICAL ASSERTIONS

The Johnson Behavioral System Theory addresses the metaparadigm concepts of person, environment, and nursing. The person is a behavioral system with seven interrelated subsystems (Figure 18-1). Each subsystem is formed of a set of behavioral responses, or responsive tendencies, or action systems that share a common drive or goal. Organized around drives (some type of intra-organismic motivational structure), these responses are differentiated, developed, and modified over time through maturation, experience, and learning. They are determined developmentally and are governed continuously by a multitude of physical, biological, and psychological factors operating in a complex and interlocking fashion.

Each subsystem can be described and analyzed in terms of structural and functional requirements. The four structural elements that have been identified include the following: (1) drive or goal—the ultimate consequence of behaviors in it; (2) set—a tendency or predisposition to act in a certain way. Set is subdivided into two types: preparatory, or what a person usually attends to, and perseverative, the habits that one maintains in a situation; (3) choice—represents the behavior a patient sees herself as being able to use in any given situation; and (4) action—or the behavior of an individual (Grubbs, 1980; Johnson, 1980). Set plays a major role both in the choices persons consider and in their ultimate behavior. Each of the seven subsystems has the same three functional requirements: (1) protection, (2) nurturance, and (3) stimulation. These functional requirements must be met through the person's own efforts, or with the outside assistance of the nurse. For the subsystems to develop and maintain stability, each must have a constant supply of these functional requirements that usually are supplied by the environment. However, during illness or when the potential for illness poses a threat, the nurse may become a source of functional requirements.

The responses by the subsystems are developed through motivation, experience, and learning and are influenced by biological, psychological, and social factors (Johnson, 1980). The behavioral system attempts to achieve balance by adapting to internal and environmental stimuli. The behavioral system is made up of "all the patterned, repetitive, and purposeful ways of behaving that characterize each man's life" (Johnson, 1980, p. 209). This functional unit of behavior "determines and limits the interaction of the person and his environment and establishes the relationship of the person with the objects, events, and situations in his environment" (Johnson, 1980, p. 209). "The behavioral system manages its relationship with its environment" (Johnson, 1980, p. 209). The behavioral system appears to be active and not passive. The nurse is external to and interactive with the behavioral system.

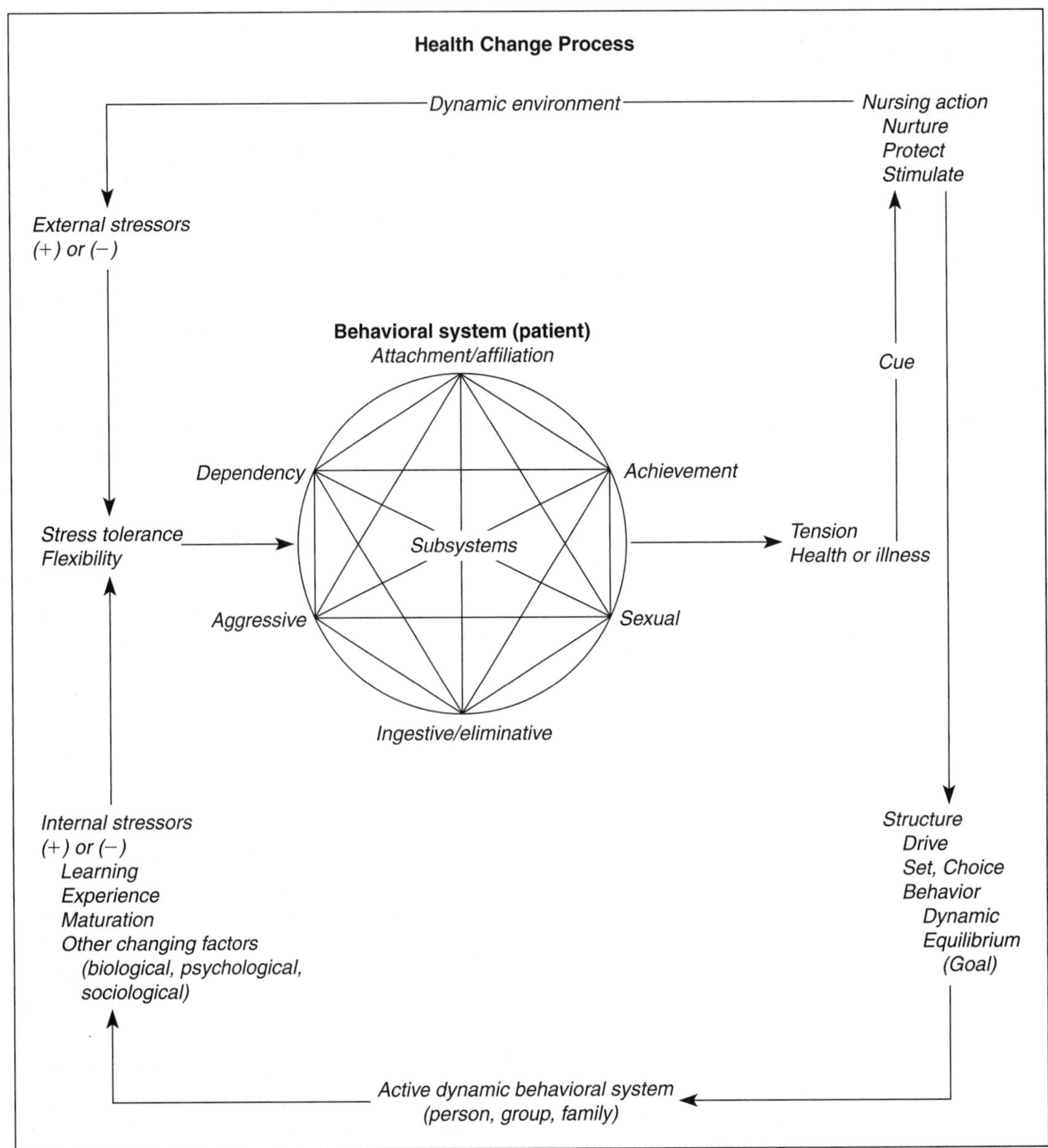

Figure 18-1 Johnson's Behavioral System Model. (Conceptualized by Jude A. Magers, Indianapolis, IN.)

Successful use of the Johnson's Behavioral System Theory in clinical practice requires the incorporation of the nursing process. The clinician must develop an assessment instrument that incorporates the components of the theory, so they are able to assess the patient as a behavioral system to determine if there is an actual or perceived threat of illness, and to determine the person's ability to adapt to illness or threat of illness without developing behavioral system imbalance. This means developing appropriate questions and observations for each of the behavioral subsystems.

A state of instability in the behavioral system results in a need for nursing intervention. Identification of the source of the problem in the system leads to appropriate nursing action that results in the maintenance or restoration of behavioral system balance (Brown, 2006). Nursing interventions can occur in such general forms as (1) repairing structural units; (2) temporarily imposing external regulatory or control measures; (3) supplying environmental conditions or resources; or (4) providing stimulation to the extent that any problem can be anticipated, and preventive nursing action is in order (Johnson, 1978). "If the source of the problem has a structural stressor, the nurse will focus on either the goal, set, choice, or action of the subsystem. If the problem is one of function, the nurse will focus on the source and sufficiency of the functional requirements since functional problems originate from an environmental excess or deficiency" (Grubbs, 1980, p. 242). The goal of nursing is to maintain or restore the person's behavioral system balance and stability, or to help the person achieve a more optimum level of behavioral system functioning when this is desired and possible (Johnson, 1978).

LOGICAL FORM

Johnson approached the task of delineating nursing's mission from historical, analytical, and empirical perspectives. Both deductive and inductive systems thinking is evident throughout the process of developing the Johnson Behavioral System Theory. A system, inasmuch as it is a whole, will lose its synergetic properties if it is decomposed. Understanding must therefore progress from the whole to its parts—a synthesis. Johnson first identified the behavioral system and then explained the properties and behavior of the system. Finally, she explained the properties and behavior of the subsystems as a part or function of the system. The analysis gave us description and knowledge, while the systems thinking (synthesis) gave us an explanation and understanding.

ACCEPTANCE BY THE NURSING COMMUNITY

Practice

The utility of the Johnson Behavioral System Theory is evident from the variety of clinical settings and age groups in which the theory has been used. It has been used in inpatient, outpatient, and community settings, as well as in nursing administration. It has been used with a variety of client populations, and several practice tools have been developed (Fawcett, 2005).

Johnson does not use the term *nursing process*. Assessment, disorders, treatment, and evaluation are concepts referred to in a variety of Johnson's works. "For the practitioner, conceptual models provide a diagnostic and treatment orientation, and thus are of considerable practical import" (Johnson, 1968, p. 2). The nursing process becomes applicable in the Behavioral System Model when behavioral malfunction occurs "that is in part disorganized, erratic, and dysfunctional. Illness or other sudden internal or external environmental change is most frequently responsible for such malfunctions" (Johnson, 1980, p. 212). "Assistance is appropriate at those times the individual is experiencing stress of a health-illness nature which disturbs equilibrium, producing tension" (Johnson, 1961a, p. 6). However, it is important to note that systems analysis is an important component of systems theory. One monitors outputs from a given subsystem in order to monitor performance. Signs of disequilibrium require one to identify the problem, to further define the problem by gathering data, and to design an intervention to restore equilibrium/balance (Miller, 1965; Jenkins, 1969).

Johnson (1959a) implied that the initial nursing assessment begins when the cue tension is observed and signals disequilibrium. Sources for assessment data include history taking, testing, and structural observations (Johnson, 1980). "The behavioral system is thought to determine and limit the interaction between the person and his environment" (Johnson, 1968, p. 3). This suggests that the accuracy and quantity of the data obtained during nursing assessment are not controlled by the nurse, but by the patient (system). The only observed part of the subsystems structure is behavior. Six internal and external regulators have been identified that "simultaneously influence and are influenced by behavior," including biophysical, psychological, developmental, sociocultural, family, and physical environmental regulators (Randell, 1991, p. 157).

The nurse must be able to access information related to goals, sets, and choices that make up the structural subsystems. "One or more of [these] subsystems is likely to be involved in any episode of illness, whether in an antecedent or a consequential way or simply in association, directly or indirectly with the disorder or its treatment" (Johnson, 1968, p. 3). Accessing the data is critical to accurate statement of the disorder.

Johnson did not define specific disorders, but she did state two general categories of disorders on the basis of their relationship to the biological system (Johnson, 1968).

> Disorders are those which are related tangentially or peripherally to disorder in the biological system; that is, they are precipitated simply by the fact of illness or the situational context of treatment; and . . . those [disorders] which are an integral part of a biological system disorder in that they are either directly associated with or a direct consequence of a particular kind of biological system disorder or its treatment (Johnson, 1968, p. 7).

The "means of management" or interventions do consist in part of the provision of nurturance, protection, and stimulation (Johnson, 1968, 1980). The nurse may provide "temporary imposition of external regulatory and control mechanisms, such as inhibiting ineffective behavioral responses, and assisting the patient to acquire new responses" (Johnson, 1968, p. 6). Johnson (1980) suggested that techniques include "teaching, role modeling, and counseling" (p. 211). If a problem or a disorder is anticipated, preventive nursing action is appropriate with adequate methods (Johnson, 1980). Nurturance, protection, and stimulation are as important for preventive nursing care or health promotion as they are for managing illness (Brown, 2006).

If the problem is a structural stressor, the nurse will focus on goal, set, choice, or action of the subsystem. The nurse could work to redirect the person's goals, change drive significance, and broaden the range of choices considered, thus altering the set, or changing the action. The nurse manipulates the structural units, or imposes temporary controls. Both types of nursing actions regulate the interaction of the subsystems.

The outcome of nursing intervention is behavioral system equilibrium. "More specifically, equilibrium can be said to have been achieved at that point at which the individual demonstrates a degree of constancy in his pattern of functioning, both internally and interpersonally" (Johnson, 1961a, p. 9). The evaluation of the nursing intervention is based on whether it made "a significant difference in the lives of the persons involved" (Johnson, 1980, p. 215).

The Behavioral System Model has been operationalized through the development of several assessment instruments. In 1974, Grubbs (1980) used the theory to develop an assessment tool and a nursing process sheet based on Johnson's seven subsystems. Questions and observations related to each subsystem provided tools with which to collect important data that assist in discovery of other choices of behavior that will enable the patient to accomplish his or her goal of health.

That same year, Holaday (1980) used the theory as a model to develop an assessment tool when caring for hospitalized children. This tool allowed the nurse to describe objectively the child's behavior and to guide nursing action. In expanding the concept of "set," Holaday also identified patterns of maternal behaviors that would indicate an inadequate or poorly functioning set that was eroding to the limited choices of action in responding to the needs of chronically ill infants (1981, 1982).

Derdiarian (1990) investigated patient and nurse satisfaction using two systematic assessment instruments. The Johnson Behavioral System Model was used to develop a self-report and observational instrument to be implemented with the nursing process. The Derdiarian Behavioral System Model instrument included assessment of the restorative subsystem and the seven subsystems advocated by Johnson. The results indicated that implementation of the instruments provided a more comprehensive and systematic approach to assessment and intervention, thereby increasing patient and nurse satisfaction with care.

Lanouette and St-Jacques (1994) used Johnson's model to compare the coping abilities and perceptions of families with premature infants with those of families with full-term infants. The results indicated that positive coping skills were relative to bonding with the infant, using resources, solving problems, and making decisions. Lanouette and St-Jacques suggested that improvement in nursing care practices in nursery, hospital, and community settings might have contributed to this outcome. This supported Johnson's (personal correspondence, 1996) statement that "the effective use of nurturance, protection, and stimulation during maternal contact at birth could significantly reduce the behavioral system problems we see today."

Case studies have documented the use and evaluation of the Johnson Behavioral System Model in clinical practice. In 1980, Rawls used the theory to assess systematically a patient who was facing the loss of function in one arm and hand. Herbert (1989) reported the outcomes of a nursing care plan developed for an elderly stroke patient. Rawls and Herbert concluded that Johnson's theory provided a theoretical base that predicted the results of nursing interventions, formulated standards for care, and administered holistic care. Fruehwirth (1989) found it equally effective in assessing and intervening with a support group for the caregivers of patients with Alzheimer's disease.

Recent studies of nursing practice using Johnson's model have focused on decision making and evaluation of outcomes. Grice (1997) found that the nurse, the patient, and the situational characteristics influenced assessment and decision making for the administration of antianxiety and antipsychotic medication to psychiatric inpatients at certain hours. Benson (1997) conducted a review of research literature on the fear of crime among older adults. The Behavioral System Model was used to describe the "hazards of fear of crime" that could cause disturbances in the ingestive, dependency, achievement, affiliative, and aggressive-protective subsystems (Benson, 1997, p. 26). Patient- and community-focused interventions were presented to improve quality of care and the quality of life of older adults. Brinkley, Ricker, and Toumey (2007) demonstrated the use of the Johnson Behavioral System Theory with a morbidly obese patient with complex needs.

Lachicotte and Alexander (1990) examined the use of Johnson's Behavioral System Model as a framework for nursing administrators to use when making decisions concerning the management of impaired nurses. They suggested that, by viewing all levels of the environment, the framework encouraged nurse administrators to assess the imbalance in the nursing system when nurse impairment exists, and evaluate the "system's state of balance in relationship to the method chosen to deal with nurse impairment" (Lachicotte & Alexander, 1990, p. 103). The results of the study indicated that nurse administrators preferred an assistive approach when dealing with nurse impairment. It was believed that "when the impaired nurse is confronted and assisted, equilibrium begins to be restored and balance brought back to the system" (Lachicotte & Alexander, 1990, p. 103).

At the University of California, Los Angeles, the Neuropsychiatric Institute and Hospital has used Johnson's Behavioral System Model for many years as the basis for their psychiatric nursing practice (Auger & Dee, 1983; Poster et al., 1997). "Patients are assessed and behavioral data are classified by subsystem. Nursing diagnoses are formulated that reflect the nature of the ineffective behavior and its relationship to the regulators in the environment" (Randell, 1991, p. 154). The use of Johnson's theory is also incorporated into the new graduate orientation program (Puntil, 2005). A study comparing the diagnostic labels generated from the Johnson Behavioral System Model with those on the North American Nursing Diagnosis Association list indicated that the Johnson Behavioral System Model was better at distinguishing the problems and the etiology (Randell, 1991).

It has become increasingly important to document nursing care and to demonstrate the effectiveness of the care on patient outcomes. Using Johnson's model, Poster and colleagues (1997) found a positive relationship between nursing interventions and the achievement of patient outcomes at discharge. They concluded that "a nursing theoretical framework made it possible to prescribe nursing care as a distinction from medical care" (Poster et al., 1997, p. 73).

Dee, van Servellen, and Brecht (1998) examined the effects of managed health care on patient outcomes, using Johnson's Behavioral System Model. Upon admission, nurses develop a behavioral profile by assessing the eight subsystems, determine the balance or imbalance of the subsystems, and rate the impact of the six regulators. This profile is used to determine the nursing diagnoses, plan of action, and evaluation of care for each patient. The results of this study indicated significant improvement in the level of functioning upon discharge for patients with shorter hospital stays.

Education

Loveland-Cherry and Wilkerson (1983) analyzed Johnson's theory and concluded that it has utility in nursing education. A curriculum based on a person as a behavioral system would have definite goals and straightforward course planning. Study would center on the patient as a behavioral system and on its dysfunction, which would require use of the nursing process. In addition to an understanding of systems theory, the student would need knowledge from the social and behavioral disciplines and the physical and biological sciences. The model has been used in practice and in educational institutions in the United States, Canada, and Australia (Derdiarian, 1981; Fleming, 1990; Grice, 1997; Hadley, 1970; Harris, 1986; Orb & Reilly, 1991; Puntil, 2005).

Research

Johnson (1968) stated that nursing research would need to "identify and explain the behavioral system disorders which arise in connection with illness, and develop the rationale for the means of management" (p. 7). Johnson believed the task for nurse scientists might follow one of two paths: (1) contributions to the basic understanding of the behavioral system of man, and (2) contributions to the understanding of behavioral system problems and treatment rationale and methodologies. She identified the important areas for research as (1) the study of the behavioral system as a whole, including such issues as stability and change, organization and interaction, and effective regulatory and control mechanisms; and (2) study of the subsystems, including the identification of additional subsystems (Class Notes, 1971). She also recommended the study of behavioral system disorders. More progress has been made in this area than in any other.

Small (1980) used Johnson's theory as a conceptual framework when caring for visually impaired children. By evaluating and comparing the perceived body image and spatial awareness of normally sighted children with those of visually impaired children, Small found that the sensory deprivation of visual impairment affected the normal development of the child's body image and his awareness of his body in space. She concluded that when the human system is subjected to excessive stress, the goals of the system cannot be maintained.

Wilkie, Lovejoy, Dodd, and Tesler (1988) examined cancer pain control behaviors using Johnson's Behavioral System Model. The results of the study demonstrated that persons used known behaviors to protect themselves from high-intensity pain. This supported the assumption that "aggressive/protective subsystem behaviors are developed and modified over time to protect the individual from pain and these behaviors represent some of the patient's pain control choices" (Wilkie et al., 1988, p. 729).

These findings were supported in a recent study that examined the "meanings associated with self-report and self-management decision-making" of cancer patients with metastatic bone pain (Coward & Wilkie, 2000, p. 101). Pain provided an incentive to seek treatment from healthcare providers; therefore, it was a protective mechanism. Yet the results indicated that most of the cancer patients did not take pain medication as often as prescribed and preferred nonpharmacological methods, such as positioning or distraction, as their pain control choices.

Believing that the model had potential in preventive care, Majesky, Brester, and Nishio (1978) used it to construct a tool to measure patient indicators of nursing care. Holaday (1980), Rawls (1980), and Stamler (1971) have conducted research using one subsystem. Derdiarian (1991) examined the relationships between the aggressive and protective subsystem and the other subsystems. Her findings supported the proposition that the subsystems are interactive, interdependent, and integrated; therefore, Derdiarian supported Johnson's contention that "changes in a subsystem resulting from illness cannot be well understood without understanding their relationship to changes in the other subsystems" (Johnson, 1980, p. 219).

Damus (1980) tested the validity of Johnson's theory by comparing serum alanine aminotransferase (ALT) values in patients who had various nursing diagnoses and had been exposed to hepatitis B. Damus correlated the physiological disorder of elevated ALT values with behavioral disequilibrium and found that disorder in one area reflected disorder in another area.

Nurse researchers have demonstrated the usefulness of Johnson's theory in clinical practice. Most of these studies have been conducted with individuals with long-term illnesses or chronic illnesses, such as those with urinary incontinence, chronic pain, cancer, acquired immunodeficiency syndrome, and psychiatric illnesses (Bhaduri & Jain, 2004; Colling, Owen, McCreedy, & Newman, 2003; Coward & Wilkie, 2000; Derdiarian, 1988; Derdiarian & Schobel, 1990; Grice, 1997; Holaday, Turner-Henson & Swan, 1996; Holaday & Turner-Henson, 1987). Studies have documented the effectiveness of using the model with children, adolescents, and the elderly population. Based on extensive practice, instrument development, and research, Holaday (1980) concluded that the user of Johnson's theory was provided with a guide for planning and giving care based on scientific knowledge

FURTHER DEVELOPMENT

Johnson (1982) acknowledged that the knowledge base for the use of her model was incomplete, and offered a challenge to researchers to complete her work. She thought that the directions provided by the model for curriculum development were clear. However, the gaps in knowledge also offered challenges for educators, as well as for practitioners. Johnson (1989) also identified a dream for nursing's growth as a scientific discipline. "Since we have specified nursing's special contribution to patient—our explicit, ideal goal in patient care, nursing's growth as a scientific discipline should be rapid—even explosive. When our scientists have the general conception of the realm in which we work, i.e., the phenomena of interest to the profession and the kinds of questions to be asked, it will be possible for them to work together in a systematic fashion to build a cumulative body of knowledge."

Primarily, the theory has been associated with individuals. However, Johnson believed that groups of individuals, such as families and communities, could be considered groups of interactive behavioral systems. Use of her theory with families and other groups needs more visibility (Johnson, 1965). The development of family and community assessment instruments based on the Johnson theory would be useful.

As a result of the current emphasis on health promotion and maintenance and illness and injury prevention, theory could be derived from the model recognizing behavioral disorders in these areas. This could be an important area for further development.

It should be noted that preventive nursing (to prevent behavioral system disorder) is not the same as preventive medicine (to prevent biological system disorders), and disorders in both cases must be identified and explicated before approaches to prevention can be developed. At this point, not even medicine has developed very many specific preventive measures (immunizations for some infectious diseases and protection against some vitamin deficiency diseases are notable exceptions). A number of general approaches to better health, including adequate nutrition, safe water, and exercise, are applicable, contributing to prevention of some disorders. It is small wonder that preventive nursing remains to be developed; this is true no matter what model or theory for nursing is used (D. Johnson, personal correspondence, 1984).

Riegel (1989) reviewed the literature to identify major factors that predict "cardiac crippled behaviors or dependency following a myocardial infarction" (p. 74). Social support, self-esteem, anxiety, depression, and perceptions of functional capacity were considered the primary factors affecting psychological adjustment to chronic coronary heart disease. This emphasized the effect of social support or nurturing on the structure and function of the dependency subsystem. Johnson stated, "If care takers were aware of how their behaviors and family behaviors interact with patients to encourage dependency behaviors at the beginning of illness, they could easily prevent many dysfunctional problems" (personal communication, 1996).

Further development could identify nursing actions that would facilitate appropriate functioning of the system toward disease prevention and health maintenance. Rather than expending energy developing nursing interventions in response to the consequences of disequilibrium, nurses need to learn how to identify precursors of disequilibrium and respond with preventive interventions.

Assuming that a community is a geographical area, a subpopulation, or any aggregate of people, and assuming that a community can benefit from nursing interventions, the behavioral system framework can be applied to community health. A community can be described as a behavioral system with interacting subsystems that have structural elements and functional requirements. For example, mothers of chronically ill children have functional requirements that are needed to maintain stability within the achievement subsystem. Environmental factors such as "economic, educational, and employment influence mothers' caretaking skills" (Turner-Henson, 1992, p. 97).

Communities have goals, norms, choices, and actions, and they need protection, nurturance, and stimulation. The community reacts to internal and external stimuli, and this leads to functional or dysfunctional behavior. An example of an external stimulus is health policy, and an example of dysfunctional behavior is a high infant mortality rate. The behavioral system consists of yet undefined subsystems that are organized, interacting, interdependent, and integrated. Physical, biological, and psychosocial factors also affect community behavior.

Finally, future development of the Johnson Behavioral System Theory needs to incorporate advances in the field of systems theory. Significant advances in the use of systems theory have occurred since Johnson developed her theory. One such advancement occurred in the area of system dynamics (Lance, 1999; Wolstenholme, 1990). System dynamics researchers, over the past four decades, have convincingly demonstrated that people's information processing capacity is limited, and that humans employ bias and heuristics (e.g., anchoring and using the available heuristic) to process information and to reduce mental effort. Groups display the same bias (Hogarth, 1987; Vennix, Gubbels, Post, & Poppen, 1990). Research in the area of cognitive maps has illustrated the restricted character of human information processing. People seem to experience difficulty in thinking in terms of causal nets. Research has demonstrated that people tend to ignore feedback processes (Dorner, 1980).

This body of research offers some useful insights for the study of the Ingestive subsystem. How do clients process information and construct the models of reality (set) that guide their decision making (choice and action)? What potential problems/deficiencies in a client's set could be identified from a nursing assessment that incorporated tenets from system dynamics? Research could lead to the development of effective assessment instruments to use in clinical settings.

The research in systems dynamics also provides some ideas for nursing interventions to test with our clients. System dynamicists have found that model building with clients (using flow charts and diagrams) is helpful in improving information processing. This is based on the premise that diagramming helps with information processing (set and choice), especially with complex topics. They have also found that using simulation and training in facilitation (asking questions that foster reflection and learning, good process structuring of questions and materials) is effective (Vennix et al., 1990; Huz, Andersen, Richardson, & Boothroyd, 1997). If a diagnosis of insufficiency or discrepancy in the Ingestive subsystem were made, would these same types of interventions be helpful?

Holden (2005) noted that complexity science builds on the tradition in nursing that views clients and nursing care from a systems perspective. Complexity science seeks to understand complex adaptive systems (Miller & Page, 2007; Rickles, Hawe, & Shiell, 2007). Complex adaptive systems are a "collection of individual agents with the freedom to act in ways that are not totally predictable and whose actions are interconnected so that one agent's actions change the context for other agents" (Plsek & Greenhaligh, 2001. p. 625). The Johnson Behavioral Systems Theory emphasized the connections and interactions within a systems paradigm. The use of complexity science could expand our understanding of the environmental context and the lifestyle-related and chronic health problems we face today. Complexity science, like Johnson's System Theory, indicates that a flexible range of interventions are essential to respond to healthcare issues. Conditions such as obesity, chronic pain, and diabetes have multiple interrelating influences such as lifestyle and social and cultural contexts, and the way forward is not easily reduced to one uniform solution. Principles form complex adaptive systems theory and Johnson's Behavioral System Theory could be used jointly to examine healthcare issues, allowing new and revised insights to emerge.

CRITIQUE

Simplicity

Johnson's theory is comprehensive and broad enough in scope to include all areas of nursing practice, as well as to provide guidelines for research and education. Yet, the theory is relatively simple in relation to the number of concepts. A person is described as a behavioral system composed of seven subsystems. Nursing is an external regulatory force. However, the theory is potentially complex because there area number of possible interrelationships among the behavioral system, its subsystems, and the environment of the potential relationships being explored therefore, more empirical work is needed (Brown, 2006).

Generality

Johnson's theory has been used extensively with people who are ill or who face the threat of illness. Its use with families, groups, and communities is limited. Johnson perceived a person as a behavioral system comprised of seven subsystems, aggregates of interactive behavioral systems. Initially, Johnson did not clearly address nonillness situations or preventive nursing (D. Johnson, curriculum vitae, 1984). In later publications, Johnson (1992) emphasized the role of nurses in preventive health care for individuals and for society. She stated, "Nursing's special responsibility for health is derived from its unique social mission. Nursing needs to concentrate on developing preventive nursing to fulfill its social obligations" (Johnson, 1992, p. 26).

Empirical Precision

Empirical precision is achieved by identifying empirical indicators for the theory because the model contains abstract concepts. Empirical precision improves when the subconcepts and the relationships between and among them become better defined, and empirical indicators are introduced to the science. The units and the relationships between the units in Johnson's theory are consistently defined and used. Thus far, an adequate degree of empirical precision has been demonstrated in research using Johnson's theory. Although some of Johnson's writings used terms such as *balance, stability,* and *equilibrium, adjustments and adaptations, disturbances, disequilibrium,* and *behavior disorders* interchangeably, the programs of research of Dee, Deridarian, Holaday, Lovejoy, and Poster operationally defined terms and were consistent in their use. The clarity of these definitions and the clarity of the definitions of the subsystems have added to the theory's empirical precision (Brown, 2006).

Derivable Consequences

Johnson's theory guides nursing practice, education, and research; generates new ideas about nursing; and differentiates nursing from other health professions. By focusing on behavior rather than biology, the theory clearly differentiates nursing from medicine, although the concepts overlap with those of the psychosocial professions.

Johnson's Behavioral System Model provides a conceptual framework for nursing education, practice, and research. The theories derived from the model have directed questions for nursing research. It has been analyzed and judged to be appropriate as a basis for the development of a nursing curriculum. Practitioners and patients have judged the resulting nursing actions to be satisfactory (Johnson, 1980). The theory has potential for continued utility in nursing to achieve valued nursing goals.

SUMMARY

Johnson's Behavioral System Model describes the person as a behavioral system with seven subsystems: the achievement, attachment-affiliative, aggressive-protective, dependency, ingestive, eliminative, and sexual subsystems. Each of the seven subsystems is interrelated with the others and with the environment and specific structural elements and functions to maintain the integrity of the behavioral system. Other nurse scholars added the restorative subsystem. The structural components of the behavioral system describe how individuals are motivated (drive) to obtain specified goals using the individual's predisposition to act in certain ways (set) and using available choices to produce an action or patterned behavior. The functional requirements/sustenal imperatives protect, nurture, and stimulate the behavioral system. When the behavioral system has balance and stability, the individual's behaviors will be purposeful, organized, and predictable. Imbalance and instability in the behavioral system occur when tension and stressors affect the relationship of the subsystems or the internal and external environments.

Nursing is an external regulatory force that acts to restore balance and stability by inhibiting, stimulating, or reinforcing certain behaviors (control mechanisms), changing the structural components (patient goals, choices, actions), or fulfilling function requirements. Health is the result of the behavioral system stability, balance, and equilibrium (Johnson, 1980).

Johnson's ultimate goals were directed toward nursing practice, a curriculum for schools of nursing, and the development of nursing science. She wanted the Johnson Behavioral System Model to successfully generate and disseminate nursing science, to systematize nursing interventions that were ethically reflective, to take into account multiple perspectives, and to be sensitive to society's values. It was her hope that the Johnson Behavioral System Model was a framework that she could leave to future generations of nurses (personal communication, 1991).

Case Study

A 67-year-old man is admitted to the hospital for diagnostic tests after experiencing severe abdominal pain and streaks of blood in his stool. He is alert and oriented. He has a history of type II diabetes and hypertension. His blood glucose level is 187 mg/dl, and blood pressure is 188/100 mm Hg. He is 5′10″ and weighs 145 pounds. He is currently taking antihypertensive, anticoagulant, antiinflammatory, and antidiabetic medications.

His recent history reveals that he had an acute cerebral vascular accident (CVA) 6 weeks ago that resulted in partial paralysis and numbness of the right arm and leg, expressive aphasia, and slurred speech. He completed 4 weeks of inpatient rehabilitation and is able to walk short distances with a cane and moderate assistance. He is weak and becomes fatigued quickly. Although he can move his right arm, he guards it because of pain with movement. He receives acetaminophen (Extra Strength Tylenol) for his right arm prior to therapy and before sleep. He also continues to exhibit slight expressive aphasia. He is anxious about continuing his therapy and indicates concern about missing his appointment with the orthopedic physician who was to evaluate his right arm. He reports that food doesn't taste right anymore, and he has no appetite. With encouragement from his family, he eats small portions of each meal and drinks fluids without difficulty.

The patient is a college graduate who recently retired. He has been married for 45 years and has two adult children who live in the same city. He is a leader in the church and social community. His family and friends visit him frequently in the hospital. He is cheerful and attempts to talk with them when they visit. When he doesn't have visitors, he sits quietly in a dark room or sleeps. He is tearful each time his family hugs him before leaving. He expresses appreciation for each visit and apologizes each time he "gets emotional."

Behavioral Assessment

Using Johnson's Behavioral System Model, the following behavioral assessment is identified:

- *Achievement:* The patient has achieved many developmental goals of adulthood. He is relearning how to do activities of daily living (ADLs), walk, and talk, as well as other cognitive-motor skills such as reading, writing, and speaking.
- *Attachment-affiliative:* The patient is married with two adult children who are supportive and live in the same city. He has many friends and social contacts who visit frequently.
- *Aggressive-protective:* The patient worries about his wife traveling to the hospital at night, and he worries that she doesn't eat well while staying with him in the hospital.
- *Dependency:* His recent stroke, resulting in decreased use of his right arm and leg, has affected his mobility and independent completion of ADLs. His potential for falling, inability to feel his arm or leg if injured, and weakness are safety concerns. His wife has taken on the financial and home maintenance responsibilities.
- *Ingestive:* Since the stroke, the patient has had a decreased appetite. He has lost 20 pounds in 6 weeks. Studies reveal no swallowing difficulties. He is able to feed himself with his left hand but needs assistance with cutting foods.
- *Eliminative:* The patient is able to urinate without difficulty in a urinal but prefers to walk to the bathroom. He becomes constipated easily because of decreased fluid and food intake.
- *Sexual:* There are changes in the patient's sexual relationship with his wife caused by pain, limited use of his right side, and fatigue.

Environmental Assessment

The assessment of internal and external environmental factors indicates that several are creating tension and are threatening the balance and stability of the behavioral system. This hospitalization and diagnostic testing add additional stress to the already weakened biological and psychological stability of the behavioral system. The stroke produced several physical and cognitive impairments that affect independence, self-care, learning, maturation, and socialization. Hospitalization at this time can delay or decrease the prognosis of the patient's physical and speech rehabilitation. He will need assistance to move safely in the hospital environment.

The patient and his wife are active in their church and participate in many social activities. The patient taught classes in Sunday school. Recent illnesses, hospitalizations, and fatigue have decreased his ability to participate in previous activities. Although he has adapted to his right-sided weakness and decreased motor function by performing his ADLs with his left hand and walking with a cane, he still needs assistance. The patient and his wife live in a suburban neighborhood. Family members installed a ramp to facilitate access to the home. His wife states that neighbors watch the house when she is away and watch for her return to be sure she is safe.

Structural Components

- *Drive or goal:* The patient seems motivated to complete the diagnostic tests and return home. He is eager to get back into his outpatient rehabilitation program. It seems equally important for him to decrease stress on his wife. His wife provides positive encouragement and support for him. He looks to her for assistance with decisions.
- *Set:* It is evident that the patient is accustomed to making his own decisions and being a leader. It is also evident that he is accustomed to conferring with his wife to ensure that she is comfortable with decisions being made.
- *Choice:* Although the patient agrees to the diagnostic tests, he is no longer in pain and has had no bleeding since his hospitalization. Therefore, he is more focused on achieving his rehabilitation goals. He initiates activities and seeks assistance from his family in walking to the bathroom, walking in the hall, and completing his ADLs.
- *Actions:* The patient socializes with visitors and family by actively participating in conversations. He requests assistance as needed for physical and cognitive needs. He asks for prayers from his family and friends for spiritual guidance in managing his illness.

Functional Requirements

The patient needs outside assistance for all three functional requirements, including protection, nurturance, and stimulation. His inability to feel his right side and his impaired mobility increase his potential for injury. Protective devices such as hand bars and a shower chair can be used. The patient needs assistance with preparing meals but has adapted to using his left hand for eating and drinking. Socialization and performance expectations at the outpatient rehabilitation facility are important methods of providing stimulation for the patient. Stimulation is also provided by friends and family who visit the patient. Continued social stimulation is vital for this patient, because he has difficulty understanding other forms of stimulation such as radio, television, and reading.

Nursing

Nursing actions are external regulatory forces that should protect, stimulate, and nurture to preserve the organization and integration of the patient's behavioral system. Nursing actions for this patient should focus on providing explanations of diagnostic tests to be performed and the results of the tests. Identification of favorite foods and encouragement of small frequent meals with sufficient fluids to prevent constipation will be needed. The nurse should advocate for inpatient physical and speech therapy to stimulate functional abilities and reinforce the patient's achievement behaviors to decrease dependency requirements. It will be equally important to encourage ongoing socialization with friends and family. The patient and his wife will need support and teaching to identify methods of adapting to and managing system imbalance and instability and to identify actions that will enhance behaviors to create system balance and stability.

CRITICAL THINKING Activities

1. Select a patient from your clinical practice and one or two of Johnson's subsystems where there is evidence of behavioral system imbalance or the threat of loss of order, and answer the following questions:
   a. What observation indicates that there is a behavioral system imbalance or the threat of the loss of order for the subsystem(s)?
   b. Consider the patient's set. What did the patient focus on in the situation?
   c. Consider the patient's choices. Did the patient consider a range of behaviors for the situation? What role did the patient's set play in his choice of behavior?
   d. What behaviors (actions) did you see and how often? What level of intensity?
   e. What were the sources of nurturance, protection, and stimulation for the

actual or desired behavior(s)? Was the source consistent and sufficient?

f. What diagnoses did you make? Describe your intervention(s).

2. After completing activity number one, reflect on the ways the model influenced your assessment, the description of the problem, and your diagnosis. What insights did using the theory provide for you about the patient?
3. Consider the use of Johnson's model for preventive care in a community setting. What strengths and limitations might you encounter?

POINTS FOR *Further Study*

- Cardinal Stritch University Library http://library.stritch.edu/research/subjects/nursingtheorists/overview.htm
- Clayton State University http://nursing.clayton.edu/eichelberger/nursing.htm
- Nursing Theory Web page—type in "Dorothy Johnson" http://www.nursingtheory.net
- Vanderbilt Medical Center http://www.mc.vanderbilt/edu/biolib/hc/biopages/djohnson.html
- Dorothy Johnson, (1988) Portraits of Excellence: The Nurse Theorists, video/DVD, available from Athens, Ohio: Fitne, Inc.
- Vanderbilt University, Eskind Biomedical Library Historical Collections, has a complete set of Dorothy Johnson's published and unpublished papers, personal correspondence, and photographs.
- Lian, H. (2007). Chinese culture versus Western medicine: Health implications for San Francisco elder Chinese immigrants with heart failure. Unpublished doctoral dissertation, Walden University. AAT 3258410.
- Holaday, B. (2006). Johnson's behavioral system model in nursing practice. In M. R. Alligood & A. M. Tomey, Eds. (pp. 157-180), Nursing theory: Utilization & application. Philadelphia; Mosby Elsevier.
- Wilmoth, M. C. (2007). Sexuality: A critical component of quality of life in chronic disease. *Nursing Clinics of North America*, 42(4): 507-514

REFERENCES

Auger, J.A. & Dee, V. (1983). A patient classification system based on the Johnson Behavioral System Model of Nursing: Part 1. *Journal of Nursing Administration*, 38-43.

Benson, S. (1997). The older adult and fear of crime. *Journal of Gerontological Nursing, 23*(10), 24-31.

Bhaduri, M. & Jain, A.G. (2004). Impact of oral cancer and related factors on the quality of life (QOL) patients. *Nursing Journal of India*, 95(6), 129-131.

Brinkley, R. Ricker, K. & Toumey, K. (2007). Esthetic knowing with a hospitalized morbidly obese patient. *Journal of Undergraduate Nursing Scholarship*, 9(1).

Brown, V. M. (2006). Behavioral system model (pp. 386-404). In A. M. Tomey & M.R. Alligood (Eds). *Nursing Theorists and Their Work*, 6th Ed. Philadelphia: Mosby/Elsevier.

Buckley, W. (Ed.) (1968). Modern systems research for the behavioral scientist: A source book, Chicago: Aldine.

Colling, J., Owen, T., McCreedy, M., & Newman, D. (2003). The effects of a continence program on frail community-dwelling elderly persons. *Urologic Nursing, 23*(2), 117-131.

Coward, D. D., & Wilkie, D. J. (2000). Metastatic bone pain: Meanings associated with self-report and self-management decision making. *Cancer Nursing, 23*(2), 101-108.

Damus, K. (1980). An application of the Johnson behavioral system model for nursing practice. In J. P. Riehl & C. Roy (Eds.), *Conceptual models for nursing practice* (2nd ed.). New York: Appleton-Century-Crofts

Dee, V., van Servellen, G., & Brecht, M. (1998). Managed behavioral health care patients and their nursing care problems, level of functioning, and impairment on discharge. *Journal of American Psychiatric Nurses Association, 4*(2), 57-66.

Derdiarian, A. K. (1981). Nursing conceptual frameworks: Implications for education, practice, and research. In D. L. Vredevae, A. K. Deridiarian, L. P. Sama, M. Eriel & J. C. Shipaoff (Eds.) Concepts of oncology nursing. (pp. 369-385). Englewood Cliffs: NJ: Prentice Hall.

Derdiarian, A. K. (1988). Sensitivity of the Derdiarian behavioral system model instrument to age, site, and stage of cancer: A preliminary validation study. *Scholarly Inquiry for Nursing Practice, 2*(2), 103-124.

Derdiarian, A. K. (1990). Effects of using systematic assessment instruments on patient and nurse satisfaction with nursing care. *Oncology Nursing Forum, 17*(1), 95-100.

Derdiarian, A. K. (1991). Effects of using a nursing model-based assessment instrument on quality of nursing care. *Nursing Administration Quarterly, 15*(3), 1-16.

Derdiarian, A, K., & Schobel, D. (1990). Comprehensive assessment of AIDS patients using the behavioral systems model for nursing practice instrument. *Journal of Advanced Nursing, 15*(4), 436-446.

Dorner, D. (1980). On the difficulties people have in dealing with complexity. Simulation and Games, 11(1), 87-106.

Fawcett, J. (2005). Contemporary nursing knowledge: Analysis and Evaluation of Nursing Models and Theories, 2nd Ed. Philadelphia: F. A. Davis.

Feshbach, S. (1970). Aggression. In P. Mussen (Ed.), *Carmichael's manual of child psychology* (3rd ed.). New York: John Wiley & Sons.

Fleming, B. H. (1990). Use of the Johnson model in nursing education (abstract). In Proceedings of the National Theory Conference (pp. 109-111). Los Angeles: UCLA Nursing Department.

Fruehwirth, S. E. S. (1989). An application of Johnson's behavioral model: A case study. *Journal of Community Health Nurse, 6*(2), 61-71.

Grice, S. L. (1997). *Nurses' use of medication for agitation for the psychiatric inpatient.* Unpublished doctoral dissertation, Catholic University of America, Washington, DC.

Grubbs, J. (1980). *An interpretation of the Johnson behavioral system model for nursing practice.* In J. P. Riehl & C. Roy (Eds.). Conceptual models for nursing practice (pp. 217-254). New York: Appleton-Century-Crofts.

Hadley, B. J. (1970). The utility of theoretical frameworks for curriculum development in nursing; the happening at Colorado. Paper presented at WIN (Western Interstate Council of Higher Education in Nursing (March). Honolulu, Hawaii.

Harris, R. B. C. (1986). Introduction of a conceptual model into a baccalaureate course. *Journal of Nursing Education,* 25(1), 66-89.

Herbert, J. (1989). A model for Anna … using the Johnson model of nursing in the care of one 75-year-old stroke patient. *The Journal of Clinical Practice, Education and Management, 3*(42), 30-34.

Hogarth, R. (1987). Judgement and choice, (2nd Ed.). Chichester, UK; Wiley.

Holaday, B. (1980). Implementing the Johnson model for nursing practice (pp. 255-263). In J. P. Riehl & C. Roy (Eds.), *Conceptual models for nursing practice* (2nd ed.). New York: Appleton-Century-Crofts.

Holaday, B. (1981). Maternal response to their chronically ill infant's attachment behavior of crying. *Nursing Research,* 30, 343-348.

Holaday, B. (1982). Maternal conceptual set development: Identifying patterns of maternal response to chronically ill infant crying. *Maternal-Child Nursing Journal,* 11, 47-69.

Holaday, B. & Turner-Henson, A. (1987). Chronically ill school-age children's use of time. *Pediatric Nursing,* 13, 411-414.

Holaday, B., Turner-Henson, A. & Swan, J. (1996). The Johnson Behavioral system model: Explaining activities of chronically ill children. In P. Hinton Walker & B. Neuman (Eds.*), Blueprint for Use of Nursing Models* (pp. 33-63). New York: NLN Press.

Holden, L. M. (2005). Complex adaptive systems: Concept analysis. *Journal of Advanced Nursing,* 52(6), 651-658.

Huz, S., Andersen, D. F, Richardson, G. P. and Boothroyd, R. (1997). A framework for evaluating systems thinking interventions: An experimental approach to mental health system change. *Systems Dynamics Review,* 13(2), 145-169.

Jenkins, G. M. (1969). The systems approach. *Journal of Systems Engineering,* 1(1), 3-49.

Johnson, D. E. (1959a). A philosophy of nursing. *Nursing Outlook, 7,* 198-200.

Johnson, D. E. (1959b). The nature of a science of nursing. *Nursing Outlook, 7,* 291-294.

Johnson, D. E. (1961a). *Nursing's specific goal in patient care.* Unpublished lecture, Faculty Colloquium, School of Nursing, University of California, Los Angeles.

Johnson, D. E. (1961b). *A conceptual basis for nursing care.* Unpublished lecture, Third Conference, C. E. Program, University of California, Los Angeles.

Johnson, D. E. (1965). *Is nursing meeting the challenge of family needs?* Unpublished lecture, Wisconsin League for Nursing, Madison, WI.

Johnson, D. E. (1968). *One conceptual model of nursing.* Unpublished lecture, Vanderbilt University, Nashville, TN.

Johnson, D. E. (1976). The Search for Truth. Paper presented at the installation of officers for the new chapter (Gamma Mu) of Sigma Theta Tau at the University of California, Los Angeles.

Johnson, D. E. (1977). The behavioral system model for nursing. Paper presented at a workshop for Sigma Theta Tau.

Johnson, D. E. (1978). Implications for research—the Johnson Behavioral System Model. Paper presented at the Second Annual Nurse Educator Conference, New York City.

Johnson, D. E. (1980). The behavioral system model for nursing. In J. P. Riehl & C. Roy (Eds.), *Conceptual models for nursing practice* (2nd ed.) (pp. 205-216). New York: Appleton-Century-Crofts.

Johnson, D. E. (1982). The behavioral system model for nursing. Paper presented at Wheeling College, West Virginia.

Johnson, D. E. (1992). Origins of behavioral system model. In F. Nightingale (Ed.), *Notes on nursing* (Commemorative edition, pp. 23-28). Philadelphia: J. B. Lippincott.

Lachicotte, J. L., & Alexander, J. W. (1990). Management attitudes and nurse impairment. *Nursing Management, 21*(9), 102-110.

Lance, D. C. (1999). Social theory and system dynamics practice. *European Journal of Operational Research,* 113(3), 501-527.

Lanouette, M., & St-Jacques, A. (1994). Premature infants and their families. *Canadian Nurse, 90*(9), 36-39.

Lorenz, K. (1966). *On aggression.* New York: Harcourt.

Loveland-Cherry, C., & Wilkerson, S. (1983). Dorothy Johnson's behavioral systems model. In J. Fitzpatrick & A. Whall (Eds.), *Conceptual models of nursing: Analysis and application.* Bowie, MD: Robert J. Brady.

Majesky, S. J., Brester, M. H., & Nishio, K. T. (1978). Development of a research tool: Patient indicators of nursing care. *Nursing Research, 27*(6), 365-371.

Miller, J. G. (1965). Living systems: Basic concepts. Behavioral Science, 10(2), 193-237.

Miller, J. G., & Page, S. E. (2007). Complex adaptive systems: An introduction to computational models of social life. Princeton, NJ: Princeton University Press.

Orb, A., & Reilly, D. E. (1991). Changing to a conceptual base curriculum. *International Nursing Review, 38*(2), 56-60.

Parsons, T. (1951). The social system. Glencoe: Free Press.

Parsons, T. (1964). Societies: Comparative and evolutionary perspectives. Englewood, NJ: Prentice Hall.

Plsek, R., & Greenhaligh, T. T. (2001). Complexity science: The challenge of complexity in health care. *British Medical Journal,* 323, (15 September). 625-628).

Poster, E. C. Dee, V., & Randell, B. P. (1997). The Johnson behavioral systems model as a framework for patient outcome evaluation. *Journal of American Psychiatric Nurses Association 3*(3), 73-80.

Puntil, C. (2005). New graduate orientation program in geriatric psychiatric inpatient setting. *Issues in Mental Health Nursing,* 56(1), 65-80.

Randell, B. P. (1991). NANDA versus the Johnson behavioral systems model: Is there a diagnostic difference? In R. M. Carroll-Johnson (Ed.), *Classification of nursing diagnosis: Proceedings of the ninth conference.* Philadelphia: J. P. Lippincott.

Rawls, A. (1980). Evaluation of the Johnson behavioral model in clinical practice: Report of a test and evaluation of the Johnson theory. *Image: The Journal of Nursing Scholarship, 12,* 13-16.

Rickles, D., Hawe, P, & Shiell, A. (2007). A simple guide to chaos and complexity. *Health,* 61(11), 933-937.

Riegel, B. (1989). Social support and psychological adjustment to chronic coronary heart disease: Operationalization of Johnson's behavioral system model. *ANS Advances in Nursing Science, 11*(2), 74-84.

Small, B. (1980). Nursing visually impaired children with Johnson's model as a conceptual framework. In J. P. Riehl & C. Roy (Eds.), *Conceptual models for nursing practice* (2nd ed.). New York: Appleton-Century-Crofts.

Stamler, C. (1971). Dependency and repetitive visits to nurses' office in elementary school children. *Nursing Research, 20*(3), 254-255.

Sterman, J. D. (1994). Learning in and about complex systems. *Systems Dynamics Review,* 10(2-3), 291-330.

Turner-Henson, A. (1992). *Chronically ill children's mothers' perceptions of environmental variables.* Unpublished doctoral dissertation, University of Alabama at Birmingham.

Vennix, J. A. M., Gubbels, J. W., Post, D., & Poppen, H. J. (1990). A structured approach to knowledge elicitation in conceptual model-building. *Systems Dynamics Review,* 6, 194-208.

Wilkie, D., Lovejoy, N., Dodd, M., & Tesler, M. (1988). Cancer pain control behaviors: Description and correlation with pain intensity. *Oncology Nursing Forum, 15*(6), 723-731.

Wilkie, D. J. (1990). Cancer pain management: State-of-the-art nursing care. *Nursing Clinics of North America, 25*(2), 331-343.

Wilmoth, M. C. (2007). Sexuality: A critical component of quality of life in chronic disease. Nursing Clinics of North America, 42(4): 507-514.

Wilmoth, M. C. & Ross, J. A. (1997). Women's perception: Breast cancer and sexuality. *Cancer Practice,* 5(6), 353-359.

Wolstenholme, E. F. (1990). Systems enquiry: A system dynamics approach. Chichester, UK: Wiley.

BIBLIOGRAPHY

Primary Sources

Book Chapters

Johnson, D. E. (1964, June). Is there an identifiable body of knowledge essential to the development of a generic professional nursing program? In M. Maker (Ed.), *Proceedings of the first interuniversity faculty work conference.* Stowe, VT: New England Board of Higher Education.

Johnson, D. E. (1973). Medical-surgical nursing: Cardiovascular care in the first person. In American Nurses Association, ANA *Clinical Sessions* (pp. 127-134). New York: Appleton-Century-Crofts.

Johnson, D. E. (1976). Foreword. In J. R. Auger (Ed.), *Behavioral systems and nursing.* Englewood Cliffs, NJ: Prentice-Hall.

Johnson, D. E. (1978). State of the art of theory development in nursing. In National League for Nursing, *Theory development: What, why, how?* (NLN Pub. No. 15-1708). New York: National League for Nursing.

Johnson, D. E. (1980). The behavioral system model for nursing. In J. P. Riehl & C. Roy (Eds.), *Conceptual models for nursing practice* (2nd ed.). New York: Appleton-Century-Crofts.

Johnson, D. E. (1990). The behavioral system model for nursing. In M. E. Parker (Ed.), *Nursing theories in practice.* New York: National League for Nursing.

Johnson, D. E. (1992). Origins of behavioral system model. In F. Nightingale (Ed.), *Notes on nursing* (Commemorative ed., pp. 23-28). Philadelphia: J. B. Lippincott.

Journal Articles

Johnson, D. E. (1943, March). Learning to know people. *American Journal of Nursing, 43* 248-252.

Johnson, D. E. (1954). Collegiate nursing education. *College Public Relations Quarterly, 5,* 32-35.

Johnson, D. E. (1959, April). A philosophy of nursing. *Nursing Outlook, 7,* 198-200.

Johnson, D. E. (1959, May). The nature of a science of nursing. *Nursing Outlook, 7*, 291-294.

Johnson, D. E. (1961, Oct.). Patterns in professional nursing education. *Nursing Outlook, 9*, 608-611.

Johnson, D. E. (1961, Nov.). The significance of nursing care. *American Journal of Nursing, 61*, 63-66.

Johnson, D. E. (1962, July/Aug.). Professional education for pediatric nursing. *Children, 9*, 153-156.

Johnson, D. E. (1964, Dec.). Nursing and higher education. *International Journal of Nursing Studies, 1*, 219-225.

Johnson, D. E. (1965, Sept.). Today's action will determine tomorrow's nursing. *Nursing Outlook, 13*, 38-41.

Johnson, D. E. (1965, Oct.). Crying in the newborn infant. *Nursing Science, 3*, 339-355.

Johnson, D. E. (1966, Jan.). Year round programs set the pace in health careers promotion. *Hospitals, 40*, 57-60.

Johnson, D. E. (1966, Oct.). Competence in practice: Technical and professional. *Nursing Outlook, 14*, 30-33.

Johnson, D. E. (1967). Professional practice in nursing. *NLN Convention Papers, 23*, 26-33.

Johnson, D. E. (1967, April). Powerless: A significant determinant in patient behavior? *Journal of Nursing Educators, 6*, 39-44.

Johnson, D. E. (1968). Critique: Social influences on student nurses in their choice of ideal and practiced solutions to nursing problems. *Communicating Nursing Research, 1*, 150-155.

Johnson, D. E. (1968, April). Toward a science in nursing. *Southern Medical Bulletin, 56*, 13-23.

Johnson, D. E. (1968, May/June). Theory in nursing: Borrowed and unique. *Nursing Research, 17*, 206-209.

Johnson, D. E. (1974). Development of theory: A requisite for nursing as a primary health profession. *Nursing Research*, 23, 372-377).

Johnson, D. E. (1974, Sept/Oct). Development of theory: A requisite for nursing as a primary health profession. *Nursing Research, 23*, 372-377.

Johnson, D. E. (1982, Spring). Some thoughts on nursing. *Clinical Nurse Specialist, 3*, 1-4.

Johnson, D. E. (1987, July/Aug.). Evaluating conceptual models for use in critical care nursing practice. *Dimensions of Critical Care Nursing, 6*, 195-197.

Johnson, D. E., Wilcox, J. A., & Moidel, H. C. (1967). The clinical specialist as a practitioner. *American Journal of Nursing, 67*, 2298-2303.

McCaffery, M., & Johnson, D. E. (1967). Effect of parent group discussion upon epistemic responses. *Nursing Research, 16*, 352-358.

*All unpublished papers are available at the Eskind Library, Vanderbilt University, Nashville, TN. Contact the Archives Division.

Secondary Sources

Books

Auger, J. R. (1976). Behavioral systems and nursing. Englewood Cliffs, NJ: Prentice Hall.

Hoeman, S. P. (1996). Conceptual bases for rehabilitation nursing. In S. P. Hoeman (Ed.), *Rehabilitation nursing: Process and application* (2nd ed., p. 7). St. Louis: Mosby.

Johnson, B. M., & Webber, P. B. (2005). An introduction to theory and reasoning in nursing. Philadelphia: Lippincott Williams & Willkins. (Johnson section pp. 141-144.)

Mc Ewin, M. & Wills, E. Mo. (2007). Theoretical basis for nursing, 2nd Ed. Philadelphia: Lippincott Williams & Willkins. (Johnson material pp. 148-152.)

Wesley, R. L. (1995). Nursing theory and models. Springhouse, PA: Springhouse. (Johnson material pp. 64-66; 152-153.

Dissertations

Aita, V. A. (1995). Toward improved practice: Formal prescriptions and informal expressions of compassion in American nursing during the 1950s. Unpublished doctoral dissertation, University of Nebraska Medical Center, Omaha, NE.

Dee, V. (1986). Validation of a patient classification instrument for psychiatric patients based on the Johnson model for nursing. *Dissertation Abstracts International, 47*, 4822B.

Devlin, S. L. (1992). The relationship between nurse managers' and staff nurses' return to school. Unpublished doctoral dissertation, D'Youville College. (ATT1347531).

Grice, S. L. (1997). *Nurses' use of medication for agitation for the psychiatric inpatient.* Unpublished doctoral dissertation, The Catholic University of America, Washington, DC.

Holaday, B. (1979). Maternal response to their chronically ill infant's attachment behavior of crying. Unpublished doctoral dissertation, University of California, San Francisco.

Huang, L. (2007). Chinese culture versus Western medicine: health implications for San Francisco elder Chinese immigrants with heart failure. Unpublished doctoral dissertation, Walden University (ATT3258410).

Litz, H. L. (1998). Smoking cessation: What works best for whom? Unpublished doctoral dissertation, Clarkson College (ATT1391123).

Lovejoy, N. C. (1981). *An empirical verification of the Johnson behavioral system model for nursing.* Unpublished doctoral dissertation, University of Alabama, Birmingham.

Naguib, H. H. (1988). Physicians', nurses' and patients' perceptions of the surgical patients' educational rights. Unpublished doctoral dissertation. University of Alexandria, United Republic of Egypt.

Riegal, B. J. (1991). *Social support and cardiac invalidism following myocardial infarction.* Unpublished doctoral dissertation, University of California, Los Angeles.

Talerico, K. A. (1999). Correlates of aggressive behavioral actions of older adults with dementia. Unpublished doctoral dissertation, University of Pennsylvania (AAT9953602).

Turner-Henson, A. (1992). *Chronically ill children's mothers' perceptions of environmental variables.* Unpublished doctoral dissertation, University of Alabama, Birmingham.

Wilkie, D. (1990). Behavioral correlates of lung cancer pain. Unpublished doctoral dissertation, University of California, San Francisco.

Wilmoth, M. D. (1993). Development and psychometric testing of the sexual behaviors questionnaire. Unpublished doctoral dissertation, University of Pennsylvania (AAT9413929).

Book Chapters

Brown, V. M. (2006). Behavioral system model (pp. 386-404). In A. M. Tomey & M. R. Alligood (Eds.), *Nursing theorists and their work,* (6th Ed.) Philadelphia: Mosby/Elsevier.

Fawcett, J. (1995). Johnson's behavioral systems model. In J. Fawcett (Ed.), *Analysis and evaluation of conceptual models of nursing* (3rd ed., pp. 67-107). Philadelphia: F. A. Davis.

Fawcett, J. (2005). Johnson's behavioral system model. In J. Fawcett (Ed.), Contemporary Nursing Knowledge. *Analysis and evaluation of contemporary knowledge: Nursing models and theories* (2nd Ed.), (pp. 60-87, 104). Philadelphia: F. A. Davis.

Fawcett, J. (2005). Johnson's behavioral system model (pp. 60-87). In J. Fawcett, *Contemporary nursing knowledge: Analysis and evaluation of nursing models and theories.* Philadelphia: F. A. Davis.

Holaday, B. (1997). Johnson's behavioral system model in nursing practice. In M. R. Alligood & A. Marriner Tomey (Eds.), *Nursing theory: Utilization & application* (pp. 49-70). St. Louis: Mosby.

Holaday, B. (2006). Dorothy Johnson's behavioral system model and its applications (pp. 79-93). In M. E. Parker (Ed.) Nursing theories and nursing practice, 2nd Ed. Philadelphia: F. A. Davis.

Holaday, B. (2006). Johnson's behavioral system model in nursing practice. (pp. 157-180). In M. R. Alligood & A. M. Tomey (Eds.). *Nursing theory: utilization and application.* Philadelphia: Mosby Elsevier.

Holaday, B., Turner-Henson, A., & Swan, J. (1996). The Johnson behavioral system model: Explaining activities of chronically ill children. In P. H. Walker & B. Neuman (Eds.), *Blueprint for use of nursing models: Education, research, practice and administration* (pp. 33-63, Pub. No. 14-2696). New York: National League for Nursing.

Lobo, M. L. (2002). Behavioral system model: Dorothy E. Johnson (pp. 155-169). In J. B. George, Nursing theories: the base for professional nursing practice, 5th Ed. Upper Saddle River, NJ: Prentice Hall.

Loveland-Cherry, D., & Wilkerson, S. (1983). Dorothy Johnson's behavioral systems model. In J. Fitzpatrick & A. Whall (Eds.), *Conceptual models of nursing: Analysis and application.* Bowie, M. D.: Robert J. Brady.

Meleis, A. (2007). Theoretical nursing: Development and progress, 4th Ed. Philadelphia: Lippincott Williams & Wilkins. (Chapter 12 – Our nursing clients – Dorothy Johnson (pp. 277-291).

Wilkerson, S. A., & Loveland-Cherry, C. J. (2005). Johnson's behavioral system model. (pp. 83-103). In J. J. Fitzpatrick & A. L. Whall, Conceptual models of nursing: Analysis and application, (4th Ed.) Upper Saddle River, NJ: Pearson/Prentice Hall.

Directional and Biographical Source

Henderson, J. (1957-1959). *Nursing studies index* (Vol. IV). Philadelphia: J. B. Lippincott

Journal Articles

Adam, E. (1987). Nursing theory: what it is and what it is not. *Nursing Papers: Perspectives in Nursing,* 19(1), 5-14.

Benson, S. (1997). The older adult and fear of crime. *Journal of Gerontological Nursing, 23*(10) 24-31.

Botha, M. E. (1989). Theory development in perspective: The role of conceptual frameworks and models in theory development. *Journal of Advanced Nursing,* 14(1), 49-55.

Colling, J., Owen, T., McCreedy, M., & Newman, D. (2003). The effects of a continence program on frail community-dwelling elderly persons. *Urologic Nursing, 23*(2), 117-131.

Coward, D. D., & Wilkie, D. J. (2000). Metastatic bone pain: Meanings associated with self-report and self-management decision making. *Cancer Nursing, 23*(2), 101-108.

Dee, V., van Servellen, G., & Brecht, M. (1998). Managed behavioral health care patients and their nursing care problems, level of functioning, and impairment on discharge. *Journal of American Psychiatric Nurses Association, 4*(2), 57-66.

Derdiarian, A. K. (1991). Effects of using a nursing model-based assessment instrument on quality of nursing care. *Nursing Administration Quarterly, 15*(3) 1-16.

Derdiarian, A. K., & Forsythe, A. B. (1983, Sept./Oct). An instrument for theory and research development using the behavioral systems model for nursing: The cancer patient. Part II. *Nursing Research, 32,* 260-266.

Derdiarian, A. K., & Schobel, D. (1990). Comprehensive assessment of AIDS patients using the behavioral systems model for nursing practice instrument. *Journal of Advanced Nursing, 15*(4), 436-446.

Dhasaradhan, I. (2001). Application of nursing theory into practice. *Nursing Journal of India, 92*(10) 224, 236.

D'Huyvetter, D. (2000). The trauma disease. *Journal of Trauma Nursing, 7*(1), 5-12.

Dimino, E. (1988). Needed: nursing research questions which test and expand our conceptual models of nursing. *Virginia Nurse,* 56(3), 43-46.

Fleming, B. H. (1990). Use of the Johnson model in nursing education (abstract). In Proceedings of the National

Theory Conference (pp. 109-111). Los Angeles: UCLA Nursing Department.

Holaday, B. (1974). Achievement behavior in chronically ill children. Nursing Research, 23, 25-30.

Keen, J. (1982). The behavioral mode. Nursing (Oxford), 2(Jul), 71-73.

Lanouette, M., & St-Jacques, A. (1994). Premature infants and their families. *Canadian Nurse, 90*(9), 36-39.

Lovejoy, N. (1983). The leukemic child's perception of family behaviors. *Oncology Nursing Forum*, 10(4), 20-25.

Lovejoy, N. C., & Moran, T. A. (1998). Selected AIDS beliefs, behaviors and informational needs of homosexual/bisexual men with AIDS or ARC. *International Journal of Nursing Studies*, 25(3), 207-216.

Ma, T., & Gandet, D. (1997). Assessing the quality of our end-stage renal disease client population. *Journal of the Canadian Association of Nephrology Nurses and Technicians 7*(2), 13-16.

Magnari, L. E. (1990). Hardiness, self-perceived health, and activity among independently functioning older adults. *Scholarly Inquiry for Nursing Practice*, 4(3), 177-188,

McCauley, K. C., Choromanski, J. D., Wallinger, C., & Liv, K. (1984). Current management of ventricular tachycardia: Symposium from the Hospital of the University of Pennsylvania. Learning to live with controlled ventricular tachycardia; Utilizing the Johnson mode. *Heart and Lung*, 13, 633-638.

Moreau, D., Poster, E. C., & Niemela, K. (1993). Implementing and evaluating an attending nurse model. *Nursing Management*, 24(6), 56-58, 60, 64.

Newman, M. A. (1994). Theory for nursing practice. *Nursing Science Quarterly, 7*(4), 153-157.

Niemela, K., Poster, E. D., & Moreau, D. (1992). The attending nurse: A new role for the advanced clinician: Adolescent inpatient unit. *Journal of Child & Adolescent Psychiatric & Mental Health Nursing*, 5(3), 5-12.

Poster, E. C., & Beliz, L. (1988). Behavioral category ratings of adolescents on an inpatient psychiatric unit. *International Journal of Adolescence and Youth,* 1, 293-303.

Poster, E. C., Dee, V., & Randell, B. P. (1997). The Johnson behavioral systems model as a framework for patient outcome evaluation. *Journal of American Psychiatric Nurses Association, 3*(3), 73-80.

Rawls, A. C. (1980, Feb.). Evaluation of the Johnson behavioral model in clinical practice. *Image: The Journal of Nursing Scholarship, 12*, 13-16.

Reynolds, W., & Cormack, D. F. S. (1991). An evaluation of the Johnson Behavioral Systems model for nursing. *Journal of Advanced Nursing*, 16(9), 1122-1130.

Urh, I. (1998). Dorothy Johnson's theory and nursing care of a pregnant woman. *OBZORNIK ZDRAVSTVENE NEGE, 32*(516), 199-203.

Wilkie, D., Lovejoy, N., Dodd, M., & Tesler, M. (1988). Cancer pain control behaviors: Description and correlation with pain intensity. *Oncology Nursing Forum, 15*(6), 723-731.

Wilmoth, M. C., & Tingle, L. R. (2001). Development and psychometric testing of the Wilmoth Sexual Behaviors Questionnaire: Female. Canadian Journal of Nursing Research, 32, 135-131.

Wilmoth, M. C., & Towsend, J. (1995). A comparison of the effects of lumpectomy versus mastectomy on sexual behaviors. *Cancer Practice*, 3(5), 279-285.

UNIT

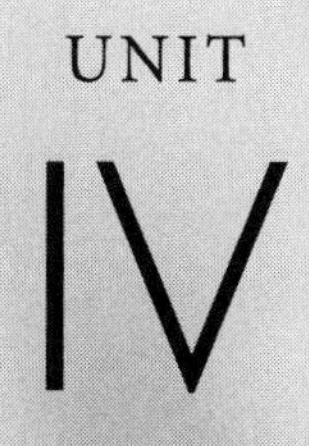

Nursing Theories

- *Nursing theories describe, explain, or predict relationships among the concepts of nursing phenomena.*
- *Theories propose relationships by framing the issue and proposing an outcome.*
- *Nursing theories are developed at various levels of abstraction.*
- *Nursing theories at a grand theory level are nearly as abstract as the nursing models from which they come, but they are theories since they propose testable outcomes.*

CHAPTER 19

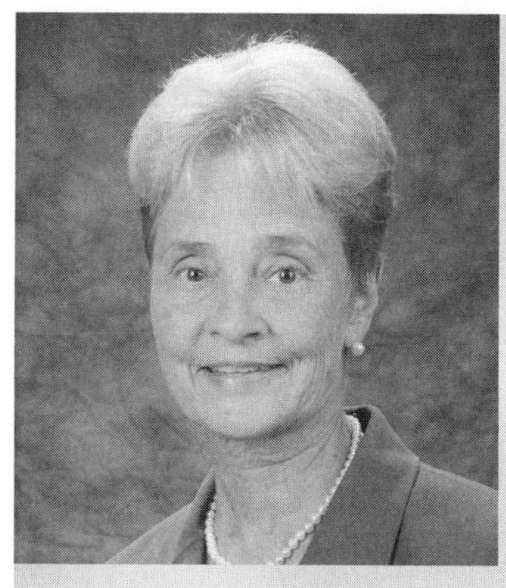

Anne Boykin

1944-present

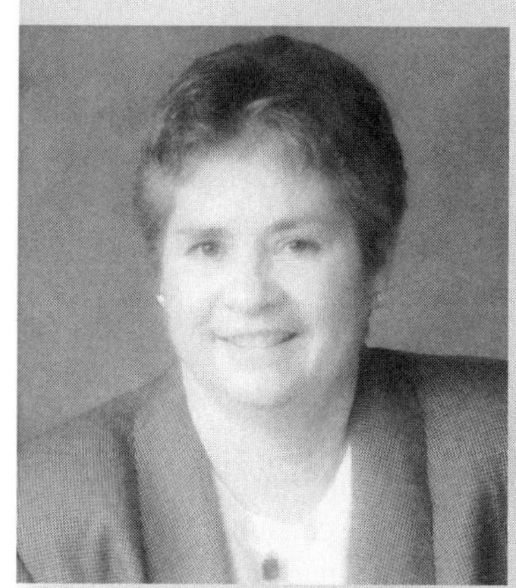

Savina O. Schoenhofer

1940-present

The Theory of Nursing as Caring: A Model for Transforming Practice

Marguerite J. Purnell

"The nature of relationships is transformed through caring" (Boykin & Schoenhofer, 2001a, p. 4).

CREDENTIALS AND BACKGROUND OF THE THEORISTS

Anne Boykin

Anne Boykin grew up in Kaukauna, Wisconsin, the eldest of six children. She began her career in nursing in 1966, graduating from Alverno College in Milwaukee, Wisconsin. She received her master's degree from Emory University in Atlanta, Georgia, and her doctorate from Vanderbilt University in Nashville, Tennessee. South Florida became her home in 1981 and, today, continues to enchant and nourish her love for the natural life. Dr. Boykin is married to Steve Staudenmeyer, and they have four children.

Anne Boykin is dean and professor of the Christine E. Lynn College of Nursing at Florida Atlantic University. She is director of the Christine E. Lynn Center for Caring, which is housed in the College of Nursing. This center was created for the purpose of humanizing care through the integration of teaching, research, and service. A new and exciting initiative is the creation of the Archives of Caring in Nursing. The goals of the Archives are to preserve the papers of caring scholars, invite the study of caring, advance caring as an essential domain of nursing knowledge, and create meaning for the practice of nursing. Boykin has a longstanding commitment to the advancement of knowledge in the discipline, especially regarding the phenomenon of caring.

Positions she has held in the International Association for Human Caring include president elect (1990 to 1993), president (1993 to 1996), and member of the nominating committee (1997 to 1999). As immediate past president, she served as coeditor of the journal, *International Association for Human Caring,* from 1996 to 1999.

Boykin's scholarly work is centered on caring as the grounding for nursing. This is evidenced in her book (coauthored with Schoenhofer), *Nursing as Caring: A Model for Transforming Practice* (1993, 2001a), and her book, *Living a Caring-Based Program* (1994b). The latter book illustrates how caring grounds the development of a nursing program by creating the environment for study through evaluation. In addition to these books, Dr. Boykin is editor of *Power, Politics and Public Policy: A Matter of Caring* (1995) and coeditor (along with Gaut) of *Caring as Healing: Renewal Through Hope* (1994). She has written numerous book chapters and articles and serves as a consultant locally, regionally, nationally, and internationally on the topic of caring.

Savina O. Schoenhofer

Savina Schoenhofer was born the second child and eldest daughter in a family of nine children and spent her formative years on the family cattle ranch in Kansas. She is named for her maternal grandfather, who was a classical musician in Kansas City, Missouri. She has a daughter, Carrie, and a granddaughter, Emma.

During the 1960s, Schoenhofer spent 3 years in the Amazon region of Brazil, working as a volunteer in community development. Her initial nursing study was completed at Wichita State University, where she earned undergraduate and graduate degrees in nursing, psychology, and counseling. She completed a PhD in educational foundations and administration at Kansas State University in 1983. In 1990, Schoenhofer co-founded *Nightingale Songs,* an early venue for communicating the beauty of nursing in poetry and prose. An early study made it apparent to Schoenhofer that caring was the service that patients overwhelmingly recognized. In addition to her work on caring, including co-authorship with Boykin of *Nursing as Caring: A Model for Transforming Practice* (1993, 2001a), Schoenhofer has written numerous articles on nursing values, primary care, nursing education, support, touch, and mentoring. Her career in nursing has been influenced significantly by three colleagues: Lt. Col. Ann Ashjian (Ret.), whose community nursing practice in Brazil presented an inspiring model of nursing; Marilyn E. Parker, PhD, a faculty colleague who mentored her in the idea of nursing as a discipline, the academic role of higher education, and the world of nursing theories and theorists; and Anne Boykin, PhD, who introduced her to caring as a substantive field of nursing study. Schoenhofer created the Theory of Nursing as Caring website, which serves as a vibrant, interactive source of information about how the theory is lived in practice and research. As Professor of Graduate Nursing at the Cora S. Balmat School of Nursing, Alcorn State University, Natchez, Mississippi, and Professor at the University of Mississippi School of Nursing in Jackson, Mississippi, Schoenhofer lives her commitment and passion for illuminating the study of nursing as caring.

THEORETICAL SOURCES

The Theory of Nursing as Caring was borne out of the early curriculum development work in the College of Nursing at Florida Atlantic University. Anne Boykin and Savina Schoenhofer were among the faculty group revising the caring-based curriculum. When the revised curriculum was instituted, each recognized the importance and human necessity of continuing to develop ideas toward a comprehensive conceptual framework that expressed the meaning and purpose of nursing as a discipline and as a profession. The point of departure from traditional thought was the acceptance that caring is the end rather than the means of nursing, and the intention of nursing rather than merely its instrument. This work led Boykin and Schoenhofer to conceptualize the focus of nursing as "nurturing persons living caring and growing in caring" (Boykin & Schoenhofer, 1993, p. 22).

Further work to identify foundational assumptions about nursing clarified the idea of the nursing situation as a shared lived experience in which the "caring between" (Boykin & Schoenhofer, 1993, p. 26) enhances personhood. Personhood is illuminated as living grounded in caring. The clarified notions of nursing situation and focus of nursing bring to life the meaning of the assumptions underlying the theory and permit the practical understanding of nursing as both a discipline and a profession. As critique and refinement of the theory and study of nursing situations progressed, the notion of nursing as being primarily concerned with health was seen as limiting. Boykin and Schoenhofer now propose that nursing is concerned with the broad spectrum of human living.

Three bodies of work significantly influenced the initial development of the theory. Paterson and Zderad's (1988) existential phenomenological theory of humanistic nursing, viewed by Boykin and Schoenhofer as the historical antecedent of Nursing as Caring, was the source for such germinal ideas as "the between," "call for nursing," "nursing response," and "personhood," and served as substantive and structural bases for their conceptualization of Nursing as Caring. Roach's (1987, 2002) thesis that caring is the human mode of being finds its natural expression and domain in the assumptions of the theory. Her "6 C's"—commitment, confidence, conscience, competence, compassion, and comportment—contribute to a language of caring (Roach, 2002).

Mayeroff's (1971) work, *On Caring,* provided rich, elemental language that facilitated the recognition and description of the practical meaning of living caring in the ordinariness of life. Mayeroff's (1971) major ingredients of caring—knowing, alternating rhythms, patience, honesty, trust, humility, hope, and courage—describe the wellspring of human living. In the Theory of Nursing as Caring, these concepts are essential for understanding living as caring, and for coming to appreciate their unique expression in the reciprocal relationship of the nurse and those nursed.

Boykin and Schoenhofer's conception of nursing as a discipline was influenced directly by Phenix (1964), King and Brownell (1976), and Orem (1979), and as a profession by Flexner's (1910) ideas. In addition to the work of these thinkers, Anne Boykin and Savina Schoenhofer are longstanding members of the community of nursing scholars whose study focuses on caring. Their collegial association and mutual support also undoubtedly brought subtle influence to bear on Boykin and Schoenhofer's work.

Nascent forms of the Theory of Nursing as Caring were first published in 1990 and 1991, with the first complete exposition of the theory presented at a theory conference in 1992 (Boykin & Schoenhofer, 1990, 1991; Schoenhofer & Boykin, 1993). These expositions were followed by the work, *Nursing as Caring: A Model for Transforming Practice,* published in 1993 (Boykin & Schoenhofer, 1993) and re-released with an epilogue in 2001 (Boykin & Schoenhofer, 2001a).

Gaut notes in Boykin and Schoenhofer (2001a) that the theory is an excellent example of growth by intension, or gradual illumination, characterized by "the development of an extant bibliography, categorization of caring conceptualizations, and the further development of human care/caring theories" (p. xii).

Major Concepts & Definitions

FOCUS AND INTENTION OF NURSING

Disciplines of knowledge are communities of scholars who develop a particular perspective on the world and what it means to be in the world (King & Brownell, 1976). Disciplinary communities hold a value system in common that is expressed in its unique focus on knowledge and practice. From the perspective of the Theory of Nursing as Caring, the focus of nursing as a discipline of knowledge and a professional practice is nurturing persons living and growing in caring. The general intention of nursing is to know persons as caring and to support and sustain them as they live caring (Boykin & Schoenhofer, 2006). This intention is expressed uniquely when the nurse enters the relationship with the nursed with the intention of knowing the other as a caring person, and affirming and celebrating the person as caring (Boykin & Schoenhofer, 2001a). Caring is an expression of nursing and is "the intentional and authentic presence of the nurse with another who is recognized as living in caring and growing in caring" (Boykin & Schoenhofer, 1993, p. 24). Sensitivity and skill in creating unique and effective ways of communicating caring are developed through the nurse's intention to care.

PERSPECTIVE OF PERSONS AS CARING

The fundamental assumption is that all persons are caring. Caring is lived by each person moment to moment and is an essential characteristic of being human. Caring is a process, and throughout life, each person grows in the capacity to express caring. Person therefore is recognized as constantly unfolding in caring. From the perspective of the theory, "fundamentally, potentially, and actually each person is caring" (Boykin & Schoenhofer, 2001a, p. 2), even though every act of the person

MAJOR CONCEPTS & DEFINITIONS—cont'd

might not be understood as caring. Knowing the person as living caring and growing in caring is foundational to the theory.

NURSING SITUATION

Caring is service that nursing offers and lives in the context of the nursing situation (Boykin & Schoenhofer, 2006). The nursing situation is the locus of all that is known and done in nursing (Boykin & Schoenhofer, 2001a) and is conceptualized as "the shared, lived experience in which caring between nurse and nursed enhances personhood" (Boykin & Schoenhofer, 1993, p. 33). Nursing situation is what is present in the mind of the nurse whenever the intent of the nurse is "to nurse" (Boykin & Schoenhofer, 2001a). It is within the nursing situation that the nurse attends to calls for caring or reaching out of the one nursed. The practice of nursing and the practical knowledge of nursing are situated in a relational locus of person being nursed with person nursing in the nursing situation. The nursing situation involves an expression of values, intentions, and actions of two or more persons choosing to live a nursing relationship. In this lived relationship, all knowledge of nursing is created and understood (Boykin & Schoenhofer, 2006).

PERSONHOOD

Personhood is a process of living that is grounded in caring. Personhood implies being who we are as authentic caring persons and being open to unfolding possibilities for caring. We are constantly living out the meaning of our caring from moment to moment. Within the nursing situation, the shared lived experience of caring within enhances personhood, and both the nurse and the nursed grow in caring. In the intimacy of caring, respect for self as person and respect for other are values that affirm personhood. "A profound understanding of personhood communicates the paradox of person-as-person and person-in-communion all at once" (Boykin & Schoenhofer, 2006, p. 336).

DIRECT INVITATION

Within the nursing situation, the direct invitation opens the relationship to true caring between the nurse and the one nursed. With the intention of truly coming to know the one nursed, the nurse risks entering the other's world and comes to know what is meaningful to them. Invitations to share what matters, such as "How might I nurse you in ways that are meaningful to you?" are communicated in the personal language of the nurse. The power of the direct invitation reaches deep into the humility of the nursing situation, uniting and guiding the intention of both the nurse and the one nursed. The focus is not on what the nurse can do for the one being nursed, but rather, the focus is on what is meaningful to the one being nursed. These uniquely expressed invitations of caring call forth responses of mutual valuing in the beauty of the caring between.

CALL FOR NURSING

Calls for nursing are calls for nurturance perceived in the mind of the nurse (Boykin & Schoenhofer, 2001a, 2001b). Intentionality (Schoenhofer, 2002a) and authentic presence open the nurse to hearing calls for nursing. The nurse responds uniquely to the one nursed with a deliberately developed knowledge of what it means to be human, acknowledging and affirming the person living caring in unique ways in the immediate situation (Boykin & Schoenhofer, 1993). Because calls for nursing are uniquely situated personal expressions, they cannot be predicted, but originate within persons who are living caring in their lives and who hold hopes and aspirations for growing in caring. "Calls for nursing are individually relevant ways of saying 'Know me as caring person in

Continued

MAJOR CONCEPTS & DEFINITIONS—cont'd

the moment and be with me as I try to live fully who I truly am'" (Boykin & Schoenhofer, 2006, p. 336).

CARING BETWEEN

When the nurse enters the world of the other person with the intention of knowing the other as a caring person, the encountering of the nurse and the one nursed gives rise to the phenomenon of caring between, within which personhood is nurtured (Boykin & Schoenhofer, 2001a). Through presence and intentionality, the nurse comes to know the other, living and growing in caring. Constant and mutual unfolding enhances this loving relation. Without the caring between the nurse and the nursed unidirectional activity or reciprocal exchange can occur but nursing in its fullest sense does not occur. It is in the context of the caring between that personhood is nurtured, each expressing self and recognizing the other as caring person (Boykin & Schoenhofer, 2001a).

NURSING RESPONSE

In responding to the nursing call, the nurse enters the nursing situation with the intention of knowing the other person as caring. This knowing of person clarifies the call for nursing and shapes the nursing response, transforming the knowledge brought by the nurse to the situation from general, to particular and unique (Boykin & Schoenhofer, 2001a). The nursing response is co-created in the immediacy of what truly matters and is a specific expression of caring nurturance to sustain and enhance the other living and growing in caring. Nursing responses to calls for caring evolve as nurses clarify their understanding of calls through presence and dialogue. Such responses are uniquely created for the moment and cannot be predicted or applied as preplanned protocols (Boykin & Schoenhofer, 1997).

STORY AS METHOD FOR KNOWING NURSING

Story is a method for knowing nursing and a medium for all forms of nursing inquiry. Nursing stories embody the lived experience of nursing situations involving the nurse and the nursed. As a repository of nursing knowledge, any single nursing situation has the potential to illuminate the depth and complexity of the experience as lived, that is, the caring that takes place between the nurse and the one nursed. The content of nursing knowledge is generated, developed, conserved, and known through the lived experience of nursing situations (Boykin & Schoenhofer, 2001a). The nursing situation as a unit of knowledge and practice is re-created in narrative or story (Boykin & Schoenhofer, 1991). Nursing situations are best communicated through aesthetic media such as storytelling, poetry, graphic arts, and dance to preserve the lived meaning of the situation and the openness of the situation through text. These media provide time and space for reflecting and for creativity in advancing understanding (Boykin & Schoenhofer, 1991, 2001a, 2006; Boykin, Parker, & Schoenhofer, 1994). Story as method re-creates and re-presents the essence of the experience, making the knowledge of nursing available for further study (Boykin & Schoenhofer, 2001a).

USE OF EMPIRICAL EVIDENCE

The assumptions of Nursing as Caring ground the practice of nursing in knowing, enhancing, and illuminating the caring between the nurse and the one nursed. As such, rather than providing empirical variables from which hypotheses and testable predictions are made, the theory *qualitatively transforms practice*. In the theory, persons are unique and unpredictable in the moment and therefore cannot and should not be manipulated or objectified as testable, researchable variables. Ellis believed that theories should reveal the knowledge that nurses must, and should, spend time pursuing (Algase & Whall, 1993). The Theory of Nursing as Caring reveals the essentiality of recognizing the caring between the nurse and the one nursed as the substantive knowledge that nurses must pursue. From this perspective, outcomes of nursing care reflect the valuing of person in ways that communicate the "value added" richness of the nursing experience (Boykin, Schoenhofer, Smith, St. Jean, & Aleman, 2003, p. 225). Characteristics of personhood essential to the theory, such as unity, wholeness, awareness, and intention, are not consonant with the objective terms of normative science that permeates the language of outcomes. In Nursing as Caring, outcomes are articulated in terms that are subjective and descriptive, rather than objective and predictive (Boykin & Schoenhofer, 1997).

MAJOR ASSUMPTIONS

Fundamental beliefs about what it means to be human undergird the Theory of Nursing as Caring. Boykin and Schoenhofer (2001a) address six major assumptions that reflect a set of values to provide a basis for understanding and explicating the meaning of nursing.

One: Persons Are Caring by Virtue of Their Humanness

The belief that persons are caring by virtue of their humanness sets forth the ontological and ethical bases on which the theory is grounded. Being a person means living caring, through which being and possibilities are known to the fullest. Each person throughout his or her life grows in the capacity to express caring. The assumption that all persons are caring does not require that each act of a person be caring, but it does require the acceptance that "fundamentally, potentially, and actually, each person is caring" (Boykin & Schoenhofer, 2001a, p. 2). Through entering, experiencing, and appreciating the life-world of other the nature of being human is understood more fully. From the perspective of Nursing as Caring, the understanding of person as caring "centers on valuing and celebrating human wholeness, the human person as living and growing in caring, and active personal engagement with others" (Boykin & Schoenhofer, 2001a, p. 5).

Two: Persons Are Whole and Complete in the Moment

Respect for the total person is communicated by the notion of person as whole or complete in the moment. Being complete in the moment signifies that there is no insufficiency, no brokenness, and no absence of something. Wholeness, or the fullness of being, is forever present. The view of person as caring and complete is intentional, offering a unifying lens for being with other that prevents segmenting into parts such as mind, body, and spirit. Through this lens, the person is at all times whole, with no insufficiency, brokenness, or absence of something. The idea of wholeness does not preclude the idea of complexity of being. Instead, from the perspective of Nursing as Caring, to encounter a person as less than whole fails to truly encounter the person.

Three: Persons Live Caring, Moment to Moment

Caring is a lifetime process that is lived moment to moment and is constantly unfolding. In the rhythm of life experiences, we continually develop expressions of ourselves as caring persons. Actualization of the potential to express caring varies in the moment. As competency in caring is developed through life, we come to understand what it means to be a caring person, to live caring, and to nurture each other as caring. This awareness of self as a caring person draws forth to consciousness the valuing of caring and becomes the moral imperative, directing the "oughts" of actions with the persistent question, "How ought I act as caring person?" (Boykin & Schoenhofer, 2001a, p. 4).

Four: Personhood Is Living Life Grounded in Caring

Personhood is a process of living caring and growing in caring: It is being authentic, demonstrating congruence between beliefs and behaviors, and living out the meaning of one's life. Personhood acknowledges the potential for unfolding caring possibilities moment to moment. From the perspective of Nursing as Caring, personhood is the universal human call. This implies that the fullness of being human is expressed in living caring uniquely day to day and is enhanced through participation in caring relationships (Boykin & Schoenhofer, 2001a).

Five: Personhood Is Enhanced Through Participating in Nurturing Relationships With Caring Others

As a process, personhood acknowledges the potential of persons to live caring and is enhanced through participation in nurturing relationships with caring others. The nature of relationships is transformed through caring. Caring is living in the context of relational responsibilities and possibilities, and acknowledges the importance of knowing person as person. "Through knowing self as caring person, I am able to be authentic to self, freeing me to truly be with others" (Boykin & Schoenhofer, 2001a, p. 4).

Six: Nursing Is Both a Discipline and a Profession

Nursing is an "exquisitely interwoven" (Boykin & Schoenhofer, 2001a, p. 6) unity of aspects of the discipline and profession of nursing. As a discipline, nursing is a way of knowing, being, valuing, and living in the world, and is envisaged as a unity of knowledge within a larger unity. The discipline of nursing attends to the discovery, creation, development, and refinement of knowledge needed for the practice of nursing. The profession of nursing attends to the application of that knowledge in response to human needs.

Nursing as caring focuses on the knowledge needed for plenary understanding of what it means to be human and the distinctive methods needed to verify this knowledge. As a human science, knowing nursing means knowing in the realms of personal, empirical, ethical, and aesthetic all at once (Carper, 1978; Phenix, 1964). These patterns of knowing provide an organizing framework for asking epistemological questions of caring in nursing.

THEORETICAL ASSERTIONS

The broad philosophical framework of the theory assures its congruence in a variety of nursing situations. As a general theory, Nursing as Caring is an appropriate model for various nursing roles, such as individual practice, group or institutional practice, and a variety of practice venues such as acute care, long-term care, nursing administration, and nursing education.

The fundamental assumptions of Nursing as Caring underpin all assertions and concepts of the theory. They are as follows: (1) To be human is to be caring, and (2) the purpose of the discipline and profession is to come to know persons and nurture them as persons living caring and growing in caring. These assumptions give rise to the concept of respect for persons as caring individuals and respect for what matters to them. The notion of respect grounds and characterizes relationships and is the starting place for all activities.

Dance of Caring Persons

The *Dance of Caring Persons* is a visual representation of the lived caring between the nurse and the nursed and expresses underlying relationships (Figure 19-1). The concept of a hierarchical ladder is inconsistent with Nursing as Caring. Instead, the egalitarian spirit of caring respect characterizes each participant in the dance of caring persons, in which the contributions of each dancer, including the one nursed, are honored.

Dancers enter the nursing situation, visualized as a circle of caring that provides organizing purpose

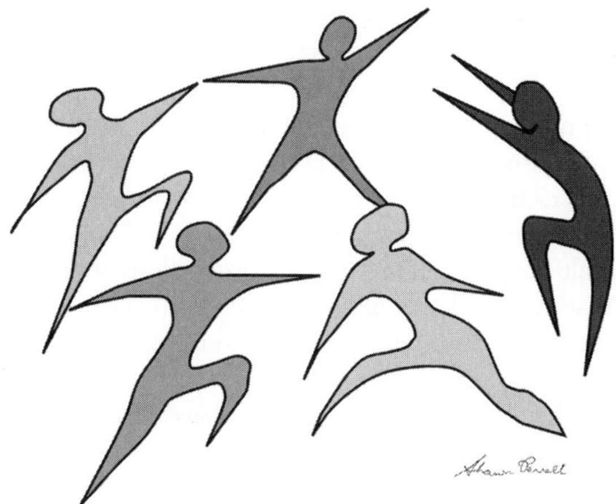

Figure 19-1 The Dance of Caring Persons. (From Boykin, A., & Schoenhofer, S. O. [2001]. *Nursing as caring: A model for transforming practice* [p. 37] [Re-release of original volume, with epilogue added]. Sudbury, MA: Jones & Bartlett; graphic created by Shawn Pennell, Florida Atlantic University, Boca Raton, FL.)

and integrated functioning (Boykin et al., 2003). Dancers move freely; some dancers touch, some dance alone, but all dance in relation to each other and to the circle. Each dancer brings special gifts as the nursing situation evolves. Some dancers may hear different notes and a different rhythm, but all harmonize in the unity of the dance and the oneness of the circle. Personal knowing of self and other is integral to the connectedness of persons in the dance, in which the nature of relating in the circle is grounded in valuing and respecting person (Boykin & Schoenhofer, 2001a). All in the nursing situation, including the nurse and the nursed, sustain the dance, being energized and resonating with the music of caring.

Outcomes of Nursing Care

The concept of outcomes of care, that is, the notion of predictable, evidence-based outcomes, is incompatible with the values experienced in caring nursing. Outcomes of nursing care are conceptualized from values experienced in the nursing relationship, and in normative documentation, these outcomes are unacknowledged. Boykin and Schoenhofer (1997) note that it is the responsibility of the courageous advanced practice nurse to "go beyond what is currently accepted in delimiting and languaging the value expressed by persons who participate in nursing situations" (p. 63). Work has begun to identify and clarify the "value added" unique outcomes of caring nursing (Thomas, Finch, Green, & Schoenhofer, 2004).

LOGICAL FORM

The theory is presented in logical form grounded in general assumptions related to persons as caring and in nursing as a discipline of knowledge and a profession. The theory is a broad-based, general theory of nursing rendered in everyday language. Mayeroff's (1971) work, *On Caring,* and Roach's (1987) "5 C's" provided language that illuminated the practical meaning of caring in nursing situations.

Key concepts of caring, nursing, intention, nursing situation, direct invitation, call for nursing as caring, caring between, and nursing response are described as general assumptions, and interrelated meanings are illustrated in the model of the dance of caring persons. The direct invitation, introduced in the 2001 edition of *Nursing as Caring: A Model for Transforming Practice,* is an elaboration of the nursing situation and further clarifies the role of the nurse in initiating and sustaining caring responses. Story, as a method for knowing, focuses on nursing situations as the locus for nursing knowledge as a fluid and logical extension of the framework.

ACCEPTANCE BY THE NURSING COMMUNITY

Practice

Nursing is a way of living caring in the world and is revealed in personal patterns of caring. Foundations for practice of the Theory of Nursing as Caring become illumined when the nurse comes to know self as caring person "in ever deepening and broadening dimensions" (Boykin & Schoenhofer, 2001a, p. 23). Practicing nursing within this framework requires the acknowledgment that knowing self as caring matters and is integral to knowing others as caring. This is especially important in light of practice environments that depersonalize and support the notion of the nurse as instrument and a means to an end. Rather than nursing practice focused on activities, the lens for practice becomes the intention to know person as caring. Often realization of the self as caring person does not occur until the story of the caring transpiring in the nursing situation is articulated and shared. When reflecting upon their caring, nurses describe "Aha!" moments, signal realizations of self as always having been caring, and rediscover freedom in caring possibilities within the nursing situation: "freedom to be, freedom to choose, and freedom to unfold" (Boykin & Schoenhofer, 2001a, p. 23). Reentering moments of caring through articulation of the nursing story allows the nurse to frame outcomes of caring in the language and substance of caring that is meaningful for practice. Honoring caring values in explicit ways reaffirms the substance of nursing and refreshes the caring intention of the nurse. Through the sharing of story, new possibilities arise for living nursing as caring.

Nursing Service Administration

In living Nursing as Caring, the nursing administrator makes decisions through a lens in which activities are infused with a concern for shaping a transformative culture that embodies the fundamental values expressed within nursing as caring. All activities of the nursing administrator must be connected to the direct work of nursing and be "ultimately directed to the person(s) being nursed" (Boykin & Schoenhofer, 2001a, p. 33). These activities include creating, maintaining, and supporting an environment open to hearing calls for nursing and to providing nurturing responses.

Boykin and Schoenhofer (2001a) point out that contrary to the perception of nurse administrators being removed from the direct care of the nursed, they are able to directly or indirectly enter the world of the nursed, respond uniquely, and assist the nurse in securing resources to nurture persons as they live and grow in caring. The nursing administrator is also able to enter the world of the nursed indirectly, through the stories of colleagues in other roles. Other activities of the nursing administrator within the interdisciplinary environment of the organization include facilitating understanding and clarity of the focus of nursing and informing other members of the interdisciplinary healthcare team of the unique contributions of nurses. Sharing the depth of nursing with others through nursing situations illuminates meanings and allows for fluid reciprocity among colleagues.

The work of the nurse administrator must also reflect the uniqueness of the discipline so that it is nursing which is being reflected, portraying respect for persons as caring and extending through mission statements, goals, objectives, standards of practice, policies, and procedures (Boykin & Schoenhofer, 2001a). The following story was related by Nancy Hilton, MSN, RN, Chief Nursing Officer, at a Florida hospital. This nurse administrator, practicing from the perspective of Nursing as Caring, reflects the complexity and intentional caring expressed in living caring uniquely and courageously:

> We are intentionally refocusing our culture from a traditional bureaucratic one to a person-centered, caring-based values organization. In 2007, our Nursing Councils at St. Lucie Medical Center selected the Theory of Nursing as Caring as the theoretical model to guide our nursing practice. As a Nursing Administrator, I pondered how I could intentionally ground our hospital environment, and the practice of the nurses within its walls, in a perspective of caring. I made a deliberate commitment to deepen our knowledge and awareness by allocating time for all of us to participate in dialogues focused on knowing ourselves as caring persons.
>
> I am able to live caring uniquely as the CNO by ministering to the nurses providing direct patient care. Many nurses were trained to focus on technology and treating symptoms. I give the nurses the freedom to care in their unique way. Our Clinical Nurse Leaders (CNLs) are transforming nursing practice at St. Lucie Medical Center by

incorporating the Theory of Nursing as Caring into bedside nursing. Through direct invitation, the CNLs are role modeling how to "hear" calls for nursing, that is, ascertaining in their own unique way "what matters most" to the patient. I have partnered with the CNLs and assisted with dialoguing with the staff. Through my honesty, I have disclosed to the nurses that I don't have all the answers. As we transform our nursing practice, we live and grow in caring together.

What I do best is utilize the art of storytelling to translate the calls for nursing into the language of the boardroom. Through the use of strategic nursing situations, I connect the administrators directly to the one nursed. While these indirect caregivers yearn for connectedness to the patient, it takes the ingredient of courage on my part to convince the administrators why it is critical to transform an entire healthcare system by intentionally grounding it in a perspective of caring.

We needed a graphic representation of how all disciplines in the hospital relate to the patient. The *Dance of Caring Persons* was the visual representation of an organizational model that supports a way of being with others that respects, honors, and celebrates each person. I have been willing to conceptualize and chart the course as well as partner with key leaders in creating an environment to embody the true values of caring.

In practicing through the lens of Nursing as Caring, the nursing administrator assists in creating a community that appreciates, supports, and nurtures persons as they live and grow in caring. Allocation of time for dialogue allows shared meanings to emerge, and demonstrates the commitment of the nursing administrator to enhance the growth of the nurse within the discipline of nursing (Boykin & Schoenhofer, 2001b). The nursing administrator interfaces with persons of many other disciplines, as well as with the one nursed, and expresses honesty and authenticity in encouraging others to live out who they are: The nature of relating with persons whose roles range from the boardroom to the bedside is grounded in a respect for and valuing of each person.

Education

The Theory of Nursing as Caring is a transformation model for all arenas, including nursing practice, nursing service organization, nursing science, and nursing education. Assumptions grounding Nursing as Caring ground the practice of nursing education and nursing education administration (Boykin & Schoenhofer, 2001a, 2001b). As expressions of the discipline, the structure and practices of the education program, including the curriculum, reflect the values and assumptions inherent in the statement of focus and the domain of the discipline, that is, nurturing persons living caring and growing in caring. Through the lens of Nursing as Caring, fundamental assumptions of the theory that honor and celebrate the uniqueness of persons as caring should be reflected. Caring, as one of the significant components of nursing knowledge, should not be limited to a single course but should be taught, studied, and infused throughout the curriculum (Schoenhofer, 2001). Through story, that is, the study of nursing situations, disciplinary and professional knowledge is accessed and nursing responses grounded in caring are conceptualized. All activities of the program of study should therefore be directed toward developing, organizing, and communicating nursing knowledge, the knowledge of nurturing persons living caring and growing in caring. Eggenberger and Keller (2008) have articulated an approach for application of the theory to the use of simulation in nursing education.

Caring has been posited as the link between spirituality and higher education and as an ethic for being in relationship (Boykin & Parker, 1997). It is therefore a framework for knowing and the moral basis for relating. Self-discovery through an ongoing search for truth prepares learners "to receive a greater understanding of his/her reality as well as the reality of others; to develop a sense of identification, connectedness and compassion with others, and a deeper understanding of truth" (Boykin & Parker, 1997, p. 32). The challenge in higher education is to create an environment that can sustain and nurture the living of caring and spirituality (Boykin & Parker, 1997).

From the perspective of Nursing as Caring, the model for organizational design of nursing education is analogous to the dance of caring persons. Faculty, students, and administrators dance together in the study of nursing. Each dancer is recognized, prized, and celebrated for the gifts he or she brings. The role of each influences how the commitment to nursing education is lived out.

The role of the dean of a caring-based nursing program is "intrinsically linked" (Boykin, 1994a, p. 17) to an understanding of nursing as both a discipline and a profession and focuses actions on developing and maintaining a caring environment in which the knowledge of the discipline can be discovered. As administrator, the dean "nurtures ideas, secures resources, communicates the nature of the discipline, models living and growing in caring, co-creates a culture in which the study of nursing can be achieved freely and fully, grounds all actions in a commitment to caring as a way of being, and treats others with the same care, concern, and understanding as those entrusted to our nursing care" (Boykin, 1994a, pp. 17-18). Such a broad scope of responsibility rests on the moral obligation inherent in the role of the dean to ensure that all actions originate in caring, and that an environment is created that fosters development of the capacity to care (Boykin, 1990).

Research Methodology

Boykin and Schoenhofer (2001a) assert that because the nature of nursing exemplified in the Nursing as Caring Theory is one of reciprocal relation, where persons are united in oneness in caring, sciencing in nursing must be commensurate with this perspective. As a human science, nursing calls for methods of inquiry that assure the dialogic circle in the nursing situation and fully encompass that which can be known of nursing. The ontology of nursing, with its locus in person as caring in community with others and with the universe, therefore requires an epistemology consonant with human science values and methods, with "methods and techniques that honor freedom, creativity, and interconnectedness" (Boykin & Schoenhofer, 2001a, p. 53). Traditional or normative methods of research derived from mathematics are not amenable for the study of the fullness of nursing situations. Likewise, phenomenology is unable to achieve a full understanding of nursing, since phenomena for study are removed from the context of the nursing situation and must be reintegrated into the nursing situation in order to be understood in a nursing context.

Boykin and Schoenhofer (2001a) have proposed that the systematic study of nursing should include a new, creative methodology that recognizes the locus of study in the nursing situation. They postulate that a methodology fully adequate to capture nursing knowledge within the nursing situation might include a "phenomenological-hermeneutical process within an action research orientation" (Boykin & Schoenhofer, 2001a, p. 62). Such a method would allow the study of nursing meaning as it is being co-created within the lived experience of the nursing situation. The idea of praxis and the theory of communicative action were explored as possible underpinnings for an emergent research methodology. Aspects of both research approaches require further consideration and development of the philosophical underpinning (Schoenhofer, 2002b).

Research Studies

Research guided by the Theory of Nursing as Caring is ongoing. The practicality of Nursing as Caring is being tested and implemented in several nursing practice settings. Executive personnel, directors of nursing, and nurse administrators are calling for practice models that speak to the essentiality of caring in nursing. Nursing practice models have been developed and are continuing to be refined in acute and long-term care settings. Several examples of use of the theory in research follow.

In separate research studies within units of two major regional hospitals, JFK Medical Center and Boca Raton Community Hospital, values and outcomes of caring were reframed and rearticulated to reflect integration of the Theory of Nursing as Caring. The significant courage of administrators collaborating in this caring research reflected a growing realization that caring for persons as persons is a value to which persons respond. Outcomes of care were documented within reframed institutional values of caring by nurses who contributed these values in their practice.

A 2-year study titled "Demonstration of a Caring-Based Model for Health Care Delivery With the Theory of Nursing as Caring" was completed at JFK Medical Center, Atlantis, Florida, and was funded by the Quantum Foundation (Boykin, Bulfin, Schoenhofer, Baldwin, & McCarthy, 2005).

A practice model based on the Theory of Nursing as Caring was implemented in a telemetry unit. Many persons from all stakeholder groups were invited to tell a story illustrating caring as it was lived in a nursing situation on the pilot unit. The model evolved from shared values of Nursing as Caring, including those expressed by patients, patients' families, nurses, other members and staff of the pilot unit, and members of the administrative team. Themes were uncovered in a narrative analysis and synthesis and served as explicit components of the model. Major themes of the nursing practice model were based on the Theory of Nursing as Caring, and strategies and operational structures were created to reflect these themes. Support for the core of the caring-based model arising from direct invitation (Boykin & Schoenhofer, 2001a, 2001b) led to a new and renewed focus on "responding to that which matters" (Boykin et al., 2003, p. 229), which nurses now recognize as integral to caring in the nursing situation.

This project demonstrated that transformation of care occurs when nursing practice is focused intentionally on coming to know person as caring, and on nurturing and supporting those nursed as they live their caring. Within this practice model, those nursed were able to articulate the experience of being cared for, patient and nurse satisfaction increased dramatically, retention increased, and the environment for care became grounded in the values and respect for person (Boykin et al., 2003). An outcome of use of the model was that nurses sought opportunities to work in a satisfying place with caring others. When nurses transferred from the demonstration unit to other floors, they carried a new focus of nursing with them.

A similar project began in 2003 (Boykin, Bulfin, Baldwin, & Southern, 2004; Bulkin et al., 2005) in the emergency department of Boca Raton Community Hospital, Boca Raton, Florida. The first phase of a model of care based on the Theory of Nursing as Caring was titled "Emergency Department: Transformation From Object Centered Care to Person Centered Care Through Caring." In creating the model, staff realized that changes were needed in conceptualizations of nursing practice. Initially, all emergency services staff, including physicians, nurses, and support services staff, were included, emulating the organization of the dance of caring persons. Evaluation began early because of the success of the model in the busy venue of the emergency department. Although integration of the Theory of Nursing as Caring at JFK Medical Center and Boca Raton Community Hospital was carried out on individual units, the theory demonstrated flexibility and broad-based application and has been integrated system-wide at St. Lucie Medical Center, Port St. Lucie, Florida.

In 2007, the decision was made by nursing staff and administrative personnel at St. Lucie Medical Center to adopt the Theory of Nursing as Caring throughout the medical center. The first step in this process began with a research study conducted to determine how best to uniquely adapt and integrate the Theory of Nursing as Caring. The caring modeled in the theory is being extended to all personnel throughout the hospital, from organization executives, to nurses, physicians, managers, technicians, therapists, and maintenance personnel. Living caring authentically and nurturing the wholeness of others within the rigors and ordinariness of daily work was studied and exemplified in all departments to be infused throughout the organization.

In a study titled "The Phenomenology of Everyday Caring," also based on the Theory of Nursing as Caring, Schoenhofer, Bingham, and Hutchins (1998) examined the lived experience of caring at the essential level of everyday life. They created an innovative research methodology that elicited a rich description of caring through a group process. Hermeneutic phenomenology, employed to illuminate the meaning of lived experience embedded in text, was coupled with guided reflection in a collaborative, developmental process. Thirteen small groups of three to five persons who shared common characteristics such as age, role, setting, or circumstance described their lived experience of caring. Participants included co-researchers who were involved in the group data generation and data synthesis process. Participants were asked to reflect on a situation in which they expressed themselves uniquely as caring persons in their everyday lives. The following essential themes emerged from the action narratives shared by the participants:

1. Caring is evidenced by empathetic understanding, actions, and patience on another's behalf.
2. Caring for one another by actions, words, and being there leads to happiness and touches the heart.
3. Caring is giving of self while preserving the importance of self (Schoenhofer et al., 1998, p. 27). A meta-theme of everyday caring emerged from the stories as "Caring is a fulfilling giving of oneself on another's behalf" (Schoenhofer et al., 1998, p. 27).

The Theory of Nursing as Caring also underpinned Schoenhofer and Boykin's (1998b) study titled "The Value of Caring Experienced in Nursing," which took place in the context of home health nursing. A client family, a nurse associated with a rural, community-based home health agency, a nursing supervisor, and an executive director of the agency participated in dialogic interviews. Caring expressed and values experienced were illuminated by the nursed, the nurse, the nursing supervisor, and the agency executive. Major themes that emerged were trust, honesty, authentic presence, commitment, intention, reciprocity-mutuality, and quality indicators of outcomes of caring (Schoenhofer & Boykin, 1998b). Schoenhofer and Boykin (1998b) noted that most of the value experienced within the nursing relationship could be categorized as patient satisfaction and nurse satisfaction, yet adequate nomenclature was not available to reflect those outcomes.

In a study titled "The Value Experienced in Relationships Involving Nurse Practitioner-Nursed Dyads," Thomas, Finch, Green, and Schoenhofer (2004) sought to describe the shared experience of caring between nurse practitioners and those they nurse, and to uncover the caring experienced in the relationship. The research approach used was praxis, in which dialogue ensued among the nurse practitioner, the nursed, and the nurse researcher, resulting in a portrait of caring relationships between the nurse practitioner and the nursed.

Kiser-Larson (2000) analyzed concepts of caring and story through the lens of Newman, Sime, and Corcoran-Perry's three nursing paradigms: particulate-deterministic, interactive-integrative, and unitary-transformative. Nursing as Caring contributed to the author's understanding of the complexity of caring in the literature and the basis for the author's thesis that "caring and story become reciprocal as caring invites story and story enhances caring" (Kiser-Larson, 2000, p. 28).

Caring from the heart (Touhy, 2004; Touhy & Boykin, 2008) is a model of practice based on the Theory of Nursing as Caring in a unit at a long-term care facility. The model of practice was designed through collaboration between project personnel and all stakeholders. All persons on the unit participated in the process to create an innovative approach that blends with the existing facility design. Major themes revolve around responding to that which matters, caring as a way of expressing spiritual commitment, devotion inspired by love for others, commitment to creating a home environment, and coming to know and respect person as person.

The major building blocks of the nursing models for acute care hospitals and the long-term care facility each reflect central themes of Nursing as Caring, but those themes are drawn out in ways unique to the setting and to the persons involved in each setting. The differences and similarities in these practice models demonstrate the power of Nursing as Caring to transform practice in a way that reflects unity without conformity and uniqueness within oneness (Touhy, 2004; Touhy & Boykin, 2008).

FURTHER DEVELOPMENT

Theory

As a general theory of nursing, Nursing as Caring serves as a broad, conceptual framework underpinning middle range theory development. Drawing on Nursing as Caring as an underlying theoretical framework, Locsin (1995) created a model of machine technologies and caring in nursing. In the model, competence in machine technology and caring is presented as nursing practice if grounded in a caring perspective, without which nursing simply becomes the practice of machine proficiency. Locsin (1998) further developed this critical understanding in the theory of *Technological Competence As Caring in Critical Care Nursing.* In this middle range theory, the intention to care and to nurture the other as caring is actualized through direct knowing, technological competence, and the medium of technologically produced data.

Dunphy and Winland-Brown (2001) presented a model on the *Circle of Caring* (Dunphy, 1998) for advanced practice nursing. The core component of the model, caring processes, focuses on ways of knowing the person as caring and of truly being with the person in advanced practice nursing situations. This core provides the crucial link of caring as the central focus of both traditional nursing and advanced practice nursing.

Purnell (2006) created a Model for Nursing Education grounded in Caring (MONEC), and Touhy and Boykin (2008) proposed caring as the central domain for nursing education. Three major aspects characterize the model for nursing education: the Theory of Nursing as Caring, the metaphor of the dance of caring persons (see Figure 19-1) as organizing construct, and intentionality in nursing with its transformative aspect of aesthetic knowing. Caring intention that guides the creation of the course and environment is understood as a vital energy that flows through and critically interconnects every aspect of the course. From this perspective, caring nursing intention in all its dimensions is essential in the shaping of teaching and learning.

Research

Research and development efforts are focused on expanding the language of caring by uncovering personal ways of living caring in everyday life (Schoenhofer et al., 1998) and on reconceptualizing nursing outcomes as "value experienced in nursing situations" (Boykin & Schoenhofer, 1997; Schoenhofer & Boykin, 1998a, 1998b). In consultation with graduate students, nursing faculties and healthcare agencies are using aspects of the theory to ground research, teaching, and practice. Developmental efforts include the following areas: (1) clarification of the concept of personhood, (2) expansion of the understanding of enhancing personhood as the general outcome of nursing, (3) illuminating understanding of the concept of direct invitation, (4) innovations in nursing research, (5) use of the theory in middle range theory work, and (6) use of the theory in the critical analysis of caring. In a development that signifies grass roots acceptance of the theory, Nursing as Caring has been translated into Japanese.

CRITIQUE

Clarity

Boykin and Schoenhofer achieve semantic clarity by developing the theory of Nursing as Caring with everyday language. The major assumptions that undergird the theory are clearly stated and interrelated. Meanings are understood intuitively and reflectively. The assumption that all persons are caring is necessary for understanding the theory, because Boykin and Schoenhofer assert that the caring between the nurse and the nursed is the source and ground of nursing. The assumption that nursing is both a discipline and a profession provides a conceptual locus for the creation of research methodologies that fluidly unite the discipline and the profession within the notion of research within praxis, or praxis as research. Schoenhofer (2002b) has asserted that a methodology fully adequate to tap nursing knowledge within the nursing situation would include a phenomenological-hermeneutical process with an action research orientation. Such a methodology permits the study of nursing meaning as it is being co-created within the lived experience of the nursing situation.

Simplicity

The simplicity of the theory rests in the everyday language and in the reciprocal nature of nursing, characterized by the fundamental grounding in person as caring. The assumptions of the theory encompass a broad sweep of human understanding and lay plainly the conceptual groundwork for living caring. In this regard, however, the theory becomes more complex, in that assumptions and concepts become richer in meaning and densely interconnected as the nurse comes to know self as caring person in ever greater dimensions (Boykin & Schoenhofer, 2001a). The lived meaning of Nursing as Caring is illuminated best in a nursing situation in which the notion of living caring enhances the knowing of self and other.

Generality

Boykin and colleagues (2003) describe the Theory of Nursing as Caring as a general or grand nursing theory that offers a broad philosophical framework with practical implications for transforming practice. From the perspective of Nursing as Caring, the focus of nursing knowledge and nursing action is nurturing persons who are living caring and growing in caring. The theory may be used to guide individual practice or to guide practice for the organizational level of institutions. The Theory of Nursing as Caring underpins middle range theory development such as Locsin's (1998) theory of technological competence as caring, Dunphy & Winland-Brown's (2001) caring model for advanced practice nursing, Purnell's (2006) model of nursing education grounded in caring, and Eggenberger and Keller's (2008) approach for simulation in caring.

Empirical Precision

The Theory of Nursing as Caring does not lend itself to research methodologies of traditional science but rather is tested in use with approaches of a human science. Because the locus of nursing inquiry is the nursing situation, the systematic study of nursing calls for a method of inquiry that can encompass the dialogic circle of understanding of persons connected in caring. Boykin and Schoenhofer (2001a) distinguish clearly between inquiry *about* nursing and inquiry *of* nursing. The fullness of the nursing situation is not amenable to study by measurement techniques, even though information derived is useful to the nurse and to the client of nursing.

Derivable Consequences

When integrated into nursing practice, the Theory of Nursing as Caring illuminates and brings into consciousness and articulation the values of nursing care. These include the direct, unmediated worth of nursing care in economic terms, the value of nursing as a social and human service, the value of nursing caring as a rich, satisfying practice for nurses, and the value of regenerative nursing for the discipline. The significance of Nursing as Caring is evidenced by the adoption of the theory at multiple levels ranging from individual practice to hospital department, to nursing administration, and now, institution-wide. Nursing values are being translated into values for general well-being, and caring is being infused into the domains of non-nursing personnel.

SUMMARY

The Theory of Nursing as Caring is a general or grand nursing theory that offers a broad philosophical framework with practical implications for transforming practice (Boykin et al., 2003). From the perspective of Nursing as Caring, the focus and aim of nursing as a discipline of knowledge and a professional service is "nurturing persons living caring and growing in caring" (Boykin & Schoenhofer, 2001a, p. 12). The theory is grounded in fundamental assumptions that (1) to be human is to be caring, and (2) the activities of the discipline and the profession of nursing coalesce in coming to know persons as caring, and nurturing them as persons living and growing in caring.

Formed intention and authentic presence guide the nurse in selecting and organizing empirically based knowledge for practical use in each unique and unfolding nursing situation. Because caring is uniquely created in the moment in response to a uniquely experienced call for nursing caring, there can be no prescribed, expected outcome. The caring that is experienced by the nursed and others in the nursing situation can, however, be described and valued (Boykin & Schoenhofer, 1997; Schoenhofer & Boykin, 1998a, 1998b), and in the theory of nursing as caring, becomes a substantive focus for study and research.

Caring in nursing is "an altruistic, active expression of love, and is the intentional and embodied recognition of value and connectedness" (Boykin & Schoenhofer, 2006, p. 336). Although caring is not unique to nursing, it is uniquely lived in nursing. The understanding of nursing as a discipline and as a profession uniquely focuses on caring as its central value, its primary interest, and the direct intention of its practice.

Models for practice are being developed in several institutional practice areas, and Nursing as Caring is being used as a conceptual basis for developing middle range theories. As the Theory of Nursing as Caring has become more widely known, consideration and referential inclusion in disciplinary journals have steadily increased. The theory has been used as a theoretical basis for master's and doctoral research (Herrington, 2002; Linden, 1996, 2000).

Case Study

A Study of the Nursing Situation

The perspective of Nursing as Caring is a study of the nursing situation; rather than a case study, for a focus on personhood as a process of living grounded in caring (Boykin & Schoenhofer, 1991; Touhy, 2004), the nursing situation is the unit of knowledge studied. The mutual relationship shared by the nurse and nursed is one of reciprocity and subjectivity. Because all nursing knowledge is found in the nursing situation, the shared, lived experience in the caring between the nurse and the nursed enhances personhood. Thus story is the method for knowing nursing.

Carper's (1978) fundamental patterns of knowing, personal, empirical, ethical, and aesthetic open useful pathways for organizing and understanding the rich content of the nursing situation. Personal knowing centers on encountering, experiencing, and knowing self and other. Empathy, the shared knowing of other, is an expression of personal knowing. Empirical knowing is impersonal and factual and addresses the science of caring in nursing. Ethical knowing is concerned with moral obligations inherent in nursing situations and what ought to be.

Each pathway transforms knowledge in the creation of aesthetic knowing. Aesthetic knowing is the subjective appreciation of phenomena as lived in the nursing situation: Nursing stories, therefore, represent both the process of aesthetic knowing (creative appreciation) and the product of aesthetic knowing (illumination and integration) (Boykin & Schoenhofer, 1991). The outcomes of nursing are the values experienced within the nursing situation.

For this study of a nursing situation, read the following story slowly, allowing yourself to be one with the nurse and with the ones nursed, sharing in the feelings of each, and dwelling in your reflections.

An Ordinary Wednesday*

> In my role as a nurse clinician, I frequently rounded in the emergency department early mornings to catch the night shift before they went home. To lend a hand to the frazzled staff, I decided to answer a call bell down the hall, where our gynecological examination rooms were located. As I entered the room, I saw a young woman sobbing quietly while her husband attempted to console her. "I think something came out of me" was all she could say.

*The author thanks Patricia "Pidge" Gooch, BSN, RN, for sharing this clinical story.

I introduced myself and proceeded to delicately lift the sheet and saw this young woman had given birth to a tiny lifeless fetus. The nurse caring for the patient joined me and told me that earlier an ultrasound had shown a robust heart rate of 150 in the fetus, but the mother's cervix appeared incompetent. The nurses were working to get her admitted upstairs as soon as possible, but nature had another plan. As many times as I have experienced this in my nursing career in the ED, I am never prepared for the sights or the emotions that accompany these circumstances.

I asked the father to stay at the bedside and went out to summon the ED physician. As the doctor clamped and cut the cord, I asked him quietly if we could wrap the fetus in a blanket and offer the mom the opportunity to see and say goodbye ... almost simultaneously, the father turned to me and said, "She wants to see the baby, but I don't think she should." I gently told him that if she wanted to see the baby, she should. Dad agreed but decided he could not be in the room for this interaction.

I wrapped this tiny bundle in a baby blanket. The fingers and toes were perfect, as were the facial features. Mom asked if we could tell what sex the baby was, and the doctor took a look and said it was really too early to tell. After everyone else had left the room and it was just she and I and her baby, I asked her what names she had planned on. She shared with me the names as she gently caressed the baby's face.

After about 10 minutes, she became very nauseous. Whether it was the Dilaudid or the experience, who knows, but her time came to say goodbye and she did so beautifully, quietly, and gracefully. She tenderly stroked the baby's head, unable to take her eyes away from the sight of her "firstborn," even as she wretched. She was so gentle, so maternal. I thought of my two healthy children at home, and my heart ached for her loss.

In a different room, after mom and dad had been reunited, another nurse and I placed the baby in the container meant for the pathology department. There was something so profoundly sad about life not even given a chance, but also profoundly amazing about the emotions that connected today. What other profession can experience this with their "clients"? How many people in the world have the internal fortitude to deal with these situations?

Intuitively, I had sensed this patient's need to see her baby. On a human level, I cried with her when she first held her baby and examined the fingers and toes, so seemingly perfect. How could something so outwardly perfect looking not survive? How could a mother bear this pain? I was reminded again how privileged I am to share these journeys with my patients and how I am so much more in tune to their needs now as I continue my formal nursing education. Later, the physician came up to me and thanked me for having the thought of letting mom say goodbye ... he said he would have overlooked that important aspect of her care.

I am proud to be a nurse every day, but this day, while I prayed for the family and the soul of that baby, I walked taller, knowing that I am a unique entity who can make a difference ... even on an ordinary Wednesday at work.

Patricia Gooch, BSN, RN
Coral Springs, Florida

CRITICAL THINKING *Activities*

A Nursing Situation Reflection

Find a comfortable space in which to pause, recall, and reflect. Close your eyes and dwell upon the meanings and the caring that took place within the nursing situation, then fully engage in the moment and in the meanings that emerge with these questions:

1. Place yourself in the nurse's shoes and see the one nursed through her eyes. Describe the calls for caring perceived by the nurse. How is the nurse expressing caring in her responses to calls for nursing?
2. In the humility of the nursing situation, how does the father live hope, humility, and trust? How is the father expressing his caring?

3. Enter into the mother's world, and be vulnerable to her pain. What were values of caring experienced in the nursing situation by the mother? How did the nurse express her compassion? How would you have responded to the mother's calls for caring?
4. Describe the empirical knowing of the nurse as captured in her poignant description of the baby. How did this influence her nurturing responses?
5. Who was being cared for when the nurse engaged in the postmortem care of the baby?
6. What difference did caring nursing make in this nursing situation? Describe the mutuality of living and growing in caring.
7. What matters most to you about your nursing? You may want to record your own story of caring in a journal and visit that story later in your career as a nurse.

POINTS FOR *Further Study*

- Archives of Caring in Nursing, Christine E. Lynn Center for Caring, College of Nursing, Florida Atlantic University http://nursing.fau.edu/index.php?main=6&nav=536
- The Theory of Nursing as Caring: A Model for Transforming Practice http://www.nursingascaring.com
- Boykin, A., & Schoenhofer, S. O. (2001). *Nursing as caring: A model for transforming practice* [Rerelease of original 1993 volume, with epilogue added]. Sudbury, MA: Jones & Bartlett Publishers.
- Touhy, T., Eggenberger, T., & Keller, K. (2008). Grounding nursing simulation in caring: An innovative approach. *International Journal for Human Caring, 12*(2), 42-49.
- Touhy, T., & Boykin, A. (2008). Caring as the central domain in nursing education. *International Journal for Human Caring, 12*(2), 8-15.
- Touhy, T. A. (2004). Dementia, personhood, and nursing: Learning from a nursing situation. *Nursing Science Quarterly, 17*(1), 43-49.

REFERENCES

Algase, D. L., & Whall, A. F. (1993). Rosemary Ellis' views on the substantive structure of nursing. *Image: The Journal of Nursing Scholarship, 25*(1), 69-72.

Boykin, A. (1990). Creating a caring environment: Moral obligations in the role of dean. In M. Leininger & J. Watson (Eds.), *The caring imperative in education* (pp. 247-254). New York: National League for Nursing.

Boykin, A. (1994a). Creating a caring environment for nursing education. In A. Boykin (Ed.), *Living a caring-based program* (pp. 11-25). New York: National League for Nursing Press.

Boykin, A. (Ed.). (1994b). *Living a caring-based program.* New York: National League for Nursing.

Boykin, A. (Ed.). (1995). *Power, politics and public policy: A matter of caring.* New York: National League for Nursing.

Boykin, A., Bulfin, S., Baldwin, J., & Southern, R. (2004). Transforming care in the emergency department. *Topics in Emergency Medicine, 26*(4), 331-336.

Boykin, A., Bulfin, S., Schoenhofer, S. O., Baldwin, J., & McCarthy, D. (2005). Living caring in practice: The transformative power of the theory of nursing as caring. *International Journal for Human Caring, 9*(3), 15-19.

Boykin, A., & Parker, M. E. (1997). Illuminating spirituality in the classroom. In M. S. Roach (Ed.), *Caring from the heart: The convergence of caring and spirituality* (pp. 21-33). Mahwah, NJ: Paulist Press.

Boykin, A., Parker, M., & Schoenhofer, S. (1994). Aesthetic knowing grounded in an explicit conception of nursing. *Nursing Science Quarterly, 7*(4), 158-161.

Boykin, A., & Schoenhofer, S. (1993). *Nursing as caring: A model for transforming practice.* New York: National League for Nursing Press.

Boykin, A., & Schoenhofer, S. O. (1990). Caring in nursing: Analysis of extant theory. *Nursing Science Quarterly, 3*(4), 149-155.

Boykin, A., & Schoenhofer, S. O. (1991). Story as link between nursing practice, ontology, and epistemology. *Image: The Journal of Nursing Scholarship, 23*(4), 245-248.

Boykin, A., & Schoenhofer, S. O. (1997). Reframing nursing outcomes. *Advanced Practice Nursing Quarterly, 1*(3), 60-65.

Boykin, A., & Schoenhofer, S. O. (2006). Nursing as caring: An overview of a general theory of nursing. In M. E. Parker (Ed.), *Nursing theories and nursing practice,* (2nd ed.) (pp. 334-348). Philadelphia: F. A. Davis.

Boykin, A., & Schoenhofer, S. O. (2001a). *Nursing as caring: A model for transforming practice* [Rerelease of original 1993 volume, with epilogue added]. Sudbury, MA: Jones & Bartlett Publishers.

Boykin, A., & Schoenhofer, S. O. (2001b). The role of nursing leadership in creating caring environments in health care delivery systems. *Nursing Administration Quarterly, 25*(3), 1-7.

Boykin, A., & Schoenhofer, S. (2006). Anne Boykin and Savina O. Schoenhofer's nursing as caring theory. In M. E. Parker (Ed.), *Nursing theories and nursing practice* (pp. 334-348). Philadelphia, PA: F. A. Davis.

Boykin, A., Schoenhofer, S. O., Smith, N., St. Jean, J., & Aleman, D. (2003). Transforming practice using a caring-based nursing model. *Nursing Administration Quarterly, 27*, 223-230.

Carper, B. A. (1978). Fundamental patterns of knowing in nursing. *ANS Advances in Nursing Science, 1*(1), 113-124.

Dunphy, L. H. (1998). *The circle of caring: A transformative model of advanced practice nursing.* 20th Research Conference of the International Association for Human Caring, Philadelphia.

Dunphy, L. H., & Winland-Brown, J. (2001). *Primary care: The art and science of advanced practice nursing.* Philadelphia: F. A. Davis.

Eggenberger, T., & Keller, K. (2008). Grounding nursing simulation in caring: An innovative approach. *International Journal for Human Caring, 12*(2), 42-49.

Flexner, A. (1910). *Medical education in the United States and Canada.* New York: The Carnegie Foundation for the Advancement of Teaching.

Gaut, D. A., & Boykin, A. (Eds.). (1994). *Caring as healing: Renewal through hope.* New York: National League for Nursing.

Herrington, C. L. (2002). *The meaning of caring: From the perspective of homeless women* (Master's thesis, University of Nevada, Reno, 2002). *Masters Abstracts International, 41*(01), 191.

King, A., & Brownell, J. (1976). *The curriculum and the disciplines of knowledge.* Huntington, NY: Robert E. Krieger Publishing.

Kiser-Larson, N. (2000). The concepts of caring and story viewed from three nursing paradigms. *International Journal for Human Caring, 4*(2), 26-32.

Linden, D. (1996). *Philosophical exploration in search of the ontology of authentic presence* (Master's thesis, Florida Atlantic University, West Palm Beach, FL, 1996). *Masters Abstracts International, 35*(2), 519.

Linden, D. (2000). The lived experience of nursing as caring. In M. E. Parker (Ed.), *Nursing theories and nursing practice* (pp. 403-407). Philadelphia, PA: F. A. Davis.

Locsin, R. C. (1995). Machine technologies and caring in nursing. *Image: The Journal of Nursing Scholarship, 27*(3), 201-203.

Locsin, R. C. (1998). Technologic competence as caring in critical care nursing. *Holistic Nursing Practice, 12*(4), 50-56.

Mayeroff, M. (1971). *On caring.* New York: Harper Collins.

Orem, D. E. (Ed.). (1979). *Concept formalization in nursing. Process and product* (2nd ed.). Boston: Little, Brown and Company.

Paterson, J.G., & Zderad, L. T. (1988).*Humanistic nursing.* New York: National League for Nursing Press.

Phenix, P. (1964). *Realms of meaning.* New York: McGraw Hill.

Purnell, M. J. (2006). Development of a model of nursing education grounded in caring and application to online nursing education. *International Journal for Human Caring, 10*(3), 8-16.

Roach, M. S. (1987). *Caring, the human mode of being.* Ottawa, Ontario, Canada: CHA Press.

Roach, M. S. (2002). *Caring, the human mode of being* (2nd revised ed.). Ottawa, Ontario, Canada: CHA Press.

Schoenhofer, S. O. (2001). Infusing the nursing curriculum with literature on caring: An idea whose time has come. *International Journal for Human Caring, 5*(2), 7-14.

Schoenhofer, S. O. (2002a). Choosing personhood: Intentionality and the theory of nursing as caring. *Holistic Nursing Practice, 16*(4), 36-40.

Schoenhofer, S. O. (2002b). Philosophical underpinnings of an emergent methodology for nursing as caring inquiry. *Nursing Science Quarterly, 15*(4), 275-280.

Schoenhofer, S. O., Bingham, V., & Hutchins, G. (1998). Giving of oneself on another's behalf: The phenomenology of everyday caring. *International Journal for Human Caring, 2*(2), 23-29.

Schoenhofer, S. O., & Boykin, A., (1998a). Discovering the value of nursing in high-technology environments: Outcomes revisited. *Holistic Nursing Practice, 12*(4), 31-39.

Schoenhofer, S. O., & Boykin, A. (1998b). The value of caring experienced in nursing. *International Journal for Human Caring, 2*(4), 9-15.

Schoenhofer, S. O., & Boykin, A. (1993). Nursing as caring: An emerging general theory of nursing. In M. E. Parker (Ed.), *Patterns of nursing theories in practice* (pp. 83-92). New York: National League for Nursing Press.

Thomas, J., Finch, L. P., Green, A., & Schoenhofer, S. O. (2004). The caring relationships created by nurse practitioners and the ones nursed: Implications for practice. *Topics in Advanced Nursing Practice, ejournal* 4(4), Retrieved March 9, 2005, from *http://www.medscape.com.*

Touhy, T. A. (2004). Dementia, personhood, and nursing: Learning from a nursing situation. *Nursing Science Quarterly, 17*(1), 43-49.

Touhy, T., & Boykin, A. (2008). Caring as the central domain in nursing education. *International Journal for Human Caring, 12*(2), 8-15.

BIBLIOGRAPHY

Primary Sources

Books

Boykin, A. (Ed.). (1994). *Living a caring-based program.* New York: National League for Nursing.

Boykin, A. (Ed.). (1995). *Power, politics and public policy: A matter of caring.* New York: National League for Nursing.

Boykin, A., & Schoenhofer, S. O. (1993). *Nursing as caring: A model for transforming practice.* New York: NLN Publications.

Boykin, A., & Schoenhofer, S. O. (2001). *Nursing as caring: A model for transforming practice* [Rerelease of original volume, with epilogue added]. Sudbury, MA: Jones & Bartlett Publishers.

Gaut, D. A., & Boykin, A. (Eds.). (1994). *Caring as healing: Renewal through hope.* New York: National League for Nursing.

Book Chapters

Beckerman, A., Boykin A., Folden S., & Winland-Brown, J. (1994). The experience of being a student in a caring-based program. In A. Boykin (Ed.), *Living a caring-based program* (pp. 79-92). New York: National League for Nursing.

Boykin A. (1990). Creating a caring environment: Moral obligations in the role of dean. In M. Leininger & J. Watson (Eds.), *The caring imperative in education* (pp. 247-254). New York: National League for Nursing.

Boykin, A. (1994). Creating a caring environment for nursing education. In A. Boykin (Ed.), *Living a caring-based program* (pp. 11-25). New York, National League for Nursing.

Boykin, A. (1998). Nursing as caring through the reflective lens. In C. Johns & D. Freshwater (Eds.), *Transforming nursing through reflective practice* (pp. 43-50). Oxford, England: Blackwell Science.

Boykin, A., & Parker, M. (1997). Illuminating spirituality in the classroom. In S. Roach (Ed.), *Caring from the heart.* Mahwah, NJ: Paulist Press.

Boykin, A., & Schoenhofer, S. O. (2000). Nursing as caring: An overview of a general theory of nursing. In M. E. Parker (Ed.), *Nursing theories and nursing practice.* Philadelphia: F. A. Davis.

Boykin, A., & Schoenhofer, S. (2006). Anne Boykin and Savina O. Schoenhofer's nursing as caring theory. In M. E. Parker (Ed.), *Nursing theories and nursing practice* (pp. 334-348). Philadelphia, PA: F. A. Davis.

Parker, M. E., & Schoenhofer, S. O. (2007). Foundations for nursing education: Nursing as a discipline. In B. A. Moyer & R. Whittman-Price (Eds.), *Nursing education: Foundations for practice and excellence,* (pp. 4-11). Philadelphia, PA: F. A. Davis.

Schoenhofer, S. O. (2001). A framework for caring in a technologically dependent nursing practice environment. In R. C. Locsin (Ed.), *Advancing technology, caring and nursing* (pp. 3-11). Westport, CT: Auburn House.

Schoenhofer, S. O. (2001). Outcomes of nurse caring in high technology practice environments. In R. C. Locsin (Ed.), *Advancing technology, caring, and nursing* (pp. 79-87). Westport, CT: Auburn House.

Schoenhofer, S. O., & Boykin, A. (1993). Nursing as caring: An emerging general theory of nursing. In M. E. Parker (Ed.), *Patterns of nursing theories in practice* (pp. 83-92). New York: National League for Nursing Press.

Schoenhofer, S. O., & Boykin, A. (2001). Caring and the advanced practice nurse. In L. Dunphy & J. Winland-Brown (Eds.), *Primary care: The art and science of advanced practice nursing.* Philadelphia: F. A. Davis.

Schoenhofer, S. O., & Coffman, S. (1993). Valuing, prizing and growing in a caring based program. In A. Boykin (Ed.), *Living a caring based program* (pp. 127-165). New York: National League for Nursing.

Journal Articles

Boykin, A., Bulfin, S., Baldwin, J., & Southern, R. (2004). Transforming care in the emergency department. *Topics in Emergency Medicine, 26*(4), 331-336.

Boykin, A., Bulfin, S., Schoenhofer, S. O., Baldwin, J., & McCarthy, D. (2005). Living caring in practice: The transformative power of the theory of nursing as caring. *International Journal for Human Caring, 9*(3), 15-19.

Boykin, A., & Dunphy, L. (2002). Reflective essay: Justice-making: Nursing's call. Florence Nightingale. *Policy, Politics and Nursing Practice, 3*(1), 14-19.

Boykin, A., Parker, M., & Schoenhofer, S. (1994). Aesthetic knowing grounded in an explicit conception of nursing. *Nursing Science Quarterly, 7*(4), 158-161.

Boykin, A., & Schoenhofer, S. O. (1990). Caring in nursing: Analysis of extant theory. *Nursing Science Quarterly, 3*(4), 149-155.

Boykin, A., & Schoenhofer, S. O. (1991). Story as link between nursing practice, ontology, and epistemology. *Image: The Journal of Nursing Scholarship, 23*(4), 245-248.

Boykin, A., & Schoenhofer, S. O. (1997). Reframing outcomes: Enhancing personhood. *Advanced Practice Nursing Quarterly, 1*(3), 60-65.

Boykin, A., & Schoenhofer, S. O. (2000). Is there really time to care? *Nursing Forum, 35*(4), 36-38.

Boykin, A., & Schoenhofer, S. O. (2001). The role of nursing leadership in creating caring environments in health care delivery systems. *Nursing Administration Quarterly, 25*(3), 1-7.

Boykin, A., Schoenhofer, S. O., Smith, N., St. Jean, J., & Aleman, D. (2003). Transforming practice using a caring-based nursing model. *Nursing Administration Quarterly, 27*, 223-230.

Boykin, A., & Winland-Brown, J. (1995). The dark side of caring: Challenges of caregiving. *Journal of Gerontological Nursing, 21*(5), 13-18.

Finch, L. P., Thomas, J. D., Schoenhofer, S. O. (2006). Research as praxis: A mode of inquiry into caring in nursing. *International Journal for Human Caring, 10*(1), 28-31.

Schoenhofer, S. O. (1989). Love, beauty, and truth: Fundamental nursing values. *Journal of Nursing Education, 28*(8), 382-384.

Schoenhofer, S. O. (1994). Transforming visions for nursing in the timeworld of Einstein's dreams. *ANS Advances in Nursing Science, 16*(4), 1-8.

Schoenhofer, S. O. (1995). Rethinking primary care: Connections to nursing. *ANS Advances in Nursing Science, 17*(4), 12-21.

Schoenhofer, S. O. (2001). Infusing the nursing curriculum with literature on caring: An idea whose time has come. *International Journal for Human Caring, 5*(2), 7-14.

Schoenhofer, S. O. (2002). Philosophical underpinnings of an emergent methodology for nursing as caring inquiry. *Nursing Science Quarterly, 15*(4), 275-280.

Schoenhofer, S. O. (2002). Choosing personhood: Intentionality and the theory of nursing as caring. *Holistic Nursing Practice, 16*(4), 36-40.

Schoenhofer, S., Bingham, V., & Hutchins, G. (1998). Giving of oneself on another's behalf: The phenomenology of everyday caring. *International Journal for Human Caring, 2*(2), 23-29.

Schoenhofer, S. O., & Boykin, A. (1998). The value of caring experienced in nursing. *International Journal for Human Caring, 2*(4), 9-15.

Schoenhofer, S. O., & Boykin, A. (1998). Discovering the value of nursing in high-technology environments: Outcomes revisited. *Holistic Nursing Practice, 12*(4), 31-39.

Schoenhofer, S. O., Dollar, C. B., & Roberson, S. (2007). Advanced practice nursing in disasters: Toward a model grounded in the theory of nursing as caring. *International Journal for Human Caring, 11*(3), 63.

Thomas, J. D., Finch, L. P., & Schoenhofer, S. O. (2004). The caring relationships created by nurse practitioners and the ones nursed: Implications for practice. *Topics in Advanced Practice Nursing, 4(4), 6.*

Touhy, T., & Boykin, A. (2008). Caring as the central domain in nursing education. *International Journal for Human Caring, 12*(2), 8-15.

Secondary Sources

Books

Locsin, R. C. (Ed.). (2001). *Advancing technology, caring, and nursing.* Westport, CT: Greenwood Publishing.

Locsin, R. C. (2005). *Technological competency as caring in nursing: A model for practice.* Indianapolis: Sigma Theta Tau International Honor Society of Nursing.

Book Chapters

George, J. (2002). Nursing as caring. Anne Boykin and Savina Schoenhofer. In J. George (Ed.), *Nursing theories.* Upper Saddle River, NJ: Prentice-Hall.

Linden, D. (2000). The lived experience of nursing as caring. In M. E. Parker (Ed.), *Nursing theories and nursing practice* (pp. 403-407). Philadelphia: F. A. Davis.

Locsin, R. C. (1995). Technology and caring in nursing. In A. Boykin (Ed.), *Power, politics, and public policy: A matter of caring* (pp. 24-36). New York: National League for Nursing.

Locsin, R., & Campling, A. (2005). Techno sapiens and post humans: Nursing, caring, and technology. In R. Locsin (Ed.), *Technological competency as caring in nursing: A model for practice* (pp. 142-155). Indianapolis: Center Nursing Press, Sigma Theta Tau International Honor Society of Nursing.

Journal Articles

Barry, C. D. (2001). Creating a quilt: An aesthetic expression of caring for nursing students. *International Journal for Human Caring, 6*(1), 25-29.

Bulfin, S., & Mitchell, G. J. (2005). Nursing as caring theory: Living theory in practice. *Nursing Science Quarterly, 18*(4), 313-319.

Carter, M. A. (1994). [Book reviews: *Nursing as caring: A model for transforming practice]. Nursing Science Quarterly, 7,* 183-184.

Kiser-Larson, N. (2000). The concepts of caring and story viewed from three nursing paradigms. *International Journal for Human Caring, 4*(2), 26-32.

Locsin, R. C. (1995). Machine technologies and caring in nursing. *Image: The Journal of Nursing Scholarship, 27*(3), 201-203.

Locsin, R. C. (1997). Expressing nursing as caring through music. *The Silliman Journal, 8*(1 & 2), 1-10.

Locsin, R. C. (1998). Music as expression of nursing: A co-created moment. *International Journal for Human Caring, 2*(3), 40-42.

Locsin, R. C. (1998). Technological competence as caring in critical care nursing. *Holistic Nursing Practice, 12*(4), 50-56.

Locsin, R. C. (2000). Technological competency as caring: Perceptions of professional nurses. *The Silliman Journal, 40* & 41, 100-104.

Locsin, R. C. (2002). Aesthetic expressions of the lived world of people waiting to know: Ebola at Mbarara, Uganda. *Nursing Science Quarterly, 15*(2), 123-130.

Locsin, R. C., & Purnell, M. J. (2007). Rapture and suffering with technology in nursing. *International Journal for Human Caring, 11*(1), 38-43.

McCance, T. V., McKenna, H. P., & Boore, J. R. P. (1999). Caring: Theoretical perspectives of relevance to nursing. *Journal of Advanced Nursing, 30,* 1388-1395.

Purnell, M. J. (2006). Development of a model of nursing education grounded in caring and application to online nursing education. *International Journal for Human Caring, 10*(3), 8-16.

Purnell, M. J., & Mead, L. J. (2007). When nurses mourn: Layered suffering. *International Journal for Human Caring, 11*(2), 47-52.

Smith, M. C. (1994). [Book review: *Nursing as caring: A model for transforming practice]. Nursing Science Quarterly, 7,* 184-185.

Smith, M. C. (1999). Caring and the science of unitary human beings. *ANS Advances in Nursing Science, 21*(4), 14-28.

Touhy, T. A. (2001). Touching the spirit of elders in nursing homes: Ordinary yet extraordinary care. *International Journal for Human Caring, 6*(1), 12-17.

Touhy, T. A. (2004). Dementia, personhood, and nursing: Learning from a nursing situation. *Nursing Science Quarterly, 17*(1), 43-49.

Winland-Brown, J. E. (1996). Can caring for critically ill patients be taught by reading a novel? *Nurse Educator, 21*(5), 23-27.

Other Sources

Herrington, C. L. (2002). The meaning of caring: From the perspective of homeless women (Master's thesis, University of Nevada, Reno, 2002). *Masters Abstracts International, 41*(01), 191.

Linden, D. (1996). Philosophical exploration in search of the ontology of authentic presence (Master's thesis, Florida Atlantic University, West Palm Beach, FL, 1996). *Masters Abstracts International, 35*(2), 519.

Touhy, T. A. (2003). *More alike than different: Caring across cultures in nursing homes.* Unpublished study of cultural harmony based on Boykin and Schoenhofer's theory of nursing as caring. Funding by Quantum Foundation, West Palm Beach, FL.

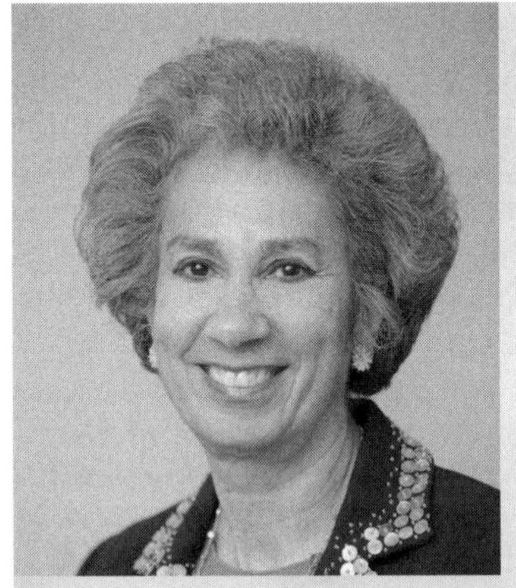

CHAPTER

20

Afaf Ibrahim Meleis

Transition Theory

Eun-Ok Im

"I believe very strongly that, while knowledge is universal, the agents for developing knowledge must reflect the nature of the questions that are framed and driven by the different disciplines about the health and well-being of individuals or populations" (Meleis, 2007, ix).

CREDENTIALS AND BACKGROUND OF THE THEORIST

Afaf Ibrahim Meleis was born in Alexandria, Egypt. In personal communications with Meleis (December 29, 2007), she reckons that nursing has been part of her life since she was born. Her mother is considered the Florence Nightingale of the Middle East; she was the first person in Egypt to obtain a BSN degree from Syracuse University, and the first nurse in Egypt who obtained an MPH and a PhD from an Egyptian university. Meleis considered nursing to be in her blood, and she admired her mother's dedication and commitment to the profession. Under the influence of her mother, Meleis became interested in nursing and loved the potential of developing the discipline. Yet, when she chose to pursue nursing, her parents objected to her choice because they knew how much nurses struggle in having a voice and affecting quality of care. However, they eventually approved of her choice and had faith that Meleis could do it.

Meleis completed her nursing degree at the University of Alexandria, Egypt. She came to the United States to pursue graduate education as a Rockefeller Fellow in order to become an academic nurse (Meleis, personal communication, December 29, 2007). From the University of California, Los Angeles, she received an MS in nursing in 1964, an MA in sociology in 1966, and a PhD in medical and social psychology in 1968.

Her career combined academic and administrative positions. After getting her doctoral degree, she worked as an acting instructor at the University of California, Los Angeles, from 1966 to 1968, and as an

Assistant Professor at the same university from 1968 to 1971. In 1971, she moved to the University of California, San Francisco (UCSF), where she spent the next 34 years, and where her Transition Theory was first developed. In 2002, she was nominated the Margret Bond Simon Dean of Nursing, and became the Dean of the School of Nursing at the University of Pennsylvania.

Meleis, a prominent nurse sociologist, is a sought-after theorist, researcher, and speaker on the topics of women's health and development, immigrant healthcare, international healthcare, and knowledge and theoretical development. She is currently on the Counsel General of the International Council on Women's Health Issues. Meleis received numerous honors and awards as well as honorary doctorates and distinguished and honorary professorships around the world. She received the Medal of Excellence for professional and scholarly achievements from Egyptian President Hosni Mubarak in 1990. In 2000, she received the Chancellor's Medal from the University of Massachusetts, Amherst. In 2001, she received the UCSF's Chancellor Award for the Advancement of Women in recognition of her role as a worldwide activist on behalf of women's issues. In 2004, she received the Pennsylvania Commission for Women Award in celebration of women's history month and the Special Recognition Award in Human Services from the Arab American Family Support Center in New York. In 2006, she was awarded the Robert E. Davies Award from the Penn Professional Women's Network for her advocacy on behalf of women.

Meleis' research focuses on global health, immigrant and international health, women's health, and the theoretical development of the nursing discipline. She authored more than 150 articles in social sciences, nursing, and medical journals; 40 chapters; and numerous monographs, proceedings, and books. Her award winning book, *Theoretical Nursing: Development and Progress* (1985, 1991, 1997, 2007), is used widely throughout the world.

The development of Transition Theory began in the mid-1960s, when Meleis was working on her PhD, and can be traced through the years of her research with students and colleagues. In her book (Meleis, 2007), describes how her theoretical journey started from her practice and research interests. In her master's and PhD dissertation research, Meleis investigated phenomena of planning pregnancies and processes involved in becoming a new parent and mastering parenting roles. She focused on spousal communication and interaction in effective or ineffective planning of the number of children in families (Meleis, 1975), and later reasoned that her earlier ideas were incomplete since she did not consider transitions.

Subsequently, her research interests were focused on people who do not make healthy transitions and discovery of interventions that would facilitate healthy transitions. For these research questions, symbolic interactionism played an important role in efforts to conceptualize the symbolic world that shapes interactions and responses. This shift in her theoretical thinking led her to role theories as were referenced in her publications in those years of the 1970s and 1980s.

Meleis' earliest work with transitions defined unhealthy transitions or ineffective transitions in relation to role insufficiency. She defined *role insufficiency* as any difficulty in the cognizance and/or performance of a role or of the sentiments and goals associated with the role behavior as perceived by the self or by significant others (Meleis, 2007). This conceptualization led Meleis to define the goal of healthy transitions as mastery of behaviors, sentiments, cues, and symbols associated with new roles and identities and non-problematic processes. Meleis believed that knowledge development in nursing should be geared toward nursing therapeutics and not toward understanding the phenomena related to responses to health and illness situations. Consequently, she initiated the development of role supplementation as a nursing therapeutic as seen in her earlier research (Meleis, 1975; Meleis & Swendsen, 1978; Jones, Zhang, & Meleis, 1978).

The gist of Meleis' works published in the 1970s defined role supplementation as any deliberate process through which role insufficiency or potential role insufficiency can be identified by the role incumbent and significant others. Thus, role supplementation includes both role clarification and role taking, which may be preventive and therapeutic.

With these changes in her theoretical thinking, role supplementation as a nursing therapeutic entered her research projects. Her main research questions were to further define the components, the processes, and the strategies related to role supplementation, which she believed would make a difference by helping patients complete a healthy transition. This led Meleis to define *health* as mastery, and she tested that definition through proxy outcome variables such as "fewer symptoms," "perceived well-being," and "ability to assume new roles."

Her theory of role supplementation was used not only in her studies on the new role of parenting (Meleis & Swendsen, 1978), but in other studies among post–myocardial infarction patients (Dracup, Meleis, Baker, & Edlefsen, 1985), elders (Kaas & Rousseau, 1983), parental caregivers (Brackley, 1992), caregivers of Alzheimer's patients (Kelley & Lakin, 1988), and women who were not successful in becoming mothers and who maintained role insufficiency (Gaffney, 1992). In these studies using role supplementation theory, Meleis began to question the nature of transitions and the human experience of transitions. Her research population interests shifted to immigrants and their health. This shift led Meleis to look back and question "transitions" as a concept. Meleis met Norma Chick from Massey University, New Zealand, and they developed transition as a concept that was published in 1985 (Chick & Meleis, 1986). This was actually Meleis' first article on transitions as a major concept of nursing.

To further develop this theoretical work, Meleis initiated extensive literature searches with Karen Schumacher, a doctoral student at the University of California, San Francisco, to discover how extensively transition was used as a concept or framework in nursing literature. Three hundred ten articles focused on transitions, so Meleis further developed the transition framework (Schumacher & Meleis, 1994) that was later further developed as a middle range theory. Publication of the transition framework was well received by nurse scholars and researchers and began to be used as a conceptual framework in a number of studies that examined the following:

- Description of immigrant transitions (Meleis, Lipson, & Dallafar, 1998)
- Women's experience of rheumatoid arthritis (Shaul, 1997)
- Recovery from cardiac surgery (Shih, et al., 1998)
- Family caregiving role for patients in chemotherapy (Schumacher, 1995)
- Early memory loss for patients in Sweden (Robinson, Ekman, Meleis, Wahlund, & Winbald, 1997)
- Aging transitions (Schumacher, Jones, & Meleis, 1999)
- African American women's transition to motherhood (Sawyer, 1997)

Using the transition framework, a middle range theory for transition was developed by the researchers who had used transition as a conceptual framework. They analyzed their findings related to transition experiences and responses, identifying similarities and differences in the use of transition; findings were compared, contrasted, and integrated through extensive reading, reviewing, and dialoguing, and in group meetings. The collective work was published in 2000 (Meleis, Sawyer, Im, Schumacher, & Messias, 2000) and has been widely used in nursing studies. See Figure 20-1 for a diagram of the middle range transition theory.

The situation-specific theories based on the transition framework that Meleis (1997) called for, with specifics in level of abstraction, degree of specificity, scope of context, and connection to nursing research and practice, were similar to the emerging midrange transition theory by Meleis et al. (Im, 2006; Im & Meleis, 1999a; Im & Meleis, 1999b; Schumacher, Jones, & Meleis, 1999). For example, Im and Meleis (1999b) developed a situation-specific theory of low-income Korean immigrant women's menopausal transition based on their research findings, while using the transition framework of Schumacher and Meleis (1994). Schumacher et al. (1999) developed

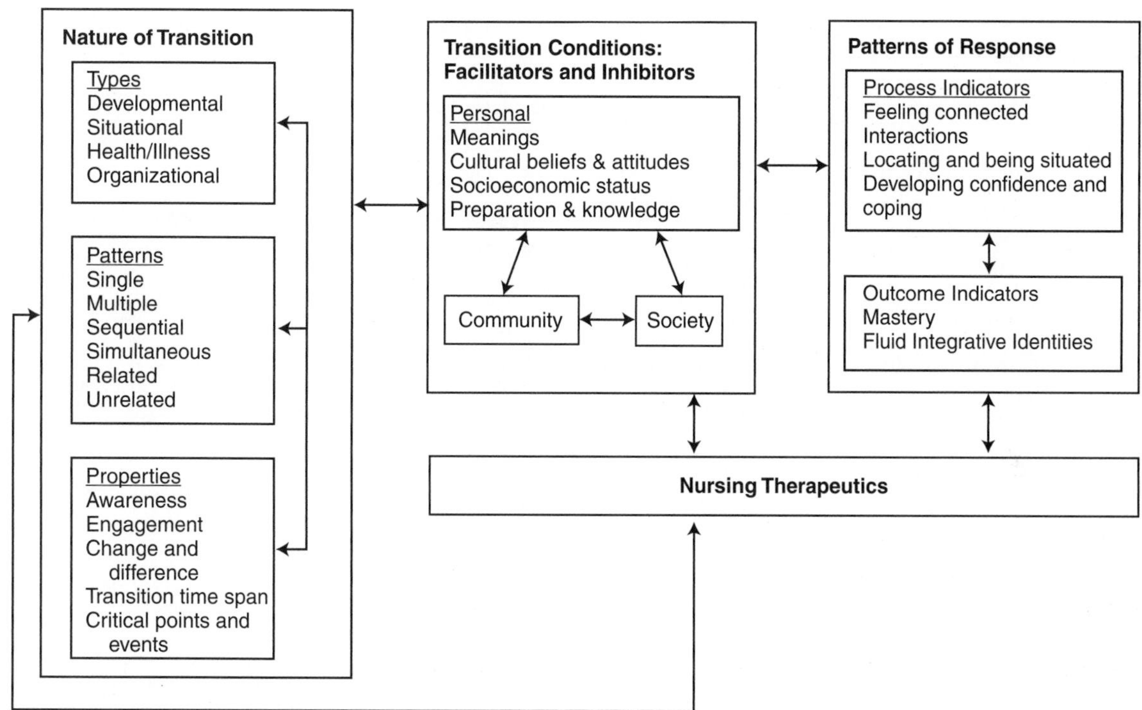

Figure 20-1 The Midrange Transition Theory. (From Meleis, A. I., Sawyer, L. M., Im, E. O., Messias, D. K. H., & Schumacher, K. [2000]. Experiencing transitions: An emerging middle range theory. *Advances in Nursing Science*, 23[1], 12-28.)

a situation-specific theory of elderly transition. Im (2006) also developed a situation-specific theory of white cancer patients' pain experience. These situation-specific theories were derivative of the middle range transition theory.

THEORETICAL SOURCES

Theoretical sources for Transition Theory are multiple. First, Meleis' background in nursing, sociology, symbolic interactionism, and role theory and her education led to the development of Transition Theory as described above. Indeed, findings and experience from research projects, educational programs, and clinical practice in hospital and community settings have been frequent sources for theoretical development in nursing (Im, 2005). A systematic, extensive literature review was another source for development of Transition Theory. A systematic, extensive literature review has been suggested as a way of compiling currently existing knowledge about a nursing phenomenon and has been used frequently as an excellent source for theory development (Walker & Avant, 1995, 2005). Finally, collaborative efforts among researchers who used the transition theoretical framework and the middle range transition theory in their studies were another source for development of Transition Theory. As Im (2005) asserted, experts in different areas of nursing who are working on the same nursing phenomenon could give different and new views/visions of the same nursing phenomenon.

MAJOR CONCEPTS & DEFINITIONS

Here, the major concepts and definitions from the most current transition theory, the middle range theory of transition suggested by Meleis et al. (2000), are presented. Some concepts that were briefly presented in the middle range theory of transition are defined in greater detail based on the transition framework by Schumacher and Meleis (1994).

Major concepts of the middle range theory of transition include the following: (a) types and patterns of transitions; (b) properties of transition experiences; (c) transition conditions (facilitators and inhibitors); (d) process indicators; (e) outcome indicators; and (f) nursing therapeutics.

TYPES AND PATTERNS OF TRANSITIONS

Types of transitions include developmental, health and illness, situational, and organizational. Developmental transition includes birth, adolescence, menopause, aging (or senescence), and death. Health and illness transitions include recovery process, hospital discharge, and diagnosis of chronic illness (Meleis & Trangenstein, 1994). Organizational transitions refer to changing environmental conditions that affect the lives of clients, as well as workers within them (Schumacher & Meleis, 1994).

Patterns of transitions include multiplicity and complexity (Meleis et al., 2000). Many people are experiencing multiple transitions at the same time rather than experiencing a single transition, which cannot be easily distinguished from the contexts of their daily lives. Indeed, in the article by Meleis et al. (2000), it was noted that each of the studies that were the basis for the theoretical development involved individuals who were experiencing at least two types of transitions at the same time, which could not be discrete or mutually exclusive. Thus, they suggested that important considerations are whether multiple transitions are sequential or simultaneous, the extent of overlap among transitions, and the nature of the relationship between the different events that are triggering transitions for a client.

PROPERTIES OF TRANSITION EXPERIENCE

Properties of the transition experience include (a) awareness; (b) engagement; (c) change and difference; (d) time span; and (e) critical points and events. Meleis et al. (2000) asserted that these properties are not necessarily discrete, but are interrelated as a complex process.

Awareness is defined as perception, knowledge, and recognition of a transition experience, and level of awareness is often reflected in the degree of congruency between what is known about processes and responses and what constitutes an expected set of responses and perceptions of individuals undergoing similar transitions (Meleis et al., 2000). While asserting that a person in transition may have some awareness of the changes that are occurring, Chick and Meleis (1986) posited that an absence of awareness of change could signify that an individual may not have initiated the transition experience; Meleis et al. (2000) later proposed that the lack of manifestation of awareness of changes does not by necessity preclude the onset of a transition experience. However, the tension between transition awareness by clients and nurses' knowledge of whether clients are in transition has not been resolved yet (Meleis et al., 2000).

Engagement is another property of transition suggested by Meleis et al. (2000). Engagement refers to the degree to which a person demonstrates involvement in the process inherent in the transition. The level of awareness is considered to influence the level of engagement in that engagement may not happen without awareness. Meleis et al. (2000) suggested that the level of engagement of a person who is aware of physical, emotional,

MAJOR CONCEPTS & DEFINITIONS—cont'd

social, or environmental changes would differ from that of a person unaware of these changes.

Changes and differences are a property of transitions (Meleis et al., 2000). Changes in identities, roles, relationships, abilities, and patterns of behavior are supposed to bring a sense of movement or direction to internal processes, as well as external processes (Schumacher & Meleis, 1994). Meleis et al. (2000) asserted that all transitions involve change, whereas not all change is related to transition. Then, they suggested that to fully understand a transition process, it is necessary to uncover and describe the effects and meanings of the changes involved and the dimensions of changes (e.g., nature, temporality, perceived importance or severity, personal, familial, and societal norms and expectations). Differences are also suggested as a property of transitions. Meleis et al. (2002) believed that confronting differences could be exemplified by unmet or divergent expectations, feeling different, being perceived as different, or seeing the world and others in different ways, and suggested that it might be useful for nurses to consider a client's level of comfort and mastery in dealing with changes and differences.

Time span is also a property of transitions—all transitions may be characterized as flowing and moving over time (Meleis et al., 2000). According to the assertion by Bridges (1980, 1991), in the middle range theory of transition, *transition* is defined as a span of time with an identifiable starting point, extending from the first signs of anticipation, perception, or demonstration of change; moving through a period of instability, confusion, and distress; to an eventual "ending" with a new beginning or period of stability. However, Meleis et al. (2000) also made the point that it might be difficult or impossible, and perhaps even counterproductive, to put boundaries on the time span of certain transition experiences.

Critical points and events are the final property of transitions suggested by Meleis et al. (2000). Critical points and events are defined as markers such as birth, death, the cessation of menstruation, or the diagnosis of an illness. Meleis et al. (2000) also acknowledge that specific marker events might not be evident for some transitions, although transitions usually have critical points and events. Critical points and events are usually associated with increasing awareness of changes or differences or more active engagement in dealing with transition experiences. Also, Transition Theory conceptualizes that there are final critical points that are characterized by a sense of stabilization in new routines, skills, lifestyles, and self-care activities, and that a period of uncertainty is marked by fluctuation, continuous change, and disruption of reality.

TRANSITION CONDITIONS

Transition conditions are those circumstances that influence the way a person moves through a transition, and that facilitate or hinder progress toward achieving a healthy transition (Schumacher & Meleis, 1994). Transition conditions include personal, community, or societal factors that may facilitate or constrain the processes and outcomes of healthy transitions.

Personal conditions include meanings, cultural beliefs and attitudes, socioeconomic status, preparation, and knowledge. Meleis et al. (2000) considered that the meanings attributed to events precipitating a transition and to the transition process itself may facilitate or hinder healthy transitions. Cultural beliefs and attitudes such as stigma attached to a transition experience (e.g., Chinese stigmatization of cancer) would influence the transition experience. Socioeconomic status could influence people's transition experiences. Anticipatory preparation or lack of preparation

Continued

MAJOR CONCEPTS & DEFINITIONS—cont'd

could facilitate or inhibit people's transition experiences. *Community conditions* (e.g., community resources) or *societal conditions* (e.g., marginalization of immigrants in the host country) could be facilitators or inhibitors for transitions. Compared with personal transition conditions, the subconcepts of community conditions and societal conditions tend to be underdeveloped.

PATTERNS OF RESPONSE *OR* PROCESS AND OUTCOME INDICATORS

Indicators of healthy transitions in the framework by Schumacher and Meleis (1994) were replaced by patterns of response in the middle range theory of transitions. Patterns of response are conceptualized as *process indicators* and *outcome indicators*. These *process indicators* and *outcome indicators* characterize healthy responses. *Process indicators* that move clients in the direction of healthy or toward vulnerability and risk allow early assessment and intervention by nurses to facilitate healthy outcomes. Also, *outcome indicators* may be used to check if a transition is a healthy one or not, but Meleis et al. (2000) warned that outcome indicators may be related to other events in people's lives if they are examined too soon in a transition process. The process indicators suggested by Meleis et al. (2000) include feeling connected, interacting, being situated, and developing confidence and coping. The need to feel and stay connected is a process indicator of a healthy transition; if immigrants make new contacts and continue old connections with extended family and friends, they are usually in a healthy transition. Through interaction, the meaning of the transition and the behaviors developed in response to the transition can be uncovered, clarified, and acknowledged, which usually leads to a healthy transition. Location and being situated in terms of time, space, and relationships are usually important in most transitions; these indicate whether the person is turned in the direction of a healthy transition. The extent to which there is a pattern indicating that the people involved are experiencing an increase in their levels of confidence is another important process indicator of a healthy transition. The outcome indicators suggested by Meleis et al. (2000) include mastery and fluid integrative identities. A healthy completion of a transition can be determined by the extent to which people demonstrate mastery of the skills and behaviors needed to manage their new situations or environments. Identity reformulation can also represent a healthy completion of a transition.

NURSING THERAPEUTICS

Schumacher and Meleis (1994) conceptualized nursing therapeutics as three measures that are widely applicable to therapeutic intervention during transitions. First, they proposed assessment of readiness as a nursing therapeutic. Assessment of readiness needs to be a multidisciplinary endeavor and requires a comprehensive understanding of the client; it requires assessment of each of the transition conditions in order to create an individual profile of client readiness, and to enable clinicians and researchers to identify various patterns of the transition experience. Second, the preparation for transition is suggested as a nursing therapeutic. The preparation of transition includes education as the primary modality for creating optimal conditions in preparation for transition. Third, role supplementation was proposed as a nursing therapeutic. Role supplementation was introduced theoretically and empirically by Meleis (1975) and was used by many researchers (Brackley, 1992; Dracup, Clark, Meleis Clyburn, Shields, & Stanley 1985; Gaffney, 1992; Meleis & Swendsen, 1978). Yet, in the middle range theory of transitions, no further development of the concept of nursing therapeutics was made.

USE OF EMPIRICAL EVIDENCE

In the development of the transition framework by Schumacher and Meleis (1994), a systematic extensive literature review of more than 300 articles related to transitions provided empirical evidence of the conceptualization and theorizing. Then, as mentioned above, the transition framework was tested in a number of studies to describe immigrants' transitions (Meleis et al., 1998), women's experiences with rheumatoid arthritis (Shaul, 1997), recovery from cardiac surgery (Shih et al., 1998), development of the family caregiving role for patients in chemotherapy (Schumacher, 1995), Korean immigrant low income women in menopausal transition (Im, 1997; Im & Meleis, 2000, 2001; Im, Meleis, & Lee, 1999), early memory loss for patients in Sweden (Robinson, Ekman, Meleis, Wahlund, & Winbald, 1997), the aging transition (Schumacher, Jones, & Meleis, 1999), African American women's transition to motherhood (Sawyer, 1997), and adult medical-surgical patients' perceptions of their readiness for hospital discharge (Weiss et al., 2007).

In the process of developing the middle range theory of transition, five research studies provided empirical evidence for conceptualization and theorizing (Sawyer, 1997; Im, 1997; Messias, Gilliss, Sparacino, Tong, & Foote, 1995; Messias, 1997; Schumacher, 1994). These studies were conducted among culturally diverse groups of people in transition, including African American mothers, Korean immigrant midlife women, parents of children diagnosed with congenital heart defects, Brazilian women immigrating to the United States, and family caregivers of persons receiving chemotherapy for cancer. Empirical findings of these five studies provided the theoretical basis for the concepts of the middle range theory of transition, and the concepts and their relationships were developed and formulated based on a collaborative process of dialogue, constant comparison of findings across the five studies, and analysis of findings. For example, one of the personal conditions, meanings, was proposed based on the findings from two studies (Im, 1997; Sawyer, 1997). According to Meleis et al. (2000), in Im's study, although Korean immigrant midlife women had ambivalent feelings toward menopause, menopause itself did not have special meaning attached to it. Im found that most of the participants did not connect any special problems they were having to their menopausal transitions. Rather, women went through their menopause without experiencing or perceiving any problems, which means that "no special meaning" might have facilitated the women's menopausal transition. Yet, Sawyer's study reported that African American women related intense enjoyment of their roles as mothers and described motherhood in terms of being responsible, protecting, supporting, and needed. Thus, Meleis et al. (2000) proposed meanings as a personal transition condition because, in both studies, neutral and positive meanings might have facilitated menopause and motherhood.

The middle range theory of transition was used recently in several studies to develop situation-specific theories (Im, 2006; Im & Meleis, 1999b; Schumacher et al., 1999) and to test the theory in a study on relatives' experience of the move to a nursing home (Davies, 2005). In turn, these studies also provide empirical evidence for the middle range theory of transition.

MAJOR ASSUMPTIONS

Based on Meleis' former works on role supplementation, the transition framework by Schumacher and Meleis (1994), and the middle range theory of transitions by Meleis et al. (2000), the following assumptions of Transition Theory could be inferred.

- Transitions are complex and multidimensional. Transitions have patterns of multiplicity and complexity.
- All transitions are characterized by flow and movement over time.
- Transition cause changes in identities, roles, relationships, abilities, and patterns of behavior.
- Transitions involve a process of movement and changes in fundamental life patterns, which are manifested in all individuals.

Change and difference are not interchangeable, nor are they synonymous with transition. Transitions both result in change and are the result of change.

- The daily lives of clients, environments, and interactions are shaped by the nature, conditions, meanings, and processes of their transition experiences.
- Vulnerability is related to transition experiences, interactions, and environmental conditions that expose individuals to potential damage, problematic or extended recovery, or delayed or unhealthy coping.
- Nurses are the primary caregivers of clients and their families who are undergoing transitions.

THEORETICAL ASSERTIONS

Theoretical assertions in transition theory were inferred in the early works of Meleis. This includes her work on role supplementation, the transition framework by Schumacher and Meleis (1994), and the middle range theory of transitions by Meleis et al. (2000). Following are the theoretical assertions made in the theoretical works:

- Developmental, health and illness, and organizational transitions are central to nursing practice.
- Patterns of transition include (a) whether the client is experiencing a single transition or multiple transitions; (b) whether multiple transitions are sequential or simultaneous; (c) the extent of overlap among transitions; and (d) the nature of the relationship between the different events that are triggering transitions for a client.
- Properties of transition experience are interrelated parts of a complex process.
- The level of awareness influences the level of engagement, in that engagement may not happen without awareness.
- Humans' perceptions of and meanings attached to health and illness situations are influenced by and in turn influence the conditions under which a transition occurs.
- Healthy transition is characterized by both process and outcome indicators.
- Negotiating successful transitions depends on the development of an effective relationship between the nurse and the client (nursing therapeutic). This relationship is a highly reciprocal process that affects both the client and the nurse.

LOGICAL FORM

Transition theory has been formulated and theorized through induction by the use of existing research (a systematic literature review and research findings). As mentioned earlier, it was initially developed as a central concept of nursing and was further developed as a middle range theory. Transition theory was formulated with the goal of integrating what is known about transition experience across different types of transitions to provide directions for nursing therapeutics for people in transition. This theory provides a framework for seeing how the results of previous research related to various types of transitions fit together more clearly, and how concepts can be manipulated for further study.

ACCEPTANCE BY THE NURSING COMMUNITY

Over the past several decades, transitions have emerged as a central concept of nursing phenomenon, and Transition Theory has been widely used throughout the world. Transition Theory was translated and used extensively in Sweden, Taiwan, and many other places.

Practice

Transition Theory can provide a comprehensive perspective on transition experience while considering the contexts within which people are experiencing a transition. Because of its comprehensiveness, applicability, and affinity with health, Transition Theory has been applied to many human phenomena of interest and concern to nurses, such as illness, recovery, birth, death, and loss, as well as immigration. Transition Theory is useful in explaining health/illness transitions such as the recovery process, hospital discharge, and diagnosis of chronic disease (Meleis & Trangenstein, 1994). Indeed, studies have indicated that Transition Theory could be applied to nursing practice with diverse groups of people, including geriatric populations, psychiatric populations, maternal populations, family caregivers, menopausal women, Alzheimer patients, immigrant women, and people with chronic illness, among others (Aroian & Prater, 1988; Brackley, 1992; Im, 1997; Kaas & Rousseau, 1983; Schumacher, Dodd, & Paul, 1993; Shaul, 1997). Transition Theory could provide direction for nursing practice with people in various types of transitions by providing a comprehensive perspective on the nature and type of transitions, transition conditions, and process and outcome indicators of patterns of response to transitions. Also, Transition Theory will lead to the development of nursing therapeutics that is congruent with the unique experience of clients and their families in transition, thus promoting healthy responses to transition.

Education

Transition Theory is used widely in graduate education and undergraduate education throughout the world (Meleis, personal communication, December 29, 2007). There is a growing international interest in integrating Transition Theory into nursing curricula across countries (Meleis, personal communication, January 2008). Transition Theory was used as a curriculum framework in a number of places, including the University of Connecticut (Meleis, personal communication, December 29, 2007). At the UCSF, an independent graduate elective course on transitions and health was taught by Meleis in order to respond to an increasing learning need of graduate students. At the University of Pennsylvania, a center called Transitions and Health was established in 2007 with a $5 million dollar endowment (Director: Mary Taylor)—this is the first center on transitions and health endowed anywhere.

Research

A number of researchers have used Transition Theory in their studies as a theoretical basis for research. Meleis' research program is naturally based on Transition Theory, and other researchers have tested the empirical precision of Transition Theory through their studies (Davies, 2005; Weiss et al., 2007). As mentioned earlier, Transition Theory was often used as a parent theory for situation-specific theories (Im & Meleis, 1999a; Im, 2006; Schumacher et al., 1999).

FURTHER DEVELOPMENT

As mentioned in the article on the middle range theory of transitions (Meleis, 2000), Transition Theory was an emerging framework that could be further developed, tested, and refined, reflecting Meleis' philosophical position on theory development as cyclic, dynamic, and evolving. Transition theory continues to be refined and tested to explain the major concepts and relationships among the major concepts with diverse groups of populations in various types of transition, which will increase its power to describe nursing phenomena. Also, because sufficient empirical support by a number of studies using Transition Theory as a theoretical basis currently exists, future studies need to aim at design and conduct of intervention studies to test Transition Theory–based interventions, through which Transition Theory will gain power to direct nursing practice. Also, as Meleis (2007) envisioned, a number of situation-specific theories could be developed based on Transition Theory.

CRITIQUE

Clarity and Simplicity

Transition Theory is simple and clear to understand. The conceptual definitions are clear and provide a comprehensive understanding of the complexity of transitions. The major concepts are logically linked, and the relationships are obvious in their theoretical assertions. The relationships among the major concepts are clearly depicted in a visually simple diagram (see Figure 3). The variables are independent of each other, yet the interactive effects among the variables are clearly depicted by arrows.

Generality

Transition Theory is a middle range theory in scope. Middle range theories have more limited scope and less abstraction than grand theories, and they address specific phenomena or concepts, which make them more easily applicable to nursing practice. Yet, because of its limited scope, Transition Theory tends to be generalizable to people in transitions. When the diverse types of transitions are considered, Transition Theory is relevant for any population in transition, depending on what type of transition the population is experiencing. The research used to derive Transition Theory was actually based on the participation of different gender and ethnic groups, in a variety of settings, which makes Transition Theory more easily applicable and generalizable, compared with other theories that were developed based on research among a specific group of people.

Empirical Precision

Transition Theory has been tested and supported by Meleis and others as a framework for explaining the transition experiences of diverse groups of populations in different types of transitions. Transition Theory continues to evolve through planned programs of research, and continued empirical research studies will further refine the theory. With the development of situation-specific theories derived from Transition Theory, its distance from the empirical world will be further reduced as well.

Derivable Consequences

Transition Theory with a focus on people in diverse types of transitions provides a comprehensive and evolving guide for all health-related disciplines. Health-related disciplines always deal with a type of transition, whether single or multiple. Especially with an increasing need for culturally competent health care for diverse groups of healthcare clients, Transition Theory could provide a more appropriate theoretical fit for current health care, because of its inherent consideration of diversities of healthcare clients and its basis in research among diverse groups of people in transition.

SUMMARY

Current healthcare systems are frequently characterized by changes, diversities, and complexities. Transition Theory that evolved from research studies among diverse groups of people in various types of transitions could adequately direct nursing practice, education, and practice in the current healthcare system. Meleis made her theoretical journey from the 1960s to now; her journey will continue, and others will follow in her footsteps. Transition Theory will continue to develop through a number of studies that are using the theory, and Meleis' visionary leadership throughout the world will continue to influence nursing practice, education, and research.

Case Study

Sue Kim, age 49, immigrated from South Korea to the United States 6 years ago. Her family came to the United States to educate their children, and moved in with family members in Los Angeles. Sue and her husband graduated from a top ranked university in South Korea, and her husband also had a master's degree in business. However, their English skills were not adequate for them to get jobs in the United States. Instead, they opened a Korean grocery store with the money that they brought from South Korea, and they managed to settle down in Los Angeles, where a number of Koreans are living. They have two children: Mina, a 25-year-old daughter who is now the manager of a local shop, and Yujun, a 21-year-old son who is a college student. Both children were born in South Korea and moved to the United States with Sue. The children had a hard time, especially Mina, who came to the United States in her senior year of high school. However, the children finally adapted to their new environment. Now, Mina is living alone in a one-bedroom apartment near downtown LA, and Yujun is living in a university dormitory. The Kim's are a religious family and attend their community's

Protestant church regularly. They are involved in many church activities.

Sue and her husband have been too busy to have regular annual checkups for the past 6 years. About 1 year ago, Sue began to have serious indigestion, nausea, vomiting, and upper abdominal pain; she took some over-the-counter medicine and tried to tolerate the pain. Last month, her symptoms became more serious; she visited a local clinic and was referred to a larger hospital. Recently, she was diagnosed with stomach cancer after a series of diagnostic tests and had surgery; she now is undergoing chemotherapy.

You are the nurse who is taking care of Sue during this hospitalization. Sue is very polite and modest whenever you approach her. Sue is very quiet and never complains about any symptoms or pain. However, on several occasions, you think that Sue is in serious pain, when considering her facial expressions and sweating forehead. You think that Sue's English skills may not allow her to adequately communicate with healthcare providers. Also, you find that Sue does not have many visitors—only her husband and two children. You frequently find Sue praying while listening to some religious songs. You also find Sue sobbing silently. About 2 weeks is left until Sue finishes her chemotherapy, and you think that you should do something for Sue, so she will not suffer through easily controlled pain and symptoms. Now, you begin some preliminary planning.

1. Describe your assessment of the transition(s) that Sue is experiencing. What types of transition(s) is Sue experiencing? What are the patterns of the transition(s)? What properties of transitions can you identify from her case?
2. Describe your assessment of the personal, community, and societal transition conditions that may have influenced Sue's experience. What are the cultural meanings attached to cancer, cancer pain, and symptoms accompanying chemotherapy, in this situation? What are Sue's cultural attitudes toward cancer and cancer patients? How is Sue's preparation for the transition(s) going? What are other factors that may facilitate her transition(s)? What are other factors that may inhibit her transition(s)?
3. Describe your assessment of the patterns of response that Sue is showing. What are the indicators of healthy transition(s)? What are the indicators of unhealthy transition(s)?
4. State how Transition Theory could help your assessment and nursing care for Sue.
5. As Sue's nurse, what would be your first action/interaction to take? Describe your plan for nursing care for Sue.

CRITICAL THINKING *Activities*

1. Consider one specific transition that you are engaged in now. Identify characteristics of the transition as defined in Transition Theory, and observable in the transition that you are experiencing. Think about other transitions that you may be engaged in now. Think about why you chose the specific transition over other transitions that you are simultaneously experiencing.
2. Analyze the changes that you are experiencing due to the specific transition. Think about how your level of awareness of these changes influences your transition experience. Think about how you have been engaged in the transition and its relationship with your level of awareness of the changes. Think about how long the transition has been, and what have been the landmark events and critical points of the transition.
3. Analyze personal, community, and societal conditions that may have influenced the transition that you are experiencing. Think about the influences of the meanings attached to the transition, cultural beliefs and attitudes related to the transition, socioeconomic status, and the level of your preparation for the transition and your knowledge of the transition.
4. Describe your responses to the transition and any patterns in the responses. Ask five friends or family members to describe what

would be their responses to the transition. Compare the descriptions given by individuals with different ages and backgrounds (e.g., ethnicity, gender, socioeconomic status).

5. Describe what would be your outcomes of the transition. What would facilitate successful outcomes of the transition? What would inhibit successful outcomes of the transition?

POINTS FOR *Further Study*

- Meleis, A. I. (2007). Theoretical Nursing: Development and Progress (4th Ed.). Philadelphia: Lippincott Williams & Wilkins.
- To respond to researchers' increasing interest in Transition Theory, a website was established at the University of Pennsylvania: http://www.nursing.upenn.edu/dean/transitions/

REFERENCES

Aroian, K., & Prater, M., (1988). Transitions entry groups: easing new patients' adjustment to psychiatric hospitalization. *Hospital and Community Psychiatry,* 39, 312-313.

Brackley, M. H. (1992). A role supplementation group pilot study: a nursing therapy for potential parental caregivers. *Clinical Nurse Specialist,* 6(1), 14-19.

Bridges, W. (1980). Transitions. Reading, MA: Addison-Wesley.

Bridges, W. (1991). Managing transition: Making the most of change. Menlo Park, CA: Addison Wesley.

Chick, N., & Meleis, A. I. (1986). Transitions: a nursing concern. In: Chin P. L. ed. Nursing Research Methodology: Issues and Implantation. Gainsburg, MD: Aspen Publishers.

Davies, S. (2005). Meleis's theory of nursing transitions and relatives' experiences of nursing home entry. *Journal of Advanced Nursing,* 52(6), 658-671.

Dracup, K., & Meleis, A. I. (1982) Compliance: an interactionist approach. *Nursing Research,* 31, 31-36.

Dracup, K., Meleis, A. T. Baker, K., & Edlefsen, P. (1985). Family-focused cardiac rehabilitation: a role supplementation program for cardiac patients and spouses. *Nursing Clinics of North America, 19*(1), 113-124.

Dracup, K., Meleis, A. I., Clark, S., Clyburn, A., Shields, L., & Staley, M. (1985). Group counseling in cardiac rehabilitation: effect on patient compliance. *Patient Education and Counseling,* 6(4), 169-177.

Gaffney, K. F. (1992). Nurse practice-model for maternal role sufficiency. *Advances in Nursing Sciences,* 15(2), 76-84.

Im, E. O. (1997). Negligence and ignorance of menopause within gender multiple transition context: Low income Korean immigrant women. Unpublished doctoral dissertation, University of California, San Francisco.

Im, E. O. (2005). Development of situation-specific theories: An integrative approach. *Advances in Nursing Science,* 28(2), 137-151.

Im, E. O. (2006). A Situation-Specific Theory of Caucasian Cancer Patients' Pain Experience. *Advances in Nursing Science,* 29(3), 232-244.

Im, E. O., & Meleis, A. I. (1999a). Situation-specific theories: Philosophical roots, properties, and approach. *Advances in Nursing Science,* 22(2), 11-24.

Im, E., & Meleis, A. I. (1999b). A situation-specific theory of Korean immigrant women's menopausal transition. *Journal of Nursing Scholarship*, 31(4), 333-338.

Im, E., & Meleis, A. I. (2000). Meanings of menopause: low-income Korean immigrant women. *Western Journal of Nursing Research,* 22(1), 84-102.

Im, E., & Meleis, A. I. (2001). Women's work and symptoms during midlife: Korean immigrant women. *Women and Health,* 33(1/2), 83-103.

Im, E., Meleis, A. I., & Lee, K. (1999). Symptom experience of low-income Korean immigrant women during menopausal transition. *Women and Health,* 29(2), 53-67.

Jones, P. S., Zhang, X. E., & Meleis, A. I. (1978). Transforming Vulnerability. *Western Journal of Nursing Research,* 25 (7), 835-853.

Kaas,.M.J., Rousseau, G. K., (1983). Geriatric sexual conformity: assessment and intervention. *Clinical Gerontologist,* 2(1), 31-44.

Kelley, L. S., Lakin, J. A. (1988). Role supplementation as a nursing intervention for Alzheimer's disease: a case study. *Public Health Nursing,* 5(3), 146-152.

Meleis, A. I. (1975). Role insufficiency and role supplementation: A conceptual framework. *Nursing Research,* 24, 264-271.

Meleis, A. I. (1985). Theoretical Nursing: Development and Progress (1st Ed). Philadelphia: Lippincott Williams & Wilkins.

Meleis, A. I. (1991). Theoretical Nursing: Development and Progress (2nd Ed). Philadelphia: Lippincott Williams & Wilkins.

Meleis, A. I. (1997). Theoretical Nursing: Development and Progress (3rd Ed). Philadelphia: Lippincott Williams & Wilkins.

Meleis, A. I. (2007). Theoretical Nursing: Development and Progress (4th Ed). Philadelphia: Lippincott Williams & Wilkins.

Meleis, A. I., Lipson, J., & Dallafar, A. (1998). The reluctant immigrant: immigration experiences among Middle Eastern groups in Northern California. In Baxter, D.

& Krulfeld, R. (Eds.), Selected Papers on Refugees and Immigrants, Vol. V, (pp. 214-230). American Anthropological Association, Arlington, VA.

Meleis, A. I., Sawyer, L., Im, E., Schumacher, K., & Messias, D. (2000) Experiencing transitions: an emerging middle range theory. *Advances in Nursing Science,* 23(1), 12-28.

Meleis, A. I., & Swendsen, L. (1978). Role supplementation: an empirical test of a nursing intervention. *Nursing Research,* 27, 11-18.

Meleis, A. I., & Trangenstein, P. A. (1994). Facilitating transitions: re-definition of the nursing mission. *Nursing Outlook,* 42, 255-259.

Messias, D. K. H. (1997). Narratives of transnational migration, work, and health: the lived experiences of Brazilian women in the United States. Unpublished doctoral dissertation, University of California, San Francisco.

Messias, D. K. H., Gilliss, C. L., Sparacino, P. S. A., Tong, E. M., & Foote, D. (1995). Stories of transition: Parents recall the diagnosis of congenital heart defects. *Family Systems Medicine,* 3(3/4), 367-377.

Robinson, P. R., Ekman, S. L., Meleis, Al, Wahlund, L. O., & Winbald, B. (1997). Suffering in silence: the experience of early memory loss. *Health Care in Later Life,* 2(2), 107-120.

Sawyer, L. (1997). Effects of racism on the transition to motherhood for African-American women. Unpublished doctoral dissertation, University of California, San Francisco.

Schumacher, K. L. (1994). Shifting patterns of self-care and caregiving during chemotherapy. Unpublished doctoral dissertation, University of California, San Francisco.

Schumacher, K. L. (1995). Family caregiver role acquisition: role-making through situated interaction. *Scholarly Inquiry for Nursing Practice,* 9, 211-271.

Schumacher, K. L., Dodd, M. J., & Paul, S. M. (1993). The stress process in family caregivers of persons receiving chemotherapy. *Research in Nursing & Health,*16, 395-404.

Schumacher, K. L., Jones, P. S., & Meleis, A. I. (1999). Helping elderly persons in transition: a framework for research and practice. In L. Swanson & T. Tripp Reimer (Eds.), Advances in Gerontological nursing: Life transitions in the older adult, (vol 3), (pp. 1-26). New York: Springer Publishing.

Schumacher, K. L., & Meleis, A. I. (1994). Transitions: a central concept in nursing. *Image: Journal of Nursing Scholarship,* 26(2), 119-127.

Shaul, M. P. (1997). Transition in chronic illness: rheumatoid arthritis in women. *Rehabilitation Nursing,* 22, 199-205.

Shih, F. J., Meleis, A. I., Yu, P. J., Hu, W. Y., Lou, M. F., & Huang, G. S. (1998). Taiwanese patients' concerns and coping strategies: transitions to cardiac surgery. *Heart and Lung,* 27(2):82-98

Walker, L. O., & Avant, K. C. (1995). Strategies for theory construction in nursing (3rd ed.). Norwalk, CT: Appleton & Lange.

Walker, L. O., & Avant, K. C. (2005). Strategies for theory construction in nursing (4th ed.). Norwalk, CT: Appleton & Lange.

Weiss, M. E., Piacentine, L. B., Lokken, L., Ancona, J., Archer, J., Gresser, S., Holmes, S. B., Toman, S., Toy, A., & Vega-Stromberg, T. (2007). Perceived readiness for hospital discharge in adult medical-surgical patients. *Clin Nurse Spec,* 21(1), 31-42.

BIBLIOGRAPHY

Primary Sources

Books

Meleis, A. I. (2007). Theoretical Nursing: Development and Progress (4th Ed). Philadelphia: Lippincott Williams & Wilkins.

Book Chapters

Brooten, D., & Naylor, M. D. (1999). Transitional Environments. In A. S. Hinshaw, S. L. Feetham, & J. Shaver (Eds), Handbook of clinical nursing research (pp. 641-654). Thousand Oaks: Sage Publications.

Chick, N., & Meleis, A. I. (1986). Transitions: a nursing concern. In P. L. Chinn (Ed.), Nursing research methodology, (pp. 237-257). Boulder, CO: Aspen Publication.

Lipson, J. G., & Meleis, A. I. (1999). Research with immigrants and refugees. In A. S. Hinshaw, S. L. Feetham, & J. Shaver (Eds), Handbook of clinical nursing research, (pp.87-106). Thousand Oaks: Sage Publications.

Meleis, A. I. (1997). On transitions and knowledge development. Nursing Beyond Art and Science: Annotated Edition. Japan: Japan Academy of Nursing Science.

Meleis, A. I. (1998). Research on role supplementation. In J. J. Fitzpatrick (Ed), Encyclopedia of Nursing Research. New Jersey: Springer Publishing.

Meleis, A. I., Lipson, J., & Dallafar, A. (1998). The reluctant immigrant: immigration experiences among Middle Eastern groups in Northern California. In D., Baxter, & Krulfeld, R. (Eds.), Selected Papers on Refugees and Immigrants, Vol. V, (pp. 214-230). American Anthropological Association, Arlington, VA.

Meleis, A. I., Lipson, J.G., Muecke, M., & Smith, G. (1998). Immigrant women and their health: an olive paper. Indianapolis: Sigma Theta Tau International Center Nursing Press.

Meleis, A. I., & Schumacher, K. L. (1998). Transitions and health. In J. J. Fitzpatrick (Ed.), Encyclopedia of Nursing Research, (pp. 570-571). New Jersey: Springer Publishing.

Meleis, A. I., & Swendsen, L. (1977). Does nursing intervention make a difference? A test of the ROSP. Communicating Nursing Research: Nursing Research Priorities: Choice or Chance, vol. 8, 308-324. Boulder, CO: Western Interstate Commission for Higher Education.

Meleis, A. I., Swendsen, L., & Jones, D. (1980). Preventive role supplementation: a grounded conceptual framework. In M.H. Miller and B. Flynn (Eds.), Current perspectives in nursing: Social issues and trends, (vol. 2), (pp. 3-14). St. Louis, MO: C.V. Mosby.

Schumacher, K. L., Jones, P. S., & Meleis, A. I. (1998). The elderly in transition: need and issues of care. In L. Swanson & T. Tripp Reimer, Advances in Gerentological Nursing. New York: Springer Publishing Comp.

Schumacher, K. L., Jones, P.S., & Meleis, A. I. (1999). Helping elderly persons in transition: a framework for research and practice. In L. Swanson & T. Tripp Reimer (Eds.), Advances in Gerontological nursing: Life transitions in the older adult, (vol 3), (pp. 1-26). New York: Springer Publishing.

Dissertations

Almendarez, B. L. (2007). Mexican American elders and nursing home transition. Unpublished doctoral dissertation, University of Texas Health Science Center at San Antonio, TX.

Batty, M. L. E. (1999). Pattern identification and expanding consciousness during the transition of "low-risk" pregnancy. A study embodying Newman's health as expanding consciousness. Unpublished doctoral dissertation, University of New Brunswick, Canada.

Fowles, E. R. (1994). The relationship between prenatal maternal attachment, postpartum depressive symptoms, and maternal role attainment. Loyola University of Chicago, Chicago, IL.

Im, E-O. (1997). Negligence and ignorance of menopause within gender multiple transition context: Low income Korean immigrant women. Unpublished doctoral dissertation, University of California, San Francisco, CA.

Kelly, C. (1997). Restructuring public health nursing: experiences in Northern California. Unpublished doctoral dissertation, University of California, San Francisco, CA.

Lenz, B. K. (2002). Correlates of tobacco use and non-use among college students at a large university: Application of a transition framework. Unpublished doctoral dissertation, University of Minnesota, MN.

McMillan, E. S. (2002). Education to practice questionnaire: A content analysis. Unpublished doctoral dissertation, Wilmington College Division of Nursing, Delaware.

Missal, B. E. (2003). The Gulf Arb woman's transition to motherhood. Unpublished doctoral dissertation, University of Minnesota.

O'Brien-Barry, P. (2003). The contribution of sex-role orientation and role commitment to interrole conflict in working first-time mothers at 6 to 9 months postpartum. Unpublished doctoral dissertation, New York University, New York.

Sawyer, L. (1997). Effects of racism on the transition to motherhood for African-American women. Unpublished doctoral dissertation, University of California, San Francisco.

Journal Articles

Aroian, K., Prater, M. (1988). Transitions entry groups: easing new patients' adjustment to psychiatric hospitalization. *Hospital and Community Psychiatry,* 39, 312-313.

Brackley, M. H. (1992). A role supplementation group pilot study: a nursing therapy for potential parental caregivers. *Clinical Nurse Specialist,* 6(1), 14-19.

Dracup, K., & Meleis, A. I. (1982). Compliance: an interactionist approach. *Nursing Research,* 31, 31-36.

Dracup, K., Meleis, Al, Baker, K., & Edlefsen, P. (1985). Family-focused cardiac rehabilitation: a role supplementation program for cardiac patients and spouses. *Nursing Clinics of North America,* 19(1), 113-124.

Dracup, K., Meleis, A. I., Clark, S., Clyburn, A., Shields, L., & Staley, M. (1985). Group counseling in cardiac rehabilitation: effect on patient compliance. *Patient Education and Counseling,* 6(4), 169-177.

Gaffney, K. F. (1992). Nurse practice-model for maternal role sufficiency. *Advances in Nursing Sciences,* 15(2), 76-84.

Im, E. O. (2006). A Situation-Specific Theory of Caucasian Cancer Patients' Pain Experience. *Advances in Nursing Science,* 29(3), 232-244.

Im, E., & Meleis, A. I. (1999). A situation-specific theory of Korean immigrant women's menopausal transition. *Journal of Nursing Scholarship,* 31(4), 333-338.

Im, E., Meleis, Al, & Lee, K. (1999). Symptom experience of low-income Korean immigrant women during menopausal transition. *Women and Health,* 29(2), 53-67.

Im, E., & Meleis, A. I. (2000). Meanings of menopause: low-income Korean immigrant women. *Western Journal of Nursing Research,* 22(1), 84-102.

Im, E., & Meleis, A. I. (2001). Women's work and symptoms during midlife: Korean immigrant women. *Women and Health,* 33(1/2), 83-103.

Kaas, M.J., Rousseau, G.K. (1983). Geriatric sexual conformity: assessment and intervention. *Clinical Gerontologist, 2*(1), 31-44.

Kelley, L.S., Lakin, J.A. (1988). Role supplementation as a nursing intervention for Alzheimer's disease: a case study. *Public Health Nursing,* 5(3), 146-152.

Meleis, A. I. (1975). Role/insufficiency and role supplementation: a conceptual framework. *Nursing Research,* 24, 264-271.

Meleis, A. I. (1987). Role transition and health. *Kango Kenkyo: The Japanese Journal of Nursing Research,* 20(1), 81, 69-89.

Meleis, A. I. (1991). Between two cultures: identity, roles, and health. *Health Care For Women International,* 12, 365-378.

Meleis, A. I. (1997). Immigrant transitions and health care: an action plan. *Nursing Outlook,* 45(1), 42.

Meleis, A. I., & Rogers, S. (1987). Women in transition: being vs. becoming or being and becoming. *Health Care for Women International,* 8, 199-217.

Meleis, A. I., Sawyer L., Im, E., Schumacher, K., & Messias, D. (2000). Experiencing transitions: an emerging middle range theory. *Advances in Nursing Science,* 23(1), 12-28.

Meleis, A. I., & Swendsen, L. (1978). Role supplementation: an empirical test of a nursing intervention. *Nursing Research,* 27, 11-18.

Meleis, A. I., & Trangenstein, P. A. (1994). Facilitating transitions: redefinition of a nursing mission. *Nursing Outlook,* 42(6), 255-259.

Messias, D. K. H. (2002). Transnational health resources, practices, and perspectives: Brazilian immigrant women's narratives. *Journal of Immigrant Health,* (4)4, 183-200.

Messias, D. K. H., Gilliss, C. L., Sparacino, P. S. A., Tong, E. M., and Foote, D. (1995). Stories of transition: Parents recall the diagnosis of congenital heart defect. *Family Systems Medicine,* 13(3;4), 367-277.

Robinson, P. R., Ekman, S. L., Meleis, AI, Wahlund, L.O., & Winbald, B. (1997). Suffering in silence: the experience of early memory loss. *Health Care in Later Life,* 2(2), 107-120.

Schumacher, K. L. (1995). Family caregiver role acquisition: role-making through situated interaction. *Scholarly Inquiry for Nursing Practice,* 9, 211-271.

Schumacher, K. L. (1996). Reconceptualizing family caregiving: family-based illness care during chemotherapy. *Research in Nursing & Health,* 19, 261-272.

Schumacher, K. L., Dodd, M. J., & Paul, S. M. (1993). The stress process in family caregivers of persons receiving chemotherapy. *Research in Nursing & Health,* 16, 395-404.

Schumacher, K. L., & Meleis, A. I. (1994). Transitions: a central concept in nursing. Image: *Journal of Nursing Scholarship,* 26(2), 119-127.

Schumacher, K. L., Stewart, B. J., & Archbold, P.G. (1998). Conceptualizing and measurement of doing family caregiving well. Image: *Journal of Nursing Scholarship,* 30(1): 63-69

Shaul, M. P. (1997). Transition in chronic illness: rheumatoid arthritis in women. *Rehabilitation Nursing,* 22, 199-205.

Shih, F. J., Meleis, A. I., Yu, P. J., Hu, W. Y., Lou, M. F., & Huang, G. S. (1998). Taiwanese patients' concerns and coping strategies: transitions to cardiac surgery. *Heart and Lung,* 27(2):82-98

Swendsen, L., Meleis, A. I., & Jones, D. (1978). Role supplementation for new parents: a role mastery plan. *The American Journal of Maternal Child Nursing,* 3, 84-91.

Secondary Sources

Books

Meleis, A. I. (2001). Guest editor of a special issue on News From The International Council On Women's Health Issues for Health Care for Women International, 22(3).

Meleis, A. I. (2001). Guest editor of a special issue on women and violence for Health Care for Women International, 22(4).

Meleis, A. I. (2001) (Ed.). Women's work, health and quality of life. Binghamton: Haworth Press, Inc.

Meleis, A. I., Isenberg, M., Koerner, J. E., Lacey, B., & Stern, P. (1995). Diversity, marginalization, and culturally competent health care: Issues in knowledge development. Washington: American Academy of Nursing.

Meleis, A. I., Lipson, J. G., Muecke, M., & Smith, G. (1998). Immigrant Women and their Health: An Olive Paper. Indianapolis, IN: Center for Nursing Press, Sigma Theta Tau.

St. Hill, P.,Lipson, J., & Meleis, A. I. (2002)(Eds.). Caring for Women Cross-Culturally: A Portable Guide, Philadelphia: F.A. Davis.

Book Chapters

Meleis, A. I. (2002). Egyptians. In P. St. Hill, J. Lipson, & A. Meleis (Eds.). Caring for Women Cross-Culturally: A Portable Guide, Philadelphia: F. A. Davis. [AJN Book of the Year Award 2004]

Meleis, A. I., Lipson, J., & Dallafar, A. The reluctant immigrant: immigration experiences among Middle Eastern groups in Northern California. In D. Baxter, & Krulfeld, R. (Eds.), Selected Papers on Refugees and Immigrants, Vol. V, (pp. 214-230). American Anthropological Association, Arlington, VA.

Journal Articles

Arruda, E. N., Larson, & Meleis A. I. (1992). Comfort: Immigrant Hispanic patients' views. *Cancer Nursing,* 15(6), 387-394.

Barnes, D., Eribes, C., Juarbe, T., Nelson, M., Proctor, S., Sawyer, L., Shaul, M., & Meleis, A. I. (1995). Primary health care and primary care: A Confusion of philosophies. *Nursing Outlook,* 43, 7-16.

Bernal, P., & Meleis, A. I. (1995). Being a mother and a "por dia" domestic worker: Companionship and deprivation. *Western Journal of Nursing Research,* 17(4), 365-382.

Bernal, P., & Meleis, A. I. (1995). Self care actions of Colombian por día domestic workers: On prevention and care. *Women and Health,* 22(4), 77-95.

Budman, C.L., Lipson, J.G. & Meleis, A. I. (1992). The cultural consultant in mental health care: The case of an Arab adolescent. *American Journal of Orthopsychiatry,* 62(3), 359-370.

Davidson, P., Meleis, A. I., Daly, J., & Douglas, M. (2003). Globalization as we enter the 21st century: Reflections and directions for nursing education, science, research and clinical practice. *Contemporary Nurse,* 15(3), 162-174.

Davis, L.H., Flaherty, S., & Meleis, A. I., et al. (1992). Culturally competent health care. *Nursing Outlook,* 40(6), 277-283.

Douglas, M. K., Meleis, A. I., Eribes, C. and Kim, S. (1996). The work of auxiliary nurses in Mexico: Stressors, satisfiers and coping strategies, *Journal of International Nursing Studies,* 33(5), 495-505.

Douglas, M. K., Meleis, A. I., & Paul, S. M. (1997). Auxiliary nurses in Mexico: Impact of multiple roles on their health. *Health Care for Women International,* 18(44), 355-368.

Dracup, K., Cronenwett, L., Meleis, A. I., & Benner, P.E. (2005). Reflections on the Doctorate of Nursing Practice. *Nursing Outlook,* 53(4), 177-182.

Dracup, K., Cronenwett, L., Meleis, A. I. & Benner, P.E. (2005). Reply to Letter to the Editor on Reflections on the Doctorate of Nursing Practice. *Nursing Outlook,* 53(6), 269.

Facione, N. C., Dodd, M., Holzemer, W., & Meleis, A. I. (1997). Help seeking for self discovered breast symptoms: Implications for early detection. *Cancer Practice,* 5(4), 220-227.

Hall, J. M., Stevens, P. E. & Meleis, A. I. (1992). Developing the construct of role integration: A narrative analysis of women clerical workers' daily lives. *Research in Nursing & Health,* 15(6), 447-457.

Hall, J. M., Stevens, P. E., & Meleis, A. I. (1992). Experiences of women clerical workers in patient care areas. *Journal of Nursing Administration,* 22(5), 11-17.

Hall, J. M., Stevens, P. E. & Meleis, A. I. (1994). Marginalization: A guiding concept for valuing diversity in nursing knowledge development. *Advances in Nursing Science,* 16(4), 23-41.

Hattar-Pollara, M. & Meleis, A. I. (1995). Stress of immigration and the daily lived experience of Jordanian immigrant women. *Western Journal of Nursing Research,* 17(5), 521-539.

Hattar-Pollara, M., & Meleis, A. I. (1995). Parenting adolescents: The experiences of Jordanian immigrant women in California. *Health Care for Women International,* 16(3), 195-211.

Hattar-Pollara, M., Meleis, A. I. & Nagib, H. (2000). A study of the spousal role of Egyptian women in clerical jobs. *Health Care For Women International,* 21(4), 305-317.

Hattar-Pollara, M., Meleis, A. I., & Nagib, H. (2003). Multiple role stress and patterns of coping of Egyptian Women in Clerical Jobs. *Transcultural Nursing,* 14(2), 125-133.

Im, E., Meleis, A. I. & Lee, K. A. (1999). Cultural competence of measurement scales of menopausal symptoms: use in research among Korean women. *International Journal of Nursing Studies,* 36 455-463.

Im, E., Meleis, A. I. & Park, Y. S. (1999). A feminist critique of the research on menopausal experience of Korean women. *Research In Nursing and Health,* 22 410-420.

Im, E., & Meleis, A. I. (2001). An international imperative for gender-sensitive theories in women's health. *Journal of Nursing Scholarship,* 33(4), 309-314.

Jones, P., & Meleis, A. I. (2002). Caregiving Between Two Cultures: An Integrative Experience. *Journal of Transcultural Nursing,* 13(3), 202-209.

Jones, P. S., Jaceldo, K. B., Lee, J. R., Zhang, X. E., & Meleis, A. I. (2001). Role integration and perceived health in Asian American women caregivers. *Research in Nursing and Health,* 24, 133-144.

Jones, P. S. & Meleis, A. I. (1993). Health is empowerment. *Advances in Nursing Science,* 15(3), 1-14.

Jones, P. S., Zhang, X. E., & Meleis, A. I. (1978). Transforming Vulnerability. Western *Journal of Nursing Research,* 25(7), 835-853.

Meleis, A. I. (1992). Community participation and involvement: Theoretical and empirical issues. *Health Services Management Research,* 5(10), 5-16.

Meleis, A. I. (1992). Directions for nursing theory development in 21st century. *Nursing Science Quarterly,* 5(3), 112-117.

Meleis, A. I. (1992). On the way to scholarship: From master's to doctorate. *Journal of Professional Nursing,* 8(6), 328-334.

Meleis, A. I. (1992, June). Nursing: A caring science with a distinct domain. *Sairaanhoitaja,* pp. 8, 10, 11 & 12.

Meleis, A. I. (1996). Culturally competent scholarship: Substance and rigor. *Advances in Nursing Science,* 19(2), 1-16.

Meleis, A. I. (2001). Small steps and giant hopes: violence on women is more than wife battering. *Health Care For Women International,* 23, 313-315 (Editorial).

Meleis, A. I. (2001). Women's work, health and quality of life: It is time we redefine women's work. *Women and Health,* 33(1/2), xv-xviii.

Meleis, A. I. (2002). Whither international research? Journal of Nursing Scholarship, First Quarter 4-5 (Editorial).

Meleis, A. I. (2003). Brain Drain or Empowerment. Journal of Nursing Scholarship, 35(2), 105. (Guest Editorial).

Meleis, A. I. (2005). Shortage of nurses means a shortage of nurse scientists. (Editorial). *Journal of Advanced Nursing,* 49, (2), 111.

Meleis, A. I. (2005). Safe womanhood is not safe motherhood: policy implications. *Health Care for Women International,* 26(2), 464-471.

Meleis, A. I. Arabs. In J. Lipson, & S. Dibble, (Eds.). (2005). Culture and Clinical Care: A Practical Guide. *San Francisco: UCSF Nursing Press.* (pp. 42-57).

Meleis, A. I. "Human Capital in Health Care: A Resource Crisis of a Caring Crisis?" (2006, June-July). Global Health Link, (139), 6-7, 21-22.

Meleis, A. I., Arruda, E.N., Lane, S. & Bernal, P. (1994). Veiled, voluminous and devalued: Narrative stories about low-income women from Brazil, Egypt & Colombia. *Advances in Nursing Science,* 17(2), 1-15.

Meleis, A. I. & Bernal, P. (1994). Domestic workers in Colombia as spouses: Security and servitude. *Holistic Nursing,* 8(4), 33-43.

Meleis, A. I. & Bernal, P. (1995). The paradoxical world of muchacha de por día in Colombia. *Human Organization,* 54, 393-400.

Meleis, A. I., Douglas, M., Eribes, C., Shih, F., & Messias, D. (1996). Employed Mexican women as mothers and partners: Valued, empowered and overloaded. *Journal of Advanced Nursing,* 23, 82-90.

Meleis, A. I. & Dracup, K. (2005, September 30). The Case Against the DNP: History, Timing, Substance, and Marginalization. Online Journal of Issues in Nursing. 10(3), Manuscript 2: www.nursingworld.org/ojin/topic28/tpc28_2.htm

Meleis, A. I. & Fishman, J. (2001). Rethinking the work in health: gendered and cultural expectations. *Health Care For Women International,* 22, 195-197 (Editorial).

Meleis, A. I., Hall, J. M. Stevens, P. E. (1994). Scholarly caring in doctoral nursing education: Promoting diversity and collaborative mentorship. Image: *Journal of Nursing Scholarship,* 26(3), 177-180.

Meleis, A. I., & Im, E. (1999). Transcending marginalization in knowledge development. *Nursing Inquiry,* 6(2), 94-102.

Meleis, A. I., & Im, E. (2002). Grandmothers and women's health: For Integrative and coherent models of women's health. *Health Care for Women International.* 23, (2), 207-224.

Meleis, A. I. & Lindgren, T. (2001). Show me a woman who does not work! Journal of Nursing, Third Quarter, 209-210.

Meleis, A. I. & Lipson, J. (2003). Cross-cultural health and strategies to lead development of nursing practice. In J. Daly, S. Speedy, & D. Jackson (Eds.). (2003). Nursing Leadership, (pp. 69-88). Philadelphia: Churchill Livingstone.

Meleis, A. I., Lipson J.G., & Paul, S.M. (1992). Ethnicity and health among five Middle Eastern immigrant groups. *Nursing Research,* 41(2), 98-103.

Meleis, A. I. & Messias, D. K. H., & Arruda, E. N. (1995). Women's work environment and health: Clerical workers in Brazil. *Research in Nursing and Health,* 19, 53-62.

Meleis, A. I. & Stevens, P. E. (1992). Women in clerical jobs: Spousal role satisfaction stress and coping. *Women & Health,* 18(1), 23-40.

Messias, D. K. H., Hall, J. M., Meleis, A. I. (1996). Voices of impoverished Brazilian women: Health implications of roles and resources. *Women and Health,* 24(1), 1-20.

Messias, D.K.H., Im, E., Page, A., Regev, H., Spiers, J., & Meleis, A. I. (1997). Defining and redefining work: Implications for women's health. *Gender and Society,* 11(3), 296-323.

Messias, D.H., Regev, H., Im, E., Spiers, J., Van, P., & Meleis, A. I. (1997). Expanding the visibility of women's work: Policy implications. *Nursing Outlook,* 45, 258-264.

Nelson, M., Proctor, S., Regev, H., Barnes, D., Sawyer, L., Messias, D., Yoder, L., & Meleis, A. I. (1996). The Cairo action plan: A challenge to nursing. Image: *Journal of Nursing Scholarship,* 28(1), 75-80.

Sawyer, L., Regev, H., Proctor, S., Nelson, M., Messias, D., Barnes, D., Meleis, A. I. (1995). Matching vs. cultural competence in research a methodological note. *Research in Nursing and Health,* 18, 531-541.

Siantz, M.L. & Meleis, A. I. (2007). Integrating Cultural Competence into Nursing Education & Practice: 21st Century Action Steps. *Journal of Transcultural Nursing,* 18(1), 86-90.

Stevens, P.E., Hall, J.M., & Meleis, A. I. (1992). Examining vulnerability of women clerical workers from five ethnic racial groups. *Western Journal of Nursing Research,* 14(6), 754-774.

Stevens, P.E., Hall, J. M. & Meleis, A. I. (1992). Narratives as a basis for culturally relevant holistic care: Ethnicity and everyday experiences of women clerical workers. *Holistic Nursing Practice,* 6(3), 49-58.

Van, P. & Meleis, A. I. (2003). Coping with grief after involuntary pregnancy loss: perspectives of African-American Women. *Journal of Obstetric, Gynecological & Neonatal Nursing,* 32(1), 28-39.

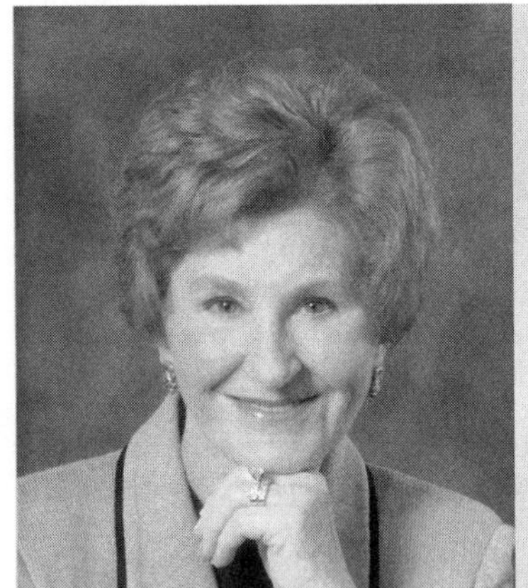

CHAPTER 21

Nola J. Pender

1941-present

Health Promotion Model

Teresa J. Sakraida

"Middle range theories that have been tested in research provide evidence for evidence-based practice, thus facilitating translation of research into practice" (Pender, personal communication, April 2008).

CREDENTIALS AND BACKGROUND OF THE THEORIST

Nola J. Pender's first encounter with professional nursing occurred at the age of 7, when she observed the nursing care given to her hospitalized aunt. "The experience of watching the nurses caring for my aunt in her illness created in me a fascination with the work of nursing," noted Pender (Pender, personal interview, May 6, 2004). This experience and her subsequent education instilled in her a desire to care for others and influenced her belief that the goal of nursing was to help people care for themselves. Pender contributes to nursing knowledge of health promotion through her research, teaching, presentations, and writings.

Pender was born August 16, 1941, in Lansing, Michigan. She was the only child of parents who were advocates of education for women. Family encouragement for her goal of becoming a registered nurse led her to attend the School of Nursing at West Suburban Hospital in Oak Park, Illinois. This school was chosen for its ties with Wheaton College and its strong Christian foundation. She received her nursing diploma in 1962 and began working on a medical-surgical unit and subsequently in a pediatric unit in a Michigan hospital (Pender, personal interview, May 6, 2004).

In 1964, Pender completed her baccalaureate in nursing at Michigan State University in East Lansing. She credits Helen Penhale, the assistant to the dean, for helping to streamline her program and foster

Previous author: Lucy Anne Tillett.

The author wishes to express appreciation to Nola J. Pender for reviewing the chapter.

her options for further education. As was common in the 1960s, Pender changed her major from nursing as she pursued her graduate degrees. She earned her master's degree in human growth and development at Michigan State University in 1965. "The M.A. in growth and development influenced my interest in health over the human life span. This background contributed to the formation of a research program for children and adolescents," stated Pender. She completed her PhD in psychology and education in 1969 at Northwestern University in Evanston, Illinois. Pender's (1970) dissertation investigated developmental changes in encoding processes of short-term memory in children. Dr. Pender credits Dr. James Hall, a doctoral program advisor, with "introducing me to considerations of how people think and how a person's thoughts motivate behavior." Several years later, she completed master's-level work in community health nursing at Rush University in Chicago (Pender, personal interview, May 6, 2004).

After earning her PhD, Pender notes a shift in her thinking toward defining the goal of nursing care as the optimal health of the individual. A series of conversations with Dr. Beverly McElmurry at Northern Illinois University and reading *High-Level Wellness* by Halpert Dunn (1961) inspired expanded notions of health and nursing. Her marriage to Albert Pender, an Associate Professor of business and economics who has collaborated with his wife in writing about the economics of health care, and the birth of a son and a daughter provided increased personal motivation to learn more about optimizing human health.

In 1975, Pender published "A Conceptual Model for Preventive Health Behavior," which was a basis for studying how individuals made decisions about their own health care in a nursing context. This article identified factors that were found in earlier research to influence decision making and actions of individuals in preventing disease. The original Health Promotion Model (HPM) was presented in the first edition of the text, *Health Promotion in Nursing Practice*, published in 1982 (Pender). Based on subsequent research, the HPM was revised and is presented in the second edition, published in 1987, and in the third edition, published in 1996. A fourth edition of *Health Promotion in Nursing Practice*, jointly authored by Pender with Carolyn L. Murdaugh (PhD) and Mary Ann Parsons (PhD), was published in 2002, and the more recent fifth edition was published in 2006.

A study funded in 1988 by National Institutes of Health was conducted at Northern Illinois University, DeKalb, Illinois, by Pender and her colleagues—Susan Walker, Karen Sechrist, and Marilyn Frank-Stromborg. The study tested the validity of the HPM (Pender, Walker, Sechrist, & Stromborg, 1988). An instrument, the Health Promoting Lifestyle Profile, was developed by the research team to study the health-promoting behavior of working adults, older adults, patients undergoing cardiac rehabilitation, and ambulatory patients with cancer (Pender et al., 2002). Results from these studies supported the HPM (Pender, personal interview, July 19, 2000). Subsequently, more than 40 studies have tested the predictive capability of the model for health-promoting lifestyle, exercise, nutrition practices, use of hearing protection, and avoidance of exposure to environmental tobacco smoke (Pender, 1996; Pender et al., 2002).

Pender provided important leadership in the development of nursing research in the United States. Her work in support of the National Center for Nursing Research in the National Institutes of Health was instrumental to its formation. She has promoted scholarly activity in nursing through her involvement with Sigma Theta Tau International, as a past president of the Midwest Nursing Research Society (1985 to 1987), and as chairperson of the Cabinet on Nursing Research of the American Nurses Association. Inducted as a fellow of the American Academy of Nursing in 1981, she served as President of the Academy from 1991 until 1993 (N. Pender, curriculum vitae, 2008). In 1998, she was appointed to a 4-year term on the U.S. Preventive Services Task Force, an independent panel charged to evaluate scientific evidence and to make age-specific and risk-specific recommendations for clinical preventive services (Pender, 2006).

A recipient of many awards and honors, Dr. Pender has served as a distinguished scholar at a number of universities. She received an honorary doctoral degree from Widener University in 1992. In 1988, she received the Distinguished Research Award from the Midwest Nursing Research Society for her contributions to research and research leadership, and in 1997, she received the American Psychological Association Award for outstanding contributions to nursing and health psychology. In 1998, the University of Michigan School of Nursing honored Pender with the Mae Edna Doyle Award for excellence in teaching (Pender, personal interview, May 24, 2004). Her widely used text, *Health Promotion in Nursing Practice* (Pender et al., 2002), was the American Nurses Association Book of the Year for contributions to community health nursing (Pender, 2006).

Pender was the Associate Dean for Research at the University of Michigan School of Nursing from 1990 to 2001. In this position, Dr. Pender facilitated external funding of faculty research, supported emerging centers of research excellence in the School of Nursing, promoted interdisciplinary research, supported translating research into science-based practice, and linked nursing research to the formulation of health policy (Pender, 2006). A child and adolescent health behavior research center initiated at the University of Michigan in 1991 represents Pender's efforts to build a large interdisciplinary research team to study and influence the health-promoting behaviors of individuals by understanding how these behaviors are established in youth (Pender, personal interview, May 24, 2000). Her current and future program of research has two major foci, as follows:

1. Understanding how self-efficacy effects the exertion and affective (activity-related affect) responses of adolescent girls to the physical activity challenge
2. Developing an interactive computer program as an intervention to increase physical activity among adolescent girls (Pender, 2006)

The Design of a Computer Based Physical Activity Counseling Intervention for Adolescent Girls is an ongoing research program led by Dr. Lorraine Robbins (Pender, personal interview, May 6, 2004).

Pender has published numerous articles on exercise, behavior change, and relaxation training as aspects of health promotion and has served as an editor for journals and books. Pender is recognized as a scholar, presenter, and consultant on health promotion topics. She has consulted with nurse scientists in Japan, Korea, Mexico, Thailand, the Dominican Republic, Jamaica, England, New Zealand, and Chile (N. Pender, curriculum vitae 2000; Pender, 2006). Her book is now available in the Japanese and Korean languages (Pender, 1997a, 1997b).

As Professor Emeritus at the University of Michigan School of Nursing, Pender is involved in influencing the nursing profession by providing leadership as a consultant to research centers and providing early scholar consultation (Pender, 2006). As a nationally and internationally known leader, Pender speaks at conferences and seminars. She collaborates with Dr. Michael O'Donnell, editor of the *American Journal of Health Promotion*, to advocate for legislation to fund health promotion research (Pender, personal interview, May 6, 2004).

Pender's future plans include continuing with travel to offer consultation and to engage in speaking opportunities. She expects to do some graduate teaching on occasion, including teaching graduate courses on the topics of theories of nursing and scientific writing as a Distinguished Professor at Loyola University in Chicago (N. Pender, personal correspondence, February 27, 2008). Pender plans to continue active mentoring through e-mail exchanges with scholars beginning research programs (Pender, personal interview, May 6, 2004).

THEORETICAL SOURCES

Pender's background in nursing, human development, experimental psychology, and education led her to use a holistic nursing perspective, social psychology, and learning theory as foundations for the HPM. The HPM (Figure 21-1) integrates several constructs. Central to the HPM is the social learning theory of Albert Bandura (1977), which postulates

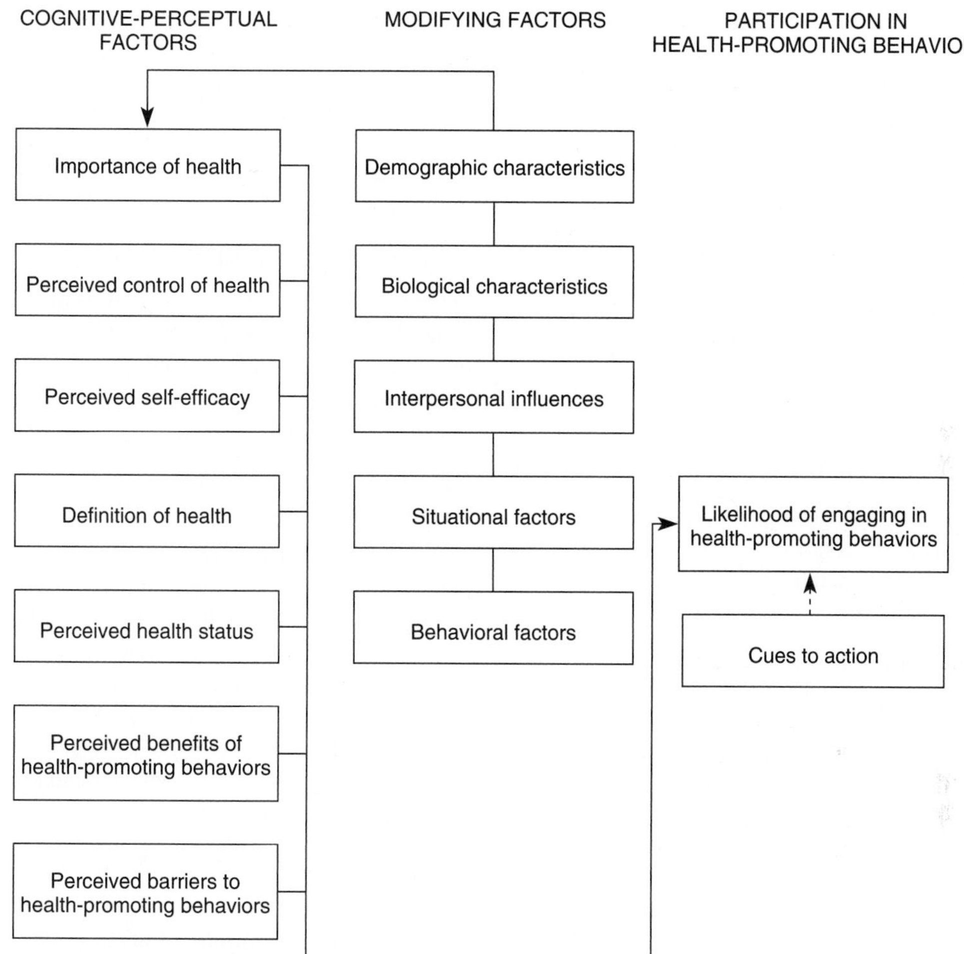

Figure 21-1 **Health Promotion Model.** (From Pender, N. J. [1987]. *Health promotion in nursing practice* [2nd ed., p. 58]. New York: Appleton & Lange. Copyright Pearson Education, Upper Saddle River, NJ.)

the importance of cognitive processes in the changing of behavior. Social learning theory, now titled social cognitive theory, includes the following self-beliefs: self-attribution, self-evaluation, and self-efficacy. Self-efficacy is a central construct of the HPM (Pender, 1996; Pender et al., 2002). In addition, the expectancy value model of human motivation that Feather (1982) described, which supports that behavior is rational and economical, is important to the model's development.

The HPM is similar in construction to the health belief model (Becker, 1974) but is not limited to explaining disease prevention behavior. The HPM differs from the health belief model in that the HPM does not include fear or threat as a source of motivation for health behavior. For this reason, the HPM expands to encompass behaviors for enhancing health and potentially applies across the life span (Pender, 1996; Pender et al., 2002).

Major Concepts & Definitions

The major concepts and definitions presented are found in the revised HPM (Pender, personal interview, May 6, 2004). The following are individual characteristics and experiences that affect subsequent health actions (Pender, curriculum vitae, 2000).

PRIOR RELATED BEHAVIOR

Frequency of the same or similar behavior in the past. Direct and indirect effects on the likelihood of engaging in health-promoting behaviors.

PERSONAL FACTORS

Categorized as biological, psychological, and sociocultural. These factors are predictive of a given behavior and are shaped by the nature of the target behavior being considered.

Personal Biological Factors

Included in these factors are variables such as age, gender, body mass index, pubertal status, menopausal status, aerobic capacity, strength, agility, and balance.

Personal Psychological Factors

These factors include variables such as self-esteem, self-motivation, personal competence, perceived health status, and definition of health.

Personal Sociocultural Factors

Factors such as race, ethnicity, acculturation, education, and socioeconomic status are included.

The following are behavioral-specific cognitions and affects that are considered of major motivational significance; these variables are modifiable through nursing actions (Pender, 1996).

PERCEIVED BENEFITS OF ACTION

Perceived benefits of action are anticipated positive outcomes that will result from health behavior.

PERCEIVED BARRIERS TO ACTION

Perceived barriers to action are anticipated, imagined, or real blocks and personal costs of undertaking a given behavior.

PERCEIVED SELF-EFFICACY

Perceived self-efficacy is judgment of personal capability to organize and execute a health-promoting behavior. Perceived self-efficacy influences perceived barriers to action, so higher efficacy results in lowered perceptions of barriers to the performance of the behavior.

ACTIVITY-RELATED AFFECT

An activity-related affect describes subjective positive or negative feelings that occur before, during, and following behavior based on the stimulus properties of the behavior itself. Activity-related affect influences perceived self-efficacy, which means the more positive the subjective feeling, the greater is the feeling of efficacy. In turn, increased feelings of efficacy can generate further positive affect.

INTERPERSONAL INFLUENCES

These influences are cognitions concerning behaviors, beliefs, or attitudes of others. Interpersonal influences include norms (expectations of significant others), social support (instrumental and emotional encouragement), and modeling (vicarious learning through observing others engaged in a particular behavior). Primary sources of interpersonal influences are families, peers, and healthcare providers.

SITUATIONAL INFLUENCES

Situational influences are personal perceptions and cognitions of any given situation or context that can facilitate or impede behavior. They include perceptions of available options, demand characteristics, and aesthetic features of the environment

MAJOR CONCEPTS & DEFINITIONS—cont'd

in which given health-promoting behavior is proposed to take place. Situational influences may have direct or indirect influences on health behavior.

The following are immediate antecedents of behavior or behavioral outcomes. A behavioral event is initiated by a commitment to action unless there is a competing demand that cannot be avoided, or a competing preference that cannot be resisted (Pender, personal interview, July 19, 2000).

COMMITMENT TO A PLAN OF ACTION

This commitment describes the concept of intention and identification of a planned strategy that leads to implementation of health behavior.

IMMEDIATE COMPETING DEMANDS AND PREFERENCES

Competing demands are alternative behaviors over which individuals have low control, because there are environmental contingencies such as work or family care responsibilities. Competing preferences are alternative behaviors over which individuals exert relatively high control, such as choice of ice cream or an apple for a snack.

HEALTH-PROMOTING BEHAVIOR

A health-promoting behavior is an end point or action outcome that is directed toward attaining positive health outcomes such as optimal well-being, personal fulfillment, and productive living. Examples of health-promoting behavior are eating a healthy diet, exercising regularly, managing stress, gaining adequate rest and spiritual growth, and building positive relationships.

USE OF EMPIRICAL EVIDENCE

The HPM, as depicted in Figure 21-1, served as a framework for research aimed at predicting overall health-promoting lifestyles and specific behaviors such as exercise and use of hearing protection (Pender, 1987). Pender and colleagues have conducted a program of research funded by the National Institute of Nursing Research to evaluate the HPM in the following four populations: (1) working adults, (2) older community-dwelling adults, (3) ambulatory patients with cancer, and (4) patients undergoing cardiac rehabilitation. These studies tested the validity of the HPM (Pender, personal interview, May 24, 2000). A summary of findings from earlier studies is included in the 1996 edition of *Health Promotion in Nursing Practice* (Pender, 1996). Additional studies testing the model are discussed in the fifth edition of *Health Promotion in Nursing Practice* (Pender et al., 2006). The fifth edition of this text includes greater emphasis on the HPM as applied to diverse and vulnerable populations and addresses evidence-based practice.

The rationale for revision of the HPM stemmed from the research studies. The process of refining the HPM, as published in 1987, led to several changes (see Figure 21-1) (Pender, 1996). First, importance of health, perceived control of health, and cues for action were deleted from the model. Second, definition of health, perceived health status, and demographic and biological characteristics were repositioned in the category of personal factors in the 1996 revision of the HPM (Pender, 1996) and are also displayed in the fourth edition of *Health Promotion in Nursing Practice* (Pender et al., 2002) (Figure 21-2). Finally, the revised HPM (see Figure 21-2) adds three new

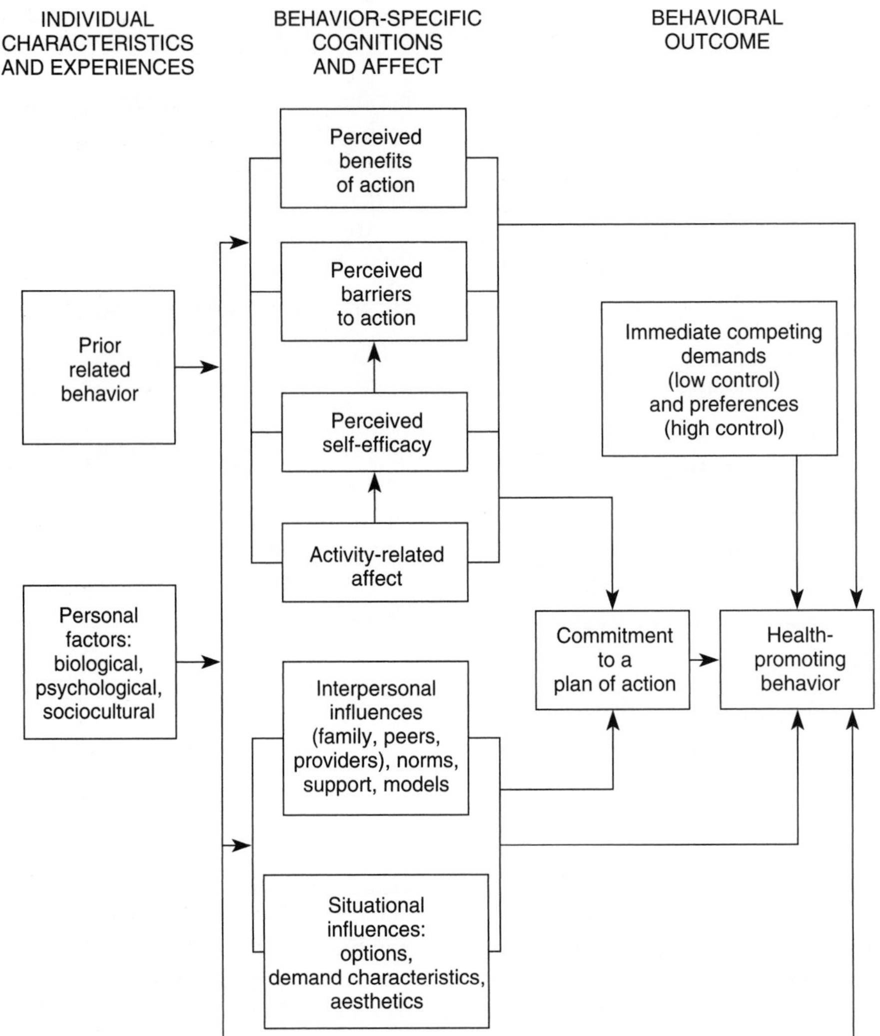

Figure **21-2** **Revised Health Promotion Model.** (From Pender, N. J., Murdaugh, C. L., & Parsons, M. A. [2002]. *Health promotion in nursing practice* [4th ed., p. 60]. Upper Saddle River, NJ: Prentice-Hall. Copyright Pearson Education, Upper Saddle River, NJ.)

variables that influence the individual to engage in health-promoting behaviors (Pender, 1996):

1. Activity-related affect
2. Commitment to a plan of action
3. Immediate competing demand and preferences

The revised HPM focuses on 10 categories of determinants of health-promoting behavior. Currently being tested empirically, the revised model identifies concepts relevant to health-promoting behaviors and facilitates the generation of testable hypotheses (Pender et al., 2002).

The HPM provides a paradigm for the development of instruments. The Health Promoting Lifestyle Profile and the Exercise Benefits-Barriers Scale

(EBBS) are two examples.* Both of these instruments serve to test the model and to further model development.

The purpose of the Health Promotion Lifestyle Profile instrument is to measure health-promoting lifestyle (Pender, 1996). The Health Promotion Lifestyle Profile II (HPLP-II), a revision of the original instrument, is used in research.† The 52-item, four-point, Likert-styled instrument consists of the following six subscales: (1) health responsibility, (2) physical activity, (3) nutrition, (4) interpersonal relations, (5) spiritual growth, and (6) stress management. Means can be derived for each subscale, or a total mean signifying overall health-promoting lifestyle (Walker, Sechrist, & Pender, 1987). The instrument provides an assessment of a health-promoting lifestyle of individuals that is clinically useful to nurses in patient support and education.

The HPM identifies cognitive and perceptual factors as major determinants of health-promoting behavior. The EBBS measures the cognitive and perceptual factors of perceived benefits and perceived barriers to exercise (Sechrist, Walker, & Pender, 1987). The 43-item, four-point, Likert-styled instrument consists of a 29-item benefits scale and a 14-item barriers scale that may be scored separately or as a whole. The higher the overall score on the 43-item instrument, the more positively the individual perceives the benefits to exercise in relation to barriers to exercise (Sechrist et al., 1987). The EBBS provides a clinically useful means for evaluating exercise perceptions.

MAJOR ASSUMPTIONS

The assumptions reflect the behavioral science perspective and emphasize the active role of the patient in managing health behaviors by modifying the environmental context. In the third edition of her book, *Health Promotion in Nursing Practice,* Pender (1996) states the major assumptions of the HPM as follows:

1. Persons seek to create conditions of living through which they can express their unique human health potential.
2. Persons have the capacity for reflective self-awareness, including assessment of their own competencies.
3. Persons value growth in directions viewed as positive and attempt to achieve a personally acceptable balance between change and stability.
4. Individuals seek to actively regulate their own behavior.
5. Individuals in all their biopsychosocial complexity interact with the environment, progressively transforming the environment and being transformed over time.
6. Health professionals constitute a part of the interpersonal environment, which exerts influence on persons throughout their life spans.
7. Self-initiated reconfiguration of person-environment interactive patterns is essential to behavioral change (pp. 54-55).

THEORETICAL ASSERTIONS

The model is an attempt to depict the multifaceted natures of persons interacting with the environment as they pursue health. Unlike avoidance-oriented models that rely upon fear or threat to health as motivation for health behavior, the HPM has a competence- or approach-oriented focus (Pender, 1996). Health promotion is motivated by the desire to enhance well-being and to actualize human potential (Pender, 1996). In her first book, *Health Promotion in Nursing Practice,* Pender (1982) asserts that complex biopsychosocial processes motivate individuals to engage in behaviors directed toward the enhancement of health. Fourteen theoretical assertions derived from the model appear in the fourth edition of the book, *Health Promotion in Nursing Practice* (Pender et al., 2002):

1. Prior behavior and inherited and acquired characteristics influence beliefs, affect, and enactment of health-promoting behavior.

*The EBBS can be obtained from the Health Promotion Research Program, Social Science Research Institute, Northern Illinois University, DeKalb, IL 60115.

†The HPLP-II can be obtained from Dr. Susan Noble Walker, EdD, RN, at the College of Nursing, University of Nebraska Medical Center, 42nd and Dewey Avenue, Omaha, NE 68105-1065. Fax: (402) 559-6379; telephone (402) 559-6561.

2. Persons commit to engaging in behaviors from which they anticipate deriving personally valued benefits.
3. Perceived barriers can constrain the commitment to action, the mediator of behavior, and the actual behavior.
4. Perceived competence or self-efficacy to execute a given behavior increases the likelihood of commitment to action and actual performance of behavior.
5. Greater perceived self-efficacy results in fewer perceived barriers to specific health behavior.
6. Positive affect toward a behavior results in greater perceived self-efficacy, which, in turn, can result in increased positive affect.
7. When positive emotions or affect is associated with a behavior, the probability of commitment and action is increased.
8. Persons are more likely to commit to and engage in health-promoting behaviors when significant others model the behavior, expect the behavior to occur, and provide assistance and support to enable the behavior.
9. Families, peers, and healthcare providers are important sources of interpersonal influences that can increase or decrease commitment to and engagement in health-promoting behavior.
10. Situational influences in the external environment can increase or decrease commitment to or participation in health-promoting behavior.
11. The greater the commitment to a specific plan of action, the more likely health-promoting behaviors are to be maintained over time.
12. Commitment to a plan of action is less likely to result in the desired behavior when competing demands over which persons have little control require immediate attention.
13. Commitment to a plan of action is less likely to result in the desired behavior when other actions are more attractive and thus preferred over the target behavior.
14. Persons can modify cognitions, affect, and the interpersonal and physical environments to create incentives for health actions (pp. 63-64).

LOGICAL FORM

The HPM has been formulated through induction by the use of existing research to form a pattern of knowledge about health behavior. Middle range theories commonly are generated through this approach. The HPM is a conceptual model that was formulated with the goal of integrating what is known about health-promoting behavior to generate questions for further testing. This model provides a framework for seeing how the results of previous research fit together more clearly, and how concepts can be manipulated for further study.

ACCEPTANCE BY THE NURSING COMMUNITY

Practice

Wellness as a nursing specialty has grown in prominence during the past decade. Current state-of-the-art clinical practice includes health promotion education. Nursing professionals find the HPM very relevant, because it applies across the life span and is useful in a variety of settings (Pender, 1996; Pender et al., 2002).

Clinical interest in health behaviors represents a philosophical shift that emphasizes the quality of lives alongside the saving of lives. In addition, there are financial, human, and environmental burdens upon society when individuals do not engage in prevention and health promotion. The HPM contributes a nursing solution to health policy and healthcare reform by providing a means for understanding how consumers can be motivated to attain personal health. Future empirical findings will be of increasing importance to nurse planners of healthcare delivery and to those who provide the care.

Education

The HPM is used widely in graduate education and is being used increasingly in undergraduate nursing education in the United States (Pender, personal interview, May 24, 2000). In the past, health promotion was placed behind illness care, because clinical education was conducted primarily in acute care settings (Pender, Baraukas, Hayman, Rice, & Anderson, 1992). Increasingly, the HPM is incorporated in nursing curricula as an aspect of health assessment, community health nursing, and wellness-focused courses (N. Pender, personal interview, May 24, 2000). Growing international efforts across a number of countries are working to integrate the HPM into nursing curricula (Pender, personal interview, May 6, 2004; Pender et al., 2002).

Research

The HPM is a tool for research. Pender's research agenda and that of other researchers have tested the empirical precision of the model. Researchers continue to report using the model as a frame of reference in their studies. The Health Promoting Lifestyle Profile, derived from the model, often serves as the operational definition for health-promoting behaviors. This model has implications for application by emphasizing the importance of the individual assessment of factors believed to influence health behavior changes.

FURTHER DEVELOPMENT

The model continues to be refined and tested for its power to explain the relationships among factors believed to influence changes in a wide array of health behaviors. Sufficient empirical support for model variables now exists for some behaviors to warrant design and conduct of intervention studies to test model-based nursing interventions. Lusk and colleagues (Lusk, Hong, Ronis, Eakin, Kerr, & Early, 1999; Lusk, Kwee, Ronis, & Eakin, 1999) used important predictors of construction workers' use of hearing protection from the HPM (self-efficacy, barriers, interpersonal influences, and situational influences) to develop an interactive, video-based program to increase use. This large, multiple-site study found that the intervention increased the use of worker hearing protection by 20% compared with the group without intervention—a statistically significant improvement from baseline (Lusk, Hong et al., 1999). Additional intervention studies represent the next step in the use of the model to build nursing science.

CRITIQUE

Simplicity

The HPM is simple to understand. The conceptual definitions provide clarity and lead to greater understanding of the complexity of health behavior phenomena. The various factors in each set are linked logically. The relationships are clarified in the theoretical assertions. The sets of factors, which are direct or indirect influences, are clearly set out in a visually simple diagram that displays their association. Factors are seen as independent, but the sets have an interactive effect that results in action.

Generality

The model is middle range in scope. It is highly generalizable to adult populations. The research used to derive the model was based on male, female, young, old, well, and ill samples. The research agenda includes application in a variety of settings. A research program tested the applicability of the model to children aged 10 to 16 years (Robbins, Gretebeck, Kazanis, & Pender, 2006). Cultural and diversity considerations support model testing in diverse populations.

Empirical Precision

The model has been supported through testing by Pender and others as a framework for explaining health promotion. The model continues to evolve through planned programs of research. Continued empirical research, especially intervention studies, will further refine the model. The Health Promoting Lifestyle Profile has emerged as an instrument used to assess health-promoting behaviors (Pender et al., 2006).

Derivable Consequences

Pender has identified health promotion as a goal for the twenty-first century, just as disease prevention was a task of the twentieth century. The model may influence the interaction between the nurse and the consumer. Pender has responded to the political, social, and personal environment of her time to clarify nursing's role in delivering health promotion services to persons of all ages.

SUMMARY

The movement to greater responsibility and accountability for successful personal health practices requires the support of the nursing profession through development of evidence-based practice. The HPM evolved from a substantive research program and continues to provide direction for better health practices. The model guides further research in various populations. Dr. Pender's visionary leadership continues to influence health promotion–related education, research, and policy.

Case Study

Thomas, a 26-year-old graduate student of Cuban descent, comes to the college health clinic to discuss his perceived weight problem. He tells you that he wants a more business-like look and wants to have more energy. He says that he is tired of having his belly fall over his belt. In your physical assessment, you find that Thomas is 5′11″, weighs 260 pounds, and has mild hypertension (132/90 mm Hg). His mother has a history of diabetes mellitus, and he tells you that high blood pressure runs in the family. His 64-year-old father had a heart attack 1 year ago. His electrocardiogram demonstrates normal sinus rhythm. He does not smoke. He says that his stress level is high, because he is working on his master's thesis. Thomas leaves to have some screening blood work and makes an appointment to see you next week. In the meantime, you begin some preliminary planning.

1. What online state-of-the-science resources would you use to help you in planning disease prevention and health promotion?
   - The Agency for Healthcare Research and Quality provides a "Guide to Clinical Preventive Services," which lists the latest available recommendations on preventive interventions: screening tests, counseling, immunizations, and medication regimens for more than 80 conditions. Age-specific periodic screenings based on gender and individual risk factors are available from the website (http://www.ahrq.gov/clinic/prevnew.htm). The consumer section for downloadable files for your personal digital assistant is another resource.
   - Go to http://www.ahrq.gov/clinic/cps3dix.htm. Look under the Clinical Category: Metabolic, Nutritional, and Endocrine Conditions to find Obesity in Adults: Screening.
   - *Healthy People 2010* includes a comprehensive set of disease prevention and health promotion objectives developed to improve the health of all people in the United States during the first decade of the twenty-first century (http://www.healthypeople.gov).
   - The U.S. Department of Health and Human Services website contains information about safety and wellness and more (http://www.hhs.gov).
2. What were some of the emotional and behavioral cues provided that suggest Thomas is ready for a weight loss management plan?
   - Thomas demonstrated self-direction, because he came to the clinic on his own.
   - He told you that he wants a more business-like look and wants to have more energy.
   - He stated that he is tired of having his belly fall over his belt.
   - He stated that his stress level is high.
3. In establishing a behavior change plan with Thomas, what are some of the interpersonal facilitators and potential barriers to change?
   - *Facilitators:* Self-direction, motivation by family medical history, desire for change.
   - *Potential barriers:* Graduate students may have limited financial resources; stress level is high, and Thomas may view self with limited time for physical activity, possibly using eating as a

coping mechanism. (Additional assessment is indicated to validate barriers.)

4. List some alternatives in the behavior change plan that you will discuss with Thomas at your next meeting. In general, discuss diet, physical activity, and stress management.
   - Complete a behavioral contract as a commitment to a plan of action. In the plan, establish a long-term weight loss goal and short-term progress goals.
   - Review kinds of foods he enjoys, while assessing dietary concerns, if any.
   - Discuss ways to increase physical activity and which of the activities he intends to carry out, and establish a calendar.
   - Provide a referral to the campus physical activity trainer.
   - Discuss stress management.
     - Establish follow-up.
   - Schedule weight checks every week.
   - Begin reward-reinforcement planning.

CRITICAL THINKING *Activities*

1. Choose one health-promoting behavior in which you personally do not engage. Identify factors, as defined in the HPM, which contribute to your decision not to participate. Include immediate competing alternatives.
2. Analyze the factors in your life that contribute to your participation in any health-promoting activity in which you currently engage. Place each factor under the appropriate label from the HPM.
3. Prepare your own description of wellness. Is absence of disease more prominent than positive, active statements of health?
4. Anticipate the health-promoting behaviors important at various stages of development across the life span. What health promotion topics do you include in your practice?

POINTS FOR *Further Study*

- Nola J. Pender University of Michigan faculty profile. Accessed July 18, 2008: http://www.nursing. umich.edu/faculty/pender_nola.html
- Pender, N. J. (2006). *Biographic sketch* (Online). Ann Arbor, MI: University of Michigan. Retrieved August 4, 2008, from: http://www.nursing.umich.edu/faculty/Pender/pender_bio.html
- Pender, N. J. (2008). Portraits of Excellence: The Nurse Theorists, Vol. 2. Athens, Ohio: Fitne, Inc.
- Pender, N. J. (1986, Oct.). *Enhancing wellness through nursing research (Videotape).* Recorded at the Nursing Conference, October 16-17, Memphis, TN. Available through University of Tennessee, Memphis, School of Nursing.
- Pender, N. J. (1989, May). *Expressing health through beliefs and actions (Videotape).* Recorded live at Discovery International, Inc.'s Nurse Theorist Conference, May 11-12, Pittsburgh. Available through Meetings Internationale, Louisville, KY.

REFERENCES

Bandura, A. (1977). Self-efficacy: Toward a unifying theory of behavioral change. *Psychology Review, 84*(2), 191-215.

Becker, M. H. (1974). *The health belief model and personal behavior.* Thorofare, NJ: Charles B. Slack.

Dunn, H. L. (1961). *High-level wellness.* Arlington, VA: Beatty.

Feather, N. T. (1982). *Expectations and actions: Expectancy-value models in psychology.* Hillsdale, NJ: Lawrence Erlbaum Associates.

Lusk, S. L., Hong, O. S., Ronis, S. L., Eakin, B. L., Kerr, M. J., & Early, M. R. (1999). Effectiveness of an intervention to increase construction worker's use of hearing protection. *Human Factors, 41*(3), 487-494.

Lusk, S. L., Kwee, M. J., Ronis, D. L., & Eakin, B. L. (1999). Applying the health promotion model to development of a worksite intervention. *American Journal of Health Promotion, 13*(4), 219-226.

Pender, N. J. (1970). A developmental study of conceptual, semantic differential, and acoustical dimensions as encoding categories in short-term memory (Doctoral dissertation Northwestern University, 1970). *Dissertation Abstracts International, A, 30*(10), 4283.

Pender, N. J. (1975). A conceptual model for preventive health behavior. *Nursing Outlook, 23*(6), 385-390.

Pender, N. J. (1982). *Health promotion in nursing practice.* New York: Appleton-Century-Crofts.

Pender, N. J. (1987). *Health promotion in nursing practice* (2nd ed.). New York: Appleton & Lange.

Pender, N. J. (1996). *Health promotion in nursing practice* (3rd ed.). Stamford, CT: Appleton & Lange.

Pender, N. J. (1997a). *Health promotion in nursing practice* (3rd ed.). Stamford, CT: Appleton & Lange. [Japanese translation].

Pender, N. J. (1997b). *Health promotion in nursing practice* (3rd ed.). Stamford, CT: Appleton & Lange. [Korean translation].

Pender, N. J. (2006). *Biographic sketch* (Online). Ann Arbor, MI: University of Michigan. Retrieved August 4, 2008, from *http://www.nursing.umich.edu/faculty/Pender/pender_bio.html.*

Pender, N. J., Baraukas, V. H., Hayman, L., Rice, V. H., & Anderson, E. T. (1992). Health promotion and disease prevention: Toward excellence in nursing practice and education. *Nursing Outlook, 40*(3), 106-120.

Pender, N. J., Murdaugh, C. L., & Parsons, M. A. (2002). *Health promotion in nursing practice* (4th ed.). Upper Saddle River, NJ: Prentice-Hall.

Pender, N. J., Murdaugh, C. L., & Parsons, M. A. (2006). *Health promotion in nursing practice* (5th ed.). Upper Saddle River, NJ: Pearson/Prentice-Hall.

Pender, N. J., Walker, S. N., Sechrist, K. R., & Stromborg, M. F. (1988). Development and testing of the health promotion model. *Cardiovascular Nursing, 24*(6), 41-43.

Robbins, L. B., Gretebeck, K. A., Kazanis, A. S., & Pender, N. J. (2006). Girls on the Move program to increase physical activity participation. *Nursing Research 55*(3), 206-216.

Sechrist, K. R., Walker, S. N., & Pender, N. J. (1987). Development and psychometric evaluation of the exercise/barriers scale. *Research in Nursing and Health, 10,* 357-365.

Walker, S. N., Sechrist, K. R., & Pender, N. J. (1987). The health-promoting lifestyle profile: Development and psychometric characteristics. *Nursing Research, 36*(2), 76-80.

BIBLIOGRAPHY

Primary Sources

Books

Pender, N. J. (1982). *Health promotion in nursing practice.* New York: Appleton-Century-Crofts.

Pender, N. J. (1987). *Health promotion in nursing practice* (2nd ed.). New York: Appleton & Lange.

Pender, N. J. (1996). *Health promotion in nursing practice* (3rd ed.). Stamford, CT: Appleton & Lange.

Pender, N. J., Murdaugh, C. L., & Parsons, M. A. (2002). *Health promotion in nursing practice* (4th ed.). Upper Saddle River, NJ: Prentice Hall.

Pender, N. J., Murdaugh, C. L., & Parsons, M. A. (2006). *Health promotion in nursing practice* (5th ed.). Upper Saddle River, NJ: Pearson/Prentice Hall.

Book Chapters

Pender, N. J. (1984). Health promotion and illness prevention. In H. Werley & J. Fitzpatrick (Eds.), *Annual review of nursing research* (pp. 83-105). New York: Springer.

Pender, N. J. (1985). Self modification. In G. Bulechek & J. McCloskey (Eds.), *Interventions: Treatments for nursing diagnosis* (pp. 80-91). Philadelphia: Saunders.

Pender, N. J. (1986). Health promotion: Implementing strategies. In B. Logan & C. Dawkins (Eds.), *Family-centered nursing in the community* (pp. 295-334). Menlo Park, CA: Addison-Wesley

Pender, N. J. (1987). Health and health promotion: The conceptual dilemmas. In M. E. Duffy & N. J. Pender (Eds.), *Conceptual issues in health promotion: Report of proceedings of a wingspread conference* (pp. 7-23). Indianapolis: Sigma Theta Tau International.

Pender, N. J. (1989). Languaging a health perspective for NANDA taxonomy on research and theory. In R. M. Carroll-Johnson (Ed.), *Classification of nursing diagnoses* (pp. 31-36). Philadelphia: Lippincott.

Pender, N. J. (1989). The pursuit of happiness, stress, and health. In S. Wald (Ed.), *Community health nursing: Issues and topics* (pp. 145-175). Englewood Cliffs, NJ: Prentice-Hall.

Pender, N. J. (1998). Motivation for physical activity among children and adolescents. In J. Fitzpatrick & J. S. Stevenson (Eds.), *Annual review of nursing research* (Vol. 16, pp. 139-172). New York: Springer.

Pender, N. J. (2004). Health promotion interventions for culturally diverse populations: Can we meet the challenge? In W. Kunaviktikul (Ed.). Improving life through health promotion: Nurse making a difference (pp.11-26). Chaing Mai, Thailand, Chotana Press.

Pender, N.J. (2005). A Global Agenda for health promotion. In W. Kunaviktikul (Ed.). Toward success in health promotion (pp. 11-23). Chaing Mai, Thailand, Chotana Press.

Pender, N. J., & Pender, A. R. (1989). Attitudes, subjective norms, and intentions to engage in health behaviors. In C. A. Tanner (Ed.), *Using nursing research* (NLN Pub. No. 15-2232, pp. 466-472). New York: National League for Nursing Publications.

Pender, N. J., & Sallis, J. (1995). Exercise counseling by health professionals. In R. Dishman (Ed.), *Exercise adherence* (2nd ed.). Champaign, IL: Human Kinetics.

Pender, N. J., Sallis, J., Long, B. J., et al. (1994). Health care provider counseling to promote physical activity. In R.K. Dishman (Ed.). Advances in exercise adherence (pp.213-235). Champaign, IL: Human Kinetics.

Pender, N. J., & Stein, K. F. (2002). Social support, the self system and adolescent health and health behaviors.

In L. L. Hayman, M. M. Mahon, J. R. Turner (Eds.). Health behavior in childhood and adolescence (pp.37-66). New York: Springer.

Dissertation

Pender, N. J. (1970). A developmental study of conceptual, semantic differential, and acoustical dimensions as encoding categories in short-term memory (Doctoral dissertation Northwestern University, 1970). *Dissertation Abstracts International, A, 30*(10), 4283.

International Journal Articles

Adeyemi, A. A., Jarad, F., Pender, N., & Higham, S. M. (2007). Assessing the efficacy of denture cleaners with quantitative light-induced fluorescence (qlf). *European Journal of Prosthodontics & Restorative Dentistry, 15*(4), 165-170.

Garcia, A. W., Broda, M. A., Frenn, M., Coviak, C., Pender, N. J., & Ronis, D. L. (1997). Gender and developmental differences in exercise beliefs among youth and prediction of their exercise behavior [Japanese translation]. *The Japanese Journal of Nursing Research, 30*(3), 51-61.

Garcia, A. W., George, T. R., Coviak, C. & Pender, N. J. (1997). Development of the child/adolescent activity log: A comprehensive and feasible measure of leisure-time physical activity. *International Journal of Behavioral Medicine, 4*(4), 323-338.

Shin, Y. H., Hur, H. K., Pender, N. J., Jang, H. J., & Kim, M. (2006). Exercise self-efficacy, exercise benefits and barriers, and commitment to a plan for exercise among Korean women with osteoporosis and osteoarthritis. *International Journal of Nursing Studies 43*(1), 3-10.

Waring, D. T., Pender, N., & Counihan, D. (2005). Mandibular arch changes following nonextraction treatment. [see comment]. *Australian Orthodontic Journal, 21*(2), 111-116.

Wu, T. Y., & Pender, N. (2005). A panel study of physical activity in Taiwanese youth: Testing the revised health-promotion model. *Family & Community Health, 28*(2), 113-124.

Wu, T. Y., Pender, N., & Noureddine, S. (2003). Gender differences in the psychosocial and cognitive correlates of physical activity among Taiwanese adolescents: A structural equation modeling approach. *International Journal of Behavioral Medicine, 10*(2), 93-105.

Journal Articles

Brimmer, P. F., Skoner, M., Pender, N. J., Williams, C. A., Fleming, J. W., & Werley, H. H. (1983). Nurses with doctoral degrees: Education and employment characteristics. *Research in Nursing and Health, 6,* 157-165.

Eden, K. B., Orleans, C. T., Mulrow, C. D., Pender, N. J., & Teutsch, S. M. (2002). Does counseling by clinicians improve physical activity? A summary of the evidence for the U. S. Preventive Services Task Force, *Annals of Internal Medicine, 137*(3), E208-E215.

Educating APHs for implementing the guidelines for adolescents in bright futures: Guidelines of health supervision of infants, children, and adolescents. *Nursing Outlook, 45*(6), 252-257

Frank-Stromborg, M., Pender, N. J., Walker, S. N., & Sechrist, K. R. (1990). Determinants of health-promoting lifestyle in ambulatory cancer patients. *Social Science and Medicine, 31*(10), 1159-1168.

Garcia, A. W., Broda, M. A. N., Frenn, M., Coviak, C., Pender, N. J., & Ronis, D. L. (1995). Gender and developmental differences in exercise beliefs among youth and prediction of their exercise behavior. *Journal of School Health, 65*(6), 213-219.

Garcia, A. W., Broda, M. A. N., Frenn, M., Coviak, C, Pender, N. J., & Ronis, D. L. (1997). Gender differences: Exercise beliefs among youth. *Reflections, 23*(1), 21-22.

Garcia, A. W., Pender, N. J., Antonakos, C. L., Ronis, D. L. (1998). Changes in physical activity beliefs and behaviors of boys and girls across the transition to junior high school. *Journal of Adolescent Health, 5,* 394-402.

Hendricks, C., Murdaugh, C., & Pender, N. (2006). The adolescent lifestyle profile: Development and psychometric characteristics. *Journal of National Black Nurses Association, 17*(2), 1-5.

Pender, N. J. (1967). The debate as a teaching and learning tool. *Nursing Outlook, 15,* 42-43.

Pender, N. J. (1971). Students who choose nursing: Are they success oriented? *Nursing Forum, 16*(1), 64-71.

Pender, N. J. (1974). Patient identification of health information received during hospitalization. *Nursing Research, 23*(3), 262-267.

Pender, N. J. (1975). A conceptual model for preventive health behavior. *Nursing Outlook, 23*(6), 385-390.

Pender, N. J. (1984). Physiologic responses of clients with essential hypertension to progressive muscle relaxation training. *Research in Nursing and Health, 7,* 197-203.

Pender, N. J. (1985). Effects of progressive muscle relaxation training on anxiety and health locus of control among hypertensive adults. *Research in Nursing and Health, 8,* 67-72.

Pender, N. J. (1987). Interview: James Michael McGinnis, MD, MPP. *Family and Community Health, 10*(2), 59-65.

Pender, N. J. (1988). Research agenda: Identifying research ideas and priorities. *American Journal of Health Promotion, 2*(4), 42-51.

Pender, N. J. (1988). Research agenda: The influences of health policy on an evolving research agenda. *American Journal of Health Promotion, 2*(3), 51-54.

Pender, N. J. (1989). Health promotion in the workplace: Suggested directions for research. *American Journal of Health Promotion, 3*(3), 38-43.

Pender, N. J. (1990). Expressing health through lifestyle patterns. *Nursing Science Quarterly, 3*(3), 115-122.

Pender, N. J. (1990). Research agenda: A revised research agenda model. *American Journal of Health Promotion, 4*(3), 220-222.

Pender, N. J. (1992). Making a difference in health policy . . . from AAN president. *Nursing Outlook, 40*(3), 104-105.

Pender, N. J. (1992). Reforming health care: Future direction . . . from AAN president. *Nursing Outlook, 40*(1), 8-9.

Pender, N. J. (1992). The NIH strategic plan: How will it affect the future of nursing science and practice? *Nursing Outlook, 40*(2), 55-56.

Pender, N. J. (1993). Creating change through partnerships . . . from AAN president. *Nursing Outlook, 41*(1), 8-9.

Pender, N. J. (1993). Health care reform: One view of the future . . . from AAN president. *Nursing Outlook, 41*(2), 56-57.

Pender, N. J. (1993). Reaching out (from AAN president. *Nursing Outlook, 41*(3), 103-104.

Pender, N. J., Barkaukas, V. H., Hayman, L., Rice, V. H., & Anderson, E. T. (1992). Health promotion and disease prevention: Toward excellence in nursing practice and education. *Nursing Outlook, 40*(3), 106-112, 120.

Pender, N. J., Bar-Or, O., Wilk, B., & Mitchell, S. (2002). Self-efficacy and perceived exertion of girls during exercise. *Nursing Research, 51*(2), 86-91.

Pender, N. J., & Pender, A. R. (1980). Illness prevention and health promotion services provided by nurse practitioners: Predicting potential consumers. *American Journal of Public Health, 70*(8), 798-803.

Pender, N. J., & Pender, A. R. (1986). Attitudes, subjective norms, and intentions to engage in health behaviors. *Nursing Research, 35*(1), 15-18.

Pender, N. J., Sechrist, K. R., Stromborg, M., & Walker, S. N. (1987). Collaboration in developing a research program grant. *Image: The Journal of Nursing Scholarship, 19*(2), 75-77.

Pender, N. J., Smith, L. C, & Vernof, J. A. (1987). Building better workers. *American Association of Occupational Health Nurses Journal, 35*(9), 386-390.

Pender, N. J., Walker, S. N., Frank-Stromborg, M., & Sechrist, K. R. (1990). Predicting health-promoting lifestyles in the workplace. *Nursing Research, 39*(6), 326-332.

Pender, N. J., Walker, S. N., Sechrist, K. R., & Frank-Stromborg, M. (1988). Development and testing of the health promotion model. *Cardiovascular Nursing, 24*(6), 41-43.

Pignone, M. P., Ammerman, A., Fernandez, L., Orleans, C. T., Pender, N., Woolf, S., et al. (2003). Counseling to promote a healthy diet in adults: A summary of the evidence for the U.S. Preventive Services Task Force. *American Journal of Preventive Medicine, 24*(1), 75-92.

Porter, C. P., Pender, N. J., Hayman, L. L., Armstrong, M. L., Riesch, S. K., & Lewis, M. A. (1997). Educating APNs for implementing the guidelines for adolescents in bright futures: Guidelines of health supervision of infants, children, and adolescents. *Nursing Outlook, 45*(6), 252-257.

Robbins, L. B., Pender, N. J., Conn, V. S., Frenn, M. D., Neuberger, G. B., Nies, M. A., et al. (2001). Physical activity research in nursing. *Journal of Nursing Scholarship, 33*(4), 315-321.

Sechrist, K. R., Walker, S. N., & Pender, N. J. (1987). Development and psychometric evaluation of the exercise benefits/barriers scale. *Research in Nursing and Health, 10* 357-365.

Shin, Y., Jang, H., & Pender, N. J. (2001). Psychometric evaluation of the Exercise Self-Efficacy Scale among Korean adults with chronic diseases. *Research in Nursing & Health, 24*(1), 68-76.

Walker, S. N., Kerr, M. J., Pender, N. J., & Sechrist, K. R. (1990). A Spanish language version of the health promoting lifestyle profile. *Nursing Research, 39*(5), 268-273.

Walker, S. N., Sechrist, K. R., & Pender, N. J. (1987). The health-promoting lifestyle profile: Development and psychometric characteristics. *Nursing Research, 36*(2), 76-81.

Walker, S. N., Volkan, K., Sechrist, K. R., & Pender, N. J. (1988). Health-promoting life styles of older adults: Comparisons with young and middle-aged adults, correlates and patterns. *ANS Advances in Nursing Science, 11*(1), 76-90.

Whitehead, D., Shin, Y., Yun, S., Pender, N. J., & Jang, H. (2005). Letter to the editor. "Test of the Health Promotion Model as a causal model of commitment to a plan for exercise among Korean adults with chronic disease" (Shin, Pender, & Yun, 2003. published in your April 2005 issue. *Research in Nursing & Health 28*(4), 357-361.

Whitlock, E. P., Orleans, C. T., Pender, N., & Allan, J. (2002). Evaluating primary care behavioral counseling interventions: An evidence-based approach. *American Journal of Preventive Medicine, 22*(4), 267-284.

Wu, T. Y., & Pender, N. (2002). Determinants of physical activity among Taiwanese adolescents: An application of the health promotional model. *Research in Nursing & Health, 25*(1), 25-36.

Wu, T. Y., Pender, N., & Yang, K. P. (2002). Promoting physical activity among Taiwanese and American adolescents. *The Journal of Nursing Research: JNR, 10*(1), 57-64.

Wu, T. Y., Ronis, D. L., Pender, N., & Jwo, J. (2002). Development of questionnaires to measure physical activity cognitions among Taiwanese adolescents. *Preventive Medicine, 35*(1), 54-64.

Secondary Sources

Dissertations and Theses

Al-Obeisat, S. M. (1999). Prenatal care utilization among Jordanian women (health care utilization, health promotion model). *Dissertation Abstracts International, 60-04B*, 1525.

Anthony, J. S. (1999). Mental health correlates of self-advocacy in health care decision-making among elderly African-Americans (Doctoral dissertation, George Mason University, 1999). *Dissertation Abstracts International, 59-12B*, 6259.

Bagwell, M. M. (1988). *Wellness in two developmental phases of employed adults.* Unpublished doctoral dissertation, Texas Woman's University, Houston.

Baker, O. G. (2003). Relationship of parental tobacco use, peer influence, self-esteem, and tobacco use among Yemeni American adolescents: Mid-range theory testing. *Dissertation Abstracts International, 64-03B*, 1175. (University Microfilms No. AAT3086416)

Barnett, F. C. (1989). *The relationship of selected cognitive-perceptual factors to health-promoting behaviors of adolescents.* Unpublished doctoral dissertation, University of Texas at Austin.

Beunting, J. A. (1990). *Psychosocial variables and gender as factors in wellness promotion.* Unpublished doctoral dissertation, State University of New York at Buffalo.

Bilderback, L. K. (1990). Health-promoting behaviors and perceived health status of rural families: A descriptive-correlational study. *Masters Abstracts International, 29-01*, 0089.

Bolio, S. M. (1999). Reported health-promoting behaviors of incarcerated males (prisoner health, family support). *Dissertation Abstracts International, 60-02B*, 0575.

Bond-Kinkade, M. A. (1999). The relationship of locus of control and participation in health-promoting behaviors among kidney transplant recipients. *Masters Abstracts International, 37-06*, 1815.

Bruna, A. C. (1998). Health promoting behaviors of rural Kansas women throughout the lifespan. *Masters Abstracts International, 37-01*, 234.

Burrill, E. B. (1998). Health conception, family health work and health promoting lifestyle practices in Latin American Mennonite families. *Masters Abstracts International, 37-01*, 239.

Butler, M. R. (1995). *Self-esteem and health-promoting lifestyle as predictors of health-risk behavior among older adolescents.* Unpublished doctoral dissertation, Texas Woman's University, Houston.

Carroll, S. A. (1995). The relationship of choice of infant feeding method and influencing factors among Hispanic mothers of the Permian basin. *Masters Abstracts International, 34-03*, 1147.

Carter, L. M. (1990). *Functional wellness among older adults: The interface of motivation, lifestyle, and capability.* Unpublished doctoral dissertation, Texas Woman's University, Houston.

Chandrasekhar, R. (1999). Cues to action which influence engagement in health-promoting behaviors among nursing students. *Masters Abstracts International, 37-02*, 0587.

Chen, C. (1995). *Physical exercise and sense of well-being among Chinese elderly in Taiwan.* Unpublished doctoral dissertation, University of Texas at Austin.

Costanzo, C. (2005). *Physical activity counseling intervention for women age 50-75 within the community.* University of Nebraska Medical Center, In ProQuest Digital Dissertations [database on-line]; available from http://www.proquest.com/ (publication number AAT: 3165167 accessed July 10, 2008).

Cunningham, G. D. (1989). Health promoting self care behaviors in an older adult community. *Dissertation Abstracts International, 50-11B*, 4968.

Dunham, K. L. (1992). Health promoting lifestyles of nursing faculty. *Masters Abstracts International, 31-02*, 0760.

Easom, L. R. (2003). Determinants of participation in health promotion activities in rural elderly caregivers. *Dissertation Abstracts International, 64-02B*, 636. (University Microfilms No. AAT3081342).

Edmonds, J. C. (2006). The relationship of weight, body image, self-efficacy, and stress to health-promoting behaviors: A study of college educated African American women. The Catholic University of America, Washington, D. C. In ProQuest Digital Dissertations [database on-line]; available from http://www.proquest.com/ (publication number AAT 3214670: accessed July 10, 2008).

Ellis, J. R. (1990). *Health status, health behavior, multidimensional health locus-of-control and factors in the development of personal control in individuals with rheumatoid arthritis.* Unpublished doctoral dissertation, University of Texas at Austin.

Fehir, J. S. (1988). Motivation, and selected demographics as determinants of health-promoting lifestyle behavior in men 35 to 64 years old: A nursing investigation. *Dissertation Abstracts International, 50-05B*, 1851.

Gabry, H. (2005). *Understanding the relationship between health behavior during pregnancy and health locus of control among Arab and non-Arab women to reduce high risk pregnancy.* George Mason University, Washington, D.C. In ProQuest Digital Dissertations [database on-line]; available from http://www.proquest.com/ (publication number AAT 3167540: accessed July 10, 2008).

Gasalberti, D. (1999). Early detection of breast cancer by self-examination: The influence of perceived barriers and health conception (cancer detection). *Dissertation Abstracts International, 60-01B*, 0129.

Gava, M. Z. (1996). *The AIDS crisis: Examining factors that influence use of condoms by young adult Zimbabwean males.* Unpublished doctoral dissertation, University of Michigan, Ann Arbor.

Gerard, M. S. (1993). *Factors related to long-term physical activity following coronary artery bypass graft surgery.* Unpublished doctoral dissertation, Rush University College of Nursing, Chicago.

Gillis, A. J. (1993). *The relationship of definition of health, perceived health status, self-efficacy, parental health-promoting lifestyle, and selected demographics to health-promoting lifestyle in adolescent females.* Unpublished doctoral dissertation, University of Texas at Austin.

Grabowski, B. J. (1997). Determinants of health promotion behavior in active duty Air Force personnel. *Masters Abstracts International, 36-01*, 0156.

Harms, J. M. (1995). Health-promoting behaviors in exercising and nonexercising seniors: A comparison. *Masters Abstracts International, 34-02*, 0719.

Harrison, R. L. (1993). *The relationship among hope, perceived health status, and health-promoting lifestyle among HIV seropositive men.* Unpublished doctoral dissertation, New York University, New York.

Hatmaker, D. D. (1993). *The effects of individual factors and health promotion during pregnancy on maternal-child health.* Unpublished doctoral dissertation, Medical College of Georgia, Augusta.

Haus, C. S. (2003). Medication management strategies used by community-dwelling older adults living alone. *Dissertation Abstracts International, 64-07B*, 3188. (University Microfilms No. AAT3097641)

Hemstron, M. M. (1993). *Relationships and differences in definition of health, perceived personal competence, perceived health status and health-promoting lifestyle profile in three elderly cohorts.* Unpublished doctoral dissertation, Rush University College of Nursing, Chicago.

Hubbard, A. B. (2002). The impact of curriculum design on health promoting behaviors at a community college in south Florida. *Dissertation Abstracts International, 63-06*, 2112.

Hubbard, D. (1987). The patterns of family interaction that promote positive child health behaviors. *Masters Abstracts International, 26-04*, 0419.

Hudak, J. W. (1988). A comparative study of the health beliefs and health-promoting behaviors of normal weight and overweight male Army personnel. *Dissertation Abstracts International, 50-06B*, 2337.

Jadalla, A. A. (2007). *Acculturation, health, and health behaviors of adult Arab Americans.* Loma Linda University, United States—California. In ProQuest Digital Dissertations [database on-line]; available from http://www.proquest.com/ (publication number AAT 3282707: accessed July 10, 2008).

Jones, C. J. (1991). *Relationship of participation in health promotion behaviors to health-related hardiness and other selected factors in older adults.* Unpublished doctoral dissertation, Texas Woman's University, Houston.

Kalampakorn, S. (2000). Stages of constructions workers use of hearing protection. *Dissertation Abstracts International, 61-07B*, 3508.

Kerr, M. J. (1994). Factors related to Mexican-American workers use of hearing protection (noise). *Dissertation Abstracts International, 50-08B*, 3238.

Kohlbry, P. W. (2006). *Exercise self-efficacy, stages of exercise change, health promotion behaviors, and physical activity in postmenopausal Hispanic women.* Unpublished Ph.D., University of Illinois at San Diego, United States—California. In *ProQuest Digital Dissertations* [database on-line]; available from http://www.proquest.com/ (publication number AAT 3218201: accessed August 1, 2008).

Kurtz, A. C. (1996). *Correlates of health-promoting lifestyles among women with rheumatoid arthritis.* Unpublished doctoral dissertation, Columbia University Teachers College, New York.

Lee, N. (1987). Health knowledge and health-promoting behavior in Chinese students. *Masters Abstracts International, 27-01*, 0086.

Lewallen, L. P. (1995). *Barriers to prenatal care in low-income women.* Unpublished doctoral dissertation, University of North Carolina at Chapel Hill.

Luther, C. H. (2003). Living the coming of osteoporosis: Health promotion behaviors of women at risk for osteoporosis in Mississippi. *Dissertation Abstracts International, 64-08B*, 3746. (University Microfilms No. AAT3101544)

Martinelli, A. M. (1996). *A study of health locus of control, self-efficacy, health promotion behaviors, and environmental factors related to the self-report of the avoidance of environmental smoke in young adults.* Unpublished doctoral dissertation, Catholic University of America, Washington, D. C.

McCullagh, M. C. (1999). Factors affecting hearing protector use among farmers. *Dissertation Abstracts International, 61-02B*, 780.

McKeon, F. M. (1997). Health-promoting behaviors: Predictors of early vs. late initiation to prenatal care. *Masters Abstracts International, 35-05*, 1390.

McMemamin, C. A. (2002). Parental perception concerning the use of peak flow meters in the child with asthma. *Masters Abstracts International, 41-05*, 1420.

Medcalf, P. L. (1988). Value placed on health and number of health promoting behaviors of adults. *Masters Abstracts International, 27-04*, 0492.

Merren, V. A. (1991). Determinants of health promotion in the elderly. *Masters Abstracts International, 29-04*, 0648.

Mitchell, M. L. (1993). *Effects of a self-efficacy intervention on adherence to antihypertensive regimens.* Unpublished doctoral dissertation, University of Rochester, Rochester, NY.

Moore, E. J. (1992). *The relationship among self-efficacy, health knowledge, self-rated health status, and selected demographics as determinants of health promoting behavior of older adults.* Unpublished doctoral dissertation, University of Akron, Akron, OH.

Oh, H. (1993). Health promoting behaviors and quality of life of Korean women with arthritis. *Dissertation Abstracts International, 54-08B*, 4083.

Phillips, P. S. (1993). Health promoting behaviors of adults attending a worksite health fair. *Masters Abstracts International, 32-05*, 1375.

Pichayapinyo, P. (2005). The relationship of perceived benefits, perceived barriers, social support, and sense of mastery on adequacy of prenatal care for first-time Thai mothers. The Catholic University of America, United States-Washington, D.C. In *ProQuest Digital Dissertations* [database on-line]; available from http://www.proquest.com/ (publication number AAT 3169867: accessed August 1, 2008).

Rothschild, S. L. (1996). *Mental health representations of attachment: Implications for health-promoting behavior and perceived stress.* Unpublished doctoral dissertation, Ohio State University, Columbus.

Rummel, C. B. (1991). *The relationship of health value and hardiness to health-promoting behavior in nurses.* Unpublished doctoral dissertation, New York University, New York.

Sakraida, T. J. (2002). Divorce transition, coping responses, and health promoting behavior of midlife women. *Dissertation Abstracts International, 62-12B*, 5646. (University Microfilms No. AAT3037817)

Sallee, A. M. (1996). The relationship of health locus of control and participation in health-promoting behaviors among older hypertensive persons. *Masters Abstracts International, 34-18*, 2349.

Sapp, C. J. (2003). Adolescents with asthma: Effects of personal characteristics and health-promoting lifestyle behaviors on health-related quality of life. *Dissertation Abstracts International, 64-05B*, 2131. (University Microfilms No. AAT3092071)

Smith Hendricks, C. K. (1992). *Perceptual determinants of early adolescent health promoting behaviors in one Alabama black belt country.* Unpublished doctoral dissertation, Boston College, Boston.

Spencer, S. A. (2007). *Effects of physiological and cognitive perceptual factors on health promotion practices in Army reservists.* Unpublished Ph.D., University of Illinois at Chicago, United States – Illinois. In *ProQuest Digital Dissertations* [database on-line]; available from http://www.proquest.com/ (publication number AAT 3267048: accessed July 16, 2008).

Stone, S. A. (1990). The relationship between self-esteem and health promoting behaviors in working women. *Masters Abstracts International, 30-04*, 1326.

Stutts, W. C. (1997). *Use of the health promotion model to predict physical activity in adults.* Unpublished doctoral dissertation, University of North Carolina at Chapel Hill.

Suwonnaroop, N. (1999). Health-promoting behaviors in older adults: The effect of social support, perceived health status, and personal factors. *Dissertation Abstracts International, 60-08B*, 3854.

Tapler, D. A. (1996). *The relationship between health value, self-efficacy, health barriers, and health behavior practices in mothers. Unpublished doctoral* dissertation, Texas Woman's University, Houston.

Tashiro, J. (1996). Health promoting lifestyle behaviors of college women in Japan: An exploratory study. *Dissertation Abstracts International, 57-04B*, 2486.

Thompson, E. M. (1995). *A descriptive study of women who successfully quit smoking.* Unpublished doctoral dissertation, Georgia State University, Atlanta.

Turner, S. J. (1989). Health protective behavior and the elderly: Hemoccult testing for early colorectal cancer detection. *Masters Abstracts International, 28-02*, 0277.

Vines, W. R. (1991). *Psychological stress reaction, coping strategies, and health promotion lifestyles among hospital nurses.* Unpublished doctoral dissertation, University of Alabama at Birmingham.

Warner, K. D. (2000). Health-related lifestyle behaviors of twins: Interpersonal and situational influences. *Dissertation Abstracts International, 61-03B*, 1331.

Warren, M. T. (1993). *The relationships of self-motivation and perceived personal competence to engaging in a health-promoting lifestyle for men in cardiac rehabilitation programs.* Unpublished doctoral dissertation, New York University, New York.

White, D. A. (1994). The relationship of intrinsic motivation and health beliefs on positive health behavior in pregnant adolescents. *Masters Abstracts International, 34-02*, 0730.

White, D. E. (2005). *Women's expectations and experiences of role performance following coronary artery bypass surgery.* Unpublished Ph.D., Georgia State University, United States—Georgia. In *ProQuestDigital Dissertations* [database on-line]; available from http://www.proquest.com/ (publication number AAT 3194604: accessed July 16, 2008).

White, J. L. (1996). *Outcomes of an individualized health promotion program for homebound older community residents.* Unpublished doctoral dissertation, Texas Woman's University, Houston.

Willis, J. L. (2001). The effect of multiple roles in the health promotion activities of college women. *Masters Abstracts International, 39-05*, 1382.

Wilson, A. H. (1991). Health promoting behaviors among married and unmarried mothers. *Dissertation Abstracts International, 52-06B*, 2999.

Wisnewski, C. A. (1996). *A study of the health-promoting behavioral effects of an exercise educational intervention in adult diabetics.* Unpublished doctoral dissertation, Texas Woman's University, Houston.

Yang, K. (2005). *Physical activities among Korean midlife immigrant women in the United States.* Unpublished Ph.D., The University of Texas at Austin, United States — Texas. In *ProQuestDigital Dissertations* [database on-line]; available from http://www.proquest.com/ (publication number AAT 3184818: accessed August 1, 2008).

Yue, S. P. (1998). Assessing the needs of the post-cardiac event population in a rural southeastern New Mexico community. *Masters Abstracts International, 36-06*, 1594.

Yuhos, J. L. (1997). Health patterns of nurses who smoke. *Masters Abstracts International, 36-01*, 0166.

Journal Articles

Agazio, J. G., Ephraim, P. M., Flaherty, N. B., & Gurney, C. A. (2002). *Health promotion in active-duty military women with children. 35*(1), 65-82.

Callaghan, D. (2005). Healthy behaviors, self-efficacy, self-care, and basic conditioning factors in older adults. *Journal of Community Health Nursing, 22*(3), 169-178.

Callaghan, D. M. (2005). The influence of spiritual growth on adolescents' initiative and responsibility for self-care. *Pediatric Nursing, 31*(2), 91-95.

Callaghan, D. (2006). Basic conditioning factors' influences on adolescents' healthy behaviors, self-efficacy, and self-care. *Issues in Comprehensive Pediatric Nursing, 29*(4), 191-204.

Callaghan, D. (2006). The influence of basic conditioning factors on healthy behaviors, self-efficacy, and self-care in adults. *Journal of Holistic Nursing, 24*(3), 178-185.

Calvert, W. J., & Bucholz, K. K. (2008). Adolescent risky behaviors and alcohol use. *Western Journal of Nursing Research, 30*(1), 147-148.

Campbell, J., & Kreidler, M. (1994). Older adults' perceptions about wellness. *Journal of Holistic Nursing, 12*(4), 437-447.

Campbell, M., & Torrance, C. (2005). Coronary angioplasty: Impact on risk factors and patients' understanding of the severity of their condition. *Australian Journal of Advanced Nursing, 22*(4), 26-31.

Chen, C., Kuo, S., Chou, Y., & Chen, H. (2007). Postpartum Taiwanese women: Their postpartum depression, social support and health-promoting lifestyle profiles. *Journal of Clinical Nursing, 16*(8), 1550-1560.

Chen, M., James, K., Hsu, L., Chang, S., Huang, L., & Wang, E. K. (2005). Health-related behavior and adolescent mothers. *Public Health Nursing, 22*(4), 280-288.

Conway, A. E., McClune, A. J., & Nosel, P. (2007). Down on the farm: Preventing farm accidents in children. *Pediatric Nursing* 2007, 33(1), 45-48.

Costanzo, C., Walker, S. N., Yates, B. C., McCabe, B., & Berg, K. (2006). Physical activity counseling for older women . . . including commentary by Pomeroy SH and Quinn ME with author response. *Western Journal of Nursing Research 28*(7), 786-810.

Daggett, L. M., & Rigdon, K. L. (2006). A computer-assisted instructional program for teaching portion size versus serving size. *Journal of Community Health Nursing, 23*(1), 29-35.

Esperat, C., Feng, D., Zhang, Y., & Owen, D. (2007). Health behaviors of low-income pregnant minority women. *Western Journal of Nursing Research, 29*(3), 284-300.

Evio, B. D. (2005). The relationship between selected determinants of health behavior and lifestyle profile of older adults. *Philippine Journal of Nursing, 75*(1), 23-31.

Guarnero, P. A. (2006). Health promotion behaviors among a group of 18-29 year old gay and bisexual men. *Communicating Nursing Research, 39*, 298.

Guarnero, P. A. (2007). Staying healthy: How are young gay and bisexual men doing? *Communicating Nursing Research, 40*, 429.

Gusain, S. (2008). Nursing and self-motivation for elderly. *Nursing Journal of India, 99*(1), 5-7.

Hageman, P. A., Walker, S. N., & Pullen, C. H. (2005). Tailored versus standard internet-delivered interventions to promote physical activity in older women. *Journal of Geriatric Physical Therapy, 28*(1).

Hensley, R. D., Jones, A. K., Williams, A. G., Willsher, L. B., & Cain, P. P. (2005). One-year clinical outcomes for Louisiana residents diagnosed with type 2 diabetes and hypertension. *Journal of the American Academy of Nurse Practitioners, 17*(9), 363-369.

Huang, T., & Dai, F. (2007). Weight retention predictors for Taiwanese women at six-month postpartum. *Journal of Nursing Research 15*(1), 11-20.

Hui, W. H. (2002). The health-promoting lifestyles of undergraduate nurses in Hong Kong. *Journal of Professional Nursing, 18*(2), 101-111.

Hulstein, P., & Berg, J. A. (2007). Premenstrual symptoms and academic stress in rural college women. *Communicating Nursing Research 40*, 540.

Johnson, R. L. (2005). Gender differences in health-promoting lifestyles of African Americans. *Public Health Nursing 22*(2), 130-137.

Johnson, R. L., & Nies, M. A. (2005). A qualitative perspective of barriers to health-promoting behaviors of African Americans. *ABNF Journal 16*(2), 39-41.

Kaewthummanukul, T., Brown, K. C., Weaver, M. T., & Thomas, R. R. (2006). Predictors of exercise participation in female hospital nurses. *Journal of Advanced Nursing 54*(6), 663-675.

Kahawong, W., Phancharoenworakul, K., Khampalikit, S., Taboonpong, S., & Chittchang, U. (2005). Nutritional health-promoting behavior among women with hyperlipidemia. *Thai Journal of Nursing Research 9*(2), 91-102.

Kerr, M. J., Lusk, S. L., & Ronis, D. L. (2002). Explaining Mexican American worker's hearing protection use with the health promotion model. *Nursing Research, 51*(2), 100-109.

Kerr, M. J., Savik, K., Monsen, K. A., & Lusk, S. L. (2007). Effectiveness of computer-based tailoring versus targeting to promote use of hearing protection. *Canadian Journal of Nursing Research 39*(1), 80-97.

Lohse, J. L. (2003). A bicycle safety education program for parents of young children. *Journal of School Nursing, 19*(2), 100-110.

Lucas, J. A., Orshan, S. A., & Cook, F. (2000). Determinants of health-promoting behavior among women ages 65 and above living in the community. *Scholarly Inquiry for Nursing Practice, 14*(1), 77-100.

Maes, C., & Louis, M. (2007). Advanced nurse practitioners and sexual history taking practices among older adults. *Communicating Nursing Research, 40*, 464.

McCullagh, M., Lusk, S. L., & Ronis, D. L. (2002). Factors influencing use of hearing protection among farmers: A test of the Pender health promotion model. *Nursing Research, 51*(1), 33-39.

McDonald, P. E., Brennan, P. F., & Wykle, M. L. (2005). Perceived health status and health-promoting behaviors of African-American and white informal caregivers of impaired elders. *Journal of National Black Nurses' Association, 16*(1), 8-17.

McMurry, T. B. (2006). A comparison of pharmacological tobacco cessation relapse rates. *Journal of Community Health Nursing 23*(1), 15-28.

Mendias, E. P., & Paar, D. P. (2007). Perceptions of health and self-care learning needs of outpatients with HIV/AIDS. *Journal of Community Health Nursing 24*(1), 49-64.

Milne, J. L., & Moore, K. N. (2006). Factors impacting self-care for urinary incontinence. *Urologic Nursing 26*(1), 41-51.

Montgomery, K. S. (2002). Health promotion with adolescents: Examining theoretical perspectives to guide research. *Research & Theory for Nursing Practice, 16*(2), 119-134.

Morowatisharifabad, M. A., & Shirazi, K. K. (2007). Determinants of oral health behaviors among preuniversity (12th-grade) students in Yazd (Iran): an application of the health promotion model. *Family & Community Health 30*(4), 342-350.

Nies, M. A., & Motyka, C. L. (2006). Factors contributing to women's ability to maintain a walking program. *Journal of Holistic Nursing 24*(1), 7-14.

Olson, A. F., & Berg, J. A. (2006). Theoretical foundations of promoting perimenopausal bone health. *Communicating Nursing Research 39*, 279.

Phuphaibul, R., Leucha, Y., Putwattana, P., Nuntawan, C., Tapsart, C., Tachudhong, A., et al. (2005). Health promoting behaviors of Thai adolescents, family health related lifestyles and parent modeling. *Thai Journal of Nursing Research 9*(1), 28-37.

Piazza, J., Conrad, K., & Wilbur, J. (2001). Exercise behavior among female occupational health nurses. Influence of self efficacy, perceived health control, and age. *AAOHN Journal, 49*(2), 79-86.

Pichayapinyo, P., O'Brien, M. E., Duffy, J. R., & Agazio, J. (2007). The relationship of perceived benefits, perceived barriers, social support, and sense of mastery on adequacy of prenatal care for first-time Thai mothers. *Thai Journal of Nursing Research 11*(2), 106-117.

Robbins, L. B., Gretebeck, K. A., Kazanis, A. S., & Pender, N. J. (2006). Girls on the Move program to increase physical activity participation. *Nursing Research 55*(3), 206-216.

Ronis, D. L., Hong, O., & Lusk, S. L. (2006). Comparison of the original and revised structures of the health promotion model in predicting construction workers' use of hearing protection. *Research in Nursing & Health 29*(1), 3-17.

Rothman, N. L., Lourie, R. J., Brian, D., & Foley, M. (2005). Temple Health Connection: a successful collaborative model of community-based primary health care. *Journal of Cultural Diversity 12*(4), 145-151.

Schlickau, J. M., & Wilson, M. E. (2005). Breastfeeding as health-promoting behaviour for Hispanic women: literature review. *Journal of Advanced Nursing 52*(2), 200-210.

Shin, K. R., Kang, Y., Park, H. J., Cho, M. O., & Heitkemper, M. (2008). Testing and developing the health promotion model in low-income, Korean elderly women. *Nursing Science Quarterly 21*(2), 173-178.

Sisk, R. J. (2000). Caregiver burden and health promotion. *International Journal of Nursing Studies, 37*(1), 37-43.

Smith, A. B., & Bashore, L. (2006). The effect of clinic-based health promotion education on perceived health status and health promotion behaviors of adolescent and young adult cancer survivors. *Journal of Pediatric Oncology Nursing 23*(6), 326-334.

Smith, S. A., & Michel, Y. (2006). A pilot study on the effects of aquatic exercises on discomforts of pregnancy. *JOGNN: Journal of Obstetric, Gynecologic, and Neonatal Nursing 35*(3), 315-323.

Srof, B. J., & Velsor-Friedrich, B. (2006). Health promotion in adolescents: a review of Pender's Health Promotion Model. *Nursing Science Quarterly 19*(4), 366-373.

Victor, J. F., de Oliveira Lopes, M. V., & Ximenes, L. B. (2005). Analysis of diagram the health promotion model of Nola J. Pender [Portuguese]. *ACTA Paulista de Enfermagem 18*(3), 235-240.

Walker, S. N., Pullen, C. H., Hertzog, M., Boeckner, L., & Hageman, P. A. (2006). Determinants of older rural women's activity and eating including commentary by Wilbur J, Zenk SN with response by Walker, Pullen, Boeckner, and Hageman. *Western Journal of Nursing Research 28*(4), 449-474.

Wang, H. H. (2001). A comparison of two models of health-promoting lifestyle in rural elderly Taiwanese women. *Public Health Nursing, 18*(3), 204-211.

Wang, W., Wang, C., Tung, Y., & Peng, J. (2007). Factors influencing adolescent second-hand smoke avoidance behavior from the perspective of Pender's health promotion model [Chinese]. *Journal of Evidence-Based Nursing 3*(4), 280-288.

Wilson, M. (2005). Health-promoting behaviors of sheltered homeless women. *Family & Community Health 28*(1), 51-63.

Yang, K., Laffrey, S. C., Stuifbergen, A., Im, E., May, K., & Kouzekanani, K. (2007). Leisure-time physical activity among midlife Korean immigrant women in the US. *Journal of Immigrant and Minority Health 9*(4), 291-298.

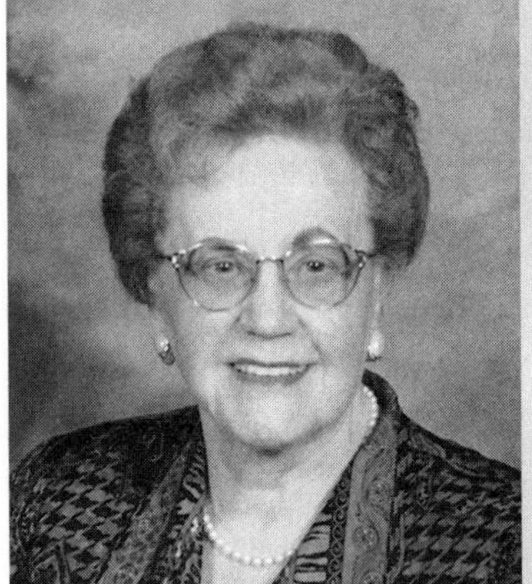
Photo credit: Kathleen Leininger, Austin, TX

CHAPTER 22

Madeleine M. Leininger

1920s-present

Culture Care Theory of Diversity and Universality

Marilyn R. McFarland

"Care is the essence of nursing and a distinct, dominant, central and unifying focus" *Madeleine Leininger (2002e, p. 192).*

CREDENTIALS AND BACKGROUND OF THE THEORIST

Madeleine M. Leininger is the founder of transcultural nursing and a leader in transcultural nursing and human care theory. She is the first professional nurse with graduate preparation in nursing to hold a PhD in cultural and social anthropology. She was born in Sutton, Nebraska, and began her nursing career after graduating from the diploma program at St. Anthony's School of Nursing in Denver, Colorado. She was in the U.S. Army Nurse Corps while pursuing the basic nursing program. In 1950, she obtained a bachelor's degree in biological science from Benedictine College in Atchison, Kansas, with a minor in philosophy and humanistic studies. After graduation, she served as an instructor, staff nurse, and head nurse on a medical-surgical unit and opened a new psychiatric unit while director of the nursing service at St. Joseph's Hospital in Omaha, Nebraska. During this time, she pursued advanced study in nursing, nursing administration, teaching and curriculum in nursing, and tests and measurements at Creighton University in Omaha, Nebraska (Leininger, 1995c, 1996b).

In 1954, Leininger obtained a master's degree in psychiatric nursing from Catholic University of America in Washington, D.C. She was then employed at the College of Health at the University of Cincinnati, Ohio, where she began the first master's level clinical specialist program in child psychiatric nursing in the world. She also initiated and directed the first graduate nursing program in psychiatric nursing at the University of Cincinnati and the

Therapeutic Psychiatric Nursing Center at the University Hospital (Cincinnati). During this time, she wrote one of the first basic psychiatric nursing texts with Hofling entitled *Basic Psychiatric Concepts in Nursing*, which was published in 1960 in 11 languages and was used worldwide (Hofling & Leininger, 1960).

While working at a child guidance home in the mid-1950s in Cincinnati, Leininger discovered that the staff lacked understanding of cultural factors influencing the behavior of children. Among these children of diverse cultural backgrounds, she observed differences in responses to care and psychiatric treatments that deeply concerned her. Psychoanalytical theories and therapy strategies did not seem to reach children who were of different cultural backgrounds and needs. She became increasingly concerned that her nursing decisions and actions, and those of other staff, did not appear to help these children adequately. Leininger posed many questions to herself and the staff about cultural differences among children and therapy outcomes. She found few staff members who were interested or knowledgeable about cultural factors in the diagnosis and treatment of clients. A short time later, Margaret Mead became a visiting professor in the Department of Psychiatry, University of Cincinnati, and Leininger discussed with Mead the potential interrelationships between nursing and anthropology. Although she did not get any direct help, encouragement, or solutions from Mead, Leininger decided to pursue her interests with focused doctoral study on cultural, social, and psychological anthropology at the University of Washington, Seattle.

As a doctoral student, Leininger studied many cultures. She found anthropology fascinating and believed it was an area that should be of interest to all nurses. She focused on the Gadsup people of the Eastern Highlands of New Guinea, where she lived alone with the indigenous people for nearly 2 years and undertook an ethnographical and ethnonursing study of two villages (Leininger, 1995c, 1996b). Not only was she able to observe unique features of the culture, she also observed a number of marked differences between Western and non-Western cultures related to caring health and well-being practices. From her in-depth study and first-hand experiences with the Gadsup, she continued to develop her Culture Care Theory of Diversity and Universality (Culture Care Theory) and the ethnonursing method (Leininger, 1978, 1981, 1991b, 1995c). Her research and theory have helped nursing students understand cultural differences in human care, health, and illness. She has been the major nurse leader to encourage many students and faculty to pursue graduate education and practice. Her enthusiasm and interest in developing this field of transcultural nursing with a human care focus have sustained her for more than 5 decades.

During the 1950s and 1960s, Leininger (1970, 1978) identified several common areas of knowledge and theoretical research interests between nursing and anthropology, formulating transcultural nursing concepts, theory, principles, and practices. The book, *Nursing and Anthropology: Two Worlds to Blend* (1970), laid the foundation for developing the field of transcultural nursing, the Culture Care Theory, and culturally based healthcare. Her next book, *Transcultural Nursing: Concepts, Theories, and Practice* (1978), identified major concepts, theoretical ideas, and practices in transcultural nursing and was the first definitive publication on transcultural nursing. During the past 50 years, Leininger has established, explicated, and used the Culture Care Theory to study many cultures within the United States and worldwide. She developed the ethnonursing qualitative research method to fit the theory and to discover the insider or emic view of cultures (Leininger, 1991b, 1995c). The ethnonursing research method was the first nursing research method developed for nurses to examine complex care and cultural phenomena. During the past 5 decades, approximately 50 nurses with doctoral degrees and many master's and baccalaureate students have been prepared in transcultural nursing and have used Leininger's Culture Care Theory (Leininger, 1990a, 1991b; Leininger & McFarland, 2002a; Leininger & Watson, 1990).

The first course in transcultural nursing was offered in 1966 at the University of Colorado, where

Leininger was a professor of nursing and anthropology. This marked the first joint appointment in the United States of a professor of nursing with another discipline. Leininger also initiated and served as the director of the first nurse scientist program (PhD) in the United States. In 1969, she was appointed Dean and Professor of Nursing and Lecturer in Anthropology at the University of Washington, Seattle. There she established the first academic nursing department on comparative nursing care systems to support master's and doctoral programs in transcultural nursing. Under her leadership, the Research Facilitation Office was established in 1968 and 1969. She initiated several transcultural nursing courses and guided the first nurses in a special PhD program in transcultural nursing. She initiated the Committee on Nursing and Anthropology with the American Anthropological Association in 1968.

In 1974, Leininger was appointed Dean and Professor of Nursing at the College of Nursing and Adjunct Professor of Anthropology at the University of Utah in Salt Lake City. At this institution, she initiated the first master's and doctoral programs in transcultural nursing and established the first doctoral program offerings at this institution (Leininger, 1978). These programs were the first in the world to offer substantive courses focused specifically on transcultural nursing. She also initiated and was director of a new research facilitation office at the University of Utah.

In 1981, Leininger was recruited to Wayne State University in Detroit, where she was Professor of Nursing and Adjunct Professor of Anthropology and Director of Transcultural Nursing Offerings until her semi-retirement in 1995. She was also Director of the Center for Health Research at this university for 5 years. While at Wayne State, she again developed several courses and seminars in transcultural nursing, caring, and qualitative research methods for baccalaureate, master's, doctoral, and postdoctoral nursing and non-nursing students. In addition to directing the transcultural course offerings at Wayne State University, Dr. Leininger taught and mentored many students and nurses in field research in transcultural nursing. One of the first nurse leaders to use qualitative research methods during the early 1960s, she has continued to teach these methods at various universities within the United States and worldwide. To date, she has studied 14 cultures and continues to consult for many research projects and institutions, especially those that are using her Culture Care Theory.

With growing interest in transcultural nursing and health care, Leininger (personal communication, 1996) has delivered keynote addresses annually and has conducted workshops and consultations both nationally and internationally since 1965. Her academic vitae includes nearly 600 conferences, keynote addresses, workshops, and services as a consultant in the United States, Canada, Europe, Pacific Island nations, Asia, Africa, Australia, and the Nordic countries. Educational and service organizations continue to request her consultation on transcultural nursing, humanistic caring, ethnonursing research, the Culture Care Theory, and futuristic trends in health care worldwide.

As the first professional nurse to complete a doctoral degree in anthropology and to initiate several master's and doctoral nursing educational programs, Leininger has many areas of expertise and interests. She has studied 14 major cultures in depth and has had experience with many other diverse cultures. In addition to transcultural nursing with care as a central focus, her areas of interest are comparative education and administration, nursing theories, politics, ethical dilemmas of nursing and health care, qualitative research methods, the future of nursing and health care, and nursing leadership. Her Culture Care Theory is now used worldwide and is growing in relevance and importance in the discovery of data from diverse cultures.

In 1974, Leininger initiated the National Transcultural Nursing Society and has been an active leader since its inception. She also established the National Research Care Conference in 1978 to help nurses focus on the study of human care phenomena (Leininger, 1981, 1984a, 1988a, 1990a, 1991b; Leininger & Watson, 1990). She initiated the *Journal of Transcultural Nursing* in 1989 and served as its editor through 1995.

Dr. Leininger has gained international recognition in nursing and related fields through her transcultural nursing and care writings, theory, research, consultation, courses, and dynamic addresses. She has worked enthusiastically to persuade nursing educators and practitioners to incorporate transcultural nursing and culture-specific care concepts based on research findings into nursing curricula and clinical practices as the new and futuristic direction of all aspects of nursing (Leininger, 1991b, 1995c; Leininger & McFarland, 2002a; Leininger & Watson, 1990). She has found time to give lectures to anthropologists, physicians, social workers, pharmacists, and educators, and to do research with colleagues. She is one of the few nurses who has kept active in two disciplines and has continued to contribute to both nursing and anthropology at national and international transcultural conferences and association meetings. Currently, Dr. Leininger resides in Omaha, Nebraska, and is semi-retired but still active in consulting, writing, and lecturing. Her present interest is to establish transcultural nursing institutes to educate and to conduct and facilitate research on transcultural nursing and health phenomena.

Leininger has written or edited more than 30 books. Some of her books include *Nursing and Anthropology: Two Worlds to Blend* (1970), *Transcultural Nursing: Concepts, Theories, Research, and Practice* (Leininger & McFarland, 2002a), *Caring: An Essential Human Need* (Leininger, 1981), *Care: The Essence of Nursing and Health* (1984a), *Qualitative Research Methods in Nursing* (1985a), *Ethical and Moral Dimensions of Care: Chapters from Conference on the Ethics and Morality of Caring* (1990a), *The Caring Imperative in Education* (Leininger & Watson, 1990), *Culture Care Diversity and Universality: A Theory of Nursing* (1991b), and *Culture Care Diversity and Universality: A Worldwide Theory of Nursing* (Leininger and McFarland, 2006), which are full accounts of her theory with the method. She has published more than 200 articles and 45 book chapters plus numerous films, videos, DVDs, and research reports focused on transcultural nursing, human care and health phenomena, the future of nursing, and related topics relevant in nursing and anthropology. She formerly served on eight editorial boards and refereed several publications, and is actively involved with the Transcultural Nursing Scholars Group and her own website (www.madeleine-leininger.com). She is known as one of the most creative, productive, innovative, and futuristic authors in nursing, always providing new and substantive research-based transcultural nursing content and ideas to advance nursing as a discipline and a profession.

Leininger has received many awards and honors for her lifetime professional and academic accomplishments. She is in *Who's Who of American Women, Who's Who in Health Care, Who's Who in Community Leaders, Who's Who of Women in Education, International Who's Who in Community Service, Who's Who in International Women,* and other such listings. Her name appears on the National Register of Prominent Americans and International Notables, International Women, and the National Register of Prominent Community Leaders. She has received several honorary degrees, such as an LHD from Benedictine College in Atchison, Kansas, a PhD from the University of Kuopio, Finland, and a DS from the University of Indiana, Indianapolis. In 1976 and 1995, she was recognized for her unique and significant contribution to the American Association of Colleges of Nursing as its first full-time president. Leininger received the Russell Sage Outstanding Leadership Award in 1995. Leininger is a fellow in the American Academy of Nursing, a fellow of the American Anthropology Society, and a fellow of the Society for Applied Anthropology. Other affiliations include Sigma Theta Tau, the national honor society for nursing; Delta Kappa Gamma, the national honor society in education; and the Scandinavian College of Caring Science in Stockholm, Sweden. She has served as a distinguished visiting scholar and lecturer at 85 universities in the United States and worldwide and has been a visiting professor at numerous foreign universities, including schools in Sweden, Wales, Japan, China, Australia, Finland, New Zealand, and the Philippines. While at Wayne State University, she received the Board of Regents' Distinguished Faculty Award, the Distinguished Research Award, the President's Excellence in Teaching, and the Outstanding Graduate Faculty Mentor Award. In 1996, Madonna University, Livonia, Michigan, honored her with the dedication of the Leininger Book Collection and a special Leininger Reading Room for her outstanding contributions to nursing and the social sciences and humanities.

THEORETICAL SOURCES

Leininger's theory is derived from the disciplines of anthropology and nursing (Leininger, 1991b, 1995c; Leininger & McFarland 2002b, 2006). She has defined *transcultural nursing* as a major area of nursing that focuses on the comparative study and analysis of diverse cultures and subcultures in the world with respect to their caring values, expressions, and health-illness beliefs and patterns of behavior.

The purpose of the theory was to discover human care diversities and universalities in relation to worldview, social structure, and other dimensions cited, and then to discover ways to provide culturally congruent care to people of different or similar cultures in order to maintain or regain their well-being or health, or to face death in a culturally appropriate way (Leininger, 1985b, 1988b, 1988c, 1988d; as cited in 1991b). The goal of the theory is to improve and to provide culturally congruent care to people that is beneficial and will fit with, and will be useful to, the client, family, or culture group healthy lifeways (Leininger, 1991b).

Transcultural nursing goes beyond an awareness state to that of using Culture Care nursing knowledge to practice culturally congruent and responsible care (Leininger, 1991b, 1995c). Leininger has stated that in time, there will be a new kind of nursing practice that reflects different nursing practices that are culturally defined, grounded, and specific to guide nursing care provided to individuals, families, groups, and institutions. She contends that because culture and care knowledge are the broadest and most holistic means to conceptualize and understand people, they are central to and imperative to nursing education and practice (Leininger, 1991b, 1995c; Leininger & McFarland, 2002a, 2006). In addition, she states that transcultural nursing has become one of the most important, relevant, and highly promising areas of formal study, research, and practice because people live in a multicultural world (Leininger, 1984a, 1988a, 1995c; Leininger & McFarland, 2002a, 2006). Leininger predicts that for nursing to be meaningful and relevant to clients and other nurses in the world, transcultural nursing knowledge and competencies will be imperative to guide all nursing decisions and actions for effective and successful outcomes (Leininger, 1991b, 1995c, 1996a, 1996b; Leininger & McFarland, 2002a, 2006).

Leininger (2002a) distinguishes between *transcultural nursing* and *cross-cultural nursing*. The former refers to nurses prepared in transcultural nursing who are prepared and committed to develop knowledge and practice in transcultural nursing, whereas cross-cultural nursing refers to nurses who use applied or medical anthropological concepts, with many nurses not committed to developing transcultural nursing theory and research-based practices (Leininger, 1995c; Leininger & McFarland, 2002a). She also identifies that international nursing and transcultural nursing are different. International nursing focuses on nurses functioning between two cultures; however, transcultural nursing focuses on several cultures with a comparative theoretical and practice base (Leininger, 1995c; Leininger & McFarland, 2002a).

Leininger describes the transcultural nurse generalist as a nurse prepared at the baccalaureate level who is able to apply transcultural nursing concepts, principles, and practices that are generated by transcultural nurse specialists (Leininger, 1989a, 1989b, 1991c, 1995c; Leininger & McFarland, 2002a). The transcultural nurse specialist prepared in graduate programs receives in-depth preparation and mentorship in transcultural nursing knowledge and practice. This specialist has acquired competency skills through post baccalaureate education. "This specialist has studied selected cultures in sufficient depth (values, beliefs, and lifeways) and is highly knowledgeable and theoretically based about care, health, and environmental factors related to transcultural nursing perspectives" (Leininger, 1984b, p. 252). The transcultural nurse specialist serves as an expert field practitioner, teacher, researcher, and consultant with respect to select cultures. This individual also values and uses nursing theory to develop and advance knowledge within the discipline of transcultural nursing, the field Leininger (1995c, 2001) predicts must be the focus of all nursing education and practice.

Leininger (1996b) holds and promotes a new and different theory from traditional theories in nursing, which usually define theory as a set of logically interrelated concepts and hypothetical propositions that can be tested for the purpose of explaining or predicting an event, phenomenon, or situation. Instead, Leininger defines theory as the systematic and creative discovery of knowledge about a domain of interest or a phenomenon that appears important to understand or to account for some unknown phenomenon. She believes that nursing theory must take into account creative discovery about individuals, families, and groups, and their caring, values, expressions, beliefs, and actions or practices based on their cultural lifeways to provide effective, satisfying, and culturally congruent care. If nursing practices fail to recognize the cultural aspects of human needs, there will be signs of less beneficial or efficacious nursing care practices and even evidence of dissatisfaction with nursing services, which limits healing and well-being (Leininger, 1991b, 1995a, 1995c; Leininger & McFarland, 2002a, 2006).

Leininger (1991b) developed her Theory of Culture Care Diversity and Universality, which is based on the belief that people of different cultures can inform and are capable of guiding professionals to receive the kind of care they desire or need from others. Culture is the patterned and valued lifeways of people that influence their decisions and actions; therefore, the theory is directed toward nurses to discover and document the world of the client and to use their emic viewpoints, knowledge, and practices with appropriate etic (professional knowledge), as bases for making culturally congruent professional care actions and decisions (Leininger, 1991b, 1995c). Indeed, Culture Care is the broadest holistic nursing theory, because it takes into account the totality and holistic perspective of human life and existence over time, including the social structure factors, worldview, cultural history and values, environmental context (Leininger, 1981), language expressions, and folk (generic) and professional patterns. These are some of the critical and essential bases for the discovery of grounded care knowledge that as the essence of nursing that can lead to the health and well-being of clients and can guide therapeutic nursing practice. The Culture Care Theory can be inductive and deductive, derived from emic (insider) and etic (outsider) knowledge. However, Leininger encourages obtaining grounded emic knowledge from the people or culture because such knowledge is most credible (1991b).

The theory is neither middle range nor macro theory but must be viewed holistically with specific domains of interest. Leininger believes the terms *middle* range and *macro* are outdated in theory development and usage (1991b, 1995c; Leininger & McFarland, 2002a, 2006).

Unique Features of the Theory

According to Leininger (2002c), the Theory of Culture Care Diversity and Universality has several distinct features, different from those of other nursing theories. It is the only theory that is focused explicitly on discovering holistic and comprehensive Culture Care, and it is a theory that can be used in Western and non-Western cultures because of the inclusion of multiple holistic factors universally found in cultures. It is the only theory focused on discovering comprehensive factors influencing human care such as worldview, social structure factors, language, generic and professional care, ethnohistory, and the environmental context. The theory has both abstract and practice dimensions that can be examined systematically to arrive at culturally congruent care outcomes. It is the only theory in nursing explicitly focused on culture and care of diverse cultures, with three theoretical practice modalities to arrive at culturally congruent care decisions and actions to support well-being, health, and satisfactory lifeways for people. The theory is designed to ultimately discover care—what is diverse and what is universally related to care and health—and has a comparative focus to identify different or contrasting transcultural nursing care practices with specific care constructs. The theory with the ethnonursing method (the first nursing research method designed to fit a theory) has enablers designed to tease out in-depth informant emic data, and these enablers can also be used for cultural health care assessments. The theory can generate new knowledge in nursing and health care to arrive at culturally congruent, safe, and responsible care.

MAJOR CONCEPTS & DEFINITIONS

Leininger has developed many terms relevant to the theory. The major ones are defined here. The reader can study her full theory from her definitive works (Leininger, 1991b, 1995c; Leininger & McFarland, 2002a, 2006).

HUMAN CARE AND CARING

The concept of human care and caring refers to the abstract and manifest phenomena with expressions of assistive, supportive, enabling, and facilitating ways to help self or others with evident or anticipated needs to improve health, a human condition, or lifeways, or to face disabilities or dying.

CULTURE

Culture refers to patterned lifeways, values, beliefs, norms, symbols, and practices of individuals, groups, or institutions that are learned, shared, and usually transmitted from one generation to another.

CULTURE CARE

Culture Care refers to the synthesized and culturally constituted assistive, supportive, enabling, or facilitative caring acts toward self or others focused on evident or anticipated needs for the client's health or well-being, or to face disabilities, death, or other human conditions.

CULTURE CARE DIVERSITY

Culture Care diversity refers to cultural variability or differences in care beliefs, meanings, patterns, values, symbols, and lifeways within and between cultures and human beings.

CULTURE CARE UNIVERSALITY

Culture Care universality refers to commonalities or similar culturally based care meanings ("truths"), patterns, values, symbols, and lifeways reflecting care as a universal humanity.

WORLDVIEW

Worldview refers to the way an individual or a group looks out on and understands the world about them as a value, stance, picture, or perspective about life and the world.

CULTURAL AND SOCIAL STRUCTURE DIMENSIONS

Cultural and social structure dimensions refer to the dynamic, holistic, and interrelated patterns of structured features of a culture (or subculture), including religion (or spirituality), kinship (social), political characteristics (legal), economics, education, technology, cultural values, philosophy, history, and language.

ENVIRONMENTAL CONTEXT

Environmental context refers to the totality of an environment (physical, geographic, and sociocultural), situation, or event with related experiences that give interpretative meanings to guide human expressions and decisions with reference to a particular environment or situation.

ETHNOHISTORY

Ethnohistory refers to the sequence of facts, events, or developments over time as known, witnessed, or documented about a designated people of a culture.

MAJOR CONCEPTS & DEFINITIONS—cont'd

EMIC

Emic refers to local, indigenous, or the insider's views and values about a phenomenon.

ETIC

Etic refers to the outsider's or more universal views and values about a phenomenon.

HEALTH

Health refers to a state of well-being or a restorative state that is culturally constituted, defined, valued, and practiced by individuals or groups and that enables them to function in their daily lives.

TRANSCULTURAL NURSING

Transcultural nursing refers to a formal area of humanistic and scientific knowledge and practices focused on holistic Culture Care (caring) phenomena and competencies to assist individuals or groups to maintain or regain their health (or well-being) and to deal with disabilities, dying, or other human conditions in culturally congruent and beneficial ways.

CULTURE CARE PRESERVATION OR MAINTENANCE

Culture Care preservation or maintenance refers to those assistive, supportive, facilitative, or enabling professional actions and decisions that help people of a particular culture to retain or maintain meaningful care values and lifeways for their well-being, to recover from illness, or to deal with handicaps or dying.

CULTURE CARE ACCOMMODATION OR NEGOTIATION

Culture Care accommodation or negotiation refers to those assistive, supportive, facilitative, or enabling professional actions and decisions that help people of a designated culture (or subculture) to adapt to or to negotiate with others for meaningful, beneficial, and congruent health outcomes.

CULTURE CARE REPATTERNING OR RESTRUCTURING

Culture Care repatterning or restructuring refers to the assistive, supportive facilitative, or enabling professional actions and decisions that help clients reorder, change, or modify their lifeways for new, different, and beneficial health outcomes.

CULTURALLY COMPETENT NURSING CARE

Culturally competent nursing care refers to the explicit use of culturally based care and health knowledge in sensitive, creative, and meaningful ways to fit the general lifeways and needs of individuals or groups for beneficial and meaningful health and well being, or to face illness, disabilities, or death.

USE OF EMPIRICAL EVIDENCE

For more than 5 decades, Leininger has held that care is the essence of nursing and the dominant, distinctive, and unifying feature of nursing (1970, 1981, 1988a, 1991b; Leininger & McFarland, 2002a, 2006). She states that care is complex, elusive, and often embedded in social structure and other aspects of culture (1991b; Leininger & McFarland, 2006). She holds that different forms, expressions, and patterns of care are diverse, and some are universal (Leininger, 1991b; Leininger & McFarland, 2002a, 2006). Leininger (1985a, 1990b) favors qualitative ethnomethods, especially ethnonursing, to study care. These methods are directed toward discovering the people-truths, views, beliefs, and patterned lifeways of people. During the 1960s, Leininger developed the ethnonursing method to study transcultural nursing phenomena specifically and systematically. This method focuses on the classification of care beliefs, values, and practices as cognitively or subjectively known by a designated culture (or cultural representatives) through their local emic people-centered language, experiences, beliefs, and value systems about actual or potential nursing phenomena such as care, health, and environmental factors (Leininger, 1991b, 1995c; Leininger & McFarland, 2002a, 2006). Although nursing has used the words *care* and *caring* for more than a century, the definitions and usage have been vague, and the terms have been used as clichés, without specific meanings to the culture of the client or nurse (Leininger, 1981, 1984a). "Indeed, the concepts about caring have been some of the least understood and studied of all human knowledge and research areas within and outside of nursing" (Leininger, 1978, p. 33). With the transcultural care theory and ethnonursing method based on emic (insider views) beliefs, a person gets close to the discovery of people-based care, because data come directly from the people and are not derived from the etic (outsider views) beliefs and practices of the researcher. An important purpose of the theory is to document, know, predict, and explain systematically through field data what is diverse and universal about generic and professional care of the cultures being studied (Leininger, 1991b).

Leininger (1984a, 1988a) holds that detailed and culturally based caring knowledge and practices should distinguish nursing's contributions from those of other disciplines. The first reason for studying care theory is that the construct of care has been critical to human growth, development, and survival for human beings from the beginning of the human species (Leininger, 1981, 1984a). The second reason is to explicate and fully understand cultural knowledge and the roles of caregivers and care recipients in different cultures to provide culturally congruent care (Leininger, 1991b, 1995c, 2002a, 2002b, 2002c). Third, care knowledge is discovered and can be used as essential to promote the healing and well-being of clients, to face death, or to ensure the survival of human cultures over time (Leininger, 1981, 1984a, 1991b). Fourth, the nursing profession needs to systematically study care from a broad and holistic cultural perspective to discover the expressions and meanings of care, health, illness, and well-being as nursing knowledge (Leininger, 1991b, 1995c, 2002a, 2002b, 2002c). Leininger (1991b, 1995c, 2002a, 2002b, 2002c) finds that care is largely an elusive phenomenon often embedded in cultural lifeways and values. However, this knowledge is a sound basis for nurses to guide their practice for culturally congruent care and specific therapeutic ways to maintain health, prevent illness, heal, or help people face death (Leininger, 1994). A central thesis of the theory is that if the meaning of care can be fully grasped, the well-being or health care of individuals, families, and groups can be predicted, and culturally congruent care can be provided (Leininger, 1991b). Leininger (1991b) views care as one of the most powerful constructs and the central phenomenon of nursing. However, such care constructs and patterns must be fully documented, understood, and used to ensure that culturally based care becomes the major guide to transcultural nursing therapy and is used to explain or predict nursing practices (Leininger, 1991b).

To date, Leininger has studied several cultures in depth and has studied many cultures with undergraduate and graduate students and faculty using qualitative research methods. She has extensively explicated care constructs throughout many cultures in which each culture has different meanings, cultural experiences, and uses by people of diverse and similar cultures (Leininger, 1991b, 1995c; Leininger & McFarland, 2002a, 2006). A new body of knowledge continues to be discovered by transcultural nurses in the development of transcultural care practices with diverse and similar cultures. In time, Leininger (1991b) believes, both diverse and universal features of care and health will be documented as the essence of nursing knowledge and practice.

Leininger stated that the goal of the care theory is to provide culturally congruent care (1991b, 1995c, 2002a, 2002b, 2002c; Leininger & McFarland, 2006). She believes that nurses must work toward explicating care use and meanings so that culture care, values, beliefs, and lifeways can provide accurate and reliable bases for planning and effectively implementing culture-specific care and for identifying any universal or common features about care. She maintains that nurses cannot separate worldviews, social structures, and cultural beliefs (folk and professional) from health, wellness, illness, or care when working with cultures, because these factors are closely linked. Social structure factors such as religion, politics, culture, economics, and kinship are significant forces affecting care and influencing illness patterns and well-being. She also emphasizes the importance of discovering generic (folk, local, and indigenous) care from the cultures and comparing it with professional care (Leininger, 1991b).

Leininger has found that cultural blindness, shock, imposition, and ethnocentrism by nurses continue to greatly reduce the quality of care offered to clients of different cultures (Leininger, 1991a, 1994, 1995c; Leininger & McFarland, 2002a, 2006). Moreover, nursing diagnoses and medical diagnoses that are not culturally based and known create serious problems for cultures that lead to unfavorable and sometimes serious outcomes (Leininger, 1990c). Culturally congruent care is what makes clients satisfied that they have received good care; it is a powerful healing force for quality health care. Quality care is what clients seek most when they come for services from nurses, and it can be realized only when culturally derived care is known and used.

MAJOR ASSUMPTIONS

Major assumptions to support Leininger's Culture Care Theory of Diversity and Universality follow. The definitions were derived from Leininger's definitive works on the theory (Leininger, 1991b; Leininger & McFarland, 2002a, 2006).

1. Care is the essence of nursing and a distinct, dominant, central, and unifying focus.
2. Culturally based care (caring) is essential for well-being, health, growth and survival, and to face handicaps or death.
3. Culturally based care is the most comprehensive and holistic means to know, explain, interpret, and predict nursing care phenomena and to guide nursing decisions and actions.
4. Transcultural nursing is a humanistic and scientific care discipline and profession with the central purpose to serve individuals, groups, communities, societies, and institutions.
5. Culturally based caring is essential to curing and healing, for there can be no curing without caring, but caring can exist without curing.
6. Culture Care concepts, meanings, expressions, patterns, processes, and structural forms of care vary transculturally with diversities (differences) and some universalities (commonalities).
7. Every human culture has generic (lay, folk, or indigenous) care knowledge and practices and usually professional care knowledge and practices, which vary transculturally and individually.
8. Culture Care values, beliefs, and practices are influenced by and tend to be embedded in the worldview, language, philosophy, religion (and spirituality), kinship, social, political, legal, educational, economic, technological, ethnohistorical, and environmental context of cultures.
9. Beneficial, healthy, and satisfying culturally based care influences the health and well-being of individuals, families, groups, and communities within their environmental contexts.
10. Culturally congruent and beneficial nursing care can occur only when care values, expressions, or patterns are known and used explicitly for appropriate, safe, and meaningful care.
11. Culture Care differences and similarities exist between professional and client-generic care in human cultures worldwide.
12. Cultural conflicts, cultural impositions practices, cultural stresses, and cultural pain reflect the lack of Culture Care knowledge to provide culturally congruent, responsible, safe, and sensitive care.
13. The ethnonursing qualitative research method provides an important means to accurately discover and interpret emic and etic embedded, complex, and diverse Culture Care data (Leininger, 1991b, pp. 44-45).

The universality of care reveals the common nature of human beings and humanity, whereas diversity of care reveals the variability and selected, unique features of human beings.

THEORETICAL ASSERTIONS

Tenets are the positions one holds or are givens that the theorist uses with a theory. In developing the theory, the following four major tenets were conceptualized and formulated with the Culture Care Theory (Leininger, 2002c, 2006):

1. Culture Care expressions, meanings, patterns, and practices are diverse, and yet there are shared commonalities and some universal attributes.
2. The worldview consists of multiple social structure factors, such as religion, economics, cultural values, ethnohistory, environmental context, language, and generic and professional care, that are critical influencers of cultural care patterns to predict health, well-being, illness, healing, and ways people face disabilities and death.
3. Generic emic (folk) and professional etic care in different environmental contexts can greatly influence health and illness outcomes.
4. From an analysis of the previously listed influencers, three major actions and decision guides were predicted to provide ways to give culturally congruent, safe, and meaningful health care to cultures. The three culturally based action and decision modes were the following: (1) Culture Care preservation or maintenance, (2) Culture Care accommodation or negotiation, and (3) Culture Care repatterning or restructuring. Decision and action modes based on culture care were predicted as key factors to arrive at congruent, safe, and meaningful care.

In conceptualizing the theory, the first major and central theoretical tenet was, "care diversities (differences) and universalities (commonalities) existed among and between cultures in the world" (Leininger, 2002c, p. 78). However, Leininger asserted that Culture Care meanings and uses had to be discovered to establish a body of transcultural knowledge. A second major theoretical tenet was "[that the] worldview, social structure factors such as religion, economics, education, technology, politics, kinship (social), ethnohistory, environment, language, and generic and professional care factors would greatly influence Culture Care meanings, expressions, and patterns in different cultures" (Leininger, 2002c, p. 78).

Leininger has maintained that documentation of these factors was necessary in order to provide meaningful and satisfying care to people, and they are predicted to be powerful influencers on culturally based care. These factors also needed to be discovered directly from the informants as influencing factors related to health, well-being, illness, and death. The third major theoretical tenet was, "both generic (emic) and professional (etic) care needs to be taught, researched, and brought together into care practices for satisfying care for clients which lead to their health and well-being" (Leininger, 2002c).

The fourth major theoretical tenet was the conceptualization of the "three major care actions and decisions, to arrive at culturally congruent care for the general health and well-being of clients, or to help them face death or disabilities" (Leininger, 2002c, p. 78). These modes are Culture Care preservation or maintenance; Culture Care accommodation and negotiation; and Culture Care repatterning or restructuring. The researcher draws upon findings from the social structure, generic and professional practices, and other influencing factors while studying culturally based care for individuals, families, and groups. These factors would need to be studied, assessed and responded to in a dynamic and participatory nurse-client relationship (Leininger 1991a, 1991b, 2002b; Leininger & McFarland, 2002a).

LOGICAL FORM

Leininger's theory (1995c) is derived from anthropology and nursing but is reformulated to become transcultural nursing theory with a human care perspective. She developed the ethnonursing research method and has emphasized the importance of studying people from their emic or local knowledge and experiences and later contrasting them with the etic (outsider) beliefs and practices. Her book, *Qualitative Research Methods in Nursing* (Leininger, 1985a), and related publications (Leininger, 1990b, 1995c, 2002c, 2006) provide substantive knowledge about qualitative methods in nursing.

In her own words, Leininger is skilled in using ethnonursing, ethnography, life histories, life stories, photography, and phenomenological methods that provide a holistic approach to study cultural behavior in diverse environmental contexts. With these qualitative methods, the researcher moves with people in their daily living activities to grasp their world. The nurse researcher inductively obtains data of documented descriptive and interpretative accounts from informants through observation and participation, or in other ways explicating care as a major challenge within the method. The qualitative approach is important to develop basic and substantive grounded data-based knowledge about cultural care to guide nurses in their work. From the beginning, ethnonursing has been grounded primarily in data from the cultures under study, which is different from the grounded theory of Glasser and Strauss (1967).

Although other methods of research such as hypothesis testing and experimental quantitative methods can be used to study transcultural care, the method of choice depends upon the researcher's purposes, the goals of the study, and the phenomena to be studied. Creativity and the willingness of the nurse researcher to use different research methods to discover nursing knowledge are encouraged. However, Leininger holds that qualitative methods are important to establish meanings and accurate cultural knowledge. Quantitative methods generally have been of limited value to study cultures and care. Combining both qualitative and quantitative methods tends to obscure the findings and is a misuse of both paradigms (Leininger, 1991b, 1995c).

Leininger developed the Sunrise Enabler (Figure 22-1) in the 1970s to depict the essential components of the theory. She has refined the sunrise to the present, and thus the evolved enabler is more definitive and valuable to study accurately the diverse elements or components of the theory, and to make culturally congruent clinical assessments. This enabler and the complete theory of cultural care diversity and universality are not fully addressed here. Only selected ideas are offered to introduce the reader to Leininger's pioneering and creative work of evolving theory over time. The sunrise enabler symbolizes the rising of the sun (care) (Leininger, 1991b, 1995c; Leininger & McFarland, 2002a, 2006). The upper half of the circle depicts components of the social structure and worldview factors that influence care and health through language, ethnohistory, and environmental context. These factors also influence the folk, professional, and nursing system(s), which are the middle part of the model. The two halves together form a full sun, which represents the universe that nurses must consider to appreciate human care and health (Leininger, 1991b, 1995c; Leininger & McFarland, 2002a, 2006). According to Leininger, nursing acts as a bridge between folk (generic) and the professional system. Three kinds of nursing care and decisions and actions are predicted in the theory: Culture Care preservation or maintenance, Culture Care accommodation or negotiation, and Culture Care repatterning or restructuring (Leininger, 1991b, 1995c; Leininger & McFarland, 2002a, 2006).

The Sunrise Enabler depicts human beings as inseparable from their cultural background and social structure, worldview, history, and environmental context as a basic tenet of Leininger's theory (Leininger, 1991b, 1995c; Leininger & McFarland, 2002a, 2006). Gender, race, age, and class are embedded in social structure factors and are studied. Biological, emotional, and other dimensions are studied from a holistic view and are not fragmented or separate. Theory generation from this model may occur at multiple levels from the micro range (small-scale specific individuals) to study groups, families, communities, or large-scale phenomena (several cultures). Leininger has also developed several enablers to facilitate studying phenomena using the four phases of qualitative data analysis. Most importantly, qualitative criteria are used to analyze the data; they are credibility, confirmability, meaning-in-context, saturation, repatterning, and transferability (Leininger, 1995c, 2002c).

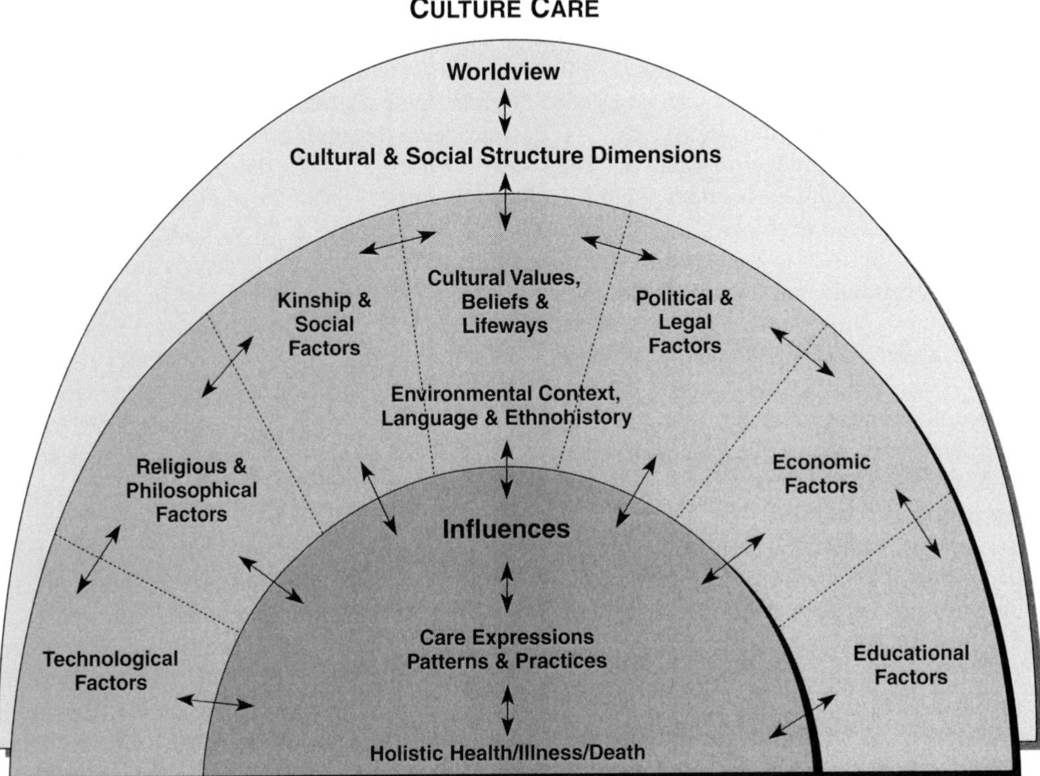

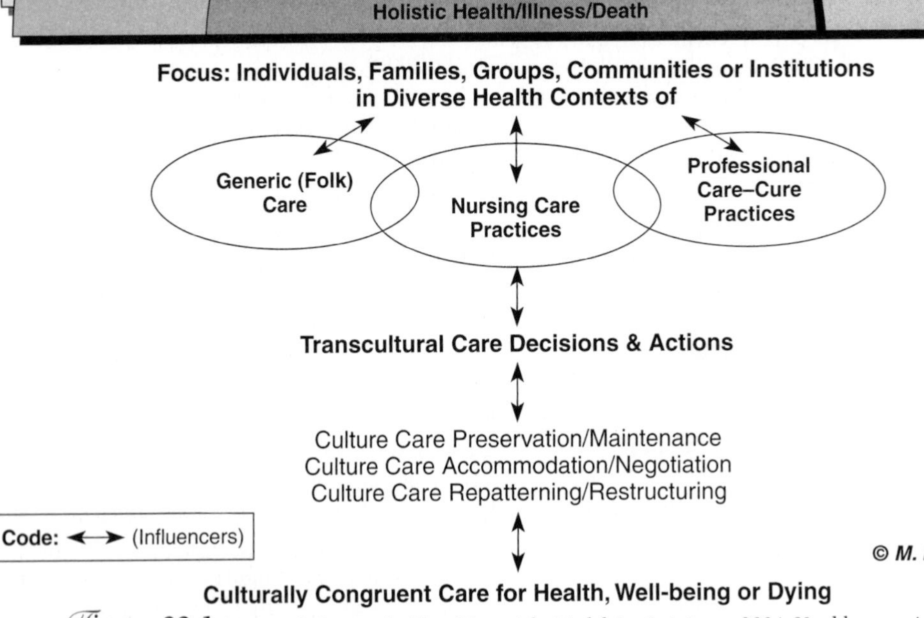

Figure 22-1 Leininger's Sunrise Enabler. (Copyright Madeleine Leininger, 2004. Used by permission.)

Quantitative criteria should not be used with qualitative methods, because the former have specific criteria to measure outcomes.

Leininger also developed four other enablers to assist nurse researchers in their use of the ethnonursing method. "Enablers sharply contrast with mechanistic devices such as tools, scales, measurement instruments, and other impersonal objective distancing tools generally used in quantitative studies. These tools are often viewed as unnatural and [are] frightening to cultural informants" (Leininger, 2002c, p. 89).

The observation participation reflection enabler is used to facilitate the researcher in entering and remaining with informants in their familiar or natural context during the study. The researcher gradually moves from the role of observer and listener, transitioning to that of participant and reflector with the informants. By moving slowly and politely with permission, the researcher does not disrupt and therefore is able to observe what is naturally occurring in the environment or with the people.

With the stranger to trusted friend enabler, the nurse researcher is able to learn much about oneself and the people and culture being studied. The goal with this guide is to become a trusted friend as one moves from distrusted stranger to trusted friend and different attitudes, behaviors, and expectations can be identified. This process is essential for the researcher to become trusted such that honest, credible, and in-depth data may be discovered from informants.

The domain of "inquiry enabler" is a process used by nurse researchers in each study to clearly establish the researcher's interest and area of focus. The domain of inquiry is a "succinct tailor made statement focused directly and specifically on Culture Care and health phenomena" (Leininger, 2002c, p. 92), stating questions or ideas related to the focus of the study, its purpose, and goals.

The acculturation health assessment enabler is another important guide used with the method. It is essential when studying cultures to assess the extent of the informants' acculturation as to whether they are more "traditionally or nontraditionally oriented in their values, beliefs, and general lifeways" (Leininger, 2002c, p. 92). This enabler is used for both cultural assessments and ethnonursing research studies.

ACCEPTANCE BY THE NURSING COMMUNITY

Practice

Leininger identifies several factors related to the slowness of nurses to recognize and value transcultural nursing and cultural factors in nursing practices and education (Leininger, 1991b; Leininger & McFarland, 2006). First, the theory was conceptualized during the 1950s, when virtually no nurses were prepared in anthropology or cultural knowledge to understand transcultural concepts, models, or theory. In the early days, most nurses had no knowledge of the nature of anthropology and how anthropological knowledge might contribute to human care and health behaviors, or serve as background knowledge to understand nursing phenomena or problems. Second, although people had longstanding and inherent cultural needs, many clients were reluctant to push health personnel to meet their cultural needs and therefore did not demand that their cultural and social needs be recognized or met (Leininger, 1970, 1978, 1995c; Leininger & McFarland, 2002a). Third, until the past decade, transcultural nursing articles submitted for publication were often rejected because editors did not know, value, or understand the relevance of cultural knowledge to transcultural nursing or as essential to nursing. Fourth, the concept of care was of limited interest to nurses until the late 1970s, when Leininger began promoting the importance of nurses studying human care, obtaining background knowledge in anthropology, and obtaining graduate preparation in transcultural nursing, research, and practice. Fifth, Leininger contends that nursing tends to remain too ethnocentric and far too involved in following medicine's interest and directions. Sixth, nursing has been slow to make substantive progress in the development of a distinct body of knowledge, because many nurse researchers have been far too dependent on quantitative research methods to obtain measurable outcomes rather than qualitative data outcomes. The recent acceptance and use of qualitative research methods in nursing will provide new insights and knowledge related to nursing and transcultural nursing (Leininger, 1991b, 1995c; Leininger & McFarland, 2002a). There is growing interest in using transcultural nursing knowledge, research, and practice by nurses worldwide.

Nurses are now realizing the importance of transcultural nursing, human care, and qualitative methods. Leininger (personal communication, April 2002) has stated:

> We are entering a new phase of nursing as we value and use transcultural nursing knowledge with a focus on human caring, health, and illness behaviors. With the migration of many cultural groups and the rise of the consumer cultural identity, and demands in culturally based care, nurses are realizing the need for culturally sensitive and competent practices. Most countries and communities of the world are multicultural today, and so health personnel are expected to understand and respond to clients of diverse and similar cultures. Immigrants and people from unfamiliar cultures expect nurses to respect and respond to values, beliefs, lifeways, and needs. No longer can nurses practice unicultural nursing.

As the world becomes more culturally diverse, nurses will find the urgent need to be prepared to provide culturally competent care. Some nurses are experiencing culture shock, conflict, and clashes as they move from one area to another and from rural to urban communities without transcultural nursing preparation. As cultural conflicts arise, families are less satisfied with nursing and medical services (Leininger, 1991b). Nurses who travel and seek employment in foreign lands are experiencing cultural stresses. Transcultural nursing education has become imperative for all nurses worldwide. Certification of transcultural nurses by the Transcultural Nursing Society has provided a major step toward protecting the public from unsafe and culturally incompetent nursing practices (Leininger, 1991a, 2001). Accordingly, more nurses are seeking transcultural certification to protect themselves and their clients. The *Journal of Transcultural Nursing* has also provided research and theoretical perspectives of more than 100 cultures worldwide to guide transcultural nurses in their practices.

Education

The inclusion of culture and comparative care in nursing curricula began in 1966 at the University of Colorado, where Leininger was professor of nursing and anthropology. Awareness of the importance of Culture Care to nursing gradually began to appear during the late 1960s, but very few nurse educators were prepared adequately to teach courses about transcultural nursing. Since the world's first master's and doctoral programs in transcultural nursing were approved and implemented in 1977 at the University of Utah, more nurses have been prepared specifically in transcultural nursing. Today, with the heightened public awareness of healthcare costs, different cultures, and human rights, there is much greater demand for comprehensive, holistic, and transcultural people care to protect and provide quality-based care and to prevent legal suits related to improper care. Leininger's demand for culture-specific care based on theoretical insights has been critical for the discovery of diverse and universal aspects of care (Leininger, 1995c, 1996a, 1996b; Leininger & McFarland, 2002b). A critical need remains for nurses to be educated in transcultural nursing in undergraduate and graduate programs. There is also a need for well-qualified faculty prepared in transcultural nursing to teach and to guide research in nursing schools within the United States and in other countries (Leininger, 1995c, 1996b; Tom-Orne, 2002).

Since 1980, an increasing number of nursing curricula are emphasizing transcultural nursing and human care. One of the early programs to focus on care was presented at Cuesta College in California during the 1970s, where care was developed as a central theme for an undergraduate program in nursing. Course titles included Caring Concepts I & II, Caring of Families, and Professional Self Care (Leininger, 1984a). During the late 1980s, four master's and four doctoral programs in the United States offered transcultural nursing courses, research experiences, and guided field study experiences (Leininger, 1995c). Leininger continues to receive numerous requests to give courses, lectures, and workshops on human care and transcultural nursing in the United States and other countries. The demand for transcultural nurses far exceeds available faculty, money, and other resources. Therefore, in 1996, Leininger put out a call for schools of nursing to offer transcultural programs to meet the worldwide demand for many nurses and cultures (Leininger, 1995a, 1995b, 1996b). These nursing programs are needed urgently for practice and preparation for certification of transcultural nurses. They are also needed for research and for worldwide consultation. At this time, there are still inadequate research funds to study transcultural nursing education and practice. Although the societal demand for transcultural nurses is evident, educational preparation remains weak and limited for many nurses worldwide. There are still graduate nursing faculty members who do not understand transcultural nursing and the Culture Care Theory and, consequently, will not permit students to study or research the phenomena, which causes great distress to nursing students (Leininger, 2002d).

Research

Many nurses today are using Leininger's Culture Care theory worldwide. This theory is the only one in nursing focused specifically on Culture Care and with a specific research method (ethnonursing) to examine the theory (Leininger, 1991b, 1995c; Leininger & McFarland, 2002a, 2006). Approximately 100 cultures and subcultures had been studied as of 1995, and more studies continue (Leininger, 1991b, 1995c, 1996a; Leininger & McFarland, 2002a). Funds to support transcultural nursing are meager and limited in most societies because biomedical and technical research funds head the priority list. Very few nursing schools in the United States receive federal support for nursing or transcultural nursing research unless they have a quantitative, objective (measurement) focus. Transcultural nurses and other nurses interested in transcultural nursing research are continuing their research despite limited or nonexistent funds. These nurses are leaders in sharing their research at conferences and instructional programs related to transcultural nursing. They have been instrumental in opening doors to transcultural nursing in many organizations. Despite societal demands for culturally competent, sensitive, responsible care, national and international organizations began to support transcultural nursing only in the 1990s. Through persistent efforts and exacting competencies of transcultural nurse specialists, progress has been forthcoming. Transcultural nurses have stimulated many other nurses to pursue research and to discover some entirely new knowledge in nursing. This knowledge will greatly reshape and transform nursing in the future.

CLINICAL APPLICATION OF THEORY TO PRACTICE

The ethnonursing study by McFarland (1995, 2002), which covered 2 years starting in the late 1980s, compared Anglo-American and African American groups living in a residence home for the elderly in one large Midwestern United States city. The research was another in-depth emic and etic culture care investigation that revealed several significant findings and the importance of using the three action and decision modes of the theory when caring for the elderly. The culturally congruent care findings were as follows:

- Anglo-American and African American elderly expect Culture Care preservation and maintenance of their lifelong generic or folk care patterns.
- Doing for other residents rather than having a self-care focus was a major care maintenance value for both cultures and was a dominant finding.
- Protective care was more important to African American than to Anglo-American elders, but nursing staff provided protective care and practiced Culture Care accommodation for both groups of elders, such as accompanying them when they desired to go for walks in the surrounding inner city neighborhood.

- African American nurses practiced culture accommodation when they linked their emic care with generic care values and practices.

Culture Care maintenance-preservation and Culture Care accommodation-negotiation were new ways for nurses to provide culturally congruent and safe lifeways care practices for the elderly of both cultures. Based on the findings of this study, several institutional Culture Care policies were developed to guide professional elderly care.

Application of the Culture Care Theory to advanced practice nursing has been explicated by McFarland and Eipperle (2008) in their article proposing the theory as a "... foundational basis for the educational preparation, primary care contextual practice, and outcomes-focused research endeavors of advanced practice nursing" using the three modes of care, the enablers, and the ethnonursing method. The authors emphasized integration of culturally congruent or sensitive care through direct and explicit approaches to be used by the nurse practitioner, who "... needs to be able to sensitively and competently integrate Culture Care into contextual routines, clinical ways, and approaches to primary care practice through role modeling, policy making, procedural performance and performance evaluation, and the use of the advance practice nursing process" (McFarland & Eipperle, 2008). Concepts and methods for integrating emic and etic care approaches into primary care practice modalities and use of the education-research-practice continuum as the basis for clinical actions and decisions are presented.

FURTHER DEVELOPMENT

Leininger predicts that all professional nurses in the world must be prepared in transcultural nursing and must demonstrate competencies in transcultural nursing (Leininger, 1981, 1995c; Leininger & McFarland, 2002a, 2006). Transcultural nursing must become an integral part of education and practice for nurses to be relevant in the twenty-first century. Currently, the demand for prepared transcultural nurses far exceeds the numbers of nurses, faculty, and clinical specialists in the world. Far more transcultural nurse theorists, researchers, and scholars are urgently needed to continue to develop a new body of transcultural knowledge and to transform nursing education and practice. By the year 2010, all nurses will need to have a basic knowledge about diverse cultures in the world and in-depth knowledge of at least two or three cultures (Leininger, 1995c, 1996a). Leininger believes that transcultural nursing research has already begun to lead to some highly promising and different ways to advance nursing education and practice (Leininger & McFarland, 2002a, 2006). All health disciplines, including medicine, pharmacy, and social work, gradually will incorporate transcultural health knowledge and practice into their programs of study in the near future. This trend will increase the demand for competent faculty in transcultural health care. Leininger (1995c) believes that the development of transcultural institutes will be essential to fill the growing need for transcultural nurses prepared to work with other disciplines.

Present and future theories and studies in transcultural nursing will be essential to meet the needs of culturally diverse people. The Culture Care Theory will grow in importance worldwide. Both universal and diverse care knowledge will be extremely important to establish a substantive body of transcultural nursing knowledge, and to make nursing a transcultural profession and discipline. Leininger's theory has already gained worldwide interest and use because it is holistic, relevant, and futuristic and deals with specific, yet abstract, care knowledge. The sunrise enabler remains invaluable as a dominant image and guide to study and assess people of diverse and similar cultural needs.

CRITIQUE

Simplicity

Transcultural nursing theory is really a broad, holistic, comprehensive perspective of human groups, populations, and species. This theory continues to generate many domains of inquiry for nurse researchers to pursue for scientific and humanistic knowledge. The theory challenges nurses to seek both universal and diverse culturally based care phenomena by diverse cultures, the culture of nursing, and the cultures of social unsteadiness worldwide. The theory is truly transcultural and global in scope; it is both complex and practical. It requires transcultural nursing knowledge and appropriate research methods to explicate the phenomena. Leininger's Culture Care Theory is relevant worldwide to help guide nurse researchers in conceptualizing the theory and research approaches and to guide practice. It is holistic and comprehensive in nature; therefore, several concepts and constructs related to social structure, environment, and language are extremely important to discover and obtain culturally based knowledge or knowledge grounded in the people's world. The theory shows multiple interrelationships of concepts and diversity of key concepts and relationships, especially to social structure factors. It requires some basic anthropological knowledge, but also considerable transcultural nursing knowledge, to be used in an accurate and scholarly fashion. Once the theory has been fully conceptualized, Leininger finds that undergraduate and graduate nursing students are excited to use the theory and discover how practical, relevant, and useful it is in their work. The use of the sunrise enabler becomes imprinted on their minds as a way of knowing.

Generality

The transcultural nursing theory does demonstrate the criterion of generality because it is a qualitatively oriented theory that is broad, comprehensive, and worldwide in scope. Transcultural nursing theory addresses nursing care from a multicultural and worldview perspective. It is useful and applicable to both groups and individuals with the goal of rendering culture-specific nursing care. The broad or generic concepts are well organized and defined for study in specific cultures. The research has led to a vast amount of expert knowledge largely unknown in the past. Many aspects of culture, care, and health are being identified, because these factors have an impact on nursing. Even more research is needed for comparative purposes from both culture-specific data and some universal care knowledge. More of the world's cultural groups need to be studied and compared to validate the caring constructs in the future. The theory is most helpful as a guide for the study of any culture and for the comparative study of several cultures. Findings from the theory are being used in client care in a variety of health and community settings worldwide to transform nursing education and service. It is being valued especially in developing a new and different approach to the traditional community nursing perspective.

Empirical Precision

The transcultural nursing theory is researchable, and qualitative research has been the primary paradigm to discover largely unknown phenomena of care and health in diverse cultures. This qualitative approach differs from the traditional quantitative research method, which renders measurement the goal of research. However, the ethnonursing research method is extremely rigorous and linguistically exacting in nature and outcomes. One hundred thirty-five care constructs have been identified, and more are being discovered each day, with a wealth of other transcultural nursing knowledge. The important attribute is that the accuracy of grounded data derived with the use of ethno methods or from an emic or people's viewpoint is leading to high credibility and confirmability, and a wealth of empirical data. Ongoing and future research will lead to additional care and health findings and implications for ethnonursing practices and education to fit specific cultures and universal features. The qualitative criteria of credibility and confirmability from in-depth studies of informants and their contexts are becoming clearly evident. Unequivocally, the body of transcultural nursing knowledge that has been established over the past decade has had a great impact on nursing and many healthcare systems (Leininger, 1995c; Leininger & McFarland 2002a, 2006).

Derivable Consequences

Transcultural nursing theory has important outcomes for nursing. Rendering culture-specific care is a necessary and essential new goal in nursing. It places the transcultural nursing theory central to the domain of nursing knowledge acquisition and use. The theory is highly useful, applicable, and essential to nursing practice, education, and research. The concept of care as the primary focus of nursing and the base of nursing knowledge and practice is long overdue and essential for advancing nursing knowledge and practices. Leininger (1991a) notes that, although nursing has always made claims to the concept of care, rigorous research on care has been limited until the past 3 decades. This theory could be the means to establish a sound and defensible discipline and profession, guiding practice to meet a multicultural world.

SUMMARY

In this chapter, the nature, importance, and major features of the Theory of Culture Care Diversity and Universality were discussed. The ethnonursing research method and the enablers were presented to show the fit between the theory and the method. Knowledge of both the theory and the method is needed before an ethnonursing study is launched. Fully understanding the theory and the method (with the enablers) leads to credible and meaningful study findings. Through complete understanding, the research becomes meaningful, exciting, and rewarding to do, and the researcher develops confidence and competence in use of the theory and the method.

As a premier theory in nursing, culture care is greatly valued worldwide. Other disciplines have found the theory and the method very helpful and valuable. Nurses who use the theory and the method frequently communicate how valuable and important it is to discover culturally based ways to know and practice nursing and health care. Practicing nurses now have holistic, culturally based research findings for use in caring for clients of diverse and similar cultures or subcultures in different countries. The theory is not difficult to use once the researcher understands it and the method and has mentor guidance. Newcomers to the theory and the method can benefit from experienced expert mentors, in addition to studying transcultural research conducted using the theory and the method. Most important, nurses often express that this theory and method are the only ones that it makes sense to use in nursing. They contend that the theory is very natural to nursing and helps one to gain fresh new insights about care, health, and well-being. Unquestionably, it is the theory of today and tomorrow and one that will grow in use in the future in our growing and increasingly multicultural world. The research and theory provide a new pathway to advance the profession of nursing and the body of transcultural knowledge for application in nursing practice, education, research, and clinical consultation worldwide.

Case Study

An elderly Arab American Muslim man who spoke little English was admitted to the hospital for increasing pain at rest in his left foot. His foot was cool and pale, and he had a history of vascular surgical procedures. He had many chronic health problems, including type 2 diabetes, hypertension, and chronic obstructive pulmonary disease. He also had had a myocardial infarction and several cerebral vascular accidents. While in the hospital, he developed abdominal pain and underwent a cholecystectomy. This elderly grandfather had a large family, including a wife, nine children, and many grandchildren. His wife insisted that all family members visit him every day while he was in the hospital. The family wanted the man's face turned toward Mecca (toward the east) while they prayed with him. They brought taped passages from the Koran, which they played at his bedside. Other families who were visiting their sick relatives complained to the nurses that the Arab family was taking up the entire waiting room, and there was no place for any one else to sit.

As a nurse, how might you use the three modes from the Theory of Culture Care Diversity and Universality to provide culturally congruent care for this elderly man and his family, as well as for the other clients and their families in the critical care unit?

CRITICAL THINKING *Activities*

1. Select four research studies reported in the *Journal of Transcultural Nursing* that used Leininger's Theory of Culture Care Diversity and Universality. Each of the studies selected should represent different cultures, different research settings, and cultures different from the student's culture.
   a. Review each of the studies and identify the relationship of the theory to the domains of inquiry, purpose, assumptions, definitions, methods, research design, data analysis, nursing decisions, and conclusions.
   b. Provide evidence that findings from these studies confirm the findings of the Theory in relation to the domain of inquiry theory tenets and derivable consequences.
2. Discuss the usefulness of the Theory of Culture Care Diversity and Universality in the twenty-first century to discover nursing knowledge and provide culturally congruent care. Take into consideration the current trends of consumers of health care, cultural diversity factors, and changes in medical and nursing school curricula. Following are some examples of trends and changes you may want to consider in your discussion:
   a. The importance of transcultural nursing knowledge in an increasingly diverse world
   b. Growth of lay support groups to provide information and sharing of experiences and support for clients, families, and groups experiencing chronic, terminal, or life-threatening illnesses or treatment modalities from diverse or similar (common) cultures
   c. Use of cultural values, beliefs, health practices, and research knowledge in undergraduate and graduate nursing curricula across the life span
   d. Inclusion of alternative or generic care in nursing curricula, such as medicine men (Native American healers, curers, and herbalists in the Southwest) and selected substantiated Chinese methods shown to be effective for the treatment of chronic disease
   e. Use of cultural caring research knowledge as the new and future direction of nursing in the twenty-first century
   f. The increased number of books, audiotapes, and videotapes published on health maintenance, alternative medicine, herbs, vitamins, minerals, and other over-the-counter medications and preparations, which demands a transcultural knowledge base
   g. Spiraling healthcare costs, forced use of health maintenance organizations, lack of health insurance, increased reliance on self-diagnosis, treatment, and care, and increased availability of diagnostic kits for acquired immunodeficiency syndrome testing, glucose monitoring, cholesterol screening, ovulation and pregnancy tests, fecal occult blood tests, and the like
   h. Problems related to cultural conflicts, stress, pain, and cultural imposition practices
3. Arrange for several observation and interview experiences at a local university student health center or public health department with people of diverse cultures. Ascertain the following:
   a. Identify the cultures represented by the clientele with the use of Leininger's theory and the sunrise enabler.
   b. What is the cultural mix of the staff (physicians, nurses, social workers, and clerics) of the center or health department? How does the cultural background of the staff differ from that of the clientele?
   c. Arrange a conference with the nursing staff, and ascertain their culture-based

attitudes, values, and beliefs, and those that are reflected in the clients using the center or department. Compare and contrast the values, attitudes, and beliefs of the staff with those of the clients. What are the cultural similarities and differences?

d. Arrange an interview with the director of the center or department, and ascertain the economic, political, legal, and other factors from Leininger's sunrise enabler that affect clients' use of the center or department.

e. Survey the printed materials such as visual aids, artifacts, and paintings in the waiting and examination rooms and in the classrooms to identify the cultures and languages that are depicted.

f. On the basis of data obtained from these exercises, how can the Theory of Culture Care Diversity and Universality be used to provide culturally sensitive and congruent care to clients using the center or department and increase the satisfaction with care received?

4. Discuss the type of prerequisite knowledge, experiences, attitudes, and skills needed to effectively use the Theory of Culture Care Diversity and Universality.
5. Discuss the relevancy of the Theory of Culture Care Diversity and Universality for nurses working in different practice settings and roles.

POINTS FOR *Further Study*

- Leininger, M. M. (2006). Envisioning the future of the culture care theory and the ethnonursing method. In M. M. Leininger and M. R. McFarland (Eds.), *Culture Care Diversity and Universality: A Worldwide Theory of Nursing* (2nd ed., pp. 389-394). Jones & Bartlett, Sudbury, MA, USA.
- Leininger, M., & McFarland, M. R. (2006). *Transcultural nursing: The theory of culture care.* DVD Set of Three.
- Morgan, M. G. (2006). Leininger's theory of culture care diversity and universality in nursing practice. In M. R. Alligood and A. M. Tomey (Eds.). *Nursing Theory: Utilization and Application, 3rd edition* (pp. 413-430), St. Louis: Mosby-Elsevier.
- Leininger, M. (1998). Transcultural Nursing Society website: www.tcns.org
- Leininger, M. M. (2007). *The evolution of transcultural nursing with breakthroughs to discipline status.* Unpublished manuscript, accessible at www.madeleine-leininger.com
- Leininger, M. M. (2008). *TCN certification: A global mandate.* Unpublished manuscript, accessible at www.madeleine-leininger.com.
- Leininger, M. (2005). *Major contributions of qualitative and quantitative criteria to evaluate research.* PowerPoint Presentation, accessible at www.madeleine-leininger.com
- Miller, J. E., Leininger, M., Leuning, C., Paquiao, D., Andrews, M., Ludwig-Beymer, P., Papadopoulos, I. (2008). Transcultural nursing society position statement on human rights. Unpublished manuscript, accessible at www.madeleine-leininger.com

REFERENCES

Glasser, B. G., & Strauss, A. L. (1967). The discovery of grounded theories: Strategies for qualitative research. Chicago: Aldine.

Hofling, C. K., & Leininger, M. (1960). Basic psychiatric concepts in nursing. Philadelphia: J. B. Lippincott.

Leininger, M. (1970). Nursing and anthropology: Two worlds to blend. New York: John Wiley & Sons.

Leininger, M. (Ed.). (1978). Transcultural nursing: Concepts, theories, and practice. New York: John Wiley & Sons.

Leininger, M. (Ed.). (1981). Caring: An essential human need. Thorofare, NJ: Charles B. Slack.

Leininger, M. (Ed.). (1984a). Care: The essence of nursing and health. Thorofare, NJ: Charles B. Slack.

Leininger, M. (1984b). Reference sources for transcultural health and nursing for teaching, curriculum, and clinical-field practice. Thorofare, NJ: Charles B. Slack.

Leininger, M. (Ed.). (1985a). Qualitative research methods in nursing. New York: Grune & Stratton.

Leininger, M. (1985b). Transcultural care diversity and universality: A theory of nursing. *Nursing and Health Care,* 6(4), 202-212.

Leininger, M. (1988a). Care: Discovery and uses in clinical and community nursing. Detroit: Wayne State University Press.

Leininger, M. (Ed.). (1988b). Care: The essence of nursing and health. Detroit: Wayne State University Press.

Leininger, M. (Ed.). (1988c). Caring: An essential human need. Detroit: Wayne State University Press.

Leininger, M. (Ed.). (1988d). Leininger's theory of nursing: Cultural diversity and universality. *Nursing Science Quarterly,* 2(4), 11-20.

Leininger, M. (1989a). Transcultural nurse specialists and generalists: New practitioners in nursing. *Journal of Transcultural Nursing,* 1, 4-16.

Leininger, M. (1989b). Transcultural nurse specialists and generalists: Imperative in today's world. *Nursing and Health Care,* 10(5), 250-256.

Leininger, M. (1990a). Ethical and moral dimensions of care: Chapters from conference on the ethics and morality of caring. Detroit: Wayne State University Press.

Leininger, M. (1990b). Ethnomethods: The philosophic and epistemic bases to explicate transcultural nursing knowledge. *Journal of Transcultural Nursing,* 1(2), 40-51.

Leininger, M. (1990c). Issues, questions, and concerns related to the nursing diagnosis cultural movement from transcultural nursing perspective. *Journal of Transcultural Nursing,* 2(1), 23-32.

Leininger, M. (1991a). Becoming aware of types of health practitioners and cultural imposition. *Journal of Transcultural Nursing,* 2(2), 32-49.

Leininger, M. (1991b). Culture care diversity and universality: A theory of nursing. New York: National League for Nursing Press.

Leininger, M. (1991c). The transcultural nurse specialist: Imperative in today's world. *Perspective in Family and Community Health,* 17, 137-144.

Leininger, M. (1994). Quality of life from a transcultural nursing perspective. *Nursing Science Quarterly,* 7(1), 22-28.

Leininger, M. (1995a). Culture care theory, research, and practice. *Nursing Science Quarterly,* 9(20), 71-78.

Leininger, M. (1995b). Editorial: Teaching transcultural nursing to transform nursing for the 21st century. *Journal of Transcultural Nursing,* 6(2), 2-3.

Leininger, M. (1995c). Transcultural nursing: Concepts, theories, and practice (2nd ed.). Columbus, OH: McGraw-Hill College Custom Series.

Leininger, M. (1996a). Major directions for transcultural nursing: A journey into the 21st century. *Journal of Transcultural Nursing,* 7(2), 37-40.

Leininger, M. (1996b). Future directions for transcultural nursing in the 21st century. *International Nursing Review,* 44(1), 19-23.

Leininger, M. (2001). Founder's focus: Certification of transcultural nurses for quality and safe consumer care. *Journal of Transcultural Nursing,* 12(3), 242.

Leininger, M. (2002a). Transcultural nursing and globalization of health care: Importance, focus, and historical aspects. In M. Leininger & M. R. McFarland (Eds.), Transcultural nursing: Concepts, theories, research, & practice (3rd ed., pp. 3-43). New York: McGraw-Hill Medical Publishing Division.

Leininger, M. (2002b). Essential transcultural nursing concepts, principles, examples, and policy statements. In M. Leininger & M. R. McFarland (Eds.), Transcultural nursing: Concepts, theories, research, & practice (3rd ed., pp. 45-69). New York: McGraw-Hill Medical Publishing Division.

Leininger, M. (2002c). Part I. The theory of culture care and the ethnonursing research method. In M. Leininger & M. R. McFarland (Eds.), Transcultural nursing: Concepts, theories, research, & practice (3rd ed., pp. 71-98). New York: McGraw-Hill Medical Publishing Division.

Leininger, M. (2002d). The future of transcultural nursing: A global perspective. In M. Leininger & M. R. McFarland (Eds.), Transcultural nursing: Concepts, theories, research, & practice (3rd ed., pp. 577-595). New York: McGraw-Hill Medical Publishing Division.

Leininger, M. (2002e). Culture care theory: A major contribution to advance transcultural nursing knowledge and practice. *Journal of Transcultural Nursing, 13*(3), 189-192.

Leininger, M., & McFarland, M. R. (2002a). Transcultural nursing: Concepts, theories, research, & practice (3rd ed.). New York: McGraw-Hill Medical Publishing Division.

Leininger, M., & McFarland, M. R. (2002b). Transcultural nursing: Curricular concepts, principles, and teaching and learning activities for the 21st century. In M. Leininger & M. R. McFarland (Eds.). Transcultural nursing: Concepts, theories, research, & practice (3rd ed., pp. 527-561). New York: McGraw-Hill Medical Publishing Division.

Leininger, M. M., & McFarland, M. R. (Eds.). (2006). Culture care diversity and universality: A worldwide theory of nursing (2nd ed.). Sudbury, MA: Jones & Bartlett.

Leininger, M., & Watson, J. (Eds.). (1990). The caring imperative in education. New York: National League for Nursing Press.

McFarland, M. R. (1995). Cultural care of Anglo and African American elderly residents within the environmental context of a long term care institution. Detroit: Wayne State University Press.

McFarland, M. R. (2002). Part II: Selected research findings from the culture care theory. In M. Leininger & M. R. McFarland (Eds.), Transcultural nursing: Concepts, theories, research, & practice (3rd ed., pp. 99-116). New York: McGraw-Hill Medical Publishing Division.

McFarland, M. R., & Eipperle, M. K. (2008 in press). Culture care theory: A proposed theory guide for nurse practitioner practice in primary care settings. *Contemporary Nurse, 28*(2).

Tom-Orne, L. (2002). Transcultural nursing and health care among Native American peoples. In M. M. Leininger & M. R. McFarland (Eds.), *Transcultural nursing: Concepts, theories, research, & practice* (3rd ed., pp. 429-440). New York: McGraw-Hill Medical Publishing Division.

BIBLIOGRAPHY

Selected Primary Sources

Books

Leininger, M. (1970). *Nursing and anthropology: Two worlds to blend.* New York: John Wiley & Sons.

Leininger, M. (1973). *Contemporary issues in mental health nursing.* Boston: Little, Brown & Co.

Leininger, M. (Ed.). (1978). *Transcultural nursing care of the elderly.* Salt Lake City, UT: University of Utah, College of Nursing.

Leininger, M. (Ed.). (1979). *Transcultural nursing care of the adolescent and middle age adult.* Salt Lake City, UT: University of Utah, College of Nursing.

Leininger, M. (Ed.). (1979). *Transcultural nursing: Proceedings from four transcultural nursing conferences.* New York: Masson.

Leininger, M. (Ed.). (1981). *Caring: An essential and human need.* Thorofare, NJ: Charles B. Slack.

Leininger, M. (Ed.). (1984). *Caring: The essence of nursing and health.* Thorofare, NJ: Charles B. Slack.

Leininger, M. (Ed.). (1984). *Reference sources for transcultural health and nursing for teaching, curriculum, and clinical-field practice.* Thorofare, NJ: Charles B. Slack.

Leininger, M. (Ed.). (1985). *Qualitative research methods in nursing.* New York: Grune & Stratton.

Leininger, M. (Ed.). (1988). *Care: Discovery and uses in clinical and community nursing.* Detroit: Wayne State University Press.

Leininger, M. (1990). *Ethical and moral dimensions of care: Chapters from conference on the ethics and morality of caring.* Detroit: Wayne State University Press.

Leininger, M. (1991). *Culture care universality and diversity: A theory of nursing.* New York: National League for Nursing Press.

Leininger, M. (1995). *Transcultural Nursing: Concepts, theories, and practice* (2nd ed.). Columbus, OH: McGraw-Hill College Custom Series.

Leininger, M., & McFarland, M. R. (2002). *Transcultural nursing: Concepts, theories, research, & practice* (3rd ed.). New York: McGraw-Hill Medical Publishing Division.

Leininger M., & McFarland, M. R. (2006). *Culture care diversity and universality: A worldwide nursing theory* (2nd ed.). Sudbury, MA: Jones & Bartlett.

Leininger, M., & Watson, J. (Eds.). (1990). *The caring imperative in education.* New York: National League for Nursing Press.

Selected Book Chapters

Leininger, M. (1988). Culture care and nursing administration. In B. Henry, C. Arndt, M. DiVincenti, & A. Marriner Tomey (Eds.), *Dimensions of nursing administration.* Boston: Blackwell Scientific.

Leininger, M. (1990). Introduction: Care: The imperative of nursing education and service. In M. Leininger & J. Watson (Eds.), *The caring imperative in education.* New York: NLN Publication, Center for Human Caring.

Leininger, M. (1992). Reflections on Nightingale with a focus on human care theory and leadership. In E. Nightingale & B. S. Barnum (Eds.), *Nightingale: Notes on nursing: What it is, and what it is not.* Philadelphia: J. B. Lippincott.

Leininger, M. (1992). Theory of culture care and uses in clinical and community contexts. In M. Parker (Ed.), *Theories on nursing* (pp. 345-372). New York: National League for Nursing Press.

Leininger, M. (1992). Transcultural mental health nursing assessment of children and adolescents. In P. West & C. Sieloff Evans (Eds.), *Psychiatric and mental health nursing with children and adolescents* (pp. 53-58). Gaithersburg, MD: Aspen Publications.

Leininger, M. (1993). Culture care theory: The comparative global theory to advance human care nursing knowledge and practice. In D. Gaut (Ed.), *A global agenda for caring* (pp. 3-18). New York: National League for Nursing.

Leininger, M. (1993). Evaluation criteria and critique of qualitative research studies. In J. Morse (Ed.), *Qualitative nursing research: A contemporary dialogue* (pp. 393-414). Newbury Park, CA: Sage Publications.

Leininger, M. (2002). Essential transcultural nursing concepts, principles, examples, and policy statements. In M. Leininger & M. R. McFarland (Eds.), *Transcultural nursing: Concepts, theories, research, & practice* (3rd ed., pp. 45-69). New York: McGraw-Hill Medical Publishing Division.

Leininger, M. (2002). Part I. The theory of culture care and the ethnonursing research method. In M. Leininger & M. R. McFarland (Eds.), *Transcultural nursing: Concepts, theories, research, & practice* (3rd ed., pp. 71-98). New York: McGraw-Hill Medical Publishing Division.

Leininger, M. (2002). The future of transcultural nursing: A global perspective. In M. Leininger & M. R. McFarland (Eds.), *Transcultural nursing: Concepts, theories, research, & practice* (3rd ed., pp. 577-595). New York: McGraw-Hill Medical Publishing Division.

Leininger, M. (2002). Transcultural nursing and globalization of health care: Importance, focus, and historical aspects. In M. Leininger & M. R. McFarland (Eds.), *Transcultural nursing: Concepts, theories, research, &*

practice (3rd ed., pp. 3-43). New York: McGraw-Hill Medical Publishing Division.

Leininger, M. M. (2006) Culture Care Diversity and Universality Theory and Evolution of the Ethnonursing Method. In M. M. Leininger and M. R. McFarland (Eds.), *Culture Care Diversity and Universality: A Worldwide Theory of Nursing* (2nd ed., pp. 1-41). Jones & Bartlett, Sudbury, MA, USA.

Leininger, M. M. (2006). Culture care of the Southern Sudanese of Africa. In M. M. Leininger and M. R. McFarland (Eds.), *Culture Care Diversity and Universality: A Worldwide Theory of Nursing* (2nd ed., pp. 255-279). Jones & Bartlett, Sudbury, MA, USA.

Leininger, M.M. (2006). Ethnonursing method and enablers. In M. M. Leininger and M. R. McFarland (Eds.), *Culture Care Diversity and Universality: A Worldwide Theory of Nursing* (2nd ed., pp. 43-81). Jones & Bartlett, Sudbury, MA, USA.

Selected Book Prefaces and Forewords

Leininger, M. (1978). Foreword. In J. Watson, *Nursing: The philosophy and science of caring.* Boston: Little, Brown & Co.

Leininger, M. (1983). Preface. In M. Leininger (Ed.), *Care: The essence of nursing and health.* Thorofare, NJ: Charles B. Slack.

Leininger, M. (1984). Preface. In M. Leininger, *Reference sources for transcultural health and nursing for teaching, curriculum, and clinical-field practice.* Thorofare, NJ: Charles B. Slack.

Leininger, M. M. (2003). Foreword. In M. R. Andrews & J. S. Boyle, Trancultural Concepts in Nursing Care (4th ed.). Lippincott: Philadelphia, PA, USA.

Leininger, M. M. (2008). Foreword. *Contemporary Nursing Journal* 28(2): in press.

Selected Journal Articles

Leininger, M. M. (1984). Qualitative research methods—to document and discover nursing knowledge. *Western Journal of Nursing Research, 6*(2), 151-152.

Leininger, M. M. (1987). Importance and uses of ethnomethods: Ethnography and ethnonursing research. *Recent Advances in Nursing, 17*, 12-36.

Leininger, M. M. (1988). Leininger's theory of nursing: Cultural care diversity and universality. *Nursing Science Quarterly, 1*(4), 152-160.

Leininger, M. (1988). Leininger's theory of nursing: Cultural care diversity and universality. *Nursing Science Quarterly, 1*(4), 152-160.

Leininger, M. M. (1989). The Journal of Transcultural Nursing has become a reality. *Journal of Transcultural Nursing, 1*(1), 1-2.

Leininger, M. M. (1989). The transcultural nurse specialist: Imperative in today's world. *Nursing and Health Care, 10*(5), 250-256.

Leininger, M. M. (1989). Transcultural nurse specialists and generalists: New practitioners in nursing. *Journal of Transcultural Nursing, 1*(1), 4-16.

Leininger, M. M., (1989). Transcultural nursing: Quo vadis (where goeth the field)? *Journal of Transcultural Nursing, 1*(1), 33-45.

Leininger, M. M. (1990). A new and changing decade ahead: Are nurses prepared? *Journal of Transcultural Nursing, 1*(2), 1.

Leininger, M. M. (1990). Ethnomethods: The philosophic and epistemic bases to explicate transcultural nursing knowledge. *Journal of Transcultural Nursing, 1*(2), 40-51.

Leininger, M. M. (1990). Issues, questions, and concerns related to the nursing diagnosis cultural movement from a transcultural nursing perspective. *Journal of Transcultural Nursing, 2*(1), 23-32.

Leininger, M. M. (1990). Leininger clarifies transcultural nursing (Letter to the Editor). *International Nursing Review, 36*(6), 356.

Leininger, M. M. (1990). The significance of cultural concepts in nursing. 1966. *Journal of Transcultural Nursing, 2*(1), 52-59.

Leininger, M. M. (1991). Transcultural nursing goals and challenges for 1991 and beyond. *Journal of Transcultural Nursing, 2*(2), 1-2.

Leininger, M. (1991). Becoming aware of the types of health practitioners and cultural imposition. *Journal of Transcultural Nursing, 2*(2), 32-39.

Leininger, M. M. (1991). Second reflection: Comparative care as central to transcultural nursing. *Journal of Transcultural Nursing, 3*(1), 2.

Leininger, M. M. (1991). Transcultural care principles, human rights, and ethical considerations. *Journal of Transcultural Nursing, 3*(1), 21-23.

Leininger, M. (1992). Transcultural nursing care values, beliefs, and practices of American (USA) gypsies. *Journal of Transcultural Nursing, 4*(1), 17-28.

Leininger, M. (1994). Nursing's agenda of health reform: Regressive or advanced—Discipline status. *Nursing Science Quarterly, 7*(2), 93-94.

Leininger, M. (1994). Reflections: Culturally congruent care: Visible and invisible. *Journal of Transcultural Nursing, 6*(1), 23-25.

Leininger, M. (1995). Culture care theory, research, and practice. *Nursing Science Quarterly, 9(2)*, 71-78.

Leininger, M. (1995). Founder's focus: Nursing theories and cultures: Fit or misfit. *Journal of Transcultural Nursing, 7*(1), 41-42.

Leininger, M. (1996). Culture care theory, research and practice. *Nursing Science Quarterly, 9*(2), 71-78.

Leininger, M. (1996). Founder's focus: Transcultural nurses and consumers tell their stories. *Journal of Transcultural Nursing, 7*(2), 32-36.

Leininger, M. (1997). Overview of the theory of culture care with the ethnonursing research method. *Journal of Transcultural Nursing, 8*(2), 32-52.

Leininger, M. (1999). Transcultural nursing: An imperative for nursing practice. *Imprint, 46*(5), 50-52.

Leininger, M. (2002). Culture care theory: A major contribution to advance transcultural nursing and practices. *Journal of Transcultural Nursing, 13*(3), 189-192.

Leininger, M. (2007). Theoretical questions and concerns: Response from the theory of Culture Care Diversity and Universality perspective. *Nursing Science Quarterly, 20(*1), 9-13.

Leininger, M., & Cummings, S. H. (1996). Nursing's new paradigm is transcultural nursing: An interview with Madeleine Leininger. *Advanced Nursing Practice Quarterly, 2*(2), 62-70.

Selected Secondary Sources

Books

Andrews, M. M., & Boyle, J. S. (2007). Transcultural concepts in nursing care (5th ed.). Lippincott: Philadelphia, PA.

Fawcett, J. (2005). Leininger's theory of culture care diversity and universality. In Analysis and evaluation of contemporary nursing knowledge: Nursing models and theories (pp. 511-547). Philadelphia: F. A. Davis Company.

Gaut, D., & Leininger, M. (1991). *Caring: The compassionate healer.* New York: National League for Nursing Press.

Meleis. A. I. (1997). *Theoretical nursing: Development and Progress* (3rd ed., pp. 245-274). Philadelphia: Lippincott.

Selected Journal Articles

Andrews, M. M. (2008). Global leadership in transcultural practice, education, and research. *Contemporary Nursing Journal, (28)*2, in press.

Berry, A. (1999). Mexican American women's expressions of the meaning of culturally congruent prenatal care. *Journal of Transcultural Nursing, 10*(3), 203-212.

Bialoskurski, M., Cox, C. L., & Hayes, J. A. (1999). The nature of attachment in a neonatal intensive care unit. *Journal of Perinatal and Neonatal Nursing, 10*(3), 66-77.

Brooke, D., & Omeri, A. (1999). Beliefs about childhood immunization among Lebanese Muslim immigrants in Australia. *Journal of Transcultural Nursing, 10*(3), 229-236.

Higgins, B. (2000). Puerto Rican cultural beliefs: Influence on infant feeding practices in western New York. *Journal of Transcultural Nursing, 11*(1), 19-30.

Hubbert, A. (2008). A partnership of a Catholic-based health system, nursing, and American Indian traditional medicine practitioners. *Contemporary Nursing Journal, (28)*2, in press.

Leuning, C. L., Swiggum, P. D., Wiegert, H. M. B., & McCullough-Zander, K. (2002). Proposed standards for transcultural nursing. *Journal of Transcultural Nursing, 13*(1), 40-46.

McFarland, M. R. (1997). Use of the culture care theory with Anglo- and African Americans in a long-term care setting. *Nursing Science Quarterly, 10*(4), 186-192.

Omeri, A. (1997). Culture care of Iranian immigrants in New South Wales, Australia: Sharing transcultural nursing knowledge. *Journal of Transcultural Nursing, 8*(2), 5-16.

Pacquiano, D. A., Archeval, L., & Shelley, E. E. (1999). Transcultural nursing study of emic and etic care in the home. *Journal of Transcultural Nursing, (10)*2, 112-119.

Ray, M.A. (1999). Transcultural caring in primary health care. *National Academies of Practice Forum, 1*(3), 177-182.

Rosenbaum, J. N. (1997). Leininger's theory of culture care diversity and universality: Transcultural critique. *The Journal of Multicultural Nursing & Health,* 3(3), 24-30.

Webbe-Alamah, H. (2008). Bridging the gap between generic and professional care practices for Muslim patients through the use of Leininger's culture care modes. *Contemporary Nursing Journal, (28)*2, in press.

*Selected Dissertations Using Leininger' Theory (*mentored by Leininger)*

*Berry, A. (1995). Culture care statements, meanings, and expressions of Mexican American women within Leininger's culture care theory. Unpublished doctoral dissertation, Wayne State University, Detroit.

*Cameron, C. (1990). An ethnonursing study of health status of elderly Anglo Canadian wives providing extended care giving to their disabled husbands. Unpublished doctoral dissertation, Wayne State University, Detroit.

*Curtis, M. (1997). Cultural care by private practice APRNs in community contexts. Unpublished doctoral dissertation, Wayne State University, Detroit.

deRuyter, L. (2008). Cultural care education and experiences of African American students in predominantly Euro American associate degree nursing programs. Unpublished doctoral dissertation, Duquesne University, Pittsburgh, PA, USA.

*Ehrmin, J. (1998). Culture care meanings and statements, and experiences of care of African American women residing in an inner city transitional home for substance abuse. Unpublished doctoral dissertation, Wayne State University, Detroit.

*Finn, J. (1993). Professional nurse and generic caregiving of childbearing women conceptualized with Leininger's theory of culture care theory. Unpublished doctoral dissertation, Wayne State University, Detroit.

*Gates, M. (1988). Care and meanings, experiences and orientations of persons dying in hospitals and hospital settings. Unpublished doctoral dissertation, Wayne State University, Detroit.

*Gelazis, R. (1994). Lithuanian care: Meanings and experiences with humor using Leininger's culture care theory. Unpublished doctoral dissertation, Wayne State University, Detroit.

*George, T. (1998). Meanings and statements and experiences of care of chronically mentally ill in a day treatment center using Leininger's culture care theory. Unpublished doctoral dissertation, Wayne State University, Detroit.

*Horton, G. (1998). Culture care by private practice APRN in a community context. Unpublished doctoral dissertation, Wayne State University, Detroit.

*Lamp, J. (1998). Generic and professional care meanings and practices of Finnish women in birth within Leininger's theory of culture care diversity and universality. Unpublished doctoral dissertation, Wayne State University, Detroit.

*Luna, L. (1989). Care and cultural context of Lebanese Muslims in an urban US community within Leininger's culture care theory. Unpublished doctoral dissertation, Wayne State University, Detroit.

*MacNeil, J. (1994). Cultural care: Meanings, patterns, and expressions for Baganda women as AIDS caregivers within Leininger's theory. Unpublished doctoral dissertation, Wayne State University, Detroit.

*McFarland, M. R. (1995). Cultural care of Anglo and African American elderly residents within the environmental context of a long term care institution. Unpublished doctoral dissertation, Wayne State University, Detroit.

*Miller, J. E. (1996). Politics and care: A study of Czech Americans within Leininger's theory of culture care diversity and universality. Unpublished doctoral dissertation, Wayne State University, Detroit.

Mixer, S. (2008). Faculty care expressions, patterns, and practices related to teaching culture care. Unpublished doctoral dissertation, University of Northern Colorado School of Nursing, Greeley, CO, USA.

*Morgan, M. (1994). African American neonatal care in northern and southern contexts using Leininger's culture care theory. Unpublished doctoral dissertation, Wayne State University, Detroit.

*Morris, E. (2004). Culture care values, meanings, and experiences of African American adolescent gang members. Unpublished doctoral dissertation, Wayne State University, Detroit.

*Omeri, A. S. (1996). Transcultural nursing care values, beliefs, and practices of Iranian immigrants in New South Wales, Australia. Unpublished doctoral dissertation, University of Sydney, Sydney, Australia.

*Rosenbaum, J. (1990). Cultural care, culture health and grief phenomena related to older Greek Canadian widows with Leininger's theory of culture care. Unpublished doctoral dissertation, Wayne State University, Detroit.

*Spangler, Z. (1991). Nursing care values and practices of Philippine American and Anglo American nurses. Unpublished doctoral dissertation, Wayne State University, Detroit.

*Stitzlein, D. (1999). The phenomenon of moral care/caring conceptualized within Leininger's theory of culture care diversity and universality. Unpublished doctoral dissertation, Wayne State University, Detroit.

*Thompson, T. (1990). A qualitative investigation of rehabilitation nursing care in an inpatient rehabilitation unit using Leininger's theory. Unpublished doctoral dissertation, Wayne State University, Detroit.

*Villarruel, A. (1993). Mexican American cultural meanings, expressions: Self care and dependent care actions associated with experiences of pain. Unpublished doctoral dissertation, Wayne State University, Detroit.

Webhe-Alamah, H. (2005). Culture care of Syrian American immigrants living in Midwestern United States. Unpublished doctoral dissertation, Duquesne University, Pittsburgh, PA, USA.

Welch, A. (1987). Concepts of health, illness, caring, aging, and problems of adjustment among elderly Filipinas residing in Hampton Roads, Virginia. Unpublished doctoral dissertation, University of Utah, Salt Lake City.

*Wenger, A. F. (1988). The phenomenon of care of old order Amish: A high context culture. Unpublished doctoral dissertation, Wayne State University, Detroit.

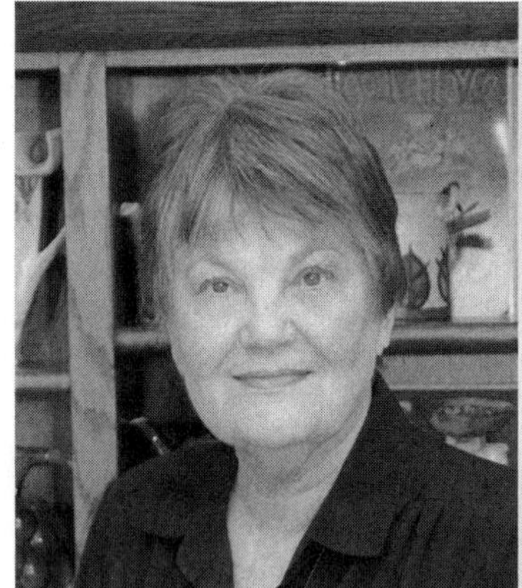
Courtesy New York University, 2009

CHAPTER 23

Margaret A. Newman

1933-present

Health as Expanding Consciousness

Janet Witucki Brown

"We have to embrace a new vision of health. Our caring must be linked with a concept of health that encompasses and goes beyond disease. The theory of health as expanding consciousness provides that perspective" (Newman, 2008, p. 2).

CREDENTIALS AND BACKGROUND OF THE THEORIST

Margaret A. Newman was born on October 10, 1933, in Memphis, Tennessee. She earned a bachelor's degree in home economics and English from Baylor University in Waco, Texas, and a second bachelor's degree in nursing from the University of Tennessee in Memphis (M. Newman, curriculum vitae, 1996). Her master's degree in medical-surgical nursing and teaching was received from the University of California, San Francisco. In 1971, she earned her PhD in nursing science and rehabilitation nursing from New York University in New York City.

After holding academic positions at the University of Tennessee, New York University, and The Pennsylvania State University, Newman was a Professor at the University of Minnesota in Minneapolis until her retirement in 1996, after which she held Professor Emeritus. She also was Director of Nursing for the Clinical Research Center at the University of Tennessee, Acting Director of the PhD Program in the Division of Nursing at New York University, and Professor-in-Charge of the Graduate Program and Research in Nursing at The Pennsylvania State University (M. Newman, curriculum vitae, 2000).

Newman has achieved numerous honors, including admission to the American Academy of Nursing in 1976; Outstanding Alumnus Award from the University of Tennessee College of Nursing in Memphis in 1975 and 2002; Distinguished Alumnus Award from the Division of Nursing at New York University in 1984; admission to the Hall of Fame

Previous authors: Snehlata Desai, M. Jan Keffer, DeAnn M. Hensley, Kimberly A. Kilgore-Keever, Jill Vass Langfitt, and LaPhyllis Peterson. The author wishes to thank Margaret A. Newman for her contributions to the chapter.

at the University of Mississippi School of Nursing in 1988; Latin-American teaching fellow in 1976 and 1977; and an *American Journal of Nursing* scholar in 1979. Additionally, she was Distinguished Faculty at the Seventh International Conference on Human Functioning at Wichita, Kansas, in 1983; received the E. Louise Grant Award for Nursing Excellence from the University of Minnesota in 1996; is listed in *Who's Who in American Women, Who's Who in America*, and *Who's Who in American Nursing*; and was included as a featured nursing theorist in the 1990 videotape series sponsored by the Helene Fuld Health Trust (M. Newman, curriculum vitae, 2000; personal correspondence, 2004). She was a Distinguished Resident at Westminster College in Salt Lake City, Utah, in 1991. She received the Distinguished Scholar in Nursing Award, New York University Division of Nursing, in 1992, the Sigma Theta Tau Founders Elizabeth McWilliams Miller Award for Excellence in Research in 1993, and the Nurse Scholar Award at Saint Xavier University School of Nursing in 1994 (M. Newman, curriculum vitae, 2000).

Newman first presented her ideas on a theory of health in 1978 at a conference on nursing theory in New York. During that time, she was also pursuing research on the relationship of movement, time, and consciousness and was expanding development of the theory of health as expanding consciousness. In 1985, as a traveling research fellow, Newman conducted workshops in New Zealand. Further, at the University of Tampere, Finland, in 1985, Newman was the major speaker for a week-long conference on the theory of consciousness as it related to nursing (M. Newman, personal correspondence, 1988).

Newman has presented many papers on topics pertaining to her theory of health as expanding consciousness. She published *Theory Development in Nursing* (1979), *Health as Expanding Consciousness* (1986, 1994), *A Developing Discipline: Selected Works of Margaret Newman* (1995a), and *Transforming Presence: The Difference That Nursing Makes* (2008). She has written numerous journal articles and book chapters.

In 1986, she did a case study analysis of practice at three sites within the Minneapolis-St. Paul area and discussed conclusions concerning changes necessary for hospital nursing practice (Newman & Autio, 1986). From 1986 to 1997, Newman investigated sequential patterns of persons with heart disease and cancer in relation to the theory of health as expanding consciousness (Newman, 1995c; Newman & Moch, 1991). Other publications reflect her passion for integration of nursing theory, practice, and research, evolving viewpoints on trends in philosophy of nursing and analysis of theoretical models of nursing practice and nursing research (Newman, 1992, 1997b, 1999, 2003). During 1989 and 1990, Newman was principal investigator of a project that explored the theory and structure of a professional model of nursing practice at Carondelet St. Mary's Community Hospitals and Health Centers in Tucson, Arizona (Newman, 1990b; Newman, Lamb, & Michaels, 1991).

Newman has been sought for consultation regarding the expansion of her theory of health in more than 40 states and numerous foreign countries. She served on several editorial review panels, including those of *Nursing Research, Western Journal of Nursing Research, Nursing and Health Care, Advances in Nursing Science,* and *Nursing Science Quarterly,* and on the advisory board of *Advances in Nursing Science* (M. Newman, personal correspondence, 2004). She was also a participating member of the nurse theorist task force from 1978 to 1982 with the North American Nursing Diagnosis Association (NANDA).

RELATIONSHIP TO METAPARADIGM CONCEPTS

Newman has designated "caring in the human health experience" (M. Newman, personal correspondence 2004; Newman, Sime, & Corcoran-Perry, 1991, p. 3) as the focus of nursing and has specified this focus as the metaparadigm of the discipline. She asserts that the interrelated concepts of nursing, person, health, and environment are inherent in this focus (M. Newman, personal correspondence, 2004). Coming from a unitary, transformative paradigm of the discipline, Newman does not see these concepts in isolation. Therefore, she does not discuss them separately in her works, but she has elaborated on some of these dimensions, particularly nursing and health, in explications of her position. In the following paragraphs, implicit definitions from Newman's work are used to discuss the four components.

Nursing

Newman emphasizes the primacy of relationships as a focus of nursing, both nurse-client relationships and relationships within clients' lives (Newman, 2008). During dialectic nurse-client relationships, clients get in touch with the meaning of their lives through identification of meanings in the process of their evolving patterns of relating (Newman, 2008). "The emphasis of this process is on knowing/caring through pattern recognition" (Newman, 2008, p. 10). Insight into these patterns provides clients with illumination of action possibilities, which then opens the way for transformation (Newman, 1990a).

The nurse facilitates pattern recognition in clients by forming relationships with them at critical points in their lives and connecting with them in an authentic way. The nurse-client relationship is characterized by "a rhythmic coming together and moving apart as clients encounter disruption of their organized, predictable state" (Newman, 1999, p. 228). She further states that the nurse will continue to connect with clients as they move through periods of disorganization and unpredictability to arrive at a higher, organized state (Newman, 1999). The nurse comes together with clients at these critical choice points in their lives and participates with them in the process of expanding consciousness. The relationship is one of rhythmicity and timing, with the nurse letting go of the need to direct the relationship or fix things. As the nurse relinquishes the need to manipulate or control, there is a greater ability to enter into this fluctuating, rhythmic partnership with the client (Newman, 1999). Newman has diagrammed this nurse-client interaction of coming together and moving apart through the processes of recognition, insight, and transformation (Figure 23-1) Nurses are seen as partners in the process of expanding consciousness, and are transformed and have their lives enhanced in the dialogical process (Newman, 2008). As a facilitator, the nurse helps an individual, family, or community to focus on patterns of relating (M. Newman, telephone interview, 2004). The nursing process is one of pattern recognition.

Newman's early suggestion (Newman, 1995b) was that the NANDA health assessment framework, based on unitary person-environment patterns of interaction, be used to facilitate clients' pattern recognition (Roy, Rogers, Fitzpatrick, Newman, & Orem, 1982). At the time, the patterns were intended to guide nurses to make holistic observations of "person-environment behaviors that together depict a very specific pattern of the whole for each person" (Newman, 1995b, p. 261). Newman (2008) has since emphasized concentrating on what is most meaningful to clients in their own stories and patterns of relating.

Within the theory, the role of the nurse in nurse-client interactions is seen as a "caring, pattern-recognizing presence" (Newman, 2008, p. 16). The nurse perceives patterns in client's stories or sequences of events, and the pattern of the individual changes with the new information. According to Newman (2008), it is important for nurses to view clients' stories comprehensively. Through active listening, nurses can enter the whole through the parts and intuit the whole from the pattern. Differences are viewed as part of a unified whole. The nurse can facilitate client insight through sharing the process of pattern recognition, thus opening action possibilities (Newman, 1987b).

Person

Throughout Newman's work, the terms *client, patient, person, individual*, and *human being* are used interchangeably. Clients are viewed as participants in the transformative process.

Persons as individuals are identified by their individual patterns of consciousness (Newman, 1986). Persons are further defined as "centers of consciousness within an overall pattern of expanding consciousness" (Newman, 1986, p. 31). The definition of *persons* has

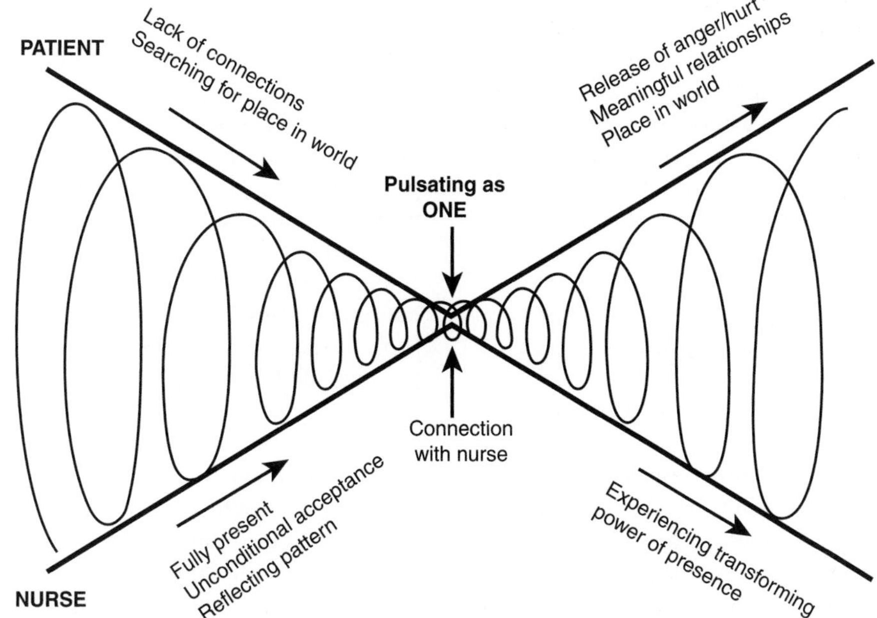

Figure 23-1 Nurse and patient coming together and moving apart in process recognition, insight, and transformation. (From Newman, M. A. [2008]. *Transforming presence: The difference that nursing makes.* Philadelphia: F. A. Davis Company.)

also been expanded to include family and community (Newman, 1994).

Environment

Although environment is not explicitly defined, it is described as being the larger whole, which contains the consciousness of the individual. The pattern of person consciousness interacts within the pattern of family consciousness and within the pattern of community interactions (Newman, 1986). A major assumption is that "consciousness is coextensive in the universe and resides in all matter" (Newman, 1986, p. 33). Client and environment are viewed as unitary evolving patterns (Newman, 2008).

Newman identifies interactions between person and environment as a key process that creates unique configurations for each individual. Patterns of person-environment evolve to higher levels of consciousness. The assumption is that all matter in the universe-environment possesses consciousness, but at different levels. Interpretation of Newman's view clarifies that health is the interaction pattern of a person with the environment. Disease in a human energy field is a manifestation of a unique pattern of person-environment interaction.

Health

Health is the major concept of Newman's theory of expanding consciousness. A fusion of disease and non-disease creates a synthesis that is regarded as health (Newman, 1979, 1991, 1992). Disease and non-disease are each reflections of the larger whole; therefore, a new concept of health, "pattern of the whole," is formed (Newman, 1986, p. 12). Newman (1999) has further elaborated her view of health by stating that "health is the pattern of the whole, and wholeness *is*" (p. 228). Further, this wholeness cannot be gained or lost. Within this perspective, becoming ill does not diminish wholeness, but wholeness takes on a different form. Newman (2008) has stated that pattern recognition is the essence of emerging health. "Manifest health, encompassing disease and non-disease can be regarded as the explication of the underlying pattern of person-environment" (Newman, 1994, p. 11). Therefore, health and evolving pattern of consciousness are the same. Specifically, health is viewed "as a transformative process to more inclusive consciousness" (Newman, 2008, p. 16).

THEORETICAL SOURCES

The theory, Health as Expanding Consciousness, stems from Rogers' (1970) science of unitary human beings. Rogers' assumptions regarding wholeness, pattern, and unidirectionality are the foundation of Newman's theory (M. Newman, personal correspondence, 2004). Hegel's process of the fusion of opposites (Acton, 1967) helped Newman to conceptualize the fusion of health and illness into a new concept of health. Bentov's (1977) explication of life as the process of expanding consciousness prompted Newman to assert that this new concept of health is the process of expanding consciousness (M. Newman, personal correspondence, 2004).

Bohm's (1980) theory of implicate order supports Newman's postulate that disease is a manifestation of the pattern of health. Newman (1994) stated that she began to comprehend "the underlying, unseen pattern that manifests itself in varying forms, including disease, and the interconnectedness and omnipresence of all that there is" (p. xxvi). Young's (1976) theory of human evolution pinpointed the role of pattern recognition for Newman. She explained that Young's ideas provided the impetus for her efforts to integrate the basic concepts of her new theory, movement, space, time, and consciousness, into a dynamic portrayal of life and health (Newman, 1994). Further, Moss' (1981) experience of love as the highest level of consciousness was important to Newman in providing affirmation and elaboration of her intuition regarding the nature of health (Newman, 1994). Newman also incorporated Prigogine's (1976) theory of dissipative structures as an explanation for the timing of nursing presence as the patient fluctuates from one level of organization to a higher level (M. Newman, personal correspondence, 2004). Although Newman (1997a) acknowledges the contributions of these theories to her theory, she has stated that her theory "was enriched by them, but was not based on them" (p. 23).

MAJOR CONCEPTS & DEFINITIONS

HEALTH

Health is the "pattern of the whole" of a person and includes disease as a meaningful manifestation of the pattern of the whole, based on the premise that life is an ongoing process of expanding consciousness (Newman, 1986). It is regarded as the evolving pattern of the person and the environment and is viewed as an increasing ability to perceive alternatives and respond in a variety of ways (Newman, 1986). Health is "a transformative process to more inclusive consciousness" (Newman, 2008, p. 16).

Using Hegel's dialectical fusion of opposites, Newman explained conceptually how disease fuses with its opposite, non-disease or absence of disease, to create a new concept of health. This new view of health is relational and is "patterned, emergent, unpredictable, unitary, intuitive, and innovative," whereas the traditional view is linear, "causal, predictive, dichotomous, rational, and controlling" (Newman, 1994, p. 13). Health and the evolving pattern of consciousness are the same. The essence of the emerging paradigm of health is recognition of pattern. Newman (1994) sees the life process as a progression toward higher levels of consciousness.

Major Concepts & Definitions—cont'd

PATTERN

Pattern is information that depicts the whole and understanding of the meaning of all of the relationships at once (M. Newman, personal correspondence, 2004). It is conceptualized as a fundamental attribute of all there is, and it gives unity in diversity (Newman, 1986). Pattern is what identifies an individual as a particular person. Examples of explicit manifestations of the underlying pattern of a person would be the genetic pattern that contains information that directs becoming, the voice pattern, and the movement pattern (Newman, 1986). Characteristics of pattern include movement, diversity, and rhythm. Pattern is further conceptualized as being somehow intimately involved in both energy exchange and transformation (Newman, 1994). According to Newman (1987b), "Whatever manifests itself in a person's life is the explication of the underlying implicate pattern . . . the phenomenon we call health is the manifestation of that evolving pattern" (p. 37).

In Health as Expanding Consciousness, Newman (1986, 1994) developed pattern as a major concept that was used to understand the individual as a whole being. Newman described a paradigm shift occurring in the field of health care: the shift from treatment of disease symptoms to the search for patterns and the meaning of those patterns. Newman (1994) stated that the patterns of interaction of person-environment constitute health. Individual life patterns according to Newman (2008) move "through peaks and troughs, variations in order-disorder that are meaningful for the person" (p. 6). An event such as a disease occurrence is part of a larger process. By interacting with the event, no matter how destructive the force might seem to be, its energy augments the person's own energy and enhances his or her own power in the situation. To see this, it is necessary to grasp the pattern of the whole (Newman, 1986).

CONSCIOUSNESS

Consciousness is both the informational capacity of the system and the ability of the system to interact with its environment (Newman, 1994). Newman asserts that an understanding of her definition of consciousness is essential to understanding the theory. Consciousness includes not only cognitive and affective awareness, but also the "interconnectedness of the entire living system which includes physicochemical maintenance and growth processes as well as the immune system" (Newman, 1990a, p. 38). In 1978, Newman identified three correlates of consciousness (time, movement, and space) as manifestations of the pattern of the whole.

The life process is seen as a progression toward higher levels of consciousness. Newman (1979) views the expansion of consciousness as what life, and therefore health, is all about. She refers to the sense of time as an indicator in the changing level of consciousness.

Newman (1986) integrates Bentov's (1977) definition of absolute consciousness as "a state in which contrasting concepts become reconciled and fused. Movement and rest fuse into one" (p. 67). Absolute consciousness is equated with love, where all opposites are reconciled and all experiences are accepted equally and unconditionally, such as love and hate, pain and pleasure, and disease and non-disease. Reed (1996) concurred that Newman's theory described the phase of evolutionary development when the person moves beyond focus on self limited by time, space, and physical concerns. Transcendence is a process through which the person moves to a high level of consciousness.

MOVEMENT-SPACE-TIME

Newman stated that it is important to examine movement-space-time together as dimensions of emerging patterns of consciousness rather than in isolation as separate concepts of the theory (M. Newman, personal correspondence, 2004).

USE OF EMPIRICAL EVIDENCE

Evidence for the theory of health as expanding consciousness emanated from Newman's early personal family experiences. Her mother's struggle with amyotrophic lateral sclerosis and her dependence on Newman, then a young college graduate, sparked an interest in nursing. From that experience evolved the idea that "illness reflected the life patterns of the person and that what was needed was the recognition of that pattern and acceptance of it for what it meant to that person" (Newman, 1986, p. 3).

Throughout Newman's writings, terms such as *call to nursing, growing conscience-like feeling, fear, power, meaning of life and health, belief of life after death, rituals of health,* and *love* are used. These terms provide a clue concerning Newman's endeavors to make a disturbing life experience logical. The life experience triggered her beginning maturation toward theory development in nursing. Within her philosophical framework, Newman began to develop a synthesis of disease-non-disease-health as recognition of the total patterning of a person.

Research has been conducted on the theoretical sources (Newman, 1987b). In 1979, Newman wrote that in order for nursing research to have meaning in terms of theory development, it must have three components. These components are as follows: (1) having as its purpose the testing of theory, (2) making explicit the theoretical framework upon which the testing relies, and (3) reexamining the theoretical underpinnings in light of the findings (Newman, 1979). She believed that if health is considered an individual personal process, research should focus on studies that explore changes and similarities in personal meaning and patterns.

MAJOR ASSUMPTIONS

The foundation for Newman's assumptions (M. Newman, telephone interview, 2000) is her definition of health, which is grounded in Rogers' 1970 model for nursing, specifically, the focus on wholeness, pattern, and unidirectionality. From this, Newman developed the following assumptions that support her theory to this day (Newman, 2008).

1. Health encompasses conditions heretofore described as illness or, in medical terms, pathology . . .
2. These "pathological" conditions can be considered a manifestation of the total pattern of the individual . . .
3. The pattern of the individual that eventually manifests itself as pathology is primary and exists prior to structural or functional changes . . .
4. Removal of the pathology in itself will not change the pattern of the individual . . .
5. If becoming "ill" is the only way an individual's pattern can manifest itself, then that is health for that person . . .

From these assumptions, Newman set forth the thesis: *Health is the expansion of consciousness* (Newman, personal correspondence, 2008).

Newman's implicit assumptions about human nature include being unitary, being an open system, being in continuous interconnectedness with the open system of the universe, and being continuously engaged in an evolving pattern of the whole (M. Newman, telephone interview, 2000). She views unfolding consciousness as a process that will occur regardless of what actions nurses perform. However, nurses can assist clients in getting in touch with what is going on and, in that way, can facilitate the process (Newman, 1994).

THEORETICAL ASSERTIONS AND DEVELOPMENT

Early Designation of Concepts and Propositions

Early writings focused heavily on the concepts of movement, space, time, and consciousness. In *Theory Development in Nursing*, Newman (1979) delineated the relationships between movement, space, time, and consciousness. One proposition was that there was a complimentary relationship between time and space (Newman, 1979, 1983). Examples of this relationship were given at the macrocosmic, microcosmic, and humanistic (everyday) levels. At the humanistic level, highly mobile individuals live in a world of expanded space and compartmentalized time. There is an inverse relationship between space and time in that when a person's life space is decreased, such as by physical or social immobility, then that person's time is increased (Newman, 1979).

Movement is a "means whereby space and time become a reality" (Newman, 1983, p. 165). Humankind is in a constant state of motion and is constantly changing internally (at the cellular level) and externally (through body movement and interaction with the environment). This movement through time and space is what gives humankind a unique perception of reality. Movement brings change and enables the individual to experience the world (Newman, 1979).

Movement was also referred to as a "reflection of consciousness" (Newman, 1983, p. 165). It is the means of experiencing reality and also the means by which an individual expresses thoughts and feelings about the reality of experiences. An individual conveys awareness of self through the movement involved in language, posture, and body movement (Newman, 1979). An indication of the internal organization of a person and of that person's perception of the world can be found in the rhythm and pattern of the person's movement. Movement patterns provide additional communication beyond that which language can convey (Newman, 1979).

The concept of time is seen as a function of movement (Newman, 1979). This assertion was supported by Newman's (1972) studies of the experience of time as related to movement and gait tempo. Newman's research demonstrated that the slower an individual walks, the less subjective time is experienced. However, when compared with clock time, time seems to "fly." Although individuals who are moving quickly subjectively feel that they are "beating the clock," they report that time seems to be dragging when checking a clock (Newman, 1972, 1979).

Time is also conceptualized as a measure of consciousness (Newman, 1979). Bentov (1977) measured consciousness with a ratio of subjective to objective time and proposed this assertion. Newman applied this measure of consciousness to subjective and objective data from her research. She found that the consciousness index increased with age. Some of her research has also supported the finding of "increasing consciousness with age" (Newman, 1982, p. 293). Newman cited this evidence as support for her position that the life process evolves toward consciousness expansion. However, she asserted that certain moods, such as depression, might be accompanied by a diminished sense of time (Newman & Gaudiano, 1984).

Synthesis of Patterns of Movement, Space-Time, and Consciousness

As the theory evolved, Newman developed a synthesis of the pattern of movement, space, time, and consciousness (M. Newman, personal correspondence, 2004, 2008). Time was not merely conceptualized as subjective or objective, but was also viewed in a holographic sense (M. Newman, telephone interview, 2000). According to Newman (1994), "Each moment has an explicate order and also enfolds all others, meaning that each moment of our lives contains all others of all time" (p. 62). Newman (1986) illustrated the centrality of space-time in the following example:

> Mrs. V. made repeated attempts to *move* away from her husband and to *move* into an educational program to become more independent. She felt she had no *space* for herself, and she tried to distance herself (space) from her husband. She felt she had no *time* for leisure (self), was overworked, and was constantly meeting other people's needs. She was submissive to the demands and criticism of her husband (p. 56).

Space, time, and movement later became linked with Newman's (1986) assertion that the intersection of movement-space-time represented the person as a center of consciousness. Further, this varied from person to person, place to place, and time to time. Newman (1986) also emphasized that the crucial task of nursing is to be able to see the concepts of movement-space-time in relation to each other, and consider them all at once, recognizing patterns of evolving consciousness.

In *Health as Expanding Consciousness* (Newman, 1986, 1994), Newman's theory encompassed the work of Young's spectrum of consciousness (Young, 1976). She saw Young's central theme as being that self and universe were of the same nature. This essential nature could not be defined but was characterized by complete freedom and unrestricted choice at both the beginning and the end of life's trajectory (Newman, 1986).

Newman established a corollary between her model of health as expanding consciousness and Young's conception of the evolution of human beings (Figure 23-2). She explained that individuals came into being from a state of consciousness, they were bound in time, found their identity in space, and through movement learned the "law" of the way that things worked; they then made choices that ultimately took them beyond space and time to a state of absolute consciousness (Newman, 1994).

Newman (1994) also stated that restrictions in movement-space-time have the effect of forcing an awareness that extends beyond the physical self. When natural movement is altered, space and time are also altered. When movement is restricted (physical or social), it is necessary for an individual to move beyond self, thereby making movement an important choice point in the process of evolving human consciousness (Newman, 1994). She assumed that the awareness corresponded to the "inward, self-generated reformation that Young [spoke] of as the turning point of the process" (Newman, 1994, p. 46). When a person progresses to the state of timelessness, there is increasing freedom from time. Finally, the last stage is absolute consciousness, which Newman asserted is equated with love (Newman, 1994).

Emphasis on Experiential Process of Nurse-Client

With the realization that the early research testing of propositional statements stemmed from a mechanistic view of movement-space-time consciousness

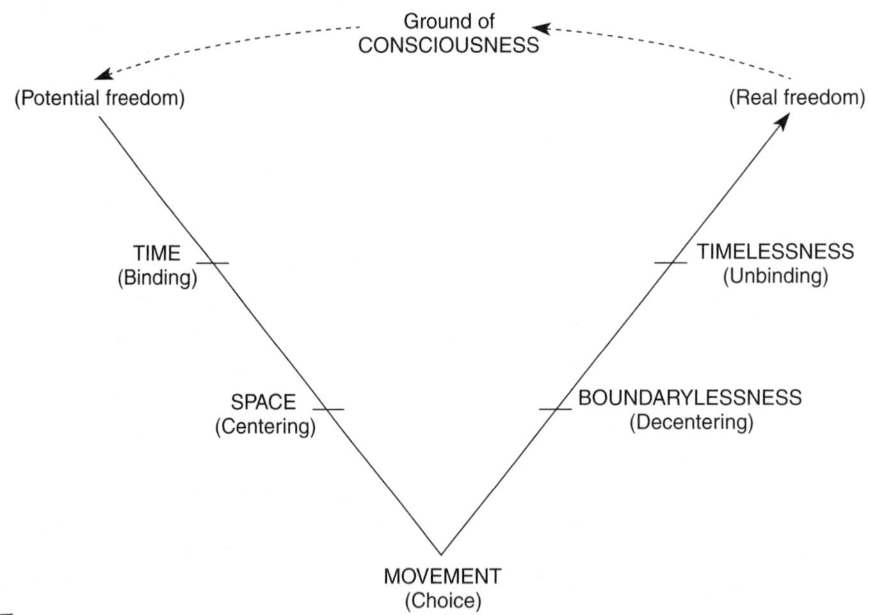

Figure 23-2 Parallel between Newman's theory of expanding consciousness and Young's stages of human evolution. (From Newman, M. A. [1990]. Newman's theory of health as praxis. *Nursing Science Quarterly*, 3[1], 37-41.)

and failed to honor the basic assumptions of her theory, Newman shifted focus to authentic involvement of the nurse researcher as a participant with the client in the unfolding pattern of expanding consciousness (Newman, 2008). The unitary, transformative paradigm demanded that the research honor and reveal the mutuality of interaction between nurse and client, the uniqueness and wholeness of pattern in each client situation, and movement of the life process toward higher consciousness. Newman (2008) states, "The nature of nursing practice is the caring, pattern-recognizing relationship between nurse and client—a relationship that is a transforming presence" (p. 52).

The protocol for this research was first started in 1994, and variations of this guide continue to be implemented in current praxis research. Litchfield (1999) explicated this process as "practice wisdom" in her work with families of hospitalized children, and Endo (1998) analyzed the phases of the process in her work with women with ovarian cancer. The data of this praxis research reveal evidence of expanding consciousness in the quality and connectedness of the client's relationships and support the importance of the nurse's creative presence in participants' insight (M. Newman, personal correspondence, 2004, 2008). Variations of the praxis research have been utilized in numerous populations and settings (Newman, 2008; Picard & Jones, 2007).

LOGICAL FORM

Newman used both inductive and deductive logic in early theory development. Inductive logic is based on observing particular instances and then relating those instances to form a whole. Newman's theory development was derived from her earlier research on time perception and gait tempo. Time and movement, with space and consciousness, were subsequently used as central components in her early conceptual framework. These concepts helped explain "the phenomena of the life process and therefore of health" (Newman, 1979, p. 59). Newman (1997a) has described the evolution of the theory as it moved from linear explication and testing of concepts of time, space, and movement to an elaboration of interacting patterns as manifestations of expanding consciousness. Evolution of the theory of health as expanding consciousness as a process of evolving, in conjunction with the research, progressed through several stages (Newman, 1997a, 1997b). These stages included testing the relationships of the concepts of movement, space, and time, identifying sequential person-environmental patterns, and recognizing the centrality of nurse-client relationships or dialogue in the clients' evolving insight and accompanying potential for action. The process actually became cyclical as the original concepts of movement-space-time emerged as dimensions in the unitary evolving process of consciousness (Newman, 1997a).

ACCEPTANCE BY THE NURSING COMMUNITY

Research/Practice

Newman believes that research within the theory of health as expanding conscious is praxis, which she defines as a "mutual process between nurse and client with the intent to help" (Newman, 2008, p. 21). Further, this process focuses "on transformation from one point to another and incorporates the guidance of an a priori theory" (Newman, 2008, p. 21). Research and practice with the theory then are interwoven.

In Newman's view, the responsibility of professional nurses is to establish a primary relationship with the client for the purpose of identifying meaningful patterns and facilitating the client's action potential and decision-making ability (Newman, 2008). Communication and collaboration with other nurses, associates, and healthcare professionals are essential (Newman, 1989). Nurses as primary care providers, focused directly and completely on relationships with clients, relate to her view of the role of professional nursing, which Newman (Newman, Lamb, & Michaels, 1991) referred to as *nursing clinician-case manager*, which is the sine qua non of the integrative model.

Relating her theory of health as expanding consciousness and acknowledging the contemporary and radical shift in philosophy of nursing that views health as a unitary human field dynamic embedded in a larger unitary field, Newman (1979) believes that "the goal of nursing is not to make people well, or to prevent their getting sick, but to assist people to utilize the power that is within them as they evolve toward higher levels of consciousness" (p. 67). The task of nursing is not to try to change the pattern of another person, but to recognize it as information that depicts the whole and relate to it as it unfolds (Newman, 1994).

From the Newman perspective, nursing is the study of "caring in the human health experience" (Newman et al., 1991, p. 3). The role of the nurse in this experience is to help clients recognize their own patterns, which results in the illumination of action possibilities that open the way for transformation to occur.

At first, Newman's theory of health was useful in the practice of nursing because it contained the concepts of movement and time that are used by the nursing profession and intrinsic to nursing interventions such as range of motion and ambulation (Newman, 1987a).

Early research with the theory manipulated concepts of space, time, and movement. In addition to Newman, several researchers conducted research about time, space, or movement. Newman and Gaudiano (1984) focused on the occurrence of depression in the elderly and decreased subjective time. Mentzer and Schorr (1986) used Newman's model of duration of time as an index to consciousness in a study of institutionalized elderly. Engle (1986) addressed the relationship between movement, time, and assessment of health. Schorr and Schroeder (1989) studied differences in consciousness with regard to time and movement, and in another study found that relationships among type A behavior, temporal orientation, and death anxiety as manifestations of consciousness had mixed results (Schorr & Schroeder, 1991). During the 1980s, Marchione, using health as expanding consciousness, investigated and reported the meaning of disabling events in families, presenting a case study in which an additional person became part of the nuclear family. The addition was a disruptive event for the family and created disturbances in time, space, movement, and consciousness, suggesting that Newman's work with patterns could be used to understand family interactions (Marchione, 1986). Marchione (1986) and Pharris (2005) both advocate application of the theory to practice with communities.

However, with evolution of the theory, the praxis research also incorporated practice, having a function of assisting clients in pattern recognition (Newman, 1990a). Schorr, Farnham, and Ervin (1991) investigated the health patterns in 60 aging women, using the theory as a framework. A study of music and pattern change in chronic pain by Schorr (1993) also supported Newman's theory of health as expanding consciousness. Fryback's (1991) dissertation revealed that persons with acquired immunodeficiency syndrome (AIDS) and human immunodeficiency virus (HIV) infection did, in fact, describe health within physical, health promotion, and spiritual domains and was consistent with Newman's theory.

The theory has been used in practice with various client populations. Kalb (1990) applied Newman's theory of health in the clinical management of pregnant women hospitalized for complications of maternal-fetal health. Smith (1995) worked with the health of rural African American women. Yamashita (1995, 1999) studied Japanese and Canadian family caregivers, and Rosa (2006) worked with persons living with chronic skin wounds. Several studies have focused on patterns of persons with rheumatoid arthritis (Brauer, 2001; Neill, 2002; Schmidt, Brauer, & Peden-McAlpine, 2003). Research studies have focused on patterns of patients with cancer as a meaningful part of health (Barron, 2005; Bruce-Barrett, 1998; Endo, 1998; Endo, Nitta, et al., 2000; Gross, 1995; Karian, Jankowski, & Beal, 1998; Kiser-Larson, 2002; Moch, 1990; Newman, 1995c; Roux, Bush & Dingley, 2001; Utley, 1999). Other studies include life patterns of persons with coronary heart disease (Newman & Moch, 1991); patterns of persons with chronic obstructive pulmonary disease (Jonsdottir, 1998; Noveletsky-Rosenthal, 1996); life patterns of people with hepatitis C

(Thomas, 2002); and patterns of expanding consciousness in persons with HIV and AIDS (Lamendola & Newman, 1994).

Litchfield (1999) described the patterning of nurse-client relationships in families with frequent illness and hospitalization of toddlers, and its use in family health. Magan, Gibbon, and Mrozek (1990) reported on implementation of the theory, as one of several theories, in the care of the mentally ill. Weingourt (1998) reported on the use of Newman's theory of health with elderly nursing home residents, and Capasso (2005) reported increased emotional and physical client healing as a result of use of the theory in nurse-client interactions.

Additional research includes studies that involved recognizing health patterns in persons with multiple sclerosis (Gulick & Bugg, 1992; Neill, 2005) and spousal caregivers of partners with dementia (Brown & Alligood, 2004; Brown, Chen, Mitchell, & Province, 2007; Schmitt, 1991), as well as patterns in adolescent males incarcerated for murder (Pharris, 2002) and life experiences of Black Caribbean women (Peters-Lewis, 2006). Additional studies have included life patterns of women who successfully lose weight and maintain weight loss (Berry, 2002); victimizing sexuality and healing patterns (Smith, 1997); meaning of the death of an adult child to an elder (Weed, 2004); experience of family members living through the sudden death of a child (Picard, 2002); nurse facilitation of health as expanding consciousness in families of children with special health care needs (Falkenstern, 2003), and health as expanding consciousness to conceptualize adaptation in burn patients (Casper, 1999).

Newman's research as praxis has also been used to describe the lived experience of life passing in middle-adolescent females (Shanahan, 1993); patterns of expanding consciousness in women in midlife (Picard, 2000) and women transitioning through menopause (Musker, 2005); pattern recognition of high-risk pregnant women (Schroeder, 1993) and low-risk pregnant women (Batty, 1999); and patterns in families of medically fragile children (Tommet, 2003). It was the framework for analysis of patterns for evidence of empowerment in community healthcare workers by Walls (1999).

Quinn (1992) reconceptualized therapeutic touch as shared consciousness. Lamb and Stempel (1994) described the role of the nurse as an insider-expert. Newman, Lamb, and Michaels (1991) described the role of the nurse case manager at St. Mary's as emanating from a philosophical and theoretical base agreeing with the unitary-transformative paradigm and exemplifying an integrated stage of professional nursing. Further, the theory of health as expanding consciousness has been proposed as beneficial for the school nurse working with adolescents with insulin-dependent diabetes (Schlotzhauer & Farnham, 1997).

Gustafson (1990) found that practice as a parish nurse supported Newman's theory of health as demonstration of pattern recognition. More recently, Endo and colleagues (2005) conducted action research involving practicing nurses and found that nurses experienced deeper meaning in their lives as a result of the transformative power of pattern recognition in their work with clients. Flanagan (2005) found that preoperative nurses working within the theory saw the effect of their presence in changing patient experiences. Additionally, Ruka (2005) developed a model of nursing home practice for use in pattern recognition with persons with dementia.

Newman states that her research over time assisted not only clients who participated, but she and fellow researchers were also assisted, in gaining a better understanding of self as a nurse researcher and understanding the limitations of previous methods used. Newman (1994) further stated that research should center on investigations that are participatory and in which client-subjects are partners and co-researchers in the search for health patterns. This method of inquiry is called *cooperative inquiry* or *interactive, integrative participation.* Newman (1989, 1990a) has developed a method to describe patterns as unfolding and evolving over time. She used the method of interviewing a subject regarding different time frames to establish a pattern for that subject (Newman, 1987b). Newman (1990a) stated that during the development of a methodology to test the theory of health, "sharing our (researcher's) perception of the person's pattern with the person was meaningful to the participants and stimulated new insights regarding their lives" (p. 37). In 1994, she described a protocol for the research and labeled it *hermeneutic dialectic.* This method allows the pattern of person-environment to reveal itself without disturbing the unity of the pattern (M. Newman, personal correspondence, 2000). From the inception of Newman's theory in the 1970s until the present, numerous nurse practitioners and scientists have used the theory to incorporate the concepts into their nursing practice or to elaborate the theory through research. Newman advocates a convergence of nursing theories as the basis of the discipline (Newman, 2003). She sees health as expanding consciousness as emerging from a Rogerian perspective, incorporating theories of caring, and projecting a transformative process (Newman, 2005).

Education

Newman (1986) stated that ideally, a new role is needed for the nurse to function in the paradigm of the evolving consciousness of the whole. "Nurses need to be free to relate to patients in an ongoing partnership that is not limited to a particular place or time" (Newman, 1986, p. 89). She suggested that nursing education should revolve around pattern as a concept, substance, process, and method. Education by this method would enable nursing to be an important resource for the continued development of health care. Newman (1986) stated that nursing is at the intersection of the focus of the healthcare industry; therefore, "nursing is in position to bring about the fluctuation within the system that will shift the system to a new higher order of functioning" (p. 90).

Newman (2008) states, "attention to the nature of transformative learning will help to establish the priorities of the discipline" (p. 73). She sees a need for student-teacher personal transformation in nursing curricula. As students and teachers directly engage together in intuitive awareness, they will resonate with each other in a transforming way (Endo, Takaki, Abe, Terashima, & Nitta, 2007). However, as the paradigm shift has taken place in nurses' views of their relationships with clients, many examples of application of the theory in traditional roles are evident (Newman, personal correspondence, 2008).

Examining the pragmatic adequacy of Newman's theory in relation to nursing education reveals that teaching the research method associated with the theory also teaches students a practice method that is congruent with the theory, and it is a means for students to experience transformation through pattern recognition (Newman, 2008). Newman sees the theory, the practice, and the research as a process rather than as separate domains of the nursing discipline. Teaching the theory of health as expanding consciousness necessitates a shift in thinking from a dichotomous view of health to a synthesized view that accepts disease as a manifestation of health. Not only that, learning to let go of the professional's control and respecting the client's choices are integral parts of practice within this framework. Students and practicing nurses who plan to use Newman's theory will face personal transformation in learning to recognize patterns through nurse-client interactions. An individual's personal experience will be the core not just of teaching and practice, but of research as well. Newman (1994) explained that the nurse would need to sense his or her own pattern of relating as an indication of the nurse-client interacting pattern. She emphasized that there needs to be a sense of the process of the relationship with clients from within, giving attention to the "we" in the nurse-client relationship (Newman, 1997b).

Newman's theory has been used in nursing education to provide some content into a model called the *healing web.* This model was designed to integrate nursing education and nursing service together with private and public education programs for baccalaureate and associate nursing degree programs in South Dakota (Bunkers, Bendtro, et al., 1992). Jacono and Jacono (1996) suggested that student creativity could be enhanced if nursing faculty applied the theory recognizing that all experience has the potential for expanding the creativity (consciousness) of individuals. Picard and Mariolis (2002, 2005) described the application of the health as expanding consciousness theory to teaching psychiatric nursing. Further, Endo and colleagues (2007) described a project in which faculty became involved with students in a project of pattern recognition, which resulted in transformation of student relationships.

FURTHER DEVELOPMENT

Previously discussed research studies have supported the theory of health as expanding consciousness, illuminating the importance of pattern recognition in the process of expanding consciousness. The theory has been used extensively in exploring and understanding the experience of health within illness, supporting a basic premise of the theory that disruptive situations may provide a catalytic effect and facilitate movement to higher levels of consciousness.

CRITIQUE

Clarity

Semantic clarity is evident in the definitions, descriptions, and dimensions of the concepts of the theory.

Simplicity

The deeper meaning of the theory of health as expanding consciousness is complex. The theory as a whole must be understood rather than isolating the concepts. If an individual wanted to use a positivist approach, Newman's original propositions would guide hypothesis development. However, researchers who have tried that approach have concluded that it is inadequate to study the theory. As Newman advocated in the 1994 edition of her book, *Health As Expanding Consciousness,* the holistic approach of the hermeneutic dialectic method is consistent with the theory and requires a high level of understanding of the theory on the part of the researcher to extend the theory in praxis research (M. Newman, telephone interview, 1996).

Generality

The concepts in Newman's theory are broad in scope because they all relate to health. The theory has been applied in several different cultures and is applicable across the spectrum of nursing care situations (M. Newman, personal correspondence, 2004). Application of the theory is universal in nature. The broad scope provides a focus for future theory development.

Empirical Precision

In early stages of development, aspects of the theory were tested with the traditional scientific mode. However, quantitative methods are inadequate to capture the dynamic, changing nature of this theory. A hermeneutic dialectic approach was developed for full explication of its meaning and application.

Derivable Consequences

The focus of Newman's theory of health as expanding consciousness provides an evolving guide for all health-related disciplines. In the quest for understanding the phenomenon of health, this unique view of health challenges nurses to make a difference in nursing practice by the application of this theory.

SUMMARY

Although Newman started with a rational, empirical approach that was both inductive and deductive, she found it restrictive and "not consistent with the paradigm from which the theory was drawn" (1997a, p. 23). Little by little, she relinquished some of the experimental control, and her work evolved to a more interactive, integrative approach that continued to be objective and controlled. When that still did not work, she shifted from the scientific paradigm with its objectivity and control and allowed the principles of her theoretical paradigm to guide her research. Then she began to see the core of pattern and process as nursing practice. She saw the evolving pattern as meaning in process that required an approach of mutual process, not just objective observation. Patterns showed that expanding consciousness was related to quality and connectedness of relationships. The nurse researcher's creative presence was important to the participant's insight. Newman (1986) concluded that individuals experience a theory in living it. She labeled her research as hermeneutic dialectic. The theory of health as expanding consciousness, along with the research as praxis method, has been used extensively in nursing practice with a variety of individuals, family and community situations, nursing education, and practice models and nursing research in the United States and several other countries. Newman continues to write, consult, and lecture, advancing her work.

Case Study

Alice is an 81-year-old widow who has lived alone in a low-income apartment complex in a small rural, Appalachian town since her husband's death 8 years ago. She has one surviving family member, a granddaughter, who lives 30 miles away. Alice has never learned to drive and depends on her granddaughter for all transportation to physician appointments and for shopping and getting medications. Her income is $824 monthly, and she requires several expensive prescriptions for arthritis, hypertension, and cardiac problems. She has osteoarthritis in her knees and requires a quad cane for support and safety when getting around her apartment. A visiting nurse stops by weekly to check her blood pressure and to give her an injection for her arthritis. The visiting nurse notes that Alice's blood pressure is elevated, and Alice states that she has been unable to get her medication because her granddaughter's car is broken. Alice also mentions that she is running low on food in the apartment because she can't get out to shop.

Alice admits that she hardly knows or speaks to her neighbors despite having lived there for 8 years, and she still feels like a stranger and doesn't want to "push myself in." She says that she hates to bother people and "won't hardly unless I just have to." She says she sometimes gets lonely for "her people," who are all deceased.

The visiting nurse, in working with Alice, recognizes the current situation as a choice point, with potential for increased interaction with others and increased consciousness. The old ways no longer work for Alice, and new ways of relating are necessary. The nurse incorporates the elements of Newman's method to assist Alice in pattern recognition for the purpose of discovering new potentials for action. As the nurse has Alice relate her story, through dialogue and interacting with Alice, she helps Alice recognize past patterns of relating and how present circumstances have changed those patterns. Alice talks about how she and her husband lived for 56 years in a rural mountain cabin with few neighbors except for two sisters and their sole daughter. They were very self-sufficient, grew large gardens, had their own livestock, and rarely went into town. All these family members are now deceased except the granddaughter, who insisted that Alice leave the cabin and move into town after the death of her husband. It is apparent that Alice's past patterns have been those of independence and limiting social contact to mainly family members.

The nurse shares her perceptions with Alice, who confirms and verifies the pattern identification. Alice states, "I just don't know how long I am going to manage by myself anymore." The nurse helps her explore sources of help, besides the granddaughter, that will help Alice remain in her apartment as independently as possible. Alice relates that there is one man, a few doors away who has stopped several times to ask if she needed anything from the grocery store, but she hasn't asked him because she hates to bother him and doesn't want "to be beholden." After further discussion, she decides that she will ask him to pick up staples and medications for her and will pay him back by baking him some bread, saying, "I just love to bake anyway and haven't had anyone much to bake for."

In subsequent weekly visits, Alice and the nurse explore the possibility of getting medications at a reduced price through the local nurse-managed clinic. Alice states that she might try getting to know some of her neighbors. The nurse helps Alice make arrangements to be picked up by the Senior Van for physician appointments. As Alice begins to build her own support system, she finds that she relies on the nurse less for help with maintaining her independence, and they resume their previous pattern of the nurse checking her blood pressure and giving her injections weekly. However, Alice and the nurse have now developed a relationship that has transformed them both, and the nurse is often met at the door with the smell of fresh-baked bread and an invitation to "have a bite." They both enjoy this new relationship.

CRITICAL THINKING Activities

1. What is the worldview of nursing? What is the nurse scientist view of nursing?
2. How does that worldview dictate or direct knowledge development for nursing?
3. What dictates the change in paradigms of health, healthcare practice, and nursing practice? Examine Newman's view about it.
4. Consider a patient you have cared for, and describe using health as expanding consciousness (pattern of the whole). Compare and contrast the characteristics of this view of the patient with the view you presently use for your practice.
5. Where and how does Newman accept or depart from Rogers' theoretical conceptual system of unitary human beings?
6. How does Newman's theory of health differ from contemporary nursing practice, education, and research?

POINTS FOR Further Study

- Newman, M. A. (2008). *Transforming presence: The difference that nursing makes.* Philadelphia: F.A. Davis Company http://www.healthasexpandingconsciousness.org
- Brown, J. W. (2006). Newman's theory of health and nursing practice. In M. R. Alligood & A. M. Tomey (Eds.), *Nursing theory: Utilization & application* (3rd ed.). St. Louis: Mosby.
- *Margaret Newman, nurse theorists: Portraits of excellence* (Videotape). (1990). Produced by Helene Fuld Health Trust. Oakland, CA: Studio Three Production. Athens, OH: Fitne, Inc.
- Newman, M. A. (1997). *Margaret Newman: Health as expanding consciousness* (CD-ROM). Available through Fuld Institute for Technology in Nursing Education (now Fitne, Inc, 5 Depot Street, Athens, OH 45701, (800) 691-8480.

REFERENCES

Acton, H. B. (1967). George Wilhelm Freidrich Hegel 1770-1831. In P. Edwards (Ed.), *The encyclopedia of philosophy* (Vols. 3 & 4). New York: Macmillan & Free Press.

Barron, A. (2005). Suffering, growth, and possibility: Health as expanding consciousness in end-of-life care. In C. Picard & D. Jones (Eds.), *Giving voice to what we know: Margaret Newman's theory of health as expanding consciousness in nursing practice, research, and education.* (pp. 43-50). Sudbury, MA: Jones & Bartlett.

Batty, M. L. E. (1999). Pattern identification and expanding consciousness during the transition of "low risk" pregnancy. A study embodying Newman's health as expanding consciousness (Margaret Newman) (Master's thesis, The University of New Brunswick, Canada, 1999). *Masters Abstracts International, 39,* 826.

Bentov, I. (1977). *Stalking the wild pendulum.* New York: E. P. Dutton.

Berry, D. C. (2002). Newman's theory of health as expanding consciousness in women maintaining weight loss (Doctoral dissertation, Boston College, 2002). *Dissertation Abstracts International, 63,* 2300.

Bohm, D. (1980). *Wholeness and the implicate order.* London: Routledge and Kegan Paul.

Brauer, D. J. (2001). Common patterns of person-environment interaction in persons with rheumatoid arthritis. *Western Journal of Nursing Research, 23,* 414-430.

Brown, J. W., & Alligood, M. R. (2004). Realizing wrongness: Stories of older wife caregivers. *Journal of Applied Gerontology, 23*(2), 104-119.

Brown, J.W., & Chen, S-L. Mitchell, C., Province, A. (2007). Help-seeking by older husbands caring for wives with dementia. *Journal of Advanced Nursing, 58*(3), 1-9.

Bruce-Barrett, C. A. (1998). Patterns of health and healing: Peer support and prostate cancer (Master's thesis, D'Youville College, 1998). *Masters Abstracts International, 37,* 0233.

Bunkers, S. S., Bendtro, M., Holmes, P. K., Howell, J., Johnson, S., Koerner, J., et al. (1992). The healing web: A transformative model for nursing. *Nursing and Health Care, 13,* 68-73.

Capasso, V. A. (2005). The theory is the practice: An exemplar. In C. Picard & D. Jones (Eds.), *Giving voice to what we know: Margaret Newman's theory of health as expanding consciousness in nursing practice, research, and education.*(pp. 65-71). Sudbury, MA: Jones & Bartlett.

Casper, S. A. (1999). Psychological adaptation as a dimension of health as expanding consciousness: Effectiveness of burn survivors support groups (Master's thesis, D'Youville College, 1999). *Masters Abstracts International, 37,* 1433.

Endo, E. (1998). Pattern recognition as a nursing intervention with Japanese women with ovarian cancer. *ANS Advances in Nursing Science, 20*(4), 49-61.

Endo, E., Miyahara, t., Sizuli, S., Ohmasa, T. (2005). Partnering of researcher and practicing nurses for transformative nursing. *Nursing Science Quarterly, 18*(2), 138-145.

Endo, E., Nitta, N., Inayoshi, M., Saito, R., Takemura, K., Minegishi, H., et al. (2000). Pattern recognition as a caring partnership in families with cancer. *Journal of Advanced Nursing, 32,* 603-610.

Endo, E., Takaki, M., Abe, K., Terashima, K. & Nitta, N. (2007). *Creating a helping model with nursing students who want to quit smoking: Patterning in a nursing student-teacher partnership based on M. Newman's theory of health.* Paper presented at The Power of Caring: The Gateway to Healing, 29th Annual International Association for Human Caring Conference. St. Louis: MO. May 16-19, 2007.

Engle, V. (1986). The relationship of movement and time to older adults' functional health. *Research in Nursing and Health, 9,* 123-129.

Falkenstern, S. K. (2003). *Nursing facilitation of health as expanding consciousness in families who have a child with special health care needs.* Unpublished doctoral dissertation, Pennsylvania State University, University Park, PA.

Flannagan, J. M. (2005). Creating a healing environment for staff and patients in a pre-surgery clinic. In C. Picard & D. Jones (Eds.), *Giving voice to what we know: Margaret Newman's theory of health as expanding consciousness in nursing practice, research, and education.* Sudbury, MA: Jones & Bartlett.

Fryback, P. B. (1991). Perceptions of health by persons with a terminal disease: Implications for nursing. *Dissertation Abstracts International, 52,* 1951.

Gross, S. W. (1995). The impact of a nursing intervention of relaxation with guided imagery on breast cancer patients' stress and health as expanding consciousness (Doctoral dissertation, University of Texas at Austin, 1995). *Dissertation Abstracts International, 56,* 5416.

Gulick, E. E., & Bugg, A. (1992). Holistic health patterning in multiple sclerosis. *Research in Nursing and Health, 15,* 175-185.

Gustafson, W. (1990). Application of Newman's theory of health: Pattern recognition as nursing practice. In M. Parker (Ed.), *Nursing theories in practice* (pp. 141-161). New York: National League for Nursing.

Jacono, B. J., & Jacono, J. J. (1996). The benefits of Newman and Parse in helping nurse teachers determine methods to enhance student creativity. *Nurse Education Today, 16,* 356-362.

Jonsdottir, H. (1998). Life patterns of people with chronic obstructive pulmonary disease: Isolation and being closed in. *Nursing Science Quarterly, 11,* 160-166.

Kalb, K. A. (1990). The gift: Applying Newman's theory of health in nursing practice. In M. Parker (Ed.), *Nursing theories in practice* (pp. 163-186). New York: National League for Nursing.

Karian, V. E., Jankowski, S. M., & Beal, J. A, (1998). Exploring the lived experience of childhood cancer survivors. *Journal of Pediatric Oncology, 15,* 153-162.

Kiser-Larson, N. (2002). Life pattern of native women experiencing breast cancer. *International Journal for Human Caring, 6*(2), 61-68.

Lamb, G. S., & Stempel, J. E. (1994). Nurse case management from the client's view: Growing as insider-expert. *Nursing Outlook, 42,* 7-13.

Lamendola, F. P., & Newman, M. A. (1994). The paradox of HIV/AIDS as expanding consciousness. *ANS Advances in Nursing Science, 16(3),* 13-21.

Litchfield, M. (1999). Practice wisdom. *ANS Advances in Nursing Science, 22*(2), 62-73.

Magan, S. J., Gibbon, E. J., & Mrozek, R. (1990). Nursing theory application: A practice model. *Issues in Mental Health Nursing, 11,* 297-312.

Marchione, J. M. (1986). Pattern as methodology for assessing family health: Newman's theory of health. In P. Winstead-Fry (Ed.), *Case studies in nursing theory.* New York: National League for Nursing.

Mentzer, C., & Schorr, J. A. (1986). Perceived situational control and perceived duration of time: Expressions of life patterns. *ANS Advances in Nursing Science, 9*(1), 13-20.

Moch, S. D. (1990). Health within the experience of breast cancer. *Journal of Advanced Nursing, 15,* 1426-1435.

Moss, R. (1981). *The I that is we.* Millbrae, CA: Celestial Arts.

Musker, K.M. (2005). *Life patterns of women transitioning through menopause* PhD dissertation. Loyola University, Chicago.

Neill, J. (2002). Transcendence and transformation in the life patterns of women living with rheumatoid arthritis. *ANS Advances in Nursing Science, 24*(4), 27-47.

Neill, J. (2005). Recognizing pattern in the lives of women with multiple sclerosis. In C. Picard & D. Jones (Eds.), *Giving voice to what we know* (pp. 153-165). Sudbury. MA: Jones & Bartlett.

Newman, M. A. (1972). Time estimation in relation to gait tempo. *Perceptual and Motor Skills, 34*, 359-366.

Newman, M. A. (1979). *Theory development in nursing.* Philadelphia: F. A. Davis.

Newman, M. A. (1982). Time as an index of expanding consciousness with age. *Nursing Research, 31*, 290-293.

Newman, M. A. (1983). Newman's health theory. In I. W. Clements & F. B. Roberts (Eds.), *Family health: A theoretical approach to nursing care.* New York: John Wiley & Sons.

Newman, M. A. (1986). *Health as expanding consciousness.* St. Louis: Mosby.

Newman, M. A. (1987a). Aging as increasing complexity. *Journal of Gerontological Nursing, 13*(9), 16-18.

Newman, M. A. (1987b). Patterning. In M. Duffy & N. J. Pender (Eds.), *Conceptual issues in health promotion.* A report of proceedings of a wingspread conference, Racine, WI, April 13-15, 1987. Indianapolis: Sigma Theta Tau.

Newman, M. A. (1989). The spirit of nursing. *Holistic Nursing Practice, 3*(3), 1-6.

Newman, M. A. (1990a). Newman's theory of health as praxis. *Nursing Science Quarterly, 3*, 37-41.

Newman, M. A. (1990b). Shifting to higher consciousness. In M. Parker (Ed.), *Nursing theories in practice* (pp. 129-139). New York: National League for Nursing.

Newman, M. A. (1991). Health conceptualizations. In J. J. Fitzpatrick, R. L. Taunton, & A. K. Jacox (Eds.), *Annual review of nursing research* (Vol. 9). New York: Springer.

Newman, M. A. (1992). Nightingale's vision of nursing theory and health. In Nightingale, F., *Notes on nursing: What it is, and what it is not* (commemorative edition, pp. 44-47). Philadelphia: Lippincott.

Newman, M. A. (1994). *Health as expanding consciousness* (2nd ed.). Sudbury MA: Jones & Bartlett (NLN Press).

Newman, M. A. (1995a). *A developing discipline: Selected works of Margaret Newman.* New York: National League for Nursing Press.

Newman, M. A. (1995b). Dialogue: Margaret Newman and the rhetoric of nursing theory. *Image: The Journal of Nursing Scholarship, 27*, 261.

Newman, M. A. (1995c). Recognizing a pattern of expanding consciousness in persons with cancer. In M. A. Newman (Ed.), *A developing discipline: Selected works of Margaret Newman* (pp. 159-171). New York: National League for Nursing Press.

Newman, M. A. (1997a). Evolution of the theory of health as expanding consciousness. *Nursing Science Quarterly, 10*, 22-25.

Newman, M. A. (1997b). Experiencing the whole. *ANS Advances in Nursing Science, 20*, 34-39.

Newman, M. A. (1999). The rhythm of relating in a paradigm of wholeness. *Image: The Journal of Nursing Scholarship, 31*, 227-230.

Newman, M. A. (2003). A world of no boundaries. *ANS Advances in Nursing Science, 26*(4), 240-245.

Newman, M. A. (2005). Foreword. In C. Picard & D. Jones (Eds.), *Giving voice to what we know: Margaret Newman's theory of health as expanding consciousness* (pp. xii-xv). Sudbury, MA: Jones & Bartlett.

Newman, M. A. (2008). *Transforming presence: The difference that nursing makes.* Philadelphia: F. A. Davis Company.

Newman, M. A., & Autio, S. (1986). *Nursing in a prospective payment system health care environment.* Minneapolis: University of Minnesota.

Newman, M. A., & Gaudiano, J. K. (1984). Depression as an explanation for decreased subjective time in the elderly. *Nursing Research, 33*, 137-139.

Newman, M. A., Lamb, G. S., & Michaels, C. (1991). Nurse case management: The coming together of theory and practice. *Nursing and Health Care, 12*, 404-408.

Newman, M. A., & Moch, S. D. (1991). Life patterns of persons with coronary heart disease. *Nursing Science Quarterly, 4*, 161-167.

Newman, M. A., Sime, M. A., & Corcoran–Perry, S. A. (1991). The focus of the discipline of nursing. *ANS Advances in Nursing Science, 14*, 1-6.

Noveletsky-Rosenthal, H. T. (1996). Pattern recognition in older adults living with chronic illness (Doctoral dissertation, Boston College). *Dissertation Abstracts International, 57*, 6180.

Peters-Lewis, A. (2006). How the strong survive: Health as expanding consciousness and the life experiences of Black Caribbean women. Doctoral Dissertation. Boston College.

Pharris, M. D. (2002). Coming to know ourselves as community through a nursing partnership with adolescents convicted of murder. *ANS Advances in Nursing Science, 24*(3), 21-42.

Pharris, M. D. (2005). Engaging with communities in a pattern recognition process. In C. Picard & D. Jones (Eds.), *Giving voice to what we know: Margaret Newman's theory of health as expanding consciousness in nursing practice, research, and education.*(pp. 83-93). Sudbury, MA: Jones & Bartlett.

Picard, C. A. (2000). Pattern of expanding consciousness in mid-life women: Creative movement and the narrative as modes of expression. *Nursing Science Quarterly, 13*, 150-158.

Picard, C. (2002). Family reflections on living through sudden death of a child. *Nursing Science Quarterly, 15*, 242-250.

Picard, C., & Jones, D. (Eds.) (2007) *Giving voice to what we know: Margaret Newman's theory of health as expanding consciousness in nursing practice, research, and education.* Sudbury, MA: Jones & Bartlett.

Picard, C., & Mariolis, T. (2002). Teaching-learning process. Praxis as a mirroring process: Teaching psychiatric nursing grounded in Newman's health as expanding consciousness. *Nursing Science Quarterly, 15*, 118-122.

Picard, C., & Mariolis, T. (2005). Praxis as a mirroring process: Teaching psychiatric nursing grounded in Newman's health as expanding consciousness. In C. Picard & D. Jones (Eds.), *Giving voice to what we know: Margaret Newman's theory of health as expanding consciousness in nursing practice, research, and education.* (pp. 169-177). Sudbury, MA: Jones & Bartlett.

Prigogine, I. (1976). Order through fluctuation: Self-organization and social system. In E. Jantsch & C. H. Waddington (Eds.), *Evolution and consciousness* (pp. 93-133). Reading, MA: Addison-Wesley.

Quinn, J. F. (1992). Holding sacred space: The nurse as healing environment. *Holistic Nursing Practice, 6*(4), 26-36.

Reed, P. G. (1996). Transcendence: Formulating nursing perspectives. *Nursing Science Quarterly, 9*, 2-4.

Rogers, M. E. (1970). Nursing, a science of unitary man. In J. P. Riehl & C. Roy (Eds.), *Conceptual models for nursing practice.* New York: Appleton-Century-Crofts.

Rosa, K. C. (2006). A process model of healing and personal transformation in persons with chronic skin wounds. *Nursing Science Quarterly, 19*(4), 359-358.

Roux, G., Bush, H. A., & Dingley, C. E. (2001). Inner strength in women with breast cancer. *Journal of Theory Construction and Testing, 5*(1), 19-27.

Roy, C., Rogers, M. C., Fitzpatrick, J. J., Newman, M., & Orem, D. E. (1982). Nursing diagnosis and nursing theory. In M. J. King & D. A. Moritz (Eds.), *Classification of nursing diagnosis* (pp. 215-231). New York: McGraw Hill.

Ruka, S. (2005). Creating balance: Rhythms and patterns in people with dementia living in a nursing home. In C. Picard & D. Jones (Eds.), *Giving voice to what we know: Margaret Newman's theory of health as expanding consciousness in nursing practice, research, and education.* Sudbury, MA: Jones & Bartlett.

Schlotzhauer, M., & Farnham, R. (1997). Newman's theory and insulin dependent diabetes mellitus in adolescence. *Journal of School Nursing, 13*(3), 20-23.

Schmidt, B. J., Brauer, D. J., & Peden-McAlpine, C. (2003). Experiencing health in the context of rheumatoid arthritis. *Nursing Science Quarterly, 16*, 155-162.

Schmitt, N. (1991). *Caregiving couples: The experience of giving and receiving social support.* Unpublished doctoral dissertation, University of Minnesota, Rochester.

Schorr, J. A. (1993). Music and pattern change in chronic pain. *ANS Advances in Nursing Science, 15*(4), 27-36.

Schorr, J. A., Farnham, R. C., & Ervin, S. M. (1991). Health patterns in aging women as expanding consciousness. *ANS Advances in Nursing Science, 13*(4), 52-63.

Schorr, J. A., & Schroeder, C. A. (1989). Consciousness as a dissipative structure: An extension of the Newman model. *Nursing Science Quarterly, 2*, 183-193.

Schorr, J. A., & Schroeder, C. A. (1991). Movement and time: Exertion and perceived duration. *Nursing Science Quarterly, 4*, 104-112.

Schroeder, C. A. (1993). Perceived duration of time and bedrest in high risk pregnancy: An exploration of the Newman model. *Dissertation Abstracts International, 54*, 1984.

Shanahan, S. M. (1993). The lived experience of life-passing in middle adolescent females. *Masters Abstracts International, 32*, 1376.

Smith, C. A. (1995). The lived experience of staying healthy in rural African American families. *Nursing Science Quarterly, 8*, 17-21.

Smith, S. K. (1997). Women's experiences of victimizing socialization. Part I: Responses related to abuse and home and family environment. *Issues in Mental Health Nursing, 18*, 395-416.

Thomas, J. A. (2002). What are the life patterns of people with hepatitis C? (Doctoral dissertation, University of Nevada, Reno). *Dissertation Abstracts International, 41*, 194.

Tommet, P. A. (2003). Nurse-parent dialogue: Illuminating the evolving pattern of families of children who are medically fragile. *Nursing Science Quarterly, 16*(3), 239-246.

Utley, R. (1999). The evolving meaning of cancer for long-term survivors of breast cancer. *Oncology Nursing Forum, 26*, 1519-1523.

Walls, P. W. (1999). Community participation in primary health care: A qualitative study of empowerment of health care workers (Doctoral dissertation, Loyola University of Chicago). *Dissertation Abstracts International, 60*, 2065.

Weed, L. D. (2004). *The meaning of the death of an adult child to an elder: A phenomenological investigation.* Unpublished doctoral dissertation, University of Tennessee, Knoxville.

Weingourt, R. (1998). Using Margaret A. Newman's theory of health with elderly nursing home residents. *Perspectives in Psychiatric Care, 34*(3), 25-30.

Yamashita, M. (1995). *Family coping with mental illness: An application of Newman's research as praxis.* Paper presented at the Midwest Nursing Research Society 19th Annual Conference, Kansas City, MO.

Yamashita, M. (1999). Newman's theory of health applied to family caregiving in Canada. *Nursing Science Quarterly, 12*, 73-79.

Young, A. M. (1976). *The reflexive universe: Evolution of consciousness.* San Francisco: Robert Briggs.

BIBLIOGRAPHY

Acton, H. B. (1967). George Wilhelm Freidrich Hegel 1770-1831. In P. Edwards (Ed.), *The encyclopedia of philosophy* (Vols. 3 & 4). New York: Macmillan & Free Press.

Barron, A. (2005). Suffering, growth, and possibility: Health as expanding consciousness in end-of-life care. In C. Picard & D. Jones (Eds.), *Giving voice to what we know: Margaret Newman's theory of health as expanding consciousness in nursing practice, research, and education.* (pp. 43-50). Sudbury, MA: Jones & Bartlett.

Batty, M. L. E. (1999). Pattern identification and expanding consciousness during the transition of "low risk" pregnancy. A study embodying Newman's health as expanding consciousness (Margaret Newman) (Master's thesis, The University of New Brunswick, Canada, 1999). *Masters Abstracts International, 39*, 826.

Bentov, I. (1977). *Stalking the wild pendulum.* New York: E. P. Dutton.

Berry, D. C. (2002). Newman's theory of health as expanding consciousness in women maintaining weight loss (Doctoral dissertation, Boston College, 2002). *Dissertation Abstracts International, 63*, 2300.

Bohm, D. (1980). *Wholeness and the implicate order.* London: Routledge and Kegan Paul.

Brauer, D. J. (2001). Common patterns of person-environment interaction in persons with rheumatoid arthritis. *Western Journal of Nursing Research, 23*, 414-430.

Brown, J. W., & Alligood, M. R. (2004). Realizing wrongness: Stories of older wife caregivers. *Journal of Applied Gerontology, 23*(2), 104-119.

Brown, J.W., & Chen, S-L., Mitchell, C., Province, A. (2007). Help-seeking by older husbands caring for wives with dementia. *Journal of Advanced Nursing, 58*(3), 1-9.

Bruce-Barrett, C. A. (1998). Patterns of health and healing: Peer support and prostate cancer (Master's thesis, D'Youville College, 1998). *Masters Abstracts International, 37*, 0233.

Bunkers, S. S., Bendtro, M., Holmes, P. K., Howell, J., Johnson, S., Koerner, J., et al. (1992). The healing web: A transformative model for nursing. *Nursing and Health Care, 13*, 68-73.

Capasso, V. A. (2005). The theory is the practice: An exemplar. In C. Picard & D. Jones (Eds.), *Giving voice to what we know: Margaret Newman's theory of health as expanding consciousness in nursing practice, research, and education.*(pp. 65-71). Sudbury, MA: Jones & Bartlett.

Casper, S. A. (1999). Psychological adaptation as a dimension of health as expanding consciousness: Effectiveness of burn survivors support groups (Master's thesis, D'Youville College, 1999). *Masters Abstracts International, 37*, 1433.

Cowling, W. R. III, Newman, M., Watson, J., & Smith, M. (2007). The power of wholeness, consciousness, and caring: a dialogue on nursing science, art, and healing. (Abstract) *International Journal for Human Caring, 11*(3), 52.

Endo, E. (1998). Pattern recognition as a nursing intervention with Japanese women with ovarian cancer. *ANS Advances in Nursing Science, 20*(4), 49-61.

Endo, E., Miyahara, t., Sizuli, S., Ohmasa, T. (2005). Caring partnering between nurse educator and practicing nurses. *Nursing Science Quarterly, 32*(3), 6-3-610.

Endo, E., Nitta, N., Inayoshi, M., Saito, R., Takemura, K., Minegishi, H., et al. (2000). Pattern recognition as a caring partnership in families with cancer. *Journal of Advanced Nursing, 32*, 603-610.

Endo, E., Takaki, M., Abe, K., Terashima, K., & Nitta, N. (2007). *Creating a helping model with nursing students who want to quit smoking: Patterning in a nursing student-teacher partnership based on M. Newman's theory of health.* Paper presented at The Power of Caring: The Gateway to Healing, 29th Annual International Association for Human Caring Conference. St. Louis: MO. May 16-19, 2007.

Engle, V. (1986). The relationship of movement and time to older adults' functional health. *Research in Nursing and Health, 9*, 123-129.

Falkenstern, S. K. (2003). *Nursing facilitation of health as expanding consciousness in families who have a child with special health care needs.* Unpublished doctoral dissertation, Pennsylvania State University, University Park, PA.

Flannagan, J. M. (2005). Creating a healing environment for staff and patients in a pre-surgery clinic. In C. Picard & D. Jones (Eds.), *Giving voice to what we know: Margaret Newman's theory of health as expanding consciousness in nursing practice, research, and education.* Sudbury, MA: Jones & Bartlett.

Fryback, P. B. (1991). Perceptions of health by persons with a terminal disease: Implications for nursing. *Dissertation Abstracts International, 52*, 1951.

Gross, S. W. (1995). The impact of a nursing intervention of relaxation with guided imagery on breast cancer patients' stress and health as expanding consciousness (Doctoral dissertation, University of Texas at Austin, 1995). *Dissertation Abstracts International, 56*, 5416.

Gulick, E. E., & Bugg, A. (1992). Holistic health patterning in multiple sclerosis. *Research in Nursing and Health, 15*, 175-185.

Gustafson, W. (1990). Application of Newman's theory of health: Pattern recognition as nursing practice. In M. Parker (Ed.), *Nursing theories in practice* (pp. 141-161). New York: National League for Nursing.

Jacono, B. J., & Jacono, J. J. (1996). The benefits of Newman and Parse in helping nurse teachers determine methods to enhance student creativity. *Nurse Education Today, 16*, 356-362.

Jonsdottir, H. (1998). Life patterns of people with chronic obstructive pulmonary disease: Isolation and being closed in. *Nursing Science Quarterly, 11*, 160-166.

Kalb, K. A. (1990). The gift: Applying Newman's theory of health in nursing practice. In M. Parker (Ed.), *Nursing theories in practice* (pp. 163-186). New York: National League for Nursing.

Karian, V. E., Jankowski, S. M., & Beal, J. A. (1998). Exploring the lived experience of childhood cancer survivors. *Journal of Pediatric Oncology, 15*, 153-162.

Kiser-Larson, N. (2002). Life pattern of native women experiencing breast cancer. *International Journal for Human Caring, 6*(2), 61-68.

Lamb, G. S., & Stempel, J. E. (1994). Nurse case management from the client's view: Growing as insider-expert. *Nursing Outlook, 42*, 7-13.

Lamendola, F. P., & Newman, M. A. (1994). The paradox of HIV/AIDS as expanding consciousness. *ANS Advances in Nursing Science, 16(3)*, 13-21.

Litchfield, M. (1999). Practice wisdom. *ANS Advances in Nursing Science, 22*(2), 62-73.

Litchfield, M. C. (1993). *The process of health patterning in families with young children who have been repeatedly hospitalized.* Unpublished master's thesis, University of Minnesota, Rochester.

Litchfield, M. C. (1997). The process of nursing partnership in family health (Doctoral dissertation, University of Minnesota). *Dissertation Abstracts International, 59*, 1802.

Magan, S. J., Gibbon, E. J., & Mrozek, R. (1990). Nursing theory application: A practice model. *Issues in Mental Health Nursing, 11*, 297-312.

Marchione, J. M. (1986). Pattern as methodology for assessing family health: Newman's theory of health. In P. Winstead-Fry (Ed.), *Case studies in nursing theory.* New York: National League for Nursing.

Mentzer, C., & Schorr, J. A. (1986). Perceived situational control and perceived duration of time: Expressions of life patterns. *ANS Advances in Nursing Science, 9*(1), 13-20.

Moch, S. D. (1990). Health within the experience of breast cancer. *Journal of Advanced Nursing, 15*, 1426-1435.

Moch, S. D. (1998). Health-within-illness: Concept development through research and practice. *Journal of Advanced Nursing, 28*, 305-310.

Moss, R. (1981). *The I that is we.* Millbrae, CA: Celestial Arts.

Musker, K. M. (2005). *Life patterns of women transitioning through menopause* PhD dissertation. Loyola University, Chicago.

Neill, J. (2002). Transcendence and transformation in the life patterns of women living with rheumatoid arthritis. *ANS Advances in Nursing Science, 24*(4), 27-47.

Neill, J. (2005). Recognizing pattern in the lives of women with multiple sclerosis. In C. Picard & D. Jones (Eds.), *Giving voice to what we know* (pp. 153-165). Sudbury. MA: Jones & Bartlett.

Newman, M. A. (1971). *An investigation of the relationship between gait tempo and time perception.* Unpublished doctoral dissertation, New York University, New York.

Newman, M. A. (1972). Time estimation in relation to gait tempo. *Perceptual and Motor Skills, 34*, 359-366.

Newman, M. A. (1979). *Theory development in nursing.* Philadelphia: F. A. Davis.

Newman, M. A. (1982). Time as an index of expanding consciousness with age. *Nursing Research, 31*, 290-293.

Newman, M. A. (1983). Newman's health theory. In I. W. Clements & F. B. Roberts (Eds.), *Family health: A theoretical approach to nursing care.* New York: John Wiley & Sons.

Newman, M. A. (1986). *Health as expanding consciousness.* St. Louis: Mosby.

Newman, M. A. (1987a). Aging as increasing complexity. *Journal of Gerontological Nursing, 13*(9), 16-18.

Newman, M. A. (1987b). Patterning. In M. Duffy & N. J. Pender (Eds.), *Conceptual issues in health promotion.* A report of proceedings of a wingspread conference, Racine, WI, April 13-15, 1987. Indianapolis: Sigma Theta Tau.

Newman, M. A. (1989). The spirit of nursing. *Holistic Nursing Practice, 3*(3), 1-6.

Newman, M. A. (1990a). Newman's theory of health as praxis. *Nursing Science Quarterly, 3*, 37-41.

Newman, M. A. (1990c). Shifting to higher consciousness. In M. Parker (Ed.), *Nursing theories in practice* (pp. 129-139). New York: National League for Nursing.

Newman, M. A. (1991). Health conceptualizations. In J. J. Fitzpatrick, R. L. Taunton, & A. K. Jacox (Eds.), *Annual review of nursing research* (Vol. 9). New York: Springer.

Newman, M. A. (1992). Nightingale's vision of nursing theory and health. In Nightingale, F., *Notes on nursing: What it is, and what it is not* (commemorative edition, pp. 44-47). Philadelphia: Lippincott.

Newman, M. A. (1994). *Health as expanding consciousness* (2nd ed.). New York: National League for Nursing Press.

Newman, M. A. (1994). Theory for nursing practice. *Nursing Science Quarterly, 7*, 153-157.

Newman, M. A. (1995). Dialogue: Margaret Newman and the rhetoric of nursing theory. *Image: The Journal of Nursing Scholarship, 27*, 261.

Newman, M. A. (1995). Recognizing a pattern of expanding consciousness in persons with cancer. In M. A. Newman (Ed.), *A developing discipline: Selected works of Margaret Newman* (pp. 159-171). New York: National League for Nursing Press.

Newman, M. A. (1997). Evolution of the theory of health as expanding consciousness. *Nursing Science Quarterly, 10*, 22-25.

Newman, M. A. (1997). Experiencing the whole. *ANS Advances in Nursing Science, 20*, 34-39.

Newman, M. A. (1999). Letters to the editor . . . a commentary on Newman's theory of health as expanding consciousness. *ANS Advances in Nursing Science, 21*(3), viii-ix.

Newman, M. A. (1999). The rhythm of relating in a paradigm of wholeness. *Image: The Journal of Nursing Scholarship, 31*, 227-230.

Newman, M. A. (2002). Caring in the human health experience. *International Journal for Human Caring, 6*(2), 8-12.

Newman, M. A. (2003). A world of no boundaries. *ANS Advances in Nursing Science, 26*(4), 240-245.

Newman, M. A. (2005). Foreword. In C. Picard & D. Jones (Eds.), *Giving voice to what we know: Margaret Newman's theory of health as expanding consciousness* (pp. xii-xv). Sudbury, MA: Jones & Bartlett.

Newman, M. A. (2008). *Transforming presence: The difference that nursing makes.* Philadelphia: F. A. Davis Company.

Newman, M. A., & Autio, S. (1986). *Nursing in a prospective payment system health care environment.* Minneapolis: University of Minnesota.

Newman, M. A., & Gaudiano, J. K. (1984). Depression as an explanation for decreased subjective time in the elderly. *Nursing Research, 33*, 137-139.

Newman, M. A., Lamb, G. S., & Michaels, C. (1991). Nurse case management: The coming together of theory and practice. *Nursing and Health Care, 12*, 404-408.

Newman, M. A., & Moch, S. D. (1991). Life patterns of persons with coronary heart disease. *Nursing Science Quarterly, 4*, 161-167.

Newman, M. A., Sime, M. A., & Corcoran-Perry, S. A. (1991). The focus of the discipline of nursing. *ANS Advances in Nursing Science, 14*, 1-6.

Noveletsky-Rosenthal, H. T. (1996). Pattern recognition in older adults living with chronic illness (Doctoral dissertation, Boston College). *Dissertation Abstracts International, 57*, 6180.

Peters-Lewis, A. (2006). How the strong survive: Health as expanding consciousness and the life experiences of Black Caribbean women. Doctoral Dissertation. Boston College.

Pharris, M.D. (2001). Margaret A. Newman, Health as Expanding Consciousness. In M. Parker (Ed.). *Nursing Theories and Nursing Practice.* Philadelphia: F. A. Davis.

Pharris, M. D. (2002). Coming to know ourselves as community through a nursing partnership with adolescents convicted of murder. *ANS Advances in Nursing Science, 24*(3), 21-42.

Pharris, M. D. (2005). Engaging with communities in a pattern recognition process. In C. Picard & D. Jones (Eds.), *Giving voice to what we know: Margaret Newman's theory of health as expanding consciousness in nursing practice, research, and education.* (pp. 83-93). Sudbury, MA: Jones & Bartlett.

Picard, C. (2002). Family reflections on living through sudden death of a child. *Nursing Science Quarterly, 15*, 242-250.

Picard, C. A. (2000). Pattern of expanding consciousness in mid-life women: Creative movement and the narrative as modes of expression. *Nursing Science Quarterly, 13*, 150-158.

Picard, C., & Jones, D. (Eds.) (2007). *Giving voice to what we know: Margaret Newman's theory of health as expanding consciousness in nursing practice, research, and education.* Sudbury, MA: Jones & Bartlett.

Picard, C., & Mariolis, T. (2002). Teaching-learning process. Praxis as a mirroring process: Teaching psychiatric nursing grounded in Newman's health as expanding consciousness. *Nursing Science Quarterly, 15*, 118-122.

Picard, C., & Mariolis, T. (2005). Praxis as a mirroring process: Teaching psychiatric nursing grounded in Newman's health as expanding consciousness. In C. Picard & D. Jones (Eds.), *Giving voice to what we know: Margaret Newman's theory of health as expanding consciousness in nursing practice, research, and education.* (pp. 169-177). Sudbury, MA: Jones & Bartlett.

Prigogine, I. (1976). Order through fluctuation: Self-organization and social system. In E. Jantsch & C. H. Waddington (Eds.), *Evolution and consciousness* (pp. 93-133). Reading, MA: Addison-Wesley.

Quinn, J. F. (1992). Holding sacred space: The nurse as healing environment. *Holistic Nursing Practice, 6*(4), 26-36.

Reed, P. G. (1996). Transcendence: Formulating nursing perspectives. *Nursing Science Quarterly, 9*, 2-4.

Rogers, M. E. (1980). Nursing, a science of unitary man. In J. P. Riehl & C. Roy (Eds.), *Conceptual models for nursing practice.* New York: Appleton-Century-Crofts.

Rosa, K. C. (2006). A process model of healing and personal transformation in persons with chronic skin wounds. *Nursing Science Quarterly, 19*(4), 359-358.

Roux, G., Bush, H. A., & Dingley, C. E. (2001). Inner strength in women with breast cancer. *Journal of Theory Construction and Testing, 5*(1), 19-27.

Roy, C., Rogers, M. C., Fitzpatrick, J. J., Newman, M., & Orem, D. E. (1982). Nursing diagnosis and nursing theory. In M. J. King & D. A. Moritz (Eds.), *Classification of nursing diagnosis* (pp. 215-231). New York: McGraw Hill.

Ruka, S. (2005). Creating balance: Rhythms and patterns in people with dementia living in a nursing home. In C. Picard & D. Jones (Eds.), *Giving voice to what we know: Margaret Newman's theory of health as expanding consciousness in nursing practice, research, and education.* Sudbury, MA: Jones & Bartlett.

Schlotzhauer, M., & Farnham, R. (1997). Newman's theory and insulin dependent diabetes mellitus in adolescence. *Journal of School Nursing, 13*(3), 20-23.

Schmidt, B. J., Brauer, D. J., & Peden-McAlpine, C. (2003). Experiencing health in the context of rheumatoid arthritis. *Nursing Science Quarterly, 16*, 155-162.

Schmitt, N. (1991). *Caregiving couples: The experience of giving and receiving social support.* Unpublished doctoral dissertation, University of Minnesota, Rochester.

Schorr, J. A. (1993). Music and pattern change in chronic pain. *ANS Advances in Nursing Science, 15*(4), 27-36.

Schorr, J. A., Farnham, R. C., & Ervin, S. M. (1991). Health patterns in aging women as expanding consciousness. *ANS Advances in Nursing Science, 13*(4), 52-63.

Schorr, J. A., & Schroeder, C. A. (1989). Consciousness as a dissipative structure: An extension of the Newman model. *Nursing Science Quarterly, 2*, 183-193.

Schorr, J. A., & Schroeder, C. A. (1991). Movement and time: Exertion and perceived duration. *Science Quarterly, 4*, 104-112.

Schroeder, C. A. (1993). Perceived duration of time and bedrest in high risk pregnancy: An exploration of the Newman model. *Dissertation Abstracts International, 54*, 1984.

Shanahan, S. M. (1993). The lived experience of life-passing in middle adolescent females. *Masters Abstracts International, 32*, 1376.

Smith, C. A. (1995). The lived experience of staying healthy in rural African American families. *Nursing Science Quarterly, 8*, 17-21.

Smith, S. K. (1997). Women's experiences of victimizing socialization. Part I: Responses related to abuse and home and family environment. *Issues in Mental Health Nursing, 18*, 395-416.

Thomas, J. A. (2002). What are the life patterns of people with hepatitis C? (Doctoral dissertation, University of Nevada, Reno). *Dissertation Abstracts International, 41*, 194.

Tommet, P. A. (2003). Nurse-parent dialogue: Illuminating the evolving pattern of families of children who are medically fragile. *Nursing Science Quarterly, 16*(3), 239-246.

Utley, R. (1999). The evolving meaning of cancer for long-term survivors of breast cancer. *Oncology Nursing Forum, 26*, 1519-1523.

Walls, P. W. (1999). Community participation in primary health care: A qualitative study of empowerment of health care workers (Doctoral dissertation, Loyola University of Chicago). *Dissertation Abstracts International, 60*, 2065.

Weed, L. D. (2004). *The meaning of the death of an adult child to an elder: A phenomenological investigation.* Unpublished doctoral dissertation, University of Tennessee, Knoxville.

Weingourt, R. (1998). Using Margaret A. Newman's theory of health with elderly nursing home residents. *Perspectives in Psychiatric Care, 34*(3), 25-30.

Yamashita, M. (1995). *Family coping with mental illness: An application of Newman's research as praxis.* Paper presented at the Midwest Nursing Research Society 19th Annual Conference, Kansas City, MO.

Yamashita, M. (1999). Newman's theory of health applied to family caregiving in Canada. *Nursing Science Quarterly, 12*, 73-79.

Young, A. M. (1976). *The reflexive universe: Evolution of consciousness.* San Francisco: Robert Briggs

Additional Suggested Readings

Brown, J. W. (2006). Newman's theory of health and nursing practice. In M. R. Alligood & A. M. Tomey (Eds.), *Nursing theory: Utilization & application* (3rd ed.). St. Louis: Mosby.

Dean, P. J. (2002). Aesthetic expression. A poem dedicated to the nursing theories of Martha Rogers and Margaret Newman. *International Journal for Human Caring, 6*, 70.

Ford-Gilboe, M. V. (1994). A comparison of two nursing models: Allen's developmental health model and Newman's theory of health as expanding consciousness. *Nursing Science Quarterly, 7*, 113-118.

Jonsdottir, H., Litchfield, M., & Pharris, M. D. (2003). Partnership in practice. *Research and Theory for Nursing Practice, 17*, 51-63.

Marchione, J. (1993). *Margaret Newman: Health as expanding consciousness.* Newbury Park, CA: Sage

Neill, J. (2002). From practice to caring praxis through Newman's theory of health as expanding consciousness: A personal journey. *International Journal for Human Caring, 6*(2), 48-54.

Nelson, M. L., Howell, J. K., Larson, J. C., & Karpiuk, K. L. (2001). Student outcomes of the healing web: Evaluation of a transformative model for nursing education. *Journal of Nursing Education, 40*, 404-413.

Newman, M. A. (1981). The meaning of health. In G. E. Laskar (Ed.), Applied systems research and cybernetics: Vol. 4. Systems research in health care, biocybernetics and ecology (pp. 1739-1743). New York: Pergamon.

Newman, M. A. (1987). Nursing's emerging paradigm: The diagnosis of pattern. In A. M. McLane (Ed.), Classification of nursing diagnoses. Proceedings of the seventh conference, North American nursing diagnosis association (pp. 53-60). St. Louis: Mosby.

Newman, M. A. (1993). Prevailing paradigms in nursing. *Nursing Outlook, 40*(1), 10-14.

Newman, M. A. (1996). Prevailing paradigms in nursing. In J. W. Kenney (Ed.), Philosophical and theoretical perspectives for advanced nursing practice (pp. 302-307). Sudbury, MA: Jones & Bartlett.

Newman, M. A. (1996). Theory of the nurse-client partnership. In E. Cohen (Ed.), Nurse case management in the 21st century (pp. 119-123). St. Louis: Mosby.

Newman, M. A. (1997). A dialogue with Martha Rogers and David Bohm about the science of unitary human beings. In M. Madrid (Ed.), Patterns of Rogerian knowing (pp. 3-10). New York: National League for Nursing Press.

Newman, M. A. (2003). The immediate applicability of nursing praxis. *Quality Nursing: The Japanese Journal of Nursing Education and Nursing Research, 9*(5), 4-6.

Yamashita, M. (1997). Family caregiving: Application of Newman's and Peplau's theories. *Journal of Psychiatric and Mental Health Nursing, 4*, 401-405.

Yamashita, M. (1998). Family coping with mental illness: A comparative study. *Journal of Psychiatric and Mental Health Nursing, 5*, 515-523.

Yamashita, M. (1998). Newman's theory of health as expanding consciousness: Research on family caregiving in mental illness in Japan. *Nursing Science Quarterly, 11*, 110-115.

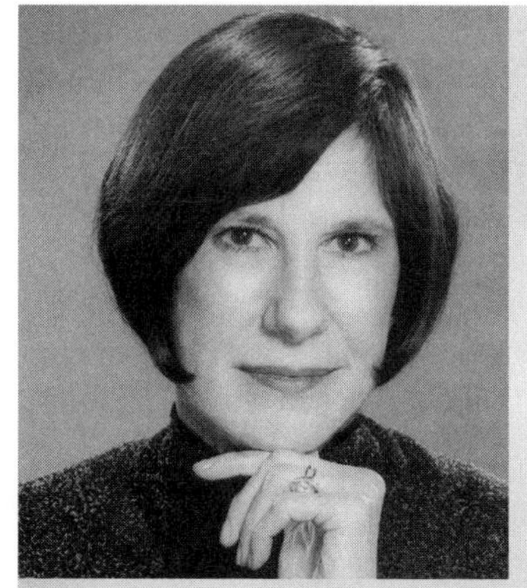

Photo copyright 1998 by Jonas, Pittsburgh.

CHAPTER 24

Rosemarie Rizzo Parse

Humanbecoming

Gail J. Mitchell and Debra A. Bournes

"The assumptions and principles of humanbecoming incarnate a deep concern for the delicate sentiments of being human and show a profound recognition of human freedom and dignity" (Parse, 2007b, p. 310).

CREDENTIALS AND BACKGROUND OF THE THEORIST

Rosemarie Rizzo Parse, a member of the American Academy of Nursing, is Distinguished Professor Emeritus at Loyola University Chicago. She is founder and editor of *Nursing Science Quarterly,* and president of Discovery International, which sponsors international nursing theory conferences. Dr. Parse is also founder of the *Institute of Humanbecoming,* where she teaches the ontological, epistemological, and methodological aspects of the humanbecoming school of thought (Parse, 1981, 1992, 1996, 1998, 2007b). She consults throughout the world with doctoral programs in nursing and with healthcare settings that are utilizing her theory as a guide to research, practice, education, and regulation of standards for quality in practice and education.

Dr. Parse is the author of many articles and books, including *Nursing Fundamentals* (1974), *Man-Living-Health: A Theory of Nursing* (1981), *Nursing Science: Major Paradigms, Theories and Critiques* (1987), *Nursing Research: Qualitative Methods* (1985) (co-authored), *Illuminations: The Human Becoming Theory in Practice and Research* (1995), *The Human Becoming School of Thought: A Perspective for Nurses and other Health Professionals* (1998), *Hope: An International Human Becoming Perspective* (1999), *Qualitative Inquiry: The Path of Sciencing* (2001b), and *Community: A Human Becoming Perspective* (2003a). *The Human Becoming School of Thought* (1998) was selected for Sigma Theta

Previous authors: Kathleen D. Pickrell, Rickard E. Lee, Larry P. Schumacher, and Prudence Twigg.
The authors wish to thank Dr. Rosemarie Rizzo Parse for reviewing the chapter.

Tau and Doody Publishing's "Best Picks" list in the nursing theory book category in 1998. *Hope: An International Human Becoming Perspective* was selected for the same list in 1999. Many of her works have been translated into Danish, Finnish, French, German, Italian, Japanese, Spanish, Swedish, Taiwanese, Korean, and other languages.

Dr. Parse graduated from Duquesne University in Pittsburgh and received her master's and doctorate from the University of Pittsburgh. She was a member of the faculty of the University of Pittsburgh, Dean of the Nursing School at Duquesne University, Professor and Coordinator of the Center for Nursing Research at Hunter College of the City University of New York (1983-1993), and Professor and Niehoff Chair at Loyola University Chicago (1993-2006). In 2001, the Unitary Research Section of the Midwest Nursing Research Society recognized Dr. Parse's contributions to the discipline by presenting her with a Lifetime Achievement Award. She also received the Lifetime Achievement Award from the Asian American Pacific Islander Nurses Association.

Parse's multiple research projects and interests are focused on lived experiences of health and human becoming. She has developed basic and applied science research methodologies (Parse, 2005) congruent with the ontology of humanbecoming and has conducted and published numerous investigations on a wide variety of phenomena, including laughter, health, aging, quality of life, joy-sorrow, contentment, feeling very tired, respect, and hope. She was principal investigator for the Hope study, which included participants and coinvestigators from nine countries (Parse, 1999). Following that, Parse (2007a) further elaborated understanding of the concept of hope in her humanbecoming hermeneutic study of hope in King's (1982) "Rita Hayworth and Shawshank Redemption." Parse's research methodologies have been used by nurse scholars in Australia, Canada, Denmark, Finland, Greece, Italy, Japan, South Korea, Sweden, Switzerland, the United Kingdom, the United States, and other countries (Doucet & Bournes, 2007). Her theory guides practice in various healthcare settings in Canada, Finland, South Korea, Sweden, Switzerland, the United Kingdom, the United States, and others. Humanbecoming is also used as a guide for education, administration, leadership, change, mentoring, and regulation in several settings on five continents.

THEORETICAL SOURCES

The humanbecoming school of thought is grounded in human science proposed by Dilthey and others over the past century (Cody & Mitchell, 2002; Mitchell & Cody, 1992; Parse, 1981, 1987, 1998, 2007b). The humanbecoming school of thought is "consistent with Martha E. Rogers' principles and postulates about unitary human beings, and it is consistent with major tenets and concepts from existential-phenomenological thought, but it is a new product, a different conceptual system" (Parse, 1998, p. 4). At the time she was developing her theory, Parse was working at Duquesne University in Pittsburgh. While she was there (during the 1960s and 1970s), Duquesne was regarded as the center of the existential-phenomenological movement in the United States. Dialogues she had with scholars in this school of thought, such as van Kaam and Giorgi, stimulated and focused her thinking on the lived experiences of human beings and their situated freedom and participation in life.

By synthesizing the science of unitary human beings, developed by Martha E. Rogers (1970, 1992), with the fundamental tenets from existential-phenomenological thought, as articulated by Heidegger, Sartre, and Merleau-Ponty, Parse secured nursing as a human science. She contends that humans cannot be reduced to component systems or parts and still be understood. Persons are living beings who are more than and different from any schemata that divide them. Parse challenges the traditional medical view of nursing and distinguishes the discipline of nursing as a unique, basic science focused on human lived experience. Parse supports the notion that nurses require a unique knowledge base that informs their practice and research, and this knowledge (of the humanuniverse process) is essential for nurses to fulfill their commitment to humankind (Parse, 1981, 1987, 1993, 2007b).

In developing her theory, Parse was especially influenced by Rogers' principles of helicy, integrality, and resonancy and by her postulates (energy field, openness, pattern, and pandimensionality) (Parse, 1981; Rogers, 1970, 1992). These ideas underpin Parse's notions about persons as open beings who relate with the universe illimitably, that is, "with indivisible, unbounded knowing extended to infinity" (Parse, 2007b, p. 308), and who are indivisible, unpredictable, everchanging, and recognized by patterns (Parse, 1981, 1998, 2007b).

From existential-phenomenological thought, Parse drew on the tenets of intentionality and human subjectivity and the corresponding concepts of coconstitution, coexistence, and situated freedom (Parse, 1981, 1998). Parse uses the prefix *co* on many of her words to denote the participative nature of persons. *Co* means *together with,* and for Parse, humans can never be separated from their relationships with the universe. Relationships with the universe include all the linkages humans have with other people and with ideas, projects, predecessors, history, and culture (Parse, 1981, 1998).

From Parse's perspective, humans are intentional beings. By this she means that human beings have an open and meaningful stance with the universe and the people, projects, and ideas that constitute lived experience. Human beings are intentional in that their involvements are not random but are chosen for reasons known and not known. Parse says that being human is being intentional and present, open, and knowing with the world. Intentionality is also about purpose and how persons choose direction and ways of thinking and acting toward projects and people. People choose attitudes and next actions from a realm of possibilities (Parse, 1981, 1998).

The basic tenet, human subjectivity, means viewing human beings not as things or objects but as beings that are indivisible, unpredictable, and everchanging (Parse, 1998), and as beings that are a mystery of being with nonbeing. Human beings live what was, is, and will be in the now moments of their intersubjective relationships with the universe. Parse posits that the human's presence in and relationship with the world are personal, and humans assign meaning to their lives and to their projects in the process of becoming who they are. As people choose meanings and projects, according to their value priorities, they coparticipate with the world in indivisible, unbounded ways (Parse, 1981, 1998, 2007b). Every person, although inseparable from the world and from others, crafts a unique relationship with the universe. Human beings have a personal relationship with the universe that is open to new possibilities and directions. The personal relationship is the person's becoming, and becoming is complex and full of explicit-implicit meanings (Parse, 1981, 1998).

Coconstitution is the idea that the meaning of any moment or situation is linked with the particulars that contribute to the moment or situation (Parse, 1981, 1998). Human beings choose meaning as they choose to see and evaluate the particular constituents of day-to-day life. Life happens, events unfold in expected and unexpected ways, and the human being coconstitutes personal meaning and significance. Coconstitution surfaces with opportunities and limitations for human beings as they live their presence with the world, and as they make choices about what things mean and how to proceed. The term *coconstitution* also links to the ways people create different meanings from the same situations. People change and are changed through their personal interpretations of life situations. Various ways of thinking and acting unite familiar patterns with newly emerging ones as people proceed with crafting their unique realities.

The term *coexistence* means "the human is not alone in any dimension of becoming" (Parse, 1998, p. 17). Human beings are always with the world of things, ideas, language, unfolding events, and cherished traditions, and they also are always with others—not only contemporaries, but also predecessors and successors. There is no individual in Parse's humanbecoming theory. There is only community that one has been cocreated with (Parse, 2003a). There is the personal and there is the intersubjective, and even the way one knows self as a human being is linked intimately to the ways others think and act around persons. Indeed, Parse posits that "without others, one would not know that one is a being" (Parse, 1998, p. 17). Persons think about themselves in relation to how they are with others and how they might be with their plans and dreams. Coexistence links with the notion of mutual process and the unity of lived experience. No objective-subjective dualities or cause-effect relationships can represent humanbecoming. Linked to the assumption of freedom, Parse describes an abiding respect for human change and possibility.

Finally, situated freedom means that human beings emerge in the context of a time and history, a culture and language, physicality, and potentiality. Parse suggests that human freedom means "reflectively and prereflectively one participates in choosing the situations in which one finds oneself as well as one's attitude toward the situations" (Parse, 1998, p. 17). Humans are always choosing. Persons decide what is important in their lives. They decide how to approach situations and what projects and people to pay attention to. Day-to-day living represents people choosing and acting on their value priorities, and value priorities shift as life unfolds. Sometimes being able to act on beliefs is as important as achieving the desired outcome. Personal integrity is linked intimately to the notion of situated freedom.

In 2007, Parse published important conceptual refinements for the humanbecoming school of thought. First, she changed human becoming and human-universe to *humanbecoming* and *humanuniverse.* These changes, according to Parse (2007b), further specify her commitment to the indivisibility of cocreation. Parse's new concepts of humanbecoming and humanuniverse demonstrate through language that there is no space for thinking that humans can be separated from becoming or the universe—these notions are irreducible.

In addition to her new conceptualizations of humanbecoming and humanuniverse, Parse (2007b) specified four postulates that permeate all principles of humanbecoming. The four postulates are illimitability, paradox, freedom, and mystery. The four postulates further specify ideas already embedded within Parse's school of thought. Illimitability better represents Parse's thinking about the indivisible, unpredictable, everchanging nature of humanbecoming. Parse (2007b) stated, "Illimitability is the 'unbounded knowing extended to infinity, the all-at-once remembering and prospecting with the moment'" (p. 308). Indivisible, unbounded knowing "is a privileged knowing accessible only to the individual living the life" (Parse, 2008b, p. 46). Paradox has always been affiliated with humanbecoming, and Parse's bringing it forth as a postulate that permeates all theoretical principles emphasizes the importance of paradox in human cocreation. She stated, "paradoxes are not opposites to be reconciled or dilemmas to be overcome but, rather, are lived rhythms . . . expressed as a pattern preference" (p. 309), "incarnating an individual's choices in day-to-day living" (Parse, 2008b, p. 46). Humans make choices about how they will be with paradoxical experiences and continuously make choices about where to focus their attention. For example, all humans live paradoxical rhythms of certainty-uncertainty, joy-sorrow, and others, and they move with the rhythm of their paradoxical experiences—at times focusing on certainty or joy, for instance, yet always having an awareness of living the uncertainty or sorrow inherent in situations. Likewise, freedom, although a cornerstone of Parse's early thinking, is positioned in a new light in her most recent thinking. Here, she (Parse, 2007b) stated that freedom is "contextually construed liberation" (p. 309). People have freedom with their situations to choose ways of being. Finally, mystery, the fourth postulate, is presented in a more specific way as something special that transcends the conceivable and as the unfathomable and unknowable that always accompanies the "indivisible, unpredictable, everchanging humanuniverse" (p. 309). Based on her latest thinking, Parse (2007b) also refined the wording of the three principles of her theory as indicated in the following.

MAJOR CONCEPTS & DEFINITIONS

Three principles constitute the humanbecoming theory flowing from these themes—meaning, rhythmicity, and transcendence (Parse, 1981, 1998, 2007b). Each principle contains three concepts that require thoughtful exploration to understand the depth of the humanbecoming theory. These principles (Parse, 2007b) are as follows:

1. Structuring meaning is the imaging and valuing of languaging.
2. Configuring rhythmical patterns of relating is the revealing-concealing and enabling-limiting of connecting-separating.
3. Cotranscending with possibles is the powering and originating of transforming (p. 309).

PRINCIPLE I: STRUCTURING MEANING

The first principle proposes that persons structure, or choose, the meaning of their realities, and this choosing happens with explicit-tacit knowing. Sometimes questions are not answerable, because people may not know why they think or feel one way or another. The first principle posits that the way people see the world, their imaging of it, is their reality, and they create this reality illimitably with others, and they show or language their reality in the ways they speak and remain silent and in the ways they move and stay still. When people language their realities, they also language their value priorities and meanings (according to the first principle). The first principle has three concepts: (1) imaging, (2) valuing, and (3) languaging.

Concept: Imaging
Paradoxes: Explicit-Tacit and Reflective-Prereflective

Imaging is the first concept of the first principle. The paradoxes of imaging are explicit-tacit and reflective-prereflective (Parse, 1998, 2007b). Imaging is an individual's view of reality. It is the shaping of personal knowledge in explicit and tacit ways (Parse, 1981, 1998). Some knowing is a reflective, deliberate process, while other knowing is prereflective and unconscious. For Parse, people are inherently curious and seek to find answers and figure things out. The answers to questions emerge as persons explore meaning in light of reality and their view of things. Imaging is a personal interpretation of meaning, possibility, and consequence. Nurses cannot completely know another's imaging, but they explore, respect, and bear witness as people struggle with the processes of shaping, exploring, integrating, rejecting, and interpreting.

Concept: Valuing
Paradox: Confirming-Not Confirming

Valuing is the second concept of the first principle. The paradox of valuing is confirming-not confirming (Parse, 1998, 2007b). This concept is about how persons confirm and do not confirm beliefs in light of a personal perspective or worldview (Parse, 1981, 1998). Persons are continuously confirming-not confirming beliefs as they are making choices about how to think, act, and feel, and these choices may be consistent with prior choices, or they may be radically different and require a shifting of value priorities. Sometimes people may think about anticipated choices and, once the choice arrives, they change their thinking and direction in life. Values reflect what is important in life to a person or a family. For Parse, living one's value priorities is how an individual expresses health and humanbecoming. Nurses learn about persons' perspectives by asking them what is most important.

Concept: Languaging
Paradoxes: Speaking-Being Silent and Moving-Being Still

Languaging is the third concept of the first principle. The paradoxes of languaging are

Continued

MAJOR CONCEPTS & DEFINITIONS—cont'd

speaking-being silent and moving-being still. Languaging is a concept that relates to how humans symbolize and express their imaged realities and their value priorities. Languaging is visible in the way people speak and remain silent and in the way they move and remain still. When languaging is visible to others, it often is expressed in patterns that are shared with those who are close. Family members or close friends often share similar patterns, such as speaking, moving, and being quiet (Parse, 1981, 1998). People disclose things about themselves when they language, even when they are silent and remain still. Nurses witness the languaging that people show, but they cannot know the meaning of the languaging. To understand languaging, nurses ask people what their words, actions, and gestures mean. It is possible that persons still may not know the meaning of their languaging, and in that case the nurse respects the process of coming to understand the meaning of a situation. Explicating meaning takes time, and people know when it is right to illuminate the meaning and significance of an event or happening.

PRINCIPLE 2: CONFIGURING RHYTHMICAL PATTERNS

The second principle of humanbecoming is "configuring rhythmical patterns of relating is the revealing-concealing and enabling-limiting of connecting-separating" (Parse, 2007b, p. 309). This principle means that human beings create patterns in day-to-day life, and these patterns tell about personal meanings and values. In the patterns of relating that people create, many freedoms and restrictions surface with choices; all patterns involve complex engagements and disengagements with people, ideas, and preferences. The second principle has three concepts: (1) revealing-concealing, (2) enabling-limiting, and (3) connecting-separating.

Concept: Revealing-Concealing
Paradox: Disclosing-Not Disclosing

Revealing-concealing is the first concept of the second principle. The paradox linked with revealing-concealing is disclosing-not disclosing (Parse, 2007b). Revealing-concealing is the way persons disclose and keep hidden, all-at-once, the persons they are becoming (Parse, 1981, 1998). There is always more to tell and more to know about ourselves as well as others. Sometimes people know what they want to say and they deliver messages with great clarity, and at other times, people may surprise themselves with the messages they give. Some aspects of reality and experience remain concealed. People also disclose-not disclose differently in different situations and with different people. Further, patterns of revealing-concealing are cocreated and intimately linked to the intentions of those persons cocreating the moment. In choosing how to be with others, nurses cocreate what happens when they are with persons.

Concept: Enabling-Limiting
Paradox: Potentiating-Restricting

Enabling-limiting is the second concept of the second principle. It is linked with the paradox potentiating-restricting (Parse, 2007b). Enabling-limiting represents the potentials and opportunities that surface with the restrictions and obstacles of everyday living. Every choice, even those made prereflectively, has potentials and restrictions. It is not possible to know all the consequences of any given choice; therefore, people make choices amid the reality of ambiguity. Every choice is pregnant with possibility in both opportunity and restriction. This is verified in practice daily when patients and families say things like, "This is the worst thing that could have happened to our family, but it has helped

Major Concepts & Definitions—cont'd

us in many ways." Enabling-limiting is about choosing from the possibilities and living with the consequences of those choices. Nurses are helpful to others as they contemplate the options and anticipated consequences of difficult choices.

Concept: Connecting-Separating
Paradox: Attending-Distancing

Connecting-separating is the third concept of the second principle. The paradox linked with connecting-separating is attending-distancing (Parse, 2007b). This concept relates to the ways persons create patterns of connecting and separating with people and projects. The patterns created reveal value priorities. Connecting-separating is about communion-aloneness and the ways people separate from some to join with others. Connecting-separating is also about the paradox attending-distancing and explains the way two people can be very close and yet separate. Sometimes there is connecting when people are separating because persons can dwell with an absent presence with great intimacy, especially when grieving for another (Bournes, 2000a; Cody, 1995b; Pilkington, 1993). Nurses learn about persons' patterns of connecting-separating by asking about their important relationships and projects.

PRINCIPLE 3: COTRANSCENDING WITH POSSIBLES

"Cotranscending with possibles is the powering and originating of transforming" (Parse, 2007b, p. 309) is the third principle of the humanbecoming theory. The meaning of this principle is that persons continuously change and unfold in life as they engage with and choose from infinite possibilities about how to be, what attitude or approach to have, whom to relate with, and what interests or concerns to explore. Their choices reflect the persons' ways of moving and changing in the process of becoming. The three concepts of this principle are as follows: (1) powering, (2) originating, and (3) transforming.

Concept: Powering
Paradoxes: Pushing-Resisting, Affirming-Not Affirming, Being-Nonbeing

Powering is the first concept of the third principle. It is connected with the paradoxes pushing-resisting, affirming-not affirming, and being-nonbeing (Parse, 1998, 2007b). Powering is a concept that conveys meaning about struggle and life and the will to go on despite hardship and threat. Parse (1981, 1998) describes powering as a pushing-resisting process that is always happening and that affirms our being in light of the possibility of nonbeing. People constantly engage being and nonbeing. Nonbeing is about loss and the risk of death and rejection. Powering is the force exerted, the pushing to act and live with purpose amid possibilities for affirming and holding what is cherished, while simultaneously living with loss and threat of nonbeing. There is always resistance with the pushing force of powering, because persons live with others who are also powering with different possibilities. Conflict, according to Parse (1981, 1998), presents opportunities to clarify meanings and values, and nurses may enhance this process by being present with persons who are exploring issues, conflicts, and options.

Concept: Originating
Paradoxes: Certainty-Uncertainty, Conforming-Not Conforming

Originating, the second concept of principle three, is about human uniqueness and holds the following two paradoxes: (1) conforming-not

Continued

MAJOR CONCEPTS & DEFINITIONS—cont'd

conforming and (2) certainty-uncertainty. People strive to be like others, and yet they also strive to be unique. Choices about originating occur with the reality of certainty-uncertainty. It is not possible to know all that may come from choosing to be different or from choosing to be like others. For some, there is greater danger in being too much like others; some may say the greater danger is in being different. Each person defines and lives originating in light of their worldview and values. Originating and creating anew is a pattern that coexists with constancy and conformity (Parse, 1981, 1998). Humans craft their unique patterns of originating as they engage the possibilities of everyday life. Nurses witness originating with persons who are in the process of choosing how they are going to be with their changing health patterns.

Concept: Transforming

Paradox: Familiar-Unfamiliar

Transforming, the third concept of the third principle, is explicated with the paradox familiar-unfamiliar. Transforming is about the continuously changing and shifting views that people have about their lives. People are always struggling to integrate the unfamiliar with the familiar in the living of everydayness. When new discoveries are made, people change their understanding and, sometimes, life patterns and worldviews can shift with insights that illuminate a familiar situation in a new light. Transforming is the ongoing change in characteristic humanuniverse and human ingenuity as people find ways to change in the direction of their cherished hopes and dreams (Parse, 1981, 1998). Nurses, in the way they are present with others, help or hinder persons' efforts to clarify their hopes, dreams, and desired directions.

USE OF EMPIRICAL EVIDENCE

Research guided by the humanbecoming theory is meant to enhance understanding of the theoretical foundation, or the knowledge contained in the principles and concepts of the humanbecoming theory. Research is not used to test Parse's theory. Nurses do not set out to test if people have unique meanings of life situations; or if persons have situated freedom; or if humans are indivisible, unpredictable, everchanging beings; or if persons relate with others and the universe in paradoxical patterns. To test these beliefs would be comparable to testing the assumption that humans are spiritual beings or that people are composed of complex systems. These statements are abstract beliefs based on experience, observation, and beliefs about the nature of reality. The foundational or ontological statements are value laden, and, as noted earlier, a nurse either has an attraction and commitment to these foundational beliefs or not. The idea of a human being who is indivisible, unpredictable, everchanging and freely choosing meaning is an assumption that is either believable or not. Assumptions about human beings are theoretical, not factual. A student or a nurse relates to one notion of human being or another. According to Parse, this is why there is a need for multiple views; the discipline of nursing can and does accommodate different views and different theories about the phenomenon of concern to nursing—the human-universe-health process. In agreement with Hall, Parse (1993) stated the following when discussing the issue of testing the humanbecoming theory:

> The human becoming theory does not lend itself to testing, since it is not a predictive theory and is not based on a cause-effect view of the human-universe process. The purpose of the research is not to verify the theory or test it but, rather, the focus

> is on uncovering the essences of lived phenomena to gain further understanding of universal human experiences. This understanding evolves from connecting the descriptions given by people to the theory, thus making more explicit the essences of being human (p. 12).

Research with Parse's theory expands understanding about humanly lived experiences and builds new knowledge about humanbecoming. Knowledge of humanbecoming contributes to the substantive knowledge of the nursing discipline. Disciplinary knowledge is different from the practical or technical knowledge that nurses use in various healthcare settings. Disciplinary knowledge is theoretical and identifies the phenomenon of concern for nurses—for Parse (1998, 2007b), humanbecoming. According to Parse (1998), "Scholarly research is formal inquiry leading to the discovery of new knowledge with the enhancement of theory" (p. 59). This idea of new knowledge with enhancement of theory requires additional attention to clarify the distinctions among different ways of thinking.

Research guided by the humanbecoming theory explores universal lived experiences with people as they live them in day-to-day life. Parse contends that there are universal human experiences, such as hope, joy, sorrow, grief, anticipation, fear, confidence, and contemplation. Further, persons experience what was, what is, and what will be—all at once. This means that research guided by the humanbecoming theory explores lived experiences as people live them. People live in the moment, and what is remembered and what is hoped for are always viewed within the reality of the now. Further, universal experiences cannot be reduced to linear time frames because lived experiences are cocreated with "indivisible, unbounded knowing" (Parse, 2007b, p. 308). A nurse researcher conducting a Parse method study invites persons to speak about a particular universal experience. For instance, a researcher might invite a participant to talk about his or her experience of grieving (Cody, 1995a, 2000; Pilkington, 1993). The researcher would not ask the participant to speak about grieving while in the hospital, for example, because lived experiences are not compartmentalized. The researcher guided by humanbecoming knows that the person's reality encompasses what is remembered and what is imagined or hoped for as it is appearing in the moment (Parse, 2007b). The researcher also assumes that the person knows his or her experience and can offer an account of the experience as he or she lives and knows it. What is shared about the experience under study is what Parse (2008b) called "truth for the moment" (p. 46). Truth for the moment is the person's description of his or her reality, an expression of "personal wisdom" (Parse, 2008b, p. 46) about the phenomenon under study in light of what is happening and known in that instant. Truth, from this perspective, is "unfolding evidence, testimony to everchanging knowing, as new insights shift meaning and truth for the moment" (Parse, 2008b, p. 46). Thus, all research evidence is "truth for the moment."

In 1987, Parse first developed a specific research method consistent with the humanbecoming theory; since then, her humanbecoming hermeneutic method has been articulated (Cody, 1995c; Parse, 1998, 2001b, 2005, 2007a). A third method, an applied science method (qualitative descriptive preproject-process-postproject) has also been articulated (Parse, 1998, 2001b). For details of all these methods, please see *The Human Becoming School of Thought: A Perspective for Nurses and Other Health Professionals* (Parse, 1998) and *Qualitative Inquiry: The Path of Sciencing* (Parse, 2001b). The Parse research method records accounts of personal experiences and systematically examines those accounts to identify the aspects of lived experiences that are shared across participants. The core concepts, or ideas shared across all participants, form a structure of the phenomenon under study. The structure as defined by Parse (2007c) is the "paradoxical living the now of remembering and prospecting all-at-once." New knowledge is embedded in the core concepts, and, once discovered, the new knowledge enhances theory and understanding in ways that go beyond the particular study. The weaving of the new knowledge with the theoretical concepts expands understanding of the content of the humanbecoming theory, and that is how the new knowledge develops disciplinary and interdisciplinary thinking and dialogue.

A metaphor of panning for gold may help describe the Parse method. The researcher gathers descriptions from participants like a person panning for gold gathers up the earth. The extraction-synthesis processes of the Parse method can be imagined to be like the gathering, sifting, swirling, seeking, and separating as when panning for gold. Researchers following the Parse method work to separate particular context from core ideas. The gathering and discovering happen over and over as context and earth are separated from the core ideas or nuggets that eventually stand out from the surrounding context or earth. Panning for gold is thought of as back-breaking work, and Parse's research method is also arduous. Both processes include excitement and anticipation of what is to be discovered. The extraction-synthesis processes of the Parse method separate the core ideas that are present in all participant descriptions. The core ideas, like gold nuggets, can be isolated but are not yet refined to a form that will make them meaningful in the world at large. Gold nuggets get refined into coins or jewelry. Core ideas are refined by being abstracted to the language of humanbecoming and nursing science, so that other nurses can see not only the gold nuggets, which are the newly discovered ideas, but also the meaningfulness of the ideas in light of a language of nursing science. Because all research is theory driven, research findings require interpretation in light of the guiding frame of reference in order to advance disciplinary knowledge.

MAJOR ASSUMPTIONS

Parse (1998) synthesized "principles, tenets, and concepts from Rogers, Heidegger, Merleau-Ponty, and Sartre . . . in the creation of the assumptions about the human and becoming, underpinning a view of nursing grounded in the human sciences. Each assumption is unique and represents a synthesis of three of the postulates and concepts drawn from Rogers' work and from existential phenomenology" (p. 19). This underscores just how firmly Parse's theoretical sources underpin her development of the humanbecoming school of thought. Parse draws upon the work of other theorists to build a solid foundation for a new nursing science. Accordingly, the assumptions underpinning the humanbecoming theory focus on beliefs about humans and about their becoming, which is health. Parse does not specify separate assumptions about the universe, because her belief is that the universe is illimitable and cocreated with humans—rather than separate from humans. This is evident in Parse's (1998, 2007d) assumptions about humans and becoming:

- The human is coexisting while coconstituting rhythmical patterns with universe (coexistence, coconstitution, and pattern).
- The human is open, freely choosing meaning with situation, bearing responsibility for decisions (situated freedom, openness, and energy field).
- The human is continuously coconstituting patterns of relating (energy field, pattern, and coconstitution).
- The human is transcending illimitably with possibles (pandimensionality, openness, and situated freedom).
- Becoming is human-living-health (openness, situated freedom, and coconstitution).
- Becoming is rhythmically coconstituting with humanuniverse (coconstitution, pattern, and pandimensionality).
- Becoming is the human's patterns of relating value priorities (situated freedom, pattern, and openness).
- Becoming is intersubjective transcending with possibles (openness, situated freedom, and coexistence).
- Becoming is the human's emerging (coexistence, energy field, and pandimensionality) (Parse, 1998, 2007d).

Parse (1998, 2007d) synthesized the original nine assumptions about humans and becoming into three assumptions about humanbecoming, as follows:

1. Humanbecoming is freely choosing personal meaning with situation, intersubjectively living value priorities.
2. Humanbecoming is configuring rhythmical patterns of relating with humanuniverse.
3. Humanbecoming is cotranscending illimitably with emerging possibles.

Three themes arise from the assumptions of the humanbecoming theory. These include (1) meaning, (2) rhythmicity, and (3) transcendence (Parse, 1998). The postulate's illimitability, paradox, freedom, and mystery (Parse, 2007b) permeate the three themes. Meaning is borne in the messages that persons give and take with others in speaking, moving, silence, and stillness (Parse, 1998). Meaning indicates the significance of something and is chosen by people. Outsiders cannot decide the meaning or significance of something for another person. Nurses cannot know what it will mean for a family to hear news of an unexpected illness or change in health until they learn the meaning it holds from the family's perspective. Sometimes people may not know the significance of something until meaning is explored and possibilities examined. Personal meanings are shared with others when people express their views, concerns, hopes, and dreams. According to Parse (1998), meaning is linked with moments of day-to-day living, as well as with the meaning or purpose of life itself.

Rhythmicity is about patterns and possibility. Parse (1981) suggests that people live unrepeatable patterns of relating with others, ideas, objects, and situations. Their patterns of relating incarnate their priorities, and these patterns are changing constantly as they integrate new experiences and ideas. For Parse, people are recognized by their unique patterns. People change their patterns when they integrate new priorities, ideas, and dreams, and when they show consistent patterns that continue like threads of familiarity and sameness throughout life.

Transcendence is the third major theme of the humanbecoming school of thought. Transcendence is about change and possibility, the infinite possibility that is humanbecoming. "The possibilities arise with . . . [humanuniverse] . . . as options from which to choose personal ways of becoming" (Parse, 1998, p. 30). To believe one thing or another, to go in one direction or another, to be persistent or let go, to struggle or acquiesce, to be certain or uncertain, to hope or despair—all these options surface in day-to-day living. Considering and choosing from these options is cotranscending with the possibles.

Nursing

Consistent with her beliefs, Parse does not write about nursing as a concept in the metaparadigm of the discipline. However, she has written extensively about her beliefs concerning nursing as a basic science. Parse (2000) wrote, "It is the hope of many nurses that nursing as a discipline will enjoy the recognition of having a unique knowledge base and the profession will be sufficiently distinct from medicine that people will actually seek nurses for nursing care, not medical diagnoses" (p. 3). For longer than 30 years, Parse has been advancing the belief that nursing is a basic science, and that nurses require theories that are different from other disciplines. Parse believes that nursing is a unique service to humankind. This does not mean that nurses do not benefit from and employ knowledge from other disciplines and fields of study. It means that nurses primarily rely on and value the knowledge of nursing theory in their practice and research activities. Parse (1992) has articulated clearly that she believes "nursing is a science, the practice of which is a performing art" (p. 35). From this view, nursing is a learned discipline, and nursing theories guide practice and research. The belief that nursing is a unique discipline requiring its own theories is often not understood, but discussions around this issue continue to clarify the opportunities nurses have by creating nursing science.

Nursing practice for those choosing Parse's theory is guided by a specific methodology that emerges directly from the humanbecoming ontology. The practice dimensions and processes are illuminating meaning (explicating), synchronizing rhythms (dwelling with), and mobilizing transcendence (moving beyond). For details of practice methodology, see *The Humanbecoming School of Thought: A Perspective for Nurses and Other Health Professionals* (Parse, 1998). "Nurses who value the humanbecoming belief system live the theory in true presence with others" (Parse, 1993, p. 12). Parse (1993) described practice in the following way:

> The nurse is in true presence with the individual (or family) as the individual (or family) uncovers the personal meaning of the situation and makes choices to move forward in the now moment with cherished hopes and dreams. The focus is on the meaning of the lived experience for the person (or family) unfolding "there with" the presence of the nurse . . . The living of the theory in practice is indeed what makes a difference to the people touched by it (p. 12).

Nursing, for Parse, is a science, and the performing art of nursing is practiced in relationships with persons (individuals, groups, and communities) in their processes of becoming. Parse (1989) has offered the following set of fundamentals as essential for practicing the art of nursing:

- Know and use nursing frameworks and theories.
- Be available to others.
- Value the other as a human presence.
- Respect differences in view.
- Own what you believe and be accountable for your actions.
- Move on to the new and untested.
- Connect with others.
- Take pride in self.
- Like what you do.
- Recognize the moments of joy in the struggles of living.
- Appreciate mystery and be open to new discoveries.
- Be competent in your chosen area.
- Rest and begin anew (p. 11).

Humanuniverse, Humanbecoming, and Health

Parse (1998, 2007b) views the concepts human, universe, and health as inseparable and irreducible. To emphasize this inseparability, she recently (Parse, 2007b) specified humanuniverse and humanbecoming as one word. For Parse, health is humanbecoming. Health is structuring meaning, configuring rhythmical patterns of relating, and cotranscending with possibles. Parse (1990) speaks of health as a personal commitment, which means, "an individual's way of becoming is cocreated by that individual, incarnating his or her own value priorities" (p. 136). For Parse (1990), health is a flowing process, a personal creation, and a personal responsibility. Personal health may be changed as commitment is changed, which "include[s] creative imagining, affirming self, and spontaneous glimpsing of the paradoxical" (Parse, 1990, p. 138).

Human beings come into the world through others and live their life cocreating patterns of communion-aloneness. This means that persons change and are changed in relating with others, ideas, objects, and events. People become known and understood as they cocreate patterns of relating with people, ideas, culture, history, meanings, and hopes. To understand human life and human beings, an individual must start from the premise that all people are interconnected with predecessors, contemporaries, and even people who are not yet present in the world. Parents may imagine and have a relationship with a child long before the child is conceived and long after a child is lost through death (Pilkington, 1993). Experience has shown that many people at various times have relationships with their parents and other loved ones who are no longer in this world. These are examples of the indivisibility and complexity of humanuniverse and humanbecoming.

THEORETICAL ASSERTIONS

Parse's (1981, 1998) principles are the assertions of the humanbecoming theory. Each principle interrelates the following nine concepts of humanbecoming: (1) imaging, (2) valuing, (3) languaging,

(4) revealing-concealing, (5) enabling-limiting, (6) connecting-separating, (7) powering, (8) originating, and (9) transforming (Figure 24-1). Research projects generate structures that further specify relationships among the theoretical concepts. For example, Wang (1999) studied hope for persons living with leprosy in Taiwan, and she presented the following theoretical structure: The lived experience of hope is imaging the connecting-separating in originating valuing. Theoretical structures can be used to enhance understanding of specific phenomena as readers consider the detailed participant descriptions that are linked to the concepts of humanbecoming theory. For more information about humanbecoming research, refer to the comprehensive overview of studies compiled by Doucet and Bournes (2007).

LOGICAL FORM

The inductive-deductive process was central to the creation of the humanbecoming theory. The theory originated from Parse's personal experiences with her readings and in nursing practice. She deductively-inductively crafted major components of humanbecoming from the science of unitary human beings and existential-phenomenological thought. With her intuitive sense, Parse methodically derived the assumptions, concepts, principles, and practice and research methodologies of the humanbecoming school of thought. Figure 24-1 shows how the principles, concepts, and theoretical structures can be linked. The figure shows the most abstract view of humanbecoming—the simplicity and the complexity of the theory are evident. Abstraction and complexity create possibility for growth, scholarship, and sustainability.

ACCEPTANCE BY THE NURSING COMMUNITY

Practice

The following bibliography demonstrates the broad scope of acceptance by the nursing community. A strong and influential group of nurse scholars is advancing humanbecoming in practice, research,

Principle 1: Structuring meaning is the imaging and valuing of languaging.

Principle 2: Configuring rhythmical patterns of relating is the revealing-concealing and enabling-limiting of connecting-separating.

Principle 3: Cotranscending with possibles is the powering and originating of transforming.

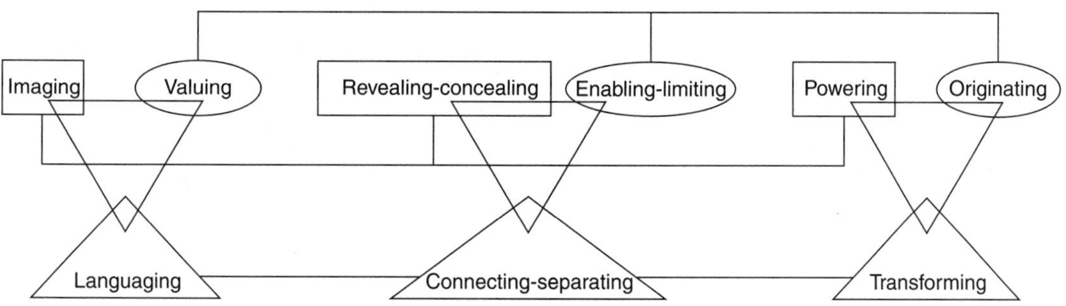

Relationship of the concepts in the squares: *Powering* is a way of *revealing and concealing imaging.*
Relationship of the concepts in the ovals: *Originating* is a manifestation of *enabling and limiting valuing.*
Relationship of the concepts in the triangles: *Transforming* unfolds in the *languaging of connecting and separating.*

Figure 24-1 Relationship of principles, concepts, and theoretical structures of the human becoming theory. (From Parse, R. R. [1981]. *Man-living-health: A theory of nursing* [p. 69]. New York: John Wiley & Sons. Principles updated from Parse, R. R. [2007]. *The humanbecoming school of thought in 2050. Nursing Science Quarterly,* 20, 308-311.)

and education. The theory has made a difference to nurses and to persons (patients) who experience humanbecoming practice. The theory informs nurses who work with older persons and with children. The theory guides practice for nurses who work with families and with persons in hospital settings, clinics, and community settings. A community-based health action model, for instance, has been developed and is receiving support from the local community and other funding agencies (Crane, Josephson, & Letcher, 1999). The theory of humanbecoming has also helped to generate controversy and scholarly dialogue about nursing as an evolving discipline and a distinct human science. It is interesting to note that the theory of humanbecoming provides a set of beliefs that can be lived by nurses who have opportunities to be with human beings. It is not a question of whether or not the theory works in any particular setting. The theory has been lived by nurses in the operating theater, in parishes, in shelters, in acute care hospitals, and in other long-term and community settings. A more important question for nurses may be, What settings consistently provide opportunities for nurses to have relationships with persons and families?

Education

The humanbecoming school of thought and the philosophical assumptions and theoretical beliefs specified by Parse have helped fuel many scholarly dialogues and comparisons about outcomes in practice, research, and education when different theories guide professional activities. In *Nursing Science Quarterly* and other journals, nurses informed by the humanbecoming theory have advanced dialogue and debate about the role of theory in nursing practice, the limitations and contributions of the medical model, the ethics of nursing diagnoses and the nurse-person relationship, paternalism and health care, the knowledge of advanced nursing practice, paradigmatic issues in nursing, the limitations of evidence-based nursing, the possibilities and politics of human science, freedom and choice, the focus of community-based nursing, the nature of truth, leadership and nursing theory, and the scope of mistakes in nursing.

Parse (2004) created a humanbecoming teaching-learning model that is consistent with the assumptions and principles of humanbecoming. The assumptions, essences, and processes of the model have been used in a variety of ways with students in academic settings (Letcher & Yancey, 2004) and practice settings (Bournes & Naef, 2006). Teachers in academic and practice settings have contributed new understanding and new processes of teaching-learning, and Parse's theory has been used as a model for explicating pros and cons of teleapprenticeship (Norris, 2002). The humanbecoming school of thought also informs nursing courses at the undergraduate and graduate levels in many schools of nursing.

In the text, *Man-Living-Health: A Theory of Nursing*, Parse (1981) presented a sample master's in nursing curriculum that incorporated the assumptions, principles, concepts, and theoretical structures of humanbecoming theory. She outlined this process-based curriculum in detail, including course descriptions and course sequencing. The curriculum plan was updated in the 1998 text, *The Humanbecoming School of Thought: A Perspective for Nurses and Other Health Professionals,* in which Parse outlined a program philosophy and goals, a conceptual framework with themes for the curriculum, program indicators, course culture content, and the evaluation process, and provided a sample curriculum plan consistent with humanbecoming.

A master's degree in nursing curriculum consistent with humanbecoming has been developed at Olivet Nazarene University in Kankakee, Illinois (Milton, 2003a). Many schools of nursing offer students some learning of humanbecoming theory. To date, most students who study the humanbecoming theory and who are guided by the theory in their practice and research activities were introduced to Parse's work at the master's level. Parse's ideas and the humanbecoming theory are increasingly being integrated into undergraduate programs, which will help to expand options for students being taught that nursing is an art and a science that supports multiple perspectives. For example, an undergraduate degree curriculum has now been designed and implemented at California Baptist University in Riverside, California (C. Milton, personal communication, March 11, 2008). In addition, undergraduate and graduate students at York University in Toronto, Ontario, Canada, have the opportunity to study humanbecoming.

Research

Humanbecoming theory has guided research studies in many different countries about numerous lived experiences, including feeling loved, feeling very tired, having courage, waiting, feeling cared for, grieving, caring for a loved one, persisting while wanting to change, feeling understood, and being listened to, as well as time passing, quality of life, health, lingering presence, hope, and contentment (see Doucet & Bournes, 2007, for examples). The Parse and the humanbecoming hermeneutic method, underpinned by the humanbecoming school of thought, generate new knowledge about universal lived experiences (Cody, 1995b, 1995c; Parse, 2001a, 2005, 2007a). For instance, research findings have helped to enhance understanding about how people experience hope, while imaging new possibilities and how people create moments of respite amid the anguish of grieving a loss. Research findings are woven with the theory so that findings can inform thinking beyond any particular study.

For instance, in several of the grieving and loss studies, researchers described a rhythm of engaging and disengaging with the one lost and with others who remind the one grieving about the one lost (Cody, 1995a; Pilkington, 1993). Women who had a miscarriage already had a relationship with their babies, and the anguish of losing the child was so intense that women invented ways to distance themselves from the reality of the lost child. When they were alone, the pain was unbearable, and when they were with others, the anguish was both eased and intensified as consoling expressions mingled with words acknowledging the reality of the lost child (Pilkington, 1993). Women described rhythms of engaging-disengaging with the lost child and close others, pain, and respite. Linking the rhythm to the theoretical concept connecting-separating means that readers can think about and be present with others' expressions of engaging-disengaging as they surface in discussions about grieving and loss. How do families in palliative care express their engaging and distancing from the one who is moving toward death? How do parents losing adult children engage and disengage with the absent children? Additional research studies about loss and grieving may further enhance understanding about the connecting-separating concept and other concepts of humanbecoming.

In 2004, Mitchell developed a framework for critiquing humanbecoming research that is expanding options for critics engaging humanbecoming-guided nursing science, and the Parse (2001b) research method continues to be refined. For example, in the text, *Qualitative Inquiry: The Path of Sciencing,* Parse introduced a process in which the researcher constructs each participant's story, including core ideas of the phenomenon under study. Most recently, Parse changed the name of the participant proposition to language-art, and she added a process that requires the researcher to select or create an artistic expression that shows how the researcher was transfigured through the research process (Parse, 2005). The artistic expression enhances understanding of what the researcher learned about the phenomenon under study. For instance, in her recent study on the experience of feeling respected, Parse (2006) reported that the 10 adult participants in her study described feeling respected as "an acknowledgement of personal worth" (p. 54). They described, for example, feeling confident, being trusted, feeling appreciated, and experiencing joy when feeling respected (Parse, 2006). Parse showed that in each case, the participant spoke about feeling respected as a "*fortifying assuredness amid potential disregard emerging with the fulfilling delight of prized alliances*" (p. 54). Parse's (2006) artistic expression for this study—that is, her depiction of her own learning about the phenomenon of feeling respected that surfaced through the research process—was the following poem:

The oak tree stands
noble on the hill
even in
cherry blossom time.

Basho (1644-1694/1962)

In describing the artistic expression, Parse (2006) wrote, "The oak tree stands noble, acknowledged as such with the potential of being disregarded amid the beauty of cherry blossoms, yet there is delight in the fortification of being known as oak tree. Oak tree and cherry blossoms live a mutuality of being prized as individually unique and uniquely together" (p. 55).

CRITIQUE

Humanbecoming is an abstract and complex school of thought that includes the humanbecoming theory (the principles). It is a theory, not a model, because its concepts and interrelationships are defined in principles that are written at an abstract level of discourse—the language of science. Readers may study various critiques of humanbecoming to clarify issues and understand the perspectives of reviewers. Ultimately, the theory's meaning and usefulness to the discipline of nursing are decided by the nurses who choose to live it, and by historians who will comment on its place in the evolution of nursing knowledge and of healthcare practices, research activities, ethics, and policies. The theory penetrates the foundations of traditional nursing and healthcare in general. That penetration may be limited to crack-like fissures or streams of activity to expand opportunities and advance thinking. This requires nurses to explore ways that are helpful to enhance the quality of life for patients.

Simplicity

In keeping with the theoretical discourse, the major concepts of humanbecoming are defined in highly abstract and philosophical terms. The abstract language has been a source of comfort and discomfort for nurses (Mitchell & Bournes, 2000). Discomfort with the language is sometimes linked more with unfamiliar beliefs and assumptions about human beings and how they relate with the universe than with abstract concepts. Also discomfiting for some are the nondirectional statements that do not specify causal or predictive relationships about humanuniverse.

The concepts of humanbecoming often resonate with people when considered at the level of lived experience. For instance, the concept of valuing when discussed at the level of lived experience focuses on the ways persons choose and act on what is important in their lives. This idea should be inherently familiar, as should the idea that people sometimes disclose intimate details about their lives and sometimes keep secrets from others (revealing-concealing). Pickrell, Lee, Schumacher, and Twigg (1998) noted that a first-time reader might be tempted to dismiss the concepts as too simple to convey the complexity inherent in the theory, but the authors caution that to do so would be a mistake. Parse's principles describe a complex and realistic picture of humanbecoming, and the picture provides a meaningful framework for understanding the illimitability, mystery, freedom, and paradox of humanuniverse.

Generality

The humanbecoming school of thought was selected as a theoretical guide by nurses and other health professionals in different settings, including acute care, long-term care, and community. The theory helped nurses be with individuals, families, and groups and was evaluated in practice settings where patients commented on the positive difference it made (Jonas, 1995a; Mitchell, Bernardo, & Bournes, 1997; Bournes & Ferguson-Paré, 2007; Northrup & Cody, 1998; Williamson, 2000). Humanbecoming has helped leaders to create beneficial change in organizational culture, and it has informed development of standards of care (Mitchell, 1998b; Mitchell & Bournes, 1998) and best-practice guidelines

(Nelligan et al., 2002; Registered Nurses Association of Ontario, 2002). The theory of humanbecoming changes what professionals see when they engage with persons in practice and research. The theory changes the thinking, acting, attitudes, and approaches that professionals rely on to fulfill their intentions with others (see, Humanbecoming/80-20: An Innovative Professional Development Program for Nurses, at: http://www.nursingchannel.org/programs.html). Indeed, the humanbecoming theory changes the intentions and purposes of professionals, and there is no limit to how this learning may contribute to meaningful practices and approaches for all professional activities linked with research, education, and leadership.

Empirical Precision

Empirical precision generally relates to the testability, relevance, and usefulness of a theory. Questions of concern include the following:

- Does evidence (taken here to mean does reality) support the theory?
- Do the principles and concepts of the humanbecoming theory make sense to nurses when they are with people in practice?
- Does the humanbecoming theory help nurses be with persons in ways that are helpful and that make a difference from the patient's perspective?
- Is the theory useful for administrators and researchers? Do research findings expand knowledge and enhance the theoretical base?

The answer to these questions is, clearly, an enthusiastic "yes." The theory is useful because it provides a meaningful foundation that is helpful for nurses who want to live certain values in practice and research (Bournes & Ferguson-Paré, 2007; Mitchell, Bournes, & Hollett, 2006). A nurse who is learning the theory might ask the following questions:

- What does humanbecoming theory say about people, and do I believe in these ideas as they are presented?
- Am I comfortable with the basic beliefs espoused in the humanbecoming theory?

The answers to the initial questions about evidence or congruence with reality often lead to a decision to pursue the more difficult task of studying the theory. A commitment to learn more requires some attraction to the basic underlying values and assumptions that Parse makes about humanuniverse and health. Additional questions that may be useful for nurses interested in the humanbecoming theory include the following:

- In my experience of reality, do different people have their own unique views about life and their health situations?
- Do people speak about what things mean on a personal level?
- Do people live their value priorities and pursue what is important to them?
- Do people make their own choices?
- Do people speak about paradoxical thoughts and feelings?
- Have I ever heard a person say something like, "On the one hand I think this way, but on the other hand I think something else," or "I know I said I feel such and such, but as soon as I said it, I realized I also feel different than that"?
- How do I believe people change? Do people make choices that help them move in the direction of their own hopes and dreams?

Derivable Consequences

Parse calls nursing a human science, and, as such, it represents particular beliefs that have been around for longer than 100 years. The humanbecoming theory has taken human science beliefs into service and knowledge development in new and important ways. The humanbecoming research and practice methodologies are generating transformations in care and a renewed sense of professional purpose. Consider these three recent developments as examples:

1. Nurses in two Canadian provinces spent longer than 12 months evaluating humanbecoming patient-centered care, and these acute care nurses reported enhanced satisfaction and purpose in their work as professional nurses (see Bournes &

Ferguson-Paré, 2007; Mitchell, Bournes, & Hollett, 2006).

2. Teams of humanbecoming researchers, practitioners, artistic writers, actors, and consumers produced a research-based drama called *I'm Still Here* about living with Alzheimer's disease. The Murray Alzheimer Research and Education Program at the University of Waterloo funded production of a DVD version of the drama, as well as an educational guide informed by humanbecoming theory, research, and self-reflective practice (Mitchell, Jonas-Simpson, & Ivonoffski, 2006). That DVD and an accompanying educational guide has been purchased by hundreds of health professionals and families in numerous countries around the globe. Researchers Mitchell, Dupuis, and Jonas-Simpson recently toured a live performance of *I'm Still Here* to complete a longitudinal study, funded by the Social Science and Humanities Council of Canada (SSHRC); this study evaluated knowledge translation through artistic performance.
3. Jonas-Simpson's work on loss for mothers who experience the loss of their baby has been informed by humanbecoming and findings presented in New York in an interactive exhibit of stories, poetry, photographs, and research-inspired paintings by artist Ann Bayly for professionals and mothers invited to share their own stories in a journal.

There are convincing indications that the humanbecoming theory is a fitting guide for practitioners who want to create respectful partnerships with people seeking assistance with health and quality of life. More than a decade ago, Phillips (1987) suggested that Parse's work would transform the knowledge base and the practice of nursing to a unitary perspective. Indeed, the humanbecoming theory is transforming practice in numerous settings, and evaluations are positive (Bournes, 2002b; Bournes & Ferguson-Paré, 2007; Jonas, 1995a; Legault & Ferguson-Paré, 1999). The humanbecoming theory directs attention to persons' meanings of health and quality of life and to their wishes, needs, concerns, and preferences for information and care. The future of health care is based on the development of theories and practices that truly honor and respect people as experts about life experience and health. At least five of the largest teaching hospitals in Canada support nurses piloting and implementing standards of practice that are explicitly informed by humanbecoming theory. University Health Network, the largest teaching hospital affiliated with the University of Toronto, supports nurses 20% of their time to participate in teaching-learning sessions informed by humanbecoming. A 2-year-long pilot study evaluated changes when a surgical unit used humanbecoming patient-centered care (Bournes & Ferguson-Paré, 2007). This pilot is being replicated on a cardiosciences unit in Regina General Hospital in Saskatchewan, Canada, and on two additional units at University Health Network in Toronto, Canada.

SUMMARY

Work with the humanbecoming theory continues to evolve, as does the theory itself. An important development happened in 1998, when Parse extended the humanbecoming school of thought and introduced the text, *Community: A Humanbecoming Perspective* (2003a), which offers new concepts about change in community. Parse is now creating humanbecoming mentoring, leading-following, and family models (Parse, 2008a; Parse, 2008c). Ongoing research expands understanding and illuminates new relationships among theoretical concepts. As schools of nursing introduce and teach the humanbecoming school of thought, more nurses explore the theory in their practice. Learning the theory requires formal study, quiet contemplation, and creative synthesis. As more nurses use the theory in practice and research, their scholarly dialogue advances the nursing discipline.

The theory of humanbecoming continues as a theory for the future. As more nurses question how they are relating with others, and as they question the knowledge base of their discipline, the humanbecoming theory provides a perspective and field of possibilities for change and growth. Persons who engage nurses and other healthcare professionals are continuing to speak and clarify not only what they want from professionals but also how they want professionals to perform for them. The predominance of the mechanistic model and its practices of assessing and diagnosing continue to lose appeal for healthcare professionals whose mandate is to relate to people as human beings living with health and illness, hope and no hope, joy and sorrow, life and death. The humanbecoming theory is an alternative to the mechanistic model for nurses and there will be even more as humankind evolves.

Case Study

Mrs. Brown, a 48-year-old woman, is living with a diagnosis of breast cancer. She has just come into the oncology clinic for her third round of chemotherapy. When asked how she is doing, Mrs. Brown starts speaking about how tired she is, and how she is feeling burdened with keeping secrets from her daughter. Mrs. Brown has not told her daughter about her cancer diagnosis because she is afraid of how her daughter might react. Mrs. Brown says she is just barely holding on to things at this time, and she cannot take much more. She is also concerned about the chemotherapy and what she can expect, because the side effects are getting more intense.

CRITICAL THINKING Activities

1. Describe how different theoretical beliefs make a difference in practice. Think about Parse's (1998) practice methodology—illuminating meaning (explicating), synchronizing rhythms (dwelling with), and mobilizing transcendence (moving beyond). Nurses live true presence with persons, and this means centering and preparing to bear witness to Mrs. Brown's reality. In order to invite Mrs. Brown to speak, the nurse may initially ask her to say more about her situation. In the cadence of speech, Mrs. Brown may pause, giving the nurse an opening to pose questions that assist Mrs. Brown's exploration of how she is feeling. The nurse may ask: What is the burden about? What does it mean? What does Mrs. Brown think will happen if her daughter gets upset? Thinking about and picturing an anticipated event is, according to Parse (1990, 1998), an opportunity to rehearse and to clarify how best to be in light of anticipated consequences. In this way, the person is helped with decisions about how best to go forward or how to change the situation. The practice dimensions and processes happen all at once as nurses honor the other's unfolding meanings, rhythms, and ways of moving forward.
2. Articulate the judgments that are called for in the humanbecoming theory. The nurse refrains from summarizing, comparing, judging, or labeling Mrs. Brown, as she struggles with the possibilities and choices in her situation. The unconditional regard called for by the humanbecoming theory is extremely challenging. It can be much easier to give advice or to try to teach, but the outcomes in the nurse-person process, the opportunities for Mrs. Brown to see her situation differently, will vary according to different nursing words and actions.
3. Where does experience lie for nurses guided by the humanbecoming theory? The nurse guided by humanbecoming theory believes that Mrs. Brown knows the best way to proceed—the nurse cannot possibly know the way for another person's quality of life. Mrs. Brown said she cannot take much more in her life and yet she is burdened with her secret. This struggle is hers to wrestle with and choose a way to move on. The mother knows her daughter, and she also knows how much upset she can take in her life. The nurse's true presence and theory-guided questions can help Mrs. Brown

to figure out how to be in light of her value priorities in the moment. The nurse also knows that Mrs. Brown's value priorities may change at any time, leading to a different course of action. The nurse may have expertise in other areas, based on her knowledge and experience, and trusts that persons will seek information when ready.

4. Think of several questions that help individuals speak about their realities. Mrs. Brown spoke about being tired. The nurse might explore this further. How does the tiredness show itself? What does Mrs. Brown find helpful? What would she like to do about it? Until these things are known, the nurse cannot know how to proceed. The nurse may discover helpful suggestions to offer. The nurse guided by humanbecoming offers information as people indicate their readiness to hear it. The nurse believes that providing information or suggestions as persons seek it in the flow of dialogue and listening is the most respectful and meaningful way of teaching.
5. Specify three benefits for humanity when nurses follow the humanbecoming theory. Humanbecoming practice is consistent with what people say they want from health professionals. Persons have indicated in numerous reports and publications that they want to be listened to, respected, involved in their care, and provided with meaningful information—when they want and need it. People want competent professionals, but if respect for the client's reality is not the foundation of the nurse-person process, it does not matter how expert or knowledgeable the professional. People do not want to be judged or labeled when it comes to their choices or ways of living. Persons want to be believed, understood, and respected. Humanbecoming theory provides a guide for nurses who want to practice in ways that clients want. It has been shown that nurses guided by the humanbecoming perspective are more vigilant, more inclined to act on client concerns, and more likely to involve clients and families in their care (Mitchell & Bournes, 1998).

POINTS FOR *Further Study*

- Parse, R. R. (2007a). Hope in "Rita Hayworth and Shawshank Redemption": A human becoming hermeneutic study. *Nursing Science Quarterly, 20,* 148-154.
- Parse, R. R. (2007b). The humanbecoming school of thought in 2050. *Nursing Science Quarterly,* 20, 308-311.
- Parse, R. R. (2008a). The humanbecoming mentoring model. *Nursing Science Quarterly, 21, 4.*
- Parse, R. R. (2008b). Truth for the moment: Personal testimony as evidence. *Nursing Science Quarterly, 21,* 45-48.
- Parse, R. R. (2008c). The humanbecoming leading-following model. *Nursing Science Quarterly,* 21, 3.
- *Parse interview. Nurse Theorists: Portraits of Excellence,* distributed by Fitne, Inc. (5 Depot Street, Athens, Ohio 45701).
- Mitchell, G. J. (2006). Parse's theory of human becoming in nursing practice. In M. R. Alligood & A. M. Tomey, (Eds.). *Nursing theory utilization & application* (3rd ed.), (pp. 431-460). St. Louis, MO: Elsevier Mosby.

www.discoveryinternationalonline.com
www.humanbecoming.org
www.nursingchannel.org/programs.html

REFERENCES

Basho. (1962). Haiku harvest. White Plains, NY: Peter Pauper Press. (Original work published 1644-1694)

Bournes, D. (2000a). A commitment to honoring people's choices. *Nursing Science Quarterly, 13,* 18-23.

Bournes, D. A. (2002b). Research evaluating human becoming in practice. *Nursing Science Quarterly, 15,* 190-195.

Bournes, D. A., & Ferguson-Paré, M. (2007). Human becoming and 80/20: An innovative professional development model for nurses. *Nursing Science Quarterly, 20,* 237-253.

Bournes, D. A., & Naef, R. (2006). Human becoming practice around the globe: Exploring the art of living true presence. *Nursing Science Quarterly, 19,* 109-115.

Cody, W. K. (1995a). The lived experience of grieving for families living with AIDS: Family-centered research using Parse's method. In R. R. Parse (Ed.), *Illuminations: The humanbecoming theory in practice and research* (pp. 197-242). New York: National League for Nursing Press.

Cody, W. K. (1995b). The meaning of grieving for families living with AIDS. *Nursing Science Quarterly, 8*, 104-114.

Cody, W. K. (1995c). Of life immense in passion, pulse, and power: Dialoguing with Whitman and Parse. A hermeneutic study. In R. R. Parse (Ed.), *Illuminations: The humanbecoming theory in practice and research* (pp. 269-308). New York: National League for Nursing Press.

Cody, W. K. (2000). The lived experience of grieving for persons living with HIV who have used injection drugs. *Journal of the Association of Nurses in AIDS Care, 11*, 82-92.

Cody, W. K., & Mitchell, G. J. (2002). Nursing knowledge and human science revisited: Practical and political considerations. *Nursing Science Quarterly, 15*, 4-13.

Crane, J., Josephson, D., & Letcher, D. (1999, Nov.). The human becoming health action model in community. Paper presented at The Seventh Annual International Colloquium on Human Becoming. Loyola University, Chicago.

Doucet, T., & Bournes, D. A. (2007). Review of research related to Parse's theory of human becoming. *Nursing Science Quarterly, 20*, 16-32.

Jonas, C. M. (1995a). Evaluation of the human becoming theory in family practice. In R. R. Parse (Ed.), *Illuminations: The human becoming theory in practice and research* (pp. 347-366). New York: National League for Nursing Press.

King, S. (1982). Rita Hayworth and Shawshank redemption. In S. King, *Different seasons* (pp. 3 101). New York: Viking Press.

Legault, F., & Ferguson-Paré, M. (1999). Advancing nursing practice: An evaluation study of Parse's theory of human becoming. *Canadian Journal of Nursing Leadership, 12*(1), 30-35.

Letcher, D. C., & Yancey, N. R. (2004). Witnessing change with aspiring nurses: A human becoming teaching-learning process in nursing education. *Nursing Science Quarterly, 17*, 36-41.

Milton, C. L. (2003a). A graduate curriculum guided by human becoming: Journeying with the possible. *Nursing Science Quarterly, 16*, 214-218.

Mitchell, G. J. (2004). An emerging framework for human becoming criticism. *Nursing Science Quarterly, 17*, 103-109.

Mitchell, G. J., Bernardo, A., & Bournes, D. (1997). Nursing guided by Parse's theory: Patient views at Sunnybrook. *Nursing Science Quarterly, 10*, 55-56.

Mitchell, G. J., & Bournes, D. A. (1998). *Finding the way: A video guide to patient focused care* (Videotape). Toronto, Ontario, Canada: Sunnybrook & Women's Health Science Centre.

Mitchell, G. J., & Bournes, D. A. (2000). Nurse as patient advocate? In search of straight thinking. *Nursing Science Quarterly, 13*, 204-209.

Mitchell, G. J., Bournes, D. A., & Hollett, J. (2006). Human becoming-guided patient centered care: New perspectives transform nursing practice. *Nursing Science Quarterly, 19*, 218-224.

Mitchell, G. J., & Cody, W. K. (1992). Nursing knowledge and human science: Ontological and epistemological considerations. *Nursing Science Quarterly, 5*, 54-61.

Mitchell, G. J., Jonas-Simpson, C., & Ivonoffski, V. (2006). Research-based theatre: The making of *I'm Still Here*. *Nursing Science Quarterly, 19*, 198-206.

Nelligan, P., Grinspun, D., Jonas-Simpson, C., McConnell, H., Peter, E., Pilkington, B. (2002, Summer). Client centered care: Making the ideal real. *Hospital Quarterly, 5*(4), 70-76.

Norris, J. R. (2002). One-to-one teleapprenticeship as a means for nurses teaching and learning Parse's theory of human becoming. *Nursing Science Quarterly, 15*, 143-149.

Northrup, D. T., & Cody, W. K. (1998). Evaluation of the human becoming theory in practice in an acute care psychiatric setting. *Nursing Science Quarterly, 11*, 23-30.

Parse, R. R. (1974). *Nursing fundamentals*. Flushing, NY: Medical Examination.

Parse, R. R. (1981). Man-living-health: A theory of nursing. New York: Wiley.

Parse, R. R. (1987). *Nursing science: Major paradigms, theories, and critiques*. Philadelphia: W. B. Saunders.

Parse, R. R. (1989). Essentials for practicing the art of nursing. *Nursing Science Quarterly, 2*, 111.

Parse, R. R. (1990). Health: A personal commitment. *Nursing Science Quarterly, 3*, 136-140.

Parse, R. R. (1992). Human becoming: Parse's theory of nursing. *Nursing Science Quarterly, 5*, 35-42.

Parse, R. R. (1993). Scholarly dialogue: Theory guides research and practice. *Nursing Science Quarterly, 6*, 12.

Parse, R. R. (Ed.). (1995). *Illuminations: The human becoming theory in practice and research*. New York: National League for Nursing Press.

Parse, R. R. (1996). The human becoming theory: Challenges in practice and research. *Nursing Science Quarterly, 9*, 55-60.

Parse, R. R. (1998). *The human becoming school of thought: A perspective for nurses and other health professionals*. Thousand Oaks, CA: Sage.

Parse, R. R. (1999). *Hope: An international human becoming perspective*. Sudbury, MA: Jones & Bartlett.

Parse, R. R. (2000). Into the new millennium. *Nursing Science Quarterly, 13*, 3.

Parse, R. R. (2001a). The lived experience of contentment: A study using the Parse research method. *Nursing Science Quarterly, 14*, 330-338.

Parse, R. R. (2001b). *Qualitative inquiry: The path of sciencing*. Boston: Jones & Bartlett.

Parse, R. R. (2003a). *Community: A human becoming perspective.* Sudbury, MA: Jones & Bartlett.

Parse, R. R. (2004). A human becoming teaching-learning model. *Nursing Science Quarterly, 17,* 33-35.

Parse, R. R. (2005). The human becoming modes of inquiry: Emerging sciencing. *Nursing Science Quarterly, 18,* 297-300.

Parse, R. R. (2006). Feeling respected: A Parse method study. *Nursing Science Quarterly, 19,* 51-56.

Parse, R. R. (2007a). Hope in "Rita Hayworth and Shawshank Redemption": A human becoming hermeneutic study. *Nursing Science Quarterly, 20,* 148-154.

Parse, R. R. (2007b). The humanbecoming school of thought in 2050. Nursing Science Quarterly, 20, 308-311.

Parse, R. R. (2007c, June). Humanbecoming modes of inquiry. Paper presented at the Institute of Humanbecoming, Pittsburgh, PA.

Parse, R. R. (2007d, June). Humanbecoming theory: Update. Paper presented at the Institute of Humanbecoming, Pittsburgh, PA.

Parse, R. R. (2008a). The humanbecoming mentoring model. *Nursing Science Quarterly,* 21,5.

Parse, R. R. (2008b). Truth for the moment: Personal testimony as evidence. *Nursing Science Quarterly, 21,* 45-48.

Parse, R. R. (2008c). The humanbecoming leading-following model. *Nursing Science Quarterly,* 21, 3.

Parse, R. R., Coyne, B., & Smith, M. J. (1985). *Nursing research: Qualitative methods.* Bowie, MD: Brady.

Phillips, J. R. (1987). A critique of Parse's man-living-health theory. In R. R. Parse (Ed.), *Nursing science: Major paradigms, theories, and critiques* (pp. 181-204). Philadelphia: W. B. Saunders.

Pickrell, K. D., Lee, R. E., Schumacher, L. P., & Twigg, P. (1998). Rosemarie Rizzo Parse: Human becoming. In A. M. Tomey & M. R. Alligood (Eds.), *Nursing theorists and their work* (4th ed., pp. 463-481). St. Louis: Mosby.

Pilkington, F. B. (1993). The lived experience of grieving the loss of an important other. *Nursing Science Quarterly, 6,* 130-139.

Pilkington, F. B. (2004). Exploring ethical implications for acting faithfully in professional relationships. *Nursing Science Quarterly, 17,* 27-32.

Registered Nurses Association of Ontario. (2002). *Client centered care: Nursing best practice guideline.* Toronto, Ontario, Canada: Registered Nurses Association of Ontario.

Rogers, M. E. (1970). *An introduction to the theoretical basis of nursing.* Philadelphia: F. A. Davis.

Rogers, M. E. (1992). Nursing science and the space age. *Nursing Science Quarterly, 5,* 27-34.

Wang, C. E. (1999). He-bung: Hope for persons living with leprosy in Taiwan. In R. R. Parse (Ed.), *Hope: An international human becoming perspective* (pp. 143-162). Sudbury, MA: Jones & Bartlett.

Williamson, G. J. (2000). The test of a nursing theory: A personal view. *Nursing Science Quarterly, 13,* 124-128.

BIBLIOGRAPHY

Primary Sources

Books

Parse, R. R. (1974). *Nursing fundamentals.* Flushing, NY: Medical Examination.

Parse, R. R. (1981). *Man-living-health: A theory of nursing.* New York: Wiley.

Parse, R. R. (1987). *Nursing science: Major paradigms, theories, and critiques.* Philadelphia: W. B. Saunders.

Parse, R. R. (Ed.). (1995). *Illuminations: The human becoming theory in practice and research.* New York: National League for Nursing Press.

Parse, R. R. (1998). *The human becoming school of thought: A perspective for nurses and other health professionals.* Thousand Oaks, CA: Sage.

Parse, R. R. (1999). *Hope: An international human becoming perspective.* Sudbury, MA: Jones & Bartlett.

Parse, R. R. (2001). *Qualitative inquiry: The path of sciencing.* Boston: Jones & Bartlett.

Parse, R. R. (2003). *Community: A human becoming perspective.* Sudbury, MA: Jones & Bartlett.

Parse, R. R., Coyne, A. B., & Smith, M. J. (1985). *Nursing research: Qualitative methods.* Bowie, MD: Brady.

Book Chapters

Parse, R. R. (1978). Rights of medical patients. In C. T. Fischer & S. L. Brodsky (Eds.), *Client participation in human services.* New Brunswick, NJ: Transaction.

Parse, R. R. (1981). Caring from a human science perspective. In M. M. Leininger (Ed.), *Caring: An essential human need* (pp. 129-132). Thorofare, NJ: Slack.

Parse, R. R. (1989). Man-living-health: A theory of nursing. In J. Riehl-Sisca (Ed.), *Conceptual models for nursing practice* (3rd ed.). Norwalk, CT: Appleton & Lange.

Parse, R. R. (1989). Parse's man-living-health model and administration of nursing service. In B. Henry, C. Arndt, M. DiVincenti, & A. M. Tomey (Eds.), *Dimensions of nursing administration: Theory, research, education, and practice.* Cambridge, MA: Blackwell Scientific.

Parse, R. R. (1989). The phenomenological research method: Its value for management science. In B. Henry, C. Arndt, M. DiVincenti, & A. M. Tomey (Eds.), *Dimensions of nursing administration: Theory, research, education, and practice.* Cambridge, MA: Blackwell Scientific.

Parse, R. R. (1991). Parse's theory of human becoming. In I. E. Goertzen (Ed.), *Differentiating nursing practice: Into the twenty-first century* (pp. 51-53). Kansas City, MO: American Academy of Nursing.

Parse, R. R. (1993). Parse's human becoming theory: Its research and practice implications. In M. E. Parker (Ed.), *Patterns of nursing theories in practice* (pp. 49-61). New York: National League for Nursing Press.

Parse, R. R. (1995). Foreword. In M. A. Frey & C. L. Sieloff (Eds.), *Advancing King's systems framework and theory of nursing*. Thousand Oaks, CA: Sage.

Parse, R. R. (1995). Man-living-health. A theory of nursing. In M. Mischo-Kelling & K. Wittneben (Eds.), *Auffassungen von pflege in theorie und praxis* (pp. 114-132). Munchen: Urban & Schwarzenberg.

Parse, R. R. (1997). The human becoming theory and its research and practice methodologies. In J. Osterbrink (Ed.), *Pflegetheorien—eine zusammenfassung der 1st international conference*. Freiburg, Germany: Verlag Hans Huber.

Parse, R. R. (1997). The language of nursing knowledge: Saying what we mean. In J. Fawcett & I. M. King (Eds.), *The language of nursing theory and metatheory* (pp. 73-77). Indianapolis: Sigma Theta Tau Monograph.

Parse, R. R. (1999). The lived experience of hope for family members of persons living in a Canadian chronic care facility. In R. R. Parse (Ed.), *Hope: An international human becoming perspective* (pp. 63-77). Sudbury, MA: Jones & Bartlett.

Parse, R. R. (2001). The human becoming school of thought in research. In M. Parker (Ed.), *Nursing theories and nursing practice* (pp. 227-238). Philadelphia: F. A. Davis.

Parse, R. R. (2006). Rosemarie Rizzo Parse's human becoming school of thought. In M. E. Parker, *Nursing theories and nursing practice* (2nd ed.; pp. 187-194). Philadelphia: F. A. Davis.

Book Reviews

Parse, R. R. (1996). [Review of the book Martha E. Rogers: Her life and her work]. Visions: The Journal of Rogerian Science, 2, 52-53.

Parse, R. R. (1997). [Review of the book Quality of life in behavioral medicine]. Women and Health, 25(3), 83-86.

Doctoral Dissertation

Parse, R. R. (1969). An instructional model for the teaching of nursing, interrelating objectives and media (Doctoral dissertation, Duquesne University, 1969). *Dissertation Abstracts International, 31*, 180A.

Journal Articles

Parse, R. R. (1967, Aug.). Advantages and disadvantages of associate degree nursing programs. *Journal of Nursing Education, 6*(15), 5-8.

Parse, R. R. (1988). Beginnings. *Nursing Science Quarterly, 1*(1), 1-2.

Parse, R. R. (1988). Creating traditions: The art of putting it together. *Nursing Science Quarterly, 1*(2), 45.

Parse, R. R. (1988). Scholarly dialogue: The fire of refinement. *Nursing Science Quarterly, 1*(4), 141.

Parse, R. R. (1988). The mainstream of science: Framing the issue. *Nursing Science Quarterly, 1*(3), 93.

Parse, R. R. (1989). Essentials for practicing the art of nursing. *Nursing Science Quarterly, 2*(3), 111.

Parse, R. R. (1989). Making more out of less. *Nursing Science Quarterly, 2*(4), 155.

Parse, R. R. (1989). Martha E. Rogers: A birthday celebration. *Nursing Science Quarterly, 2*(2), 55.

Parse, R. R. (1989). Qualitative research: Publishing and funding. *Nursing Science Quarterly, 2*(1), 1-2.

Parse, R. R. (1990). A time for reflection and projection. *Nursing Science Quarterly, 3*(4), 143.

Parse, R. R. (1990). Health: A personal commitment. *Nursing Science Quarterly, 3*(3), 136-140.

Parse, R. R. (1990). Nursing theory–based practice: A challenge for the 90s. *Nursing Science Quarterly, 3*(2), 53.

Parse, R. R. (1990). Parse's research methodology with an illustration of the lived experience of hope. *Nursing Science Quarterly, 3*(1), 9-17.

Parse, R. R. (1990). Promotion and prevention: Two distinct cosmologies. *Nursing Science Quarterly, 3*(3), 101.

Parse, R. R. (1991). Electronic publishing: Beyond browsing. *Nursing Science Quarterly, 4*(1), 1.

Parse, R. R. (1991). Growing the discipline of nursing. *Nursing Science Quarterly, 4*(4), 139.

Parse, R. R. (1991). Mysteries of health and healing: Two perspectives. *Nursing Science Quarterly, 4*(3), 93.

Parse, R. R. (1991). Phenomenology and nursing. *Japanese Journal of Nursing, 17*(2), 261-269.

Parse, R. R. (1991). The right soil, the right stuff. *Nursing Science Quarterly, 4*(2), 47.

Parse, R. R. (1992). Human becoming: Parse's theory of nursing. *Nursing Science Quarterly, 5*(1), 35-42.

Parse, R. R. (1992). Moving beyond the barrier reef. *Nursing Science Quarterly, 5*(3), 97.

Parse, R. R. (1992). Nursing knowledge for the 21st century: An international commitment. *Nursing Science Quarterly, 5*(1), 8-12.

Parse, R. R. (1992). The performing art of nursing. *Nursing Science Quarterly, 5*(4), 147.

Parse, R. R. (1992). The unsung shapers of nursing science. *Nursing Science Quarterly, 5*(2), 47.

Parse, R. R. (1993). Cartoons: Glimpsing paradoxical moments. *Nursing Science Quarterly, 6*(1), 1.

Parse, R. R. (1993). Critical appraisal: Risking to challenge. *Nursing Science Quarterly, 6*(4), 163.

Parse, R. R. (1993). Nursing and medicine: Two different disciplines. *Nursing Science Quarterly, 6*(3), 109.

Parse, R. R. (1993). Plant now; reap later. *Nursing Science Quarterly, 6*(2), 55.

Parse, R. R. (1993). Scholarly dialogue: Theory guides research and practice. *Nursing Science Quarterly, 6*(1), 12.

Parse, R. R. (1993). The experience of laughter: A phenomenological study. *Nursing Science Quarterly, 6*(1), 39-43.

Parse, R. R. (1994). Charley Potatoes or mashed potatoes? *Nursing Science Quarterly, 7*(3), 97.

Parse, R. R. (1994). Laughing and health: A study using Parse's research method. *Nursing Science Quarterly, 7*(2), 55-64.

Parse, R. R. (1994). Martha E. Rogers: Her voice will not be silenced. *Nursing Science Quarterly, 7*(2), 47.

Parse, R. R. (1994). Quality of life: Sciencing and living the art of human becoming. *Nursing Science Quarterly, 7*(1), 16-21.

Parse, R. R. (1994). Scholarship: Three essential processes. *Nursing Science Quarterly, 7*(4), 143.

Parse, R. R. (1995). Again: What is nursing? *Nursing Science Quarterly, 8*(4), 143.

Parse, R. R. (1995). Building the realm of nursing knowledge. *Nursing Science Quarterly, 8*(2), 51.

Parse, R. R. (1995). Commentary: Parse's theory of human becoming: An alternative to nursing practice for pediatric oncology nurses. *Journal of Pediatric Oncology Nursing, 12*(3), 128.

Parse, R. R. (1995). Nursing theories and frameworks: The essence of advanced practice nursing. *Nursing Science Quarterly, 8*(1), 1.

Parse, R. R. (1995). Nursing theory based research and practice. A conference coming to Japan. Tokyo, Japan: Igacu Shoin. *Medical News Weekly*.

Parse, R. R. (1996). Building knowledge through qualitative research: The road less traveled. *Nursing Science Quarterly, 9*(1), 10-16.

Parse, R. R. (1996). Critical thinking: What is it? *Nursing Science Quarterly, 9*(3), 138.

Parse, R. R. (1996). Hear ye, hear ye: Novice and seasoned authors! *Nursing Science Quarterly, 9*(1), 1.

Parse, R. R. (1996). Nursing theories: An original path. *Nursing Science Quarterly, 9*(2), 85.

Parse, R. R. (1996). Quality of life for persons living with Alzheimer's disease: A human becoming perspective. *Nursing Science Quarterly, 9*(3), 126-133.

Parse, R. R. (1996). Reality: A seamless symphony of becoming. *Nursing Science Quarterly, 9*(4), 181-183.

Parse, R. R. (1996). The human becoming theory: Challenges in practice and research. *Nursing Science Quarterly, 9*(1), 55-60.

Parse, R. R. (1997). Concept inventing: Unitary creations. *Nursing Science Quarterly, 10*(2), 63-64.

Parse, R. R. (1997). Investing the legacy: Martha E. Rogers' voice will not be silenced. *Visions: The Journal of Rogerian Science, 5*, 7-11.

Parse, R. R. (1997). Joy-sorrow: A study using the Parse research method. *Nursing Science Quarterly, 10*(2), 80-87.

Parse, R. R. (1997). Leadership: The essentials. *Nursing Science Quarterly, 10*(3), 109.

Parse, R. R. (1997). New beginnings in a quiet revolution. *Nursing Science Quarterly, 10*(1), 1.

Parse, R. R. (1997). The human becoming theory: The was, is, and will be. *Nursing Science Quarterly, 10*(1), 32-38.

Parse, R. R. (1997). Transforming research and practice with the human becoming theory. *Nursing Science Quarterly, 10*(4), 171-174.

Parse, R. R. (1998). Moving on. *Nursing Science Quarterly, 11*(4), 135.

Parse, R. R. (1998). The art of criticism. *Nursing Science Quarterly, 11*(2), 43.

Parse, R. R. (1998). Will nursing exist tomorrow? A reprise. *Nursing Science Quarterly, 11*(1), 1.

Parse, R. R. (1999). Authorship: Whose responsibility? *Nursing Science Quarterly, 12*(2), 99.

Parse, R. R. (1999). Community: An alternative view. *Nursing Science Quarterly, 12*(2), 119-124.

Parse, R. R. (1999). Expanding the vision: Tilling the field of nursing knowledge. *Nursing Science Quarterly, 12*(1), 3.

Parse, R. R. (1999). Integrity and the advancement of nursing knowledge. *Nursing Science Quarterly, 12*(3), 187.

Parse, R. R. (1999). Nursing science: The transformation of practice. *Journal of Advanced Nursing, 30*(6), 1383-1387.

Parse, R. R. (1999). Nursing: The discipline and the profession. *Nursing Science Quarterly, 12*(4), 275.

Parse, R. R. (1999). Witnessing as true presence. *Illuminations: Newsletter for the International Consortium of Parse Scholars, 8*(3), 1.

Parse, R. R. (2000). Into the new millennium. *Nursing Science Quarterly, 13*(1), 3.

Parse, R. R. (2000). Language: Words reflect and cocreate meaning. *Nursing Science Quarterly, 13*(3), 187.

Parse, R. R. (2000). Obfuscating: The persistent practice of misnaming. *Nursing Science Quarterly, 13*(2), 91-92.

Parse, R. R. (2000). Paradigms: A reprise. *Nursing Science Quarterly, 13*(4), 275-276.

Parse, R. R. (2001). Contributions to the discipline. *Nursing Science Quarterly, 14*(1), 5.

Parse, R. R. (2001). Nursing: Still in the shadow of medicine. *Nursing Science Quarterly, 14*(3), 181.

Parse, R. R. (2001). The lived experience of contentment: A study using the Parse research method. *Nursing Science Quarterly, 14*, 330-338.

Parse, R. R. (2001). The universe is flat. *Nursing Science Quarterly, 14*(2), 93.

Parse, R. R. (2002). 15th anniversary celebration. *Nursing Science Quarterly, 15*, 3.

Parse, R. R. (2002). Aha! a! hha! Discovery, wonder, laughter. *Nursing Science Quarterly, 15*, 273.

Parse, R. R. (2002). Mentoring moments. *Nursing Science Quarterly, 15*, 97.

Parse, R. R. (2002). Transforming healthcare with a unitary view of human. *Nursing Science Quarterly, 15*, 46-50.

Parse, R. R. (2002). Words, words, words: Meanings, meanings, meanings! *Nursing Science Quarterly, 15*, 183.

Parse, R. R. (2003). A call for dignity in nursing. *Nursing Science Quarterly, 16*, 193.

Parse, R. R. (2003). Research approaches: Likenesses and differences. *Nursing Science Quarterly, 16*, 5.

Parse, R. R. (2003). Silos and schools of thought. *Nursing Science Quarterly, 16*, 101.

Parse, R. R. (2003). The lived experience of feeling very tired: A study using the Parse research method. *Nursing Science Quarterly, 16*, 319-325.

Parse, R. R. (2003). What constitutes nursing research? *Nursing Science Quarterly, 16*, 287.

Parse, R. R. (2004). A human becoming teaching-learning model. *Nursing Science Quarterly, 17*, 33-35.

Parse, R. R. (2004). New directions. *Nursing Science Quarterly, 17*, 5.

Parse, R. R. (2004). Power in position. *Nursing Science Quarterly, 17*, 101.

Parse, R. R. (2004). A human becoming teaching-learning model. *Nursing Science Quarterly, 17*, 33-35.

Parse, R. R. (2004). Quality of life: A human becoming perspective. *Japanese Journal of Nursing Research, 37*(5), 21-26.

Parse, R. R. (2004). Person-centered care. *Nursing Science Quarterly, 17*, 193.

Parse, R. R. (2004). The many meanings of unitary: A plea for clarity. *Nursing Science Quarterly, 17*, 293.

Parse, R. R. (2004). The ubiquitous nature of unitary: Major change in human becoming language. *Illuminations: Newsletter for the International Consortium of Parse Scholars, 13*(1), 1.

Parse, R. R. (2004). Another look at vigilance. *Illuminations: Newsletter for the International Consortium of Parse Scholars, 13*(2), 1.

Parse, R. R. (2005). A community of scholars. *Nursing Science Quarterly, 18*, 119.

Parse, R. R. (2005). Attentive reverence. *Illuminations: Newsletter for the International Consortium of Parse Scholars, 14*(2), 1.

Parse, R. R. (2005). Challenges for global nursing. *Nursing Science Quarterly, 18*, 285.

Parse, R. R. (2005). Choosing a doctoral program in nursing: What to consider. *Nursing Science Quarterly, 18*, 5.

Parse, R. R. (2005). Nursing and medicine: Continuing challenges. *Nursing Science Quarterly, 18*, 5.

Parse, R. R. (2005). Parse's criteria for evaluation of theory with a comparison of Parse and Fawcett. *Nursing Science Quarterly, 18*, 135-137.

Parse, R. R. (2005). Scientific standards: A renewed alert. *Nursing Science Quarterly, 18*, 97.

Parse, R. R. (2005). Symbols and meanings in academia. *Nursing Science Quarterly, 18*, 197.

Parse, R. R. (2005). The human becoming modes of inquiry: Emerging sciencing. *Nursing Science Quarterly, 18*, 297-300.

Parse, R. R. (2005). The meaning of freely choosing. *Illuminations: Newsletter for the International Consortium of Parse Scholars, 14*(1), 1-2.

Parse, R. R. (2006). Concept Inventing: Continuing Clarification. *Nursing Science Quarterly, 19*, 289.

Parse, R. R. (2006). Feeling respected: A Parse method study. *Nursing Science Quarterly, 19*, 51-57.

Parse, R. R. (2006). Nursing and medicine: Continuing challenges. *Nursing Science Quarterly, 19*, 5.

Parse, R. R. (2006). Outcomes: Saying what you mean. *Nursing Science Quarterly, 19*, 189.

Parse, R. R. (2006). Research findings evince benefits of nursing theory-guided practice. *Nursing Science Quarterly, 19*, 87.

Parse, R. R. (2007). A human becoming perspective on quality of life. *Nursing Science Quarterly,* 20, 217.

Parse, R. R. (2007). Building a research culture. *Nursing Science Quarterly,* 20, 197.

Parse, R. R. (2007). Data-based articles and duplicate publication. *Nursing Science Quarterly,* 20, 301.

Parse, R. R. (2007). Hope in "Rita Hayworth and Shawshank Redemption": A human becoming hermeneutic study. *Nursing Science Quarterly, 20*, 148-154.

Parse, R. R. (2007). Nursing knowledge and health policy. *Nursing Science Quarterly, 20*, 105.

Parse, R. R. (2007). The humanbecoming school of thought in 2050. *Nursing Science Quarterly,* 20, 308

Parse, R. R. (2007). Twenty years of commitment to nursing's uniqueness as a discipline. *Nursing Science Quarterly, 20*, 5.

Parse, R. R. (2008). Is there a tipping point for congruence in nursing knowledge? *Nursing Science Quarterly, 21*(3).

Parse, R. R. (2008). Nursing knowledge development: Who's to say how? *Nursing Science Quarterly,* 21(2).

Parse, R. R. (2008). Proliferation of degrees in nursing: A call for clarity. *Nursing Science Quarterly,* 21, 5.

Parse, R. R. (2008). The humanbecoming leading-following model. *Nursing Science Quarterly, 21*(4).

Parse, R. R. (2008). The humanbecoming mentoring model. *Nursing Science Quarterly, 21*(3).

Parse, R. R. (2008). Truth for the moment: Personal testimony as evidence. *Nursing Science Quarterly, 21*, 45-48.

Parse, R. R., Bournes, D. A., Barrett, E. A. M., Malinski, V. M., & Phillips, J. R. (1999). A better way: 10 things health professionals can do to move toward a more personal and meaningful system. *On Call: A Magazine for Nurses and Healthcare Professionals, 2*(8), 14-17.

Secondary Sources

Book Chapters About Parse's Theory of Human Becoming

Allchin-Petardi, L. (1999). Hope for American women with children. In R. R. Parse (Ed.), *Hope: An international human becoming perspective* (pp. 273-285). Sudbury, MA: Jones & Bartlett.

Banonis, B. C. (1995). Metaphors in the practice of the human becoming theory. In R. R. Parse (Ed.), *Illuminations: The human becoming theory in practice and research* (pp. 87-95). New York: National League for Nursing Press.

Baumann, S. L. (1999). The lived experience of hope: Children in families struggling to make a home. In R. R. Parse (Ed.), *Hope: An international human becoming perspective* (pp. 191-210). Sudbury, MA: Jones & Bartlett.

Bunkers, S. S. (1999). The lived experience of hope for those working with homeless persons. In R. R. Parse (Ed.), *Hope: An international human becoming perspective* (pp. 227-250). Sudbury, MA: Jones & Bartlett.

Bunkers, S. S. (1999). Translating nursing conceptual frameworks and theory for nursing practice. In A. Solari-Twadell & M. A. McDermott (Eds.), *Parish nursing: Promoting whole person health within faith communities* (pp. 205-214). Thousand Oaks, CA: Sage.

Bunkers, S. S., & Daly, J. (1999). The lived experience of hope for Australian families living with coronary disease. In R. R. Parse (Ed.), *Hope: An international human becoming perspective* (pp. 45-61). Sudbury, MA: Jones & Bartlett.

Cody, W. K. (1995). Of life immense in passion, pulse, and power: Dialoguing with Whitman and Parse. A hermeneutic study. In R. R. Parse (Ed.), *Illuminations: The human becoming theory in practice and research* (pp. 269-307). New York: National League for Nursing Press.

Cody, W. K. (1995). The lived experience of grieving for families living with AIDS: Family-centered research using Parse's method. In R. R. Parse (Ed.), *Illuminations: The human becoming theory in practice and research* (pp. 197-242). New York: National League for Nursing Press.

Cody, W. K. (1995). The view of the family within the human becoming theory. In R. R. Parse (Ed.), *Illuminations: The human becoming theory in practice and research* (pp. 9-26). New York: National League for Nursing Press.

Cody, W. K. (1995). True presence with families living with HIV disease. In R. R. Parse (Ed.), *Illuminations: The human becoming theory in practice and research* (pp. 115-133). New York: National League for Nursing Press.

Cody, W. K., & Filler, J. E. (1999). The lived experience of hope for women residing in a shelter. In R. R. Parse (Ed.), *Hope: An international human becoming perspective* (pp. 211-225). Sudbury, MA: Jones & Bartlett.

Cody, W. K., Hudepohl, J. H., & Brinkman, K. S. (1995). True presence with a child and his family. In R. R. Parse (Ed.), *Illuminations: The human becoming theory in practice and research* (pp. 135-146). New York: National League for Nursing Press.

Daly, J. (1995). The lived experience of suffering. In R. R. Parse (Ed.), *Illuminations: The human becoming theory in practice and research* (pp. 253-268). New York: National League for Nursing Press.

Daly, J. (1995). The view of suffering within the human becoming theory. In R. R. Parse (Ed.), *Illuminations: The human becoming theory in practice and research* (pp. 45-59). New York: National League for Nursing Press.

Daly, J., & Watson, J. (1996). Parse's human becoming theory of nursing. In J. Greenwood (Ed.), *Nursing theory in Australia: Development and application* (pp. 177-200). Pymble, NSW, Australia: Harper Educational Publishers.

Jonas, C. M. (1995). Evaluation of the human becoming theory in family practice. In R. R. Parse (Ed.), *Illuminations: The human becoming theory in practice and research* (pp. 347-366). New York: National League for Nursing Press.

Jonas, C. M. (1995). True presence through music for persons living their dying. In R. R. Parse (Ed.), *Illuminations: The human becoming theory in practice* (pp. 97-104). New York: National League for Nursing Press.

Kelley, L. S. (1995). The house-garden-wilderness metaphor: Caring frameworks and the human becoming theory. In R. R. Parse (Ed.), *Illuminations: The human becoming theory in practice and research* (pp. 61-76). New York: National League for Nursing Press.

Kelley, L. S. (1999). Hope as lived by Native Americans. In R. R. Parse (Ed.), *Hope: An international human becoming perspective* (pp. 251-272). Sudbury, MA: Jones & Bartlett.

Mitchell, G. J. (1991). Distinguishing practice with Parse's theory. In I. E. Goertzen (Ed.), *Differentiating nursing practice into the twenty-first century* (pp. 55-58). New York: American Nurses Association Publication.

Mitchell, G. J. (1993). Parse's theory in practice. In M. E. Parker (Ed.), *Patterns of nursing theories in practice* (pp. 62-80). New York: National League for Nursing Press.

Mitchell, G. J. (1995). Evaluation of the human becoming theory in practice in an acute care setting. In R. R. Parse (Ed.), *Illuminations: The human becoming theory in practice and research* (pp. 367-399). New York: National League for Nursing Press.

Mitchell, G. J. (1995). The lived experience of restriction-freedom in later life. In R. R. Parse (Ed.), *Illuminations: The human becoming theory in practice and research* (pp. 159-195). New York: National League for Nursing Press.

Mitchell, G. J. (1995). The view of freedom within the human becoming theory. In R. R. Parse (Ed.), *Illumination: The human becoming theory in practice and research* (pp. 27-43). New York: National League for Nursing Press.

Mitchell, G.J. (2002). Parse's theory of human becoming and nursing practice. In M. R. Alligood & A. Marriner-Tomey (Eds.), *Nursing theory: Utilization and application* (2nd ed.), (pp. 403-428). St. Louis, MO: Mosby-Year Book Inc.

Mitchell, G.J. (2002). Rosemarie Rizzo Parse: Human becoming. In M. R. Alligood & A. Marriner-Tomey, (Eds.), *Nursing theorists and their work* (5th ed), (pp. 227-259). St. Louis, MO: Mosby.

Mitchell, G.J. (2004). Leading and enhancing patient-focused care: The human becoming theory in action. In J. Daly, S. Speedy, & D. Jackson (Eds.), *Nursing leadership* (pp. 299-312). Marrickville, New South Wales: Elsevier Australia.

Mitchell, G. J. (2006). Parse's theory of human becoming and nursing practice. In M. Alligood and A. Marriner-Tomey (Eds.), *Nursing theory: Utilization & application* (3rd ed) (pp. 431-460). PA: Elsevier.

Mitchell, G. J. (2006). Rosemarie Rizzo Parse: Human becoming. In A. Marriner-Tomey & M. R. Alligood, (Eds.), *Nursing theorists and their work* (6th ed.) (pp. 522-559). St. Louis, MO: Mosby-Year Book.

Mitchell, G. J. (2007). Parse's theory of human becoming and nursing practice. In M. Alligood and A. Marriner-Tomey (Eds.), *Nursing theory: Utilization & application* (3rd ed) (pp. 431-460). PA: Elsevier. C. Calamandrei, Italian translation. Milano, Italy: McGraw-Hill. (2006).

Mitchell, G. J., Bunkers, S. S., & Bournes, D. A. (2006). Applications of Parse's human becoming school of thought. In M. E. Parker, *Nursing theories and nursing practice* (2nd ed.; pp. 194-216). Philadelphia: F. A. Davis.

Pickrell, K. D., Lee, R. E., Schumacher, L. P., & Twigg, P. (1998). Rosemarie Rizzo Parse: Human becoming. In A. M. Tomey & M. R. Alligood (Eds.), *Nursing theorists and their work* (4th ed.). St. Louis: Mosby.

Pilkington, F. B., & Millar, B. (1999). The lived experience of hope with persons from Wales, UK. In R. R. Parse (Ed.), *Hope: An international human becoming perspective* (pp. 163-189). Sudbury, MA: Jones & Bartlett.

Rasmusson, D. L. (1995). True presence with homeless persons. In R. R. Parse (Ed.), *Illuminations: The human becoming theory in practice and research* (pp. 105-113). New York: National League for Nursing Press.

Santopinto, M. D. A., & Smith, M. C. (1995). Evaluation of the human becoming theory in practice with adults and children. In R. R. Parse (Ed.), *Illuminations: The human becoming theory in practice and research* (pp. 309-346). New York: National League for Nursing Press.

Smith, M. J. (1989). Research and practice application related to man-living-health. In J. Riehl-Sisca (Ed.), *Conceptual models for nursing practice* (3rd ed., pp. 267-276). Norwalk, CT: Appleton & Lange.

Takahashi, T. (1999). Kibou: Hope for persons in Japan. In R. R. Parse (Ed.), *Hope: An international human becoming perspective* (pp. 115-128). Sudbury, MA: Jones & Bartlett.

Toikkanen, T., & Muurinen, E. (1999). Toivo: Hope for persons in Finland. In R. R. Parse (Ed.), *Hope: An international human becoming perspective* (pp. 79-96). Sudbury, MA: Jones & Bartlett.

Wang, C. E. H. (1999). He-Bung: Hope for persons living with leprosy in Taiwan. In R. R. Parse (Ed.), *Hope: An international human becoming perspective* (pp. 45-61). Sudbury, MA: Jones & Bartlett.

Willman, A. (1999). Hopp: The lived experience for Swedish elders. In R. R. Parse (Ed.), *Hope: An international human becoming perspective* (pp. 129-142). Sudbury, MA: Jones & Bartlett.

Zanotti, R., & Bournes, D. A. (1999). Speranza: A study of the lived experience of hope with persons from Italy. In R. R. Parse (Ed.), *Hope: An international human becoming perspective* (pp. 97-114). Sudbury, MA: Jones & Bartlett.

Journal Articles About Parse's Theory

Allchin-Petardi, L. (1998). Weathering the storm: Persevering through a difficult time. *Nursing Science Quarterly, 11*(4), 172-177.

Andrus, K. (1995). Parse's nursing theory and the practice of perioperative nursing. *Canadian Operating Room Nursing Journal, 13*(3), 19-22.

Aquino-Russell, C. E. (2006). A phenomenological study: The lived experience of persons having a different sense of hearing. *Nursing Science Quarterly, 19*, 339-348.

Aquino-Russell, K., Struby, F. V. M., & Reviczky, K. (2007). Living attentive presence and changing perspectives with a web-based nursing theory course. *Nursing Science Quarterly, 20*, 128-134.

Arndt, M. J. (1995). Parse's theory of human becoming in practice with hospitalized adolescents. *Nursing Science Quarterly, 8*(2), 86-90.

Arrigo, B., & Cody, W. K. (2004). A dialogue on existential-phenomenological thought in psychology and in nursing. *Nursing Science Quarterly, 17*, 6-11.

Banonis, B. C. (1989). The lived experience of recovering from addiction: A phenomenological study. *Nursing Science Quarterly, 2*(1), 37-43.

Baumann, S. (1994). No place of their own: An exploratory study. *Nursing Science Quarterly, 7*(4), 162-169.

Baumann, S. (1995). Two views of children's art: Psychoanalysis and Parse's human becoming theory. *Nursing Science Quarterly, 8*(2), 65-70.

Baumann, S. (1996). Feeling uncomfortable: Children in families with no place of their own. *Nursing Science Quarterly, 9*(4), 152-159.

Baumann, S. (1996). Parse's research methodology and the nurse-researcher-child process. *Nursing Science Quarterly, 9*(1), 27-32.

Baumann, S. (1997). Contrasting two approaches in a community-based nursing practice with older adults: The medical model and Parse's nursing theory. *Nursing Science Quarterly, 10*(3), 124-130.

Baumann, S. L. (1997). Qualitative research with children as participants. *Nursing Science Quarterly, 10*(2), 68-69.

Baumann, S. L. (1999). Art as a path of inquiry. *Nursing Science Quarterly, 12*(2), 106-110.

Baumann, S. L. (2003). The lived experience of feeling very tired: A study of adolescent girls. *Nursing Science Quarterly, 16*, 326-333.

Baumann, S., & Braddick, M. (1999). Out of their element: Fathers of children who are "not the same." *Journal of Pediatric Nursing, 14*(6), 269-278.

Baumann, S. L., Dyches, T. T., & Braddick, M. (2005). Being a sibling. *Nursing Science Quarterly, 18*, 51-58.

Baumann, S. L., & Englert, R. (2003). A comparison of three views of spirituality in oncology nursing. *Nursing Science Quarterly, 16*, 52-59.

Baumann, S. L. & Söderhamn, O. (2005). Considering and enjoying tomorrow: Global aging through a human becoming lens. *Nursing Science Quarterly, 18*, 353-358.

Benedict, L. L., Bunkers, S. S., Damgaard, G. A., Duffy, C. E., Hohman, M. L., & Vander Woude, D. L. (2000). The South Dakota board of nursing theory–based regulatory decisioning model. *Nursing Science Quarterly, 13*(2), 167-171.

Bernardo, A. (1998). Technology and true presence in nursing. *Holistic Nursing Practice, 12*(4), 40-49.

Bournes, D. A. (2000). A commitment to honoring people's choices. *Nursing Science Quarterly, 13*(1), 18-23.

Bournes, D. A. (2000). Concept inventing: A process for creating a unitary definition of having courage. *Nursing Science Quarterly, 13*(2), 143-149.

Bournes, D. A. (2002). Having courage: A lived experience of human becoming. *Nursing Science Quarterly, 15*, 220-229.

Bournes, D. A. (2002). Research evaluating human becoming in practice. *Nursing Science Quarterly,* 15, 190-195.

Bournes, D. A. (2006). Human becoming-guided practice. *Nursing Science Quarterly, 19*, 329-330.

Bournes, D. A. (2007). Rosemarie Rizzo Parse over the years. *Nursing Science Quarterly*, 20, 305.

Bournes, D. A., Bunkers, S. S., & Welch, A. J. (2004). Human becoming: Scope and challenges. *Nursing Science Quarterly, 17*, 227-232.

Bournes, D. A., & Das Gupta, T. L. (1997). Professional practice leader: A transformational role that addresses human diversity. *Nursing Administration Quarterly, 21*(4), 61-68.

Bournes, D. A., & Ferguson-Paré, M. (2005). Persevering through a difficult time during the SARS outbreak in Toronto. *Nursing Science Quarterly, 18*, 324-333.

Bournes, D. A., & Ferguson-Paré, M. (2007). Human becoming and 80/20: An innovative professional development model for nurses. *Nursing Science Quarterly, 20*, 237-253.

Bournes, D. A., & Flint, F. (2003). Mis-takes: Mistakes in the nurse-person process. *Nursing Science Quarterly, 16*, 127-130.

Bournes, D. A., & Linscott, J. (1998). Patient-focused care: A process of discovery. *Theoria, 7*(4), 3-5.

Bournes, D. A., & Mitchell, G. J. (2002). Waiting: The experience of persons in a critical care waiting room. *Research in Nursing & Health, 25*, 58-67.

Bournes, D. A., & Naef, R. (2006). Human becoming practice around the globe: Exploring the art of living true presence. *Nursing Science Quarterly, 19*, 109-115.

Bunkers, S. S. (1998). A nursing theory–guided model of health ministry: Human becoming in parish nursing. *Nursing Science Quarterly, 11*(1), 7-8.

Bunkers, S. S. (1998). Considering tomorrow: Parse's theory-guided research. *Nursing Science Quarterly, 11*(2), 56-63.

Bunkers, S. S. (1999). Commentary on Parse's view of community. *Nursing Science Quarterly, 12*(2), 121-124.

Bunkers, S. S. (1999). Emerging discoveries and possibilities in nursing. *Nursing Science Quarterly, 12*(1), 26-29.

Bunkers, S. S. (1999). Learning to be still. *Nursing Science Quarterly, 12*, 172-173.

Bunkers, S. S. (1999). The meaning of new age: The judging and misjudging of values and beliefs. *Nursing Science Quarterly, 12*(2), 100-105.

Bunkers, S. S. (1999). The teaching-learning process and the theory of human becoming. *Nursing Science Quarterly, 12*(3), 227-232.

Bunkers, S. S. (2002). Lifelong learning: A human becoming perspective. *Nursing Science Quarterly, 15*, 294-300.

Bunkers, S. S. (2003). Comparison of three Parse method studies on feeling very tired. *Nursing Science Quarterly, 16*, 340-344.

Bunkers, S. S. (2003). Understanding the stranger. *Nursing Science Quarterly, 16*, 305-309.

Bunkers, S. S. (2004). The lived experience of feeling cared for: A human becoming perspective. *Nursing Science Quarterly, 17*, 63-71.

Bunkers, S. S. (2006). Reflections of the prairie as a creative teaching-learning process. *Nursing Science Quarterly, 19*, 25-29.

Bunkers, S. S. (2007). The experience of feeling unsure for women at end of life. *Nursing Science Quarterly, 20*, 56-63.

Bunkers, S. S., Michaels, C., & Ethridge, P. (1997). Advanced practice nursing in community: Nursing's opportunity. *Advanced Practice Nursing Quarterly, 2*(4), 79-84.

Butler, M. J. (1988). Family transformation: Parse's theory in practice. *Nursing Science Quarterly, 1*(2), 68-74.

Butler, M. J., & Snodgrass, F. G. (1991). Beyond abuse: Parse's theory in practice. *Nursing Science Quarterly, 4*(2), 76-82.

Carson, M. G., & Mitchell, G. J. (1998). The experience of living with persistent pain. *Journal of Advanced Nursing, 28*(6), 1242-1248.

Chan, E. A. (2005). The influence of the human becoming theory on teaching-learning stories in Hangzhou, China. *Nursing Science Quarterly, 18*, 306-312.

Chapman, J. S., Mitchell, G. J., & Forchuk, C. (1994). A glimpse of nursing theory-based practice in Canada. *Nursing Science Quarterly, 7*(3), 104-112.

Cody, W. K. (1991). Grieving a personal loss. *Nursing Science Quarterly, 4*, 61-68.

Cody, W. K. (1991). Multidimensionality: Its meaning and significance. *Nursing Science Quarterly, 4*, 140-141.

Cody, W. K. (1993). Norms and nursing science: A question of values. *Nursing Science Quarterly, 6*(3), 110-112.

Cody, W. K. (1994). Meaning and mystery in nursing science and art. *Nursing Science Quarterly, 7*(2), 48-51.

Cody, W. K. (1994). Nursing theory–guided practice: What it is and what it is not. *Nursing Science Quarterly, 7*(4), 144-145.
Cody, W. K. (1994). Radical health care reform: The person as case manager. *Nursing Science Quarterly, 7*(4), 180-182.
Cody, W. K. (1995). All those paradigms: Many in the universe, two in nursing. *Nursing Science Quarterly, 8*(4), 144-147.
Cody, W. K. (1995). The meaning of grieving for families living with AIDS. *Nursing Science Quarterly, 8*(3), 104-114.
Cody, W. K. (1996). Drowning in eclecticism. *Nursing Science Quarterly, 9*, 86-88.
Cody, W. K. (1996). Occult reductionism in the discourse of theory development. *Nursing Science Quarterly, 9*(4), 140-142.
Cody, W. K. (1997). The many faces of change: Discomfort with the new. *Nursing Science Quarterly, 10*(2), 65-67.
Cody, W. K. (1998). Critical theory and nursing science: Freedom in theory and practice. *Nursing Science Quarterly, 11*(2), 44-46.
Cody, W. K. (1999). Affirming reflection. *Nursing Science Quarterly, 12*(1), 4-6.
Cody, W. K. (1999). Middle-range theories: Do they foster the development of nursing science? *Nursing Science Quarterly, 12*(1), 9-14.
Cody, W. K. (2000). Paradigm shift or paradigm drift? A meditation on commitment and transcendence. *Nursing Science Quarterly, 13*(2), 93-102.
Cody, W. K. (2000). The challenge of unitary conceptualizations: An exemplar. *Nursing Science Quarterly, 13*(1), 4.
Cody, W. K. (2003). Diversity and becoming: Implications of human existence as coexistence. *Nursing Science Quarterly, 16*, 195-200.
Cody, W. K., & Mitchell, G. J. (1992). Parse's theory as a model for practice: The cutting edge. *ANS Advances in Nursing Science, 15*(2), 52-65.
Costello-Nickitas, D. M. (1994). Choosing life goals: A phenomenological study. *Nursing Science Quarterly, 7*(2), 87-92.
Daly, J., & Jackson, D. (1999). On the use of nursing theory in nursing education, nursing practice, and nursing research in Australia. *Nursing Science Quarterly, 12*(4), 342-345.
Daly, J., Mitchell, G. J., & Jonas-Simpson, C. M. (1996). Quality of life and the human becoming theory: Exploring discipline-specific contributions. *Nursing Science Quarterly, 9*(4), 170-174.
Damgaard, G., & Bunkers, S. S. (1998). Nursing science-guided practice and education: A state board of nursing perspective. *Nursing Science Quarterly, 11*(4), 142-144.
Davis, C., & Cannava, E. (1995). The meaning of retirement for communally-living retired performing artists. *Nursing Science Quarterly, 8*(1), 8-16.
Doucet, T., & Bournes, D. A. (2007). Review of research related to Parse's theory of human becoming. *Nursing Science Quarterly, 20*, 16-32.
Fawcett, J. (2001). The nurse theorists: 21st-century updates—Rosemarie Rizzo Parse. *Nursing Science Quarterly, 14*, 126-131.
Fisher, M. A., & Mitchell, G. J. (1998). Patients' views of quality of life: Transforming the knowledge base of nursing. *Clinical Nurse Specialist, 12*(3), 99-105.
Florczak, K. L. (2006). The lived experience of sacrificing something important. *Nursing Science Quarterly, 19*, 133-141.
Futrell, M., Wondolowski, C., & Mitchell, G. J. (1994). Aging in the oldest old living in Scotland: A phenomenological study. *Nursing Science Quarterly, 6*(4), 189-194.
Gates, K. M. (2000). The experience of caring for a loved one: A phenomenological study. *Nursing Science Quarterly, 13*(1), 54-59.
Hamalis, P. (1999). Reaching out. *Nursing Science Quarterly, 12*(4), 346.
Hansen-Ketchum, P. (2004). Parse's theory in practice. *Journal of Holistic Nursing, 22*, 57-72.
Heine, C. (1991). Development of gerontological nursing theory: Applying man-living-health theory of nursing. *Nursing and Health Care, 12*, 184-188.
Hodges, H. F., Keeley, A. C., & Grier, E. C. (2001). Masterworks of art and chronic illness experiences in the elderly. *Journal of Advanced Nursing, 36*, 389-398.
Huch, M. H. (2002). Response to: Critical review of R. R. Parse's "The human becoming school of thought. A perspective for nurses and other health professionals." *Journal of Advanced Nursing, 37*, 217.
Huch, M. H., & Bournes, D. A. (2003). Community dwellers' perspectives on the experience of feeling very tired. *Nursing Science Quarterly, 16*, 334-339.
Huchings, D. (2002). Parallels in practice: Palliative nursing practice and Parse's theory of human becoming. *American Journal of Hospice and Palliative Care, 19*, 408-414.
International Consortium of Parse Scholars. (1999). A nursing position on global healthcare: Our commitment to humankind. *Nursing Science Quarterly, 12*(4), 347.
Jacono, B. J., & Jacono, J. J. (1996). The benefits of Newman and Parse in helping nurse teachers determine methods to enhance student creativity. *Nursing Education Today, 16*, 356-362.
Janes, N. M., & Wells, D. L. (1997). Elderly patients' experiences with nurses guided by Parse's theory of human becoming. *Clinical Nursing Research, 6*, 205-224.
Jonas, C. M. (1992). The meaning of being an elder in Nepal. *Nursing Science Quarterly, 5*(4), 171-175.
Jonas-Simpson, C. M. (1996). The patient-focused care journey: Where patients and families guide the way. *Nursing Science Quarterly, 9*(4), 145-146.
Jonas-Simpson, C. (1997). Living the art of the human becoming theory. *Nursing Science Quarterly, 10*(4), 175-179.
Jonas-Simpson, C. M. (1997). The Parse research method through music. *Nursing Science Quarterly, 10*(3), 112-114.

Jonas-Simpson, C. M. (2001). Feeling understood: A melody of human becoming. *Nursing Science Quarterly, 14*, 222-230.

Jonas-Simpson, C. M. (2003). The experience of being listened to: A human becoming study with music. *Nursing Science Quarterly, 16*, 232-238.

Jonas-Simpson, C. J. (2006). The possibility of changing meaning in light of space and place. *Nursing Science Quarterly, 19*, 89-94.

Jonas-Simpson, C., & McMahon, E. (2005). The language of loss when a baby dies prior to birth: Cocreating human experience. *Nursing Science Quarterly, 18*, 124-130.

Kagan, P. N. (2008). Feeling listened to: A lived experience of humanbecoming. *Nursing Science Quarterly, 21*, 59-67.

Karnick, P. M. (2005). Human becoming theory with children. *Nursing Science Quarterly, 18*, 221-226.

Karnick, P. M. (2007). Nursing practice: Imaging the possibles. *Nursing Science Quarterly, 20*, 44-47.

Kelley, L. S. (1991). Struggling with going along when you do not believe. *Nursing Science Quarterly, 4*(3), 123-129.

Kelley, L. S. (1995). Parse's theory in practice with a group in the community. *Nursing Science Quarterly, 8*(3), 127-132.

Kelley, L. S. (1999). Evaluating change in quality of life from the perspective of the person: Advanced practice nursing and Parse's goal of nursing. *Holistic Nursing Practice, 13*(4), 61-70.

Kim, M. S., Shin, K. R., & Shin, S. R. (1998). Korean adolescents' experiences of smoking cessation: A prelude to research with the human becoming perspective. *Nursing Science Quarterly, 11*(3), 105-109.

Kruse, B. G. (1999). The lived experience of serenity: Using Parse's research method. *Nursing Science Quarterly, 12*(2), 143-150.

Lee, O. J., & Pilkington, F. B. (1999). Practice with persons living their dying: A human becoming perspective. *Nursing Science Quarterly, 12*(4), 324-328.

Legault, F., & Ferguson-Paré, M. (1999). Advancing nursing practice: An evaluation study of Parse's theory of human becoming. *Canadian Journal of Nursing Leadership, 12*(1), 30-35.

Letcher, D. C., & Yancey, N. R. (2004). Witnessing change with aspiring nurses: A human becoming teaching-learning process in nursing education. *Nursing Science Quarterly, 17*, 36-41.

Liehr, P. R. (1989). The core of true presence: A loving center. *Nursing Science Quarterly, 2*(1), 7-8.

Linscott, J., Spee, R., Flint, F., & Fisher, A. (1999). Creating a culture of patient-focused care through a learner-centered philosophy. *Canadian Journal of Nursing Leadership, 12*(4), 5-10.

Liu, S. L. (1994). The lived experience of health for hospitalized older women in Taiwan. *Journal of National Taipei College of Nursing, 1*, 1-84.

Markovic, M. (1997). From theory to perioperative practice with Parse. *Canadian Operating Room Nursing Journal, 15*(1), 13-16.

Mattice, M. (1991). Parse's theory of nursing in practice: A manager's perspective. *Canadian Journal of Nursing Administration, 4*(1), 11-13.

Mattice, M., & Mitchell, G. J. (1990). Caring for confused elders. *The Canadian Nurse, 86*(11), 16-18.

Melnechenko, K. L. (2003). To make a difference: Nursing presence. *Nursing Forum, 38*, 18-24.

Milton, C. L. (2000). Beneficence: Honoring the commitment. *Nursing Science Quarterly, 13*(2), 111-115.

Milton, C. L. (2003). A graduate curriculum guided by human becoming: Journeying with the possible. *Nursing Science Quarterly, 16*, 214-218.

Milton, C. L. (2003). The American Nurses Association Code of Ethics: A reflection on the ethics of respect and human dignity with nurse as expert. *Nursing Science Quarterly, 16*, 301-304.

Milton, C. L., & Buseman, J. (2002). Cocreating anew in public health nursing. *Nursing Science Quarterly, 15*, 113-116.

Mitchell, G. J. (1986). Utilizing Parse's theory of man-living-health in Mrs. M's neighborhood. *Perspectives, 10*(4), 5-7.

Mitchell, G. J. (1988). Man-living-health: The theory in practice. *Nursing Science Quarterly, 1*(3), 120-127.

Mitchell, G. J. (1990). Struggling in change: From the traditional approach to Parse's theory-based practice. *Nursing Science Quarterly, 3*(4), 170-176.

Mitchell, G. J. (1990). The lived experience of taking life day-by-day in later life: Research guided by Parse's emergent method. *Nursing Science Quarterly, 3*(1), 29-36.

Mitchell, G. J. (1991). Diagnosis: Clarifying or obscuring the nature of nursing. *Nursing Science Quarterly, 4*(2), 52-53.

Mitchell, G. J. (1991). Human subjectivity: The cocreation of self. *Nursing Science Quarterly, 4*(3), 144-145.

Mitchell, G. J. (1991). Nursing diagnosis: An ethical analysis. *Image: The Journal of Nursing Scholarship, 23*(2), 99-103.

Mitchell, G. J. (1992). Parse's theory and the multi-disciplinary team: Clarifying scientific values. *Nursing Science Quarterly, 5*(3), 104-106.

Mitchell, G. J. (1993). Living paradox in Parse's theory. *Nursing Science Quarterly, 6*(1), 44-51.

Mitchell, G. J. (1993). The same-thing-yet-different phenomenon: A way of coming to know—Or not? *Nursing Science Quarterly, 6*(2), 61-62.

Mitchell, G. J. (1993). Time and a waning moon: Seniors describe the meaning to later life. *The Canadian Journal of Nursing Research, 25*(1), 51-66.

Mitchell, G. J. (1994). Discipline-specific inquiry: The hermeneutics of theory-guided nursing research. *Nursing Outlook, 42*(5), 224-228.

Mitchell, G. J. (1994). The meaning of being a senior: A phenomenological study and interpretation with Parse's theory of nursing. *Nursing Science Quarterly, 7*, 70-79.

Mitchell, G. J. (1996). Clarifying contributions of qualitative research findings. *Nursing Science Quarterly, 9*(4), 143-144.

Mitchell, G. J. (1996). Pretending: A way to get through the day. *Nursing Science Quarterly, 9*(2), 92-93.

Mitchell, G. J. (1997). Retrospective and prospective of practice applications: Views in the fog. *Nursing Science Quarterly, 10*(1), 8-9.

Mitchell, G. J. (1997). Theory and practice in long term care: The acorn doesn't fall far from the tree. *Long Term Care, 7*(4), 31-34.

Mitchell, G. J. (1998). Living with diabetes: How understanding expands theory for professional practice. *Canadian Journal of Diabetes Care, 22*(1), 30-37.

Mitchell, G. J. (1998). Standards of nursing and the winds of change. *Nursing Science Quarterly, 11*(3), 97-98.

Mitchell, G. J. (2003). Abstractions and particulars: Learning theory for practice. *Nursing Science Quarterly, 16*, 310-314.

Mitchell, G. J. (2004). An emerging framework for human becoming criticism. *Nursing Science Quarterly, 17*, 103-109.

Mitchell, G. J. (2006). Human becoming criticism—a critique of Florczak's study on the lived experience of sacrificing something important. *Nursing Science Quarterly, 19*, 142-146.

Mitchell, G. J., Bernardo, A., & Bournes, D. (1997). Nursing guided by Parse's theory: Patient views at Sunnybrook. *Nursing Science Quarterly, 10*(1), 55-56.

Mitchell, G. J., Bournes, D. A., & Hollett, J. (2006). Human becoming-guided patient centered care: New perspectives transform nursing practice. *Nursing Science Quarterly, 19*, 218-224.

Mitchell, G. J., & Bunkers, S. S. (2003). Engaging the abyss: A mis-take of opportunity? *Nursing Science Quarterly, 16*, 121-125.

Mitchell, G. J., & Cody, W. K. (1993). The role of theory in qualitative research. *Nursing Science Quarterly, 6*(4), 170-178.

Mitchell, G. J., & Cody, W. K. (1999). Human becoming theory: A complement to medical science. *Nursing Science Quarterly, 12*(4), 304-310.

Mitchell, G. J., & Cody, W. K. (1992). Nursing knowledge and human science: Ontological and epistemological considerations. *Nursing Science Quarterly, 5*(2), 54-61.

Mitchell, G. J., & Cody, W. K. (2002). Ambiguous opportunity: Toiling for truth of nursing art and science. *Nursing Science Quarterly, 15*, 71-79.

Mitchell, G. J., & Copplestone, C. (1990). Applying Parse's theory to perioperative nursing: A nontraditional approach. *AORN Journal, 51*(3), 787-798.

Mitchell, G. J., & Halifax, N. D. (2005). Feeling respected-not respected: The embedded artist in Parse method. *Nursing Science Quarterly, 18*, 105-112.

Mitchell, G. J., & Heidt, P. (1994). The lived experience of wanting to help another. *Nursing Science Quarterly, 7*(3), 119-127.

Mitchell, G. J., Jonmas-Simpson, C., & Ivonoffski, V. (2006). Research-based theatre: The making of *I'm Still Here! Nursing Science Quarterly, 19*, 198-206.

Mitchell, G. J., & Lawton, C. (2000). Living with the consequences of personal choices for person with diabetes: Implications for educators and practitioners. *Canadian Journal of Diabetes Care, 24*(2), 23-31.

Mitchell, G. J., & Pilkington, F. B. (1990). Theoretical approaches in nursing practice: A comparison of Roy and Parse. *Nursing Science Quarterly, 3*(2), 81-87.

Mitchell, G. J., & Pilkington, F. B. (1999). A dialogue on the comparability of research paradigms—And other theoretical things. *Nursing Science Quarterly, 12*(4), 283-289.

Mitchell, G. J., & Pilkington, F. B. (2000). Comfort-discomfort with ambiguity: Flight and freedom in nursing practice. *Nursing Science Quarterly, 13*(1), 31-36.

Mitchell, G. J., & Santopinto, M. D. A. (1988). An alternative to nursing diagnosis. *The Canadian Nurse, 84*(10), 25-28.

Mitchell, G. J., & Santopinto, M. D. A. (1988). The expanded role nurse: A dissenting viewpoint. *Canadian Journal of Nursing Administration, 4*(1), 8-14.

Mitchell, M. G. (2002). Patient-focused care on a complex continuing care dialysis unit: Rose's story. *CAANT Journal—Canadian Association of Nephrology Nurses & Technicians, 12*, 48-49.

Nokes, K. M., & Carver, K. (1991). The meaning of living with AIDS: A study using Parse's theory of man-living-health. *Nursing Science Quarterly, 4*(4), 175-179.

Norris, J. R. (2002). One-to-one teleapprenticeship as a means for nurses teaching and learning Parse's theory of human becoming. *Nursing Science Quarterly, 15*, 143-149.

Northrup, D. T. (2002). Time passing: A Parse research method study. *Nursing Science Quarterly, 15*, 318-326.

Northrup, D. T., & Cody, W. K. (1998). Evaluation of the human becoming theory in practice in an acute care psychiatric setting. *Nursing Science Quarterly, 11*(1), 23-30.

Ortiz, M. R. (2003). Lingering presence: A study using the human becoming hermeneutic method. *Nursing Science Quarterly, 16*, 146-154.

Paille, M., & Pilkington, F. B. (2002). The global context of nursing: A human becoming perspective. *Nursing Science Quarterly, 15*, 165-170.

Pilkington, F. B. (1993). The lived experience of grieving the loss of an important other. *Nursing Science Quarterly, 6*(3), 130-139.

Pilkington, F. B. (1999). An ethical framework for nursing practice: Parse's human becoming theory. *Nursing Science Quarterly, 12*(1), 21-25.

Pilkington, F. B. (1999). A qualitative study of life after stroke. *Journal of Neuroscience Nursing, 31*(6), 336-347.

Pilkington, F. B. (2000). A unitary view of persistence-change. *Nursing Science Quarterly, 13*(1), 5-11.

Pilkington, F. B. (2004). Exploring ethical implications for acting faithfully in professional relationships. *Nursing Science Quarterly, 17*, 27-32.

Pilkington, F. B. (2005). Grieving a loss: The experience for elders residing in an institution. *Nursing Science Quarterly, 18*, 233-242.

Pilkington, F. B. (2005). Myth and symbol in nursing theories. *Nursing Science Quarterly, 18*, 198-203.

Pilkington, F. B. (2005). The concept of intentionality in human science nursing theories. *Nursing Science Quarterly, 18*, 98-104.

Pilkington, F. B. (2006). Developing nursing knowledge on grieving: A human becoming perspective. *Nursing Science Quarterly, 19*, 299-303.

Pilkington, F. B. (2006). On joy-sorrow: A paradoxical pattern of human becoming. *Nursing Science Quarterly, 19*, 290-291.

Pilkington, F. B., Frederickson, K., & Velsasco-Whetsell, M. (2006). The glass menagerie as heuristic for explicating nursing theory. *Nursing Science Quarterly, 19*, 190-196.

Pilkington, F. B., & Mitchell, G. J. (2004). Quality of life for women living with a gynecological cancer. *Nursing Science Quarterly, 17*, 147-155.

Profile: Rosemarie Rizzo Parse. (1991). *The Japanese Journal of Nursing, 55*(8), 744.

Quiquero, A., Knights, D., & Meo, C. O. (1991). Theory as a guide to practice: Staff nurses choose Parse's theory. *Canadian Journal of Nursing Administration, 4*(1), 14-16.

Ramey, S. L. & Bunkers, S. S. (2006). Teaching the abyss: Living the art-science of nursing. *Nursing Science Quarterly, 19*, 311-315.

Rasmusson, D. L., Jonas, C. M., & Mitchell, G. J. (1991). The eye of the beholder: Applying Parse's theory with homeless individuals. *Clinical Nurse Specialist Journal, 5*(3), 139-143.

Rendon, D. C., Sales, R., Leal, I., & Pique, J. (1995). The lived experience of aging in community-dwelling elders in Valencia, Spain: A phenomenological study. *Nursing Science Quarterly, 8*(4), 152-157.

Ross, J. R. L. (1997). A paradigm shift: What a difference a day makes. *Perspectives, 21*(4), 2-6.

Saltmarche, A., Kolodny, V., & Mitchell, G. J. (1998). An educational approach for patient-focused care: Shifting attitudes and practice. *Journal of Nursing Staff Development, 14*(2), 81-86.

Santopinto, M. D. A. (1989). The relentless drive to be ever thinner: A study using the phenomenological method. *Nursing Science Quarterly, 2*(1), 29-36.

Smith, M. C. (1990). Struggling through a difficult time for unemployed persons. *Nursing Science Quarterly 3*(1), 18-28.

Smith, M. K. (2002). Human becoming and women living with violence: The art of practice. *Nursing Science Quarterly, 15*, 302-307.

Spenceley, S. M. (1995). The CNS in multidisciplinary pulmonary rehabilitation: A nursing science perspective. *Clinical Nurse Specialist, 9*, 192-198.

Stanley, G. D., & Meghani, S. H. (2001). Reflections on using Parse's theory of human becoming in a palliative care setting in Pakistan. *Canadian Nurse, 97*, 23-25.

Thornburg, P. (2002). "Waiting" as experienced by women hospitalized during the antepartum period. *MCN, American Journal of Maternal Child Nursing, 27*, 245-248.

Walker, C. A. (1996). Coalescing the theories of two nurse visionaries: Parse and Watson. *Journal of Advanced Nursing, 24*, 988-996.

Wang, C. E. (2000). Developing a concept of hope from a human science perspective. *Nursing Science Quarterly, 13*, 248-251.

Wang, C. H. (1997). Quality of life and health for persons living with leprosy. *Nursing Science Quarterly, 10*(3), 144-145.

Welch, A. J. (2007). The phenomenon of taking life day-by-day: Using Parse's research method. *Nursing Science Quarterly*, 20, 265-272.

Williamson, G. J. (2000). The test of a nursing theory: A personal view. *Nursing Science Quarterly, 13*(2), 124-128.

Wimpenny, P. (1993). The paradox of Parse's theory. *Senior Nurse, 13*(5), 10-13.

Wing, D. M. (1999). The aesthetics of caring: Where folk healers and nurse theorists converge. *Nursing Science Quarterly, 12*(13), 256-262.

Wondolowski, C., & Davis, D. K. (1988). The lived experience of aging in the oldest old: A phenomenological study. *The American Journal of Psychoanalysis, 48*, 261-270.

Wondolowski, C., & Davis, D. K. (1991). The lived experience of health in the oldest old: A phenomenological study. *Nursing Science Quarterly, 4*(3), 113-118.

Woude, D. V. (1998). Nursing theory-based regulatory decisioning model in South Dakota. *Issues, 19*(3), 14.

Woude, D. V., Damgaard, G., Hegge, M. J., Soholt, D., & Bunkers, S. S. (2003). The unfolding: Scenario planning in nursing. *Nursing Science Quarterly, 16*, 27-35.

Woude, D. V., & Letcher, D. C. (2005). Becoming a living-learning organization. *Nursing Science Quarterly, 18*, 24-30.

Yancy, N. R. (2005). The experience of the novice nurse: A human becoming perspective. *Nursing Science Quarterly, 18*, 215-220.

Book Chapters and Journal Articles by Others Critiquing Parse's Theory

Cowling, W. R. (1989). Parse's theory of nursing. In J. J. Fitzpatrick & A. L. Whall (Eds.), *Conceptual models of nursing: Analysis and application* (2nd ed., pp. 385-399). Norwalk, CT: Appleton & Lange.

Hickman, J. S. (1990). Rosemarie Rizzo Parse. In J. B. George (Ed.), *Nursing theories: The base for professional nursing practice* (3rd ed., pp. 311-332). Norwalk, CT: Appleton & Lange.

Lee, R. E., & Schumacher, L. P. (1989). Rosemarie Rizzo Parse: Man-living-health. In A. Marriner Tomey (Ed.), *Nurse theorists and their work* (2nd ed., pp. 174-186). St. Louis: Mosby.

Phillips, J. (1987). A critique of Parse's man-living-health theory. In R. R. Parse (Ed.), *Nursing science: Major paradigms, theories, and critiques* (pp. 181-204). Philadelphia: W. B. Saunders.

Pugliese, L. (1989). The theory of man-living-health: An analysis. In J. Riehl-Sisca (Ed.), *Conceptual models for nursing practice* (3rd ed., pp. 259-265). Norwalk, CT: Appleton & Lange.

Smith, M. C., & Hudepohl, J. H. (1988). Analysis and evaluation of Parse's theory of man-living-health. *The Canadian Journal of Nursing Research: Nursing Papers, 20*(4), 43-58.

Winkler, S. J. (1983). Parse's theory of nursing. In J. J. Fitzpatrick & A. L. Whall (Eds.), *Conceptual models of nursing: Analysis and application* (pp. 275-294). Bowie, MD: Brady.

Reviews of Parse's Books

[Review of the book Man-living-health: A theory of nursing]. (1981). International Journal of Rehabilitation Research, 4, 449.

Clarke, P. N. (1996). [Review of the book Illuminations: The human becoming theory in practice and research]. *Nursing Science Quarterly,* 9(2), 81-82.

Fawcett, J. (1996). [Review of the book Illuminations: The human becoming theory in practice and research]. *Nursing Science Quarterly,* 9(2), 82-83.

Fawcett, J., & Phillips, J. R. (1999). [Review of the book The human becoming school of thought: A perspective for nurses and other health professionals]. *Nursing Science Quarterly,* 12(1), 85-89.

Jacobs-Kramer, M. K., Levine, M. E., & Menke, E. M. (1988). Three perspectives on a scholarly work [Review of the book Nursing science: Major paradigms, theories, and critiques]. *Nursing Science Quarterly,* 1(4), 182-186.

Jonas-Simpson, C. (2004). Community: A human becoming perspective [Reviewed by K. Egenes, S. H. Gueldner, & L. S. Kelley]. *Nursing Science Quarterly,* 17, 177-182.

Limandri, B. J. (1982). [Review of the book Man-living-health: A theory of nursing]. *Western Journal of Nursing Research,* 4(1), 105-106.

Rawnsley, M. M. (1988). Quest for quality: A comparative review [Review of the book Nursing research: Qualitative methods]. *Nursing Science Quarterly,* 1(1), 40-41.

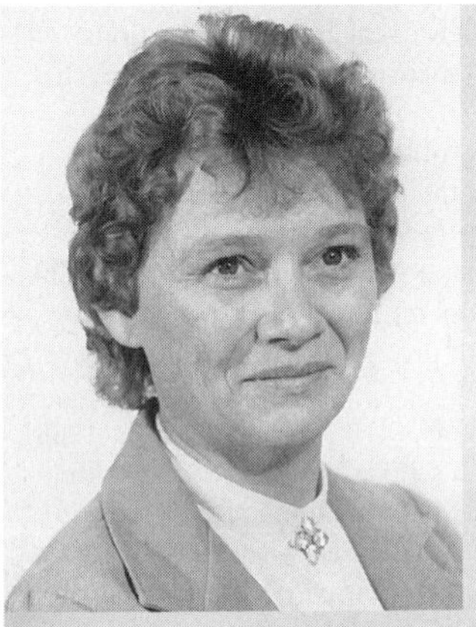

CHAPTER 25

Helen C. Erickson

1937-present

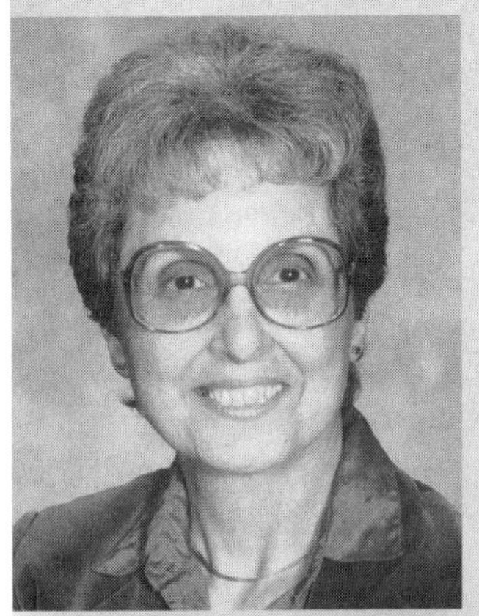

Evelyn M. Tomlin

1929-present

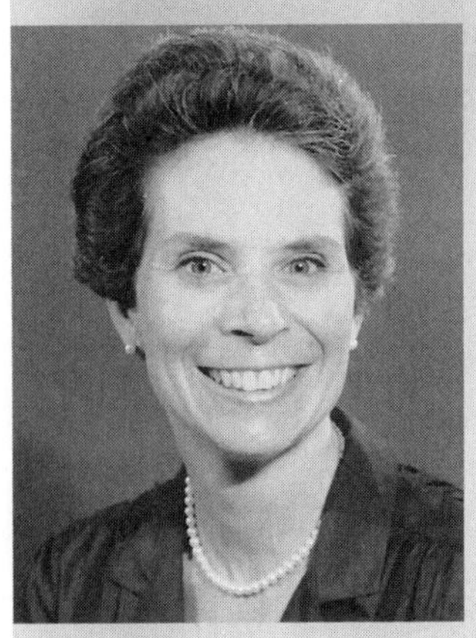

Mary Ann P. Swain

1941-present

Modeling and Role-Modeling

Margaret E. Erickson

"Unconditional acceptance of the person as a human in the process of Being and Becoming is basic to the Modeling and Role-Modeling paradigm. It is a prerequisite to facilitating holistic growth ... Unconditional acceptance of the person as a human being who has an inherent need for dignity and respect from others, and for connectedness—that kind of Unconditional Acceptance is based on Unconditional Love" (Erickson, 2006, p. 343).

CREDENTIALS AND BACKGROUND OF THE THEORISTS

Helen C. Erickson

Helen C. Erickson received a diploma from Saginaw General Hospital, Saginaw, Michigan, in 1957. Her degrees include a baccalaureate in nursing in 1974, dual master's degrees in psychiatric nursing and medical-surgical nursing in 1976, and a doctor of educational psychology in 1984, all from the University of Michigan.

Erickson's professional experience began in the emergency room of the Midland Community Hospital in Midland, Texas, where she was Head Nurse for 2 years. She then worked in Mount Pleasant, Michigan, as Night Supervisor of Nursing in the Michigan State Home for the Mentally Impaired and Handicapped. In 1960, she moved to Puerto Rico with her husband and assumed the position of Director of Health Services at the Inter-American University in San German, Puerto Rico, until 1964. On her return to the United States, she worked as a staff nurse at both St. Joseph's Hospital and University Hospital in Ann Arbor, Michigan. Erickson later served as a psychiatric nurse consultant to the Pediatric Nurse Practitioner Program at the University of Michigan and the University of Michigan Hospitals–Adult Care.

Her academic career began as an assistant instructor in the RN Studies Program at the University of Michigan School of Nursing, where she later served as Chairperson of the Undergraduate Program and Dean for Undergraduate Studies. Erickson was Assistant Professor of Nursing at the University of Michigan from 1978 to 1986. In 1986, she left Michigan to go to the University of South Carolina College of Nursing. Initially, she served as Associate Professor and Assistant Dean for Academic Programs; later, she held the position of Associate Dean for Academic Affairs. In 1988, she moved to Austin, Texas, and served as Professor of Nursing and Chair of Adult Health at the University of Texas at Austin School of Nursing. In addition, she served as Special Assistant to the Dean, Graduate Programs. Since 1997, she has been an Emeritus Professor at the University of Texas at Austin. Erickson has maintained an independent nursing practice since 1976.

Erickson is a member of the American Nurses Association, American Nurses Foundation, the Charter Club, American Holistic Nurses Association, Texas Nurses Association, Sigma Theta Tau, and the Institute for the Advancement of Health. In addition, she served as President of the Society for the Advancement of Modeling and Role-Modeling from 1986 to 1990. She was the Chairperson of the

---

Previous authors: Margaret E. Erickson, Jane A. Caldwell-Gwin, Lisa A. Carr, Brenda Kay Harmon, Karen Hartman, Connie Rae Jarlsberg, Judy McCormick, and Kathryn W. Noone.

The authors express appreciation to Helen C. Erickson, Evelyn M. Tomlin, and Mary Ann P. Swain for critiquing earlier editions of this chapter.

First National Symposium on Modeling and Role-Modeling in 1986 and served on the planning committee for the second, third, fourth, fifth, sixth, seventh, eighth, ninth, and tenth national conferences in 1988, 1990, 1992, 1994, 1996, 1998, 2000, 2002, 2004, and 2006, respectively.

Erickson has been listed in *Who's Who Among University Students* and is a member of Phi Kappa Phi. She received the Sigma Theta Tau Rho Chapter Award of Excellence in Nursing in 1980 and the Amoco Foundation Good Teaching Award in 1982, and was accepted into ADARA (a University of Michigan honor society for women in leadership) in 1982. In 1990, she received the Faculty Teaching Award, University of Texas at Austin, School of Nursing. She received a founders award from the Sigma Theta Tau International Honor Society in Nursing, Excellence in Education Award by the Epsilon Theta Chapter in 1993; she received the Graduate Faculty Teaching Award, University of Texas at Austin School of Nursing in 1995; and she was inducted as a Fellow into the American Academy of Nursing in 1996. The Helen Erickson Endowed Lectureship in Holistic Health Nursing was established in her honor in 1997 at the University of Texas at Austin. She received the Distinguished Faculty citation from Humboldt State University in California in 2001.

Erickson continues to research actively the Modeling and Role-Modeling Theory and has presented numerous seminars, conferences, and papers on various aspects of the theory, both nationally and internationally. She has served as a consultant in the implementation of the theory in clinical practice at the University of Michigan Medical Center in the surgical area, at Brigham and Women's Hospital in Boston, at the Oregon Health Science University Hospital in Portland, and at the University of Pittsburgh hospitals. She has consulted with faculty members who have adopted the theory into their curricula and practice in various schools of nursing and service agencies. Humboldt University School of Nursing in Arcata, California, was the first school to use the Modeling and Role-Modeling Theory as its conceptual base. Metropolitan State University at St. Paul, Minnesota, has adopted the Modeling and Role-Modeling Theory for its RN and baccalaureate and master's in nursing programs. St. Catherine's College, St. Paul, Minnesota, has also adopted it for the associate degree in nursing program. The University of Texas at Austin has adopted concepts as a foundation for the alternative entry program, and the University of Texas at Galveston has adopted core concepts for the academic and service model at the University of Texas Medical Branch in Galveston (H. Erickson, personal correspondence, July 1992).

Erickson has been an invited speaker at many national and international conferences. She has participated in numerous workshops, including several congresses on Ericksonian approaches to hypnosis sponsored by the Erickson Foundation and several conferences sponsored by the National Institute for the Clinical Application of Behavioral Medicine. She has also been involved in activities sponsored by the American Holistic Nurses' Association. She served as a content expert for certification curricula and was included in a book featuring nurse healers (H. Erickson, personal correspondence, July 1992). Although retired from the University of Texas at Austin, Erickson continues to be actively involved in the promotion of holistic nursing. She became Chairman for the board of directors of the American Holistic Nurses' Certification Corporation in 2002, provides consultation and educational programs, and is actively involved in the Society for the Advancement of Modeling and Role-Modeling (H. Erickson, personal correspondence, June 10, 2000).

Evelyn M. Tomlin

Evelyn M. Tomlin's nursing education began in Southern California. She attended Pasadena City College, Los Angeles County General Hospital School of Nursing, and the University of Southern California, where she received her bachelor of science in nursing. She received a master of science in psychiatric nursing from the University of Michigan in 1976.

Tomlin's professional experiences are varied. She began as a clinical instructor at Los Angeles County General Hospital School of Nursing in surgical nursing and maternal and premature infant nursing. She later lived in Kabul, Afghanistan, where she taught English at the Afghan Institute of Technology. She then served as a school nurse and practiced family nursing in the overseas American and European communities where she lived, a role that included participating in more than 46 home deliveries with a certified nurse-midwife. After the establishment of medical services at the United States Embassy Hospital, she functioned as a relief staff nurse. Upon returning to the United States, she was employed by the Visiting Nurse Association (VNA) as a staff nurse in Ann Arbor, Michigan. At the VNA, she acted as the coordinator and clinical instructor for student practical nurses. In addition, she was a staff nurse in a coronary care unit for 5 years, worked in the respiratory intensive care unit, and was Head Nurse of the emergency department at St. Joseph's Mercy Hospital in Ann Arbor. For the next 8 years, she taught the fundamentals of nursing as Assistant Professor of Nursing in the RN Studies Program at the University of Michigan School of Nursing. During that time, she also served as mental health consultant to the pediatric nurse practitioner program at the University of Michigan.

Tomlin was among the first 16 nurses in the United States to be certified by the American Association of Critical Care Nurses. With several colleagues, she opened one of the first offices for independent nursing practice in Michigan. She continued her independent practice until 1993.

She is a member of Sigma Theta Tau Rho Chapter, the California Scholarship Federation, and the Philomathian Society. She has presented programs incorporating a variety of nursing topics based on the Modeling and Role-Modeling Theory and paradigm, with an emphasis on clinical applications.

In 1985, she moved to Big Rock, Illinois, where she enjoyed teaching small community and nursing groups and working in a community shelter serving the women and children of Fox Valley. Later she moved to Geneva, Illinois, where she currently resides with her husband. Tomlin has had inquiries from staff nurses for help in integrating the framework into practice. She believes that elements of the theory and paradigm can be introduced easily in many settings and can be very valuable for practicing nurses (E. Tomlin, telephone interview, 1992). She was first editor for the newsletter of the Society for the Advancement of Modeling and Role-Modeling (E. Tomlin, curriculum vitae, 1992).

Tomlin identifies herself as a Christian in retirement from nursing for pay, but not from nursing practice. She is pursuing her interest in the practice of healing prayer, stating that she has always been interested in the interface of the Modeling and Role-Modeling Theory and Judeo-Christian principles. She is on the board of directors and works as a volunteer at Wayside Cross Ministries in Aurora, Illinois, where she teaches and counsels homeless women, most of whom are single mothers. She is semi-retired but continues to help them develop skills necessary to live healthier, happier lives (E. Tomlin, telephone interview, July 10, 1996).

Mary Ann P. Swain

Mary Ann P. Swain's educational background is in psychology. She received her bachelor of arts degree in psychology from DePauw University in Greencastle, Indiana, and her master of science and doctoral degrees from the University of Michigan, both in the field of psychology.

Swain taught psychology, research methods, and statistics as a teaching assistant at DePauw University and later as a lecturer and Professor of Psychology and Nursing Research at the University of Michigan. She became the Director of the Doctoral Program in Nursing in 1975 and served in that capacity for 1 year. She was Chairperson of Nursing Research from 1977 to 1982. In 1983, she became Associate Vice President for Academic Affairs at the University of Michigan (M. Swain, curriculum vitae, February 1988).

She is a member of the American Psychological Association and an associate member of the Michigan Nurses Association. She developed and taught classes in psychology, research, and nursing research methods. She also collaborated with nurse researchers on various projects, including health promotion among diabetic patients and ways to influence compliance among patients with hypertension. She helped Erickson publish a model that assessed an individual's potential to mobilize resources and adapt to stress, which is significant to the Modeling and Role-Modeling Theory.

Swain received the Alpha Lambda Delta, Psi Chi, Mortar Board, and Phi Beta Kappa awards while at DePauw University. In 1981, she was recognized by the Rho Chapter of Sigma Theta Tau for Contributions to Nursing and, in 1983, became an honorary member of Sigma Theta Tau. In 1994, she moved to Appalachia, New York, with her husband, when she accepted the position of Provost for Binghamton University.

THEORETICAL SOURCES

The theory and paradigm Modeling and Role-Modeling was developed using a retroductive process. The original model was derived inductively from the primary author's clinical and personal life experiences. The works of Maslow, Erikson, Piaget, Engel, Selye, and M. Erickson were then integrated and synthesized into the original model to label, further articulate, and refine a holistic theory and paradigm for nursing. Erickson (1976) argued that people have mind-body relations and an identifiable resource potential that predicts their ability to contend with stress. She also articulated a relationship between needs status and developmental processes, satisfaction with needs and attachment objects, loss and illness, and health and need satisfaction. Tomlin and Swain validated and affirmed Erickson's practice model and helped to expand and articulate labeled phenomena, concepts, and theoretical relationships.

The authors used Maslow's theory of human needs to label and articulate their personal observations that "all people want to be the best that they can possibly be; unmet basic needs interfere with holistic growth whereas satisfied needs promote growth" (Erickson, Tomlin, & Swain, 2002, p. 56; Jensen, 1995). The authors further integrated the model to state that unmet basic needs create need deficits, which can lead to initiation or aggravation of physical or mental distress or illness. At the same time, need satisfaction creates assets that provide resources needed to contend with stress and promote health, growth, and development.

Piaget's theory of cognitive development provides a framework for understanding the development of thinking. On the other hand, integration of Erik Erikson's work on the stages of psychosocial development through the life span provides a theoretical basis for understanding the psychosocial evolution of the individual. Each of his eight stages represents developmental tasks. As an individual resolves each task, he or she gains strengths that contribute to character development and health. Furthermore, as an outcome of each stage, people develop a sense of their own worth and, therefore, a projection of themselves into the future. "The utility of Erikson's theory is the freedom we may take to view aspects of people's problems as uncompleted tasks. This perspective provides a hopeful expectation for the individual's future since it connotes something still in progress" (Erickson et al., 2002, pp. 62-63).

The works of Winnicott, Klein, Mahler, and Bowlby on object attachment were integrated with the original model to develop and articulate the concept of affiliated-individuation (AI). Object relations theory proposes that an infant initially forms an attachment to his or her caregiver after having repeated positive contacts. As the child grows and begins to move toward a more separate and individuated state, a sense of autonomy develops. During this time, he or she usually transfers some attachment to an inanimate object such as a cuddly blanket or a teddy bear. Later, the child may attach to a favorite baseball glove, doll, or pet, and finally onto more abstract things in adulthood, such as an educational degree, professional role, or relationship. On the basis of the work of these individuals, a theoretical relationship was identified between object attachment and need satisfaction. According to the theorists, when an object repeatedly meets an individual's basic needs, attachment or connectedness to that object occurs. After further synthesis of these theoretical linkages and research findings, the authors identified a new concept, AI. They defined AI as the inherent need to be connected with significant others at the same time that there is a sense of separateness from them that enhances their uniqueness. AI runs across the life span from birth to death. Research supports that AI and object attachment are essential to need satisfaction, adaptive coping, and healthy growth and development.

The authors further state, "object loss results in basic need deficits" (Erickson et al., 2002, p. 88). Loss is real, threatened, or perceived; it may be a normal part of the developmental process, or it may be situational. Loss always results in grief; normal grief is resolved in approximately 1 year. When only inadequate or inappropriate objects are available to meet needs, morbid grief results. Morbid grief interferes with the individual's ability to grow and develop to maximal potential. The work of Selye and Engel, as cited by Erickson, Tomlin, and Swain (1983), provided an additional conceptual basis for the beliefs the theorists hold regarding loss and an individual's stress responses to that loss or losses. Selye's theory pertains to an individual's biophysical responses to stress, whereas Engel's work explores the psychosocial responses to stressors.

The synthesis of these theories, with the integration of the primary author's clinical observations and lived experiences, resulted in the development of the Adaptive Potential Assessment Model (APAM). The APAM focuses on the individual's ability to mobilize resources when confronted with stressors, rather than the adaptation process. This model was first developed by Erickson (1976) and was later described in publication by Erickson and Swain (1982).

Erickson credits Milton H. Erickson with influencing her clinical practice and providing inspiration and direction in the development of this theory. Initially, he articulated the formulation of the Modeling and Role-Modeling Theory when he urged Erickson to "model the client's world, understand it as they do, then role-model the picture the client has drawn, building a healthy world for them" (H. Erickson, telephone interview, November 1984).

Major Concepts & Definitions

The theory and paradigm Modeling and Role-Modeling contains multiple concepts.

MODELING

The act of Modeling, then, is the process the nurse uses as she develops an image and an understanding of the client's world—an image and understanding developed within the client's framework and from the client's perspective . . . The art of Modeling is the development of a mirror image of the situation from the client's perspective . . . The science of Modeling is the scientific aggregation and analysis of data collected about the client's model (Erickson et al., 2002, p. 95).

Modeling occurs as the nurse accepts and understands her client (Erickson et al., 2002, p. 96).

ROLE-MODELING

The art of Role-Modeling occurs when the nurse plans and implements interventions that are unique for the client. The science of Role-Modeling occurs as the nurse plans interventions with respect to her theoretical base for the practice of nursing . . . Role-Modeling is . . . the essence of nurturance . . . Role-Modeling requires an unconditional acceptance of the person as the person is while gently encouraging the facilitating growth and development at the person's own pace and within the person's own model (Erickson et al., 2002, p. 95).

Role-Modeling starts the second the nurse moves from the analysis phase of the nursing process to the planning of nursing interventions (Erickson et al., 2002, p. 95).

Continued

MAJOR CONCEPTS & DEFINITIONS—cont'd

NURSING

Nursing is the holistic helping of persons with their self-care activities in relation to their health. This is an interactive, interpersonal process that nurtures strengths to enable development, release, and channeling of resources for coping with one's circumstances and environment. The goal is to achieve a state of perceived optimum health and contentment (Erickson et al., 2002, p. 49).

NURTURANCE

Nurturance fuses and integrates cognitive, physiological, and affective processes, with the aim of assisting a client to move toward holistic health. Nurturance implies that the nurse seeks to know and understand the client's personal model of his or her world, and to appreciate its value and significance for that client from the client's perspective (Erickson et al., 2002, p. 48).

UNCONDITIONAL ACCEPTANCE

Being accepted as a unique, worthwhile, important individual—with no strings attached—is imperative if the individual is to be facilitated in developing his or her own potential. The nurse's use of empathy helps the individual learn that the nurse accepts and respects him or her as is. The acceptance will facilitate the mobilization of resources needed as this individual strives for adaptive equilibrium (Erickson et al., 2002, p. 49).

PERSON

People are alike because they have holism, lifetime growth and development, and their need for AI. They are different because they have inherent endowment, adaptation, and self-care knowledge (Erickson et al., 1983).

HOW PEOPLE ARE ALIKE

Holism

Human beings are holistic persons who have multiple interacting subsystems. Permeating all subsystems are the inherent bases. These include genetic makeup and spiritual drive. Body, mind, emotion, and spirit are a total unit and they act together. They affect and control one another interactively. The interaction of the multiple subsystems and the inherent bases creates holism: Holism implies that the whole is greater than the sum of the parts (Erickson et al., 2002, pp. 44-45).

Basic Needs

All human beings have basic needs that can be satisfied, but only from within the framework of the individual (Erickson et al., 2002, p. 58).

Basic needs are met only when the individual perceives that they are met (Erickson et al., 2002, p. 57).

Lifetime Development

Lifetime development evolves through psychological and cognitive stages, as follows:

- Psychological Stages

Each stage represents a developmental task or a decisive encounter resulting in a turning point, a moment of decision between alternative basic attitudes (e.g., trust versus mistrust or autonomy versus shame and doubt). As a maturing individual negotiates or resolves each age-specific crisis or task, the individual gains enduring strengths and attitudes that contribute to the character and health of the individual's personality in his or her culture (Erickson et al., 2002, p. 61).

- Cognitive Stages

Consider how thinking develops rather than what happens in psychosocial or affective development . . . Piaget believed that cognitive learning develops in a sequential manner, and he has identified several periods in this process. Essentially, there are four periods: sensorimotor, preoperational, concrete operations, and formal operations (Erickson et al., 2002, pp. 63-64).

MAJOR CONCEPTS & DEFINITIONS—cont'd

Affiliated-Individuation

Individuals have an instinctual need for affiliated-individuation. They need to be able to be dependent on support systems while simultaneously maintaining independence from these support systems. They need to feel a deep sense of both the "I" and the "we" states of being, and to perceive freedom and acceptance in both states (Erickson et al., 2002, p. 47).

HOW PEOPLE ARE DIFFERENT

Inherent Endowment

Each individual is born with a set of genes that will to some extent predetermine appearance, growth, development, and responses to life events . . . Clearly, both genetic makeup and inherited characteristics influence growth and development. They might influence how one perceives oneself and one's world. They make individuals different from one another, each unique in his or her own way (Erickson et al., 2002, pp. 74-75).

Adaptation

Adaptation occurs as the individual responds to external and internal stressors in a health-directed and growth-directed manner. Adaptation involves mobilizing internal and external coping resources. No subsystem is left in jeopardy when adaptation occurs (Erickson et al., 2002).

The individual's ability to mobilize resources is depicted by the APAM. The APAM identifies three different coping potential states: (1) arousal, (2) equilibrium (adaptive and maladaptive), and (3) impoverishment. Each of these states represents a different potential to mobilize self-care resources. "Movement among the states is influenced by one's ability to cope [with ongoing stressors] and the presence of new stressors" (Erickson et al., 2002, pp. 80-81).

Nurses can use this model to predict an individual's potential to mobilize self-care resources in response to stress.

Mind-Body Relationships

We are all biophysical, psychosocial beings who want to develop our potential, this is, to be the best we can be (Erickson et al., 2002, p. 70).

Self-Care

Self-care involves the use of knowledge, resources, and actions, as follows:

- Self-Care Knowledge

At some level, a person knows what has made him or her sick, lessened his or her effectiveness, or interfered with his or her growth. The person also knows what will make him or her well, optimize his or her effectiveness or fulfillment (given circumstances), or promote his or her growth (Erickson et al., 2002, p. 48).

- Self-Care Resources

Self-care resources are "the internal resources, as well as additional resources, mobilized through self-care action that help gain, maintain, and promote an optimum level of holistic health" (Erickson et al., 2002, pp. 254-255).

- Self-Care Action

Self-care action is "the development and utilization of self-care knowledge and self-care resources" (Erickson et al., 2002, p. 254).

USE OF EMPIRICAL EVIDENCE

Several studies have provided initial evidence for philosophical premises and theoretical linkages implied in the original book by Erickson, Tomlin, and Swain (1983), and later specified by Erickson (1990b). The APAM (Figures 25-1 and 25-2) has been tested as a classification model (Barnfather, 1987; Erickson, 1976; Kleinbeck, 1977) and as a predictor for health status (Barnfather, 1990b) and for length of hospital

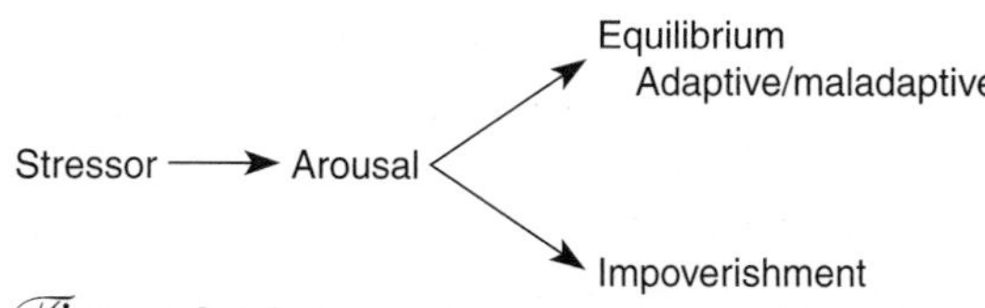

Figure 25-1 Adaptive Potential Assessment Model. (From Erickson, H. C., Tomlin, E. M., & Swain, M. A. P. [1983]. *Modeling and role-modeling: A theory and paradigm for nursing.* Englewood Cliffs, NJ: Prentice Hall.)

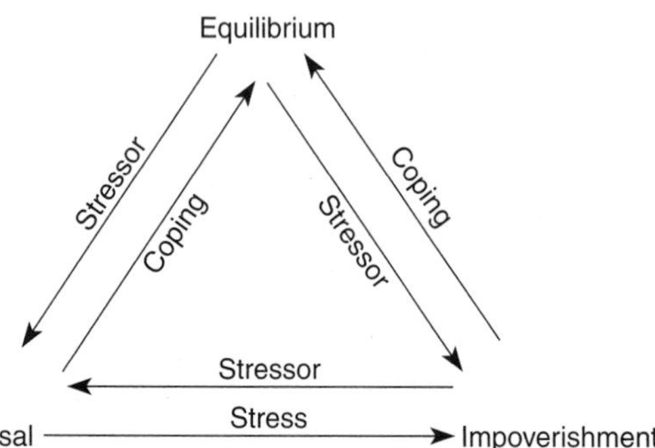

Figure 25-2 Dynamic relationship among the states of the Adaptive Potential Assessment Model. (From Erickson, H. C., Tomlin, E. M., & Swain, M. A. P. [1983]. *Modeling and role-modeling: A theory and paradigm for nursing.* Englewood Cliffs, NJ: Prentice Hall.)

stay (Erickson & Swain, 1982), as it relates to basic need status (Barnfather, 1993). Findings from these studies provide beginning evidence for the proposed three-state model across populations, a relationship between health and ability to mobilize resources, and an ability to mobilize resources and needs status. Two other studies have shown relationships among stressors (measured as life events) and propensity for accidents (Babcock & Mueller, 1980) and resource state and ability to take in and use new information (Clementino & Lapinske, 1980). Finally, Benson (2003) has studied the APAM as applied to small groups.

Relationships among self-care knowledge, resources, and activities have been demonstrated in several studies (Acton, 1993; Baas, 1992; Irvin, 1993; Jensen, 1995; Miller, 1994). The self-care knowledge construct, first studied by Erickson (1985), was replicated and found to be significantly associated with perceived control (Cain & Perzynski, 1986) and quality of life (Baas, Fontana, & Bhat, 1997). Self-directedness, need for harmony (affiliation), and need for autonomy (individuation) were found when multidimensional scaling was used to explore relationships among self-care knowledge, resources, and actions. The author concluded that a positive attitude was a major factor when health-directed self-care actions were assessed (Rosenow, 1991). Physical activity in patients after myocardial infarction was shown to be affected by life satisfaction (not physical condition); life satisfaction was predicted by availability of self-care resources and resources needed. Furthermore, resources needed served as a suppressor for resources available (Baas, 1992). In a sample of caregivers, social support predicted for stress level and self-worth had an indirect effect on hope through self-worth (Irvin, 1993; Irvin & Acton, 1997), whereas persons with diabetes with spiritual well-being were better able to cope (Landis, 1991).

When the Modeling and Role-Modeling Theory was used as a guideline, interviews were used to determine the client's model of the world. The following seven themes emerged (Erickson, 1990a):

1. Cause of the problem, which was unique to the individual
2. Related factors, also unique to the individual
3. Expectations for the future
4. Types of perceived control
5. Affiliation
6. Lack of affiliation
7. Trust in the caregiver

Each model was unique and each warranted individualized interventions. Other qualitative studies on self-care knowledge showed that acutely ill patients perceived monitoring, caring, presence, touch, and voice tones as comforting (Kennedy, 1991); healthy adults sought need satisfaction from the nurse practitioner in primary care (Boodley, 1990, 1986); and hospice patients benefited from nurse empathy (Raudonis, 1991). Studies also showed relationships among mistrust and length of stay in hospitalized subjects (Finch, 1990); perceived enactment of autonomy, self-care, and holistic health in the elderly (Anschutz, 2000; Hertz & Anschutz, 2002); perceived support, control, and well being in the elderly (Chen, 1996); and loss, morbid grief, and onset of symptoms of Alzheimer's disease (Erickson, Kinney et al., 1994; Irvin & Acton, 1996).

Other studies addressed linkages between role-modeled interventions and outcomes (Erickson, et al., 1994; Hertz, 1991; Irvin, 1993; Jensen, 1995; Kennedy, 1991). College level students who perceived satisfaction of needs were more successful in school. Seven nursing students who perceived that they were supported were more able to attain their goals for advanced education (Smith, 1980), the elderly who felt supported reported higher need satisfaction and were better able to cope (Keck, 1989), adolescent mothers who felt supported and perceived need satisfaction had a more positive maternal-infant attachment (Erickson, M., 2006; Erickson, M., 1996a; Erickson, M., 1996b), those with a strong social network reported better health (Doornbos, 1983), and persons convicted of sexual offenses and then were provided with support to remodel their worlds were able to develop new behaviors and move on with their lives (Scheela, 1991). Families and post–myocardial infarction patients who were able to participate in planning their own care through contracting had less anxiety and better perceived control and perceived support (Holl, 1992), and caregivers of adults with dementia who experienced theory-based nursing using the Modeling and Role-Modeling Theory perceived that their needs were met and that they were healthier (Hopkins, 1995). They also reported feeling that they were encouraged, which helped them accept the situation and transcend the experience of caregiving (Hopkins, 1995). Self-care resources, measured as needs, are related to perceived support and coping in women with breast cancer (Keck, 1989), physical well-being in persons with chronic obstructive pulmonary disease (Kline, 1990, 1988), and anxiety in hospitalized patients who have had cardiac surgery and their families (Holl, 1992). Finally, when AI was tested as a buffer between stress and well-being, a mediation effect was found (Acton, 1997; Acton, 1993; Acton, Irvin, Jensen, Hopkins, & Miller, 1997).

Other studies that operationalized self-care resources by measuring developmental residuals have shown that identity resolution in adolescents with facial disfiguration can be predicted by previous developmental residual (Miller, 1986). Chen (1996) found that feelings of control over one's health (health control orientation) status in elderly individuals with hypertension correlated highly with self-efficacy and self-care. In addition, her work supported that health control orientation, self-efficacy, and self-care were associated with well-being. Through interviews of older adults living independently, Hertz, Rossetti, and Nelson (2006) were able to identify categories of self-care actions that encompassed important self-care activities.

Other researchers found that trust predicts for adolescent clients' involvement in the prescribed medical regimen (Finch, 1987), perceived support and adaptation are related to developmental residual in families with newborn infants (Darling-Fisher, 1987; Darling-Fisher & Leidy 1988), mistrust predicts length of hospital stay, and positive residual serves as a buffer (Finch, 1987). Positive residual in the intimacy stage of healthy adults predicts for health behaviors (MacLean, 1992, 1990, 1987), developmental residual predicts for hope, trust-mistrust residual predicts for generalized hope, autonomy-shame and doubt residual predicts for particularized hope in the elderly (Curl, 1992), and negative residual is related to speed and impatience behaviors in a healthy sample of military personnel (Kinney, 1992). Case study methods have been used to show relationships among needs, attachment, and developmental residual (Kinney, 1990, 1992; Kinney & Erickson, 1990) and needs and coping (Jensen, 1995), and two unpublished studies have shown relationships between healthy adults and need status (Erickson, Kinney, Stone, & Acton, 1990).

Studies have also been used to explore self-care knowledge in informants in the hospital (Erickson, 1985), perceived enactment of autonomy and life satisfaction in the elderly (Anschutz, 2000), the experience of persons 85 and older as they manage their health (Beltz, 1999), perceptions of hope in elementary school children (Baldwin, 1996), the experiential meaning of well-being and the lived experience in employed mothers (Weber, 1995, 1999), developmental growth in adults with heart failure (Baas, Beery, Fontana, & Wagoner, 1999), the individual's ability to mobilize coping resources and basic needs (Barnfather, 1990a), the relationship between basic need satisfaction and emotionally motivated eating (Timmerman & Acton, 2001), relations among hostility, self-esteem, self-concept, and psychosocial residual in persons with coronary heart disease (Sofhauser, 1996), and the human-environment relationship when healing from an episodic illness (Bowman, 1998). Studies have explored the relationship between spiritual well-being and heart failure (Beery, Baas, Fowler, & Allen, 2002), spirituality in caregivers of family members with dementia (Acton & Miller, 1996), the implementation of a mind, body, spirit self-empowerment program for adolescents (Nash, 2007) and women with breast cancer (Kinney, Rodgers, Nash, & Bray, 2003), the meaning and impact of suffering in people with rheumatoid arthritis (Dildy, 1992), and the relationship between experiences of prolonged family suffering and evolving spiritual identity (Clayton, 2001). Studies with cardiovascular have continued as Baas (2004) studied self-care resources and quality of life in patients following myocardial infarction, and Baas et al. (2004) explored body awareness in heart failure or transplant patients. Similarly, Beery, Baas, Mathews, Burrough, and Henthorn (2005) developed an adjustment scale to measure self-report with implanted devices in cardiac patients, and Beery, Baas, and Henthorn (2007) reported on patient adjustments to the devices.

Tools that have been developed to test the Modeling and Role-Modeling Theory include the Basic Needs Satisfaction Inventory (Kline, 1988), the Erikson Psychosocial Stage Inventory (Darling-Fisher & Leidy, 1988), the Perceived Enactment of Autonomy tool designed to measure a prerequisite to self-care actions in the elderly (Hertz, 1991, 1999; Hertz & Anschutz, 2002), the Self-Care Resource Inventory (Baas, 1992), the Robinson Self-Appraisal Inventory designed to measure denial (the first stage in the grief process) in patients after myocardial infarction (Robinson, 1992), the Erickson Maternal Bonding-Attachment Tool designed to measure self-care knowledge as motivational style (deficit or being motivation) and self-care resource (Erickson, M., 1996b), a theory-based nursing assessment (Finch, 1990), and the Hopkins Clinical Assessment of the APAM (Hopkins, 1995).

MAJOR ASSUMPTIONS

Nursing

"The nurse is a facilitator, not an effector. Our nurse-client relationship is an interactive, interpersonal process that aids the individual to identify, mobilize, and develop his or her own strengths to achieve a perceived optimal state of health and well-being" (H. Erickson, personal correspondence, 2004). Rogers (1996) has defined this relationship as facilitative-affiliation. The five aims of nursing interventions are to build trust, affirm and promote client strengths, promote positive orientation, facilitate perceived control, and set health-directed mutual goals (Erickson et al., 2002).

Person

A differentiation is made between patients and clients in this theory. A patient is given treatment and instruction; a client participates in his or her own care. "Our goal is for nurses to work with clients" (Erickson et al., 2002, p. 21). "A client is one who is considered to be a legitimate member of the decision-making team, who always has some control over the planned regimen, and who is incorporated into the planning and implementation of his or her own care as much as possible" (Erickson et al., 1990, p. 20; Erickson et al., 2002, p. 253).

Health

"Health is a state of physical, mental, and social wellbeing, not merely the absence of disease or infirmity. It connotates a state of dynamic equilibrium among the various subsystems [of a holistic person]" (Erickson et al., 2002, p. 46).

Environment

"Environment is not identified in the theory as an entity of its own. The theorists see environment in the social subsystems as the interaction between self and others both cultural and individual. Biophysical stressors are seen as part of the environment" (H. Erickson, telephone interview, March 30, 1988).

THEORETICAL ASSERTIONS

The theoretical assertions of the Modeling and Role-Modeling Theory are based on the linkages between completion of developmental tasks and basic need satisfaction; among basic need satisfaction, object attachment and loss, and developmental tasks; and between the ability to mobilize coping resources and need satisfaction. Three generic theoretical assertions that constitute several theoretical linkages implied in the theory, but are delineated less specifically, are as follows:

1. "The degree to which developmental tasks are resolved is dependent on the degree to which human needs are satisfied" (Erickson et al., 2002, p. 87).
2. "The degree to which needs are satisfied by object attachment depends on the availability of those objects and the degree to which they provide comfort and security as opposed to threat and anxiety" (Erickson et al., 1983, p. 90).
3. "An individual's potential for mobilizing resources, the person's state of coping according to the APAM, is directly associated with the person's need satisfaction level" (Erickson et al., 2002, p. 91).

LOGICAL FORM

The Modeling and Role-Modeling Theory was formulated by the use of retroductive thinking. The theorists went through four levels of theory development and then recycled from inductive to deductive to inductive to deductive reasoning (H. Erickson, telephone interview, March 30, 1988). Theoretical sources were used to validate clinical observations. Clinical observations were tested in light of the theoretical bases. These sources were synthesized with their observations, which enabled Erickson, Tomlin, and Swain to develop a "multidimensional new theory and paradigm—modeling and role-modeling" (H. Erickson, telephone interview, November 1984).

Modeling and Role-Modeling may be viewed as a theory and a paradigm. Although most commonly referred to as a theory or a model, it also meets the functions of a paradigm identified by Merton (1968), who said that paradigms "provide a compact arrangement of central concepts and their interrelations that are utilized for description and analysis" (p. 70).

ACCEPTANCE BY THE NURSING COMMUNITY

Practice

The book, *Modeling and Role-Modeling: A Theory and Paradigm for Nursing* (Erickson et al., 2002), chapters in several nursing theory books, and research studies based on the theory have exposed practicing nurses to this theory. Nurses on surgical units at the University of Michigan Medical Center are using an assessment tool based on the Modeling and Role-Modeling Theory. The tool is used to gather information to identify the client's need assets, deficits, developmental residual, attachment-loss and grief status, and potential therapeutic interventions (see Appendix at the end of this chapter) (Bowman, 1998; H. Erickson, personal correspondence, 1988).

Helen Erickson has lectured extensively on their theory and has held one-on-one consultations that exposed nurses (nationally and internationally) from various practice and educational backgrounds to the theory. Nurses in adult health, case management, community health, critical and intensive care, infant, adolescent, and family health, gerontology, mental health, emergency rooms, and hospices are using the theory. Erickson noted that what seemed to be a revolutionary idea as recently as 1972 (calling for the client to be the head of the healthcare team) has gained acceptance, as has the notion that nurses can practice independently (H. Erickson, telephone interview, November 1984). According to Erickson, negative responses to the theory came from individuals who cannot accept the idea of listening to the client first, or who do not take the concept of holism seriously (H. Erickson, telephone interview, November 1984).

Brigham and Women's Hospital in Boston has used the Modeling and Role-Modeling Theory as a theoretical basis for the professional practice model for the past several years. The nurses use the theory as a framework to structure care planning and conduct case conferences. Jenny James, the former vice president for nursing, stated that "consistency of language, the way care is talked about and planned" is one of the major advantages of using this theoretical basis (J. James, telephone interview, July 6, 1992). The basic fundamentals of the theory are easy to apply in practice, and with a small amount of knowledge, an individual can begin to apply the theory. Nurses at Brigham and Women's Hospital use an adaptation of the assessment tool developed at the University of Michigan Medical Center. It was at the Fourth National Conference on Modeling and Role-Modeling (Boston, October 1992) that implementation of the professional practice model at Brigham and Women's Hospital and case studies were presented by the staff nurses (J. James, telephone interview, July 6, 1992). Nurses at the University of Pittsburgh Medical Center, Children's Hospital of the University of Wisconsin at Madison, University of Tennessee Medical Center in Knoxville, Oregon Health Sciences University Hospital, and other hospitals and state agencies across the United States have also adopted the Modeling and Role-Modeling Theory as the foundation for their professional practice.

Education

The Modeling and Role-Modeling Theory is introduced into the curriculum during the sophomore year at the University of Michigan School of Nursing and is required for returning registered nursing students as well. Faculty members at several nursing schools have contacted Erickson regarding the use of the theory in their curricula. Many use the theory for specific courses. Others, such as those at Humboldt State University in Arcata, California, selected Modeling and Role-Modeling as the conceptual framework for their curriculum. Students are taught theory-based practice throughout the program. Other nursing programs that use the Modeling and Role-Modeling Theory as a basis for curriculum include Metropolitan State University in St. Paul, Minnesota; St. Catherine's University in St. Paul, Minnesota; the Alternate Entry Master's nursing program at the University of Texas at Austin; and Foo Yin College of Nursing and Medical Technology in Taiwan.

Research

Nurses throughout the world continue to base their research on Modeling and Role-Modeling. Research activity continues to support and validate the self-care knowledge construct and the importance of support and control. The initial study provided evidence that psychosocial factors are significantly related to physical health problems (Erickson, 1976). A follow-up study in 1988 conducted by Erickson, Lock, and Swain (H. Erickson, curriculum vitae, February 1988) supported these findings, and subsequent research has provided for expansion and enrichment of the concepts. Key concepts include perceived support, perceived control, hope for the future, and satisfaction with daily life. The theorists identified several other research projects that have tested the theory. Several master's and doctoral students at the University of Michigan School of Nursing, the University of Texas at Austin, and other universities have pursed various research questions based on this theory. Campbell, Finch, Allport, Erickson, and Swain (1985) conducted a research study at the University of Michigan Medical Center and hypothesized that the length of hospital stay correlated with stages of development. They used a nursing assessment tool adapted from the assessment model to measure a patient's psychosocial development and to relate developmental status to the length of hospitalization and the number of health problems identified during hospitalization. Results indicated that the balance of trust-mistrust accounts for a large percentage of the variance in the length of hospitalization. No significant relationship was evident between psychosocial coping skills and the number of health problems identified.

Erickson was the principal investigator of a research project, Modeling and Role-Modeling with Alzheimer's Patients, funded by the National Institutes of Health, National Center for Nursing Research. This research project included 10 other investigators. Results supported the constructs of self-care knowledge and affiliated individuation (H. Erickson, personal correspondence, July 1, 1992).

Numerous graduate students have used the Modeling and Role-Modeling Theory as a basis for their theses and dissertations. In addition, extensive work has been published that substantiates many of the major constructs and theoretical linkages of the theory (Erickson, 1990a). Hertz, Baas, Curl, and Robinson (1994) conducted an integrative review of research from 1982 to 1992 using Modeling and Role-Modeling as a theoretical basis. Empirical evidence has provided bases for validation, refinement, and revision of the theory. Research will continue to expand the Modeling and Role-Modeling Theory.

FURTHER DEVELOPMENT

As this theory is practiced, explored, examined, and researched, much potential exists for further development. The theory continues to gain national and international attention. One reason for this increased attention is the founding of the Society for the Advancement of Modeling and Role-Modeling. The society was formed to develop a network of colleagues who could advance the development and application of the Modeling and Role-Modeling Theory. One of the society's goals is to promote continued research related to the theory. The society held its first national symposium in 1986 and has met biennially thereafter. At the 1988 conference, held at Hilton Head, South Carolina, the membership chair announced that society members came from 12 states (H. Erickson, personal correspondence, 1988). By the 1990 conference in Austin, Texas, members represented more than 33 states (H. Erickson, personal correspondence, July 1, 1992). These conferences provide a forum for researchers, educators, and practitioners to disseminate knowledge pertaining to the Modeling and Role-Modeling Theory and paradigm (H. Erickson, personal correspondence, 1988).

The Fourth National Conference on Modeling and Role-Modeling Theory and Paradigm for Professionals, held in Boston in October 1992, demonstrated the breadth and depth of the use and research for the Modeling and Role-Modeling Theory. Presentations included studies based in critical care units and community-based practice, in multiple types of educational settings, and across the age span. The biennial conferences held throughout the country continue to provide an opportunity for nurses to discuss interrelationships among nursing practice, theory, research, and education. The twelfth national conference was held in Bloomington, Illinois in 2008. The 2010 conference will be held in San Antonio, Texas.

Many of the research data related to the theory are yet to be published. Erickson stated, "Every part of it [the theory] needs further development... There are a thousand research questions in that book... You can take any one statement we make and ask a research question about it... Modeling and Role-Modeling has only begun" (H. Erickson, telephone interview, November 1984).

CRITIQUE

Clarity

Erickson, Tomlin, and Swain present their theory clearly. Definitions in the theory are denotative, with the concepts explicitly defined. They use everyday language and offer many examples to illustrate their meaning. Their definitions and assumptions are consistent, and there is a logical progression from assumptions to assertions.

Simplicity

The theory appears simple at first. However, on closer inspection, its complexity appears. It is based on biological and psychological theories and on several of the theorists' own assumptions. The interactions among the major concepts, assumptions, and assertions add depth to the theory and increase its complexity.

Generality

Major assumptions that deal with developmental tasks, basic needs satisfaction, object attachment and loss, and adaptive potential are broad enough to be applicable in diverse nursing situations; therefore, the theory is generalizable to all nursing and patient situations. The theorists cite numerous examples of the applicability of their concepts in the educational setting, clinical practice, and research. It may be argued that the theory lacks applicability in nonverbal or comatose populations. However, the theorists believe that the theory is also applicable in these situations, although it may require creativity of the clinician. The Modeling and Role-Modeling Theory is generalizable to all aspects and settings of professional nursing practice.

Empirical Precision

Empirical precision is increased if the theory has operationally defined concepts, identifiable subconcepts, and denotative definitions. The major concepts, Modeling and Role-Modeling, are reality based, which makes them more empirical than general. Definitions in the theory are denotative, making it possible to test the concepts identified empirically. The theorists provide an outline for collecting, analyzing, and synthesizing data and guidelines for implementing their theory based on the client's model. These explicit guidelines increase the empirical precision of the theory by allowing any practitioner to test the theory using these tools.

Chinn and Kramer (2004) proposed that empirical precision increases with research testing as data reflecting research testing of the theory continue to support the theory. The Modeling and Role-Modeling Theory gains greater empirical precision as new and ongoing studies become available for critical analysis. The theorists recognize the need for continued research of their theory and encourage practicing nurses to do it.

Derivable Consequences

One of the many challenges facing the profession of nursing is recognition of its unique, scientific knowledge base. A major aid in this process is the use of nursing theory as a basis for professional practice. The Modeling and Role-Modeling Theory provides the stimulus to accomplish this goal. Although this theory is relatively young, it has gained recognition in the nursing community. As interest has grown, additional research supporting its theoretical statements has been generated. Numerous nurses have engaged in research based on this theory. Additional publications of the findings lend more and more credence to the theoretical propositions.

Chinn and Kramer (2004) state that a theory should be evaluated in terms of its derivable consequences. The derivable consequences are determined by examining whether the theory guides research, directs practice, generates new ideas, and differentiates nursing from other professions. In terms of these criteria, this theory possesses inherent value and research that supports its wide extensive scope.

SUMMARY

Nurses have the opportunity to share in important, intimate life experiences with their clients. We have the ability and responsibility to facilitate healing and achieve our clients' perceived maximal state of health and well-being. The Modeling and Role-Modeling Theory provides nurses with a practice-based theoretical framework that allows us to attain these goals, in any setting, with any population. Data from numerous research studies, as well as ongoing scientific work, provide empirical support for this nursing theory. As the theory matures, the extent of its merit and worth will become evident.

Case Study

Robert, a 75-year-old rancher with a history of chronic obstructive pulmonary disease (COPD), is admitted with shortness of breath, angina, and nausea (unmet physiological needs). It is his fourth admission in 6 months (he is having difficulty adapting to stressors in his life). The nurse introduces herself in a quiet, calm voice and tells him she will be his primary nurse during his stay (interventions designed to establish trust and a sense of safety and security and to facilitate a sense of connectedness). She asks him why he came in (he is the primary source of data). He states, "I can't breath and my chest hurts." After he is stabilized (physiological needs are met, so the nurse can focus on his other needs), she says, "I notice that you have had multiple admissions in the last few months. Why do you think you are here today?" (the nurse seeks information from the client who is the primary data source and facilitates a sense of client control). He replies, "My wife of 49 years died a few months ago; she took care of me and my heart is broken. My life no longer has meaning" (he is experiencing unmet needs, is having problems with the developmental stage of generativity, and is grieving the loss of his wife).

During her assessment, the nurse discovers that Robert lives on a ranch by himself, his nearest neighbor is 4 miles away, his son lives out of state, he has no help with his daily living activities, he is housebound because he no longer can drive, he has no support system, and he feels unable to get on with his life without his wife. The nurse asks him what he needs to feel better and to help him get through the next few weeks (promoting positive future orientation). He replies, "I need to be closer to my friends and the hospital. I am so lonely and afraid out there by myself" (unmet love and belonging and safety and security needs).

After a lengthy discussion, they decide together to implement a plan of care (the nurse is facilitating client control, affirming his strengths and his self-care knowledge that he knows what will make him heal). Robert calls and speaks to his son, who plans to come and visit (this action facilitates his sense of perceived support and AI). His minister is called, and grief counseling is arranged (support is perceived, facilitation of grief resolution is initiated, client is facilitated in being future focused). A social worker visits, and Robert decides that he will move to town into a senior citizen apartment that provides meals and other services. This will help him feel safer and more secure, because he will be closer to the hospital and other people if he needs them. His love and belonging needs can be met, because he can choose when to visit with friends or participate in social activities that are offered at the complex (facilitates client's sense of control). He can also receive assistance with basic physiological needs when needed (meals, housekeeping services). The nurse provides him with her phone number, so he can call if he needs anything or if he just wants to check in (support and love and belonging needs are met). This action facilitates the client's trust and AI. His control is maintained, and his strengths and self-care knowledge are affirmed (he will know and be able to call when he needs assistance, or will be connected to the nurse). Arrangements are made for him to have help with the moving process. Finally, the nurse schedules regular phone calls (based on the client's schedule) to check in on him to see how he is doing and to address any concerns or questions he has. This action facilitates trust, and his safety and security and love and belonging needs are met.

CRITICAL THINKING Activities

1. Interview a client and use the theory to interpret the data. Identify nursing diagnoses based on the interpretations.
2. Given the findings, propose a nursing plan of care. Identify what predictions can be made if the care is not given.
3. Assuming that the goal is to promote the client's health and development, predict the outcome on the basis of the proposed nursing plan of care.
4. Assess the client from primary, secondary, and tertiary sources. Compare for congruency among the three types of sources.

POINTS FOR *Further Study*

- http://www.mrmnursingtheory.org/
- Research and conceptual references are available on the website on mid range theories, major constructs, and philosophical assumptions of the MRM theory.
- Erickson, H. (Ed.) (2006). Modeling and Role-Modeling: A View From the Client's World. Cedar Park, TX: Unicorns Unlimited.
- Erickson, H. C., Tomlin, E. M., & Swain, M. A. (2002). Modeling and role-modeling: A theory and paradigm for nursing. Cedar Park, TX: Est. Co. (Original work published 1983, Englewood Cliffs, NJ: Prentice-Hall.)

REFERENCES

Acton, G. (1993). The relationships among stressors, stress, affiliated-individuation, burden, and well-being in caregivers of adults with dementia: A test of the theory and paradigm for nursing, modeling and role-modeling. Unpublished doctoral dissertation, University of Texas, Austin.

Acton, G. (1997). The mediating effect of affiliated-individuation in caregivers of adults with dementia. *Journal of Holistic Nursing,* 15(4), 336-357.

Acton, G. J., Irvin, B. L., Jensen, B. A., Hopkins, B. A., & Miller, E. W. (1997). Explicating midrange theory through methodological diversity. *Advances in Nursing Science,* 19(3), 78-85.

Acton, G. J., & Miller, E. W. (1996). Affiliated individuation in caregivers of adults with dementia. *Issues in Mental Health Nursing,* 17, 245-260.

Anschutz, C. A. (2000). Perceived enactment of autonomy and life satisfaction: An elderly perspective. Unpublished master's thesis, Fort Hays State University, Hays, KS.

Baas, L. S. (1992). The relationships among self-care knowledge, self-care resources, activity level and life satisfaction in persons three to six months after a myocardial infarction. *Dissertation Abstracts International,* 53, 1780B.

Baas, L. S. (2004). Self-care resources and activity as predictors of quality of life in persons after myocardial infarction. *Dimensions of Critical Care Nursing,* 23(3), 131-138.

Baas, L. S., Beery, T. A., Allen, G. A., Wizer, M., & Wagoner, L. E. (2004). An exploratory study of body awareness in persons with heart failure or transplant. *Journal of Cardiovascular Nursing,* 19(1), 32-40.

Baas, L. S., Beery, T. A., Fontana, J. A., & Wagoner, L. E. (1999). An exploratory study of developmental growth in adults with heart failure. *Journal of Holistic Nursing,* 17(2), 117-138.

Baas, L. S., Fontana, J. A., & Bhat, G. (1997). Relationships between self-care resources and the quality of life of persons with heart failure: A comparison of treatment groups. *Progress in Cardiovascular Nursing,* 12(1), 25-38.

Babcock, M., & Mueller, P. (1980). Accidents and life stress. Unpublished master's thesis, University of Michigan, Ann Arbor, MI.

Baldwin, C. M. (1996). Perceptions of hope: Lived experiences of elementary school children in an urban setting. *The Journal of Multicultural Nursing & Health,* 2(3), 41-45.

Barnfather, J. S. (1987). Mobilizing coping resources related to basic need status in healthy, young adults. *Dissertation Abstracts International,* 49/02-B, 0360.

Barnfather, J. S. (1990a). An overview of the ability to mobilize coping resources related to basic needs. In H. Erickson & C. Kinney (Eds.), Modeling and role-modeling: Theory, practice and research (Vol. 1). Austin, TX: Society for the Advancement of Modeling and Role-Modeling.

Barnfather, J. S. (1990b). Mobilizing coping resources related to basic need status. In H. Erickson & C. Kinney (Eds.), Modeling and role-modeling: Theory, practice and research (Vol. 1). Austin, TX: Society for the Advancement of Modeling and Role-Modeling.

Barnfather, J. (1993). Testing a theoretical proposition for modeling and role-modeling: A basic need and adaptive potential status. *Issues in Mental Health Nursing,* 13, 1-18.

Beery, T. A., Baas, L. S., Fowler, C., & Allen, G. (2002). Spirituality in persons with heart failure. *Journal of Holistic Nursing,* 20(10), 5-30.

Beery, T., Baas, L. S., & Henthorn R. (2007). Self reported adjustment to implanted cardiac devices. *Journal of Cardiovascular Nursing,* 22(6), 516-524

Beery, T., Baas, L. S., & Mathews, H., Burrough, J. & Henthorn R. (2005). Development of the Implanted Devices Adjustment Scale. *Dimensions of Critical Care Nursing,* 24(5), 242-248.

Beltz, S. (1999). How persons 85 years and older, living in congregate housing, experience managing their health: Preservation of self. Unpublished doctoral dissertation, University of Texas, Austin, TX.

Benson, D. (2003). Adaptive potential assessment model as applied to small groups. Unpublished doctoral dissertation, University of LaVerne, LaVerne CA.

Boodley, C. A. (1990). The experience of having a healthy examination. In H. Erickson & C. Kinney (Eds.), Modeling and role-modeling: Theory, practice and research (Vol. 1). Austin, TX: Society for the Advancement of Modeling and Role-Modeling.

Boodley, C. A. (1986). A nursing study of the experience of having a health examination. Unpublished doctoral dissertation, University of Michigan, Ann Arbor, Michigan.

Bowman, S. S. (1998). The human-environment relationship in self-care when healing from episodic illness.

Unpublished doctoral dissertation, University of Texas, Austin, TX.

Cain, E., & Perzynski, K. (1986). Utilization of the self-care knowledge model with wife caregivers. Unpublished master's thesis, University of Michigan, Ann Arbor, MI.

Campbell, J., Finch, D., Allport, C., Erickson, H. C., & Swain, M. A. (1985). A theoretical approach to nursing assessment. *Journal of Advanced Nursing,* 10, 111-115.

Chen, Y. (1996). Relationships among health control orientation, self-efficacy, self-care, and subjective well-being in the elderly with hypertension. Unpublished doctoral dissertation, University of Texas, Austin, TX.

Chinn, P. L., & Kramer M. K. (2004). Integrated Knowledge Development in Nursing (6th ed.) St. Louis: Mosby.

Clayton, D. (2001). Journeys through chaos: Experiences of prolonged family suffering and evolving spiritual identity. Unpublished doctoral dissertation, University of Texas, Austin, TX.

Clementino, D., & Lapinske, M. (1980). The effects of different preparatory messages on distress from a bronchoscopy. Unpublished master's thesis, University of Michigan, Ann Arbor, MI.

Curl, E. D. (1992). Hope in the elderly: Exploring the relationship between psychosocial developmental residual and hope. *Dissertation Abstracts International,* 47, 992B.

Darling-Fisher, C. S. (1987). The relationship between mothers' and fathers' Eriksonian psychosocial attributes, perceptions of family support, and adaptation to parenthood. Unpublished doctoral dissertation, University of Michigan, Ann Arbor, Michigan.

Darling-Fisher, C., & Leidy, N. (1988). Measuring Eriksonian development of the adult: The modified Erikson psychosocial stage inventory. *Psychological Reports,* 62, 747-754.

Dildy, S. M. P. (1992). A naturalistic study of the meaning and impact of suffering in people with rheumatoid arthritis. Unpublished doctoral dissertation, University of Texas, Austin, TX.

Doornbos, M. (1983). The relationship of the social network to emotional health in the aged. Unpublished master's thesis, University of Michigan, Ann Arbor, MI.

Erickson, H. (1985). Self-care knowledge: Relations among the concepts support, hope, control, satisfaction with life, and physical health. In Sigma Theta Tau International Proceedings, Social support and health: New directions for theory development and research. Rochester, NY: University of Rochester.

Erickson, H. (1990a). Modeling and role-modeling with psychophysiological problems. In J. K. Zeig & S. Gilligan (Eds.), Brief therapy: Myths, methods, and metaphors. New York: Brunner/Mazel.

Erickson, H. (1990b). Theory based nursing. In H. Erickson & C. Kinney (Eds.), Modeling and role-modeling: Theory, practice and research (Vol. 1). Austin, TX: Society for the Advancement of Modeling and Role-Modeling.

Erickson, H. C. (1976). Identification of states of coping utilization physiological and psychological data. Unpublished master's thesis, University of Michigan, Ann Arbor, MI.

Erickson, H. C., Kinney, C., Becker, H., Acton, G., Irvin, B., Hopkins, R., et al. (1994). Modeling and role-modeling with Alzheimer's patients (National Institutes of Health funded grant). Unpublished manuscript, University of Texas, Austin, TX.

Erickson, H. C., Kinney, C., Stone, D., & Acton, G. (1990). Self-care activities, knowledge, and resources related to physical health. Unpublished manuscript, University of Texas, Austin, TX.

Erickson, H. C., & Swain, M. A. (1982). A model for assessing potential adaptation to stress. Research in Nursing and Health, 5, 93-101.

Erickson, H. C., Tomlin, E. M., & Swain, M. A. P. (1983). Modeling and role-modeling: A theory and paradigm for nursing. Englewood Cliffs, NJ: Prentice Hall.

Erickson, H., Tomlin, E., & Swain, M. (2002). Modeling and role-modeling: A theory and paradigm for nursing. Cedar Park, TX: Est. Co.

Erickson, M. (1996a). Factors that influence the mother-infant dyad relationships and infant well-being. *Issues in Mental Health Nursing,* 17, 185-200.

Erickson, M. (1996b). Relationships among support, needs satisfaction, and maternal attachment in the adolescent mother. Unpublished doctoral dissertation, University of Texas, Austin, TX.

Erickson, M. (2006). Attachment, Loss, and Reattachment. In Erickson, H. (Ed). Modeling and role-modeling: A view from the client's world. Cedar Park, TX Unicorns Unlimited Books.

Finch, D. (1987). Testing a theoretically based nursing assessment. Unpublished doctoral dissertation, University of Michigan, Ann Arbor, MI.

Finch, D. A. (1990). Testing a theoretically based nursing assessment. In H. Erickson & C. Kinney (Eds.), Modeling and role-modeling: Theory, practice and research (Vol. 1). Austin, TX: Society for the Advancement of Modeling and Role-Modeling.

Hertz, J. E. (1999). Testing two self-care measures in elderly home care clients. In S. H. Gueldner & L. W. Poon (Eds.), Gerontological nursing issues for the 21st century (pp. 195-205). Indianapolis: Center Nursing Press.

Hertz, J. E. G. (1991). The perceived enactment of autonomy scale: Measuring the potential for self-care action in the elderly. Dissertation Abstracts International, 52, 1953B.

Hertz, J. E., & Anschutz, C. A. (2002). Relationships among perceived enactment of autonomy, self-care, and holistic health in community-dwelling older adults. *Journal of Holistic Nursing,* 20(2), 166-186.

Hertz, J., Baas, L., Curl, E., & Robinson, K. (1994). An integrative review of research for modeling and role-modeling theory: 1982-1992. Unpublished manuscript, University of Illinois at Urbana-Champaign, Champaign, IL.

Hertz, J. E., Rossetti, J. & Nelson, C. M. (2006). Self-care activities reported by older adults living in senior apartments. Unpublished manuscript, Northern Illinois University, DeKalb, IL.

Holl, R. M. (1992). The effect of role-modeled visiting in comparison to restricted visiting on the well-being of clients who had open heart surgery and their significant family members in the critical care unit. *Dissertation Abstracts International,* 53, 4030B.

Hopkins, B. A. (1995). Adaptive potential of caregivers of adults with dementia. Paper presented at the meeting of Sigma Theta Tau International, Detroit.

Irvin, B. L. (1993). Social support, self-worth and hope as self-care resources for coping with caregiver stress. *Dissertation Abstracts International,* 54(06), B2995.

Irvin, B. L., & Acton, G. (1996). Stress mediation in caregivers of cognitively impaired adults: Theoretical model testing. *Nursing Research,* 45(3), 160-166.

Irvin, B. L., & Acton G. J. (1997). Stress, hope and well-being of women caring for family members with Alzheimer's disease. *Holistic Nursing Practices,* 11(2), 69-79.

Jensen, B. (1995). Caregiver responses to a theoretically based intervention program: Case study analysis. Unpublished doctoral dissertation, University of Texas, Austin, TX.

Keck, V. E. (1989). Perceived social support, basic needs satisfaction, and coping strategies of the chronically ill. *Dissertation Abstracts International,* 50, 3921B.

Kennedy, G. T. (1991). A nursing investigation of comfort and comforting care of the acutely ill patient. *Dissertation Abstracts International,* 52, 6318B.

Kinney, C. (1992). Psychosocial developmental correlates of coronary prone behavior in healthy adults. Unpublished manuscript, University of Texas at Austin, Austin, TX.

Kinney, C. K. (1990). Facilitating growth and development: A paradigm case for modeling and role-modeling. *Issues in Mental Health Nursing,* 11, 375-395.

Kinney, C., & Erickson, H. (1990). Modeling the client's world: A way to holistic care. *Issues in Mental Health Nursing,* 11, 93-108.

Kinney, C. K., Rodgers, D. R., Nash, K., & Bray, C. (2003). Holistic Healing for Women with Breast Cancer Through a Mind, Body, and Spirit Self-Empowerment Program. *Journal of Holistic Nursing,* 21, 260-279.

Kleinbeck, S. (1977). Coping states of stress. Unpublished master's thesis, University of Michigan, Ann Arbor, MI.

Kline Leidy, N. (1990). A structural model of stress, psychosocial resources, and symptomatic experience in chronic physical illness. *Nursing Research,* 39, 230-236.

Kline, N. W. (1988). Psychophysiological processes of stress in people with a chronic physical illness. *Dissertation Abstracts International,* 49, 2129B.

Landis, B. J. (1991). Uncertainty, spiritual well-being, and psychosocial adjustment to chronic illness. *Dissertation Abstracts International,* 52, 4124B.

MacLean, T. T. (1987). Health behaviors, developmental residual and stressors. In H. Erickson & C. Kinney (eds). Modeling and role-modeling: Theory, practice and research (Vol 1, No 1; pp.147-155). Austin: The Society for the Advancement of Modeling and Role-Modeling.

MacLean, T. T. (1990). Erikson's development and stressors as factors in healthy lifestyle. *Dissertation Abstracts International,* 48, 1710A.

MacLean, T. T. (1992). Influence of psychosocial development and life events on the health practices of adults. *Issues in Mental Health,* 13, 403-414.

Merton, R. K. (1968). Social theory and social structure. New York: The Free Press.

Miller, E. W. (1994). The meaning of encouragement and its connection to the inner-spirit as perceived by caregivers of the cognitively impaired. Unpublished doctoral dissertation, University of Texas, Austin, TX.

Miller, S. H. (1986). The relationship between psychosocial development and coping ability among disabled teenagers. *Dissertation Abstracts International,* 47, 4113B.

Nash, K. (2007). Evaluation of the empower peer support and education program for middle school-aged adolescents. *Journal of Holistic Health,* 25, 26-36.

Raudonis, B. (1991). A nursing study of empathy from the hospice patient's perspective. Unpublished doctoral dissertation, University of Texas, Austin, TX.

Robinson, K. R. (1992). Developing a scale to measure responses of clients with actual or potential myocardial infarctions. *Dissertation Abstracts International,* 53, 6226B.

Rogers, S. (1996). Facilitative affiliation: Nurse-client interactions that enhance healing. *Issues in Mental Health Nursing,* 17, 171-184.

Rosenow, D. J. (1991). Multidimensional scaling analysis of self-care actions for reintegrating holistic health after a myocardial infarction: Implications for nursing. *Dissertation Abstracts International,* 53, 1789B.

Scheela, R. (1991). The remodeling process: A grounded study of adult male incest offenders' perceptions of the treatment process. Unpublished doctoral dissertation, University of Texas, Austin, TX.

Smith, K. (1980). Relationship between social support and goal attainment. Unpublished master's thesis, University of Michigan, Ann Arbor, MI.

Sofhauser, C. (1996). The relations among hostility, self-esteem, self-concept, psychosocial residual in persons with coronary heart disease. Dissertations Abstracts International 5B/01-B.

Timmerman, G., & Acton, G. (2001). The relationship between basic need satisfaction and emotional eating. *Issues in Mental Health Nursing,* 22(7), 691-701.

Weber, G. J. (1999). The experiential meaning of well-being for employed mothers. *Western Journal of Nursing Research,* 21(6), 785-795.

Weber, G. J. T. (1995). Employed mothers with pre-school-aged children: An exploration of their lived experiences and the nature of their well-being. *Dissertation Abstracts International,* 56-06(B), 3131.

BIBLIOGRAPHY

Primary Sources

Books

Erickson, H. (1986). Synthesizing clinical experiences: A step in theory development. Ann Arbor, MI: Biomedical Communications.

Erickson, H. (Ed.) (2006). Modeling and Role-Modeling: A View From the Client's World. Cedar Park, TX: Unicorns Unlimited.

Erickson, H. C., Tomlin, E. M., & Swain, M. A. (2002). Modeling and role-modeling: A theory and paradigm for nursing. Cedar Park, TX: Est. Co. (Originally work published 1983, Englewood Cliffs, NJ: Prentice-Hall.)

Erickson, H., & Kinney, C. (Eds.). (1990). Modeling and role-modeling: Theory, practice and research (Vol. 1). Austin, TX: Society for the Advancement of Modeling and Role-Modeling.

Book Chapters

Erickson, H. (1977). Communication in nursing. In H. Erickson (Ed.), *Professional nursing matrix: A workbook* (pp. 1-150). Ann Arbor, MI: Media Library, University of Michigan.

Erickson, H. (1985). Modeling and role-modeling: Ericksonian approaches with physiological problems. In J. Zeig & S. Langton (Eds.), *Ericksonian psychotherapy: The state of the art.* New York: Brunner/Mazel.

Erickson, H. (1990). Modeling and role-modeling with psychophysiological problems. In J. K. Zeig & S. Gilligan (Eds.), *Brief therapy: Myths, methods, and metaphors* (pp. 473-491). New York: Brunner/Mazel.

Erickson, H. (1990). Self-care knowledge: An exploratory study. In C. Kinney & H. Erickson (Eds.), *Modeling and role-modeling: Theory, practice and research* (Vol. 1, pp. 178-202). Austin, TX: Society for the Advancement of Modeling and Role-Modeling.

Erickson, H. (1990). Theory based nursing. In C. Kinney & H. Erickson (Eds.), *Modeling and role-modeling: Theory, practice and research* (Vol. 1, pp. 1-27). Austin, TX: Society for the Advancement of Modeling and Role-Modeling.

Journal Articles

Barnfather, J., Swain, M. A., & Erickson, H. (1989). Construct validity of an aspect of the coping process: Potential adaptation to stress. *Issues in Mental Health Nursing, 10,* 23-40.

Barnfather, J., Swain, M. A., & Erickson, H. (1989). Evaluation of two assessment techniques. *Nursing Science Quarterly, 4,* 172-182.

Campbell, J., Finch, D., Allport, C., Erickson, H., & Swain, M. (1985). A theoretical approach to nursing assessment. *Journal of Advanced Nursing, 10,* 111-115.

Erickson, H. (1983, March). Coping with new systems. *Journal of Nursing Education, 22*(3), 132-135.

Erickson, H. (1991). Modeling y role-modeling con psychophysiological problemas. *Rapport: Hipnosis de Milton H. Erickson—Revista del Instituto Milton H. Erickson de Buenos Aires* (Argentina), *1*(1), 41-53.

Erickson, H., & Swain, M. A. (1982). A model for assessing potential adaptation to stress. *Research in Nursing and Health, 5,* 93-101.

Erickson, H., & Swain, M. A. (1990). Mobilizing self-care resources: A nursing intervention for hypertension. *Issues in Mental Health Nursing, 11,* 217-236.

Erickson, M. (1996). Factors that influence the mother infant dyad relationships and infant well-being. *Issues in Mental Health Nursing, 17,* 185-200.

Secondary Sources

Books

Bowlby, J. (1969). *Attachment.* New York: Basic Books.

Bowlby, J. (1973). *Separation.* New York: Basic Books.

Bowlby, J. (1980). *Loss.* New York: Basic Books.

Engel, G. S. (1962). *Psychological development in health and disease.* Philadelphia: W. B. Saunders.

Erikson, E. (1963). *Childhood and society.* New York: W. W. Norton.

Haley, J. (1973). *Uncommon therapy: The psychiatric techniques of Milton H. Erickson, M.D.* New York: W. W. Norton.

Mahler, M. S., & Furer, M. (1968). *On human symbiosis and the vicissitudes of individuation* (Vol. I). *Infantile psychosis.* New York: International Universities Press.

Maslow, A. H. (1968). *Toward a psychology of being* (2nd ed.). New York: D. Von Nostrand.

Maslow, A. H. (1970). *Motivation and personality* (2nd ed.). New York: Harper & Row.

Merton, R. K. (1968). *Social theory and social structure.* New York: The Free Press.

Piaget, J. (1952). *The origins of intelligence in children.* New York: International Universities Press.

Piaget, J., & Inhelder, B. (1969). *The psychology of the child.* New York: Basic Books.

Rossi, E. (1986). *The psychobiology of mind-body healing.* New York: W. W. Norton.

Selye, H. (1974). *Stress without distress.* Philadelphia: J. B. Lippincott.

Selye, H. (1976). *The stress of life* (2nd ed.). New York: McGraw-Hill.

Book Chapters

Barnfather, J. (1990). An overview of the ability to mobilize coping resources related to basic needs. In H. Erickson & C. Kinney (Eds.), *Modeling and role-modeling: Theory, practice and research* (Vol. 1, pp. 156-169). Austin, TX: Society for the Advancement of Modeling and Role-Modeling.

Bowlby, J. (1960). Child care and the growth of love. In M. Haimowitz & N. Haimowitz (Eds.), *Human development* (2nd ed., pp. 155-166). New York: Thomas Y. Crowell.

Erikson, E. (1960). Identity versus self-diffusion. In M. Haimowitz & N. Haimowitz (Eds.), *Human development* (2nd ed., pp. 766-770). New York: Thomas Y. Crowell.

Erikson, E. (1960). The case of Peter. In M. Haimowitz & N. Haimowitz, *Human development* (2nd ed., pp. 355-359). New York: Thomas Y. Crowell.

Hassan, A., & Hassan, B. M. (1987). Interpersonal development across the life span: Communion and its interaction with agency in psychosocial development. In L. A. Meachem (Ed.), *Contributions to human development* (Vol. 18, pp. 102-127). Basel: Werner Druck AG.

Klein, M. (1952). Some theoretical conclusions regarding the emotional life of the infant. In J. Riviere (Ed.), *Developments in psychoanalysis* (pp. 198-236). London: Hogarth Press.

Piaget, J. (1974). The pathway between subjects' recent life changes and their near-future illness reports: Representative results and methodological issues. In B. S. Dohrenwend & B. P. Dohrenwend (Eds.), *Stressful life events: Their nature and effects* (pp. 73-86). New York: John Wiley & Sons.

Winnicott, D. W. (1965). The theory of the parent-infant relationship. In D. W. Winnicott (Ed.), *The maturational processes and the facilitating environment.* London: Hogarth Press.

Journal Articles

Acton, G., & Miller, E. (1996). Affiliated-individuation in caregivers of adults with dementia. *Issues in Mental Health Nursing, 17,* 245-260.

Adamson, J., & Schmale, A. (1965). Object loss, giving up, and the onset of psychiatric disease. *Psychosomatic Medicine, 27*(6), 557-576.

Baas, L. S., Fontana, J. A., & Bhat, G. (1997). Relationships between self-care resources and the quality of life of persons with heart failure: A comparison of treatment groups. *Progress in Cardiovascular Nursing, 12*(1), 25-38.

Barnfather, J. (1993). Testing a theoretical proposition for modeling and role-modeling: A basic need and adaptive potential status. *Issues in Mental Health Nursing, 13,* 1-18.

Bartholomew, K. (1990). Avoidance of intimacy: An attachment perspective. *Journal of Social and Personal Relationships, 7,* 147-178.

Beery, T., & Baas, L. (1996). Medical devices and attachment: Holistic healing in the age of invasive technology. *Issues in Mental Health Nursing, 17,* 233-243.

Bowlby, J. (1958). The nature of the child's tie to his mother. *International Journal of Psychoanalysis, 39,* 89-97.

Bowlby, J. (1961). Childhood mourning and its explications for psychiatry. *American Journal of Psychiatry, 118,* 481-498.

Bowlby, J. (1961). Process of mourning. *International Journal of Psychoanalysis, 42,* 317-340.

Bowlby, J., Robertson, J., & Rosenbluth, D. (1952). A two-year-old goes to the hospital. *Psychoanalytic Study of the Child, 7,* 89-94.

Engel, G. (1968). A life setting conducive to illness: The giving-up-given-up complex. *Annuals of Internal Medicine, 69*(2), 293-300.

Hertz, J. (1996). Conceptualization of perceived enactment of autonomy in the elderly. *Issues in Mental Health Nursing, 17,* 261-273.

Irvin, B., & Acton, G. (1996). Stress mediation in caregivers of cognitively impaired adults: Theoretical model testing. *Nursing Research, 45*(3), 160-166.

Irvin, B., & Acton, G. (1997). Stress, hope and well-being of women caring for family members with Alzheimer's disease. *Holistic Nursing Practice, 11*(2), 69-79.

Kinney, C. (1996). Transcending breast cancer: Reconstructing one's self. *Issues in Mental Health Nursing, 17,* 201-216.

Landis, B. J. (1996). Uncertainty, spiritual well-being, and psychosocial adjustment to chronic illness. *Issues in Mental Health Nursing, 17,* 217-231.

Leidy, N. (1994). Operationalizing Maslow's theory: Development and testing of the Basic Needs Satisfaction Inventory. *Issues in Mental Health Nursing, 15,* 277-295.

Leidy, N. K., & Traver, G. A. (1995). Psychophysiological factors contribution to functional performance in people with COPD: Are there gender differences? *Research in Nursing and Health, 18,* 535-546.

Mahler, M. S. (1967). On human symbiosis and the vicissitudes of individuation. *Journal of the American Psychoanalytic Association, 15,* 740-763.

Maslow, A. H. (1936). The need to know and the fear of knowing. *Journal of General Psychology, 68,* 111-125.

Miller, E. W. (1995). Encouraging Alzheimer's caregivers. *Journal of Christian Nursing, 12*(4), 7-12.

Robinson, K. R. (1994). Developing a scale to measure denial levels of clients with actual or potential myocardial infarctions. *Heart and Lung, 23,* 36-44.

Rogers, S. (1996). Facilitative affiliation: Nurse-client interactions that enhance healing. *Issues in Mental Health Nursing, 17,* 171-184.

Sappington, J., & Kelley, J. H. (1996). Modeling and role-modeling theory: A case study of holistic care. *Journal of Holistic Nursing, 14*(2), 130-141.

Walsh, K. K., Vanden Bosch, T. M., & Boehm, S. (1989). Modeling and role-modeling: Integrating nursing theory into practice. *Journal of Advanced Nursing, 14*, 755-761.

Theses

Kirk, L. (1996). *A descriptive study of level of hope in cancer patients.* Unpublished master's thesis, University of Texas, San Antonio, TX.

Kleinbeck, S. (1977). *Coping states of stress.* Unpublished master's thesis, University of Michigan, Ann Arbor, MI.

Dissertations

Acton, G. (1993). Relationships among stressors, stress, affiliated-individuation, burden, and well-being in caregivers of adults with dementia: A test of the theory and paradigm for nursing, modeling and role-modeling. Unpublished doctoral dissertation, University of Texas, Austin, TX.

Baas, L. S. (1992). The relationships among self-care knowledge, self-care resources, activity level and life satisfaction in persons three to six months after a myocardial infarction. *Dissertation Abstracts International,* 53, 1780B.

Barnfather, J. S. (1987). Mobilizing coping resources related to basic need status in healthy, young adults. *Dissertation Abstracts International,* 49, 360B.

Beltz, S. (1999). How persons 85 years and older, living in congregate housing, experience managing their health: Preservation of self. Unpublished doctoral dissertation, University of Texas, Austin, TX.

Benson, D. (2003). Adaptive potential assessment model as applied to small groups. Unpublished doctoral dissertation, The University of LaVerne, LaVerne, CA.

Chen, Y. (1996). Relationships among health control orientation, self-efficacy, self-care, and subjective well-being in the elderly with hypertension. Unpublished doctoral dissertation, University of Texas, Austin, TX.

Curl, E. D. (1992). Hope in the elderly: Exploring the relationship between psychosocial developmental residual and hope. *Dissertation Abstracts International,* 47, 992B.

Daniels, R. (1994). Exploring the self-care variables that explains a wellness lifestyle in spinal cord injured wheelchair basketball athletes. Unpublished doctoral dissertation, University of Texas, Austin, TX.

Darling-Fisher, C. S. (1987). The relationship between mothers' and fathers' Eriksonian psychosocial attributes, perceptions of family support, and adaptation to parenthood. *Dissertation Abstracts International,* 48, 1640B.

Erickson, M. (1996). Relationships among support, needs satisfaction, and maternal attachment in the adolescent mother. Unpublished doctoral dissertation, University of Texas, Austin, TX.

Hertz, J. E. G. (1991). The perceived enactment of autonomy scale: Measuring the potential for self-care action in the elderly. *Dissertation Abstracts International,* 52, 1953B.

Hopkins, B. (1994). Assessment of adaptive potential. Unpublished doctoral dissertation, University of Texas, Austin, TX.

Irvin, B. L. (1993). Social support, self-worth and hope as self-care resources for coping with caregiver stress. *Dissertation Abstracts International,* 54(06), B2995.

Jensen, B. (1995). Caregiver responses to a theoretically based intervention program: Case study analysis. Unpublished doctoral dissertation, University of Texas, Austin, TX.

Kline, N. W. (1988). Psychophysiological processes of stress in people with a chronic physical illness. *Dissertation Abstracts International,* 49, 2129B.

Landis, B. J. (1991). Uncertainty, spiritual well-being, and psychosocial adjustment to chronic illness. *Dissertation Abstracts International,* 52, 4124B.

MacLean, T. T. (1987). Erikson's development and stressors as factors in healthy lifestyle. Dissertation Abstracts International, 48, 1710A.

Miller, E. W. (1994). The meaning of encouragement and its connection to the inner-spirit as perceived by caregivers of the cognitively impaired. Unpublished doctoral dissertation, University of Texas, Austin, TX.

Nash, K. (2003). Evaluation of a holistic peer support and education program aimed at facilitating self-care resources in adolescents (Unpublished doctoral dissertation). The University of Texas at Galveston, Galveston, TX.

Raudonis, B. (1991). A nursing study of empathy from the hospice patient's perspective. Unpublished doctoral dissertation, University of Texas, Austin, TX.

Robinson, K. R. (1992). Developing a scale to measure responses of client with actual or potential myocardial infarctions. *Dissertation Abstracts International,* 53, 6226B.

Sofhauser, C. (1996). The relations among hostility, self-esteem, self-concept, psychosocial residual in persons with coronary heart disease. *Dissertation Abstracts International* 5B/01-B.

Weber, G. (1995). Employed mothers with pre-schoolaged children: An exploration of their lived experiences and the nature of their well-being. *Dissertation Abstracts International* 56/06-B3/31.

APPENDIX

ASSESSMENT TOOL BASED ON MODELING AND ROLE-MODELING*

I. Description of the situation
   A. Overview of the situation
   B. Etiology
      1. Eustressors
      2. Stressors
      3. Distressors
   C. Therapeutic needs
II. Expectations
   A. Immediate
   B. Long term
III. Resource potential
   A. External
      1. Social network
      2. Support system
      3. Healthcare system
   B. Internal
      1. Strengths
      2. Adaptive potential
         a. Feeling states
         b. Physiological parameters
IV. Goals and life tasks
   A. Current
   B. Future

DATA INTERPRETATION TOOL BASED ON MODELING AND ROLE-MODELING†

I. Interpret data for ability to mobilize resources (APAM)
II. Interpret data for needs status (assets and deficits related to type of need), attachment objects, loss, grief (normal or morbid), life tasks (developmental: actual and chronological)

DATA ANALYSIS TOOL BASED ON MODELING AND ROLE-MODELING‡

I. Step one
   A. Articulate relationships between stressors and needs status
   B. Articulate relationships between needs status and ability to mobilize resources
   C. Articulate relationships between needs status and loss of attachment
   D. Articulate relationships between loss and type of grief response
   E. Articulate relationships between type of need assets and deficits and developmental residual
   F. Articulate relationships between chronological developmental task and developmental residual
II. Step two
   A. Articulate relationships among stressors, resource potential, needs status, loss, grief status, developmental residual, chronological task, and attachment potential
   B. Articulate relationships among needs, status, potential resources, developmental residual, and personal goals

AI, Affiliated-individuation; *APAM,* Adaptive Potential Assessment Model.

*Interview questions and thoughts that guide critical thinking are suggested in Erickson, H. C., Tomlin, E. M., & Swain, M. A. (1983). *Modeling and role-modeling: A theory and paradigm for nursing* (pp. 116-168). Englewood Cliffs, NJ: Prentice-Hall. Suggestions for interviewing techniques are found in Erickson, H. C. (1990). Self-care knowledge. In H. C. Erickson & C. Kinney (Eds.), *Modeling and role-modeling: Theory, practice and research* (Vol. 1). Austin, TX: Society for the Advancement of Modeling and Role-Modeling.

†Critical thinking guidelines for data interpretation are suggested in Erickson, H. C., Tomlin, E. M., & Swain, M. A. (1983). *Modeling and role-modeling: A theory and paradigm for nursing* (pp. 148-166). Englewood Cliffs, NJ: Prentice-Hall; and Erickson, H. C. (1990). Theory based nursing. In H. C. Erickson & C. Kinney (Eds.), *Modeling and role-modeling: Theory, practice and research* (Vol. 1). Austin, TX: Society for the Advancement of Modeling and Role-Modeling.

‡Critical thinking guidelines for data analysis are suggested in Erickson, H. C., Tomlin, E. M., & Swain, M. A. (1983). *Modeling and role-modeling: A theory and paradigm for nursing* (pp. 148-166). Englewood Cliffs, NJ: Prentice-Hall; and Erickson, H. C. (1990). Theory-based nursing. In H. C. Erickson & C. Kinney (Eds.), *Modeling and role-modeling: Theory, practice and research* (Vol. 1). Austin, TX: Society for the Advancement of Modeling and Role-Modeling.

APPENDIX—cont'd

PLANNING TOOL BASED ON MODELING AND ROLE-MODELING§

I. Aims of interventions
   A. Build trust
   B. Promote positive orientation
   C. Promote client control
   D. Promote strengths
   E. Set health-directed goals

II. Intervention goals
   A. Develop a trusting and functional relationship between yourself and your client
   B. Facilitate a self-projection that is futuristic and positive
   C. Promote AI with the minimal degree of ambivalence possible
   D. Promote a dynamic, adaptive, and holistic state of health
   E. Promote and nurture a coping mechanism that satisfies basic needs and permits growth-need satisfaction
   F. Facilitate congruent actual and chronological developmental stages

§Critical thinking guidelines for planning are suggested in Erickson, H. C., Tomlin, E. M., & Swain, M. A. (1983). *Modeling and role-modeling: A theory and paradigm for nursing* (pp. 169-220). Englewood Cliffs, NJ: Prentice-Hall; and Erickson, H. C. (1990). Theory-based nursing. In H. C. Erickson & C. Kinney (Eds.), *Modeling and role-modeling: Theory, practice and research* (Vol. 1). Austin, TX: Society for the Advancement of Modeling and Role-Modeling.

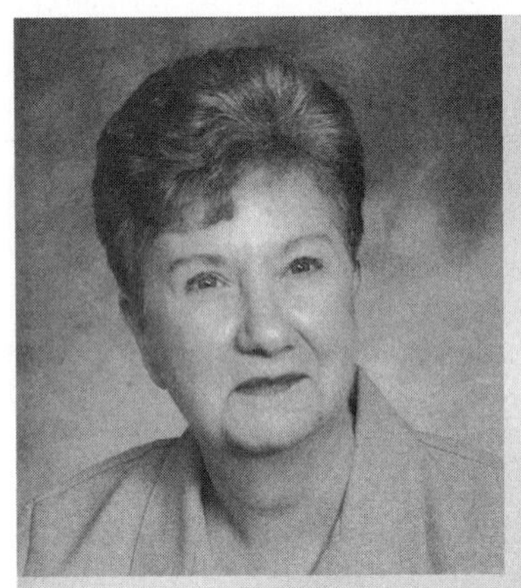

CHAPTER

26

Gladys L. Husted

1941-present

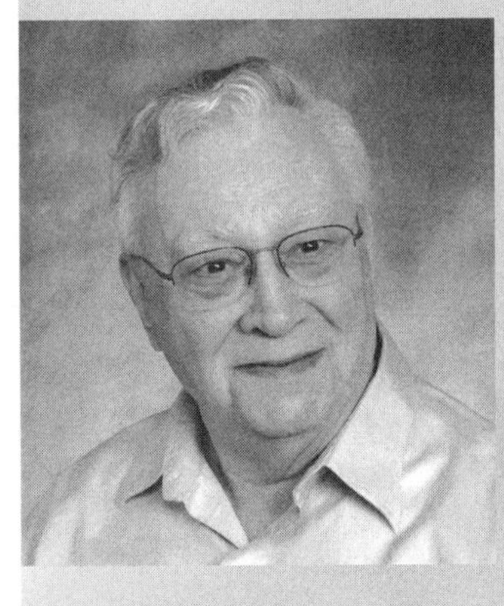

James H. Husted

1931-present

Symphonological Bioethical Theory

Carrie Scotto

"Symphonology (from 'symphonia,' a Greek word meaning agreement) is a system of ethics based on the terms and preconditions of an agreement". (Husted & Husted, n.d.)

CREDENTIALS AND BACKGROUND OF THE THEORISTS

Gladys Husted was born in Pittsburgh, where her life, practice, education, and teaching continue to influence the nursing profession. Husted received a Bachelor of Science in Nursing degree from University of Pittsburgh in 1962 and began practice in public health and acute in-patient medical-surgical care. Observations of interactions between nurses and patients initiated her interest in ethical issues. In 1968, she earned a master's degree in nursing education while teaching at the Louise Suyden School of Nursing at St. Margaret's Memorial Hospital in Pittsburgh. Her love of teaching prompted doctoral study that resulted in a terminal degree from the University of Pittsburgh Department of Curriculum and Supervision.

G. Husted is currently professor emeritus at Duquesne University School of Nursing, where in 1998 she was awarded the title of School of Nursing Distinguished Professor. She continues to teach part time and direct dissertations. The school has also recognized her teaching excellence at all levels of the curriculum through the Duquesne University School of Nursing Recognition Award for Excellence 1990/1991 and the Faculty Award for Excellence in Teaching 1994/1995. The Medical College of Ohio chose Husted as the Distinguished Lecturer in 2000. She is a member of Sigma Theta Tau International, Phi Kappa Phi, and National League for Nursing.

G. Husted served as a consultant for Western Pennsylvania Hospital Nursing Division regarding the development of an ethics committee, including education of staff and management, and providing guidance for the newly formed committee. She also provided consultation for the Allegheny General Medical Center for staff development and the National Nursing Ethics Advisory Group for the Department of Veterans Affairs. She served as curriculum consultant for several schools of nursing. In addition, G. Husted has presented at many national level conferences.

James Husted was born in Kingston, Pennsylvania, and has had a lifelong interest in philosophy. While in the Army in Germany, he became interested in ethics, particularly the work of Benedict Spinoza, through conversations with a former ethics professor.

His post-Army career focused on sales and hiring and training agents for health insurance companies. However, he continued to read and develop his philosophical and ethical ideas. During the 1980s, J. Husted joined the high-IQ societies, Mensa and Intertel, serving as a philosophy expert for Mensa and a regional director for Intertel.

The theorists met and were married in 1974, establishing and cultivating a dialogue that brought about the theory of Symphonology. They are coauthors of several editions of *Ethical Decision Making in Nursing*. Their book was selected as one of Nursing and Health Care's Notable Books of 1991, 1995a, and 2001. It also won the Nursing Society Award in 2001. Their regular column, "A Practice Based Bioethic," appeared in *Advanced Practice Nursing Quarterly* 1997-1998. In addition to publishing books, book chapters, and journal articles, they have presented their ethical theory at conferences and workshops.

The Husteds reside in Pittsburgh and continue to develop and disseminate their work through teaching, writing, and presenting at conferences and workshops and serving as consultants for ethics committees.

THEORETICAL SOURCES

The authors define Symphonology as "the study of agreements and the elements necessary to forming agreements," (Husted & Husted, 2008, p. xv). In health care, it is the study of agreements between health care professionals and patients. An agreement is based on the nature of the relationship between the parties involved. In its ethical dimensions, it outlines the commitments and obligations of each. Although the theory developed from the observation of nurses and nursing practice, it later expanded to include all healthcare professionals (HCPs). The development of this theory has led to the construction of a practice-based decision-making model that assists in determining when and what actions are appropriate for HCPs and patients. The name of the theory is derived from the Greek word for agreement, *symphonia.*

Ethics is "a system of standards to motivate, determine, and justify actions directed to the pursuit of vital and fundamental goals" (Husted & Husted, 2008, p. 8). Ethics examines what ought to be done, within the realm of what can be done, to preserve and enhance human life. The Husteds, therefore, described ethics as the science of living well.

Bioethics is concerned with the ethics of interactions between a patient and an HCP, what ought to be done to preserve and enhance human life within the healthcare arena. Within the past century, the expanding knowledge base and growth of technology altered existing healthcare practice and created threatening and confusing circumstances not previously encountered. Increasing numbers and types of treatment options allowed patients to survive conditions they would not have in the past. However, the morbidity of the survivors brought new questions: Who should receive treatment? What is the appropriateness of treatments under particular circumstances? Who should decide what treatments are appropriate? In this way, bioethics became a central issue in what previously had been a prescriptive environment. It became essential to consider ethical concerns, as well as scientific solutions, to questions of health (Jecker, Jonsen, & Pearlman, 1997). Through personal experience and observation of nurses, the Husteds recognized the increasingly complex nature of bioethical dilemmas and the failure of the healthcare system to adequately address the problem.

To clarify the reasons for the deficiency of the healthcare system in addressing the issue of delivering ethical care, the Husteds examined traditional ideas and concepts used to guide ethical behavior. These ideas include deontology, utilitarianism, emotivism, and social relativism. Deontology is a duty-based ethic in which the consequences of one's actions are irrelevant. One acts in accordance with preset standards regardless of the outcome. The inappropriateness of this type of guideline is obvious in relation to HCPs, because they are responsible for foreseeing the effects of their actions and acting only in ways that benefit a patient. Utilitarian thought would have HCPs acting to bring about the greatest good for the greatest number of people. This is inconsistent with the practice of HCPs who act as agents for individual patients. Emotivism promotes ethical actions in accordance with the emotions of those involved. Rational thought has no place in emotive choices, making this type of decision-making process inappropriate in the healthcare arena. Social relativism imposes the beliefs of a society onto the individual. This approach is absurd when one considers the diversity of our emerging global society. The authors recognized that the inappropriateness of traditional methods of ethical reasoning brought about the failure of the healthcare system to successfully address bioethical issues.

Because traditional models proved inadequate to guide ethical behavior for HCPs, the Husteds began to conceive and develop a method by which HCPs might determine appropriate ethical actions. The theory was based on logical thinking, emphasizing the provision of holistic, individualized care. They drew from the work of Aristotle, Benedict Spinoza, and Michael Polanyi. These philosophers adhere to rational thought and value persons as individuals. Aristotle was a student of Plato who advanced his teacher's work by recognizing that there is more to understanding phenomena than simple rationality. He believed that one must develop insight and perception to recognize how principles can be applied to each situation (McKeon, 1941).

The Dutch philosopher, Spinoza, examined the nature of humans and human knowledge. He recognized that, although the process and outcomes of reasoning may be comparable for each person, intuitive and discerning thought is unique to each. Spinoza believed that reason must be coupled with intuitive thought for true understanding (Lloyd, 1996). Spinoza was noted for taking well-worn philosophical concepts and transforming them into new and engaging ideas. This is true of the Husteds' development of Symphonology, particularly in the evolution of the meaning of the bioethical standards.

Polanyi proposed that understanding is derived from awareness of the entirety of a phenomenon, that the lived experience is greater than separate, observable parts. Tacit knowledge, that which is implied, is necessary to understand and interpret that which is explicit (Polanyi, 1964). These concepts, the uniqueness of the individual and the extension of reason and rationality with insight and discernment to create true understanding, are the foundations of the symphonological method.

MAJOR CONCEPTS & DEFINITIONS

AGENCY

Agency is the capacity of an agent to initiate action toward a chosen goal. The shared goal of a nurse and a patient is to restore the patient's agency (Husted & Husted, 2008).

CONTEXT

The "context is the interweaving of the relevant facts of a situation" (Husted & Husted, 2008, p. 84). There are three interrelated elements of context: the context of the situation and the context of knowledge, and the context of an agent's awareness. The context of the situation includes all aspects of the situation that provide understanding of the situation and promote the ability to act effectively within it. The context of knowledge is an agent's preexisting knowledge that includes factors usually found within the situation. The context of awareness is where the first two contexts are interwoven. It is an agent's present awareness of all the relevant aspects (knowledge and circumstances) of the situation necessary to understand and act effectively within it (Husted & Husted, 2008).

ENVIRONMENT-AGREEMENT

The environment established by Symphonology is formed by agreement within a context. Agreement is a shared state of awareness on the basis of which interaction occurs (Husted & Husted, 2008). Agreement creates the realm in which nursing and all other human interactions occur. Every agreement is aimed toward a final value to be attained through interactions made possible by understanding.

The HCP-patient agreement is formed by a meeting of the professional's and the patient's needs. Their agreement is one in which the needs and desires of the patient are central. The professional's commitment is defined in terms of the patient's needs. Without this agreement, there would be no context for interaction between the two; the relationship would be unintelligible to both (Husted & Husted, 1999).

HEALTH

Health is a concept applicable to every potential of a person's life. Health involves not only thriving of the physical body, but also happiness.

Continued

MAJOR CONCEPTS & DEFINITIONS—cont'd

Happiness is realized as individuals pursue and progress toward the goals of their chosen life plan (Husted & Husted, 2001). Health is evident when individuals experience, express, and engage in the fundamental bioethical standards.

NURSING

A nurse acts as the agent of the patient, doing for her patient what he would do for himself if he were able (Husted & Husted, 2008). The nurse's ethical responsibility is to encourage and strengthen those qualities in the patient that serve life, health, and well-being through their interaction (Fedorka & Husted, 2001).

PERSON-PATIENT

A person is an individual with a unique character structure, possessing the right to pursue vital goals as he chooses (Husted & Husted, 2001). These characteristics are unique to an individual, and also may be shared by others (Husted & Husted, 2008). Vital goals are related to survival and the enhancement of life. A person takes on the role of patient when he has lost or experienced a decrease in agency resulting in his inability to take the actions required for survival or happiness (Husted & Husted, 1998).

RIGHTS

The product of an implicit agreement among rational beings, by virtue of their rationality, not to obtain actions or the product of actions from others except through voluntary consent, objectively gained (Husted & Husted, 2001). The term *rights* is a singular term that represents the critical agreement of nonaggression among rational people (Husted & Husted, 1997b).

USE OF EMPIRICAL EVIDENCE

Study and dialogue between the two theorists, coupled with experience of the overall evolution of health care and observation of individual nurse-patient relationships, provided the impetus to develop Symphonology theory. G. Husted's dissertation focused on the effect of teaching ethical principles on a student's ability to use these in practical ways through case studies. J. Husted was very instrumental in the selection of the dissertation topic and was used as a consultant during the process. Development of G. Husted's doctoral work led to numerous publications and presentations before the first edition of the book *Ethical Decision Making in Nursing* was published in 1991. This first edition presented their work as a conceptual model only. As they continued to develop their ideas, incorporating feedback from graduate students, the Symphonological theory emerged. Before publication of the second edition, the Husteds (1995a) continued to clarify the theoretical concepts and developed the model for practice.

Beginning in 1990, Duquesne University offered a course devoted to this bioethical theory. The authors continued to seek critique and examples about their work from students, practitioners, and other experts. The third edition of the book, *Ethical Decision Making in Nursing and Healthcare: The Symphonological Approach* (Husted & Husted, 2001), offered a clarified description of the theory with advanced concepts separated from the basic concepts. In addition, the model was redrawn to better represent the nonlinear nature of the theory in practice. The 4th edition offers further clarification of concepts and the integration of concepts in the theory as a whole. In addition, the text is rearranged to present the concepts from simple to more complex.

As the theory emerged, the need for an emphasis on the individual became apparent and essential. In recent years, it has become accepted practice in the literature to designate patients and nurses as he/she, or simply use the plural form, referring to nurses and their patients. The authors recognized that these awkward and anonymous terms distract readers from thinking in terms of real people within the context of a particular situation. Therefore, they chose to refer to individuals as *he*, in the case of patients, and *she*, in the case of HCPs in particular situations and examples. This chapter will continue with this practice.

MAJOR ASSUMPTIONS

The assumptions from this theory arise from the practical reasoning. The model is meant to provide nurses and other HCPs with a logical method of determining appropriate ethical actions. Although many of the terms are familiar to nurses and HCPs, some have been redefined to support the reality of human interaction and ethical delivery of health care.

Nursing

Symphonology holds that a nurse or any other HCP acts as the agent of the patient. Using her education and experience, a nurse does for her patient what he would do for himself if he were able. Nursing cannot occur without both nurse and patient. "A nurse takes no actions that are not interactions" (Husted & Husted, 2001, p. 37). The nurse's ethical responsibility is to encourage and strengthen those qualities in the patient that serve life, health, and well-being through their interaction (Fedorka & Husted, 2001).

Agency is the capacity of an agent to take action toward a chosen goal. A nurse as agent takes action for a patient, one who cannot act on his own behalf. The shared goal of a nurse and a patient is to restore the patient's agency. The nurse acts with and for the patient toward this end.

Person or Patient

The Husteds define a person as an individual with a unique character structure possessing the right to pursue vital goals as he chooses (Husted & Husted, 2001). Vital goals are concerned with survival and the enhancement of life. A person takes on the role of patient when he has lost or experienced a decrease in agency resulting in his inability to take the actions required for survival or happiness. The inability to take action may result from physical or mental problems, or from a lack of knowledge or experience (Husted & Husted, 1998).

Health

The authors do not address or define health directly. The entire theory is driven by the concept of health in the broadest, most holistic sense. Health is a concept applicable to every potential of a person's life. Health involves not only thriving of the physical body, but also happiness. Happiness is realized as individuals pursue and progress toward the goals of their chosen life plan (Husted & Husted, 2001). Health is evident when individuals experience, express, and engage in the fundamental bioethical standards.

Environment-Agreement

The environment established by Symphonology is formed by agreement. "Agreement is a shared state of awareness on the basis of which interaction occurs" (Husted & Husted, 2001, p. 61). Agreement creates the realm in which nursing and all other human interactions occur. Every agreement is aimed toward a final value to be attained through interactions made possible by understanding.

The HCP-patient agreement is formed by a meeting of the professional's and the patient's needs. Their agreement is one in which the needs and desires of the patient are central. The professional's commitment is defined in terms of the patient's needs. Without this agreement, there would be no context for interaction between the two. The relationship would be unintelligible to both (Husted & Husted, 1999).

Symphonology theory is not a compilation of traditional cultural platitudes. It is a method of determining what is practical and justifiable in the ethical dimensions of professional practice. Symphonology recognizes that what is possible and desirable in the agreement is dependent on the context.

The context is the interweaving of the relevant facts of a situation—the facts that are necessary to act upon to bring about a desired result (Husted & Husted, 2001). There are three interrelated elements of context: the context of the situation, the context of knowledge, and the context of awareness. The context of the situation includes all facts relevant to the situation that provide understanding of the situation and promote the ability to act effectively within it. The context of knowledge is an agent's preexisting knowledge of the relevant facts of the situation. The context of awareness represents an integration of the agent's awareness of the facts of the situation and her preexisting knowledge about how to most effectively deal with these facts (Husted & Husted, 2008).

THEORETICAL ASSERTIONS

Symphonology is classified as a grand theory because of its broad scope. Grand theories explicate a worldview related to a specific discipline (Walker & Avant, 1995). Grand theories are developed through astute, perceptive, discerning consideration of existing ideas in regard to a general discipline (Fawcett, 1995). The authors developed Symphonology theory not from natural progression of other work, but from the recognition of a need for theoretical guidelines related to the ethical delivery of health care. The understanding and use of this theory are based on a fundamental ethical element that describes the rational relationship between human beings: human rights.

Rights

The Husteds describe rights as the fundamental ethical element. Traditionally, rights are viewed as a list of options to which one is entitled, such as a list of items or actions to which one has a just claim. Symphonology holds rights as a singular concept. It is the implicit, species-wide agreement that one will not force another to act, or take by force the products of another's actions. Rights are viewed as the critical agreement among rational people, the agreement of nonaggression (Husted & Husted, 1997a). This agreement emerged as humans became rational and developed a civilized social structure. A nonaggression agreement is preconditional to all human interaction. It serves as a foundation on which all other agreements rest. The formal definition is as follows: "the product of an implicit agreement among rational beings, held by virtue of their rationality, not to obtain actions or the products of actions from others except through voluntary consent, objectively gained" (Husted & Husted, 2001, p. 4). The operation of this is evident in human interaction.

According to the Husteds, Symphonology theory can ensure ethical action in the provision of health care. Agreement is the foundation of Symphonology. Agreements can occur based on the implicit understanding of human rights. The understanding of nonaggression that exists among rational persons constitutes human rights. This understanding makes negotiation and cooperation among individuals possible.

Ethical Standards

Ethical standards have been the benchmarks of ethical behavior. The standards include terms familiar to HCPs such as beneficence, veracity, and confidentiality. However, the authors have conceived new meanings for ethical standards that correspond to the foundational concepts of Symphonology: the person as a unique individual and the use of insight and discernment in addition to reason and rationality in order to achieve a deeper understanding.

Traditionally, bioethical concepts have been used to guide ethical action by mandating concrete directives for action. For instance, the concept of beneficence conventionally maintains that one must see that no harm comes to a patient. However, it is not always possible to predict how and when harm will occur, making adherence to this directive an unrealistic goal. The concept of beneficence, viewed as a mandate, could also imply that defending yourself against a physical attack is unethical. Similarly, veracity, or truth telling, holds that one must always speak the truth regardless of the consequences. Therefore, it is unethical to withhold potentially harmful information, regardless of the consequences. Adhering to veracity may interfere with one's commitment to beneficence. Clearly, ethical standards taken as concrete directives do not allow for the consideration of context.

The authors have redefined the ethical standards, not as concrete rules, but as human qualities or character structures that can and must be recognized and respected in the individual (Husted & Husted, 1995b). For example, in Symphonological terms, beneficence includes the idea of acting in the patient's best interest, but it begins with the patient's evaluation of what is beneficial. In this way, ethical standards are presuppositions in the HCP-patient agreement and ethical guides to decision making. The participants work together with the implicit understanding that each is possessed of human characteristics. The description and names of the bioethical standards have changed over time based on feedback from practitioners. Symphonological theory holds that patients have a right to receive the benefits specified in the bioethical standards. Box 26-1 provides definitions and examples of bioethical standards.

Just as the bioethical standards are not to be considered as concrete directives, so too, they are not distinct entities. Each standard blends with the others as representative of the unique character structure of the individual (J. Husted, personal communication, March 5, 2004). As stated earlier, recognition of these standards is preconditional to the implicit patient-HCP agreement. When recognized and respected in each individual, these human qualities and capabilities form the basis for ethical interaction. When they are disregarded, the context of the situation is lost. Interaction is then based on whatever is served by concrete directives or on the whim of the participants.

Box 26-1 *Bioethical Standards*

AUTONOMY

Autonomy is the uniqueness of the individual, the singular character structure of the individual. Every person has the right to act on his or her unique and independent purposes.

BENEFICENCE

Beneficence is the capability to act to acquire desired benefits and necessary life requirements. Each person may act to obtain those things that he or she needs and prefers.

FIDELITY

Fidelity is an individual's faithfulness to his or her own uniqueness. Each person manages, maintains, and sustains his unique life. For the HCP, fidelity in agreement means the commitment to the obligations accepted in the professional role.

FREEDOM

Freedom is the capability and right to take action based on the agent's own evaluation of the situation. Every person may choose his or her course of action.

OBJECTIVITY

Objectivity is the right to achieve and sustain the exercise of objective awareness. Every person has an awareness and understanding of the universe outside himself or herself. Every person has the right to manage, maintain, and sustain that understanding as he or she chooses.

SELF-ASSERTION

Self-assertion is the right and capability to control one's time and effort. Each person has the right to pursue chosen courses of action without interference.

Certainty

There are circumstances in health care when a patient is unable to communicate his unique character structure, as in the case of an infant or a comatose patient. HCPs also interact with individuals from different cultures for whom a common language is lacking. In these cases, the bioethical standards can provide a measure of certainty when knowledge of an individual's unique character is unobtainable.

> If you know nothing whatever about an individual's uniqueness, then you are justified in acting on the basis that, as a member of the human species, he shares much in common with every other individual (Fedorka & Husted, 2001, p. 58).

These commonalities are the bioethical standards. Each person needs the power to sustain his unique nature, the power to be objectively aware of his surroundings, and the power to control his time and effort, to pursue benefit, and to avoid harm. Lacking other information, nurses and HCPs are justified to do all they can to restore these powers to the individual.

Decision-Making Model

Figure 26-1 demonstrates the way the concepts of the theory interact with direct decision making. The elements of ethical decision making interact in the following way:

- A person is a rational being with a unique character structure. Each person has the right to choose and pursue, without interference, a course of action in accordance with his needs and desires.
- Agreements between individuals are demonstrated by a shared state of awareness directed toward a goal.
- The HCP-patient agreement is directed toward preserving and enhancing the life of the patient.
- Context is the basis for determining what actions are ethical within the HCP-patient agreement. "Context is the interweaving of the relevant facts of the situation—the facts that are necessary to act upon to bring about a desired result, an agent's awareness of these facts, and the knowledge an agent has of how to deal most effectively with these facts" (Husted & Husted, 2008, p. 84). In this way, there are no universal ethical principles.
- Ethical decisions are the result of reasoning from the context to a decision rather than applying a decision or principle to a situation without regard for the context.

The Husteds described the ultimate application and practice of these assumptions by HCPs in the following way. The professional will come to understand and work from the philosophy that:

> My patient's virtues (autonomy) are such that he is moving (self-assertion) toward his goal (freedom) in these circumstances (objectivity) for this reason (beneficence). My virtues (autonomy) are such that I must act with him (interactive self-assertion) to assist him (his freedom) within the possibilities (of beneficence) in his circumstances to achieve every possible benefit that can be discovered (by objective awareness) (Husted & Husted, 2001, p. 154).

An interactive model can be found at: http://www.nursing.duq.edu/faculty/husted/index.html

LOGICAL FORM

Abductive reasoning, like induction and deduction, follows a pattern:

- A is a collection of data (the process of discerning ethical action).
- B (if true) explains A (Symphonology).
- No other hypothesis explains A as well as B does (traditional methods).
- Therefore B is probably correct.

The strength of an abductive conclusion depends on how solidly B can stand by itself, how clearly B exceeds alternatives, how comprehensive was the search for alternatives, the cost of B being wrong and the benefits of being right, and how strong the need is to come to a conclusion at all (Josephson & Josephson, 1994).

The abductive method is evident in the inception and evolution of Symphonology. The strength of this theory is evident as well. The concepts of Symphonology clearly can be observed not only in health care but also in other walks of life. It is clear that ethical action based on the context of an individual's particular circumstances is far superior to the imposition of concrete directives that often contradict each other or have little

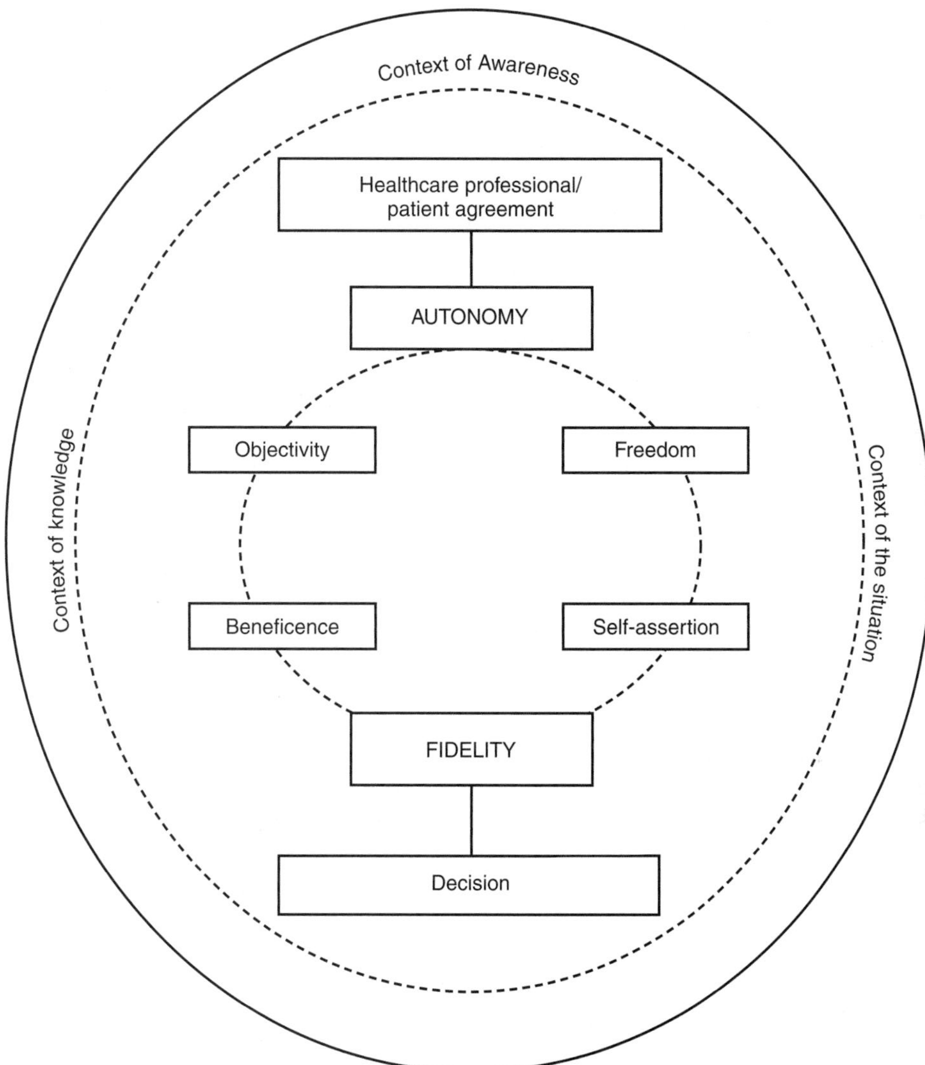

Figure 26-1 Bioethical Decision-Making Model. (Husted, J. H., & Husted, G. L. [2008]. Ethical decision making in nursing and health care: The symphonological approach [4th ed.]. New York: Springer.)

relationship to the situation at hand. The authors' extensive study of the philosophy of knowledge, science, and the human condition attests to the comprehensive search for alternative answers. The benefit to patients and HCPs of receiving practice-based ethical care would be immeasurable. Finally, the need to address the problem of how to achieve ethical action in health care could not be more critical.

Since the initial development of Symphonology, inductive reasoning based on observation and feedback from practitioners has provided for refinement of the concepts and clarification of the relationships among concepts.

ACCEPTANCE BY THE NURSING COMMUNITY

Practice

The Husted Symphonological model for ethical decision making (Husted & Husted, 2001, p. 201) was developed as a practice model for applying the concepts of Symphonology. This model, stressing the centrality of the individual and the necessity of reason directed by context, is vital in existing and emerging healthcare systems. The model provides a philosophical framework to ensure ethical care delivery by nurses and all other disciplines of health care. Unlike traditional models, the Symphonological model provides for logically justifiable ethical decision making. The North Memorial Medical Center in Robbinsdale, Minnesota, has adopted the model for use by their nursing ethics committee.

The call to care in nursing is central to the profession. Hartman (1998) asserted that caring is demonstrated when nurses recognize that the bioethical standards are so intertwined with caring that together they provide a perfect circle of ethical justification. Symphonology offers a practice-based approach to care, as follows:

> A practice-based approach is derived from, and therefore is intended to be appropriate to, the situation of a patient, the purpose of the health care setting, and the role of the nurse. The more an ethical system restricts practice based on abstract principles the more nurse and patient become alienated from each other (Husted & Husted, 1997b, p. 14).

Many nurses practice within systems bound by protocols and critical pathways. Using a symphonological approach can ensure that nursing practice remains ethical and does not become prescriptive.

Offering culturally sensitive care is essential as our healthcare systems change in response to a global society. Although cultural factors can be helpful in directing caring for a patient, nurses must also consider the individual's personal commitment to the traditions and beliefs of his culture. In this way, a nurse provides care for the patient rather than the culture (Zoucha & Husted, 2000). Using the Husted model, care is directed within the context of the individual's circumstances. Imposition of a false context, cultural or otherwise, is avoided.

Brown (2001b) advocated the use of Symphonology theory to direct discussion and education of patients regarding advance directives. Bioethical standards are used to guide discussion about what types of treatment an individual would or would not want, given particular circumstances. Hardt (2004) has proposed an intervention for nurses in ethical dilemmas.

The emergence of healthcare teams as a method of delivering comprehensive care brings many disciplines together to serve patients' needs. Overlapping roles and disparate goals can cause confusion among team members. Symphonological theory, with its patient-centered focus, can serve as common ground to initiate and promote collaboration among HCPs of all disciplines.

Education

As Symphonology is disseminated, it is easy to envision its use in nursing education. Currently, ethics is often addressed in nursing curricula as a topic separate from nursing. Frequently, the study and application of ethical concepts are reserved for advanced students. The broad applicability for Symphonology makes it an excellent framework for nursing curricula. Beginning students can easily grasp and apply the theoretical concepts. Using this theory as a basis for nursing interactions would direct the student in ethical practice from the beginning of learning and practice. The concept of context can be used as the basis for assessment. The bioethical standards will direct the student in choosing appropriate approaches, timing, and type of interventions for each patient. Because of the holistic approach and central concern for the patient, Symphonology can be incorporated easily in existing nursing curricula.

Brown (2001a) addressed the importance of ethical interaction between nurse educator and student.

The agreement in this case is more explicit, because both parties are more aware of the commitments and responsibilities. Recognizing the bioethical standards in both the educator and the student serves to direct ethical actions between them. Above all, the educator and student recall that the educator-student-patient agreement is central to the learning process.

Steckler (1998) agreed with Brown's application of Symphonology in the educational process and recommended incorporating the theory in continuing education. The Husted model not only identifies and organizes professional values and ethical principles for learners, but helps the educator to develop a consistent professional ethical orientation.

Administration

Health care administrators make decisions at several levels. They have responsibility to the community at large and the financial viability of the institution within the community, the employees, and those receiving care. Hardt and Hopey (2001) described how administrators use the principles of Symphonology to guide their decision making to produce ethically justifiable outcomes.

With regard to issues at the community and institutional levels, one considers the needed services provided by the institution. In cases in which the services needed would not be feasible for the institution, resources within the community can be shared and supported by the institution so that needed services are available with the least amount of loss to the institution. At the employee level, the administrators are concerned with care delivery as well as interpersonal relations. Symphonology guides decision making into equitable rather than equal solutions. For example, an employer may choose to forego use of a harsh sanction for absenteeism when the employee is able to show extenuating circumstances that prevented his attendance. This is also true for the development of policy regarding employees' behavior. Ethical policy provides guidelines for examining situations rather than prescribed rules with concrete directives for action. With regard to individual patients, administrators act as role models and consultants when addressing ethical issues.

Hardt and Hopey (2001) also described the problematic situations that occur within managed care systems. Difficulties that have been identified include the refusal of the organization to provide care deemed appropriate by HCPs and the inappropriate demands of patients and families. Using the principles of Symphonology, HCPs can examine the context and determine appropriate ethical actions within the implicit and explicit agreements.

Research

Symphonology in research is useful in relation to the researcher-subject agreement. The HCP-patient relationship is to some extent implicit, but the relationship between a researcher and a subject must be thoroughly explicit. Brown (2001c) suggested using the bioethical standards to develop an ethical informed consent protocol. Particularly in cases where the research involves vulnerable populations, the consent of surrogates is made more acceptable and is obtained more easily if the good of the individual is made central by using the bioethical standards.

FURTHER DEVELOPMENT

Initial testing of Symphonological theory included two phases. First, a qualitative study examined the perceptions and satisfaction of nurses and patients and their significant others as they engaged in ethical decision making for health care issues (Husted, 2001). The themes that emerged from this study were used to develop visual analog tools to measure these feelings in nurses and patients. In the second phase, a pilot study to test the tool was completed. The Cronbach alpha for the nurse's tool was reported as 0.74, and 0.82 for the patient's tool (Husted, 2004).

Irwin (2004) used a sample of 30 participants involved in a variety of decisions about health care and treatment during hospitalization in an acute care setting. The study included a decision support intervention for patients to determine the following: (1) whether key concepts of Symphonological theory describe the experience of individuals making healthcare decisions, and (2) whether application of the decision-making framework will enable nurses and patients to make ethically justifiable decisions. Results confirmed that patients expressed all the concepts of Symphonology when discussing their experiences with healthcare decision making. Statistical analysis of pretest and posttest Bioethical Decision Making Preference Scale for Patients scores demonstrated that subjects had a more positive experience of being involved in decision making ($p = 0.02$) and felt more sufficiency of knowledge ($p = 0.013$), less frustration ($p = 0.014$), and more sense of power ($p = 0.009$) after the intervention. These findings support the validity of Symphonology theory. The theory can be used to describe the experience of being involved in decision making, and Symphonology has utility as a model for assisting patients through the decision-making process.

A former graduate student used the nursing visual analog tool to discover how nurses felt when dealing with disclosure issues with patients. The Cronbach alpha for that study was 0.82 (Bavier, 2003). Further testing of this theory is by doctoral students is planned.

CRITIQUE

Clarity

In *Ethical Decision Making in Nursing* (Husted & Husted, 1995a), the authors presented the emerging concepts of Symphonology and the relationships among the concepts. The book may be difficult for beginning nurses to read because deeper concepts meant for advanced practitioners are included along with basic ideas. The third edition, *Ethical Decision Making in Nursing and Healthcare: The Symphonological Approach,* begins with the basic concepts for understanding and using the theory, moving more advanced concepts to later sections (Husted & Husted, 2001). Along with this improved organization, the third edition shows the emergence of increasing clarity for all concepts, the bioethical standards in particular. The fourth edition provides yet further clarity using tables and figures and includes a user-friendly teacher manual.

This work challenges traditional methods of thought and requires the reader to develop a new understanding of familiar concepts. Storytelling and examples provide the opportunity to recognize and understand the importance of alternative and extended meanings for familiar terms. The conversational tone of the writing is appealing and creates a comfortable atmosphere for a complex subject.

Simplicity

The authors first challenge the truth and efficacy of traditional ideas about ethical behavior and decision making. This is a simple matter if the reader is willing to make the effort to be open-minded. Once the reader is beyond the challenge, the simplicity of the theory is evident. There are few concepts, and the relational statements flow logically from the definitions. The model clearly demonstrates the elements of the process of ethical reasoning and the manner in which those elements interact.

Generality

Symphonology is applicable at all levels of nursing practice and in all areas of the healthcare field. These principles can be applied between nurse and patient, researcher and subject, manager and employee, and educator and student. HCPs of all types can use this method to determine appropriate ethical behaviors in practice. This theory can also be applied to the process of establishing healthcare policy that is ethical in nature. Indeed, these principles can be applied in all walks of life, depending on the nature of the agreement between the parties involved.

Empirical Precision

Complex theories lend themselves more easily to producing empirical evidence. The research projects in progress will likely add to the reported findings that support this theory. Symphonology is a theory based in reality. Although evidence is gathered to support the theory, the reality of the usefulness of the theory in practice is evident. Nurses and other HCPs can easily understand the concepts and apply them in all situations. The result of using the Symphonological model is a patient-centered, ethically justifiable decision.

Derivable Consequences

Being able to identify ethical actions in health care is of vital importance to patients, HCPs, and the health care industry itself. Before a nurse or any HCP takes action, regardless of how effective that action has proved in the past, the action must be justified as ethical with regard to the particular patient at hand. Reliance on concrete directives to guide action serves the directives, but only by chance serves the patient. Therefore, the pursuit of a practice-based ethical theory is essential for all of health care.

SUMMARY

The Husteds recognized that traditional methods of decision making were insufficient to address the bioethical problems emerging in the evolving healthcare system. They developed a theory of ethics and a decision-making model based on rational thought combined with insight and understanding. The theory is founded on the singular concept of human rights, the essential agreement of nonaggression among rational people that forms the foundation of all human interaction. Upon that foundation, HCPs and patients enter into an agreement to act to achieve the patient's goals. Preconditional to that agreement are recognition and respect for each person's unique character structure and the attendant properties of that structure: freedom, objectivity, beneficence, self-assertion, and fidelity. Ethical decisions are established within the context of a particular situation, using knowledge pertaining to the situation. Symphonological theory and the model for practice ensure ethically justifiable, individualized decisions.

POINTS FOR *Further Study*

- Husted, G. L., & Husted, J. H. (2008). Ethical decision making in nursing and healthcare: The symphonological approach (4th ed.). New York: Springer.
- Husted & Husted's Theory website http://www.nursing.duq.edu/faculty/husted/details.html

Case Study

Alvin, 66, has been in the hospital for 12 weeks with multiple trauma following a motor vehicle accident. His condition worsens each day, and his prognosis is very grave. He is not alert, but he grimaces and withdraws from stimulation. Prior to his injury, Alvin signed a living will and discussed with his family his desire not to be kept alive in the event he was ill or injured and recovery was not possible. The healthcare team tells his family that, despite aggressive treatment, many of Alvin's body systems are failing. Even if Alvin survives, there is no hope that he will be able to live without a ventilator because of extensive lung damage. The team suggests supportive care for Alvin and a do-not-resuscitate order. Most of the family members express the desire to ensure Alvin's comfort. Two family members believe Alvin will survive and recover. They refuse the team's suggestion and demand that Alvin receive every available treatment to keep him alive.

Analysis

- Autonomy: Alvin's desires should be given priority over his family members' desires.
- Freedom: Not to honor Alvin's wishes is a violation of his freedom.
- Objectivity: The subjective feelings of two family members are in conflict with objective reality. Only the patient's feelings are considered in ethical decisions.
- Self-assertion: It is not justifiable to substitute family members' values for the patient's.

- **Beneficence: The patient's goals cannot be obtained by aggressive treatment; however, aggressive treatment may well cause the patient further harm.**
- **Fidelity: The HCP's agreement with Alvin was to act as his agent in pursuing goals that are possible to attain.**

CRITICAL THINKING *Activities*

Using the Husted model, analyze this situation and those that follow from an ethical perspective.

1. Christina, 46, has been in the hospital for 2 weeks following a traumatic injury. Her condition was very grave, but she is beginning to show signs of recovery. The healthcare team suggests that a blood transfusion will provide the necessary support to continue her improvement. Christina and her family practice a religious faith that does not permit blood transfusions. Christina's husband and religious leader insist that she not be given the transfusion regardless of the consequences. When the visitors leave, Christina tells the nurse that she would like to receive the transfusion, but only if it could be kept secret from her family. What should the nurse do?
2. Angela, 34, is dying of lung cancer. Despite counseling and support, she is very frightened. When her death is imminent, she screams over and over, "Don't let me die! Don't let me die!" Despite all efforts, Angela succumbs before her husband arrives. He asks, "How was she? Was she afraid?" What should the nurse say?
3. Johnny, 7, is a psychiatric in-patient with a diagnosis of trichomania (hair pulling). His parents are very concerned about stopping his destructive behavior and have developed a series of punishments for incidents of hair pulling. Johnny has been seen pulling his hair out several times during the day. His parents arrive and ask how many times Johnny pulled his hair. What should the nurse say?
4. Eugene, 47, has several chronic illnesses. Despite education and support, Eugene declines to adhere to prescribed healthcare practices. Mark, a home healthcare nurse, has been seeing Eugene for several months and has made no progress in helping Eugene to improve his health. While discussing the situation, Eugene tells Mark that he has no intention of changing any of his behaviors. Is Mark justified in asking the physician to discontinue home health visits?
5. Agnes is a nurse on a busy medical nursing unit. Mr. Brown frequently asks Agnes to interrupt her work to answer questions and perform nonemergent tasks for him. Agnes' other patients complain of neglect. What should Agnes do and how can she justify her actions?
6. Burt, 34, has a diagnosis of manic depression. He lives in a group home with several others like himself. Several times a year, Burt stops taking his medication and disappears for weeks at a time. Occasionally Burt is arrested for vagrancy, but he has never been violent with himself or others. He states he enjoys his "vacations" because his medicine makes his life seem boring, dull, and difficult. Burt's family calls the director of the group home and insists that Burt be required to take his medicine each morning under supervision. What should the director say and how could he justify various courses of action?

REFERENCES

Bavier, A. (2003). *Types of disclosure discussion between oncology nurses and their patients/families: An exploratory study.* Unpublished manuscript, Duquesne University, Pittsburgh.

Brown, B. (2001a). The educator student/patient agreement. In G. L. Husted & J. H. Husted, *Ethical decision making in nursing and healthcare: The symphonological approach* (3rd ed., pp. 215-217). New York: Springer.

Brown, B. (2001b). The professional/patient agreement and advanced directives. In G. L. Husted & J. H. Husted (Eds.), *Ethical decision making in nursing and healthcare: The symphonological approach* (3rd ed., pp. 233-237). New York: Springer.

Brown, B. (2001c). The researcher/subject agreement. In G. L. Husted & J. H. Husted (Eds.), *Ethical decision making in nursing and healthcare: The symphonological approach* (3rd ed., pp. 229-231). New York: Springer.

Fawcett, J. (1995). *Analysis and evaluation of conceptual models of nursing* (3rd ed.). Philadelphia: F. A. Davis.

Fedorka, P., & Husted, G. L. (2001). Ethical decision making in clinical emergencies. *Topics in Emergency Medicine, 26*, 52-60.

Hardt, M. (2004). *Efficacy of a symphonological intervention in promoting a positive experience for nurses and patients experiencing bioethical dilemmas.* Unpublished manuscript, Duquesne University, Pittsburgh.

Hardt, M., & Hopey, K. (2001). The administrator/health professional/patient agreement. In G. L. Husted & J. H. Husted (Eds.), *Ethical decision making in nursing and healthcare: The symphonological approach* (3rd ed., pp. 219-227). New York: Springer.

Hartman, R. (1998). Revisiting the call to care: An ethical perspective. *Advanced Practice Nursing Quarterly, 4*(2), 14-18.

Husted & Husted's Symphonological Bioethcial Theory. (n.d.). Retrieved July 3, 2008, from http://www.nursing.duq.edu/faculty/husted/details.html

Husted, G. L. (2001). The feelings nurses and patients/families experience when faced with the need to make bioethical decisions. *Nursing Administration Quarterly, 25*(3), 1-9.

Husted, G. L. (2004). *The feelings of nurses and patients/families involved in the bioethical decision making process: The psychometric testing of two instruments.* Unpublished manuscript, Duquesne University, Pittsburgh.

Husted, G. L., & Husted, J. H. (1991). *Ethical decision making in nursing.* St. Louis: Mosby.

Husted, G. L., & Husted, J. H. (1995a). *Ethical decision making in nursing* (2nd ed.). St. Louis: Mosby.

Husted, G. L., & Husted, J. H. (1995b). The bioethical standards: The analysis of dilemmas through the analysis of persons. *Advanced Practice Nursing Quarterly, 1*(2), 69-76.

Husted, G. L., & Husted, J. H. (1997a). An ethical defense against the plague of cloning. *Advanced Practice Nursing Quarterly, 3*(2), 82-84.

Husted, G. L., & Husted, J. H. (1997b). Is a return to a caring perspective desirable? *Advanced Practice Nursing Quarterly, 3*(1), 14-17.

Husted, G. L., & Husted, J. H. (2001). *Ethical decision making in nursing and healthcare: The symphonological approach* (3rd ed.). New York: Springer.

Husted, G. L., & Husted, J. H. (2008). *Ethical decision making in nursing and healthcare: The symphonological approach* (4th ed.). New York: Springer.

Husted, J. H., & Husted, G. L. (1998). The role of the nurse in ethical decision making. In G. DeLoughery (Ed.), *Issues and trends in nursing* (pp. 216-242). St. Louis: Mosby.

Husted, J. H., & Husted, G. L. (1999). Agreement: The origin of ethical action. *Critical Care Nursing, 22*(3), 12-18.

Irwin, M. (2004). *Effect of Symphonology on patients' experience of involvement in health care decision making: A qualitative and quantitative study.* Unpublished dissertation, Duquesne University, Pittsburgh.

Jecker, N., Jonsen, A., & Pearlman, R. (1997). *Bioethics: An introduction to the history, methods and practice.* Sudbury, MA: Jones & Bartlett.

Josephson, J., & Josephson, S. (1994). *Abductive inference: Computation, philosophy, technology.* New York: Cambridge University Press.

Lloyd, G. (1996). *Spinoza and the ethics.* New York: Routledge.

McKeon, R. (Ed.). (1941). *The basic works of Aristotle.* New York: Random House.

Polanyi, M. (1964). *Personal knowledge.* New York: Harper & Row.

Steckler, J. (1998). Examination of ethical practice in nursing continuing education using the Husted model. *Advanced Practice Nursing Quarterly, 4*(2), 59-64.

Walker, L., & Avant, K. (1995). *Strategies of theory construction in nursing* (3rd ed.). Norwalk, CT: Appleton & Lange.

Zoucha, R., & Husted, G. (2000). The ethical dimensions of delivering cultural congruent nursing and health care. *Issues in Mental Health Nursing, 21*, 325-340.

BIBLIOGRAPHY

Primary Sources

Books

Husted, G. L., & Husted, J. H. (1991). *Ethical decision making in nursing.* St. Louis: Mosby.

Husted, G. L., & Husted, J. H. (1995). *Ethical decision making in nursing* (2nd ed.). St. Louis: Mosby.

Husted, G. L., & Husted, J. H. (2001). *Ethical decision making in nursing and healthcare: The Symphonological approach* (3rd ed.). New York: Springer.

Husted, G. L., & Husted, J. H. (2008). *Ethical decision making in nursing and healthcare: The Symphonological approach* (4th ed.). New York: Springer.

Book Chapters

Husted, G. L., & Husted, J. H. (1999). Strength of character through the ethics of nursing. In S. Osgood (Ed.), *Essential readings in nursing managed care* (pp. 102-106). Gaithersburg, MD: Aspen.

Husted, G. L., & Husted, J. H. (2004). Ethics and the advanced practice nurse. In L. A. Joel (Ed.), *Advanced practice nursing* (pp. 639-661). Philadelphia: F. A. Davis.

Husted, G. L., & Husted, J. H. (2005). The ethical experience of caring for vulnerable populations: The symphonological approach. In M. DeChesnay (Ed.), *Caring for vulnerable populations* (pp. 71-79). St. Louis: Mosby.

Husted, J. H., & Husted, G. L. (1998). The role of the nurse in ethical decision making. In G. DeLoughery (Ed.), *Issues and trends in nursing* (pp. 216-242). St. Louis: Mosby.

Journal and Other Articles

Fedorka, P., & Husted, G. L. (2001). Ethical decision making in clinical emergencies. *Topics in Emergency Medicine, 26*, 52-60.

Husted, G. L. (2001). The feelings nurses and patients/families experience when faced with the need to make bioethical decisions. *Nursing Administration Quarterly, 25*(3), 1-9.

Husted, G. L., & Husted, J. H. (1995). The bioethical standards: The analysis of dilemmas through the analysis of persons. *Advanced Practice Nursing Quarterly, 1*(2), 69-76.

Husted, G. L., & Husted, J. H. (1996). Ethical dilemmas: Time and fidelity. *American Journal of Nursing, 96*(11), 74.

Husted, G. L., & Husted, J. H. (1997). A modest proposal concerning policies. *Advanced Practice Nursing Quarterly, 3*(3), 17-19.

Husted, G. L., & Husted, J. H. (1997). An ethical defense against the plague of cloning. *Advanced Practice Nursing Quarterly, 3*(2), 82-84.

Husted, G. L., & Husted, J. H. (1997). An ethical examination of in-vitro fertilization and cloning. *AORN, 65*(6), 1-2.

Husted, G. L., & Husted, J. H. (1997). Is a return to a caring perspective desirable? *Advanced Practice Nursing Quarterly, 3*(1), 14-17.

Husted, G. L., & Husted, J. H. (1997). Is cloning moral? *Nursing and Health Care: Perspectives on Community, 18*, 168-169.

Husted, G. L., & Husted, J. H. (1998). Ethical balance versus ethical anomaly. *Advanced Practice Nursing Quarterly, 4*(1), 51-53.

Husted, G. L., & Husted, J. H. (1998). Strength of character through the ethics of nursing. *Advanced Practice Nursing Quarterly, 3*(4), 23-25.

Husted, G. L., & Husted, J. H. (1998). With the ethical agreement: Where are you now? *Advanced Practice Nursing Quarterly, 4*(2), 34-35.

Husted, J. H., & Husted, G. L. (1999). Agreement: The origin of ethical action. *Critical Care Nursing, 22*(3), 12-18.

Husted, J. H., & Husted, G. L. (2000). When is a health care system not an ethical health care system? Suspending the do-not-resuscitate order in the operating room. *Critical Care Nursing Clinics of North America, 12*, 157-163.

Husted, G. L., Miller, M. C., & Brown, B. (1999). Test of an educational brochure on advance directives designed for the well-elderly. *Journal of Gerontological Nursing, 25*(1), 34-40.

Husted, G. L., Miller, M. C., Zaremba, J. A., Clutter, S. L., Jennings, K. R., & Stainbrook, D. (1997). Advance directives and what attracts elderly people to particular brochures. *Journal of Gerontological Nursing, 23*(2), 41-45.

Zoucha, R., & Husted, G. L. (2000). Is delivering culturally congruent psychosocial healthcare ethical? *Issues in Mental Health Nursing, 21*, 325-340.

Zoucha, R. D., & Husted, G. L. (2002). The ethical dimensions of delivering culturally congruent nursing and health care. *Review Series Psychiatry, Sweden, 3*, 10-11.

Secondary Sources

Books

Burkhardt, M. A., & Nathaniel, A. K. (2002). *Ethics and issues in contemporary nursing* (2nd ed.). Clifton Park, NJ: Delmar.

Daly, J., Speedy, S., & Jackson, D. (2005). Professional Nursing: Concepts, Issues, and Challenges. New York: Springer.

de Chesnay, M., & Anderson, B. (2008). Caring for the Vulnerable: Perspectives in Nursing Theory, Practice, and Research. Sudbury, Mass.: Jones & Bartlett.

Fry, S., & Johnstone, M. (2002). Ethics in Nursing Practice: A Guide to Ethical Decision Making. Malden, MD: Blackwell Science.

Lauritzen, P. (Ed.). (2001). *Cloning and the future of human embryo research.* London: Oxford University Press.

Lipe, S. K., & Beasley, S. (2004). *Critical thinking in nursing: A cognitive skills workbook.* Philadelphia: Lippincott Williams & Wilkins.

Spencer, E. M. (Ed.). (2000). *Organizational ethics in health care.* London: Oxford University Press.

Thomson Learning Series. (2001). *Surgical technology for surgical technologists: A positive care approach.* Clifton Park, NJ: Delmar.

Journal and Other Articles

Anderson, J., Biba, S., & Hartman, R. L. (1996). Ethical case comment. To tell or not to tell . . . the case for ethical analysis. *DCCN-Dimensions of Critical Care Nursing, 15*(6), 318-323.

Bavier, A. (2003). *Types of disclosure discussion between oncology nurses and their patients/families: An exploratory study.* Unpublished manuscript, Duquesne University, Pittsburgh.

Baldonado, A. (1996). Ethnicity and morality in a multicultural world. *Journal of Cultural Diversity* 3(4), 105-108.

Best, J. T. (2001). Effective teaching for the elderly: Back to basics. *Orthopedic Nursing, 20*(3), 46-52.

Bridger, J. C. (1997). A study of nurses' views about the prevention of nosocomial urinary tract infections. *Journal of Clinical Nursing, 6*(5), 379-387.

Brown, B. (2003). Historical perspectives. The history of advance directives: a literature review. *Journal of Gerontological Nursing 29*(9), 4-14.

Burcham, J. L. R. (2002). Cultural competence: An evolutionary perspective. *Nursing Forum, 37*(4), 5-15.

Caitlin, A. (1997). Pediatric ethics, issues, & commentary. Creating a beginning ethics library. Pediatric Nursing 23(5), 495-496.

Chenowethm, L. (2006). Cultural competency and nursing care: an Australian perspective. *International Nursing Review 53*(1), 34-40.

Cioffi, R. (2003). Communicating with culturally and linguistically diverse patients in an acute care setting: nurses' experiences. *International Journal of Nursing Studies 40*(3), 299-306.

Claassen, M. (2000). A handful of questions: supporting parental decision making. *Clinical Nurse Specialist, 14*(4), 189-195.

DeLikkis, A., & Sauer, R. (2004). Respect as ethical foundation for communication in employee relations. *Laboratory Medicine 35*(5), 262-266.

Dennis, B. (1999). The origin and nature of informed consent: Experiences among vulnerable groups. *Journal of Professional Nursing 15*(5), 281-287.

Enns, C., & Gregory, D. (2007). Lamentation and loss: Expressions of caring by contemporary surgical nurses. *Journal of Advanced Nursing, 55*(4), 339-347.

Goldblatt, D. (2001). A messy necessary end—Health care proxies need our support. *Neurology 56*(2), 148-152.

Greipp, M. E. (1995). A survey of ethical decision making models in nursing. *Journal of Nursing Science, 1*(1/2), 51-60.

Groupp, E. (2005). Recruiting seniors with chronic low back pain for a randomized controlled trial of a self-management program. *Journal of Manipulative & Physiological Therapeutics 28*(2), 97-102.

Hardt, M. (2001). Core then care: the nurse leader's role in "caring". *Nursing Administration Quarterly 25*(3), 37-45.

Hardt, M. (2004). *Efficacy of a symphonological intervention in promoting a positive experience for nurses and patients experiencing bioethical dilemmas.* Unpublished manuscript, Duquesne University, Pittsburgh.

Hunt, S. (1996). Ethics of resource distribution: Implications for palliative care services. *International Journal of Palliative Nursing 2*(4), 222-226.

Irwin, M. (2004). *Effect of Symphonology on patients' experience of involvement in health care decision making: A qualitative and quantitative study.* Unpublished dissertation, Duquesne University, Pittsburgh.

Jeffery, D. (2005). Adapting de-escalation techniques with deaf service users. *Nursing Standard 19*(49), 41-47.

Jirwe, M. (2006). The theoretical framework of cultural competence. *Journal of Multicultural Nursing & Health 12*(3), 6-16.

Johnson, J. E. (2002). Six steps to ethical leadership in health care. *Patient Care Management, 18*(2), 5-9.

Kinion, E. S., Jonke, N. L., & Paradise, N. (1995). Descriptive ethics and neuroleptic dose reduction. *Perspectives in Psychiatric Care, 31*(2), 11-14.

Lorys, F., Oddi, V., Cassidy, R., & Fisher, C. (1995). Nurses' sensitivity to the ethical aspects if clinical practice. *Nursing Ethics 2,* 197.

Mariano, C. (2001). Holistic ethics. *American Journal of Nursing, 101*(1 part 1), Hospital Extra: 24A-C.

Martindale, A., & Collins, D. (2005). Professional judgment and decision making: The role of intention for impact. *Sport Psychologist 19*(3), 303-313.

McFadden, E. A. (1996). Moral development and reproductive health decisions. *Journal of Obstetric, Gynecologic, & Neonatal Nursing, 25*(6), 507-512.

Oberle, K., & Tenove, S. (2000). Ethical issues in public health nursing. *Nursing Ethics: An International Journal for Health Care Professionals, 7*(5), 425-438.

Oddi, L. F., Cassidy, V. R., & Fisher, C. (1995). Nurses' sensitivity to the ethical aspects of clinical practice. *Nursing Ethics: An International Journal for Health Care Professionals, 2*(3), 197-209.

Perry, J. (2006). Resisting vulnerability: the experiences of families who have kin in hospital—a feminist ethnography. *International Journal of Nursing Studies 43*(2), 173-184.

Reveillere, C., Pham, T., Masclet, G., Nandrino, J. L., & Beaune, D. (2000). The relationship between burnout and personality in care-givers in a palliative care unit. *Annals Medico Psychologiques, 158*(9), 716-721.

Rice, V. H., Beck, C., & Stevenson, J. S. (1997). Ethical issues relative to autonomy and personal control in independent and cognitive impaired elders. *Nursing Outlook, 45*(1), 27-34.

Roberson, D. (2007). Inequities in screening for sexually transmitted infections in African American adolescents: can health policy help? *Journal of Transcultural Nursing 18*(3), 286-291.

Saulo, M. (1996). How good case managers make tough choices: Ethics and mediation. Part I. *Journal of Care Management, 2*(1), 8, 10, 12 passim.

Scotto, C. (2003). A new view of caring. *Journal of Nursing Education, 42*(7), 289-291.

Scotto, C. (2005). Symphonological Bioethical theory. In A. M. Tomey & M. R. Alligood (Eds.), *Nursing Theorists and Their Work* (6th ed, pp. 584-601). St. Louis: Mosby.

Sellar, B. Subjective leisure experiences of older Australians. *Australian Occupational Therapy Journal 53*(3), 211-219.

Simko, L. (1999). Adults with congenital heart disease: Utilizing quality of life and Husted's nursing theory as a conceptual framework. *Critical Care Nursing Quarterly, 22*(3), 1-11.

Steckler, J. (1998). Examination of ethical practices in nursing continuing education using the Husted model. *Advanced Practice Nursing Quarterly, 4*(2), 59-64.

Szirony, T., Price, J., Wolfe, E., Telljohann, S., Dake, J. (2004). Perceptions of nursing faculty regarding ethical issues in nursing research. *Journal of Nursing Education 43*(6), 270-279.

Thomas, A. (1997). Patient autonomy and cancer treatment decisions. *International Journal of Palliative Nursing 3*(6), 317-323.

Thompson, L. W. (1998). Nursing ethics: The ANA code for nurses. *Tennessee Nurse, 61*(6), 23, 25-29.

Troskie, R. (1998). Ethical decision making in a transcultural context. *Health SA Gesondheid, 3*(1), 3-8.

Tschudin, V. (1994). Nursing ethics IV: Theories and principles. *Nursing Standard 9*(2), 51-55.

Viney, C. (1996). A phenomenological study of ethical decision-making experiences among senior intensive care nurses and doctors concerning withdrawal of treatment. *Nursing in Critical Care 4,* 182-187.

Von Post, I. (1996). Exploring ethical dilemmas in perioperative nursing practice through critical incidents. *Nursing Ethics: An International Journal for Health Care Professionals, 3*(3), 236-249.

Weiner, C., Tabak, N., & Bergman, R. (2001). The use of physical restraints for patients suffering from dementia. *Nursing Ethics, 56*(2), 148-152.

Wilmot, S. (2000). Nurses and whistleblowing: The ethical issues. *Journal of Advanced Nursing, 32*(5), 1051-1057.

Wilson, D. M. (1998). Administrative decision making in response to sudden health care agency funding reductions: Is there a role for ethics? *Nursing Ethics: an International Journal for Health Care Professionals, 5*(4), 319-329.

Wurzbach, M. E. (1999). Acute care nurses' experiences of moral certainty. *Journal of Advanced Nursing, 30*(2), 287-293.

Zoucha, R. Considering culture in understanding interpersonal violence. *Journal of Forensic Nursing 2*(4), 195-196.

UNIT

V

Middle Range Theories

- *Middle range theories are the least abstract and are at the practice level.*
- *Middle range theories are specific to practice outcomes.*
- *Middle range theories specify characteristics of nursing situations.*
- *Middle range theories indicate the following about the nursing situation:*
  - *The situation or health condition*
  - *Client population or age-group*
  - *Location or area of practice (e.g., community)*
  - *Action of the nurse or intervention*
  - *The patient outcome that is anticipated*

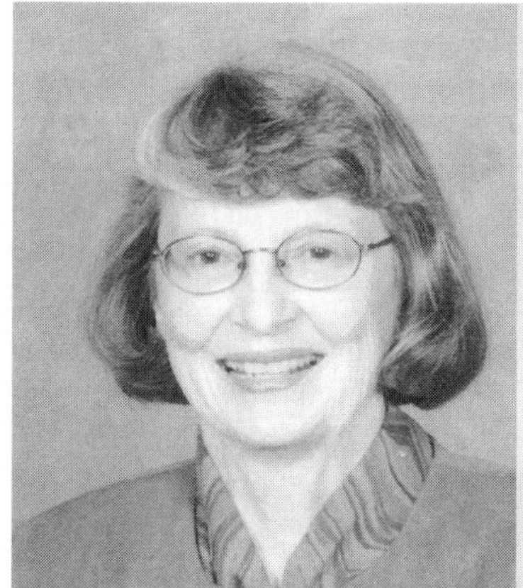
Photo credit: Marie Cox, M&M Studios, San Francisco

CHAPTER 27

Ramona T. Mercer

1929-present

Maternal Role Attainment—Becoming a Mother

Molly Meighan

"The process of becoming a mother requires extensive psychological, social, and physical work. A woman experiences heightened vulnerability and faces tremendous challenges as she makes this transition. Nurses have an extraordinary opportunity to help women learn, gain confidence, and experience growth as they assume the mother identity." (Mercer, 2006, p. 649)

CREDENTIALS AND BACKGROUND OF THE THEORIST

Ramona T. Mercer began her nursing career in 1950, when she received her diploma from St. Margaret's School of Nursing in Montgomery, Alabama. She graduated with the L.L. Hill Award for Highest Scholastic Standing. She returned to school in 1960 after working as a staff nurse, head nurse, and instructor in the areas of pediatrics, obstetrics, and contagious diseases. She completed a bachelor's degree in nursing in 1962, graduating with distinction from the University of New Mexico, Albuquerque. She went on to earn a master's degree in maternal-child nursing from Emory University in 1964 and completed a Ph.D. in maternity nursing at the University of Pittsburgh in 1973.

After receiving a Ph. D., Mercer moved to California and accepted the position of assistant professor in the Department of Family Health Care Nursing at the University of California, San Francisco. She was promoted to associate professor in 1977, and in 1983 she was promoted to professor. She remained in that role until her retirement in 1987. Currently, Dr. Mercer is Professor Emeritus in Family Health Nursing at the

Previous authors: Mary M. (Molly) Meighan, Alberta M. Bee, Denise Legge, and Stephanie Oetting.

University of California, San Francisco (R. Mercer, curriculum vitae, 2002).

Mercer received awards throughout her career. In 1963, while working and pursuing studies in nursing, she received the Department of Health, Education, and Welfare Public Health Service Nurse Trainee Award at Emory University and was inducted into Sigma Theta Tau. She received this award again during her years at the University of Pittsburgh. She also received the Bixler Scholarship for Nursing Education and Research, Southern Regional Board, for doctoral study. In 1982, she received the Maternal Child Health Nurse of the Year Award from the National Foundation of the March of Dimes and American Nurses Association, Division of Maternal Child Health Practice. She was presented with the Fourth Annual Helen Nahm Lecturer Award at the University of California, San Francisco School of Nursing, in 1984. Mercer's research awards include the American Society for Psychoprophylaxis in Obstetrics (ASPO)/Lamaze National Research Award in 1987; the Distinguished Research Lectureship Award, Western Institute of Nursing, Western Society for Research in Nursing in 1988; and the American Nurses Foundation's Distinguished Contribution to Nursing Science Award in 1990 (R. Mercer, curriculum vitae, 2002). Mercer has authored numerous articles, editorials, and commentaries. In addition, she has published six books and six book chapters.

In early research efforts, Mercer focused on the behaviors and needs of breastfeeding mothers, mothers with postpartum illness, mothers bearing infants with defects, and teenage mothers. Her first book, *Nursing Care for Parents at Risk* (1977), received an *American Journal of Nursing* Book of the Year Award in 1978. Her study of teenage mothers over the first year of motherhood resulted in the 1979 book, *Perspectives on Adolescent Health Care*, which also received an *American Journal of Nursing* Book of the Year Award in 1980. Preceding research led Mercer to study family relationships, antepartal stress as related to familial relationships and the maternal role, and mothers of various ages. In 1986, Mercer's research on three age groups of mothers was drawn together in her third book, *First-Time Motherhood: Experiences From Teens to Forties* (1986a). Mercer's fifth book, *Parents at Risk*, published in 1990, also received an *American Journal of Nursing* Book of the Year Award. *Parents at Risk* (1990) focused on strategies for facilitating early parent-infant interactions and promoting parental competence in relation to specific risk situations. Mercer's sixth book *Becoming a Mother: Research on Maternal Identity From Rubin to the Present* was published by Springer Publishing Company of New York in 1995. This book contains a more complete description of Mercer's Theory of Maternal Role Attainment and her framework for studying variables that impact the maternal role.

Since her first publication in 1968, Mercer has written numerous articles for both nursing and nonnursing journals. She published several online courses for *Nurseweek* during the 1990s and through early 2000, including "Adolescent Sexuality and Childbearing," "Transitions to Parenthood," and "Helping Parents When the Unexpected Occurs."

Mercer has maintained membership in several professional organizations, including the American Nurses Association and the American Academy of Nursing, and has been an active member on many national committees. From 1983 to 1990, she was the associate editor of *Health Care for Women International*. She has served on the review panel for *Nursing Research* and *Western Journal of Nursing Research* and the editorial board of the *Journal of Adolescent Health Care*, and was on the executive advisory board of *Nurseweek*. She has also served as a reviewer for numerous grant proposals. Additionally, she has been actively involved with regional, national, and international scientific and professional meetings and workshops (R. Mercer, curriculum vitae, 2002). She was honored as a Living Legend by the American Academy of Nursing during the Annual Meeting and Conference in Carlsbad, California, in November 2003. Mercer was honored by University of New Mexico in 2004, receiving the first College of Nursing Distinguished Alumni Award. In 2005, she was recognized as among the most outstanding alumni and faculty, and her name appears on the Wall of Fame at University of California, San Francisco.

THEORETICAL SOURCES

Mercer's Theory of Maternal Role Attainment was based on her extensive research on the topic beginning in the late 1960s. Mercer's professor and mentor, Reva Rubin at the University of Pittsburgh, was a major stimulus for both research and theory development. Rubin (1977, 1984) was well known for her work in defining and describing maternal role attainment as a process of binding-in, or being attached to, the child and achieving a maternal role identity or seeing oneself in the role and having a sense of comfort about it. Mercer's framework and study variables reflect many of Rubin's concepts.

In addition to Rubin's work, Mercer based her research on both role and developmental theories. She relied heavily on an interactionist approach to role theory, using Mead's (1934) theory on role enactment and Turner's (1978) theory on the core self. In addition, Thornton and Nardi's (1975) role acquisition process helped shape Mercer's theory, as did the work of Burr, Leigh, Day, and Constantine (1979). Werner's (1957) developmental process theories also contributed. In addition, Mercer's work was influenced by von Bertalanffy's (1968) general system theory. Her model of maternal role attainment depicted in Figure 27-1 uses Bronfenbrenner's (1979) concepts of nested circles as a means of portraying interactional environmental influences on the maternal role. The complexity of her research interest led Mercer to rely on several theoretical sources to identify and study variables that affect maternal role attainment. Although much of her work involved testing and extending Rubin's theories, she has consistently looked to the research of others in the development and expansion of her theory.

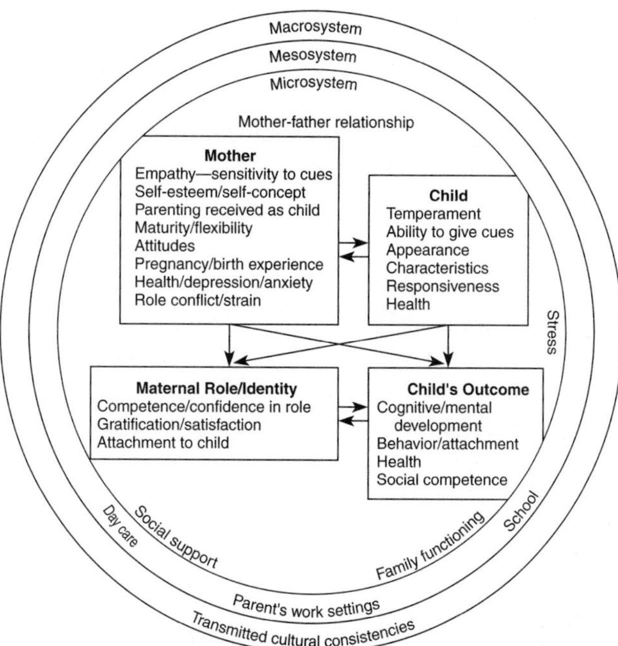

Figure 27-1 Model of Maternal Role Attainment. (Modified from Mercer, R. T. [1991]. *Maternal role: Models and consequences.* Paper presented at the International Research Conference sponsored by the Council of Nurse Researchers and the American Nurses Association, Los Angeles, CA. Copyright Ramona T. Mercer, 1991. NOTE: This figure has been modified based on personal communication with R. T. Mercer [January 4, 2003]. The word *exosystem* was replaced with the word *mesosystem* to be more consistent with Bronfenbrenner's [1979] model on which it is based.)

MAJOR CONCEPTS & DEFINITIONS

Mercer uses the concepts outlined below in her theory.

MATERNAL ROLE ATTAINMENT

Maternal role attainment is an interactional and developmental process occurring over time in which the mother becomes attached to her infant, acquires competence in the caretaking tasks involved in the role, and expresses pleasure and gratification in the role (Mercer, 1986a). "The movement to the personal state in which the mother experiences a sense of harmony, confidence, and competence in how she performs the role is the end point of maternal role attainment—maternal identity" (Mercer, 1981, p. 74).

MATERNAL IDENTITY

Maternal identify is defined as having an internalized view of the self as a mother (Mercer, 1995).

PERCEPTION OF BIRTH EXPERIENCE

A woman's perception of her performance during labor and birth is her perception of the birth experience (Mercer, 1990).

SELF-ESTEEM

Mercer, May, Ferketich, and DeJoseph (1986) describe self-esteem as "an individual's perception of how others view oneself and self-acceptance of the perceptions" (p. 341).

SELF-CONCEPT (SELF-REGARD)

Mercer (1986a) outlines self-concept, or self-regard, as "The overall perception of self that includes self-satisfaction, self-acceptance, self-esteem, and congruence or discrepancy between self and ideal self" (p. 18).

FLEXIBILITY

Roles are not rigidly fixed; therefore, who fills the roles is not important (Mercer, 1990). "Flexibility of childrearing attitudes increases with increased development . . . Older mothers have the potential to respond less rigidly to their infants and to view each situation in respect to the unique nuances" (Mercer, 1986a, p. 43; 1990, p. 12).

CHILDREARING ATTITUDES

Childrearing attitudes are maternal attitudes or beliefs about childrearing (Mercer, 1986a).

HEALTH STATUS

Health status is defined as "The mother's and father's perception of their prior health, current health, health outlook, resistance-susceptibility to illness, health worry concern, sickness orientation, and rejection of the sick role" (Mercer et al., 1986, p. 342).

ANXIETY

Mercer and colleagues (1986) describe anxiety as "a trait in which there is specific proneness to perceive stressful situations as dangerous or threatening, and as a situation-specific state" (p. 342).

DEPRESSION

According to Mercer and colleagues (1986), depression is "having a group of depressive symptoms, and in particular the affective component of the depressed mood" (p. 342).

ROLE STRAIN–ROLE CONFLICT

Role strain is the conflict and difficulty felt by the woman in fulfilling the maternal role obligation (Mercer, 1985a).

GRATIFICATION-SATISFACTION

Mercer (1985b) describes gratification as "the satisfaction, enjoyment, reward, or pleasure that a woman experiences in interacting with her infant, and in fulfilling the usual tasks inherent in mothering."

Major Concepts & Definitions—cont'd

ATTACHMENT

Attachment is a component of the parental role and identity. It is viewed as a process in which an enduring affectional and emotional commitment to an individual is formed (Mercer, 1990).

INFANT TEMPERAMENT

An easy versus a difficult temperament is related to whether the infant sends hard-to-read cues, leading to feelings of incompetence and frustration in the mother (Mercer, 1986a).

INFANT HEALTH STATUS

Infant health status is illness causing maternal-infant separation, interfering with the attachment process (Mercer, 1986a).

INFANT CHARACTERISTICS

Characteristics include infant temperament, appearance, and health status (Mercer, 1981).

INFANT CUES

Infant cues are infant behaviors that elicit a response from the mother (R. T. Mercer, personal communication, September 3, 2003).

FAMILY

Mercer and colleagues (1986) define family as "a dynamic system that includes subsystems—individuals (mother, father, fetus/infant) and dyads (mother-father, mother-fetus/infant, and father-fetus/infant) within the overall family system" (p. 339).

FAMILY FUNCTIONING

Family functioning is the individual's view of the activities and relationships between the family and its subsystems and broader social units (Mercer & Ferketich, 1995).

FATHER OR INTIMATE PARTNER

The father or intimate partner contributes to the process of maternal role attainment in a way that cannot be duplicated by any other person (R. T. Mercer, personal communication, January 4, 2003). The father's interactions help diffuse tension and facilitate maternal role attainment (Donley, 1993; Mercer, 1995).

STRESS

Stress is made up of positively and negatively perceived life events and environmental variables (Mercer, 1990).

SOCIAL SUPPORT

According to Mercer and colleagues (1986), social support is "the amount of help actually received, satisfaction with that help, and the persons (network) providing that help" (p. 341).

Four areas of social support are as follows:

1. Emotional support: "Feeling loved, cared for, trusted, and understood" (Mercer, 1986a, p. 14)
2. Informational support: "Helping the individual help herself by providing information that is useful in dealing with the problem and/or situation" (Mercer, 1986a, p. 14)
3. Physical support: A direct kind of help (Mercer, Hackley, & Bostrom, 1984)
4. Appraisal support: "A support that tells the role taker how she is performing in the role; it enables the individual to evaluate herself in relationship to others' performance in the role" (Mercer, 1986a, p. 14)

MOTHER-FATHER RELATIONSHIP

The mother-father relationship is the perception of the mate relationship that includes intended and actual values, goals, and agreements between the two (Mercer, 1986b). The maternal attachment to the infant develops within the emotional field of the parent's relationship (Donley, 1993; Mercer, 1995).

USE OF EMPIRICAL EVIDENCE

Mercer selected both maternal and infant variables for her studies on the basis of her review of the literature and findings of researchers in several disciplines. She found that many factors may have a direct or indirect influence on the maternal role, adding to the complexity of her studies. Maternal factors in Mercer's research included age at first birth, birth experience, early separation from the infant, social stress, social support, personality traits, self-concept, childrearing attitudes, and health. She included the infant variables of temperament, appearance, responsiveness, health status, and ability to give cues. Mercer (1995) and Ferketich and Mercer (1995a, 1995b, 1995c) also noted the importance of the father's role and applied many of Mercer's previous findings in studying the paternal response to parenthood. Her research required numerous instruments to measure the variables of interest.

Mercer has studied the influence of these variables on parental attachment and competence over several intervals, including the immediate postpartum period and 1 month, 4 months, 8 months, and 1 year following birth (Mercer & Ferketich, 1990a, 1990b). In addition, she has included adolescents, older mothers, ill mothers, mothers dealing with congenital defects, families experiencing antepartal stress, parents at high risk, mothers who had cesarean deliveries, and fathers in her research (Mercer, 1989; Mercer & Ferketich, 1994, 1995; Mercer, Ferketich, & DeJoseph, 1993). As a recent step, she compared her findings and the basis for her original theory with current research. As a result, Mercer (2004) has proposed that the term *maternal role attainment* be replaced with *becoming a mother*, because this more accurately describes the continued evolvement of the role across the woman's life span. In addition, she proposed using more recent nursing research findings to describe the stages and process of becoming a mother.

MAJOR ASSUMPTIONS

For maternal role attainment, Mercer (1981, 1986a, 1995) stated the following assumptions:

- A relatively stable core self, acquired through lifelong socialization, determines how a mother defines and perceives events; her perceptions of her infant's and others' responses to her mothering, with her life situation, are the real world to which she responds (Mercer, 1986a).
- In addition to the mother's socialization, her developmental level and innate personality characteristics also influence her behavioral responses (Mercer, 1986a).
- The mother's role partner, her infant, will reflect the mother's competence in the mothering role through growth and development (Mercer, 1986a).
- The infant is considered an active partner in the maternal role-taking process, affecting and being affected by the role enactment (Mercer, 1981).
- The father's or mother's intimate partner contributes to role attainment in a way that cannot be duplicated by any other supportive person (Mercer, 1995).
- Maternal identity develops concurrently with maternal attachment and each depends on the other (Mercer, 1995; Rubin, 1977).

Nursing

Mercer (1995) stated that, "Nurses are the health professionals having the most sustained and intense interaction with women in the maternity cycle" (p. xii). Nurses are responsible for promoting the health of families and children; nurses are pioneers in developing and sharing assessment strategies for these patients, she explained. Her definition of nursing provided in a personal communication is as follows:

> Nursing is a dynamic profession with three major foci: health promotion and prevention of illness, providing care for those who need professional assistance to achieve their optimal level of health and functioning, and research to enhance the knowledge base for providing excellent nursing care. Nurses provide health care for individuals, families, and communities. Following assessment of the client's

situation and environment, the nurse identifies goals with the client, provides assistance to the client through teaching, supporting, providing care the client is unable to provide for self, and interfacing with the environment and the client (R. Mercer, personal communication, March 21, 2004).

In her writing, Mercer (1995) refers to the importance of nursing care. Although she does not specifically mention nursing care, in her book, *Becoming a Mother: Research on Maternal Identity From Rubin to the Present*, Mercer emphasizes that the kind of help or care a woman receives during pregnancy and over the first year following birth can have long-term effects for her and her child. Nurses in maternal-child settings play a sizable role in providing both care and information during this period.

Person

Mercer (1985a) does not specifically define person, but refers to the self or core self. She views the self as separate from the roles that are played. Through maternal individuation, a woman may regain her own personhood as she extrapolates her self from the mother-infant dyad (Mercer, 1985b). The core self evolves from a cultural context and determines how situations are defined and shaped (Mercer, 1985a). The concepts of self-esteem and self-confidence are important in attainment of the maternal role. The mother as a separate person interacts with her infant and with the father or her significant other. She is both influential and is influenced by both of them (Mercer, 1995).

Health

In her theory, Mercer defines health status as the mother's and father's perception of their prior health, current health, health outlook, resistance-susceptibility to illness, health worry or concern, sickness orientation, and rejection of the sick role. Health status of the newborn is the extent of disease present and infant health status by parental rating of overall health (Mercer, 1986b). The health status of a family is affected negatively by antepartum stress (Mercer, Ferketich, DeJoseph, May, & Sollid, 1988; Mercer, May, Ferketich, & DeJoseph, 1986). Health status is an important indirect influence on satisfaction with relationships in childbearing families. Health is also viewed as a desired outcome for the child. It is influenced by both maternal and infant variables. Mercer (1995) stresses the importance of health care during the childbearing and childrearing processes.

Environment

Mercer conceptualized the environment from Bronfenbrenner's definition of the ecological environment and based her earliest model in Figure 27-1 on it (Mercer, 1995; R. Mercer, personal communication, June 24, 2000). This model illustrates the ecological interacting environments in which maternal role attainment develops. During a personal communication on January 4, 2003, Mercer explained, "Development of a role/person cannot be considered apart from the environment; there is a mutual accommodation between the developing person and the changing properties of the immediate settings, relationships between the settings, and the larger contexts in which the settings are embedded." Stresses and social support within the environment influence both maternal and paternal role attainment and the developing child.

THEORETICAL ASSERTIONS

Mercer's original Theory and Model of Maternal Role Attainment were first introduced in 1991 during a symposium at the International Research Conference sponsored by the Council of Nursing Research and American Nurses Association in Los Angeles, California (Mercer, 1995). It was refined and was presented more clearly in her 1995 book, *Becoming a Mother: Research on Maternal Identity From Rubin to the Present* (see Figure 27-1).

Mercer's (2004) more recent revision of her theory focuses on the woman's transition in becoming a mother. It involves an extensive change in her life space that requires her ongoing development. According to Mercer, becoming a mother is more extensive than just assuming a role. It is unending and continuously evolving. Therefore she proposed that the term *maternal role attainment* be retired. Her recommendations are based partly on the work of Walker, Crain, and Thompson (1986a, 1986b), Koniak-Griffin (1993), and McBride and Shore (2001), who have examined the process of mothering and have raised questions about the appropriateness of maternal role attainment as an end point in the process.

Maternal Role Attainment: Mercer's Original Model

Mercer's Model of Maternal Role Attainment was placed within Bronfenbrenner's (1979) nested circles of the microsystem, mesosystem, and macrosystem (see Figure 27-1). The original model proposed by Mercer was altered in 2000, changing the term *exosystem* originally found in the second circle and replacing it with the term *mesosystem*. Mercer (personal communication, January 4, 2003) explained that this change made the model more consistent with Bronfenbrenner's terminology, as follows:

1. The microsystem is the immediate environment in which maternal role attainment occurs. It includes factors such as family functioning, mother-father relationships, social support, economic status, family values, and stressors. The variables contained within this immediate environment interact with one or more of the other variables in affecting the transition to motherhood. The infant as an individual is embedded within the family system. The family is viewed as a semi-closed system maintaining boundaries and control over interchange between the family system and other social systems (Mercer, 1990).

   The microsystem is the most influential on maternal role attainment (Mercer, 1995; R. Mercer, personal communication, January 4, 2003). In 1995, Mercer expanded her earlier concepts and model to emphasize the importance of the father in role attainment, stating that he helps "diffuse tension developing within the mother-infant dyad" (p. 15). Maternal role attainment is achieved through the interactions of father, mother, and infant. Figure 27-2, first introduced in Mercer's (1995) sixth book, *Becoming a Mother: Research on Maternal Identity From Rubin to the Present*, depicts this interaction. The layers *a* through *d* represent the stages of maternal role attainment from anticipatory to personal (role identity) and the infant's growth and developmental stages (Mercer, 1995).
2. The mesosystem encompasses, influences, and interacts with persons in the microsystem. Mesosystem interactions may influence what happens to the developing maternal role and the child. The mesosystem includes day care, school, work setting, places of worship, and other entities within the immediate community.
3. The macrosystem refers to the general prototypes existing in a particular culture or transmitted cultural consistencies. The macrosystem includes the social, political, and cultural influences on the other two systems. The health care environment and the current health care system policies that affect maternal role attainment originate in this system (Mercer, 1995). National laws regarding women and children and health priorities that influence maternal role attainment are within the macrosystem.

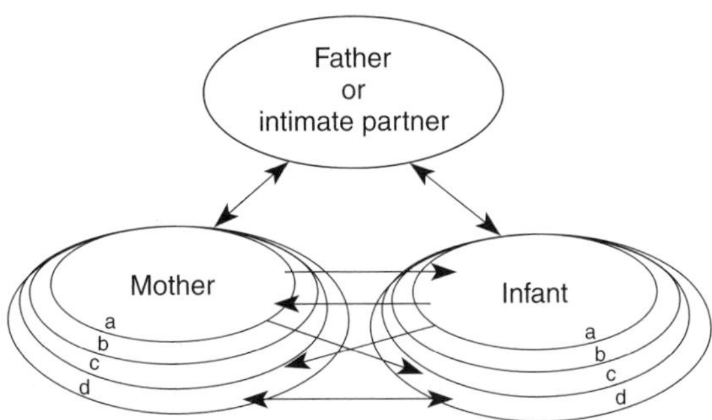

Figure 27-2 **A microsystem within the evolving model of maternal role attainment.** (From Mercer, R. T. [1995]. Becoming a mother: Research on maternal identity from Rubin to the present. New York: Springer; used by permission.)

Maternal role attainment is a process that follows four stages of role acquisition; these stages have been adapted from Thornton and Nardi's 1975 research. The following stages are indicated in Figure 27-2 as the layers *a* through *d*:

a. Anticipatory: The anticipatory stage begins during pregnancy and includes the initial social and psychological adjustments to pregnancy. The mother learns the expectations of the role, fantasizes about the role, relates to the fetus in utero, and begins to role play.

b. Formal: The formal stage begins with the birth of the infant and includes learning and taking on the role of mother. Role behaviors are guided by formal, consensual expectations of others in the mother's social system.

c. Informal: Begins as the mother develops unique ways of dealing with the role not conveyed by the social system. The woman makes her new role fit within her existing lifestyle based on past experiences and future goals.

d. Personal: The personal or role-identity stage occurs as the woman internalizes her role. The mother experiences a sense of harmony, confidence, and competence in the way she performs the role, and the maternal role is achieved.

Stages of role attainment overlap and are altered as the infant grows and develops. A maternal role identity may be achieved in a month, or it can take several months (Mercer, 1995). The stages are influenced by social support, stress, family functioning and also by the relationship between mother and father or significant other.

Traits and behaviors of both the mother and the infant may influence maternal role identity and child outcome. Maternal traits and behaviors included in Mercer's model are empathy, sensitivity to infant cues, self-esteem and self-concept, parenting received as a child, maturity and flexibility, attitudes, pregnancy and birth experience, health, depression, and role conflict. Infant traits having an impact on maternal role identity include temperament, ability to send cues, appearance, general characteristics, responsiveness, and health. Examples of the infant's developmental responses that interact with mother's developing maternal identity—depicted as *a* through *d* in Figure 27-2—include the following:

a. Eye contact with the mother as she talks to her or him, grasp reflex

b. Smile reflex and quieting behavior in response to mother's care

c. Consistent interactive behaviors with mother

d. Eliciting responses from the mother; increasingly more mobile

According to Mercer (1995):

> The personal role identity stage is reached when the mother has integrated the role into her self system with a congruence of self and other roles; she is secure in her identity as mother, is emotionally committed to her infant, and feels a sense of harmony, satisfaction, and competence in the role (p. 14).

Using Burke and Tully's (1977) work, Mercer (1995) stated that a role identity has internal and external components: the identity is the internalized view of self (recognized maternal identity), and role is the external, behavioral component.

Becoming a Mother: A Revised Model

Mercer has continued to use both her own research and the research of others as building blocks for her theory. In 2003, she began reexamining the Theory of Maternal Role Attainment, proposing that the term *becoming a mother* more accurately reflects the process based on recent research. According to Mercer (2004), the concept of role attainment suggests an end point rather than an ongoing process and may not address the continued expansion of the self as a mother. Mercer's conclusions are based largely on current nursing research about the cognitive and behavioral dimensions of women becoming mothers. Walker, Crain, and Thompson's (1986a, 1986b) questions about maternal role attainment as a continuing process contributed to Mercer's reexamination of her theory. Koniak-Griffin (1993) also questioned the behavioral and cognitive dimensions of maternal role attainment. Hartrick (1997) reported that women in her study of mothers of children from 3 to 16 years old undergo a continual process of self-definition. McBride and Shore (2001) in their research on mothers and grandmothers suggested that there may be a need to retire the term *maternal role attainment* because "it implies a static situation rather than fluctuating process" (p. 79). Finally, in a synthesis of nine qualitative studies, Nelson (2003) described continued growth and transformation in women as they become mothers. Mercer (2004) acknowledged that new challenges in motherhood require making new connections to regain confidence in the self and proposed replacing the term *maternal role attainment* with *becoming a mother*.

Qualitative studies have identified stages of maternal role attainment using the descriptive terms of participants. A compilation of the results of several of these studies has led Mercer (2004, 2006) to the following proposed changes in the names of stages leading to maternal role identity:

- Commitment and preparation (pregnancy)
- Acquaintance, practice, and physical restoration (first 2 weeks)
- Approaching normalization (second week to 4 months)
- Integration of maternal identity (approximately 4 months)

These stages parallel the original stages in Mercer's theory, but they embrace the maternal experience more completely and use terminology derived from new mothers' descriptions of their experiences.

Theory building, according to Mercer (personal communication, September 3, 2003), is a continual process as research provides evidence for clarifying concepts, additions, and deletions. Although many of the more recent studies support the findings of both Rubin and Mercer, Mercer (2004) recognized the evidence for needed changes in her original theory for greater clarity and consistency. It is with this insight that she proposed retiring the term *maternal role attainment*. Mercer (2004) acknowledges that becoming a mother, which connotes continued growth in mothering, is more descriptive of the process, which is much larger than a role. Although some roles may be terminated, motherhood is a lifelong commitment.

Mercer has continued to use Bronfenbrenner's concept of interacting nested ecological environments. However, she renamed them to reflect the living environments: family and friends, community, and society at large (Figure 27-3). The new model places the interactions between mother, infant, and father at the center of the interacting, living environments (R. Mercer, personal communication, September 3, 2003; Mercer & Walker, 2006). Variables within the family and friends environment include physical and social support, family values, cultural guidelines for parenting, knowledge and skills, family functioning, and affirmation as a mother. The community environment includes day care, places of worship, schools, work setting, health care facilities, recreational facilities, and support groups. Within the society at large, influences come from laws affecting woman and children, evolving reproductive and neonatal science, national health care programs, various social programs, and funding for research promoting becoming a mother.

LOGICAL FORM

Mercer used both deductive and inductive logic in developing the theoretical framework for studying factors that influence maternal role attainment during the first year of motherhood and in her theory. Deductive logic is demonstrated in Mercer's use of works from other researchers and disciplines. Role and developmental theories and the work of Rubin on maternal role attainment provided a base for the original framework. Mercer also used inductive logic in the development of her Theory of Maternal Role Attainment. Through practice and research, she observed adaptation to motherhood from a variety of circumstances. She noted that differences existed in adaptation to motherhood when maternal illness complicated the postpartum period, when a child with a defect was born, and when a teenager became a mother. These observations directed the

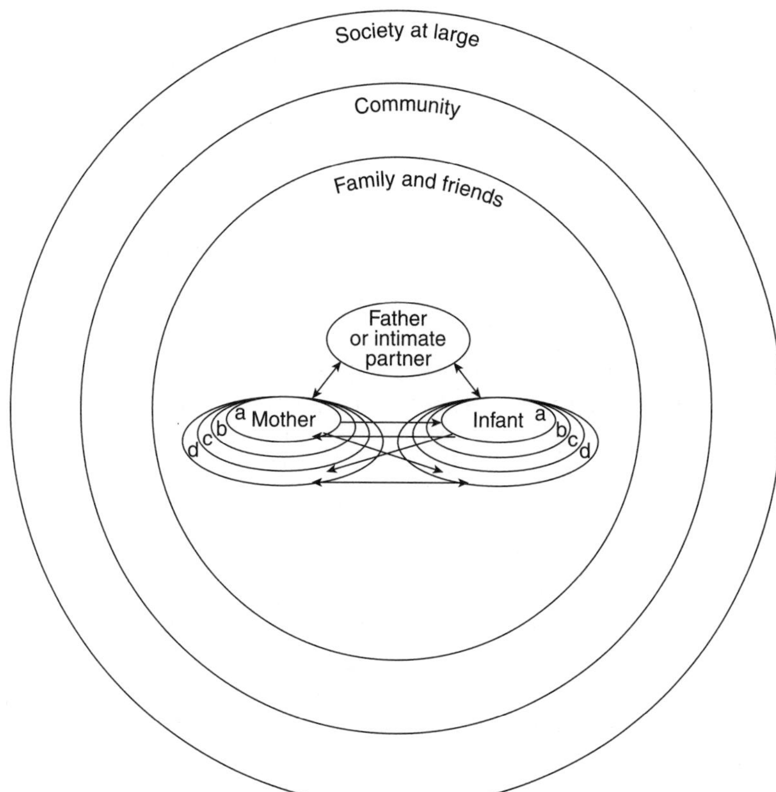

Figure 27-3 **Becoming a mother: A revised model.** (From R. T. Mercer, personal communication, September 3, 2003.)

research about those situations and the subsequent development of her theory. Changes to her original theory have been based on more recent research and deductive reasoning coupled with her belief in continually improving the clarity and usefulness of her theory.

ACCEPTANCE BY THE NURSING COMMUNITY

Practice

Mercer's theory is highly practice oriented. The concepts in her theory have been cited in many obstetrical textbooks and have been used in practice by nurses and those in other disciplines. Both the theory and the model are capable of serving as a framework for assessment, planning, implementing, and evaluating nursing care of new mothers and their infants. The utility of Mercer's theory in nursing practice is described by Meighan (2005) in the third edition of *Nursing Theory: Utilization & Application* by Alligood and Marriner Tomey. Mercer's theory is useful to practicing nurses across many maternal-child settings. Mercer (1986a, 1986b) linked her research findings with nursing practice at each interval from birth through the first year, making her theory applicable in a variety of pediatric settings.

In addition, Mercer's theory has been used in organizing patient care. Concepts in the research conducted by Neeson, Patterson, Mercer, and May (1983), "Pregnancy Outcome for Adolescents Receiving Prenatal Care by Nurse Practitioners in

Extended Roles," were used in setting up a clinical practice. Clark, Rapkin, Busen, and Vasquez (2001) used Mercer's theory to establish and test a parent education curriculum for substance-abusing women in a residential treatment facility. Meighan and Wood (2005) used the theory of maternal role attainment to explore the impact of hyperemesis gravidarum on maternal role assumption.

Education

Mercer's work has appeared extensively in both maternity and pediatric nursing texts. Many of the current concepts in maternal-child nursing are based on Mercer's research. Her theory and model help simplify the very complex process of becoming a parent. The Theory of Maternal Role Attainment is credited with enhancing understanding and making Mercer's contribution extremely valuable to nursing education. The Theory of Maternal Role Attainment provides a framework for students as they learn to plan and provide care for parents in a wide variety of settings. The Theory of Becoming a Mother has rapidly gained acceptance since its introduction in 2004. Mercer's theory and research have also been used in other disciplines as they relate to parenting and maternal role attainment. It has been shown to be helpful to students in psychology, sociology, and education.

Research

Mercer advocated the involvement of students in faculty research. During her tenure at the University of California, San Francisco, she chaired committees and was a committee member for numerous graduate theses and dissertations. Collaborative research with a graduate student and junior faculty member in 1977 and 1978 led to the development of a highly reliable, valid instrument to measure mothers' attitudes about the labor and delivery experience. Numerous researchers have requested permission to use the instrument.

Mercer's work has served as a springboard for other researchers. Her theoretical framework for a correlational study exploring differences between three age groups of first-time mothers (ages 15 to 19, 20 to 29, and 30 to 42) has been tested in part by others, including Walker and colleagues (1986a, 1986b). Sank (1991) used Mercer's theory in her doctoral dissertation research at the University of Texas, Austin, entitled *Factors in the Prenatal Period That Affect Parental Role Attainment During the Postpartum Period in Black American Mothers and Fathers.* Mercer's Theory of Maternal Role Attainment also served as the framework for Washington's (1997) dissertation, *Learning Needs of Adolescent Mothers When Identifying Fever and Illnesses in Infants Less Than Twelve Months of Age* at the University of Miami. Bacon (2001), a student at the Chicago School of Professional Psychology, used Mercer's theory in her dissertation, *Maternal Role Attainment and Maternal Identity in Mothers of Premature Infants.* Dilmore (2003) based her study, *A Comparison of Confidence Levels of Postpartum Depressed and Non-Depressed First Time Mothers,* on Mercer's research.

McBride (1984) wrote the following:

> Maternal role attainment has been a fundamental concern of nursing since the pioneering work of Mercer's mentor, Rubin, almost two decades ago. It is now becoming the research-based, theoretically sound construct that nurse researchers have been searching for in their analysis of the experience of new mothers (p. 72).

FURTHER DEVELOPMENT

Mercer used her initial research as a building block for other studies. In later research, Mercer aimed at identifying predictors of maternal-infant attachment on the basis of maternal experience with childbirth and maternal risk status. She also examined paternal competence on the basis of experience with childbirth and pregnancy risk status. In another study, she developed and tested a causal model to predict partner relationships in high-risk and low-risk pregnancy. More work and refinement of the original model and theory have taken place during the past few years, as described earlier.

She included the importance of the father in maternal role attainment, adding this to her model and theory in a section of her 1995 book, *Becoming a Mother: Research on Maternal Identity from Rubin to the Present*.

In her book, *First-Time Motherhood: Experiences from Teens to Forties*, Mercer (1986a) presented a model of the following four phases occurring in the process of maternal role attainment during the first year of motherhood:

1. The physical recovery phase, occurring from birth to 1 month
2. The achievement phase, from 2 to 4 or 5 months
3. The disruptions phase, occurring from 6 to 8 months
4. The reorganization phase, from after the eighth month and still in process at 1 year

Additionally, adaptation to the maternal role was proposed to occur at three levels (biological, psychological, and social), which are interacting and interdependent throughout the phases. These phases and levels of adaptation were described briefly and were applied to her research. In 2003, additional changes to the theory were proposed by Mercer (2004), that included abandoning *maternal role attainment* for the term *becoming a mother*. Changes to the model and adoption of the following four descriptive phases to the process of becoming a mother were also proposed:

1. Commitment and preparation (pregnancy)
2. Acquaintance, practice, and physical restoration (first 2 weeks)
3. Approaching normalization (second week to 4 months)
4. Integration of maternal identity (approximately 4 months)

These changes were based on the research studies by other nurses and are evidence of Mercer's continued scrutiny and critique of her theory to improve its utility in practice and research.

According to Mercer and Walker (2006), research into specific nursing interventions that foster becoming a mother is needed. They encourage the involvement of nursing staff, students, and faculty in the development and testing of assessment guidelines and instruments to measure outcomes of nursing interventions that support maternal role identity and the process of becoming a mother. Mercer and Walker also encourage further research in dealing with mothers who face special challenges, including childbirth complications, low social and economic resources, adolescents, and mothers with high-risk infants. According to Mercer and Walker, development and testing of nursing interventions that support and empower parents are warranted. They encourage research to determine how best to foster becoming a mother in culturally diverse groups, explaining that each culture has customs and values attached to childbearing that have an impact on the transition to motherhood.

Mercer's concern for the utility and applicability of her theory is evident in her continued work toward clarity and usefulness. Her revisions to her theory in 2003, although based on nursing research, have not been completely tested in other studies. Mercer's (2004) proposal of abandoning maternal role attainment for the term *becoming a mother* is argued logically, but few studies put it to use in practice or research. Although qualitative research to describe the phases of becoming a mother uses the exact words of women experiencing this transition, these phases have not been confirmed among women in other cultures or in different circumstances.

CRITIQUE

Clarity

The concepts, variables, and relationships have not always been defined explicitly, but they were described and implied in Mercer's earlier work. However, the concepts were defined theoretically and operationalized consistently. Work toward improving clarity is evident. Concepts, assumptions, and goals have been organized into a logical and coherent whole, so that understanding the interrelationships among the concepts is relatively easy. Some interchanging of terms and labels used to identify concepts, such as adaptation and attainment, social support, and support network, is potentially confusing for the reader. Additionally, maternal role attainment has not been defined consistently, which can obstruct clarity. Maternal identity, a term that Mercer defines as the final stage of role attainment (personal or role identity stage), is sometimes substituted for maternal role attainment. According to Mercer (1995), when the maternal role has been attained, the mother has achieved a maternal identity, the internalized role of mother. However, the terms *attainment* and *role identity* are sometimes confusing.

Mercer has continued to work toward greater clarity. She has proposed using terms derived from nursing researchers that would be understood more clearly by users of her theory. She has questioned the use of the term *maternal role attainment,* because it connotes a static state rather than the continuously evolving role as a mother. She has also examined qualitative research containing the exact words of women experiencing motherhood and has favored using these words to describe the stages of becoming a mother.

Simplicity

Despite numerous concepts and relationships, the theoretical framework for maternal role attainment or becoming a mother organizes a rather complex phenomenon into an easily understood and useful form. The theory is predictive in nature and readily lends itself to guide practice. Concepts are not specific to time and place and are abstract, but they are described and operationalized to the extent that meanings are not easily misinterpreted. However, it should be noted that the research to define and support the theoretical relationships was very complex, which was due largely to the great number of concepts. The process of becoming a mother is multifaceted and varies considerably according to the individual and to environmental influences. Mercer's theory provides a framework for understanding this complex, multidimensional process.

Generality

Mercer's theory is derived from and is specific to parent-child nursing but has been used by other disciplines concerned with mothering and parenting. The theory can be generalized to all women during pregnancy through the first year after birth, regardless of age, parity, or environment. It is among the few theories applicable to high-risk perinatal patients and their families. As previously mentioned, it can be applied to a variety of pediatric settings. Mercer (1995) has also respecified her theory to study and predict parental attachment, including that of the pregnant woman's partner. Therefore, it is useful in both studying and working with family members following birth. Mercer's work has done much to broaden the range of application of previously existing theories on maternal role attainment, because her studies have spanned various developmental levels and situational contexts, a quality that many other studies do not share.

Empirical Precision

Mercer's work has evolved from extensive research efforts. The concepts, assumptions, and relationships are grounded predominantly in empirical observations and are congruent. The degree of concreteness and the completeness of operational definitions further increase the empirical precision. The theoretical framework for exploring differences among age groups of first-time mothers lends itself well to further testing and is being used by others for this purpose. The continued scrutiny by Mercer herself has continually improved her theory and solidified her concepts. Mercer's most recent proposed changes to improve clarity of concepts are based on research studies of others within the discipline of nursing.

Derivable Consequences

The theoretical framework for maternal role attainment during the first year has proved to be useful, practical, and valuable to nursing. Mercer's work is used repeatedly in research, practice, and education. The framework is also readily applicable to any discipline that works with mothers and children during the first year of motherhood. McBride (1984) wrote, "Dr. Mercer is the one who developed the most complete theoretical framework for studying one aspect of parental experience, namely, the factors that influence the attainment of the maternal role in the first year of motherhood" (p. 72).

Throughout her career, Mercer consistently has linked research to practice. Implications for nursing or nursing interventions are addressed and provide the bond between research and practice in most of her works. She believes that nursing research is the "bridge to excellence" in nursing practice (Mercer, 1984, p. 47).

SUMMARY

The Theory of Maternal Role Attainment has been shown to be useful in both research and practice for nurses, as well as other disciplines concerned with parenting. Mercer's continued devotion to improving the usefulness and clarity of her theory and model is evident and has served well those who use her theory. Mercer's use of both her own research and the research of others strengthens her work. Her proposal to adopt the Theory of Becoming a Mother is based solidly on the research process. Motherhood and attainment of the parenting role is a very complex, multilevel process. Mercer's theory and her work make this process logical and understandable and provide a solid foundation for practice, education, and research.

Case Study

Susan, a 19-year-old woman, delivered her first infant prematurely 5 days ago. Although her postpartum course has been relatively uneventful, the infant has had difficulty and must remain hospitalized. Susan and her young husband visit the nursery every afternoon to be with the baby, but they ask very few questions. In talking with the couple, the nurse learns that the only living grandparents of the baby live a great distance away. Susan will not have any family or friends to turn to when she takes the baby home.

In this high-risk perinatal case, Mercer's framework should be useful for nursing assessment and intervention to facilitate maternal role attainment. How would you use it as a guide in planning care for Susan?

CRITICAL THINKING Activities

1. In your own practice, consider Mercer's Theory and Model of Maternal Role Attainment as a guide. In what ways is it useful?
2. High-risk families often continue to experience problems for years after the birth of a child with a congenital problem. Can Mercer's theory be adapted to help in assessment and intervention for these mothers and their families beyond the first year? What areas need further research and development?
3. Consider the current health care environment. Does the model proposed by Mercer adequately address current changes in health care delivery and the impact on the family? What changes in Mercer's model, if any, would you suggest?
4. Mercer has proposed changing her theory from Maternal Role Attainment to Becoming a Mother to address the evolving role of motherhood. Do you agree or disagree with this change? Would this alter the theory's use in the clinical setting in any way?

POINTS FOR Further Study

Publications

- Mercer, R.T. (2006). Nursing support of the process of becoming a mother. *JOGNN 35* (5), 649-651.
- Mercer, R.T., & Walker, L. O. (2006). A review of nursing interventions to foster becoming a mother. *JOGNN 35* (5), 568-582.

- Meighan, M. (2006). Mercer's maternal role theory and nursing practice. In M. R. Alligood & A. Marriner Tomey (Eds.), *Nursing theory: Utilization & application* (3rd ed., pp. 393-411). St. Louis: Mosby.

Web Sites

- BioInfoBank Library: RT Mercer, Accessed February 7, 2008: http://lib.bioinfo.pl/auth:Mercer,RT
- Cardinal Stritch University Library. (2004). Model and theories of nursing. Ramona T. Mercer: Maternal role attainment. Milwaukee, WI: Cardinal Stritch University. Accessed February 7, 2008: http://library.stritch.edu/nursingtheroies/mercer
- Nurses for Nurses Everywhere. (2004). Nurse information: Ramona T. Mercer. Melbourne, Australia: Nurses.info. Accessed February 7, 2008: http://www.nurses.info/nursing_theory_midrange_theories_ramona_mercer.htm
- Nurses for Nurses Everywhere. (2004). Nurse information: Reva Rubin. Melbourne, Australia: Nurses.info. Accessed February 7, 2008: http://www.nurses.info/nursing_theory_midrange_theories_reva_rubin.htm
- The Nursing Theory Network. (2005). Role Attainment: Ramona T. Mercer Accessed February 7, 2008: http://www.nursingtheory.net/mr_roleattainment.html
- The Nursing Theory Network. (2005). Maternal Identity: Reva Rubin Accessed February 7, 2008: http://www.nursingtheory.net/mr_maternalidentity.html

REFERENCES

Bacon, A. C. (2001). Maternal role attainment and maternal identity in mothers of premature infants (Doctoral dissertation, Chicago School of Professional Psychology, Chicago, 2001). *Dissertation Abstracts International, 61*, 8-B. (University Microfilms No. 2001-95004-447)

Bronfenbrenner, U. (1979). *The ecology of human development: Experiment by nature and design.* Cambridge, MA: Harvard University Press.

Burke, P. J., & Tully, J. C. (1977). The measurement of role identity. *Social Forces, 55*, 881-897.

Burr, W. R., Leigh, G. K., Day, R. D., & Constantine, J. (1979). Symbolic interaction and the family. In W. R. Burr, R. Hill, F. I. Nye, & I. L. Reiss (Eds.), *Contemporary theories about the family* (Vol. 2, pp. 42-111). New York: Free Press.

Clark, B. S., Rapkin, D., Busen, N. H., & Vasquez, E. (2001). Nurse practitioners and parent education: A partnership for health. *Journal of the American Academy of Nurse Practitioners, 13*(7), 310-316.

Dilmore, D. L. (2003) A comparison of confidence levels of postpartum depressed and non-depressed first time mothers. Unpublished thesis, University of Florida.

Donley, M. G. (1993). Attachment and the emotional unit. *Family Process, 32*, 3-20.

Ferketich, S. L., & Mercer, R. T. (1995a). Paternal-infant attachment of experienced and inexperienced fathers during infancy. *Nursing Research, 44*, 31-37.

Ferketich, S. L., & Mercer, R. T. (1995b). Predictors of paternal role competence by risk status. *Nursing Research, 43*, 80-85.

Ferketich, S. L., & Mercer, R. T. (1995c). Predictors of role competence for experienced and inexperienced fathers. *Nursing Research, 44*, 89-95.

Hartrick, G. A. (1997). Women who are mothers: The experience of defining self. *Health Care for Women International, 18*, 263-277.

Koniak-Griffin, D. (1993). Maternal role attainment. *Image: The Journal of Nursing Scholarship, 25*, 257-262.

McBride, A. B. (1984). The experience of being a parent. *Annual Review of Nursing Research, 2*, 63-81.

McBride, A. B., & Shore, C. P. (2001). Women as mothers and grandmothers. *Annual Review of Nursing Research, 19*, 63-85.

Mead, G. H. (1934). *Mind, self and society.* Chicago: University of Chicago Press.

Meighan, M. (2005). Mercer's maternal role theory and nursing practice. In M. R. Alligood & A. Marriner Tomey (Eds.), *Nursing theory: Utilization & application* (3rd ed., pp. 393-411). St. Louis: Mosby.

Meighan, M. & Wood, A. F. (2005). The Impact of Hyperemesis Gravidarum on Maternal Role Assumption. *JOGNN, 34*(2), 172-179.

Mercer, R. T. (1977). *Nursing care for parents at risk.* Thorofare, NJ: Charles B. Slack.

Mercer, R. T. (1979). *Perspectives on adolescent health care.* Philadelphia: J. B. Lippincott.

Mercer, R. T. (1981). A theoretical framework for studying factors that impact on the maternal role. *Nursing Research, 30*, 73-77.

Mercer, R. T. (1984). Nursing research: The bridge to excellence in practice. *Image: The Journal of Nursing Scholarship, 16*(2), 47-51.

Mercer, R. T. (1985a). The process of maternal role attainment over the first years. *Nursing Research, 34*, 198-204.

Mercer, R. T. (1985b). The relationship of age and other variables to gratification in mothering. *Health Care for Women International, 6*, 295-308.

Mercer, R. T. (1986a). *First-time motherhood: Experiences from teens to forties.* New York: Springer.

Mercer, R. T. (1986b). The relationship of developmental variables to maternal behavior. *Research in Nursing Health, 9*, 25-33.

Mercer, R. T. (1989). Responses to life-span development: A review of theory and practice for families with chronically ill members. *Scholarly Inquiry for Nursing Practice: An International Journal, 3*, 23-26.

Mercer, R. T. (1990). *Parents at risk.* New York: Springer.

Mercer, R. T. (1995). *Becoming a mother: Research on maternal identity from Rubin to the present.* New York: Springer.

Mercer, R. T. (2000, June 24) Personal communication.

Mercer, R. T. (2002). Curriculum vitae.

Mercer, R. T. (2003, Jan. 4) Personal correspondence.

Mercer, R. T. (2003, Sep. 3) Personal correspondence.

Mercer, R. T. (2004). Becoming a mother versus maternal role attainment. *Journal of Nursing Scholarship, 36*(3), 226-232.

Mercer, R. T. (2004, Mar. 21) Personal correspondence.

Mercer, R. T. (2006). Nursing support of the process of becoming a mother. *JOGNN 35*(5), 649-651.

Mercer, R. T., & Ferketich, S. L. (1990a). Predictors of family functioning eight months following birth. *Nursing Research, 39*, 76-82.

Mercer, R. T., & Ferketich, S. L. (1990b). Predictors of parental attachment during early parenthood. *Journal of Advanced Nursing, 15*, 268-280.

Mercer, R. T., & Ferketich, S. L. (1994). Maternal-infant attachment of experienced and inexperienced mothers during infancy. *Nursing Research, 43*, 344-350.

Mercer, R. T., & Ferketich, S. L. (1995). Experienced and inexperienced mothers' maternal competence during infancy. *Research in Nursing Health, 18*, 333-343.

Mercer, R. T., Ferketich, S. L., & DeJoseph, J. F. (1993). Predictors of partner relationships during pregnancy and infancy. *Research in Nursing Health, 16*, 45-56.

Mercer, R. T., Ferketich, S. L., DeJoseph, J., May, K. A., & Sollid, D. (1988). Effects of stress on family functioning during pregnancy. *Nursing Research, 37*, 268-275.

Mercer, R. T., Hackley, K. C., & Bostrom, A. (1984). Social support of teenage mothers. *Birth Defects: Original Article Series, 20*(5), 245-290.

Mercer, R. T., May, K. A., Ferketich, S., & DeJoseph, J. (1986). Theoretical models for studying the effect of antepartum stress on the family. *Nursing Research, 35*, 339-346.

Mercer, R. T, & Walker, L. O. (2006). A review of nursing interventions to foster becoming a mother. *Journal of Obstetric, Gynecologic, and Neonatal Nursing, 35* (5), 568-582.

Neeson, J. D., Patterson, K. A., Mercer, R. T., & May, K. A. (1983). Pregnancy outcome for adolescents receiving prenatal care by nurse practitioners in extended roles. *Journal of Adolescent Health Care, 4*, 94-99.

Nelson, A. M. (2003). Transition to motherhood. *Journal of Obstetric, Gynecologic, & Neonatal Nursing, 32*, 465-477.

Rubin, R. (1977). Binding-in in the postpartum period. *Maternal Child Nursing Journal, 6*, 67-75.

Rubin, R. (1984). *Maternal identity and the maternal experience.* New York: Springer.

Sank, J. C. (1991). Factors in the prenatal period that affect parental role attainment during the postpartum period in black American mothers and fathers (Doctoral dissertation, University of Texas, Austin, Texas, 1991). (University Microfilms No. 1993-155453)

Thornton, R., & Nardi, P. M. (1975). The dynamics of role acquisition. *American Journal of Sociology, 80*, 870-885.

Turner, J. H. (1978). *The structure of sociological theory* (Revised ed.). Homewood, IL: Dorsey Press.

von Bertalanffy, L. (1968). *General system theory.* New York: George Braziller.

Walker, L. O., Crain, H., & Thompson, E. (1986a). Maternal role attainment and identity in the postpartum period: Stability and change. *Nursing Research, 35*(2), 68-71.

Walker, L. O., Crain, H., & Thompson, E. (1986b). Mothering behavior and maternal role attainment during the postpartum period. *Nursing Research, 35*(6), 322-325.

Washington, L. J. (1997). Learning needs of adolescent mothers when identifying fever and illnesses in infants less than twelve months of age (Doctoral dissertation, University of Miami, Miami). *Dissertation Abstracts International, 57*, (12-B). (University Microfilms No. 1997-95012-208)

Werner, H. (1957). The concept of development from a comparative and organismic point of view. In D. H. Harris (Ed.), *The concept of development* (pp. 125-148). Minneapolis: University of Minnesota.

BIBLIOGRAPHY

Primary Sources

Books

Mercer, R. T. (1977). *Nursing care for parents at risk.* Thorofare, NJ: Charles B. Slack.

Mercer, R. T. (1979). *Perspectives on adolescent health care.* Philadelphia: J. B. Lippincott.

Mercer, R. T. (1986). *First-time motherhood: Experiences from teens to forties.* New York: Springer.

Mercer, R. T. (1990). *Parents at risk.* New York: Springer.

Mercer, R. T. (1995). *Becoming a mother: Research on maternal identity from Rubin to the present.* New York: Springer.

Journal Articles

Ferketich, S. L., & Mercer, R. T. (1995). Paternal-infant attachment of experienced and inexperienced fathers during infancy. *Nursing Research, 44*, 31-37.

Ferketich, S. L., & Mercer, R. T. (1995). Predictors of role competence for experienced and inexperienced fathers. *Nursing Research, 44*, 89-95.

Mercer, R. T. (1995). A tribute to Reva Rubin. *Maternal Child Nursing, 20*, 184.

Mercer, R. T. (1997). Chronically ill children: How families adjust. *Nurseweek, 10*(9), 14-15, 17.

Mercer, R. T. (1997). The employed mother's challenges. *Nurseweek, 10*(17), 10-11, 15.

Mercer, R. T. (2000). Response to "Life-span development: A review of theory and practice for families with chronically ill members." *Scholarly Inquiry for Nursing Practice, 14*(4), 375-378.

Mercer, R. T., & Ferketich, S. L. (1995). Experienced and inexperienced mothers' maternal competence during infancy. *Research in Nursing Health, 18*, 333-343.

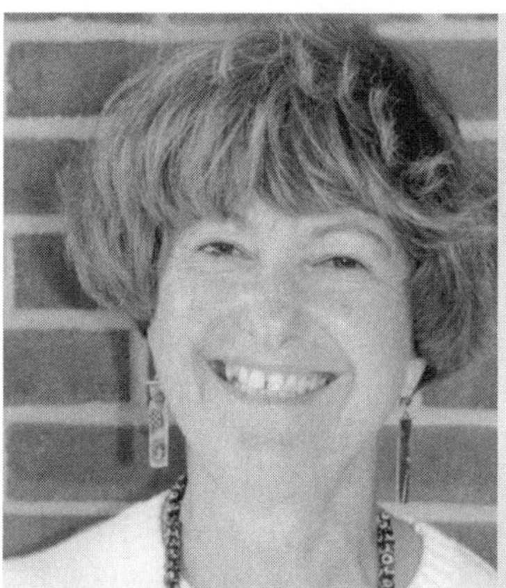

Photo credit: Dr. Michael Belyea, University of North Carolina, Chapel Hill, NC.

CHAPTER

28

Merle H. Mishel

1939-present

Uncertainty in Illness Theory

Donald E. Bailey, Jr. and Janet L. Stewart

"My theory can be applied to both practice and research. It has been used to explain clinical situations and design interventions that lead to evidence-based practice. Current and future nurse scientists have and will continue to extend the theory to different patient populations. This work has the potential to transform health care."(Mishel, personal communication, May 28, 2008)

CREDENTIALS AND BACKGROUND OF THE THEORIST

Merle H. Mishel was born in Boston, Massachusetts. She graduated from Boston University with a B.A. in 1961 and received her M.S. in psychiatric nursing from the University of California in 1966. Mishel completed her M.A. and Ph.D. in social psychology at the Claremont Graduate School, Claremont, California, in 1976 and 1980, respectively. Her dissertation research, supported by an individual National Research Service Award, was the development and testing of the Perceived Ambiguity in Illness Scale, later renamed the Mishel Uncertainty in Illness Scale (MUIS-A). The original scale has been used as the basis for the following three additional scales:

1. A community version (MUIS-C) for chronically ill individuals who are not hospitalized or receiving active medical care
2. A measure of parents' perceptions of uncertainty (PPUS) with regard to their child's illness experience
3. A measure of uncertainty in spouses or other family members when another member of the family is acutely ill (PPUS-FM)

Early in her professional career, Mishel practiced as a psychiatric nurse in acute care and community settings. While pursuing her doctorate, she

The authors wish to think Dr. Merle Mishel for her review and input for this chapter.

was on faculty in the Department of Nursing at the California State University at Los Angeles, rising from assistant to full professor. In addition, she practiced as a nurse therapist in both community and private practice settings from 1973 to 1979. After completing her doctorate in social psychology, she relocated to the University of Arizona College of Nursing in 1981 as an associate professor and was promoted to professor in 1988. She served as Division Head of Mental Health Nursing from 1984 to 1991. While at the University of Arizona, Mishel received numerous intramural and extramural research grants that supported the continued development of the theoretical framework of uncertainty in illness. During this period, she continued practicing as a nurse therapist, working with the heart transplant program at the University Medical Center. She was inducted as a fellow in the American Academy of Nursing in 1990.

Mishel returned to the East Coast in 1991 and joined the faculty as a professor in the School of Nursing, University of North Carolina at Chapel Hill, and was awarded the endowed Kenan Professor of Nursing Chair in 1994. Friends of the National Institute of Nursing Research presented her with a Research Merit Award in 1997 and invited her to present her research as an exemplar of federally funded nursing intervention studies at a Congressional Breakfast in 1999. She is the Director of the T-32 Institutional National Research Service Award Training Grant, Interventions for Preventing and Managing Chronic Illness. The T-32 awards predoctoral and postdoctoral fellowships to nurses interested in developing interventions for a variety of underserved chronically ill patients. Currently she serves as the Director of Doctoral and Post-doctoral Programs at the School. Mishel also maintains a prolific program of nursing intervention research with several cancer populations. Of note is that Mishel's research program has been funded continually by the NIH since 1984, such that each research grant has built upon findings from prior studies in order to move systematically toward theoretically derived, scientifically tested nursing interventions.

In addition to the awards previously identified, Mishel was the recipient of a Sigma Theta Tau International Sigma Xi Chapter Nurse Research Predoctoral Fellowship from 1977 to 1979 and received the Mary Opal Wolanin Research Award in 1986. In 1987, Mishel was first alternate for the Fulbright Award. She has been a visiting scholar at many institutions throughout North America, including University of Nebraska, University of Texas at Houston, University of Tennessee at Knoxville, University of South Carolina, University of Rochester, Yale University, and McGill University. She served as doctoral program consultant for the University of Cincinnati College of Nursing from 1991 to 1992 and Rutgers University School of Nursing in 1993. In 2004, Mishel received the Linnea Henderson Research Fellowship Program Award, from Kent State University, School of Nursing. Over the last 15 years, Mishel has presented more than 80 invited addresses at schools of nursing throughout the United States and Canada. Reflecting the growing international interest in her theory and measurement models, Mishel conducted an International Symposium on Uncertainty at Kyungpook National University in Daegu, South Korea, served as a visiting scholar at Mahidol University in Bangkok, Thailand, and recently delivered the keynote address at the annual convention of the Japanese Society of Nursing Research, in Sapporo, Japan.

Mishel is a member of a number of professional organizations. They include the American Academy of Nursing, Sigma Theta Tau International, American Psychological Association, American Nurses Association, Society of Behavioral Medicine, Oncology Nursing Society, Southern Nursing Research Society, and the Society for Education and Research in Psychiatric Nursing. She has served as a grant reviewer for the National Cancer Institute, National Center for Nursing Research, and National Institute on Aging and was a charter member of the study section on human immunodeficiency virus (HIV) at the National Institute of Mental Health.

THEORETICAL SOURCES

When Mishel began her research into uncertainty, the concept had not previously been applied in the health and illness context. Her original Uncertainty in Illness Theory (Mishel, 1988) drew from existing information-processing models (Warburton, 1979) and personality research (Budner, 1962) from the psychology discipline, which characterized uncertainty as a cognitive state resulting from insufficient cues with which to form a cognitive schema or internal representation of a situation or event. Mishel attributes the underlying stress-appraisal-coping-adaptation framework in the original theory to the work of Lazarus and Folkman (1984). The unique aspect was her application of this framework to uncertainty as a stressor in the context of illness, which made the framework particularly meaningful for nursing.

With the reconceptualization of the theory, Mishel (1990) recognized that the Western approach to science supported a mechanistic view in its emphasis on control and predictability. By using critical social theory, Mishel recognized the bias inherent in the original theory, an orientation toward certainty and adaptation. Mishel then incorporated tenets from chaos theory, and because of its focus on open systems, allowed for a more accurate representation of how chronic illness creates disequilibrium and how people ultimately can incorporate continual uncertainty to find new meaning in illness.

MAJOR CONCEPTS & DEFINITIONS

UNCERTAINTY

Uncertainty is the inability to determine the meaning of illness-related events, occurring when the decision maker is unable to assign definite value to objects or events, or is unable to predict outcomes accurately (Mishel, 1988).

COGNITIVE SCHEMA

Cognitive schema is a person's subjective interpretation of illness, treatment, and hospitalization (Mishel, 1988).

STIMULI FRAME

Stimuli frame is the form, composition, and structure of the stimuli that a person perceives, which are then structured into a cognitive schema (Mishel, 1988).

Symptom Pattern

Symptom pattern is the degree to which symptoms occur with sufficient consistency to be perceived as having a pattern or configuration (Mishel, 1988).

Event Familiarity

Event familiarity is the degree to which a situation is habitual or repetitive, or contains recognized cues (Mishel, 1988).

Event Congruence

Event congruence refers to the consistency between the expected and the experienced in illness-related events (Mishel, 1988).

STRUCTURE PROVIDERS

Structure providers are the resources available to assist the person in the interpretation of the stimuli frame (Mishel, 1988).

Credible Authority

Credible authority is the degree of trust and confidence a person has in his or her healthcare providers (Mishel, 1988).

Continued

MAJOR CONCEPTS & DEFINITIONS—cont'd

Social Supports

Social supports influence uncertainty by assisting the individual to interpret the meaning of events (Mishel, 1988).

COGNITIVE CAPACITIES

Cognitive capacities are the information-processing abilities of a person, reflecting both innate capabilities and situational constraints (Mishel, 1988).

INFERENCE

Inference refers to the evaluation of uncertainty using related, recalled experiences (Mishel, 1988).

ILLUSION

Illusion refers to beliefs constructed out of uncertainty (Mishel, 1988).

ADAPTATION

Adaptation reflects biopsychosocial behavior occurring within persons' individually defined range of usual behavior (Mishel, 1988).

NEW VIEW OF LIFE

New view of life refers to the formulation of a new sense of order, resulting from the integration of continual uncertainty into one's self-structure, in which uncertainty is accepted as the natural rhythm of life (Mishel, 1988).

PROBABILISTIC THINKING

Probabilistic thinking refers to a belief in a conditional world in which the expectation of continual certainty and predictability is abandoned (Mishel, 1988).

USE OF EMPIRICAL EVIDENCE

The Uncertainty in Illness Theory grew out of Mishel's dissertation research with hospitalized patients, for which she used both qualitative and quantitative findings to generate the first conceptualization of uncertainty in the context of illness. Beginning with the publication of Mishel's Uncertainty in Illness Scale (Mishel, 1981), there has been extensive research into adults' experiences with uncertainty related to chronic and life-threatening illnesses. Considerable empirical evidence has accumulated to support Mishel's theoretical model in adults. Several recent integrative reviews of uncertainty research have comprehensively summarized and critiqued the current state of the science (Mast, 1995; Mishel, 1997a, 1999; Stewart & Mishel, 2000). The authors include studies here that directly support the elements of Mishel's uncertainty model.

Most empirical studies have focused predominantly on two of the antecedents of uncertainty, stimuli frame and structure providers, and the relationship between uncertainty and psychological outcomes. Mishel tested other elements of the model, such as the mediating roles of appraisal and coping, early in her program of research (Mishel & Braden, 1987; Mishel, Padilla, Grant, & Sorenson, 1991; Mishel & Sorenson, 1991), but these model elements, along with cognitive capacity as an antecedent to uncertainty, have generated less research attention.

Several studies have shown that objective or subjective indicators of the severity of life-threat or illness symptoms were associated positively with uncertainty (Braden, 1990; Grootenhuis & Last, 1997; Hinds, Birenbaum, Clarke-Steffen, Quargnenti, Kreissman, Kazak, et al., 1996; Janson-Bjerklie, Ferketich, & Benner, 1993; Tomlinson, Kirschbaum, Harbaugh, & Anderson, 1996). Across a sustained illness trajectory, unpredictability in symptom onset, duration, and intensity has been related to perceived uncertainty (Becker, Jason-Bjerklie, Benner, Slobin, & Ferketich, 1993; Brown & Powell-Cope, 1991; Jessop & Stein, 1985; Mishel & Braden, 1988; Murray, 1993). Similarly, the ambiguous nature of illness symptoms and the consequent difficulty in determining the significance of physical sensations frequently have been identified as sources of uncertainty (Cohen, 1993; Comaroff & Maguire, 1981; Hilton, 1988; Nelson, 1996; Weitz, 1989).

Mishel and Braden (1988) found that social support had a direct impact on uncertainty by reducing perceived complexity and an indirect impact through its effect on the predictability of symptom pattern. The perception of stigma associated with some conditions, particularly HIV infection (Regan-Kubinski & Sharts-Hopko, 1995; Weitz, 1989) and Down's syndrome (Van Riper & Selder, 1989), served to create uncertainty when families were unsure about how others would respond to the diagnosis. Family members have been shown consistently to experience high levels of uncertainty as well, which may further reduce the amount of support experienced by the patient (Brown & Powell-Cope, 1991; Hilton, 1996; Wineman, O'Brien, Nealon, & Kaskel, 1993). In addition, uncertainty was heightened by interactions with healthcare providers in which patients and family members received unclear information or simplistic explanations that did not fit their experience, or perceived that care providers were not expert or responsive enough to help them manage the intricacies of the illness (Becker et al., 1993; Comaroff & Maguire, 1981; Mason, 1985; Sharkey, 1995).

Numerous studies have reported the negative impact of uncertainty on psychological outcomes, characterized variously as anxiety, depression, hopelessness, and psychological distress (Failla, Kuper, Nick, & Lee, 1996; Grootenhuis & Last, 1997; Jessop & Stein, 1985; Miles, Funk, & Kasper, 1992; Mishel & Sorenson, 1991; Schepp, 1991; Wineman, 1990). Uncertainty has also been shown to negatively impact quality of life (Braden, 1990; Padilla, Mishel, & Grant, 1992), satisfaction with family relationships (Wineman et al., 1993), satisfaction with healthcare services (Green & Murton, 1996; Turner, Tomlinson, & Harbaugh, 1990), and family caregivers' maintenance of their own self-care activities (Brett & Davies, 1988; Lang, 1987; O'Brien, Wineman, & Nealon, 1995).

Mishel reconceptualized the uncertainty theory in 1990 to accommodate responses to uncertainty over time in people with chronic conditions. The original theory was expanded to include the idea that uncertainty may not be resolved but may become part of an individual's reality. In this context, uncertainty is reappraised as an opportunity and prompts the formation of a new, probabilistic view of life. To adopt this new view of life, the patient must be able to rely on social resources and healthcare providers who themselves accept the idea of probabilistic thinking (Mishel, 1990). If uncertainty can be framed as a normal part of life, it can become a positive force for multiple opportunities with resulting positive mood states (Gelatt, 1989; Mishel, 1990).

Support for the reconceptualized Uncertainty in Illness Theory has been found in predominantly qualitative studies of people with a variety of chronic and life-threatening illnesses. The process of formulating a new view of life has been described by women with breast cancer and cardiac disease as a revised life perspective (Hilton, 1988), new life goals (Carter, 1993), new ways of being in the world (Mast, 1998; Nelson, 1996), growth through uncertainty (Pelusi, 1997), and new levels of self-organization (Fleury, Kimbrell, & Kruszewski, 1995). In studies of predominantly men with chronic illness or their caregivers, the process has been described as transformed self-identity and new goals for living (Brown & Powell-Cope, 1991), a more positive perspective on life (Katz, 1996), reevaluating what is worthwhile (Nyhlin, 1990), contemplation and self-appraisal (Charmaz, 1995), uncertainty viewed as opportunity (Baier, 1995), and redefining normal and building new dreams (Mishel & Murdaugh, 1987).

MAJOR ASSUMPTIONS

Mishel's original Uncertainty in Illness Theory, first published in 1988, included several major assumptions (Figure 28-1). The first two reflect how uncertainty was conceptualized originally within the psychology discipline's information-processing models, as follows:

1. Uncertainty is a cognitive state, representing the inadequacy of an existing cognitive schema

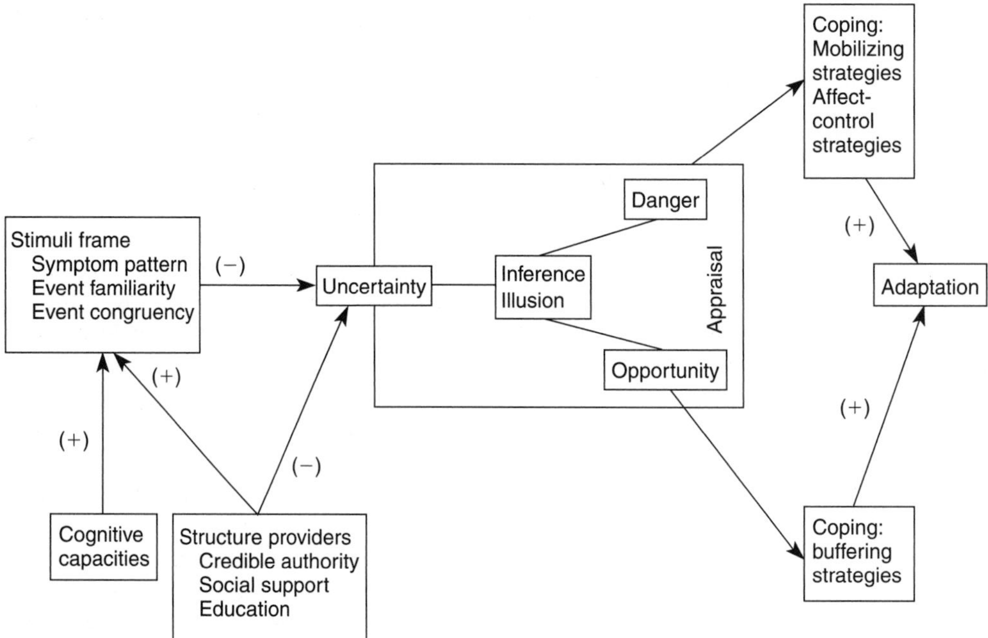

Figure 28-1 **Model of perceived uncertainty in illness.** (From Mishel, M. H. [1988, Winter]. Uncertainty in illness. *Image: The Journal of Nursing Scholarship, 20*, 226.)

to support the interpretation of illness-related events.

2. Uncertainty is an inherently neutral experience, neither desirable nor aversive until it is appraised as such.

Two more assumptions reflect the uncertainty theory's roots in traditional stress and coping models that posit a linear stress → coping → adaptation relationship as follows:

3. Adaptation represents the continuity of an individual's usual biopsychosocial behavior and is the desired outcome of coping efforts to either reduce uncertainty appraised as danger or maintain uncertainty appraised as opportunity.
4. The relationships among illness events, uncertainty, appraisal, coping, and adaptation are linear and unidirectional, moving from situations promoting uncertainty toward adaptation.

Mishel herself challenged these last two assumptions in her reconceptualization of the theory, published in 1990. The reconceptualization came about as a result of contradictory findings when the theory was applied to people with chronic illnesses. The original formulation of the theory held that uncertainty typically is appraised as an opportunity only in conditions that represent a known downward trajectory; in other words, uncertainty is appraised as opportunity when it is the alternative to negative certainty. Mishel and others found that people also appraised uncertainty as an opportunity in situations without a certain downward trajectory, particularly in long-term chronic illnesses, and that in this context people often developed a new view of life.

Dissatisfied with the traditional linear models that informed the original theory, Mishel turned to the more dynamic chaos theory to explain how prolonged uncertainty could function as a catalyst to change a person's perspective on life and illness. Chaos theory contributed two of the following theoretical assumptions, which replace the linear stress → coping → adaptation outcome portion of the model as follows:

- People, as biopsychosocial systems, typically function in far-from-equilibrium states.

- Major fluctuations in a far-from-equilibrium system enhance the system's receptivity to change.
- Fluctuations result in repatterning, which is repeated at each level of the system.

In Mishel's reconceptualized model, neither the antecedents to uncertainty nor the process of cognitive appraisal of uncertainty as danger or opportunity changes. However, uncertainty over time, associated with a serious illness, functions as a catalyst for fluctuation in the system by threatening one's preexisting cognitive model of life as predictable and controllable. Because uncertainty pervades nearly every aspect of a person's life, its effects become concentrated and ultimately challenge the stability of the system. In response to the confusion and disorganization created by continued uncertainty, the system ultimately must change in order to survive.

Ideally, under conditions of chronic uncertainty, a person gradually moves away from an evaluation of uncertainty as aversive to adopt a new view of life that accepts uncertainty as a part of reality (Figure 28-2). Thus uncertainty, especially in chronic or life-threatening illness, can result in a new level of organization and a new perspective on life, incorporating the growth and change that can result from uncertain experiences.

THEORETICAL ASSERTIONS

Mishel asserted the following (1988, 1990):

- Uncertainty occurs when a person cannot adequately structure or categorize an illness-related event because of the lack of sufficient cues.
- Uncertainty can take the form of ambiguity, complexity, lack of or inconsistent information, or unpredictability.

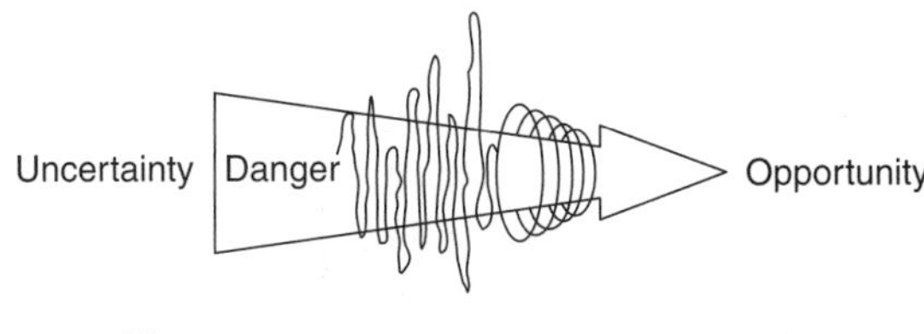

Figure 28-2 Reconceptualized model of uncertainty in chronic illness. (Copyright Merle Mishel, 1990.)

- As symptom pattern, event familiarity, and event congruence (stimuli frame) increase, uncertainty decreases.
- Structure providers (credible authority, social support, and education) decrease uncertainty directly by promoting interpretation of events, and indirectly by strengthening the stimuli frame.
- Uncertainty appraised as danger prompts coping efforts directed at reducing the uncertainty and managing the emotional arousal generated by it.
- Uncertainty appraised as opportunity prompts coping efforts directed at maintaining the uncertainty.
- The influence of uncertainty on psychological outcomes is mediated by the effectiveness of coping efforts to reduce uncertainty appraised as danger or to maintain uncertainty appraised as opportunity.
- When uncertainty appraised as danger cannot be reduced effectively, coping strategies can be employed to manage the emotional response.
- The longer uncertainty continues in the illness context, the more unstable the individual's previously accepted mode of functioning becomes.
- Under conditions of enduring uncertainty, individuals may develop a new, probabilistic perspective on life, which accepts uncertainty as a natural part of life.
- The process of integrating continual uncertainty into a new view of life can be blocked or prolonged by structure providers who do not support probabilistic thinking.
- Prolonged exposure to uncertainty appraised as danger can lead to intrusive thoughts, avoidance, and severe emotional distress.

LOGICAL FORM

As a middle range theory both derived from and applicable to clinical practice, Mishel's Uncertainty in Illness Theory is a classic example of the multiple steps required to develop theory with both heuristic and practical value. Neither purely inductive nor deductive, Mishel's theoretical work initially arose from asking questions about the nature of an important clinical problem, followed by systematic qualitative and quantitative inquiry and careful application of theoretical models borrowed from other disciplines. Since publication of the original theory in 1988, Mishel and others have carried out numerous empirical tests of the relationships among the major constructs in the model, applying and largely confirming the theory in many illness contexts. Mishel's reconceptualization of the theory in 1990 was deductive, in that it was generated from principles of chaos theory, and was confirmed by empirical evidence from qualitative studies that suggested that people's responses to uncertainty changed over time within the context of serious chronic illnesses. Thus Mishel's theory represents the bidirectional process by which theory both informs and is shaped by research.

ACCEPTANCE BY THE NURSING COMMUNITY

Practice

Mishel's theory describes a phenomenon experienced by acute and chronically ill individuals and their families. The theory has its beginning in Mishel's own experience with her father's battle with cancer. During his illness, he began to focus on events that seemed unimportant to those around him. When asked why he had chosen to focus on such events, he replied that when these activities were being done, he understood what was happening to him. Mishel believed this was her father's way of taking control and making sense out of an overwhelming situation. She knew early in the development of her concept and theory that nurses could identify the phenomenon from their experiences in caring for patients.

Several nurses have moved the theory from research to practice. Writing for an audience of critical care nurses, Hilton (1992) applied the theory in prescribing how to assess and intervene with patients experiencing uncertainty. Using examples of patients recovering from a cardiac event, Hilton explained how patients who misinterpret unclear physical symptoms may overprotect themselves by limiting physical activity that could be essential to their recovery. She further delineated how uncertainty can activate various types of coping to manage the situation, and described appropriate nursing interventions based on a thorough assessment of the patient's or family member's uncertainty.

Wurzbach (1992), writing for medical-surgical nurses, exemplified the experience of a woman hospitalized with a lump in her breast. Focusing on the woman's family history of breast cancer and no previous experience with hospitalization, Wurzbach counseled nurses to assess for certainty as well as uncertainty. Based on this assessment, management strategies in the form of nursing interventions were prescribed. Wurzbach cautioned nurses that intervention may not be appropriate in situations in which the patient experiences a moderate or optimal level of certainty-uncertainty. In these circumstances, patients may feel hopeful and may not require nursing intervention.

Mishel's Uncertainty in Illness Theory has also been applied to the practice of enterostomal therapy (ET) nursing. Righter (1995) described how trust in the ET nurse's knowledge and experiences helps patients develop a cognitive schema for the ostomy experience. Functioning as a credible authority, an antecedent of uncertainty, an ET nurse is able to intervene with patients to promote effective coping strategies.

Based on review of the database of the Managing Uncertainty in Illness Scale users (Mishel, 1997b), many are master's prepared clinicians seeking to understand the experience of uncertainty in a variety of clinical settings with different patient populations. The scale and theory were both used by clinicians from eight countries other than the United States.

Education

The theory has been widely used by graduate students as the theoretical framework for their theses and dissertations, as the topic of concept analysis, and for the critique of middle range nursing theory. Mishel uses the theory as an exemplar of how theory guides the development of nursing interventions in her doctoral level courses. Mishel is frequently an invited guest at schools of nursing seminars and symposia nationally and internationally, presenting both her empirical findings and the process of theory development for audiences of faculty and students.

Research

As described above, a large body of knowledge has been generated by researchers using the Uncertainty in Illness Theory and scales. With her colleagues at the University of Arizona, Mishel tested and confirmed the major components of the theoretical model, predominantly in samples of women with cancer. Currently her program of research encompasses testing psychoeducational nursing interventions derived from the theoretical model in samples of adults with breast and prostate cancer. The scales and theory are used by nurse researchers as well as by scientists from other disciplines to describe and explain the psychological responses of people experiencing uncertainty due to illness. The scales have been translated into 12 languages and applied in research throughout the world. Mishel (1997a, 1999) has reviewed the research conducted on uncertainty in both acute and chronic illness and has coauthored a review of the research on uncertainty in childhood illness (Stewart & Mishel, 2000). However, she notes that although many investigators have used one of the scales derived from the theory, most studies have not used the uncertainty in illness framework to guide their research.

FURTHER DEVELOPMENT

Mishel and her colleagues have used the original theory as the framework for seven federally funded nursing intervention studies. The intervention has proved effective in increasing cancer knowledge, reducing symptom burden, and improving quality of life in Mexican-American, white, and African-American women with breast cancer, and in African-American and white men with localized, advanced, or recurrent prostate cancer and their family members (Gil, Mishel, Belyea, Germino, Porter et al., 2004; Gil, Mishel, Belyea, Germino, Porter, et al., 2006; Gil, Mishel, Germino, Porter, Carlton-LaNey, et al., 2005; Mishel, Belyea, Germino, Stewart, Bailey, Robertson, et al., 2002; Mishel, Germino, Belyea, Stewart, Bailey, Mohler, et al., 2003). Data analysis is under way for the continuation study that extended the intervention to African-American and white men newly diagnosed with early stage prostate cancer and their primary support persons to aid in decision making. The applicability of the theory to the context of serious childhood illness has been supported in parents of children with HIV infection (Santacroce, Deatrick, & Ledlie, 2002) and in children undergoing treatment for cancer (Stewart, 2003). Bailey is using the theory to support research with a new and often silent disease, chronic hepatitis C (Bailey, Landerman, Barroso, Bixby, Mishel, et al., in press), and is preparing to test the intervention in patients awaiting liver transplant.

From qualitative data supporting the reconceptualized theory, Mishel and Fleury (1994) developed the Growth Through Uncertainty Scale (GTUS) to measure the new view of life that can emerge from continual uncertainty. The reconceptualized theory has also been used by researchers to understand the uncertainty experience of long-term survivors of breast cancer (Mast, 1998) and individuals with schizophrenia and their family members (Baier, 1995). The reconceptualized theory serves as the foundation for Mishel and colleagues' most recent nursing intervention study with women under 50 years of age facing the enduring uncertainties inherent in surviving breast cancer. Bailey has also used the theory, along with data from qualitative interviews with older men electing watchful waiting as treatment for their prostate cancer, to develop a nursing intervention helping men integrate uncertainty into their lives, view their lives in a positive perspective, and improve their quality of life (Bailey, Wallace, & Mishel, 2007). In the first trial of the Uncertainty Management Intervention for Watchful Waiting, men did come to see their lives in a new and positive light, reported their quality of life as higher than did the control group, and expected it to be high in the future (Bailey, Mishel, Belyea, Stewart, & Mohler, 2004). Wallace and Bailey are beginning to develop and pilot test a web based version of the intervention for men with prostate cancer undergoing active surveillance (previously referred to as watchful waiting) (Wallace, Bailey, Latini, Carroll, Klein, & Albertsen, 2007).

Mishel believes the most important product of her research program is the return of knowledge to practice. Toward that end, plans are under way to move the theoretically derived intervention into current practice, allowing nurses responsible for different types of patient populations to incorporate uncertainty assessment and intervention into their plans of care.

CRITIQUE

Clarity

Clarity refers to how well the theory is understood and how consistently the concepts are presented and conceptualized. Uncertainty is the primary concept of this theory and is defined as a cognitive state in which individuals are unable to determine the meaning of illness-related events (Mishel, 1988). The original theory postulates that managing uncertainty is critical to adaptation during illness and explains how individuals cognitively process illness-associated events and construct meaning from them.

The original theory's concepts are organized in a linear model around the following three major themes:

1. Antecedents of uncertainty
2. Process of uncertainty appraisal
3. Coping with uncertainty

The framework is easy to follow and is clear in all sections of the model. The antecedents of uncertainty include the stimuli frame, cognitive capacities, and structure providers. In the linear model, these antecedent variables have both a direct and indirect inverse relationship with uncertainty.

The second conceptual component of the model is appraisal. Uncertainty is seen as a neutral state, neither positive nor negative, until it has been appraised by the individual. Appraisal of uncertainty involves the following two processes: (1) inference and (2) illusion. Inference is constructed from the individual's personality disposition and includes learned resourcefulness, mastery, and locus of control. These characteristics contribute to an individual's confidence in the ability to handle life events. Illusion is defined as a belief constructed from uncertainty that considers the favorable aspects of a situation. Based on the appraisal process, uncertainty is viewed as either a danger or an opportunity. Uncertainty viewed as a danger results when the individual considers the possibility of a negative outcome. Uncertainty is viewed as an opportunity primarily through the use of illusion, but inference also can lead to the individual appraising the situation as having a positive outcome. In this situation, uncertainty is preferred and the individual remains hopeful.

Coping is the third theme of the original model of uncertainty. Coping occurs in two forms with the end result of adaptation. If uncertainty is appraised as a danger, then coping includes direct action, vigilance, and seeking information from mobilizing strategies, and it affects management using faith, disengagement, and cognitive support. If uncertainty is appraised as an opportunity, coping offers a buffer to maintain the uncertainty.

The original theory was reconceptualized in 1990 to incorporate the idea that chronic illness unfolds over time, possibly years, and with that, uncertainty is reappraised. The person is viewed as an open system exchanging energy within his or her environment, and rather than seeking a return to a stable state, chronically ill individuals may move toward a complex world orientation, thus forming a new meaning for their lives. If uncertainty can be framed as a normal view of life, it can become a positive force for multiple opportunities with resulting positive mood states. To achieve this, the individual must develop probabilistic thinking, which allows one to examine a variety of possibilities and to consider numerous ways of achieving them. The individual envisions a variety of responses to situations and realizes that life can change from day to day.

Mishel described this process as a new view of life in which uncertainty shifts from being seen as a danger to being viewed as an opportunity. To adopt this new view of life, the patient must be able to rely on social resources and healthcare providers who accept probabilistic thinking. The relationship between the healthcare provider and the patient must focus on recognizing continual uncertainty and teaching the patient how to use the uncertainty to generate different explanations for events. Hence the importance of structure providers, introduced in the original theory, is maintained in the reconceptualized model.

Despite the complexity and dimensionality of the two models, they are presented clearly and conceptualized comprehensively. Mishel published her measurement model in 1981, her original theoretical model in 1988, and her reconceptualized theory in 1990, and these publications fully explicate the model so that it is applied easily in clinical and research contexts.

Simplicity

The two uncertainty-in-illness models contain concepts comprising relationships that range from simple to complex and direct to indirect. Eleven major concepts are found in the three themes of the original theory, and several new concepts are introduced in the reconceptualized model. The antecedents of uncertainty are concise and their definitions are clear and simple. The appraisal component is complex because it considers cognitive processes along with beliefs and values held by the individual. The coping phase of the theory is also complex because it is dependent on the appraisal portion of the model and again involves different kinds of strategies targeted toward adaptation. The outcome portion of the model is differentiated into two conceptualizations of the theory, the first relating to patients with acute illness and the second representing an expansion of the model to accommodate patients with chronic illness. Although the models can hardly be called simple, overall the concept definitions and relationships are well operationalized and easily understood.

Generality

The theory explains how individuals construct meaning from illness-related events. It is broad and generalizable and can be used with individuals experiencing their own illnesses, as well as with spouses and parents of people experiencing illness-related uncertainty. The concept of credible authority can be applied to physicians, nurses, and other healthcare workers. The theory can be applied to many areas of nursing practice and has been used by clinicians for acute and chronic illnesses such as cancer, cardiac disease, and multiple sclerosis.

Empirical Precision

Mishel derived both theoretical models from her own program of research and that of others. Many of the concepts, assumptions, and relationships among variables draw support from empirical investigation. The concepts are well described and their relationships precisely constructed such that operational definitions have been written and tested. Testing of the theory has occurred in both research and clinical settings. The theory has allowed for development and testing of nursing interventions to manage uncertainty.

Derivable Consequences

Derivable consequences are determined by examining whether a theory guides research, informs practice, generates new ideas, and differentiates the focus of nursing from other professions. Mishel's work represents an exemplar of middle range theory that informs clinical practice within the encompassing context of acute and chronic illness. The theory has likewise generated considerable empirical research in adults dealing with their own illness or that of a family member and continue to stimulate new research directions, such as uncertainty in ill children, in older men electing watchful waiting as their treatment for prostate cancer, and in healthcare providers informing patients of treatment choices in conditions with uncertain prognoses. Mishel believes that by defining and conceptualizing an important clinical problem, her work supports and enriches nursing practice. The Uncertainty in Illness Theory and its reconceptualization represent frameworks derived from and for practice, a process that is essential to nursing as a practice discipline.

SUMMARY

The Uncertainty in Illness Theory provides a comprehensive framework within which to view the experience of acute and chronic illness and to organize nursing interventions to promote optimal adjustment. The theory helps explain the stresses associated with the diagnosis and treatment of a major illness or chronic condition, the processes by which individuals assess and respond to the uncertainty inherent in an illness experience, and the importance of professional caregivers in providing information and supporting individuals in understanding and managing uncertainty. The reconceptualized theory addresses the unique context of continual uncertainty and thereby expands the original theory to encompass the ongoing uncertain trajectory of many life-threatening and chronic illnesses. The original theory and its reconceptualization are well explicated, derive support from both sound theoretical foundations and extensive empirical confirmation, and can be applied in many illness contexts to support evidence-based nursing practice.

Case Study

Part 1: Original Theory

Rosie, a 45-year-old mother of three, has been diagnosed with stage III breast cancer. A mass was detected in her left breast during her annual gynecological appointment and she has undergone an extensive diagnostic workup, including mammography and sentinel node biopsy. She was referred by her primary physician to a comprehensive breast cancer program at a regional medical center that was two hours from her home. The multidisciplinary team has recommended that Rosie undergo preoperative chemotherapy, followed by partial mastectomy and reconstructive surgery. Rosie's husband has accompanied her to most of her medical encounters but was unable to attend the final conference, where the treatment recommendations were made.

Lily, the advanced practice nurse coordinating Rosie's care (structure provider-credible authority), directs her interventions toward addressing the many sources of uncertainty for Rosie and her family, including lack of information about treatment options and outcomes (event familiarity), unfamiliarity with the treatment environment (event familiarity), expectations for chemotherapy side effects and postoperative recovery (symptom pattern), impact of treatment on family relationships, and prognosis. In particular, Lily addresses Rosie's many questions about why her treatment plan is different from what her primary physician told her to expect (event congruence) and how she will manage her family life while undergoing treatment. Lily provides an audiotape of the treatment conference so that Rosie's husband (structure provider-social support) can hear what took place and can support Rosie in asking questions and understanding the information provided. Lily's support for Rosie and her family continues throughout Rosie's treatment course, and she periodically reassesses the sources of uncertainty and the strategies that Rosie and her family use to manage them.

Part 2: Reconceptualized Theory

Two years after her breast cancer diagnosis, Rosie returns to the center for a follow-up appointment. Lily asks Rosie to reflect on her cancer experience. Although Rosie describes the time of diagnosis and treatment as chaotic and dominated by uncertainty, she wonders how she and her family got through it, but she tells Lily that gradually she came to see the cancer experience as providing new meaning to her life and helping her set priorities. She left a job she was dissatisfied with and now directs her energy toward her relationships with her teen-age children. Rosie and her husband recently enjoyed a long-postponed second honeymoon trip to Hawaii. She tells Lily that she now embraces each day as an opportunity to live life and enrich the lives of her children.

CRITICAL THINKING *Activities*

1. Imagine that you are interviewing a client who is new to your practice. Think about the kind of questions you would ask to assess the level of uncertainty about the health issue that brought the client to you. What would you want to know about this person's perceptions of the current situation, supportive relationships, and previous experiences with health and illness?
2. You are working with a young woman who has been living with multiple sclerosis for 6 years. During an exacerbation of her disease, she focuses on her plans for going to law school. One of your colleagues suggests that she may be in denial about the severity of her illness. How might you use the reconceptualized Uncertainty in Illness Theory to propose an alternative interpretation of her perspective?

POINTS FOR *Further Study*

- Mishel, M. (2008). Portraits of Excellence: The Nurse Theorist Series, Vol 2, Fitne, Inc., Athens, Ohio.
- Managing Uncertainty in Cancer Website: http://nursing.unc.edu/muic/index.html
- Research Tested Interventions for Practice (RTIP), NCI. Managing Uncertainty in Older Long-term Breast Cancer Survivors Website: http://rtips.cancer.gov/rtips/index.do and click on "survivorship" link

REFERENCES

Baier, M. (1995). Uncertainty of illness for persons with schizophrenia. *Issues in Mental Health Nursing, 16*, 201-212.

Bailey, D. E., Landerman, L, Barroso, J., Bixby, P., Mishel, M. H., Muir, A., Strickland, L., &. Clipp, E. (in press). Uncertainty, symptoms and quality of life in persons with chronic hepatitis C undergoing watchful waiting. *Psychosomatics.*

Bailey, D. E., Mishel, M. H., Belyea, M., Stewart, J. L., & Mohler, J. (2004). Uncertainty intervention for watchful waiting in prostate cancer. *Cancer Nursing, 27*(5), 339-346.

Bailey, D. E., Wallace, M., & Mishel, M. H. (2007). Watching, waiting, and uncertainty in prostate cancer. *Journal of Clinical Nursing, 16*, 734-741.

Becker, G., Jason-Bjerklie, S., Benner, P., Slobin, K., & Ferketich, S. (1993). The dilemma of seeking urgent care: Asthma episodes and emergency service use. *Social Science and Medicine, 37*, 305-313.

Braden, C. J. (1990). A test of the self-help model: Learned response to chronic illness experience. *Nursing Research, 39*, 42-47.

Brett, K. M., & Davies, E. M. B. (1988). "What does it mean?" Sibling and parental appraisals of childhood leukemia. *Cancer Nursing, 11*, 329-338.

Brown, M. A., & Powell-Cope, G. M. (1991). AIDS family caregiving: Transitions through uncertainty. *Nursing Research, 40*, 338-345.

Budner, S. (1962). Intolerance of ambiguity as a personality variable. *Journal of Personality, 30*, 29-50.

Carter, B. J. (1993). Long-term survivors of breast cancer. *Cancer Nursing, 16*(5), 354-361.

Charmaz, K. (1995). Identity dilemmas of chronically ill men. In D. Sobo & D. F. Gordon (Eds.), *Men's health and illness: Gender, power, and the body* (pp. 266-291). Thousand Oaks, CA: Sage.

Cohen, M. H. (1993). The unknown and the unknowable—Managing sustained uncertainty. *Western Journal of Nursing Research, 15*, 77-96.

Comaroff, J., & Maguire, P. (1981). Ambiguity and the search for meaning: Childhood leukaemia in the modern clinical context. *Social Science and Medicine, 15B*, 115-123.

Failla, S., Kuper, B. C., Nick, T. G., & Lee, F. A. (1996). Adjustment of women with systemic lupus erythematosus. *Applied Nursing Research, 9*, 87-96.

Fleury, J., Kimbrell, L. C., & Kruszewski, C. (1995). Life after cardiac event: Women's experience in healing. *Heart & Lung, 24*, 474-482.

Gelatt, H. B. (1989). Positive uncertainty: A new decision-making framework for counseling. *Journal of Consulting & Clinical Psychology, 36*, 252-256.

Gil, K. M., Mishel, M. H., Belyea, M., Germino, B., Porter, L. S., Stewart, J. L., et al. (2004). Triggers of uncertainty about recurrence and long term treatment side effects in older African American and Caucasian breast cancer survivors. *Oncology Nursing Forum, 31*, 633-639.

Gil, K. M., Mishel, M. H., Belyea, M., Germino, B., Porter, L. S., et al. (2006). Benefits of the uncertainty management intervention for African American and white older breast cancer survivors: 20-month outcomes. *International Journal of Behavioral Medicine, 13*, 286-294.

Gil, K. M., Mishel, M. H., Germino, B., Porter, L. S., Carlton-LaNey, I., et al. (2005). Uncertainty management intervention for older African American and Caucasian long-term breast cancer survivors. *Journal of Psychosocial Oncology, 23*, 2-3, 3-21.

Green, J. M., & Murton, F. E. (1996). Diagnosis of Duchenne muscular dystrophy: Parents' experiences and satisfaction. *Child: Care, Health, and Development, 22*, 113-128.

Grootenhuis, M. A., & Last, B. L. (1997). Parents' emotional reactions related to different prospects for the survival of their children with cancer. *Journal of Psychosocial Oncology, 15*, 43-61.

Hilton, B. A. (1988). The phenomenon of uncertainty in women with breast cancer. *Issues in Mental Health Nursing, 9*, 217-238.

Hilton, B. A. (1992). Perceptions of uncertainty: Its relevance to life-threatening and chronic illness. *Critical Care Nurse, 12*, 70-73.

Hilton, B. A. (1996). Getting back to normal: The family experience during early stage breast cancer. *Oncology Nursing Forum, 23*, 605-614.

Hinds, P. S., Birenbaum, L. K., Clarke-Steffen, L., Quargnenti, A., Kreissman, S., Kazak, A., et al. (1996). Coming to terms: Parents' response to a first cancer recurrence in their child. *Nursing Research, 45*, 148-153.

Janson-Bjerklie, S., Ferketich, S., & Benner, P. (1993). Predicting the outcomes of living with asthma. *Research in Nursing and Health, 16*, 241-250.

Jessop, D. J., & Stein, R. E. K. (1985). Uncertainty and its relation to the psychological and social correlates of chronic illness in children. *Social Science and Medicine, 20*, 993-999.

Katz, A. (1996). Gaining a new perspective of life as a consequence of uncertainty in HIV infection. *JANAC, 7*, 51-60.

Lang, A. (1987). Nursing of families with an infant who requires home apnea monitoring. *Issues in Comprehensive Pediatric Nursing, 10*, 123-133.

Lazarus, R. S., & Folkman, S. (1984). *Stress, appraisal, and coping.* New York: Springer Publishing.

Mason, C. (1985). The production and effects of uncertainty with special reference to diabetes mellitus. *Social Science and Medicine, 21*, 1329-1334.

Mast, M. E. (1995). Adult uncertainty in illness: A critical review of the literature. *Scholarly Inquiry for Nursing Practice, 9*, 3-24.

Mast, M. E. (1998). Survivors of breast cancer: Illness uncertainty, positive reappraisal, and emotional distress. *Oncology Nursing Forum, 25*, 555-562.

Miles, M. S., Funk, S. G., & Kasper, M. A. (1992). The stress response of mothers and fathers of preterm infants. *Research in Nursing and Health, 15*, 261-269.

Mishel, M. H. (1981). The measurement of uncertainty in illness. *Nursing Research, 30*, 258-263.

Mishel, M. H. (1988). Uncertainty in illness. *Image: The Journal of Nursing Scholarship, 20*, 225-231.

Mishel, M. H. (1990). Reconceptualization of the uncertainty in illness theory. *Image: The Journal of Nursing Scholarship, 22*, 256-262.

Mishel, M. H. (1997a). Uncertainty in acute illness. *Annual Review of Nursing Research, 15*, 57-80.

Mishel, M. H. (1997b). *Uncertainty in illness scales manual.* Available upon request from the author at http://nursing.unc.edu/music/instruments.html

Mishel, M. H. (1999). Uncertainty in chronic illness. *Annual Review of Nursing Research, 17*, 269-294.

Mishel, M. H., Belyea, M., Germino, B. B., Stewart, J. L., Bailey, D. E., Robertson, C, et al. (2002). Helping patients with localized prostate carcinoma manage uncertainty and treatment side effects—Nurse-delivered psychoeducational intervention over the telephone. *Cancer, 94*, 1854-1866.

Mishel, M. H., & Braden, C. J. (1987). Uncertainty: A mediator between support and adjustment. *Western Journal of Nursing Research, 9*, 43-57.

Mishel, M. H., & Braden, C. J. (1988). Finding meaning: Antecedents of uncertainty in illness. *Nursing Research, 37*, 98-103.

Mishel, M. H., & Fleury, J. (1994). *Psychometric testing of the growth through uncertainty scale.* Unpublished data, University of North Carolina at Chapel Hill.

Mishel, M. H., Germino, B. B., Belyea, M., Stewart, J. L., Bailey, D. E., Mohler, J., et al. (2003). Moderators of an uncertainty management intervention for men with localized prostate cancer. *Nursing Research, 52*, 89-97.

Mishel, M. H., & Murdaugh, C. L. (1987). Family adjustment to heart transplantation: Redesigning the dream. *Nursing Research, 36*, 332-338.

Mishel, M. H., Padilla, G., Grant, M., & Sorenson, D. S. (1991). Uncertainty in illness theory: A replication of the mediating effects of mastery and coping. *Nursing Research, 40*, 236-240.

Mishel, M. H., & Sorenson, D. S. (1991). Coping with uncertainty in gynecological cancer: A test of the mediating function of mastery and coping. *Nursing Research, 40*, 167-171.

Murray, J. (1993). Coping with the uncertainty of uncontrolled epilepsy. *Seizure, 2*, 167-178.

Nelson, J. P. (1996). Struggling to gain meaning: Living with the uncertainty of breast cancer. *ANS Advances in Nursing Science, 18*(3), 59-76.

Nyhlin, K. T. (1990). Diabetic patients facing long-term complications: Coping with uncertainty. *Journal of Advanced Nursing, 15*, 1021-1029.

O'Brien, R. A., Wineman, N. M., & Nealon, N. R. (1995). Correlates of the caregiving process in multiple sclerosis. *Scholarly Inquiry for Nursing Practice, 9*, 323-342.

Padilla, G. V., Mishel, M. H., & Grant, M. M. (1992). Uncertainty, appraisal, and quality of life. *Quality of Life Research, 1*, 155-165.

Pelusi, J. (1997). The lived experience of surviving breast cancer. *Oncology Nursing Forum, 24*, 1343-1353.

Regan-Kubinski, M. J., Sharts-Hopko, N. (1995). Illness cognition of HIV-infected mothers. *Issues in Mental Health Nursing, 16*, 327-344.

Righter, B. M. (1995). Ostomy care: Uncertainty and the role of the credible authority during an ostomy experience. *Journal of Wound, Ostomy, and Continence Nurses Society, 22*, 100-104.

Santacroce, S. J., Deatrick, J. A., & Ledlie, S. W. (2002). Redefining treatment: How biological mothers manage their children's treatment for perinatally acquired HIV. *AIDS Care, 14*, 47-60.

Schepp, K. G. (1991). Factors influencing the coping effort of mothers of hospitalized children. *Nursing Research, 40*, 42-46.

Sharkey, T. (1995). The effects of uncertainty in families with children who are chronically ill. *Home Healthcare Nurse, 13*(4), 37-42.

Stewart, J. L. (2003). "Getting used to it": Children finding the ordinary and routine in the uncertain context of cancer. *Qualitative Health Research, 13*, 394-407.

Stewart, J. L., & Mishel, M. H. (2000). Uncertainty in childhood illness: A synthesis of the parent and child literature. *Scholarly Inquiry for Nursing Practice, 14*, 299-320.

Tomlinson, P. S., Kirschbaum, M., Harbaugh, B., & Anderson, K. H. (1996). The influence of illness severity and family resources on maternal uncertainty during critical pediatric hospitalization. *American Journal of Critical Care, 5*, 140-146.

Turner, M. A., Tomlinson, P. S., & Harbaugh, B. L. (1990). Parental uncertainty in critical care hospitalization of children. *Maternal Child Nursing Journal, 19*, 45-62.

Van Riper, M., & Selder, F. E. (1989). Parental responses to the birth of a child with Down syndrome. *Loss, Grief, & Care, 3*(3-4), 59-76.

Wallace, M., Bailey, D., Latini, D. M., Carroll, P. R., Klein, E. A., & Albertsen, P. E. (2007). Active surveillance for older men with prostate cancer: Experiences, measurement & interventions. *The Gerontologist 47 (Special Issue I)* pp. 753-754

Warburton, D. M. (1979). Physiological aspects of information processing and stress. In V. Hamilton & D. M. Warburton (Eds.), *Human stress and cognition: An information processing approach* (pp. 33-65). New York: John Wiley & Sons.

Weitz, R. (1989). Uncertainty and the lives of persons with AIDS. *Journal of Health and Social Behavior, 30*, 270-281.

Wineman, N. (1990). Adaptation to multiple sclerosis: The role of social support, functional disability, and perceived uncertainty. *Nursing Research, 39*, 294-299.

Wineman, N. M., O'Brien, R. A., Nealon, N. R., & Kaskel, B. (1993). Congruence in uncertainty between individuals with multiple sclerosis and their spouses. *Journal of Neuroscience Nursing, 25*, 356-361.

Wurzbach, M. E. (1992). Assessment and intervention for certainty and uncertainty. *Nursing Forum, 27*, 29-35.

BIBLIOGRAPHY

Primary Sources

Book Chapters

Mishel, M. H. (1993). Living with chronic illness: Living with uncertainty. In S. G. Funk, E. M. Tornquist, M. T. Champagne, & R. A. Weise (Eds.), Key aspects of caring for the chronically ill, hospital and home (pp. 46-58). New York: Springer.

Mishel, M. H. (1998). Methodological studies: Instrument development. In P. Brink & M. Woods (Eds.), Advanced design in nursing research (pp. 235-282) (2nd Ed.). Beverly Hills, CA: Sage Press.

Mishel, M. H. (2008). Conducting evidence-based intervention. In *Advancing Oncology Nursing Science.* Pittsburgh, PA: Oncology Nursing Society Publications.

Mishel, M. H., & Clayton, M. F. (2008). Uncertainty in illness theories. In M. J. Smith & P. Liehr (Eds.), *Middle range theory in advanced practice nursing* (pp. 55-84) New York: Springer Publishing.

Mishel, M. H., Germino, B. G., Belyea, M., Harris, L., Stewart, J., Bailey, D. E. Jr., Mohler, J., & Robertson, C. (2001). Helping patients with localized prostate cancer: Managing after treatment. In S. G. Funk, E. M. Tornquist, J. Leeman, M. S. Miles, & J. S. Harrell (Eds.), Key aspects of preventing and managing chronic illness (pp. 235-246). New York: Springer Publishing.

Journal Articles

Amoako, E. P., Skelly, A. H., & Mishel, M. M. (2004). Identifying intervention strategies for older African-American women to manage uncertainty in diabetes. *Diabetes, 53*, A513.

Badger, T. A., Braden, C. J., Longman, A. J., Mishel, M. H. (1999). Depression burden, self-help interventions, and social support in women receiving treatment for breast cancer. *Journal of Psychosocial Oncology, 17*(2), 17-35.

Badger, T. A., Braden, C. J., & Mishel, M. H. (2001). Depression burden, self-help interventions, and side effect experience in women receiving treatment for breast cancer. *Oncology Nursing Forum, 28*, 567-574.

Badger, T. A., Braden, C. J., Mishel, M. H., & Longman, A. (2004). Depression burden, psychological adjustment, and quality of life in women with breast cancer: Patterns over time. *Research in Nursing & Health, 27*, 19-28.

Bailey, D., Stewart, J., & Mishel, M. (2005). Watchful waiting in prostate cancer: Where can older men find support? *Oncology Nursing Forum, 32*, 177.

Bailey, D. E., Mishel, M. H., Belyea, M., Stewart, J. L., & Mohler, J. (2004). Uncertainty intervention for watchful waiting in prostate cancer. *Cancer Nursing, 27*, 339-346.

Bailey, D. E., Wallace, M., & Mishel, M. H. (2007). Watching, waiting, and uncertainty in prostate cancer. *Journal of Clinical Nursing, 16*, 734-741.

Braden, C. J., & Mishel, M. H. (2000). Highlights of the self-help intervention project (SHIP): Health-related quality of life during breast cancer treatment. *Innovations in Breast Cancer Care, 5*, 51-54.

Braden, C. J., Mishel, M. H., Longman, A. J., & Burns, L. R. (1998). Self-help intervention project: Women receiving treatment for breast cancer. *Cancer Practice, 6*, 87-98.

Clayton, M. F., Mishel, M. H., & Belyea, M. (2006). Testing a model of symptoms, communication, uncertainty and well-being, in older breast cancer survivors. *Research in Nursing and Health, 29*, 18-39.

Gil, K. M., Mishel, M. H., Belyea, M., Germino, B., Porter, L. S., et al. (2004). Triggers of uncertainty about recurrence and long term treatment side effects in older African American and Caucasian breast cancer survivors. *Oncology Nursing Forum, 31*, 633-639.

Gil, K. M., Mishel, M. H., Belyea, M., Germino, B., Porter, L. S., et al. (2006). Benefits of the uncertainty management intervention for African American and white older breast cancer survivors: 20-month outcomes. *International Journal of Behavioral Medicine, 13*, 286-294.

Gil, K. M., Mishel, M. H., Germino, B., Porter, L. S., Carlton-LaNey, I, et al. (2005). Uncertainty management intervention for older African American and Caucasian long-term breast cancer survivors. *Journal of Psychosocial Oncology, 23*, 2-3, 3-21.

Germino, B. B., Mishel, M. H., Belyea, M., Harris, L., Ware, A., & Mohler, J. (1998). Uncertainty in prostate cancer: Ethnic and family patterns. *Cancer Practice, 6*, 107-113.

Harris, L., Belyea, M., Mishel, M., & Germino, B. (2003). Issues in revising research instruments for use with Southern populations. *Journal of the National Black Nurses Association, 14*, 44-50.

Longman, A., Braden, C. J., & Mishel, M. H. (1997). Pattern of association over time of side-effects burden, self-help and self-care in women with breast cancer. *Oncology Nursing Forum, 24*, 1555-1560.

Mishel, M. H. (1981). The measurement of uncertainty in illness. *Nursing Research, 30*, 258-263.

Mishel, M. H. (1983). Parents' perception of uncertainty concerning their hospitalized child: Reliability and validity of a scale. *Nursing Research, 32*, 324-330.

Mishel, M. H. (1988). Uncertainty in illness. *Image: Journal of Nursing Scholarship 20*, 225-232.

Mishel, M. H. (1990). Reconceptualization of the Uncertainty in Illness Theory. *Image: Journal of Nursing Scholarship, 22*, 256-262.

Mishel, M. H. (1997). Uncertainty in acute illness. *Annual Review of Nursing Research, 15*, 57-80.

Mishel, M. H. (1999). Uncertainty in chronic illness. *Annual Review of Nursing Research, 17*, 269-294.

Mishel, M. H., Belyea, M., Germino, B. B., Stewart, J. L., Bailey, D. E., Robertson, C., et al. (2002). Helping patients with localized prostate carcinoma manage uncertainty and treatment side effects—Nurse-delivered psychoeducational intervention over the telephone. *Cancer, 94*, 1854-1866.

Mishel, M. H., Germino, B. B., Belyea, M., Stewart, J. L., Bailey, D. E., Mohler, J., et al. (2003). Moderators of an uncertainty management intervention for men with localized prostate cancer. *Nursing Research, 52*, 89-97.

Mishel, M. H., Germino, B. B., Gilk, K. M., Belyea, M., LaNey, I. C., et al. (2005). Benefits from an uncertainty management intervention for African-American and Caucasian older long-term breast cancer survivors. *Psychooncology, 14*, 962-978.

Porter, L. S., Clayton, M. R., Belyea, M., Mishel, M., Gil, K. M., et al. (2006). Predicting negative mood state and personal growth in African American and white long-term breast cancer survivors. *Annals of Behavioral Medicine, 31*, 195-204.

Porter, L. S., Mishel, M., Neelon, V., Belyea, M., Pisano, E., et al. (2003). Cortisol levels and responses to mammography screening in breast cancer survivors: A pilot study. *Psychosomatic Medicine, 65*, 842-848.

Schroeder, J. C., Bensen, J. T., Su, L. J., Mishel, M., Ivanova, A., et al. (2006). The North Carolina Louisiana Prostate Cancer Project (PCaP): Methods and design of a multidisciplinary population-based cohort study of racial differences in prostate cancer outcomes. *Prostate, 66*, 1162-1176.

Stewart, J. L., Lynn, M. R., & Mishel, M. H. (2005). Evaluating content validity for children's self-report instruments using children as content experts. *Nursing Research, 54*, 414-418.

Stewart, J. L., & Mishel, M. H. (2000). Uncertainty in childhood illness: A synthesis of the parent and child literature. *Scholarly Inquiry for Nursing Practice, 14*, 299-320.

Secondary Sources

Selected Recent Publications Citing Mishel's Work

Amoako, E., & Skelly, A. H. (2007). Managing uncertainty in diabetes: an intervention for older African American women. *Ethnicity & Disease, 17*(3), 515-521.

Anderson, G. (2007). Patient decision-making for clinical genetics. *Nursing Inquiry, 14*(1), 13-22.

Apostolo, J. L. A., Viveiros, C. S. C., Nunes, H. I. R., & Domingues, H. R. F. (2007). Illness uncertainty and treatment motivation in type 2 diabetes patients. *Revista Latino-Americana De Enfermagem, 15*(4), 575-582.

Bailey, D. E., Jr., & Wallace, M. (2007). Critical review: Is watchful waiting a viable management option for older men with prostate cancer? *American Journal of Men's Health, 1(1),* 18-28.

Baty, B. J., Dudley, W. N., Musters, A., & Kinney, A. Y. (2006). Uncertainty in BRCAI cancer susceptibility testing. *American Journal of Medical Genetics Part C-Seminars in Medical Genetics, 142C*(4), 241-250.

Bishop, M., Stenhoff, D. M., & Shepard, L. (2007). Psychosocial adaptation and quality of life in multiple sclerosis: Assessment of the disability centrality model. *Journal of Rehabilitation, 73*(1), 3-12.

Boehmke, M. M., & Dickerson, S. S. (2006). The diagnosis of breast cancer: Transition from health to illness. *Oncology Nursing Forum, 33*(6), 1121-1127.

Bonner, M. J., Hardy, K. K., Guill, A. B., McLaughlin, C., Schweitzer, H., & Carter, K. (2006). Development and validation of the parent experience of child illness. *Journal of Pediatric Psychology, 31*(3), 310-321.

Brashers, D. E., Neidig, J. L., & Goldsmith, D. J. (2004). Social support and the management of uncertainty for people living with HIV or AIDS. *Health Communication, 16*(3), 305-331.

Brown, R. T., Fuemmeler, B., Anderson, D., Jamieson, S., Simonian, S., Hall, R. K., et al. (2007). Adjustment of children and their mothers with breast cancer. *Journal of Pediatric Psychology, 32*(3), 297-308.

Bunkers, S. S. (2007). The experience of feeling unsure for women at end-of-life. *Nursing Science Quarterly, 20*(1), 56-63.

Carpentier, M. Y., Mullins, L. L., Wagner, J. L., Wolfe-Christensen, C., & Chaney, J. M. (2007). Examination of the cognitive diathesis-stress conceptualization of the hopelessness theory of depression in children with chronic illness: The moderating influence of illness uncertainty. *Childrens Health Care, 36*(2), 181-196.

Chung, B. P. M., Wong, T. K. S., Suen, E. S. B., & Chung, J. W. Y. (2005). SARS: Caring for patients in Hong Kong. *Journal of Clinical Nursing, 14*(4), 510-517.

Dale, W., Bilir, P., Han, M., & Meltzer, D. (2005). The role of anxiety in prostate carcinoma: A structured review of the literature. *Cancer, 104*(3), 467-478.

Davidson, P. M., Dracup, K., Phillips, J., Padilla, G., & Daly, J. (2007). Maintaining hope in transition: A Theoretical framework to guide interventions for people with heart failure. *Journal of Cardiovascular Nursing, 22*(1), 58-64.

Dillard, J. P., & Carson, C. L. (2005). Uncertainty management following a positive newborn screening for cystic fibrosis. *Journal of Health Communication, 10*(1), 57-76.

Donovan-Kicken, E., & Bute, J. J. (2008). Uncertainty of social network members in the case of communication—debilitating illness or injury. *Qualitative Health Research, 18*(1), 5-18.

Eggly, S., Penner, L., Albrecht, T. L., Cline, R. J. W., Foster, T., Naughton, M., et al. (2006). Discussing bad news in the outpatient oncology clinic: Rethinking current communication guidelines. *Journal of Clinical Oncology, 24*(4), 716-719.

Elphee, E. E. (2008). Understanding the concept of uncertainty in patients with indolent lymphoma. *Oncology Nursing Forum. 35(3),* 449-454.

Flattery, M. P., Pinson, J. M., Savage, L., & Salyer, J. (2005). Living with pulmonary artery hypertension: Patients' experiences. *Heart & Lung, 34*(2), 99-107.

Flemme, I., Edvardsson, N., Hinic, H., Jinhage, B. M., Dalman, M., & Fridlund, B. (2005). Long-term quality of life and uncertainty in patients living with an implantable cardioverter defibrillator. *Heart & Lung, 34*(6), 386-392.

Gill, E. A., & Babrow, A. S. (2007). To hope or to know: Coping with uncertainty and ambivalence in women's magazine breast cancer articles. *Journal of Applied Communication Research, 35*(2), 133-155.

Giske, T., & Artinian, B. (2008). Patterns of 'balancing between hope and despair' in the diagnostic phase: a grounded theory study of patients on a gastroenterology ward. *Journal of Advanced Nursing 62*(1), 22-31.

Giske, T., & Gjengedal, E. (2007). "Preparative waiting" and coping theory with patients going through gastric diagnosis. *Journal of Advanced Nursing, 57*(1), 87-94.

Haugh, K. H., & Salyer, J. (2007). Needs of patients and families during the wait for a donor heart. *Heart & Lung, 36*(5), 319-329.

Hebert, R. S., Prigerson, H. G., Schulz, R., & Arnold, R. M. (2006). Preparing Caregivers for the death of a loved one: A theoretical framework and suggestions for future research. *Journal of Palliative Medicine, 9*(5), 1164-1171.

Helgeson, V. S., Snyder, P., & Seltman, H. (2004). Psychological and physical adjustment to breast cancer over 4 years: Identifying distinct trajectories of change. *Health Psychology, 23*(1), 3-15.

Iseri, P. K., Ozten, E., & Aker, A. T. (2006). Posttraumatic stress disorder and major depressive disorder is common in parents of children with epilepsy. *Epilepsy & Behavior, 8*(1), 250-255.

Johnson, L. M., Zautra, A. J., & Davis, M. C. (2006). The role of illness uncertainty on coping with fibromyalgia symptoms. *Health Psychology, 25*(6), 696-703.

Jordan, A. L., Eccleston, C., & Osborn, M. (2007). Being a parent of the adolescent with complex chronic pain: An interpretative phenomenological analysis. *European Journal of Pain, 11*(1), 49-56.

Jurgens, C. Y. (2006). Somatic awareness, uncertainty, and delay in care-seeking in acute heart failure. *Research in Nursing & Health, 29*(2), 74-86.

Kagan, I., & Bar-Tal, Y. (2008). The effect of preoperative uncertainty and anxiety on short-term recovery after elective arthroplasty. *Journal of Clinical Nursing, 17*(5), 576-583.

Kang, Y. (2005). Effects of uncertainty on perceived health status in patients with atrial fibrillation. *Nursing in Critical Care 10*(4), 184-191.

Kang, Y. (2006). Effect of uncertainty on depression in patients with newly diagnosed atrial fibrillation. *Progress in Cardiovascular Nursing 21*(2), 83-88.

Kang, Y., Daly, B. J., & Kim, J. S. (2004). Uncertainty and its antecedents in patients with atrial fibrillation. *Western Journal of Nursing Research, 26*(7), 770-783.

Kasper, J., Geiger, F., Freiberger, S., & Schmidt, A. (2008). Decision-related uncertainties perceived by people with cancer: modeling the subject of shared decision making. *Psycho-Oncology, 17*(1), 42-48.

Lee, Y. L., Santacroce, S. J., & Sadler, L. (2007). Predictors of healthy behaviour in long-term survivors of childhood cancer. *Journal of Clinical Nursing, 16*(11C), 285-295.

Lemaire, G. S. (2004). More than just menstrual cramps: Symptoms and uncertainty among women with endometriosis. *Jognn-Journal of Obstetric Gynecologic and Neonatal Nursing, 33*(1), 71-79.

Lenhard, W., Breitenbach, E., Ebert, H., Schindelhauer-Deutscher, H. J., & Henn, W. (2005). Psychological benefit of diagnostic certainty for mothers of children with disabilities: Lessons from Down syndrome. *American Journal of Medical Genetics Part A, 133A*(2), 170-175.

Liu, L. N., Li, C. Y., Tang, S. T., Huang, C. S., & Chiou, A. F. (2006). Role of continuing supportive cares in increasing social support and reducing perceived uncertainty among women with newly diagnosed breast cancer in Taiwan. *Cancer Nursing, 29*(4), 273-282.

Livneh, H., & Antonak, R. F. (2005). Psychosocial adaptation to chronic illness and disability: A primer for counselors. *Journal of Counseling and Development, 83*(1), 12-20.

Lockwood-Rayermann, S. (2006). Survivorship issues in ovarian cancer: A review. *Oncology Nursing Forum, 33*(3), 553-562.

Malbasa, T., Kodish, E., & Santacroce, S. J. (2007). Adolescent adherence to oral therapy for leukemia: A focus group study. *Journal of Pediatric Oncology Nursing, 24*(3), 139-151.

Martens, T. Z., & Emed, J. D. (2007). The experiences and challenges of pregnant women coping with thrombophilia. *Jognn-Journal of Obstetric Gynecologic and Neonatal Nursing, 36*(1), 55-62.

McCormick, K. M., Naimark, B. J., & Tate, R. B. (2006). Uncertainty, symptom distress, anxiety, and functional status in patients awaiting coronary artery bypass surgery. *Heart & Lung, 35*(1), 34-45.

McNulty, K., Livneh, H., & Wilson, L. M. (2004). Perceived uncertainty, spiritual well-being, and psychosocial adaptation in individuals with multiple sclerosis. *Rehabilitation Psychology, 49*(2), 91-99.

Mu, P. F. (2005). Paternal reactions to a child with epilepsy: uncertainty, coping strategies, and depression. *Journal of Advanced Nursing, 49*(4), 367-376.

Mullins, L. L., Wolfe-Christensen, C., Pai, A. L. H., Carpentier, M. Y., Gillaspy, S., Cheek, J., et al. (2007). The relationship of parental overprotection, perceived child vulnerability, and parenting stress to uncertainty in youth with chronic illness. *Journal of Pediatric Psychology, 32*(8), 973-982.

Pai, A. L. H., Mullins, L. L., Drotar, D., Burant, C., Wagner, J., & Chaney, J. M. (2007). Exploratory and confirmatory factor analysis of the child uncertainty in illness scale among children with chronic illness. *Journal of Pediatric Psychology, 32*(3), 288-296.

Penrod, J. (2007). Living with uncertainty: concept advancement. *Journal of Advanced Nursing, 57*(6), 658-667.

Persson, E., Severinsson, E., & Hellstrom, A. L. (2004). Spouses' perceptions of and reactions to living with a partner who has undergone surgery for rectal cancer resulting in a stoma. *Cancer Nursing, 27*(1), 85-90.

Pickles, T., Ruether, J. D., Weir, L., Carlson, L., & Jakulj, F. (2007). Psychosocial barriers to active surveillance for the management of early prostate cancer and a strategy for increased acceptance. *BJU International, 100*(3), 544-551.

Politi, M. C., Han, P. K. J., & Col, N. F. (2007). Communicating the uncertainty of harms and benefits of medical interventions. *Medical Decision Making, 27*(5), 681-695.

Puterman, J., & Cadell, S. (2008). Timing is everything: The experience of parental cancer for young adult daughters—A pilot study. *Journal of Psychosocial Oncology, 26*(2), 103-121.

Reich, J. W., Johnson, L. M., Zautra, A. J., & Davis, M. C. (2006). Uncertainty of illness relationships with mental health and coping processes in fibromyalgia patients. *Journal of Behavioral Medicine, 29*(4), 307-316.

Rosen, N. O., Knauper, B., & Sammut, J. (2007). Do individual differences in intolerance of uncertainty affect health monitoring? *Psychology & Health, 22*(4), 413-430.

Rybarczyk, B., Grady, K. L., Naftel, D. C., Kirklin, J. K., White-Williams, C., Kobashigawa, J., et al. (2007). Emotional adjustment 5 years after heart transplant: A multisite study. *Rehabilitation Psychology, 52*(2), 206-214.

Santacroce, S. J., & Lee, Y. L. (2006). Uncertainty, posttraumatic stress, and health behavior in young adult childhood cancer survivors. *Nursing Research, 55*(4), 259-266.

Scordo, K. A. (2005). Mitral valve prolapse syndrome health concerns, symptoms, and treatments. *Western Journal of Nursing Research, 27*(4), 390-405.

Shaha, M., Cox, C. L., Talman, K., & Kelly, D. (2008). Uncertainty in breast, prostate, and colorectal cancer: implications for supportive care. *Journal of Nursing Scholarship. 40(1),* 60-67.

Shaida, N., Jones, C., Ravindranath, N., Das, T., Wilmott, K., Jones, A., & Malone, P. R. (2007). Patient satisfaction with nurse-led telephone consultation for the follow-up of patients with prostate cancer. Prostate Cancer & Prostatic Diseases. *10*(4), 369-373.

Shih, F. J., Gau, M. L., Kao, C. C., Yang, C. Y., Lin, Y. S., Liao, Y. C., et al. (2007). Dying and caring on the edge: Taiwan's surviving nurses' reflections on taking care of patients with severe acute respiratory syndrome. *Applied Nursing Research, 20*(4), 171-180.

Sossong, A. (2007). Living with an implantable cardioverter defibrillator: Patient outcomes and the nurse's role. *Journal of Cardiovascular Nursing, 22*(2), 99-104.

Stiegelis, H. E., Hagedoorn, M., Sanderman, R., Bennenbroek, F. T. C., Buunk, B. P., Van den Bergh, A. C. M., et al. (2004). The impact of an informational self-management intervention on the association between control and illness uncertainty before and psychological distress after radiotherapy. *Psycho-Oncology, 13*(4), 248-259.

Van Pelt, J. C., Mullins, L. L., Carpentier, M. Y., & Wolfe-Christensen, C. (2006). Brief report: Illness uncertainty and dispositional self-focus in adolescents and young adults with childhood-onset asthma. *Journal of Pediatric Psychology, 31*(8), 840-845.

Wallace, M. (2005). Finding more meaning: the antecedents of uncertainty revisited. *Journal of Clinical Nursing, 14*(7), 863-868.

Wonghongkul, T., Dechaprom, N., Phumivichuvate, L., & Losawatkul, S. (2006). Uncertainty appraisal coping and quality of life in breast cancer survivors. *Cancer Nursing, 29*(3), 250-257.

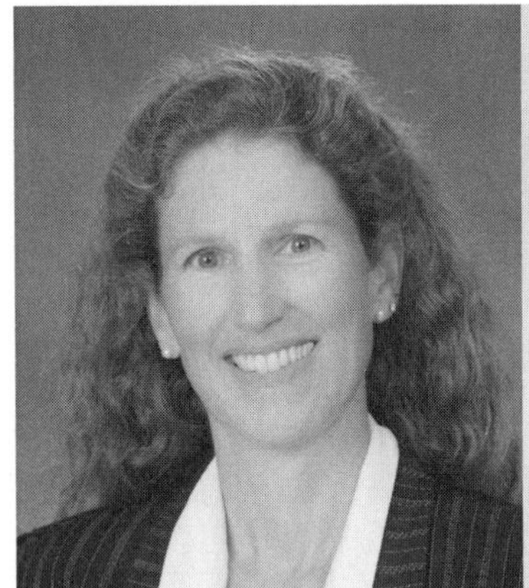

Photo credit: Mark Thaler, Biomedical Communications Department, University of Arizona Health Sciences Center, Tucson, Arizona

CHAPTER 29

Pamela G. Reed

1952-present

Self-Transcendence Theory

Doris D. Coward

"The quest for nursing is to understand the nature of and to facilitate nursing processes in diverse contexts of health experiences." (Reed, 1997a, p. 77)

CREDENTIALS OF THE THEORIST

Pamela G. Reed was born in Detroit, Michigan. She married her husband, Gary, in 1973, and they have two daughters. Reed graduated with her baccalaureate from Wayne State University in Detroit, Michigan, in 1974 and earned her M.S.N. in psychiatric-mental health of children and adolescents and in nursing education in 1976. She began doctoral study at that institution in 1979 and received her Ph.D. in 1982 with a concentration in nursing theory and research, and a minor in adult development and aging. Her dissertation research was directed by Joyce J. Fitzpatrick and focused on the relationship between well-being and spiritual perspectives on life and death in terminally ill and well individuals.

Reed is on the faculty at The University of Arizona College of Nursing in Tucson, where she has taught, conducted research, and served in administrative roles, including Associate Dean for Academic Affairs since January 1983. Reed has received several awards for her teaching focused on nursing theory development and metatheory. Her major fields of research include well-being and aging. She was a pioneer in nursing research into spirituality. She developed two widely used research instruments, the *Spiritual Perspectives Scale* and the *Self-Transcendence Scale.* Her research studies, financed by both intramural and extramural funding, are reported in many

The author expresses her appreciation to Pamela G. Reed for her insights over the years and particularly for her support during the development of this chapter.

scholarly journals. Her current research and scholarship address family caregiver wisdom in palliative care, in addition to her abiding focus on knowledge development and theory in nursing. Reed became co-editor of *Perspectives on Nursing Theory* for the 4th and 5th editions.

Reed is a fellow in the American Academy of Nursing and is a member of a number of professional organizations, including Sigma Theta Tau International, the American Nurses Association, and the International Society of Rogerian Scholars. She has served on the editorial review boards of numerous journals and as Contributing Editor for a *Nursing Science Quarterly* column, Scholarly Dialogue.

Reed's influence is evident not only in her own research and publications. The impact of her work is reflected in the research of more than 50 students whose theses and dissertations she has directed, in undergraduate student projects and in the work of other scientists who have applied her theory or her two measurement scales in their research. Her theoretical ideas are supported and extended by the many nurses Reed mentored.

THEORETICAL SOURCES

Reed (1991a) developed her theory of self-transcendence using the strategy of "deductive reformulation." This strategy, among other theory development approaches that deliberately utilize nursing models, originated with Reed's professors, notably Ann Whall and Joyce Fitzpatrick of Wayne State University. (See Fitzpatrick, Whall, Johnston, & Floyd, 1982; Shearer & Reed, 2004; and Whall, 1986 for applications of this strategy.) Deductive reformulation in constructing middle range theory uses knowledge derived from non-nursing theory that is reformulated deductively from a nursing conceptual model. The primary non-nursing theory sources were life span theories on adult social-cognitive and transpersonal development (e.g., Alexander & Langner, 1990; Commons, Richards, & Armon, 1984; Wilber, 1980, 1981, 1990). Principles from life-span theories were reformulated using the nursing perspective of Martha E. Rogers' conceptual system of unitary human beings (Rogers, 1970, 1980, 1990).

Reed describes her theory as originating from three sources (Reed, 2003, 2008). The first source was the conceptualization of human development (Lerner, 2002) as a lifelong process that extended beyond the attainment of adulthood throughout the aging and dying processes. This emerging belief in the ongoing potential for development was a paradigm shift from previously held views that both physical growth and mental development ended at adolescence (Reed, 1983).

The second source for the theory was the early work of nursing theorist Martha E. Rogers (Rogers, 1970, 1980, 1990). Rogers' three principles of homeodynamics were congruent with the key principles of the evolving life span developmental theory. Rogers' integrality principle identified development as a function of both human and contextual factors; it also identified disequilibrium between person and environment as an important trigger of development. Similarly, developmental theorist Riegel (1976) proposed that asynchrony in development among physical, emotional, environmental, and social dimensions was necessary for developmental progress. Rogers' helicy principle characterized human development as innovative and unpredictable. This principle is similar to life span principles that identified development as nonlinear, continuous throughout the life span, and evident in variability within and across individuals and groups. Rogers' resonancy principle described human development as a process of movement that, although unpredictable, had pattern and purpose. Life span theorists also proposed that the process of development displayed patterns of complexity and organization. Thus knowledge gained from the non-nursing life span developmental perspective was reformulated, using an appropriate nursing conceptual system.

The third source for the theory was evidence from clinical experience and research indicating that clinically depressed older persons reported fewer developmental resources to sustain their sense of well-being in the face of decreased physical and cognitive abilities than did a matched group of mentally healthy older adults (Reed, 1986b). In addition, development in elderly and in "oldest-old" adults was found not be a linear process of gain and subsequent loss, but a process of transforming old perspectives and behaviors, and integrating new views and activities (Reed, 1989, 1991b).

MAJOR CONCEPTS & DEFINITIONS

VULNERABILITY

Vulnerability is defined as one's awareness of personal mortality (Reed, 2003). In Reed's earlier work, the phrase "awareness of one's personal mortality" was the context for development or maturation in later adulthood or at the end of life. Self-transcendence was a pattern associated with advanced development within that context (Reed, 1991b). The concept of vulnerability broadens the awareness of personal mortality situations to include life crises such as disability, chronic illness, childbirth, and parenting.

SELF-TRANSCENDENCE

Self-transcendence initially was defined by Reed (1991b) as "expansion of self-conceptual boundaries multidimensionally: inwardly (e.g., through introspective experiences), outwardly (e.g., by reaching out to others), and temporally (whereby past and future are integrated into the present)" (p. 71). Reed (1997b) provided a more comprehensive definition, as follows, in a later publication:

> Self-transcendence refers to a fluctuation of perceived boundaries that extends the person (or self) beyond the immediate and constricted views of self and the world. This fluctuation is pandimensional, that is, outward (toward others and the environment), inward (toward greater awareness of one's own beliefs, values, and dreams), and temporal (toward integration of past and future in a way that enhances the relative present) (p. 192).

In 2003, another pattern of boundary expansion was incorporated so that self-transcendence is also the capacity to expand one's self-boundaries "transpersonally (to connect with dimensions beyond the typically discernible world)" (Reed, 2003, p. 147). Because self-transcendence is pandimensional, it is possible that other dimensions may be added to describe the capacities for boundary expansion (P. Reed, personal communication, June 17, 2004).

WELL-BEING

Well-being is defined as "the sense of feeling whole and healthy, in accord with one's own criteria for wholeness and well-being" (Reed, 2003, p. 148). In her earlier work, Reed did not explicitly define well-being but linked the concept to mental health, which was dependent on salient issues of development within a given phase of life (Reed, 1989, 1991b). Reed also described the underlying mechanisms of well-being in a 1997 article. In that article (Reed, 1997a, p. 76), she proposed nursing to be "the study of the nursing processes of well being." Well-being as a nursing process, then, was described in terms of a synthesis of two kinds of change: changes in complexity in a life (i.e., the increasing frailness of advanced aging or the loss of a beloved spouse) tempered by changes in integration (i.e., constructing meaning from such life events).

MODERATING-MEDIATING FACTORS

A wide variety of personal and contextual variables and their interactions may influence the process of self-transcendence as it contributes to well-being. Examples of such variables are age, gender, cognitive ability, life experiences, spiritual perspectives, social environment, and historical events. These personal and contextual variables may strengthen or weaken relationships between vulnerability and self-transcendence and between self-transcendence and well-being (Reed, 2003).

Major Concepts & Definitions—cont'd

POINTS OF INTERVENTION

There are two points of intervention in self-transcendence theory. Both points interface in some way with the process of self-transcendence. Nursing actions may focus directly on a person's inner resource for self-transcendence, or indirectly on personal and contextual factors that affect the relationships between vulnerability and self-transcendence and between self-transcendence and well-being (Reed, 2003).

USE OF EMPIRICAL EVIDENCE

Self-transcendence theory was grounded in belief in the developmental nature of older adults and the necessity of continued development to maintain mental health and a sense of well-being during the process of aging (Reed, 1983). Therefore, the initial research in theory building was conducted with older adults (Reed, 1986b, 1989, 1991b).

In the first study, Reed (1986b) examined patterns of developmental resources and depression over time in 28 mentally healthy and 28 clinically depressed older adults (mean age, 67.4 years). Levels of developmental resources were measured 3 times (6 weeks apart) with the 36-item Developmental Resources of Later Adulthood (DRLA) scale, previously developed and tested by Dr. Reed. The healthy adults perceived higher levels of resources across time than did the depressed adults. Scores on the Center for Epidemiological Studies Depression (CES-D) scale (Radloff, 1977) were significantly higher in depressed individuals across time than were those of the mentally healthy. Strong relationships between DRLA scores and subsequent CES-D scores indicated that developmental resources influenced mental health outcomes in the healthy group; the reverse relationship found in the depressed group indicated that depression negatively influenced developmental resources in terms of the ability to explore new outlooks on life, to share wisdom and experience with others, and to find spiritual meaning.

In the second study, Reed (1989) explored the degree to which key developmental resources of later adulthood were related to mental health in 30 hospitalized clinically depressed older adults (mean age, 67 years). Participants completed the DRLA and CES-D measures and rated the importance in their current lives of each developmental resource reflected in the DRLA items. An inverse correlation was found between the level of resources and depression. Participants also reported that the resources represented by the DRLA items were highly important in their lives. In addition, key reasons given by participants for their psychiatric hospitalization were congruent with self-transcendence issues significant in later adulthood (e.g., physical health concerns, relationships with adult children, questions about life and death).

During the initial DRLA instrument development and testing, a factor labeled *transcendence* accounted for 45.2% of the variance in DRLA scores. In the second study (Reed, 1989), the 15-item transcendence factor was also more highly correlated with the CES-D than was the entire DRLA. Therefore, a recommendation for future research was to examine further the psychometric properties of the instrument, with one goal being to shorten the DRLA to facilitate ease of administration in clinical settings.

A third study explored patterns of self-transcendence and mental health in 55 independent-living elders (ranging in age from 80 to 97 years) (Reed, 1991b). In this study, self-transcendence was defined as "the expansion of one's conceptual boundaries inwardly through introspective activities, outwardly through concerns about other's welfare, and temporally by integrating perceptions of one's past and future to enhance the present"

(Reed, 1991b, p. 5). Self-transcendence was measured by the newly developed Self-Transcendence Scale (STS), derived from the previously identified transcendence factor in the original DRLA scale. The STS score was correlated inversely with both CES-D and Langner Scale of Mental Health Symptomatology (MHS) scores. The MHS is an index of general mental health on which higher scores indicate impairment in mental health in nonpsychiatric populations (Langner, 1962). In addition, the four patterns of self-transcendence identified by participants (generativity, introjectivity, temporal integration, and body-transcendence) were congruent with Reed's definition of the concept.

In summary, Reed's three studies provided evidence for the theoretical idea that self-transcendence views and behaviors were, in fact, present in older adults. Her data also indicated that such views and behaviors were related strongly to mental health. The findings thus supported a conceptualization of mental health in later adulthood that included the importance of resources that expanded self-concept boundaries beyond a preoccupation with the physical and cognitive declines of aging.

MAJOR ASSUMPTIONS

Early in her theoretical work, Reed (1986a, 1987) proposed a process model approach for constructing conceptual frameworks that would guide nurses and nursing education in clinical specialties. In that model, health was proposed as the central concept, or axis, around which revolved nursing activity, person, and environment. The assumption of the model was that the focus of the nursing discipline was on building and engaging knowledge to promote health processes.

Health

Health, in that early process model, was defined implicitly as a life process of both positive and negative experiences from which individuals create unique values and environments that promote well-being.

Nursing

The role of nursing activity was to assist persons (through interpersonal processes and therapeutic management of their environments) with the skills required for promoting health and well-being.

Person

Persons were conceived as developing over their life span in interaction with other persons and within an environment of changing complexity and vibrancy that could both positively and negatively contribute to health and well-being.

Environment

Family, social networks, physical surroundings, and community resources were environments that significantly contributed to health processes that nurses influenced through "managing therapeutic interactions among people, objects, and [nursing] activities" (Reed, 1987, p. 26).

This metaparadigmatic approach to conceptual framework development for a nursing specialty was innovative and foundational to Reed's own future work with the concepts of spirituality and self-transcendence. Self-transcendence theory evolved from the perspective that self-transcendence is one of many processes related to health, and that the overall goal of the theory was to provide nurses with another perspective on the human capacity for well-being.

In her initial explication of the emerging self-transcendence theory, Reed (1991a) identified one key assumption based on Rogers' conceptual system. This assumption was that persons are open systems who impose conceptual boundaries upon themselves to define their reality and to provide a sense of wholeness and connectedness within themselves and their environment. Reed (2003) reaffirmed this assumption in a later publication, restating Rogers' basic assumption that "human beings are integral with their environment" (p. 146). Self-conceptual boundaries fluctuate in form across the life span and are associated with human health and development. Self-transcendence was proposed as an important indicator of a person's conceptual self-boundaries that could be assessed at specific times.

A second assumption identified in the later description of the theory was that self-transcendence is a developmental imperative (Reed, 2003), that is, self-transcendence must be expressed like any other developmental capacity in life for a person to realize a continuing sense of wholeness and connectedness. This assumption is congruent with Frankl's (1969) and Maslow's (1971) conceptualizations of self-transcendence as an innate human characteristic that, when actualized, gives purpose and meaning to a person's existence.

THEORETICAL ASSERTIONS

There are three basic concepts in the theory of self-transcendence: vulnerability, self-transcendence, and well-being (Reed, 2003, 2008). Vulnerability is the awareness of personal mortality that arises with aging and other life phases, or during health events and life crises (Reed, 2003). Although vulnerability was not explicitly identified as a concept in Reed's earlier writings, it was not a new idea. The concept of vulnerability clarifies that the context within which self-transcendence is realized is not only when confronting end-of-own-life issues but includes life crises such as disability, chronic illness, childbirth, and parenting. Self-transcendence refers to the fluctuations in perceived boundaries that extend persons beyond their immediate and constricted views of self and the world. The fluctuations are pandimensional: outward (toward awareness of others and the environment), inward (toward greater insight into one's own beliefs, values, and dreams), temporal (toward integration of past and future in a way that enhances the relative present), and transpersonal (toward awareness of dimensions beyond the typically discernible world) (Reed, 1997b, 2003, 2008). Well-being means "feeling whole and healthy, in accord with one's own criteria for wholeness and well-being" (Reed, 2003, p. 148).

Additional concepts in the theory are moderating-mediating factors and points of intervention. Moderating-mediating factors are personal and contextual variables such as age, gender, life experiences, and social environment that can influence the relationships between vulnerability and self-transcendence and between self-transcendence and well-being. Points of intervention are nursing activities that facilitate self-transcendence.

Three major propositions were developed using the three basic concepts. The first proposition of the theory is that self-transcendence is greater in persons facing end-of-own-life issues than in persons not facing such issues. End-of-own-life issues are interpreted broadly, as they arise with life events, illness, aging, and other experiences that increase awareness of personal mortality.

The second proposition of the theory is that conceptual boundaries are related to well-being (Reed, 1991a). Depending on their nature, fluctuations in conceptual boundaries influence well-being positively or negatively across the life-span. For example, an increase in self-transcendence views and behaviors is expected to be positively related to mental health as an indicator of well-being in persons confronting end-of-life issues. A specific example of a negative influence is that the inability to reach out for or to accept friendship would be expected to be related to depression as an indicator of mental health.

Given the key assumption about the person-environmental process (Reed, 1991a), a third set of propositions was identified by Reed in 2003. Personal and environmental factors function as correlates, moderators, or mediators of the relationships between vulnerability, self-transcendence, and well-being.

In summary, the 2003 model of the self-transcendence theory proposes the following three sets of relationships (Figure 29-1):

1. Increased vulnerability is related to increased self-transcendence.
2. Self-transcendence is positively related to well-being.
3. Personal and contextual factors may influence the relationship between vulnerability and self-transcendence and between self-transcendence and well-being.

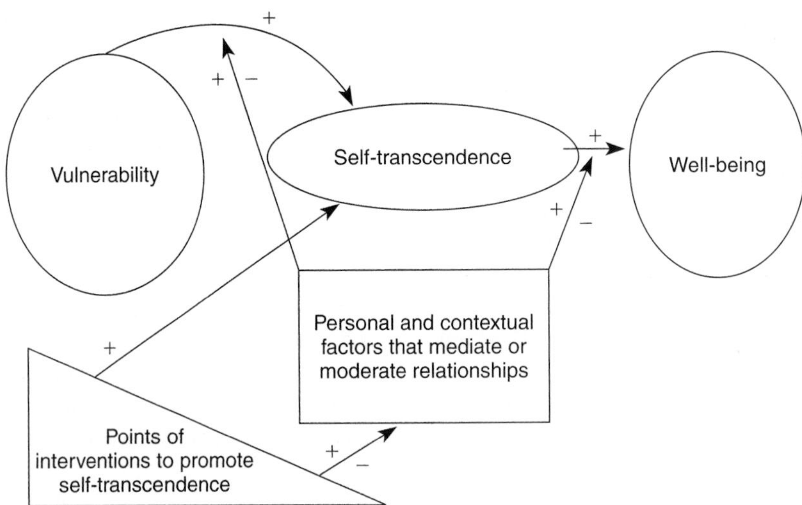

Figure 29-1 Model of self-transcendence theory. (From Reed, P. G. [2003]. The theory of self-transcendence. In M. J. Smith & P. Liehr [Eds.], *Middle range theory for nursing* [p. 150]. New York, Springer. Used by permission.)

LOGICAL FORM

Reed's empirical middle range theory was constructed using the strategy of deductive reformulation to enhance understanding of the end-of-life phenomenon of self-transcendence (Reed, 1991a). The logic used is primarily deduction, to ensure that the middle range theory was congruent with Rogerian and life span principles. Analogical reasoning was also used to work from other theories of life span development, drawing comparisons between psychology and nursing about human development and potential for well-being at all phases of life. The key concepts of the theory are related in a clear and logical manner, while still allowing for creativity in the way the theory is applied, tested, and further developed. Reed's strategy of constructing a nursing theory—from non-nursing theories, a nursing conceptual model, research, and clinical and personal experiences—piqued nurses' interest in this phenomenon of developmental maturity and provided impetus for further theorizing and research into the variety of situations in which awareness of personal mortality occurs.

ACCEPTANCE BY THE NURSING COMMUNITY

The quest for nursing is to facilitate human well-being through what Reed called "nursing processes," of which self-transcendence is one example (Reed, 1997a). Toward this end, self-transcendence theory has been used in practice, education, and research.

Practice

Reed's (1986a, 1987) process model for clinical specialty education and psychiatric–mental health nursing practice articulated the relationships between the metaparadigm constructs of health, persons and their environments, and nursing activity. Self-transcendence theory delineates specific concepts derived from process model constructs of health (i.e., well-being), person (i.e., self-transcendence), and environment (i.e., vulnerability) and proposes relationships among those concepts to provide direction for nursing activities. Reed (1991a) and Coward and Reed (1996) suggested a variety of nursing activities that facilitate expansion of self-conceptual boundaries—journaling, meditation, life review, and religious expression, to name a few.

Self-transcendence may be integral to healing in many life situations. Nurse activities that promote the perspectives and activities of self-reflection, altruism, hope, and faith in vulnerable persons are associated with an increased sense of well-being. Group psychotherapy (Stinson & Kirk, 2006; Young & Reed, 1995) and breast cancer support groups (Coward, 1998, 2003; Coward & Kahn 2004; 2005) are interventions that nurse researchers have used to provide clients with opportunity for examining their values, for reaching out to share experience with and help similar others, and for finding meaning from their health situations. Others have suggested similar strategies to facilitate well-being in caregivers of persons with dementia (Acton & Wright, 2000) and in bereaved individuals (Joffrion & Douglas, 1994). Acton and Wright (2000) suggest arranging respite care for caregivers so that they have time and energy for transpersonal activities. McGee (2000) suggests that recovery in alcoholism involves a process of self-transcendence, as facilitated by a nurse-designed environment that supports the 12 steps and 12 traditions of Alcoholics Anonymous. Walsh and her students are using applications of creative art therapy to promote self-transcendence in nursing students and long-term care residents (Chen & Walsh, 2009).

Education

Themes of self-transcendence are found in the writings of nurse theorists influential in nursing education. Sarter (1988) analyzed the philosophical roots of four contemporary nursing theories (Rogers' Science of Unitary Human Beings, 1970, 1980; Newman's theory of expanding consciousness, 1986; Watson's theory of caring, 1979, 1985; and Parse's theory of man-living-health, 1981). These theories share a common view in identifying self-transcendence as an appropriate philosophical foundation for the discipline. Modeling and Role-Modeling Theory, which contains concepts similar to self-transcendence that are associated with development and health, guides the curricula of several undergraduate programs (Erickson, 2002; Erickson, Tomlin, & Swain, 1983).

Reed describes self-transcendence as "both a human capacity and a human struggle that can be facilitated by nursing" (Reed, 1996, p. 3). Reed (1997a) went on to define nursing succinctly as "an inherent human process of well-being, manifested by complexity and integration" (p. 76), with self-transcendence as an important factor in the process of well-being. Given this link between well-being and self-transcendence, it seems imperative that nurses be educated to understand and to promote self-transcendence views and behaviors in their clients. Self-transcendence is also a pathway for helping the healer, or healing the healer, so that nurses themselves maintain a healthy lifestyle as they care for others (Conti-O'Hare, 2002).

Research

A large number of research studies provide evidence that supports the association between self-transcendence and increased well-being in populations that typically are confronted with an awareness of their own personal mortality. The initial research studies relating self-transcendence to depression were conducted with elders (Reed, 1986b, 1989, 1991a). More recent research reported similar relationships in depressed older adults (Klaas, 1998; Stinson & Kirk, 2006; Young & Reed, 1995), middle-aged adults (Ellermann & Reed, 2001), and individuals who lost loved ones from HIV/AIDS (Kausch & Amer, 2007). Buchanan, Ferran, and Clark (1995) examined self-transcendence and suicidal thought in older adults. Upchurch (1993, 1999) and Upchurch & Mueller (2005) explored the relationship between self-transcendence and activities of daily living in non-institutionalized older adults. Two studies explored self-transcendence and elders' perceptions of positive physical and mental health (Bickerstaff, Grasser, & McCabe, 2005; Nygren et al., 2005). Walton, Shultz, Beck, and Walls (1991) identified an inverse relationship between self-transcendence and loneliness in healthy older adults. Decker and Reed (2005) found that integrated moral reasoning, completion of a living will, and prior experience with a life-threatening illness, but not level of self-transcendence, were related to elders' desire for less aggressive treatment at end-of-life.

An impressive number of studies have demonstrated a positive relationship between self-transcendence and well-being or quality of life in persons with HIV or AIDS (Coward, 1994, 1995; Coward & Lewis, 1993; McCormick, Holder, Wetsel, & Cawthon, 2001; Mellors, Erlen, Coontz, & Lucke, 2001; Mellors, Riley, & Erlen, 1997; Stevens, 1999). Several studies have described self-transcendence or related concepts in women with breast cancer (Carpenter, Brockopp, & Andrykowski, 1999; Coward, 1990a, 1990b, 1991; Coward & Kahn, 2004, 2005; Kamienski, 1997; Kinney, 1996; Matthews, 2000; Pelusi, 1997; Taylor, 2000). The positive effect of a self-transcendence theory–based cancer support group intervention on self-transcendence and well-being in newly diagnosed women also was documented by Coward (1998, 2003).

Self-transcendence in caregivers of persons with dementia was explored by Acton (2003) and Acton & Wright (2000) and was studied in caregivers of terminally ill patients who had died within the previous year (Enyert & Burman, 1999; Reed & Rousseau, 2007). Other populations studied include healthy middle-aged adults (Coward, 1996), elderly men with prostate cancer (Chin-A-Loy & Fernsler, 1998), female nursing students and faculty (Kilpatrick, 2002), nurses (Hunnibell, 2006; McGee, 2004); homeless adults (Runquist & Reed, 2007), elders with chronic heart failure (Gusick, 2005), and liver transplant recipients (Bean & Wagner, 2006; Wright, 2003). Other studies reported positive relationships between transcendence and transformation and finding meaning among elders (Klaas, 1998) and women with rheumatoid arthritis (Neill, 2002).

In addition, Reed has mentored a number of master's and doctoral students in research on self-transcendence. Research results from these studies, some of which are cited above, provide additional empirical support for the theory. See the bibliography for a more complete listing.

FURTHER DEVELOPMENT

Reed's initial conceptualization of self-transcendence focused on later adulthood and identified the importance of personal resources that expand self-boundaries beyond the concerns generated by physical and cognitive decline. More recent studies by Reed and others have extended the scope of the theory to include additional populations of adolescent and adult age groups, patients and non-patients, who may have increased awareness of personal mortality.

Diverse personal and contextual variables impact the relationship between self-transcendence and well-being. Although a number of studies have associated older age with increased self-transcendence, many younger research participants report self-transcendence views and behaviors and score high on self-transcendence measures. A variety of human experiences, such as childbirth and parenting, illness and disability, caregiving, creating a work of art or literature, and spiritual perspectives, all may, over a long or short period in one's life, evoke the pandimensional views and behaviors indicative of self-transcendence. Continued research into these and other personal and contextual factors will increase understanding of the role they play in the theoretical propositions (Reed, 2003, 2008).

Continued development of the theory will include further examination of points of intervention to facilitate self-transcendence perspectives and behaviors in persons who express a need for increased sense of wholeness and well-being. One such intervention, a self-transcendence theory–based support group, had a small positive effect on self-transcendence variables in women with newly diagnosed breast cancer (Coward, 2003; Coward & Kahn, 2004, 2005). Young and Reed (1995) found group psychotherapy effective in facilitating self-transcendence in a small sample of elder adults. As the theory of self-transcendence evolves, nursing will learn more about new potentials for well-being in health experiences over the life span.

Reed received funding to study self-transcendence as it relates to end-of-life decisions and well-being in patients and their family caregivers. People facing the end of life represent some of the most vulnerable individuals to whom nurses may provide care. Although an abundance of lay literature exists about the developmental and transcendent experiences of end of life and dying, there is a dearth of systematic research into this human experience. The theory of self-transcendence can guide initial questions and may undergo further refinement as this inquiry progresses.

Other forms of inquiry may occur in reference to the theory, particularly in view of Reed's recent reconceptualization of nursing. Through her philosophical writings, Reed (1997a) clarified a more foundational definition of nursing that shifted the source of nursing activity from that of external agent (i.e., the "nurse") to viewing nursing as an inner human process. Specifically, Reed defines nursing as a process of well-being that exists within and among human systems. The process of nursing is characterized by changing complexity and integration. From this, she presented self-transcendence as a nursing process. Further explorations into mechanisms of changing complexity and integration may help achieve new theoretical explanations about how self-transcendence emerges and functions in human lives.

CRITIQUE

Clarity and Consistency

Clarity and consistency are key criteria in the description of and critical reflection on a theory (Chinn & Kramer, 2004). Theory clarity is evaluated by how clearly defined are the concepts (semantic clarity) and by how understandable are the connections among the concepts and the reasoning within the theory (structural clarity). Semantic consistency is evaluated by how well the concepts are used in ways that are consistent with their definitions and the basic assumptions of the theory. Structural consistency evaluation involves assessing how congruent are the assumptions, theory purpose, concept definitions, and connections among the concepts.

Theoretical sources for development of the theory are described clearly in several publications (Reed, 1991b, 1996, 1997b, 2003). However, the definitions and assumptions about the concepts derived from life span developmental theory and Rogers' Science of Unitary Human Beings have sometimes been difficult for nurses to grasp. In attempting to clarify concepts such as health and self-transcendence, Reed has presented slightly varying definitions and numerous examples that, although theoretically consistent, may confuse some readers. In terms of structural clarity, some relationships in the schematic model of the theory (see Figure 29-1) are not yet fully defined and described in Reed's writings, except in the publication in which that diagram appears (Reed, 2003). Structural consistency is good in that the identified relationships are logical and consistent.

It is not unusual to find these issues about clarity in definitions when a theory incorporates concepts that are somewhat abstract. In addition, some clarity and consistency may be challenged because theorizing is an ongoing process that develops over time, and theories may outgrow some of the initial ideas of the theorist (Malinski, 2006). Overall, however, Reed's theoretical thinking has remained congruent with the original Rogerian and life span conceptual views and assumptions underlying her knowledge development, and she has conceptualized a theory that can be understood by both nurse clinicians and nurse researchers.

Simplicity

Simplicity, referring to having a minimal number of concepts and interrelationships (Chinn & Kramer, 2004), is valued in a middle range theory developed to guide nursing practice. Reed's theory is strong on simplicity, with three major concepts (vulnerability, self-transcendence, and well-being), along with two other concepts (personal and environmental factors, and points of intervention). The theory likely will increase in complexity somewhat as specific personal and environmental factors and their relationships to the major concepts are identified. Overall, the major concepts and the number of relationships generated by these concepts are minimal while still being meaningful and fairly comprehensive.

Generality

The scope and purpose of Reed's theory are such that the theory can be applied to a wide variety of human health situations. The purpose of the theory is to enhance nurses' understanding about well-being (Reed, 2003, 2008). When presented initially, Reed's work focused on developmental resources in persons confronted by challenges of later adulthood as related to indicators of mental health symptomatology (specifically, clinical depression) (Reed, 1983, 1986b, 1991a). In linking self-transcendence (an indicator of developmental maturity, but not necessarily associated with aging) to mental health (an indicator of overall well-being), the scope of the emerging theory expanded to include persons other than elders who were facing end-of-own-life issues (Reed, 1991b). Further development and testing of the theory led to the specification of the additional concepts of vulnerability, points of intervention, and personal and contextual variables (Reed, 2003, 2008). The theory is now broader in scope and is more congruent with a life span perspective, because the major concepts can be applied to anyone who is confronted with life events ranging from childbirth and caregiving to long-term care contexts, life-threatening illness, and dying. Broadening the scope and purpose of the theory from explaining mental health to explaining well-being increased its generality and resulted in a theory that is applicable in the many situations that involve both health and healing.

Empirical Precision

Empirical precision refers to how well the concepts are linked to observed or observable reality, particularly in contexts relevant to nursing practice. Chinn and Kramer (2004) refer to this criterion in terms of the accessibility of the theory. Although the theory's concepts are somewhat abstract (vulnerability, self-transcendence, and well-being), empirical indicators of subconcepts (e.g., the impact of life-threatening illness, reaching out to others, and depression, respectively) have been identified and studied by numerous researchers. In particular, measurement of self-transcendence has been honed through development and refinement of Reed's Self-Transcendence Scale. Well-being has been measured by a variety of empirical indicators.

Researchers may use different approaches and empirical indicators to measure self-transcendence because the concept lends itself to a variety of approaches and measures that fit the clinical nursing context of interest. Research findings that support a strong relationship among self-transcendence and various indicators of well-being, as hypothesized by the theory, also attest to the theory's empirical precision.

Derivable Consequences

Self-transcendence theory is a middle range theory that leads to valued goals in nursing education, practice, and research. The theory, grounded in nursing philosophy, research, and practice and tested in subsequent research, has led to new knowledge that is useful in nursing practice. The theory provides insight into the developmental nature of humans as related to health situations relevant to nursing care. Nurses and patients often face events that challenge personal mortality; knowledge of developmental resources (i.e., self-transcendence) that can be engaged by or for the person expands the nursing repertoire for facilitating well-being in times of increased vulnerability. The abstract yet definable nature of self-transcendence facilitates the development of many interventions that may be tested as strategies that ultimately promote well-being in a variety of nurse-patient encounters.

SUMMARY

Self-transcendence theory was developed initially using the strategy of deductive reformulation from life span developmental theories, Rogers' conceptual system of unitary human beings, empirical research, and clinical and personal experiences of the theorist. Although the theoretical concepts are abstract, more concrete subconcepts have been developed and studied extensively in a number of populations. Exploratory, descriptive correlational, and quasi-experimental studies support the hypothesized relationship between self-transcendence views and behaviors and indicators of well-being. Such research findings increase nurses' understanding that, no matter how desperate a health situation, people retain a capacity for personal development that is associated with feelings of well-being.

Research findings also have suggested ways in which nurses can promote self-transcendence views and behaviors in themselves and in their clients. Further research will examine interventions to promote self-transcendence and study the personal and contextual factors that modify relationships among the theory concepts. In addition, qualitative research approaches may assist in gaining further understanding of the concept of self-transcendence as a nursing process and as it expresses the depth and changing complexity of human beings.

Case Study

Mr. Jones is a 65-year-old gentleman whose wife died 6 months ago after a long illness. The couple was married 45 years, and they were devoted to each other. They had three children who are now in their 30s. Two of the children live several hundred miles away, but one son lives with his wife, and two preschool children less than a mile from the Jones' home.

Mr. Jones provided much of the care for his wife during her illness. Although her care was time consuming and fatiguing and kept him at home much of the time, he was grateful that he could care for her. He now is alone in their home, is very lonely, is uninterested in preparing meals or eating, and lacks energy to return to his former community and social activities or even to interact with his son and family.

The hospice nurse contacted Mr. Jones for follow-up bereavement counseling. She told him that although he had "passed" a routine physical examination the week before, she was concerned about his continuing sadness and lack of energy. The nurse reassured him that it was not uncommon to grieve for many months after a major loss. She asked him if he thought his wife would have had a similar experience if he had been the first to die. His response was that his wife would have had an even more difficult time adjusting. The nurse and Mr. Jones then spent some time reflecting on and talking about his response. The nurse's initial question and Mr. Jones' resulting insight that his grief was not as bad as his wife's would have been helped him transcend his immediate experience of loss and to find some meaning in his grief.

This illustration is an example of an inward expansion of self-conceptual boundaries indicative of self-transcendence. Other expressions of self-transcendence might help Mr. Jones facilitate his own healing and regain a measure of well-being.

In terms of outward expansion, Mr. Jones, with some encouragement, might reach out to his son's family to begin to reconnect to the world outside himself. Walking to and from his home to theirs could expand his sensory world and provide opportunities to interact with other people and with nature along the way. Spending time with his grandchildren could be enlivening through the joy young children can bring to an older person, as could a sense of satisfaction derived from being helpful to his son and daughter-in-law.

Offering at a future time to use the skills he learned while caring for his wife through volunteering with hospice would be an example of transcending temporally. Integrating his memories of Mrs. Jones into his current life would be another example of temporal self-transcendence.

Transpersonal self-transcendence is another important experience for Mr. Jones. Although he was unable to attend church services for several years, he had in the past found worshiping with others a source of comfort. His spiritual life might even be expanded to consider new spiritual dimensions such as that found in the possibility of "being with" his wife again someday or in some way experiencing her presence in the present. Returning to church or to addressing spiritual

dimensions outside of organized worship that relates Mr. Jones' understanding of death to some greater or divine design is another example of transpersonal self-transcendence.

CRITICAL THINKING *Activities*

1. Considering the pandimensional aspect of self-transcendence, list a few examples of when you experienced expanded boundaries in your own life. Reflect on how this expanded awareness influences your health or sense of well-being.
2. What are some personal and contextual factors in your life that negatively or positively influence your own experience of self-transcendence?
3. What might you do to facilitate self-transcendence and a sense of wholeness in a woman with acquired immunodeficiency syndrome who is dying?
4. How could you apply the theory of self-transcendence to help a frail 95-year-old person living in a nursing home maintain or gain a sense of well-being?

POINTS FOR *Further Study*

- Reed, P. G. (2008). The theory of self-transcendence. In M. J. Smith & P. R. Liehr (Eds.), *Middle range theory for nursing* (2nd ed.) (pp. 163-200). New York: Springer.
- Reed, P. G. (1991a). Toward a nursing theory of self-transcendence: Deductive reformulation using developmental theories. *ANS Advances in Nursing Science, 13*(4), 64-77.
- Coward, D. D., & Reed, P. G. (1996). Self-transcendence: A resource for healing at the end-of-life. *Issues in Mental Health Nursing, 17*(3), 275-288.
- Reed, P. G. (2007). Scholarly reflections on nursing practice: Undergraduate student discoveries from four case studies. *Journal of Undergraduate Nursing Scholarship*, <www.juns.nursing.arizona.edu>

REFERENCES

Acton, G. (2003). Self-transcendent views and behaviors: Exploring growth in caregivers of adults with dementia. *Journal of Gerontological Nursing, 28*(12), 22-30.

Acton, G., & Wright, K. (2000). Self-transcendence and family caregivers of adults with dementia. *Journal of Holistic Nursing, 18*(2), 143-158.

Alexander, C. N., & Langner, E. J. (1990). *Higher stages of human development: Perspectives on adult growth.* New York: Oxford University Press.

Bean, K., & Wagner, K. (2006). Self-transcendence, illness distress, and quality of life among liver transplant recipients. *Journal of Theory Construction & Testing, 10(2),* 47-53.

Bickerstaff, K. A., Grasser, C. M., & McCabe, B. (2005). How elderly nursing home residents transcend losses of later life. *Holistic Nursing Practice, 17*(3), 159-165.

Buchanan, D., Ferran, C., & Clark, D. (1995). Suicidal thought and self-transcendence in older adults. *Journal of Psychosocial Nursing and Mental Health Services, 33*(10), 31-34, 42-43.

Carpenter, J. S., Brockopp, D., & Andrykowski, M. (1999). Self-transformation as a factor in the self-esteem and well-being of breast cancer survivors. *Journal of Advanced Nursing, 29*(6), 1042-1411.

Chen, S., & Walsh, S. (2009). A creative-bonding intervention model to promote nursing students' self-transcendence and positive attitudes toward elders. *Research in Nursing and Health, 32*(2), 204-216

Chin-A-Loy, S. S., & Fernsler, J. I. (1998). Self-transcendence in older men attending a prostate cancer support group. *Cancer Nursing, 21*(5), 358-363.

Chinn, P. L., & Kramer, M. K. (2004). *Integrated knowledge development in nursing* (6th ed.). St. Louis: Mosby.

Commons, M. L., Richards, F. A., & Armon, C. (Eds.). (1984). *Beyond formal operations: Late adolescent and adult cognitive development.* New York: Praeger.

Conti-O'Hare, M. (2002). *The nurse as wounded healer: From trauma to transcendence.* Sudbury, MA: Jones & Bartlett.

Coward, D. D. (1990a). The lived experience of self-transcendence in women with advanced breast cancer. *Nursing Science Quarterly, 3*, 162-169.

Coward, D. D. (1990b). Correlates of self-transcendence in women with advanced breast cancer. *Dissertation Abstracts International, B 52*(01). (University Microfilms No. 9108416)

Coward, D. D. (1991). Self-transcendence and emotional well-being in women with advanced breast cancer. *Oncology Nursing Forum, 18*, 857-863.

Coward, D. D. (1994). Meaning and purpose in the lives of persons with AIDS. *Public Health Nursing, 11*(5), 331-336.

Coward, D. D. (1995). Lived experience of self-transcendence in women with AIDS. *Journal of Obstetrics, Gynecologic, & Neonatal Nursing, 24*, 314-318.

Coward, D. D. (1996). Correlates of self-transcendence in a healthy population. *Nursing Research, 45*(2), 116-121.

Coward, D. D. (1998). Facilitation of self-transcendence in a breast cancer support group. *Oncology Nursing Forum, 25*, 75-84.

Coward, D. D. (2003). Facilitation of self-transcendence in a breast cancer support group II. *Oncology Nursing Forum, 30*(Part 1 of 2), 291-300.

Coward, D. D., & Kahn, D. L. (2004). Resolution of spiritual disequilibrium in women newly diagnosed with breast cancer (Online exclusive). *Oncology Nursing Forum, 31*(2), E24-E31.

Coward, D. D., & Kahn, D. L. (2005). Transcending breast cancer: Making meaning from diagnosis and treatment. *Journal of Holistic Nursing, 23*(3), 264-283.

Coward, D. D., & Lewis, F. M. (1993). The lived experience of self-transcendence in gay men with AIDS. *Oncology Nursing Forum, 20*, 1363-1369.

Coward, D. D., & Reed, P. G. (1996). Self-transcendence: A resource for healing at the end-of-life. *Issues in Mental Health Nursing, 17*(3), 275-288.

Decker, I. M., & Reed, P. G. (2005). Developmental and contextual correlates of elders' anticipated end-of-life decisions. *Death Studies, 29*, 827-846.

Ellermann, C. R., & Reed, P. G. (2001). Self-transcendence and depression in middle-aged adults. *Western Journal of Nursing Research, 23*(7), 698-713.

Enyert, G., & Burman, M. E. (1999). A qualitative study of self-transcendence in caregivers of terminally ill patients. *American Journal of Hospice and Palliative Care, 16*(2), 455-462.

Erickson, H. C., Tomlin, E. M., & Swain, M. A. P. (1983). *Modeling and role-modeling: A theory and paradigm for nursing.* Englewood Cliffs, NJ: Prentice-Hall.

Erickson, M. (2002). Modeling and role-modeling. In A. M. Tomey & M. R. Alligood (Eds.), *Nursing theorists and their work* (5th ed., pp. 443-464). St. Louis: Mosby.

Fitzpatrick, J. J., Whall, A. L., Johnston, R. L., & Floyd, J. A. (1982). *Nursing models and their psychiatric mental health applications.* Bowie, MD: Robert J. Brady.

Frankl, V. (1969). *The will to meaning.* New York: New American Library.

Gusick, G. M. (2005). Factors affecting the symptom burden in chronic heart failure. *Dissertation Abstracts International B66(03)* (University Microfilms No. 3166193).

Hunnibell, L. S. (2006). Self-transcendence and the three aspects of burnout syndrome in hospice and oncology nurses. *Dissertation Abstracts International B 68(02)* (University Microfilms No. 3253704).

Joffrion, L. P., & Douglas, D. (1994). Grief resolution: Facilitating self-transcendence in the bereaved. *Journal of Psychosocial Nursing, 32*(3), 13-19.

Kamienski, M. C. (1997). An investigation of the relationship among suffering, self-transcendence, and social support in women with breast cancer. *Dissertation Abstracts International, B 58*(04). (University Microfilms No. ATT9729588)

Kausch, K. D., & Amer, K. (2007). Self-transcendence and depression among AIDS Memorial Quilt panel Makers. *Journal of Psychosocial Nursing & Mental Health Services, 45*(6), 44-53.

Kilpatrick, J. A. W. (2002). Spiritual perspective, self-transcendence, and spiritual well-being in female nursing students and female nursing faculty. *Dissertation Abstracts International, B63*(02). (University Microfilms No. ATT 3044802)

Kinney, C. (1996). Transcending breast cancer: Reconstructing one's self. *Issues in Mental Health Nursing, 17*(3), 201-216.

Klaas, D. (1998). Testing two elements of spirituality in depressed and non-depressed elders. *The International Journal of Psychiatric Nursing Research, 4*, 452-462.

Langner, T. S. (1962). A twenty-two item screening score of psychiatric symptoms indicating impairment. *Journal of Health and Human Behavior, 3*, 269-276.

Lerner, R. (2002). *Concepts and theories of human development (3rd ed.).* Mahwah, NJ: Lawrence Erlbaum Associates.

Malinski, V. M. (2006). Rogerian science-based nursing theories. *Nursing Science Quarterly, 19*(1), 7-12.

Maslow, A. H. (1971). *Farther reaches of human nature.* New York: Viking Press.

Matthews, E. E. (2000). Optimism and emotional well-being in women with breast cancer: The role of mediators. *Dissertation Abstracts International, B61*(03) (University Microfilms No. 9967106).

McCormick, D. P., Holder, B., Wetsel, M., & Cawthon, T. (2001). Spirituality and HIV disease: An integrated perspective. *Journal of the Association of Nurses in AIDS care, 12*(3), 58-65.

McGee, E. (2000). Alcoholics Anonymous and nursing: Lessons in holism and spiritual care. *Journal of Holistic Nursing, 18*(1), 11-26.

McGee, E. M. (2004). *I'm better for having known you: An exploration of self-transcendence in nurses.* Unpublished doctoral dissertation, Boston College, Boston.

Mellors M. P., Erlen, J. A., Coontz, P. D., & Lucke, K. T. (2001). Transcending the suffering of AIDS. *Journal of Community Health Nursing, 18*(4), 235-246.

Mellors, M. P., Riley, T. A., & Erlen, J. A. (1997). HIV, self-transcendence, and quality of life. *Journal of the Association of Nurses in AIDS Care, 8*(2), 59-69.

Neill, J. (2002). Transcendence and transformation in life patterns of women living with rheumatoid arthritis. *ANS Advances in Nursing Science, 24*(2), 27-47.

Newman, M. A. (1986). *Health as expanding consciousness.* St. Louis: Mosby.

Nygren, B., Alex, L., Jonsen, E., Gustafson, Y., Norberg, A. & Lundman, B. (2005). Resilience, sense of coherence, purpose in life and self-transcendence in relation to perceived physical and mental health among the oldest old. *Aging & Mental Health, 9*(4), 354-362.

Parse, R. R. (1981). *Man-living-health: A theory of nursing.* New York: John Wiley & Sons.

Pelusi, J. (1997). The lived experience of surviving breast cancer. *Oncology Nursing Forum, 24*(3), 1343-1353.

Radloff L. S. (1977). The CES-D scale: A self-report depression scale for research in the general population. *Applied Psychological Measurement, 1*, 385-401.

Reed, P. G. (1983). Implications of the life span developmental framework for well-being in adulthood and aging. *ANS Advances in Nursing Science, 6*(1), 18-25.

Reed, P. G. (1986a). A model for constructing a conceptual framework for education in the clinical specialty. *Journal of Nursing Education, 25*(7), 295-299.

Reed, P. G. (1986b). Developmental resources and depression in the elderly. *Nursing Research, 35*(6), 368-374.

Reed, P. G. (1987). Constructing a conceptual framework for psychosocial nursing. *Journal of Psychosocial Nursing, 25*(2), 24-28.

Reed, P. G. (1989). Mental health of older adults. *Western Journal of Nursing Research, 11*, 143-163.

Reed, P. G. (1991a). Toward a nursing theory of self-transcendence: Deductive reformulation using developmental theories. *ANS Advances in Nursing Science, 13*(4), 64-77.

Reed, P. G. (1991b). Self-transcendence and mental health in the oldest-old adults. *Nursing Research, 40*(1), 5-11.

Reed, P. G. (1996). Transcendence: Formulating nursing perspectives. *Nursing Science Quarterly, 9*(1), 2-4.

Reed, P. G. (1997a). Nursing: The ontology of the discipline. *Nursing Science Quarterly, 10*(2), 76-79.

Reed, P. G. (1997b). The place of transcendence in nursing's science of unitary human beings: Theory and research. In M. Madrid (Ed.), *Patterns of Rogerian knowing* (pp. 187-196). New York: National League for Nursing.

Reed, P. G. (2003). The theory of self-transcendence. In M. J. Smith & P. R. Liehr (Eds.), *Middle range theory for nursing* (pp. 145-165). New York: Springer.

Reed, P. G. (2008). The theory of self-transcendence. In M. J. Smith & P. R. Liehr (Eds.), *Middle range theory for nursing* (2nd ed., pp. 163-200). New York: Springer.

Reed, P. G., & Rousseau, E. (2007). Spiritual inquiry and well-being in life limiting illness. *Journal of Religion, Spirituality, & Aging, 19*(4), 81-98.

Riegel, K. (1976). The dialectics of human development. *American Psychologist, 31*, 689-699.

Rogers, M. E. (1970). *An introduction to the theoretical basis of nursing.* Philadelphia: F. A. Davis.

Rogers, M. E. (1980). A science of unitary man. In J. Riehl & C. Roy (Eds.), *Conceptual models for nursing practice* (2nd ed., pp. 329-338). New York: Appleton-Century-Crofts.

Rogers, M. E. (1990). Nursing: Science of unitary, irreducible, human beings: Update 1990. In E. A. M. Barrett (Ed.), *Visions of Rogers' science based nursing* (pp. 5-12). New York: National League for Nursing Press.

Runquist. J. J., & Reed, P. G. (2007). Self-transcendence and well-being in homeless adults. *Journal of Holistic Nursing, 25*(1), 5-13.

Sarter, B. (1988). Philosophical sources of nursing theory. *Nursing Science Quarterly, 1*(2), 52-59.

Shearer, N. B. C., & Reed, P. G. (2004). Empowerment: Reformulation of a non-Rogerian concept. *Nursing Science Quarterly, 17*(3), 253-259.

Stevens, D. D. (1999). Spirituality, self-transcendence and depression in young adults with AIDS (Immune deficiency). *Dissertation Abstracts International, B61(02)* (University Microfilms No. 9961253).

Stinson, C. K. & Kirk, E. (2006). Structured reminiscence: an intervention to decrease depression and increase self-transcendence in older women. *Journal of Clinical Nursing, 15*, 208-218.

Taylor, E. J. (2000). Transformation of tragedy among women surviving breast cancer. *Oncology Nursing Forum, 27*, 781-788.

Upchurch, S. L. (1993). Self-transcendence, health status, and selected variables as determinants of the ability to perform activities of daily living in non-institutionalized adults. *Dissertation Abstracts International, B55*(01) (University Microfilms No. 9407736).

Upchurch, S. L. (1999). Self-transcendence and activities of daily living: The woman with the pink slippers. *Journal of Holistic Nursing, 17*(3), 251-266.

Upchurch, S. L., & Mueller, W. H. (2005). Spiritual influences on ability to engage in self-care activities among older African Americans. *International Journal of Aging & Human Development, 60*(1), 77-94.

Walton, C., Shultz, C., Beck, C., & Walls, R. (1991). Psychological correlates of loneliness in the older adult. *Archives of Psychiatric Nursing, 5*(3), 165-170.

Watson, J. (1979). *Nursing: The philosophy and science of caring.* Boston: Little, Brown & Co.

Watson, J. (1985). *Nursing: Human science and human care: A theory of nursing.* Norwalk, CT: Appleton-Century-Crofts.

Whall, A. L. (1986). *Family therapy theory for nursing: Four approaches.* East Norwalk, CT: Appleton-Century-Crofts.

Wilber, K. (1980). *The Atman project: A transpersonal view of human development.* Wheaton, IL: Quest.

Wilber, K. (1981). *Up from Eden: A transpersonal view of human evolution.* Garden City, NY: Theosophical Publishing House.

Wilber, K. (1990). *Eye to eye: The quest for the new paradigm* (2nd ed.). Boston: Shambhala.

Wright, K. (2003). Quality of life, self-transcendence, illness distress, and fatigue in liver transplant recipients. *Dissertation Abstracts International, B64(12)* (University Microfilms No. 3116238).

Young, C. A., & Reed, P. G. (1995). Elders' perceptions of the role group psychotherapy in fostering self-transcendence. *Archives of Psychiatric Nursing, 9*(6), 338-347.

BIBLIOGRAPHY

Primary Sources

Book

Reed, P. G., & Shearer, N. B. C. (2008). *Perspectives on nursing theory* (5th ed). New York: Lippincott Williams & Wilkins.

Reed, P. G., Shearer, N. B. C., & Nicoll, L. H., (Eds.) (2004). *Perspectives on nursing theory* (4th ed). New York: Lippincott Williams & Wilkins.

Book Chapters

Reed, P. G. (1985). Early and middle adulthood. In D. L. Critchley & J. T. Maurin (Eds.), *The clinical specialist in psychiatric-mental health nursing: Theory, research, and practice* (pp. 135-154). New York: John Wiley & Sons.

Reed, P. G. (1986). The developmental conceptual framework: Nursing reformulations and applications for family theory. In A. Whall (Ed.), *Family therapy theory for nursing: Four approaches* (pp. 69-92). New York: Appleton-Century-Crofts.

Reed, P. G. (1992). Nursing theorizing as an ethical endeavor. In L. Nicoll (Ed.), *Perspectives on nursing theory* (2nd ed., pp. 168-175). New York: Lippincott.

Reed, P. G. (1996). Peplau's interpersonal relations model. In J. J. Fitzpatrick & A. L. Whall (Eds.), *Conceptual models of nursing: Analysis and application* (3rd ed., pp. 55-76). Norwalk: Appleton & Lange.

Reed, P. G. (1997). The place of transcendence in nursing's science of unitary human beings: Theory and research. In M. Madrid (Ed.), *Patterns of Rogerian knowing* (pp. 187-196). New York: National League for Nursing Press.

Reed, P. G. (1998). Nursing theoretical models. In J. Fitzpatrick (Ed.), *Encyclopedia of nursing research* (pp. 385-387). New York: Springer.

Reed, P. G. (1998). The re-enchantment of health care: A paradigm of spirituality. In M. Cobb & V. Robshaw (Eds.), *The spiritual challenge of health care* (pp. 35-55). Edinburgh, Scotland: Churchill Livingstone.

Reed, P. G. (2003). The theory of self-transcendence. In M. J. Smith & P. Liehr (Eds.), *Middle range theory for nursing* (pp. 145-165). New York: Springer.

Reed, P. G. (2005). Peplau's nursing theory of interpersonal relations. In J. Fitzpatrick & A. L. Whall (Eds.), *Conceptual models of nursing: Analysis and application* (4th ed., pp. 46-67). Englewood Cliffs, NJ: Prentice Hall.

Reed, P. G. (2008). The theory of self-transcendence. In M. J. Smith & P. Liehr (Eds.), *Middle range theory for nursing* (2nd ed., pp. 163-200). New York: Springer.

Reed, P. G., & Johnston, R. L. (1983). Peplau's model: The interpersonal process. In J. J. Fitzpatrick & A. Whall (Eds.), *Conceptual models of nursing: Analysis and application* (pp. 27-46). Bowie, MD: Brady.

Reed, P. G., & Johnston, R. L. (1989). Peplau's model: The interpersonal process. In J. J. Fitzpatrick & A. Whall (Eds.), *Conceptual models of nursing: Analysis and application* (2nd ed., pp. 49-68). Norwalk, CT: Appleton & Lange.

Reed, P. G., & Larson, C. (2006). Spirituality. In J. J. Fitzpatrick & M. Wallace (Eds.), *Encyclopedia for nursing research* (2nd ed., pp. 565-567). New York: Springer.

Reed, P. G., & Shearer, N. C. (2006). Peplau's theoretical model. In J. J. Fitzpatrick & M. Wallace (Eds.), *Encyclopedia for nursing research* (2nd ed., pp. 459-461). New York: Springer.

Reed, P. G., & Zurakowski, T. (1983). Nightingale: A visionary model for nursing. In J. J. Fitzpatrick & A. Whall (Eds.), *Conceptual models of nursing: Analysis and application* (pp. 12-26). Bowie, MD: Brady.

Reed, P. G., & Zurakowski, T. (1989). Nightingale: A visionary model for nursing revisited. In J. J. Fitzpatrick & A. Whall (Eds.), *Conceptual models of nursing: Analysis and application* (2nd ed., pp. 33-48). Norwalk, CT: Appleton & Lange.

Reed, P. G., & Zurakowski, T. L. (1996). Florence Nightingale: Foundations of nursing theory, education, research, and practice. In J. J. Fitzpatrick & A. L. Whall (Eds.), *Conceptual models of nursing: Analysis and application* (3rd ed., pp. 27-54). Norwalk, CT: Appleton & Lange.

Shearer, N., & Reed, P. G. (1998). Peplau's theoretical model. In J. Fitzpatrick (Ed.), *Encyclopedia of nursing research.* New York: Springer.

Journal Articles

Coward, D. D., & Reed, P. G. (1996). Self-transcendence: A resource for healing at the end of life. *Issues in Mental Health Nursing, 17*, 275-288.

Decker, I. M., & Reed, P. G. (2005). Developmental and contextual correlates of elders' anticipated end-of-life decisions. *Death Studies, 29*, 827-846.

Ellermann, C., & Reed, P. G. (2001). Self-transcendence and depression in middle-aged adults. *Western Journal of Nursing Research, 23*(7), 698-713.

Felton, G., Reed, P. G., & Perla, S. (1981). Measurement of nursing students' and nurses' attitudes toward cancer. *Western Journal of Nursing Research, 3*(1), 62-75.

Fitzpatrick, J. J., & Reed, P. G. (1980). Stress in the crisis experience: Nursing intervention. *Occupational Health Nursing, 28*(12), 19-21.

Jesse, E., & Reed, P. G. (2004). Effects of spirituality and psychosocial well-being on health risk behaviors among pregnant women from Appalachia. *Journal of Obstetric, Gynecologic, & Neonatal Nursing, 33*(6), 739-747.

Moore, I. K., & Reed, P. G. (2000). Stress-response sequence model in pediatric oncology nurses: Theory critique and commentary. *Journal of Pediatric Oncology Nursing, 17*(2), 72-75.

Reed, P. G. (1982). On Smith's definition of health (Editorial). *ANS Advances in Nursing Science, 4*, ix-x.

Reed, P. G. (1983). Implications of the life span developmental framework for well-being in adulthood and aging. *ANS Advances in Nursing Science, 6*, 18-25.

Reed, P. G. (1984). The developmental concept (Editorial). *ANS Advances in Nursing Science, 6*, vii.

Reed, P. G. (1985). Strategies for teaching nursing research: Theory and metatheory in an undergraduate course. *Western Journal of Nursing Research, 7*, 482-486.

Reed, P. G. (1986). A model for constructing a conceptual framework for education in the clinical specialty. *Journal of Nursing Education, 25*(7), 295-299.

Reed, P. G. (1986). Death perspectives and temporal variables in terminally ill and healthy adults. *Death Studies, 10*, 443-454.

Reed, P. G. (1986). Developmental resources and depression in the elderly: A longitudinal study. *Nursing Research, 35*, 368-374.

Reed, P. G. (1986). Religiousness among terminally ill and healthy adults. *Research in Nursing and Health, 9*, 35-42.

Reed, P. G. (1987). Constructing a conceptual framework for psychosocial nursing practice. *Journal of Psychosocial Nursing, 25*(2), 24-28.

Reed, P. G. (1987). Liberal arts and professional nursing education: Integration for knowledge and wisdom. *Nursing Educator, 12*(4), 37-40.

Reed, P. G. (1987). Spirituality and well-being in terminally ill hospitalized adults. *Research in Nursing and Health, 10*(5), 335-344.

Reed, P. G. (1988). Promoting research productivity in new faculty: A developmental perspective of the early postdoctoral years. *Journal of Professional Nursing, 4*(2), 119-125.

Reed, P. G. (1989). Mental health of older adults [includes commentaries and author's response]. *Western Journal of Nursing Research, 11*(2), 143-163.

Reed, P. G. (1989). Nursing theorizing as an ethical endeavor. *ANS Advances in Nursing Science, 11*(3), 1-9.

Reed, P. G. (1991). Preferences for spiritually-related nursing interventions among terminally ill and nonterminally ill hospitalized adults and well adults. *Applied Nursing Research, 4*(3), 122-128.

Reed, P. G. (1991). Response to "Serenity: Caring with perspective." *Scholarly Inquiry for Nursing Practice, 5*(2), 143-147.

Reed, P. G. (1991). Self-transcendence and mental health in oldest-old adults. *Nursing Research, 40*, 7-11.

Reed, P. G. (1991). Spirituality and mental health of older adults: Extant knowledge for nursing. *Family and Community Health, 14*(2), 14-25.

Reed, P. G. (1991). Toward a theory of self-transcendence: Deductive reformulation using developmental theories. *ANS Advances in Nursing Science, 13*(4), 64-77.

Reed, P. G. (1992). An emerging paradigm for the investigation of spirituality in nursing. *Research in Nursing and Health, 15*, 349-357.

Reed, P. G. (1994). The spirituality factor: Response to "The relationship between spiritual perspective, social support, and depression in care giving and non-care giving wives." *Scholarly Inquiry for Nursing Practice: An International Journal, 8*(4), 391-396.

Reed, P. G. (1995). A treatise on nursing knowledge development for the 21st century: Beyond postmodernism. *ANS Advances in Nursing Science, 17*(3), 70-84.

Reed, P. G. (1996). Transcendence: Formulating nursing perspectives. *Nursing Science Quarterly, 9*(1), 2-4.

Reed, P. G. (1996). Transforming knowledge into nursing knowledge through the scholarship of practice: A revisionist analysis of Peplau. *Image: The Journal of Nursing Scholarship, 28*(1), 29-33.

Reed, P. G. (1997). Nursing: The ontology of the discipline. *Nursing Science Quarterly, 10*(2), 76-79.

Reed, P. G. (1998). A holistic view of nursing concepts and theories in practice. *Journal of Holistic Nursing, 16*(4), 4415-4419.

Reed, P. G. (1998). Response to commentary on "The ontology of the discipline of nursing": Breaking through a breakdown in logic. *Nursing Science Quarterly, 11*(4), 146-148.

Reed, P. G. (1999). Commentary: Spirituality in older women who have osteoarthritis. *Graduate Research in Nursing* (Online publication), *1*(1). Retrieved November 12, 2004, from http://www.graduateresearch.com/reed.htm

Reed, P. G. (1999). Response to "Attentively-embracing story: A middle range theory with practice and research implications." *Scholarly Inquiry for Nursing Practice, 13*(2), 205-210.

Reed, P. G. (2000). Nursing reformation: Historical reflections and philosophic foundations. *Nursing Science Quarterly, 13*(2), 129-136.

Reed, P. G. (2001). Commentary: Spiritual care provided by parish nurses. *Western Journal of Nursing Research, 23*, 456-458.

Reed, P. G. (2006). Neomodernism and evidence based nursing: The production of nursing knowledge. *Nursing Outlook, 54*(1), 36-38.

Reed, P. G. (2006). The practice turn in nursing epistemology. *Nursing Science Quarterly, 19*(1), 36-38.

Reed, P. G. (2006). Theory and nursing practice. *Nursing Science Quarterly, 19*(2),116.

Reed. P. G. (2008). The practice of nursing science: Crossing boundaries. *Nursing Science Quarterly, 21*(1), 37-39.

Reed, P. G. (2008). Spiritual care as nursing care: Commentary on 'Spiritual care perspectives of Danish registered nurses.' *Journal of Holistic Nursing*. 26, 15-16.

Reed, P. G., & Leonard, V. E. (1989). An analysis of the concept of self-neglect. *ANS Advances in Nursing Science, 12*(1), 39-53.

Reed, P. G., & Rolfe, G. (2006). Nursing knowledge and nurses' knowledge: A reply to Mitchell and Bournes. *Nursing Science Quarterly, 19*(2), 120-122.

Reed, P. G., & Runquist, J. (2007). Reformulation of a methodological concept in grounded theory. *Nursing Science Quarterly, 20*(2), 118-122.

Reed, P. G., & Verran, J. (1988). Cross-lag panel correlation analysis assumptions: Stationarity, synchronicity, stability. *Western Journal of Nursing Research, 10*(5), 671-676.

Book Reviews

Reed, P. G. (1999). Nursing theorists and their work by M. Tomey & M. Alligood. *Nursing Science Quarterly, 12*(3), 266-268.

Reed, P. G. (1999). Theory and nursing: Integrated knowledge development by P. Chinn & M. Kramer. *Nursing Leadership Forum, 4*(2), 2-3.

Reed, P. G. (2001). Nursing as a spiritual practice: A contemporary application of Florence Nightingale's views by Janet Macrae. *Nursing Leadership Forum, 6*(2), 90.

Reed, P. G. (2003). Nursing theories and nursing practice by Marilyn Parker. *Nursing Science Quarterly, 16*(2), 175-176.

Reed, P. G. (2005). Giving voice to what we know: Margaret Newman's theory of health as expanding consciousness in nursing practice, research, and education by Carol Picard and Dorothy Jones. *Nursing Science Quarterly, 18,* 272-273.

Dissertation

Reed, P. G. (1982). Well-being and perspectives on life and death among death-involved and non-death-involved individuals. Unpublished doctoral dissertation, Wayne State University, Detroit.

Secondary Sources

Selected Book Chapters

Coward, D. D. (2000). Making meaning within the experience of life-threatening illness. In G. Reker & K. Chamberlain (Eds.), *Existential meaning: Optimizing human development across the life span* (pp. 157-170). Thousand Oaks, CA: Sage.

Haase, J., Britt, T., Coward, D., Kline Leidy, N., & Penn, P. (2000). Simultaneous concept analysis: A strategy for developing multiple interrelated concepts. In B. Rodgers & K. Knafl (Eds.), *Concept development in nursing: Foundations, techniques, and applications* (2nd ed., pp. 209-229). Philadelphia: W. B. Saunders.

Selected Journal Articles (not included in REFERENCES)

Budin, W. C. (2001). Birth and death: Opportunities for self-transcendence. Journal of Perinatal Education, 10(2), 38-42.

Chen, K., & Snyder, M. (1999). A research-based use of Tai Chi/movement therapy as a nursing intervention. *Journal of Holistic Nursing, 17*(3), 267-279.

Chiu, L. (2000). Lived experience of spirituality in Taiwanese women with breast cancer. *Western Journal of Nursing Research, 22,* 29-53.

Chiu, L., Emblen, J., van Hofwegen, L., Sawatzky, R., & Meyerhoff, H. (2004). An integrative review of the concept of spirituality in the health sciences. *Western Journal of Nursing Research, 26*(4), 405-428.

Coward, D. D. (1996). Self-transcendence: Making meaning from the cancer experience. *Quality of Life—A Nursing Challenge, 4*(2), 53-58.

Haase, J. E., Britt, T., Coward, D. D., Leidy, N. K., & Penn, P. E. (1992). Simultaneous concept analysis of spiritual perspective, hope, acceptance, and self-transcendence. Image: *The Journal of Nursing Scholarship, 24*(2), 141-147.

Hall, B. (1997). Spirituality in terminal illness: An alternative view of theory. *Journal of Holistic Nursing, 15*(1), 82-96.

Phillips-Salimi, C. R., Haase, J. E., Kintner, E. K., Monahan, P. O., & Azzouz, F. (2007). Psychometric properties of the Herth Hope Index in adolescents and young adults with cancer. *Journal of Nursing Measurement, 15*(1), 3-23.

Ramer, L., Johnson, D., Chan, L., & Barrett, M. T. (2006). The effect of HIV/AIDS disease progression on spirituality and self-transcendence in a multicultural population. *Journal of Transcultural Nursing. 17*(3), 280-289.

Rawnsley, M. (2000). Response to Reed's nursing reformulation: Historical and philosophic foundations. *Nursing Science Quarterly, 13*(2), 134-136.

Reese, C. G., & Murray, R. B. (1996). Transcendence: The meaning of great-grandmothering. *Archives of Psychiatric Nursing, 10*(4), 245-251.

Runquist, J. J. (2006). Persevering through postpartum fatigue. *Journal of Obstetric, Gynecological & Neonatal Nursing, 36*(1), 28-37.

Shearer, N. B. (2007). Toward a nursing theory of Health Empowerment in Homebound Older Women. *Journal of Gerontological Nursing, 33*(12), 38-45.

Teixeira, M. E. (2008). Self-Transcendence: a concept for nursing practice. *Holistic Nursing Practice 22*(1), 25-31.

Thorne, S., & Paterson, B. (1998). Shifting images of chronic illness. *Image: The Journal of Nursing Scholarship, 30*(2), 173-178.

Walker, C. A. (2002). Transformative aging: How mature adults respond to growing older. *Journal of Theory Construction & Testing, 6*(2), 109-116.

Selected Master's Theses and Dissertations

Billard, A. (2001). The impact of spiritual transcendence on the well-being of aging Catholic sisters. *Dissertation Abstracts International, B61*(12) (University Microfilms No. 9999061).

Bouwkamp, C. I. (1996). *The relationships among depression, quality of life, and spirituality in older adults.* Unpublished master's thesis, University of Arizona, Tucson, AZ.

Brauchler, D. S. (1992). *An empirical study of the relationship between spiritually-related variables and depression in hospitalized adults.* Unpublished master's thesis, University of Arizona, Tucson, AZ.

Britt, T. (1989). *The relationship of self-transcendence, spirituality, and hope to positive personal death perspectives in healthy older adults.* Unpublished master's thesis, University of Arizona, Tucson, AZ.

Brown, M. L. (1995). *The relationship of spirituality and self-transcendence to life satisfaction among chronically ill Euro-American and Mexican-American older adults.* Unpublished master's thesis, University of Arizona, Tucson, AZ.

Campesino-Flenniken, M. (2003). Voces de las madres: Traumatic bereavement after gang-related homicide. *Dissertation Abstracts International, B64*(09) (University Microfilms No. 3106975).

Cookman, C. A. (1992). Attachment structures of older adults. *Dissertation Abstracts International, B53*(07) (University Microfilms No. 9234901).

Coward, D. (1990). Correlates of self-transcendence in women with advanced breast cancer. *Dissertation Abstracts International, B52*(01) (University Microfilms No. 9108416).

Decker, I. (1998). Moral reasoning, self-transcendence, and end-of-life decisions in a group of community dwelling elders. *Dissertation Abstracts International, B59*(11) (University Microfilms No. 9912131).

Egan, S. R. (1996). *The relationship of meaning of death field patterns to well-being, spiritual perspective and perception of health in healthy older adults.* Unpublished master's thesis, University of Arizona, Tucson, AZ.

Ellermann, C. (1998). *Depression and self-transcendence in middle-aged adults.* Unpublished master's thesis, University of Arizona, Tucson, AZ.

Forbes, M. A. R. (1998). Testing a causal model of hope and its antecedents among chronically ill older adults. *Dissertation Abstracts International, B59*(08) (University Microfilms No. 9901665).

Gallup, J. R. (1985). *The relationship of death anxiety to developmental resources and perceived distance to personal death in later adulthood.* Unpublished master's thesis, University of Arizona, Tucson, AZ.

Gross, D. (1994). *Harvesting the wisdom of the elders: A study of the lives of seven exemplary aged women.* Unpublished doctoral dissertation, Institute of Transpersonal Psychology, Palo Alto, CA.

Gusick, G. M. (2005). Factors affecting the symptom burden in chronic heart failure. *Dissertation Abstracts International B66(03)* (University Microfilms No. 3166193).

Hunnibell, L. S. (2006). Self-transcendence and the three aspects of burnout syndrome in hospice and oncology nurses. *Dissertation Abstracts International B 68(02)* (University Microfilms No. 3253704).

Jacobs, M. L. (1995). *Spiritual perspective and death acceptance as correlates of the aggressiveness of elders' end-of-life treatment choices.* Unpublished master's thesis, University of Arizona, Tucson, AZ.

Kamienski, M. C. (1997). An investigation of the relationship among suffering, self-transcendence, and social support in women with breast cancer. *Dissertation Abstracts International, B58*(04) (University Microfilms No. 9729588).

Kim, S. (Graduating in May 2008). *Family interdependence of spirituality and self-transcendence and well-being among Korean elders and family caregivers.* Unpublished doctoral dissertation, University of Arizona, Tucson, AZ.

Kelley, M. G. (1999). *The lived experience of spiritual healing touch in older women with chronic pain.* Unpublished master's thesis, University of Arizona, Tucson, AZ.

Kilpatrick, J. A. W. (2002). Spiritual perspective, self-transcendence, and spiritual well-being in female nursing students and female nursing faculty. *Dissertation Abstracts International, B63*(02) (University Microfilms No. 3044802).

Klaas, D. J. K. (1996). The experience of depression, meaning in life and self-transcendence in two groups of elders. *Dissertation Abstracts International, B58*(02) (University Microfilms No. 9720690).

Larson, C. D. (1998). *The relationship of spiritual perspective and functional status to morale in adults with chronic pulmonary disease.* Unpublished master's thesis, University of Arizona, Tucson, AZ.

Larson, C. D. (2004). *Spiritual, psychosocial, and physical correlates of well-being across the breast cancer experience.* Unpublished doctoral dissertation, University of Arizona, Tucson, AZ.

Malcolm, J. D. (1989). *Self-transcendence, chronic illness and depression in later adulthood.* Unpublished master's thesis, Arizona State University, Tempe, AZ.

Matthews, E. E. (2000). Optimism and emotional well-being in women with breast cancer: The role of mediators. *Dissertation Abstracts International, B61*(03) (University Microfilms No. 9967106).

McGaffic, C. M. (1996). Patterns of spirituality and health. *Dissertation Abstracts International, B57*(03). (Unavailable from University Microfilms International). University of Arizona, Tucson, AZ.

McGee, E. M. (2004). *I'm better for having known you: An exploration of self-transcendence in nurses.* Unpublished doctoral dissertation, Boston College, Boston.

Nielson, S. T. P. (1992). *Life events as determinants of wisdom in older adults.* Unpublished doctoral dissertation, University of Arizona, Tucson, AZ.

Rieck, S. B. (2000). The relationship between the spiritual dimension of the nurse-patient relationship and patient well-being. *Dissertation Abstracts International, B61*(08) (University Microfilms No. 9983908).

Rosdahl, D. (2004). The effect of mindfulness meditation on tension headaches and secretory immunoglobulin A in saliva. *Dissertation Abstracts International, B65*(01) (University Microfilms No. 3119979).

Rose, S. S. (2003). Catastrophic injury and illness in the elderly. *Dissertation Abstracts International, B64*(05) (University Microfilms No. 3090018).

Runquist, J. J. (2006). Persevering through postpartum fatigue. *Dissertation Abstracts International, B67*(01) (University Microfilms No. 3205369).

Sabre, L. K. (1997). *Perceived insomnia, life-events and self-transcendence in middle and older adults.* Unpublished master's thesis, University of Arizona, Tucson, AZ.

Scharpf, S. S. (1996). *Self-transcendence in older men with prostate cancer.* Unpublished master's thesis, University of Delaware, Newark.

Shearer, N. B. C. (2000). Facilitators of health empowerment in women. *Dissertation Abstracts International, B61*(03) (University Microfilms No. 9965911).

Stevens, D. D. (1999). Spirituality, self-transcendence and depression in young adults with AIDS (Immune deficiency). *Dissertation Abstracts International, B61*(02) (University Microfilms No. 9961253).

Suzuki, M. (1999). *The relationship of depression and self-transcendence among community-living Japanese elders.* Unpublished master's thesis, University of Arizona, Tucson, AZ.

Upchurch, S. L. (1993). Self-transcendence, health status, and selected variables as determinants of the ability to perform activities of daily living in non-institutionalized adults. *Dissertation Abstracts International, B55*(01) (University Microfilms No. 9407736).

Van Lent, D. (1988). *The relationship of spirituality, self-transcendence, and social support to morale in chronically ill elderly.* Unpublished master's thesis, University of Arizona, Tucson, AZ.

Walker, C. A. (2000). Aging among baby boomers. *Dissertation Abstracts International, B61*(11) (University Microfilms No. 9993966).

Wright, K. (2003). Quality of life, self-transcendence, illness distress, and fatigue in liver transplant recipients. *Dissertation Abstracts International, B64*(12) (University Microfilms No. 3116238).

Young, C. (1994). *Older adults group members' perceptions of the role of outpatient group psychotherapy in enhancing self-transcendence.* Unpublished master's thesis, University of Arizona, Tucson, AZ.

CHAPTER 30

Carolyn L. Wiener

1930-present

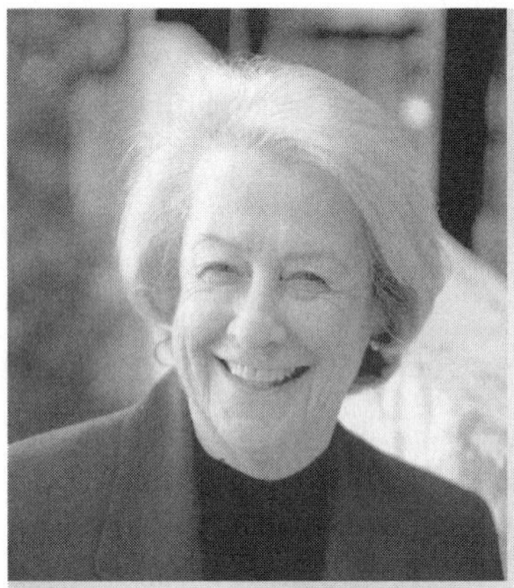

Photo credit: Robert Foothorap. From (2001). The UCSF School of Nursing Annual Publication, *The Science of Caring, 13*(1), 7.

Marylin J. Dodd

1946-present

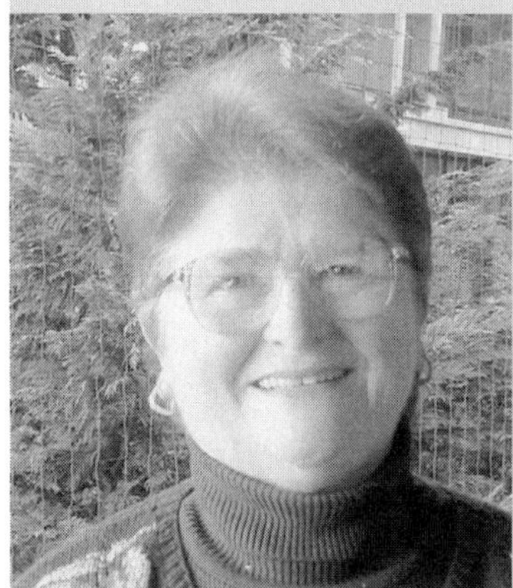

Photo credit: Craig Carlson.

Theory of Illness Trajectory

Janice Penrod, Lisa Kitko, and Chin-Fang Liu

"The uncertainty surrounding a chronic illness like cancer is the uncertainty of life writ large. By listening to those who are tolerating this exaggerated uncertainty, we can learn much about the trajectory of living." (Wiener & Dodd, 1993, p. 29)

CREDENTIALS OF THE THEORISTS

Carolyn L. Wiener

Carolyn L. Wiener was born in 1930 in San Francisco. She earned her bachelor's degree in interdisciplinary social science from San Francisco State University in 1972. Wiener received her master's degree in sociology from the University of California, San Francisco (UCSF) in 1975. She returned to UCSF to pursue her doctorate in sociology and completed her Ph.D. in 1978. After receiving a Ph.D., Wiener accepted the position of assistant research sociologist at UCSF.

Wiener is an adjunct professor and research sociologist in the Department of Social and Behavioral Sciences at the School of Nursing at UCSF. Her research focuses on organization in healthcare institutions, chronic illness, and health policy. She teaches qualitative research methods and has conducted numerous seminars and workshops on the grounded theory method.

Throughout her career, Wiener's excellence has earned for her several meritorious awards and honors. Her intense collaborative relationship with the late Anselm Strauss (co-originator of grounded theory methods) and prolific experience in grounded theory methods are evidenced by her invited presentations at the Celebration of the Life and Work of Anselm Strauss at UCSF in 1996 and at a conference entitled *Anselm Strauss, a Theoretician: The Impact of His Thinking on German and European Social Sciences* in Magdeburg, Germany, in 1999. She is highly sought as a methodological consultant to researchers and students from a variety of specialties.

Dissemination of research findings and methodological papers is a hallmark of Wiener's work. She has produced a steady stream of research and theory articles since the mid-1970s. In addition, she has authored or coauthored several books (Strauss, Fagerhaugh, Suczek, & Wiener, 1997; Wiener, 1981, 2000; Wiener & Strauss, 1997; Wiener & Wysmans, 1990). In her early efforts, Wiener focused on illness trajectories, biographies, and the evolving medical technology scene. From the late 1980s to 1990s, Wiener focused on coping, uncertainty, and accountability in hospitals. Then she completed a study examining the quality management and redesign efforts in hospitals and the interplay between agencies and hospitals around the issue of accountability (Wiener, 2000). All of this work is grounded in her strong methodological expertise and sociological perspective.

Marylin J. Dodd

Marylin J. Dodd was born in 1946 in Vancouver, Canada. She qualified as a registered nurse after studying at the Vancouver General Hospital, British

Columbia, Canada. She continued her education, earning a bachelor's and a master's degree in nursing from the University of Washington in 1971 and 1973, respectively. Dodd worked as an instructor in nursing at University of Washington following graduation with her master's degree. By 1977, Dodd returned to academe and completed a Ph.D. in nursing from Wayne State University. She then accepted the position of assistant professor at UCSF. During her tenure there, Dodd has advanced to the rank of full professor, serving as the director for the Center for Symptom Management at UCSF. In 2003, she was awarded the Sharon A. Lamb Endowed Chair in Symptom Management at the School of Nursing, UCSF.

Her exemplary program of research is focused in oncology nursing, specifically, self-care and symptom management. Dodd's outstanding record of funded research provides evidence of the superiority and significance of her work. She has skillfully woven modest internal and external funding with 23 years of continuous National Institutes of Health funding to advance her research. Her research trajectory has advanced impeccably as she progressively utilized both descriptive studies and intervention studies employing randomized clinical trial methodologies to extend an understanding of complex phenomena in cancer care.

Dodd's research was designed to test self-care interventions (PRO-SELF Program) to manage the side effects of cancer treatment (mucositis) and symptoms of cancer (fatigue, pain). This research entitled The PRO-SELF: Pain Control Program—An Effective Approach for Cancer Pain Management was published in *Oncology Nursing Forum* (West, Dodd, Paul, Schumacher, Tripathy et al., 2003). Currently, she teaches in the Oncology Nursing Specialty. In 2002, she instituted two new courses ("Biomarkers I and II") developed by the Center for Symptom Management Faculty Group.

Dodd's illustrious career has merited several prestigious awards. Among these honors, she was recognized as a fellow of the American Academy of Nursing (1986). Her continued excellence and significant contributions to oncology nursing are evidenced by her having been awarded the Oncology Nursing Society/Schering Excellence in Research Award (1993, 1996), the Best Original Research Paper in *Cancer Nursing* (1994, 1996), the Oncology Nursing Society Bristol-Myers Distinguished Researcher Career Award (1997), and the Oncology Nursing Society/Chiron Excellence of Scholarship and Consistency of Contribution to the Oncology Nursing Literature Career Award (2000). In 2005, Dodd received the prestigious Episteme Laureate (the Nobel Prize in Nursing) Award from the Sigma Theta Tau International Honor Society of Nursing. This impressive partial listing of awards provides a sense of the magnitude of professional respect and admiration that Dodd has garnered throughout her career.

Dodd's record in research dissemination is equally illustrious. Her volume of original publications began in 1975. By the early 1980s, she was publishing multiple, focused articles each year, and that pace has only accelerated. She has authored or coauthored 130+ data-based peer-reviewed journal articles, seven books and many book chapters, and numerous editorials, conference proceedings, and review papers (1978, 1987, 1988, 1991, 1997, 2001). Her many presentations at scientific gatherings around the world accentuate this work. Dodd has been an invited speaker throughout North America, Australia, Asia, and Europe.

Her active service to the university, School of Nursing, Department of Physiological Nursing, and to numerous professional and public organizations and journal review boards augments her outstanding record of service to the profession of nursing. Despite the breadth and volume of these activities, Dodd is an active teacher and mentor. She is the faculty member on record for several graduate courses and carries a significant advising load in the master's, doctoral, and postdoctoral programs at UCSF. With this brief overview of but a few highlights in an amazing career, it is clear that Dodd is an exemplar of excellence in nursing scholarship.

THEORETICAL SOURCES

Being ill creates a disruption in normal life. Such disruption affects all aspects of life, including physiological functioning, social interactions, and conceptions of self. Coping is the response to such disruption. Although coping with illness has been of interest to social scientists and nursing scholars for decades, Weiner and Dodd clearly explicate that formerly implicit theoretical assumptions have limited the utility of this body of work (Wiener & Dodd, 1993, 2000). Because the processes surrounding the disruption of illness are played out in the context of living, coping responses are inherently situated in sociological interactions with others and biographical processes of self. Coping is often described as a compendium of strategies used to manage the disruption, attempts to isolate specific responses to one event that is lived within the complexity of life context, or assigned value labels (e.g., good or bad) to the responsive behaviors that are described collectively as coping. Yet, the complex interplay of physiological disruption, interactions with others, and the construction of biographical conceptions of the self warrants a more sophisticated perspective of coping.

The Theory of Illness Trajectory* addresses these theoretical pitfalls by framing this phenomenon within a sociological perspective of a trajectory that emphasizes the experience of disruption related to illness within the changing contexts of interactional and sociological processes that ultimately influence the person's response to such disruption. This theoretical approach defines this theory's significant contribution to nursing: coping is not a simple stimulus-response phenomenon that can be isolated from the complex context of life. Because life is centered in the living body, the physiological disruptions of illness permeate other life contexts to create a new way of being, a new sense of self. Responses to the disruptions caused by illness are interwoven into the various contexts encountered in one's life and the interactions with other players in those life situations.

From this perspective, coping is best viewed as change over time that is highly variable in relation to biographical and sociological influences. The trajectory is this course of change, of variability, that cannot be confined to or modeled in linear phases or stages. Rather, the trajectory of illness organizes insights to better understand the dynamic interplay of the disruption of illness within the changing contexts of life.

Within this sociological framework, Wiener and Dodd address serious concerns regarding conceptual overattribution of the role of uncertainty in the framework of understanding responses to living with the disruptions of illness (Wiener & Dodd, 1993). An old adage tells us that nothing in life is certain, except death and taxes. Living is fraught with uncertainty, yet illness (especially chronic illness) compounds this uncertainty in profound ways. Being chronically ill exaggerates the uncertainties of living within being for those who are compromised (i.e., by illness) in their capability to respond to these uncertainties. Thus, although the concept of uncertainty provides a useful theoretical lens for understanding the illness trajectory, it cannot be theoretically positioned so as to overshadow conceptually the dynamic context of living with chronic illness.

In other words, the trajectory of illness is driven by the illness experience lived within contexts that are inherently uncertain and involve both the self and others. The dynamic flow of life contexts (both biographical and sociological) creates a dynamic flow of uncertainties that take on different forms, meanings, and combinations when living with chronic illness. Thus, tolerating uncertainty is a critical theoretical strand in the illness trajectory theory.

*The Theory of Illness Trajectory is used herein to refer to theoretical formulations regarding coping with uncertainty through the cancer illness trajectory. It is important to note that this work extends preexisting theory on illness trajectories, biographies, and related concepts (identity, temporality, and body) that were developed through an extensive 4-year research project. Readers are advised to refer to the original works of Corbin, Fagerhaugh, Strauss, Suczek, and Wiener for further explication of the larger theory.

MAJOR CONCEPTS & DEFINITIONS

Life is situated in a biographical context. Conceptions of self are rooted in the physical body and are formulated based on the perceived capability to perform usual or expected activities to accomplish the objectives of varied roles. Interactions with others are a major influence on the establishment of the conception of self. As varied role behaviors are enacted, the person monitors reactions of others and a sense of self in an integrated process of establishing meaning. Identity, temporality, and body are key elements in the biographical context, as follows:

- *Identity:* the conception of self at a given time that unifies multiple aspects of self and is situated in the body
- *Temporality:* biographical time reflected in the continuous flow of the life course events; perceptions of the past, present, and possible future interwoven into the conception of self
- *Body:* activities of life and derived perceptions based in the body

Illness, particularly cancer, disrupts the usual or everyday conception of self and is compounded by the perceived actions and reactions of others in the sociological context of life. This disruption permeates the interdependent elements of biography: identity, temporality, and body. This disruption or sense of disequilibrium is marked by a sense of a loss of control, resulting in states of uncertainty.

As life contexts continually unfold, dimensions of uncertainty are manifest, not in a linear sequence of stages or phases, but in an unsettling intermingling of perceptions of the uncertain body, uncertain temporality, and uncertain identity. The experience of illness always is placed within the biographical context, that is, illness is experienced in the continual flow of the life. The domains of illness-related uncertainty vary in dominance across the illness trajectory (Table 30-1) through a dynamic flow of perceptions of self and interactions with others.

The activities of life and of living with an illness are forms of work. The sphere of work includes the person and all others with whom he or she interacts, including family and healthcare providers. This network of players is called the *total organization.* The ill person (or patient) is the central worker; however, all work takes place within and is influenced by the total organization. Types of work are organized around the following four lines of trajectory work performed by patients and families:

1. *Illness-related work:* diagnostics, symptom management, care regimen, and crisis prevention
2. *Everyday-life work:* activities of daily living, keeping a household, maintaining an occupation, sustaining relationships, and recreation
3. *Biographical work:* the exchange of information, emotional expressions, and the division of tasks through interactions within the total organization
4. *Uncertainty abatement work:* activities enacted to lessen the impact of temporal, body, and identity uncertainty

The balance of these types of work is dynamically responsive, fluctuating across time, situations, perceptions, and varied players in the total organization in order to gain some sense of equilibrium (i.e., a sense of control). This interplay among the types of work creates a tension that is marked by shifts in the dominance of types of work across the trajectory. Recall, however, that the biographical context is rooted in the body. As the body changes through the course of illness and treatment, the capacity to perform certain types of work and, ultimately, one's identity are transformed.

A major contribution of this work was the delineation of types of uncertainty abatement work (Table 30-2). These activities were enacted to lessen the impact of the varied states of uncertainty induced by undergoing cancer chemotherapy. These strategies were highly dynamic and responsive and

MAJOR CONCEPTS & DEFINITIONS—cont'd

occurred in varied combinations and configurations across the trajectory of illness for different players in the organization. Those enacting these strategies affected the conception of self as they monitored others' responses to the strategy as they attempted to manage living with illness.

Table 30-1 *Illness Trajectory: States of Uncertainty*

Domain	Sources of Uncertainty	Dimensions of Uncertainty
UNCERTAIN TEMPORALITY	Life is perceived to be in a constant state of flux related to illness and treatment.	Loss of temporal predictability prompts concerns surrounding:
Taken-for-granted expectations regarding the flow of life events are disrupted A temporal disjunction in the biography	The self of the past is viewed differently (e.g., the way it used to be). Expectations of the present self are distorted by illness and treatment.	■ *Duration:* how long ■ *Pace:* how fast ■ *Frequency:* how often the experience of time is distorted (i.e., stretched out, constrained, or limitless)
	Anticipation of the future self is altered.	
UNCERTAIN BODY	Faith in the body is shaken (body failure).	Ambiguity in reading body signs Concerns surrounding:
Changes related to illness and treatment centered in one's ability to perform usual activities, involving appearance, physiological functions, and response to treatment	The conception of the former body (the way it used to be) comingles with the altered state of the body at present and the changed expectations for how the body may perform in the future.	■ What is being done to the body ■ Jeopardized body resistance ■ Efficacy and risks of treatment ■ Disease recurrence
UNCERTAIN IDENTITY Interpretation of self is distorted as the body fails to perform in usual ways, and expectations related to the flow of events (temporality) are altered by disease and treatment.	Body failure and difficulty reading the new body upset the former conception of self. Skewed temporality impairs the expected life course.	Expected life course is shattered. Evidence gleaned from reading the body is not interpretable within the usual frame of understanding. Hope is sustained despite changing circumstances.

USE OF EMPIRICAL EVIDENCE

The Theory of Illness Trajectory was expanded through a secondary analysis of qualitative data collected during a prospective longitudinal study that examined family coping and self-care during 6 months of chemotherapy treatment. The sample for the larger study included 100 patients and their families. Each patient had been diagnosed with cancer (including breast, lung, colorectal, gynecological, or lymphoma) and was in the process of receiving

Table 30-2 *Uncertainty Abatement Work*

Type of Activity	Behavioral Manifestations
Pacing	Resting or changing usual activities
Becoming "professional" patients	Using terminology related to illness and treatment Directing care Balancing expertise with super-medicalization
Seeking reinforcing comparisons	Comparing self with persons who are in worse condition to reassure self that it is not as bad as it could be
Engaging in reviews	Looking back to reinterpret emergent symptoms and interactions with others in the organization
Setting goals	Looking toward the future to achieve desired activities
Covering up	Masking signs of illness or related emotions Bucking up to avoid stigma or to protect others
Finding a safe place to let down	Establishing a place where, or people with whom, true emotions and feelings could be expressed in a supportive atmosphere
Choosing a supportive network	Selective sharing with individuals deemed to be positive supporters
Taking charge	Asserting the right to determine the course of treatment

chemotherapy for initial disease treatment or for recurrence. Subjects in the study designated at least one family member who was willing to participate in the study.

Although both quantitative and qualitative measures were used in data collection for the larger study, this theory was derived through analysis of the qualitative data. Interviews were structured around family coping and were conducted at three points during chemotherapeutic treatment. The patients and the family members were asked to recall the previous month and then discuss the most important problem or challenge with which they had to deal, the degree of distress created by that problem within the family, and their satisfaction with the management of that concern.

Meticulous attention was paid to consistency in data collection: family members were consistent and present for each interview, the interview guide was structured, and the same nurse-interviewer conducted each data collection point for a given family. Audiotaping the interview proceedings, verbatim transcription, and having a nurse-recorder present at each interview to note key phrases as the interview progressed further enhanced methodological rigor. The resultant data set consisted of 300 interviews (three interviews for each of 100 patient-family units) that were obtained at varied points in the course of chemotherapeutic treatment for cancer.

As the data for the larger study were analyzed, it became apparent to Dodd (principal investigator) that the qualitative interview data held significant insights that could further inform the study. Wiener, a grounded theorist who collaborated with Anselm Strauss, one of the method's founders, was subsequently recruited to conduct a secondary analysis of interview data. It should be noted that traditional grounded theory methods typically involve a concurrent, reiterative process of data collection and analysis (Glaser, 1978; Glaser & Strauss, 1965). As theoretical insights are identified, sampling and the focus of subsequent data collection theoretically are driven to flesh out emergent concepts, dimensions, variations, and negative cases. However, in this project, the data were collected previously using a structured interview guide; this was a secondary analysis of an established data set.

Wiener's expertise in grounded theory methods permitted the adaptation of grounded theory methods for application to secondary data that proved successful. In essence, the principles under-girding analysis (i.e., the coding paradigm) were applied to the preexisting data set. The analytical inquiry proceeded inductively to reveal the core social-psychological process around which the theory is explicated: tolerating the uncertainty of living with cancer. Dimensions of the uncertainty, management processes, and consequences were further explicated to reveal the internal consistency of the theoretical perspective of illness trajectory.

When considering the authors' use of adapted grounded theory methods to analyze preexisting empirical evidence, several insights may be useful to support the integrity of this work. First, Wiener was certainly well prepared to advance new applications of the method by her training and experience as a grounded theorist. The methodological credibility of this researcher supports her extension of a traditional research method into a new application within her disciplinary perspective (sociology). Further, it is important to recall the size of this data set: 100 patients and families were interviewed 3 times each, for a total of 300 interviews. This is a very large data set for a qualitative inquiry. Oberst pointed out that given this volume of data, some semblance of theoretical sampling (within the full data set) would likely be permitted by the researchers (Oberst, 1993). But the sheer size of the data set does not tell the whole story.

Sampling patients who had a relatively wide range of types of cancers (ranging from gynecological cancers to lung cancer) and both patients undergoing initial chemotherapeutic treatment and those receiving treatment for recurrence contributed significantly to variation in the data set. These sampling strategies ultimately contributed to establishing an appropriate sample, especially for revealing a trajectory perspective of change over time. Finally, despite the structured format of the interview, it is important to note that the patients and families dialogued about the previous month's events in a form of "brainstorming" (Wiener & Dodd, 1993, p. 18). This technique would allow the subjects to introduce almost any topic that was of concern to them (regardless of the subsequent structure of the interview). The audiotaping and verbatim transcription of these dialogues contributed to the variation and appropriateness of the resultant data set. Given these insights, it may be concluded that the empirical evidence culled through the interviews conducted during the larger study provided adequate and appropriate data for a secondary analysis using expertly adapted grounded theory methods.

MAJOR ASSUMPTIONS

Wiener and Dodd's Theory of Illness Trajectory explicates major assumptions that reflect its derivation within a sociological perspective (Wiener & Dodd, 1993). Closer examination of each assumption reveals several related basic premises undergirding the theory. In contrast to other nursing theories, the constructs of nursing, person, health, and environment are not explicitly addressed; however, the following discussion of theoretical assumptions sheds some light on the theoretical interpretation of these constructs.

The trajectory model encompasses not only the physical components of the disease, but the "total organization of work done over the course of the disease" (Wiener & Dodd, 1993, p. 20). An illness trajectory is theoretically distinct from the course of an illness. In this theory, the illness trajectory is not limited to the person who suffers the illness. Rather, the total organization involves the person with the illness, family, and healthcare professionals who render health care.

Also, notice the use of the term *work*. "The varied players in the organization have different types of work; however, the patient is the 'central worker' in the illness trajectory" (Wiener & Dodd, 1993, p. 20). This statement reaffirms an earlier assertion found in illness trajectory literature (Fagerhaugh, Strauss, Suczek, & Wiener, 1987; Strauss, Corbin, Fagerhaugh, Glaser, Maines, Suczek, et al., 1984). The work of living with an illness produces certain consequences or impacts that permeate the lives of the people involved. In turn, consequences and reciprocal consequences ripple throughout the organization, enmeshing the total organization with the central worker (i.e., the patient) through the trajectory of living with the illness. The relationship among the workers in the trajectory is a critical attribute that "affects both the management of that course of illness, as well as the fate of the person who is ill" (Wiener & Dodd, 1993, p. 20).

THEORETICAL ASSERTIONS

The focus on the social context for work and the social relationships affecting the work of living with illness in the Theory of Illness Trajectory is based in the seminal work of Corbin and Strauss (1988). As the central worker, actions are undertaken by the person to manage the impact of living with illness within a range of contexts, including the biographical (conception of self) and the sociological (interactions with others). From this perspective, managing disruptions (or coping with uncertainty) involves interactions with the various players in the organization as well as external sociological conditions. Given the complexity of such interactions across multiple contexts and with the numerous players experienced throughout the trajectory of illness, coping is a highly variable and dynamic process.

Originally, it was anticipated that the trajectory of living with cancer had discernible phases or stages that could be identified by major shifts in reported problems, challenges, and activities. This was the rationale for collecting qualitative data at three points during the chemotherapy treatment. In fact, this conjecture did not hold true: the physical status of the patient with cancer and the social-psychological consequences of illness and treatment were the central themes at all points of measurement across the trajectory.

The authors conceptually equate uncertainty with loss of control, described as "the most problematic facet of living with cancer" (Wiener & Dodd, 1993, p. 18). This theoretical assertion is reflected further in the identification of the core social-psychological process of living with cancer, "tolerating the uncertainty that permeates the disease" (p. 19). Factors that influenced the degree of uncertainty expressed by the patient and family were based in the theoretical framework of the total organization and external sociological conditions, including the nature of family support, financial resources, and the quality of assistance from healthcare providers.

LOGICAL FORM

The primary logical form employed to produce this grounded theory was inductive reasoning. Analytical reading of the interviews provided insights that led to the identification of the core process that unifies the theoretical assertions: tolerating uncertainty. Systematic coding processes were applied to define further the dimensions of uncertainty and of management processes used to deal with the disease and its consequences. Then, given these insights, the findings were examined for their fit within extant theoretical writings to extend our understanding of the trajectory of illness. The resultant qualitatively derived theory was well grounded in the reported experiences of the participants and skillfully integrated with what was known of trajectories of illness to advance the state of the science.

ACCEPTANCE BY THE NURSING COMMUNITY

Practice

The importance of the Theory of Illness Trajectory for nursing practice is in providing a framework for understanding how cancer patients tolerate uncertainty manifested as a loss of control. The identification of types of uncertainty abatement work is especially useful in revealing the strategies commonly employed by oncology patients as they attempt to manage their lives as normally as possible in the wake of the uncertainty created by a diagnosis of cancer. Awareness of these themes of uncertainty and related management strategies faced by patients undergoing chemotherapy and their family members could have a significant impact on how nurses subsequently intervene with these compromised patient systems who are managing the work of their illness to "facilitate a less troubled trajectory course for some patients and their families" (Wiener & Dodd, 1993, p. 29). An example of such an intervention was described by Horner as she recommended that nurses explore family assumptions about health care experiences to open a dialogue about the work that surrounds the uncertainties faced in the illness trajectory (Horner, 1997).

Education

Wiener and Dodd are highly respected educators who share their ongoing work through international conferences, seminars, consultations, graduate thesis advising, and course offerings. Incorporation of this work into these presentations not only advances knowledge related to the utility of illness trajectory models but, perhaps more importantly, demonstrates how such data-based theoretical advancement contributes to an evolving program of research in cancer care (Dodd, 1997, 2001). The recent reprinting of the theory in a nursing text on research and theory in chronic illness will increase exposure of the work to nursing scholars (Wiener & Dodd, 2000).

Research

The theory has been referenced in a limited number of concept analyses or state-of-the-science papers addressing uncertainty (McCormick, 2002; Mishel, 1997; Parry, 2003). Mishel (1997) has praised the broad theoretical focus maintained through the qualitative approach to theory derivation. Much of the work in coping with illness is constrained by the application of Lazarus and Folkman's framework of problem-based or emotion-based coping; however, in this study, inductive reasoning produced data-based theory that identifies a broad range of strategies related to tolerating and abating uncertainty (Lazarus & Folkman, 1984; Mishel, 1997). The variation and range of abatement strategies identified in this theory are a unique and significant contribution to the body of research in coping with the uncertainty of illness.

FURTHER DEVELOPMENT

In a response article to the original publication, Oberst (1993) took issue with the delimitation of the concept of uncertainty to loss of control. This criticism has been echoed by McCormick (2002), who theoretically positions loss of control as a component in the uncertainty cycle rather than as a manifestation of a state of uncertainty. Further research into the concept of control is warranted to untangle the conceptual boundaries and linkages between control and uncertainty throughout the illness trajectory.

Other researchers have criticized the implicit assertion that uncertainty (or loss of control) is always a negative event that requires some form of abatement (Oberst, 1993; Parry, 2003). Oberst (1993) suggests that further investigation is needed to differentiate work related to tolerating uncertainty from abatement work in order to reveal how effective strategies in each type of work affect the sense of uncertainty throughout the trajectory. Parry (2003) studied survivors of childhood cancer and revealed that although uncertain states may be a problematic stressor for some, a more universal theme of embracing uncertainty toward transformational growth was evident in these survivors.

Penrod (2007) helped to clarify the concept of uncertainty with a phenomenological investigation that advanced the concept of uncertainty. Penrod (2007) identified different types of uncertainty. The experience of living with uncertainty was dynamic in nature with changes in the types and modes of uncertainty. The various types of uncertainty were guided by the primary tenets of confidence and a sense of control.

These insights demonstrate an evolving body of research related to uncertainty, control, and the illness trajectory. Inquiry must not be constrained by an assumption that uncertainty is necessarily a negative aspect of life; researchers must remain open to positive transformational outcomes of living through uncertainty. Wiener and Dodd's original recommendation to expand the scope of the illness trajectory framework remains salient (Wiener & Dodd, 1993). The illness trajectory theoretical framework would be especially useful for understanding variations in uncertainty and control across a fuller perspective of the illness trajectory in cancer and other conditions in which the significance of uncertainty and control may vary.

CRITIQUE

Clarity

One concern in the clarity in Wiener and Dodd's Theory of Illness Trajectory is the delimitation of the concept of uncertainty to a loss of control. This limited conceptual perspective of uncertainty is clearly set forth in the work; therefore, this issue does not create a significant or fatal flaw in the work. The theory is delineated clearly and is well supported by previous work in illness trajectories. Propositional clarity is achieved in the logical presentation of relationships and the linkages between concepts discussed in the theory. The conceptual derivation of managing illness as work is well developed and provides unique insights into the meaning of living through chemotherapy during cancer treatment. The application of the trajectory model is used consistently to demonstrate the dynamic fluctuations in coping, not in clearly demarcated stages or phases, but in situation-specific contexts of the work of managing illness. The dynamic flow of work contexts, players within the organization of work, and situation in cancer treatment make diagramming or modeling of the theory impractical.

Simplicity

This complex theory is interpreted in a highly accessible manner. The Theory of Illness Trajectory adopts a sociological framework that is applied to a phenomenon of concern to nursing: chemotherapeutic treatment of cancer patients and their families. The sense of understanding imparted by the theory is highly relevant to oncology nursing. The descriptions of patient and family behaviors and insights are congruent with clinical experiences. The theory presents an eloquent and parsimonious interpretation of the complexity of this phenomenon using key concepts with adequate definition; however, in order to comprehend fully the theoretical assertions of the theory, further study of previous work in trajectory models would be very helpful.

Generality

The authors have limited carefully the scope of this theory to patients and families progressing through chemotherapy for initial treatment or recurrence of cancer. The Theory of Illness Trajectory is well defined within this context. The integration of this middle range theory with other work in trajectories of illness and uncertainty theory indicates that there is an emergent fit with other models of illness trajectories and uncertainty. Further theory-building work may produce higher levels of theory with broader scope that may permit the application of these theoretical propositions in other contexts of illness trajectories.

Empirical Precision

Grounded theory methods rely on the dominance of inductive reasoning, that is, drawing abstractions or generalities from examples of specific situations. Thus, the derived theory is rooted in the experiences expressed in the hundreds of interviews with cancer patients and their families. The integration of data-based evidence (e.g., quotes) in the formal description of the theory supports the linkages between the theoretical abstractions and empirical observations. The empirical evidence is presented in a logical and consistent manner that rings true to clinical experiences. Thus, the theory is relevant and useful to clinicians and holds promise for further research application.

Derivable Consequences

The significance of the theoretical contributions made by this work, especially the types of work and uncertainty abatement strategies used during chemotherapy, has been established. The utility of this theory is apparent in cancer treatment and, with further theoretical development, the theory may be further generalizable to other contexts within cancer care or even other illness trajectories. Yet, there is limited evidence of directly derived consequences related to the application of the Theory of Illness Trajectory in practice-based studies in nursing.

This issue remains problematic. The sociological perspective reflected in the work should not inhibit nurse scholars. Applicability of this theory to phenomena of concern to nursing has been established by the authors' focus on cancer chemotherapy. The potential utility of the theory for guiding nursing practice is perhaps best demonstrated by the integration of the theory into Dodd's exemplary program of research in cancer care (Dodd & Miaskowski, 2000; Dodd, 2001; 2004; Miaskowski, Dodd, & Lee, 2004; Jansen, Miaskowski, Dodd, & Dowling, 2007).

SUMMARY

Wiener and Dodd's Theory of Illness Trajectory is at once complex, yet eloquently simple. The sociological perspective of defining the work of managing illness is especially relevant to the context of cancer care. The theory provides new ways of understanding how patients and families tolerate uncertainty and work strategically to abate uncertainty throughout a dynamic flow of illness events, treatment situations, and varied players who become involved in the organization of care. The theory is pragmatic and relevant to nursing. The merits of this work warrant further attention to using the theory to produce more direct practice implications that could change the way nurses interpret and facilitate the management of an illness.

Case Study

Mr. Miller is a 67-year-old man who has metastatic cancer. His primary caregiver is his wife, Mrs. Miller. Early in the course of treatment in your outpatient cancer care center, the couple focused their questions on the course of the disease, treatment options, and potential side effects of varied treatment options. They were proud of their ability to maintain "normal life" as Mr. Miller continued to work throughout aggressive treatment, taking time off only when the discomforts of treatment were so debilitating that he was physically unable to get to his office. Mr. and Mrs. Miller expressed little emotion throughout the course of treatment; they frequently praised each other's strength and fortitude. During recent visits, Mrs. Miller has become extremely focused on laboratory values and test results, using highly technical language. She has also become adamant that certain staff members must perform certain tasks because "she does it better than anyone."

The Theory of Illness Trajectory helps the clinician to interpret these behaviors and to intervene to help ease transitions across this trajectory. For example, clinicians can identify easily with patients and families who have become "professional patients" as they learn to use complex technical jargon about their treatment, laboratory values, or illness (Wiener & Dodd, 1993). These "junior doctors" attempt to earn a modicum of control as they manage treatment by requesting particular staff members to perform specific tasks (Dodd, 1997, p. 988). Care providers have a tendency to view this behavior as a positive hallmark of assuming self-care and, therefore, often reinforce such behaviors.

Deeper consideration of the theoretical assertions of the Theory of Illness Trajectory reveals that these behavioral strategies are efforts to tolerate the uncertainty of the illness experience. The confidence built through these socially reinforced behaviors can be converted to guilt very quickly when situations beyond the expertise of the patient or family go awry. Given this perspective, the limitation of this management strategy becomes clear, and intervention is indicated: if patients and families are to manage care effectively, they must be educated proactively to do so (Dodd, 1997, 2001).

In proactively educating the patient-family system, consider the varied domains of uncertainty and the varied forms of uncertainty abatement work. To understand the patient-family trajectory, assessment data are critical. For example, although well-developed protocols for symptom management or palliation are available, such protocols are useless if patients or caregivers fail to describe the extent of symptoms because they perceive these "hassles" or "bothers" as trivial in the face of life-threatening disease. Compounding this issue, nurses may fall into a pattern of focusing on illness-related work, thereby diverting important attention from the other forms of work faced by these patients and their families. Understanding of the varied domains of uncertainty and forms of uncertainty abatement work facilitates a more open dialogue regarding these key areas of concern, allowing the nurse to encourage the patient and caregiver to share more about their experiences in an effort to help them through this difficult time.

CRITICAL THINKING *Activities*

1. How does a trajectory of illness differ from a course of illness? Differentiate how the application of each perspective may yield different foci for intervention for a selected health condition. Which perspective is most congruent with your paradigmatic views of nursing?
2. Considering your clinical experiences, give examples of how patients and their families have experienced health-related uncertainty. Is uncertainty always related to a loss of control? Are there different conditions under which health-related uncertainty is perceived as a negative life event versus those in which the uncertainty is positioned as a growth-enhancing event?
3. As a clinician, you are intimately involved in the work of managing an illness. Based on your understanding of the work of illness management espoused in the Theory of Illness Trajectory, what nursing behaviors may exacerbate feelings of loss of control or uncertainty in your patients? What factors (personal, environmental, or organizational) may contribute to these behaviors? What interventions would you suggest to create a less troubling trajectory for your patients and their families?

POINTS FOR *Further Study*

- Dodd, M. J. (2001). Managing the side effects of chemotherapy and radiation therapy: A guide for patients and their families (4th ed.). San Francisco: UCSF School of Nursing Press.
- Dodd, M. J., Miaskowski, C. (2000). The PRO-SELF program: A self care intervention program for patients receiving cancer treatment. *Seminars in Oncology, 16*(4), 300-308.
- Jansen, C. E., Miaskowski, C. A., Dodd, M. J., & Dowling, G. A. (2007). A meta-analysis of the sensitivity of various neuropsychological tests used to detect chemotherapy-induced cognitive impairment in patients with breast cancer. *Oncology Nursing Forum, 34*(5), 997-1005.
- Penrod, J. (2007). Living with uncertainty: Concept advancement. *Journal of Advanced Nursing, 57*(6), 658-667.
- West, C. M., Dodd, M. J., Paul, S. M., Schumacher, K., Tripathy, D., Koo, P., et al. (2003). The PRO-SELF: Pain control program—An effective approach for cancer pain management. *Oncology Nursing Forum, 30,* 65-73.
- Dodd, M. (2004). The pathogenesis and characterization of oral mucositis associated with cancer therapy. Oncology Nursing Forum, 31(4 Suppl), 5-11.

REFERENCES

Corbin, J., & Strauss, A. (1988). *Unending work and care.* San Francisco: Jossey Bass.

Dodd, M. J. (1978). *Oncology nursing case studies.* New York: Medical Publication Co.

Dodd, M. J. (1987). *Managing the side effects of chemotherapy and radiation therapy: A guide for patients and nurses.* Norwalk, CT: Appleton & Lange.

Dodd, M. J. (1988). *Monograph of the advanced research session at the 13th Annual Oncology Nursing Society's Congress.* Pittsburgh: Oncology Nursing Society Press.

Dodd, M. J. (1991). *Managing the side effects of chemotherapy and radiation: A guide for patients and their families* (2nd ed.). Englewood, NJ: Prentice-Hall.

Dodd, M. J. (1997). *Managing the side effects of chemotherapy and radiation therapy: A guide for patients and their families* (3rd ed.). San Francisco: UCSF School of Nursing Press.

Dodd, M. J. (2001). *Managing the side effects of chemotherapy and radiation therapy: A guide for patients and their families* (4th ed.). San Francisco: UCSF School of Nursing Press.

Dodd, M. (2004). The pathogenesis and characterization of oral mucositis associated with cancer therapy. *Oncology Nursing Forum, 31*(4 Suppl), 5-11.

Dodd, M. J., Miaskowski, C. (2000). The PRO-SELF program: A self care intervention program for patients receiving cancer treatment. *Seminars in Oncology, 16* (4), 300-308.

Fagerhaugh, S., Strauss, A., Suczek, B., & Wiener, C. (1987). *Hazards in hospital care: Ensuring patient safety.* San Francisco: Jossey-Bass.

Glaser, B. (1978). *Theoretical sensitivity.* Mill Valley, CA: Sociology Press.

Glaser, B., & Strauss, A. (1965). *Awareness of dying.* Chicago: Aldine.

Horner, S. D. (1997). Uncertainty in mothers' care for their ill children. *Journal of Advanced Nursing, 26*, 658-663.

Jansen, C. E., Miaskowski, C. A., Dodd, M. J., & Dowling, G. A. (2007). A meta-analysis of the sensitivity of various neuropsychological tests used to detect chemotherapy-induced cognitive impairment in patients with breast cancer. *Oncology Nursing Forum, 34*(5), 997-1005.

Lazarus, R. S., & Folkman, S. (1984). *Stress, appraisal, and coping.* New York: Springer.

McCormick, K. M. (2002). A concept analysis of uncertainty in illness. *Journal of Nursing Scholarship, 34*(2), 127-131.

Miaskowski, C., Dodd, M., & Lee, K. (2004). Symptom clusters: The new frontier in symptom management research. *Journal of the National Cancer Institute Monographs, 32*, 17-21.

Mishel, M. H. (1997). Uncertainty in acute illness. *Annual Review of Nursing Research, 15*, 57-80.

Oberst, M. T. (1993). Response to "Coping amid uncertainty: An illness trajectory perspective." *Scholarly Inquiry for Nursing Practice: An International Journal, 7*(1), 33-35.

Parry, C. (2003). Embracing uncertainty: An exploration of the experiences of childhood cancer survivors. *Qualitative Health Research, 13*(1), 227-246.

Penrod, J. (2007). Living with uncertainty: Concept advancement. *Journal of Advanced Nursing, 57*(6), 658-667.

Strauss, A., Corbin, J., Fagerhaugh, S., Glaser, B., Maines, D., Suczek, B., et al. (1984). *Chronic illness and the quality of life.* St. Louis: Mosby.

Strauss, A., Fagerhaugh, S., Suczek, B., & Wiener, C. (1997). *Social organization of medical work.* New Brunswick, NJ: Transaction Books.

West, C. M., Dodd, M. J., Paul, S. M., Schumacher, K., Tripathy, D., Koo, P., et al. (2003). The PRO-SELF: Pain control program—An effective approach for cancer pain management. *Oncology Nursing Forum, 30*, 65-73.

Wiener, C. (1981). *The politics of alcoholism: Building an arena around a social problem.* New Brunswick, NJ: Transaction Books.

Wiener, C. (2000). *The elusive quest: Accountability in hospitals.* New York: Aldine deGruyter.

Wiener, C. L., & Dodd, M. J. (1993). Coping amid uncertainty: An illness trajectory perspective. *Scholarly Inquiry for Nursing Practice: An International Journal, 7*(1), 17-31.

Wiener, C. L., & Dodd, M. J. (2000). Coping amid uncertainty: An illness trajectory perspective. In R. Hyman & J. Corbin (Eds.), *Chronic illness: Research and theory for nursing practice* (pp. 180-201). New York: Springer.

Wiener, C., & Strauss, A. (1997). *Where medicine fails* (5th ed.). New Brunswick, NJ: Transaction Books.

Wiener, C., & Wysmans, W. M. (1990). *Grounded theory in medical research: From theory to practice.* Amsterdam: Sivets and Zeitlinger.

BIBLIOGRAPHY

Primary Sources

Books

Dodd, M. J. (2001). Managing the side effects of chemotherapy and radiation therapy: A guide for patients and their families (4th ed.). San Francisco: UCSF School of Nursing Press.

Wiener, C. (2000). The elusive quest: Accountability in hospitals. New York: Aldine deGruyter.

Wiener, C. (2004). Grounded theory in medical research from theory to practice. Oxfordshire, United Kingdom: Routledge.

Wiener, C., & Strauss, A. (1997). Where medicine fails (5th ed.). New Brunswick, NJ: Transaction Books.

Wiener, C., & Wysmans, W. M. (1990). Grounded theory in medical research: From theory to practice. Amsterdam: Sivets and Zeitlinger.

Book Chapters

Dodd, M. J. (1997). Measuring self-care activities. In M. Frank-Stromborg & S. J. Olsen (Eds.), *Instruments for clinical health-care research* (pp. 378-385). Wilsonville, OR: Jones & Bartlett.

Dodd, M. J. (1999). Self-care and patient/family teaching. In S. L. Groenwald, M. H. Frogge, M. Goodman, & C. H. Yarbro (Eds.), *Cancer symptom management* (2nd ed., pp. 20-29). Wilsonville, OR: Jones & Bartlett.

Dodd, M. J., & Miaskowski, C. (2003). Symptom management, the PRO-SELF Program: A self-care intervention program. In B. Given, C. Given, & V. Champion (Eds.), *Evidence-based behavioral interventions for cancer patients: State of the knowledge across the cancer care trajectory* (pp. 218-241). New York: Springer.

Journal Articles

Baggott, C., Beale, I. L., Dodd, M. J., & Kato, P. M. (2004). A survey of self-care and dependent-care advice given by pediatric oncology nurses. *Journal of Pediatric Oncology, 21*(4), 214-222.

Chen, L., Miaskowski, C., Dodd, M., & Pantilat, S. (2008). Concepts within the Chinese culture that influence the cancer pain experience. *Cancer Nursing, 31*(2), 103-108.

Cho, M. H., Dodd, M. J., Lee, K. A., Padilla, G., & Slaughter, R. (2006). Self-reported sleep quality in family caregivers of gastric cancer patients who are receiving chemotherapy in Korea. *Journal of Cancer Education, 21*(1 Suppl), S37-S41.

Chou, F., Dodd, M., Abrams, D., & Padilla, G. (2007). Symptoms, self-care, and quality of life of Chinese American patients with cancer. *Oncology Nursing Forum, 34*(6), 1162-1167.

Cotanch, P., & Dodd, M. J. (1990). *Monograph of the advanced research sessions at the 14th Annual Oncology Nursing Society's Congress.* Pittsburgh: Oncology Nursing Society Press.

Dibble, S. L., Padilla, G. V., Dodd, M. J., & Miaskowski, C. (1998). Gender differences in the dimensions of quality of life. *Oncology Nursing Forum, 25*(3), 577-583.

Dodd, M. (2000). Cancer-related fatigue. *Cancer Investigation, 18*(1), 97.

Dodd, M. (2004). The pathogenesis and characterization of oral mucositis associated with cancer therapy. *Oncology Nursing Forum, 31*(4 Suppl), 5-11.

Dodd, M. J. (2002). Defining clinically meaningful outcomes in the evaluation of new treatments for oral mucositis: A commentary. *Cancer Investigation, 20*(5-6), 851-852.

Dodd, M. J., Cho, M. H., Cooper, B., Miaskowski, C., Lee, K. A., & Bank, K. (2005). Advancing our knowledge of symptoms clusters. *Journal of Supportive Oncology, 3*(6 Suppl 4), 30-31.

Dodd, M. J., Dibble, S., Miaskowski, C., Paul, S., Cho, M., MacPhil, L., Greenspan, D., & Shiba, G. (2001). A comparison of the affective state and quality of life of chemotherapy patients who do and do not develop chemotherapy-induced oral mucositis. *Journal of Pain and Symptom Management, 21*(6), 498-505.

Dodd, M. J., Dibble, S. L., Miaskowski, C., MacPhil, L., Greenspan, D., Paul, S. M., Shiba, G., & Larson, P. (2000). Randomized clinical trial of the effectiveness of 3 commonly used mouthwashes to treat chemotherapy-induced mucositis. *Journal of Oral Surgery, Oral Medicine, Oral Pathology, Oral Radiology, and Endodontics, 90*(1), 39-47.

Dodd, M. J., Janson, S., Facione, N., Faucett, J., Froelicher, E. S., Humphreys, J., et al. (2001). Advancing the science of symptom management. *Journal of Advanced Nursing, 33*(5), 668-676.

Dodd, M. J., & Miaskowski, C. (2000). The PRO-SELF program: A self-care intervention program for patients receiving cancer treatment. *Seminars in Oncology, 16*(4), 300-308.

Dodd, M. J., Miaskowski, C., Dibble, S. L., Paul, S. M., MacPhil, L., Greenspan, D., & Shiba, G. (2000). Factors influencing oral mucositis in patients receiving chemotherapy. *Cancer Practice, 8*(6), 291-297.

Dodd, M. J., Miaskowski, C., Greenspan, D., MacPhil, L., Shis, A. S., Shiba, G., Facione, N., & Paul, S. M. (2003). Radiation-induced mucositis: A randomized clinical trial of micronized sucralfate versus salt & soda mouthwashes. *Cancer Investigation, 21*(1), 21-33.

Dodd, M. J., Miaskowski, C., & Lee, K. A. (2004). Occurrence of symptom clusters. *Journal of the National Cancer Institute Monographs, 32,* 76-78.

Dodd, M. J., Miaskowski, C., & Paul, S. M. (2001). Symptom clusters and their effect on the functional status of patients with cancer. *Oncology Nursing Forum, 28*(3), 465-470.

Dodd, M. J., Miaskowski, C., Shiba, G. H., Dibble, S. L., Greenspan, D., MacPhil, L., Paul, S. M., & Larson, P. (1999). Risk factors for chemotherapy-induced oral mucositis: Dental appliances, oral hygiene, previous oral lesions, and history of smoking. *Cancer Investigation, 17* (4), 278-284.

Dowling, G. A., & Wiener, C. L. (1997). Roadblocks encountered in recruiting patients for a study of sleep disruption in Alzheimer's disease. *Image: Journal of Nursing Scholarship, 29*(1), 59-64.

Edrington, J., Miaskowski, C., Dodd, M., Wong, C., & Padilla, G. (2007). A review of the literature on the pain experience of Chinese patients with cancer. *Cancer Nursing, 30*(5), 335-346.

Edrington, J. M., Paul, S., Dodd, M., West, C., Facione, N., Tripathy, D., Koo, P., Schumacher, K., & Miaskowski, C. (2004). No evidence for sex differences in the severity and treatment of cancer pain. *Journal of Pain and Symptom Management, 28*(3), 225-232.

Facione, N. C., Miaskowski, C., Dodd, M. J., & Paul, S. M. (2002). The self-reported likelihood of patient delay in breast cancer: New thoughts for early detection. *Preventative Medicine, 34*(4), 397-407.

Fletcher, B. S., Dodd, M. J., Schumacher, K. L., & Miaskowski, C. (2008). Symptom experience of family caregivers of patients with cancer. *Oncology Nursing Forum, 35*(2), E23-E44.

Fletcher, B. S., Paul, S. M., Dodd, M. J., Schumacher, K., West, C., Cooper, B., Lee, K., Aouizerat, B., Swift, P., Wara, W., & Miaskowski, C.A. (2008). Prevalence, severity, and impact of symptoms on female family caregivers of patients at the initiation of radiation therapy for prostate cancer. *Journal of Clinical Oncology, 26*(4), 599-605.

Hilton, J. F., MacPhil, L. A., Pascasio, L., Sroussi, H. Y., Cheikh, B., LaBao, M. E., Malvin, K., Greenspan, D., & Dodd, M. J. (2004). Self-care intervention to reduce oral candidiasis recurrence in HIV-seropositive persons: A pilot-study. Community *Dentistry and Oral Epidemiology, 32*(3), 190-200.

Hinds, P. S., Baggott, C., DeSwarte-Wallace, J., Dodd, M., Haase, J., Hockenberry, M., Hooke, C., McGuire-Cullen, P., Moore, I., Roll, L., & Ruccione, K. (2003). Functional integration of nursing research into a pediatric oncology cooperative group: Finding common ground. *Oncology Nursing Forum, 30*(6), E121-E126.

Jansen, C. E., Miaskowski, C., Dodd, M., & Dowling, G. (2005). Chemotherapy-induced cognitive impairment in women with breast cancer: A critique of the literature. *Oncology Nursing Forum, 32*(2), 329-342.

Jansen, C. E., Miaskowski, C., Dodd, M., Dowling, G., & Kramer, J. (2005). A metaanalysis of studies of the effects of cancer chemotherapy on various domains of cognitive functioning. *Cancer, 104*(10), 2222-2233.

Jansen, C. E., Miaskowski, C., Dodd, M., Dowling, G., & Kramer, J. (2005). Potential mechanisms for chemotherapy-induced impairments in cognitive function. *Oncology Nursing Forum, 32* (6), 1151-1163.

Jansen, C. E., Miaskowski, C. A., Dodd, M. J., & Dowling, G. A. (2007). A meta-analysis of the sensitivity of various neuropsychological tests used to detect chemotherapy-induced cognitive impairment in patients with breast cancer. *Oncology Nursing Forum, 34*(5), 997-1005.

Katapodi, M. C., Facione, N. C., Humphreys, J. C., & Dodd, M. J., (2005). Perceived breast cancer risk: Heuristic reasoning and search for a dominance structure. *Social Science and Medicine, 60*(2), 421-432.

Katapodi, M. C., Facione, N. C., Miaskowski, C., Dodd, M. J., & Waters, C. (2002). The influence of social support on breast cancer screening in a multicultural community sample. *Oncology Nursing Forum, 29* (5), 845-852.

Katapodi, M. C., Lee, K. A., Facione, N. C., & Dodd, M. J. (2004). Predictors of perceived breast cancer risk and the relation between perceived breast cancer screening: A meta-analytic review. *Preventative Medicine, 38*(4), 388-402.

Kim, J. E., Dodd, M., West, C., Paul, S., Facione, N., Schumacher, K., Tripathy, D., Koo, P., & Miaskowski, C. (2004). The PRO-SELF pain control program improves patients' knowledge of cancer pain management. *Oncology Nursing Forum, 31*(6), 1137-1143.

Krasnoff, J. B., Vintro, A. Q., Ascher, N. L., Bass, N. M., Dodd, M. J., & Painter, P. L. (2005). Objective measures of health-related quality of life over 24 months post-liver transplantation. *Clinical Transplantation 19*(1), 1-9.

Krasnoff, J. B., Vintro, A. Q., Ascher, N. L., Bass, N. M., Paul, S. M., Dodd, M. J., & Painter, P. L. (2006). A randomized trial of exercise and dietary counseling after liver transplantation. *American Journal of Transplantation, 6*, 1896-1905.

Kris, A. E., & Dodd, M. J. (2004). Symptom experience of adult hospitalized medical-surgical patients. *Journal of Symptom Management, 28*(5), 451-459.

Larson, P., Dodd, M. J., & Aksamit, I. (1998). A symptom-management program for patients undergoing cancer treatment: The PRO-SELF Program. *Journal of Cancer Education, 13*(4), 248-252.

Larson, P. J., Miaskowski, C., MacPhil, L., Dodd, M. J., Greenspan, D., Dibble, S. L., Paul, S. M., & Ignoffo, R. (1998). The PRO-SELF Mouth Aware program: An effective approach for reducing chemotherapy-induced mucositis. *Cancer Nursing, 21*(4), 263-268.

Lee, K., Cho, M., Miaskowski, C., & Dodd, M. (2004). Impaired sleep and rhythms in persons with cancer. *Sleep Medicine Reviews, 8*(3), 199-212.

Lovely, M. P., Miaskowski, C., & Dodd, M. (1999). Relationship between fatigue and quality of life in patients with glioblastoma multiforme. *Oncology Nursing Forum, 25* (5), 921-925.

Mandrell, B. N., Ruccione, K., Dodd, M. J., Moore, J., Nelson, A. E., Pollock, B., et al. (2000). Consensus statements. Applying the concept of self-care to pediatric oncology patients. *Seminars in Oncology Nursing, 16*(4), 315-316.

McLemore, M. R., Miaskowski, C., Aouizerat, B. E., Chen, L. E., & Dodd, M. (2008). Rules of cell development and their application to biomarkers for ovarian cancer. *Oncology Nursing Forum, 35*(3), 403-409.

Miaskowski, C., Cooper, B. A., Paul, S. M., Dodd, M., Lee, K., Aouizerat, B. E., West, C., Cho, M., & Bank, A. (2006). Subgroups of patients with cancer with different symptoms experiences and quality-of-life outcomes: A cluster analysis. *Oncology Nursing Forum, 33*(5), E79-E89.

Miaskowski, C., Dodd, M., & Lee, K. (2004). Symptom clusters: The new frontier in symptom management research. *Journal of the National Cancer Institute Monographs, 32*, 17-21.

Miaskowski, C., Dodd, M., West, C., Paul, S. M., Schumacher, K., Tripathy, D., & Koo, P. (2007). The use of a responder analysis to identify differences in patient outcomes following a self-care intervention to improve cancer pain management. *Pain, 129*, 55-63.

Miaskowski, C., Dodd, M., West, C., Paul, S. M., Tripathy, D., Koo, P., Schumacher, K. (2001). Lack of adherence with the analgesic regimen: A significant barrier to effective cancer pain management. *Journal of Clinical Oncology, 19* (23), 4275-4279.

Miaskowski, C., Dodd, M., West, C., Schumacher, K., Paul, S. M., Tripathy, D., & Koo, P. (2004). Randomized clinical trial of the effectiveness of a self-care interventions to improve cancer pain management. *Journal of Clinical Oncology, 22*(90), 1713-1720.

Miaskowski, C., Mack, K. A., Dodd, M., West, C., Paul, S. M., Tripathy, D., Koo, P., Schumacher, K., & Facione, N. (2002). Oncology outpatients with pain from bone metastasis require more than around-the-clock dosing of analgesics to achieve adequate pain control. *The Journal of Pain, 3*(1), 12-20.

Molfenter, T., Zetts, C., Dodd., M., Owens, B., Ford, J., & Mccarty, D. (2005). Reducing errors of omission in chronic disease management. *Journal of Interprofessional Care, 19*(5), 521-523.

Schumacher, K. L., Koresawa, S., West, C., Dodd, M., Paul, S. M., Tripathy, D., Koo, P., & Miaskowski, C. (2002). The usefulness of a daily pain management diary for outpatients with cancer-related pain. *Oncology Nursing Forum, 29*(9), 1304-1313.

Schumacher, K. L., Koresawa, S., West, C., Dodd, M., Paul, S. M., Tripathy, D., Koo, P., & Miaskowski, C. (2005). Qualitative research contribution to a randomized clinical trial. *Research in Nursing & Health, 28,* 268-280.

Schumacher, K. L., Koresawa, S., West, C., Hawkins, C., Johnson, C., Wais, E., Dodd, M., Paul, S. M., Tripathy, D., Koo, P., & Miaskowski, C. (2002). Putting cancer pain management regimens into practice at home. *Journal of Pain and Symptom Management, 23*(5), 369-382.

Schumacher, K. L., Stewart, B., Archbold, P., Dodd, M., & Dibble, S. (2000). Family caregiving skill: Development of the concept. *Research in Nursing & Health, 23,* 191-203.

Schumacher, K. L., West, C., Dodd, M., Paul, S. M., Tripathy, D., Koo, P., & Miaskowski, C. A. (2002). Pain management autobiographies and reluctance to use opioids for cancer pain management. *Cancer Nursing, 25*(2), 125-133.

Shih, A., Miaskowski, C., Dodd, M. J., Stotts, N. A., & MacPhil, L. (2002). A research review of the current treatments for radiation-induced oral mucositis in patients with head and neck cancer. *Oncology Nursing Forum, 29*(7), 1063-1080.

Shih, A., Miaskowski, C., Dodd, M. J., Stotts, N. A., & MacPhil, L. (2003). Mechanisms for radiation-induced oral mucositis and the consequences. *Cancer Nursing, 26* (3), 222-229.

Tierney, D. K., Facione, N., Padilla, G., Blume, K., & Dodd, M. (2007). Altered sexual health and quality of life in women prior to hematopoietic cell transplantation. *European Journal of Oncology Nursing, 11*(4), 298-308.

Tierney, D. K., Facione, N., Padilla, G., & Dodd, M. (2007). Response shift: A theoretical exploration of quality of life following a hematopoietic cell transplantation. *Cancer Nursing, 30*(2), 125-138.

Villars, P., Dodd, M., West, C., Koetters, T., Paul, S. M., Schumacher, K., Tripathy, D., Koo, P., & Miaskowski, C. (2007). Differences in the prevalence and severity of side effects based on type of analgesic prescriptions in patients with chronic cancer pain. *Journal of Pain and Symptom Management, 33*(1), 67-77.

Voss, J. G., Dodd, M., Portillo, C., & Holzemar, W. (2006). Theories of fatigue: Application in HIV/AIDS. *The Journal of the Association of Nurses in AIDS Care, 17*(1), 37-50.

Voss, J., Portillo, C. J., Holzemer, W. L., & Dodd, M. J. (2007). Symptom cluster of fatigue and depression in HIV/AIDS. *Journal of Prevention and Intervention in the Community, 33*(1-2), 19-34.

West, C. M., Dodd, M. J., Paul, S. M., Schumacher, K., Tripathy, D., Koo, P., & Miaskowski, C. (2003). The PRO-SELF(c): Pain control program—an effective approach for cancer pain management. *Oncology Nursing Forum, 30*(1), 65-73.

Wiener, C., Fagerhaugh, S., Strauss, A., & Suczek, B. (1979). Trajectories, biographies and the evolving medical technology scene: Labor and delivery and the intensive care nursery. *Sociology of Health and Illness, 1*, 261-283. (Reprinted in A. Strauss & J. Corbin [Eds.]. [1997]. *Grounded theory in practice* [pp. 229-250]. Thousand Oaks, CA: Sage.)

Wiener, C., Fagerhaugh, S., Strauss, A., & Suczek, B. (1982). What price chronic illness? *Society, 19*, 22-30. (Reprinted in C. Wiener & A. Strauss [Eds.]. [1987]. *Where medicine fails* [5th ed., pp. 25-42]. New Brunswick, NJ: Transaction Books.)

Wiener, C. L. (2000). Applying the Straussian framework of action, negotiation, and social arenas to a study of accountability in hospitals. *Sociological Perspectives, 43*, S59-S71.

Wiener, C. L. (2004). Holding American hospitals accountable: Rhetoric and reality. *Nursing Inquiry, 11*(2), 82-90.

Wong, P. C., Dodd, M. J., Miaskowski, C., Paul, S. M., Bank, S. A., Shiba, G. H., & Facione, N. (2006). Mucositis pain induced by radiation therapy: Prevalence, severity, and use of self care behaviors. *Journal of Pain and Symptom Management, 32*(1), 27-37.

Wood, K. A., Wiener, C. L., & Kayser-Jones, J. (2007). Supraventricular tachycardia and the struggle to be believed. *European Journal of Cardiovascular Nursing, 6* (4), 293-302.

Secondary Sources

Horner, S. D. (1997). Uncertainty in mothers' care for their ill children. *Journal of Advanced Nursing, 26*, 658-663.

McCormick, K. M. (2002). A concept analysis of uncertainty in illness. *Journal of Nursing Scholarship, 34*(2), 127-131.

Mishel, M. H. (1997). Uncertainty in acute illness. *Annual Review of Nursing Research, 15*, 57-80.

Oberst, M. T. (1993). Response to "Coping amid uncertainty: An illness trajectory perspective." *Scholarly Inquiry for Nursing Practice: An International Journal, 7*(1), 33-35.

Parry, C. (2003). Embracing uncertainty: An exploration of the experiences of childhood cancer survivors. *Qualitative Health Research, 13*(1), 227-246.

Penrod, J. (2007). Living with uncertainty: Concept advancement. *Journal of Advanced Nursing, 57*(6), 658-667.

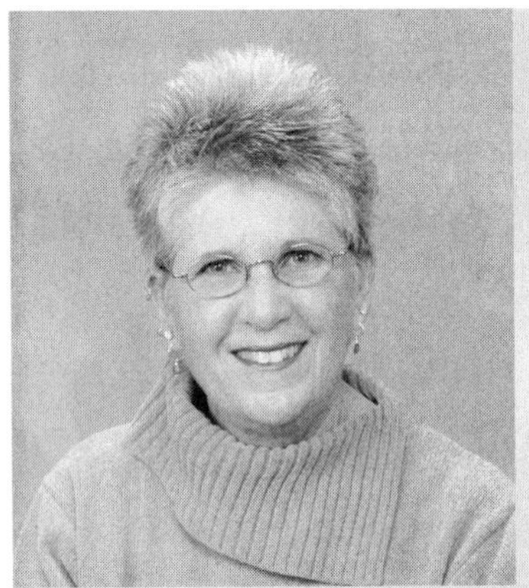

Photo credit: Center for Health Sciences Communication, Brody School of Medicine, East Carolina University, Greenville, NC.

CHAPTER 31

Georgene Gaskill Eakes

1945-present

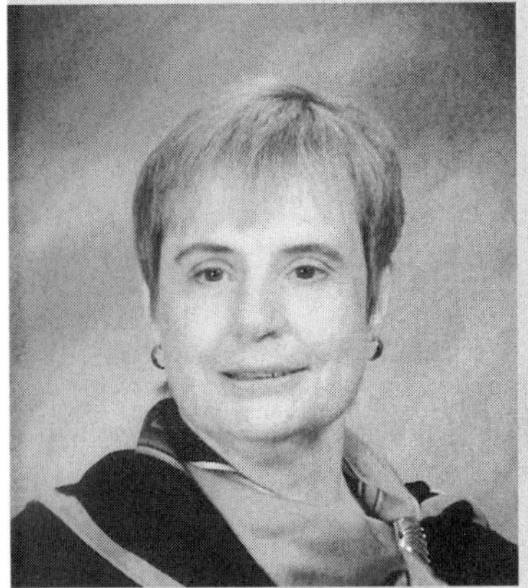

Photo credit: Olan Mills Portrait Studio, Centerdale, RI.

Mary Lermann Burke

1941-present

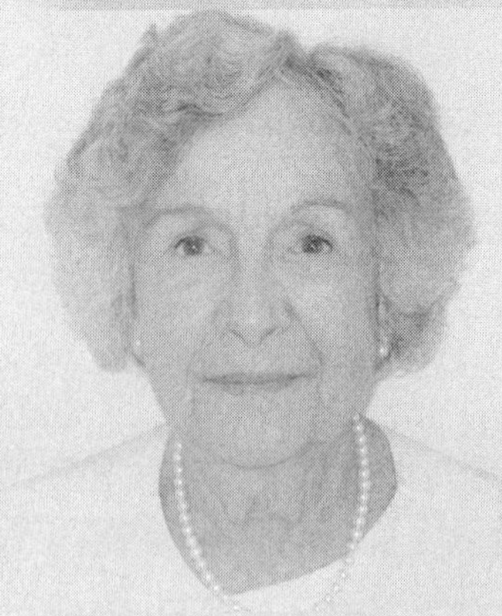

Photo credit: Shawn Hainsworth, New York.

Margaret A. Hainsworth

1931-present

Theory of Chronic Sorrow

Ann M. Schreier and Nellie S. Droes

"Chronic sorrow is the presence of pervasive grief-related feelings that have been found to occur periodically throughout the lives of individuals with chronic health conditions, their family caregivers and the bereaved." (Burke, Eakes, & Hainsworth, 1999, p. 374)

CREDENTIALS OF THE THEORISTS

Georgene Gaskill Eakes

Georgene Gaskill Eakes was born in New Bern, North Carolina. She received a Diploma in Nursing from Watts Hospital School of Nursing in Durham, North Carolina, in 1966, and in 1977, she graduated Summa Cum Laude from North Carolina Agricultural and Technical State University with a baccalaureate in nursing. Eakes completed an M.S.N. at the University of North Carolina at Greensboro in 1980, and an Ed.D. from North Carolina State University in 1988. Eakes was awarded a federal traineeship for her graduate study at the master's level and a graduate fellowship from the North Carolina League for Nursing to support her doctoral studies. She was inducted into Sigma Theta Tau International Honor Society of Nurses in 1979 and Phi Kappa Phi Honor Society in 1988.

Early in her professional career, Eakes worked in both acute and community-based psychiatric and mental health settings. In 1980, she joined the faculty at East Carolina University School of Nursing, Greenville, North Carolina, and continues there today.

Eakes' interest in issues related to death, dying, grief, and loss dates to the 1970s, when she sustained life-threatening injuries in an automobile crash. Her near-death experience heightened her awareness of how ill prepared healthcare professionals and lay people are to deal with individuals facing their mortality and the general lack of understanding of grief reactions experienced in response to loss situations. Motivated by this insight, she directed her early research efforts to the investigation of death anxiety among nursing personnel in long-term care settings and to the exploration of grief resolution among hospice nurses.

In 1983, Eakes established, as a community service, a twice-monthly support group for individuals diagnosed with cancer and their significant others, which she continues to co-facilitate. Her involvement with this group alerted her to the ongoing nature of grief reactions associated with diagnosis of potentially life-threatening, chronic illness. While presenting her dissertation research at a Sigma Theta Tau International research conference in Taipei, Taiwan, in 1989, she attended a presentation on chronic sorrow by Mary Lermann Burke and immediately made the connection between Burke's description of chronic sorrow in mothers of children with a myelomeningocele disability and her observations of grief reactions among the cancer support group members.

After the conference, Eakes contacted Burke to explore the possibility of collaborative research endeavors. Subsequent to their discussions, they scheduled a meeting that included Burke and her colleague, Margaret A. Hainsworth, and Carolyn Lindgren, a colleague of Hainsworth. The Nursing Consortium for Research on Chronic Sorrow (NCRCS) was an outcome of this first meeting in the summer of 1989.

Subsequent to NCRCS's establishment, members conducted numerous collaborative qualitative research studies on populations of individuals affected with chronic or life-threatening conditions, on family caregivers, and on bereaved individuals. Eakes focused her individual studies on those diagnosed with cancer, family caregivers of adult mentally ill children, and individuals who have experienced the death of a significant other. From 1992 through 1997, Eakes received three research grant awards from East Carolina University School of Nursing and two research grants from Beta Nu Chapter of Sigma Theta Tau International to support her research endeavors.

In addition to her professional publications, Eakes has conducted numerous presentations on issues related to grief-loss and death and dying to professionals and lay groups at the local, state, national, and international levels. She has been heavily involved with the training of sudden infant death syndrome counselors for North Carolina and local and regional hospice volunteers. Eakes is also active in efforts to improve the quality of care at the end of life and, toward that end, serves as a member of the Board of Directors of the End of Life Care Coalition of Eastern North Carolina.

In 2002, Eakes received the East Carolina University Scholar Teacher Award in recognition of excellence in the integration of research into teaching practices. In 1999, Eakes received the Best of Image award for theory publication presented by Sigma Theta Tau International Honor Society of Nursing for the publication, "Middle-Range Theory of Chronic Sorrow." She was a finalist in the *Oncology Nursing Forum* Excellence in Writing Award in 1994. Other honors and awards include selection as North Carolina Nurse Educator of the Year by the North Carolina Nurses Association in 1991 and as Outstanding Researcher by Beta Nu Chapter of Sigma Theta Tau International Honor Society for Nurses in 1994 and 1998. Eakes also serves as a reviewer for *Qualitative Health Research*, an international, interdisciplinary journal.

Eakes is a professor in the Department of Family and Community Nursing at East Carolina University School of Nursing, where she teaches undergraduate courses in psychiatric and mental health nursing and nursing research, a master's level course in nursing education, and an interdisciplinary graduate course titled "Perspectives on Death/Dying." Her current research efforts are directed toward further development of the Burke/Eakes Chronic Sorrow Assessment Tool, a quantitative instrument designed to assess for evidence of chronic sorrow and to identify effective coping mechanisms (G. Eakes, personal communication, 2005).

Mary Lermann Burke

Mary Lermann Burke was born in Sandusky, Ohio, where she received her elementary and secondary education. She was awarded her initial nursing diploma from Good Samaritan Hospital School of Nursing in Cincinnati in 1962, followed later that year by a postgraduate certification, from Children's Medical Center in District of Columbia. After several years of work experience in pediatric nursing, Burke graduated Summa Cum Laude from Rhode Island College, Providence, with a bachelor's degree in nursing. In 1982, she received her master's degree in parent-child nursing from Boston University. During this program, she was also awarded a Certificate in Parent-Child Nursing and Interdisciplinary Training in Developmental Disabilities from the Child Development Center of Rhode Island Hospital and the Section on Reproductive and Developmental Medicine, Brown University, in Providence. Her doctorate of nursing science in the Family Studies Cognate from Boston University followed this in 1989.

Burke was inducted as a member of Theta Chapter, Sigma Theta Tau, during her master's program at Boston University in 1981 and as a charter member of Delta Upsilon Chapter-at-Large of Sigma Theta Tau at Rhode Island College in 1988. She received a Doctoral Student Scholarship Award from the Theta Chapter in 1988. She received the 1996 Delta Upsilon Chapter-at-Large Louisa A. White Award for Research Excellence.

During the period from 1991 through 1996, Burke received four Rhode Island College Faculty Research Grants for studies in the area of chronic sorrow. In 1998, she was awarded a grant from the Delta Upsilon Chapter-at-Large for initial quantitative instrument development for the study of chronic sorrow. Burke was principal investigator on the Transition to Adult Living Project, funded by a grant from the Department of Health and Human Services, Maternal and Child Health Bureau, Genetics Services Branch, from 1992 through 1995. A New England Regional Genetics Group Special Projects Grant, The Transition to Adult Living Project—System Dissemination of Information, supplemented this in 1995. Burke was co-principal investigator.

In her early career, Burke practiced in the pediatric nursing specialty in both acute and primary settings. She joined the faculty of Rhode Island College Department of Nursing as a clinical instructor in 1980 and became a full-time instructor in 1982, assistant professor in 1987, associate professor in 1991, and professor in 1996. During this period, she taught pediatric nursing in both theory and clinical courses. She also developed and taught a foundation nursing curriculum course encompassing nutrition, pharmacology, and pathophysiology. She retired from her Rhode Island College faculty position in December 2002.

Burke became interested in the concept of chronic sorrow during her master's degree program while engaged in a clinical practicum at the Child Development Center of Rhode Island Hospital. While working there with children with spina bifida and their parents, she developed the clinical hunch that the emotions displayed by the parents were consistent with chronic sorrow as first described by Olshansky (1962). Her master's thesis, *The Concerns of Mothers of Preschool Children with Myelomeningocele*, identified emotions similar to chronic sorrow. She then developed the Burke Chronic Sorrow Questionnaire for conducting her doctoral dissertation research, *Chronic Sorrow in Mothers of School-Age Children With Myelomeningocele.*

In June 1989, Burke presented her dissertation research at the Sigma Theta Tau International Research Congress in Taipei, Taiwan, where she interacted with Dr. Eakes of East Carolina University and Dr. Hainsworth of Rhode Island College. Subsequently, this group became the NCRCS, joined briefly by Dr. Carolyn Lindgren of Wayne State University. Together they developed a modified Burke/NCRCS Chronic Sorrow Questionnaire and conducted individually a series of studies that were analyzed collaboratively. Burke's individual studies in this series focused on chronic sorrow in infertile couples, adult children of parents with chronic conditions, and bereaved parents. The collaboratively analyzed studies resulted in the development of a middle range Theory of Chronic Sorrow, published in 1998. Members of the Consortium, both individually and collaboratively, presented numerous papers on chronic sorrow at local, state, national, and international conferences and wrote 10 articles published in refereed journals, receiving the Best of Image Award in the Theory Category from Sigma Theta Tau International for their article, "Middle-Range Theory of Chronic Sorrow." Most recently, Burke has collaborated with Dr. Eakes in the development of the Burke/Eakes Chronic Sorrow Assessment Tool.

Burke is active in numerous professional and community organizations. She is a member of the St. Joseph's Health Services of Rhode Island Board of Trustees. She has been awarded the Outstanding Alumna Award for Contributions in Nursing Education by Rhode Island College Department of Nursing and the Rhode Island College Alumni Honor Roll Award (L. Burke, personal communication, 2005).

Margaret A. Hainsworth

Margaret A. Hainsworth was born in Brockville, Ontario, Canada. She received her early elementary and secondary education in her hometown of Prescott, Ontario. Following high school graduation in 1949, she entered the diploma school of nursing at the Brockville General Hospital, Brockville, Ontario, graduating in 1953. In 1959, she immigrated to the United States to attend George Peabody College for Teachers in Nashville, Tennessee, receiving a diploma in public health nursing. In 1974, she continued her education at Salve Regina College, Newport, Rhode Island, and received a baccalaureate degree in nursing in 1973 and a master's degree in psychiatric and mental health nursing from Boston College in 1974. She received a doctoral degree in education administration from the University of Connecticut in 1986. In 1988, she was board certified as a clinical specialist in psychiatric and mental health nursing.

She was inducted into Sigma Theta Tau, Alpha Chi Chapter in 1978 and Delta Upsilon Chapter-at-Large in 1989. In 1976, she was awarded an outstanding faculty award at Rhode Island College. In 1992, she was selected to attend the Technical Assistance Workshop and Mentorship for Nurses in Implementation of the National Plan for Research in Child and Adolescent Mental Disorders that was sponsored by the National Institutes of Health. In 1991, she was selected to review manuscripts for the journal, *Qualitative Health Research, an Interdisciplinary Journal*, a Sage publication. In 1999, Hainsworth was accepted at the Royal Melbourne Institute of Technology in Melbourne, Australia, as a visiting fellow on a faculty exchange program.

Her practice in nursing was in the specialties of public health and psychiatric and mental health nursing. In 1974, she was accepted as a lecturer in the Department of Nursing at Rhode Island College and was promoted to full professor in 1992. Her major area of teaching was psychiatric care that consisted of both classroom lectures and clinical practice. She taught a course entitled "Death and Dying" that became an elective in the college's general studies program. Hainsworth always maintained her practice and was employed for 13 years as a consultant at the Visiting Nursing Association. She entered into a private practice at Bay Counseling Association in 1993 and maintained this practice for 5 years.

Her interest in chronic illness and its relationship to sorrow began in her practice as a facilitator for a support group for women with multiple sclerosis. This practice led to her dissertation work, *An Ethnographic Study of Women With Multiple Sclerosis Using a Symbolic Interaction Approach.* This research was accepted for a presentation at the Sigma Theta Tau Research Congress in Taipei, Taiwan, in 1989. At this conference, she became familiar with the research on chronic sorrow after attending a presentation by Burke.

Building on Burke's work, the NCRCS was established in 1989 to expand the understanding of chronic sorrow. Hainsworth was one of the four co-founders and remained an active member until 1996. The research began with four studies that focused on chronic sorrow in individuals in chronic life situations, and the members of the consortium analyzed the data collaboratively. During the 7 years that she was a member, the consortium published 13 manuscripts and presented the findings from their studies at international, state, and regional conferences. In 1999, they were awarded the Best of Image Award in Theory from Sigma Theta Tau International (M. Hainsworth, personal communication, 2005).

THEORETICAL SOURCES

The NCRCS based the middle range Theory of Chronic Sorrow on two main sources. The work of Olshansky in 1962 was cited as the basis of the original concept of chronic sorrow (Eakes, Burke, & Hainsworth, 1998). Lazarus and Folkman's (1984) model of stress and adaptation formed the foundation for the conceptualization of how persons cope with chronic sorrow.

The concept of chronic sorrow originated with the work of Olshansky in 1962 (Lindgren, Burke, Hainsworth, & Eakes, 1992). The NCRCS theorists cite Olshansky's observations of parents with mentally retarded children that indicated these parents experienced recurrent sadness and his coining the term *chronic sorrow.* This original concept was described as "a broad, simple description of psychological reaction to a tragic situation" (Lindgren et al., 1992, p. 30).

During the 1980s, other researchers began to examine the experience of parents of children who were either physically or mentally disabled. This work validated a recurrent sadness and a never-ending nature of grief experienced by these parents. Previous to this work, grief was conceptualized as a process that resolves over time, and if unresolved, grief is abnormal according to Bowlby and Lindemann's work (Lindgren et al., 1992). In contrast to this time-bound conceptualization, inherent in the concept of chronic sorrow is that recurrent sadness is a normal experience, according to Wikler, Wasow, and Hatfield (Lindgren et al., 1992). Burke, in her study of children with spina bifida, defined chronic sorrow as "pervasive sadness that is permanent, periodic and progressive in nature" (Hainsworth, Eakes, & Burke, 1994, p. 59).

The NCRCS did not confine its theory to the existence of chronic sorrow but sought to examine the response to the grief. This group incorporated Lazarus and Folkman's 1984 work on stress and adaptation as the basis for effective management methods described in its model (Eakes et al., 1998). The disparity encountered and the response to regrief stimulate individual coping mechanisms. There are categories of coping styles or management. Internal coping strategies include action-oriented, cognitive reappraisal and interpersonal behaviors (Eakes et al., 1998). Thus, the middle range Theory of Chronic Sorrow extended the theoretical base of chronic sorrow to not only the experience of chronic sorrow in certain situations but also the coping responses to the phenomenon.

USE OF EMPIRICAL EVIDENCE

Chronic Sorrow

The empirical evidence supporting NCRCS's initial conceptual definition of chronic sorrow was derived from interviews with mothers of children with spina bifida, which Burke conducted as part of her dissertation work. Through this research, Burke was able to define chronic sorrow as a pervasive sadness and found that the experience was permanent, periodic, and potentially progressive (Eakes, Burke, Hainsworth, & Lindgren, 1993). Burke's initial work provided the foundation for subsequent series of studies, including the basis for interview guides used in these studies.

MAJOR CONCEPTS & DEFINITIONS

CHRONIC SORROW

Chronic sorrow is the ongoing disparity resulting from a loss characterized by pervasiveness and permanence. Symptoms of grief recur periodically, and these symptoms are potentially progressive.

LOSS

Loss occurs as a result of disparity between the "ideal" and real situations or experiences. For example, there is a "perfect child" and a child with a chronic condition who differs from that ideal.

TRIGGER EVENTS

Trigger events are situations, circumstances, and conditions that highlight the disparity or the recurrent loss and initiate or exacerbate feelings of grief.

MANAGEMENT METHODS

Management methods are means by which individuals deal with chronic sorrow. These may be internal (personal coping strategies) or external (health care practitioner or other persons' interventions).

Ineffective Management

Ineffective management results from strategies that increase the individual's discomfort or heighten the feelings of chronic sorrow.

Effective Management

Effective management results from strategies that lead to increased comfort of the affected individual.

These NCRCS studies involved the following:

- Individuals with cancer (Eakes, 1993), infertility (Eakes et al., 1998), multiple sclerosis (Hainsworth, Burke, Lindgren, & Eakes, 1993; Hainsworth, 1994), and Parkinson's disease (Lindgren, 1996)
- Spouse caregivers of persons with chronic mental illness (Hainsworth, Busch, Eakes, & Burke, 1995), multiple sclerosis (Hainsworth, 1995), and Parkinson's disease (Lindgren, 1996)
- Parent caregivers of adult children with chronic mental illness (Eakes, 1995)

Based on these studies, the theorists postulated that chronic sorrow occurs in any situation in which the loss is unresolved. These studies did not demonstrate consistently that the associated emotions worsened over time. However, the theorists concluded that the studies did support the "potential for progressivity and intensification of chronic sorrow over time" (Eakes et al., 1998, p. 180).

The NCRCS theorists extended their studies to individuals experiencing a single loss (bereaved). They found that this population experienced these same feelings of chronic sorrow (Eakes, Burke, & Hainsworth, 1999).

Based on this extensive empirical evidence, the NCRCS theorists refined the definition of chronic sorrow as the "periodic recurrence of permanent, pervasive sadness or other grief-related feelings associated with ongoing disparity resulting from a loss experience" (Eakes et al., 1998, p. 377).

Triggers

Using the empirical data from these series of studies, the NCRCS theorists identified primary events or situations that precipitated the re-experience of initial grief feelings. These events were labeled *chronic sorrow triggers* (Eakes et al., 1993). The NCRCS compared and contrasted the triggers of chronic sorrow in individuals with chronic conditions, family caregivers, and bereaved persons (Burke, Eakes, & Hainsworth, 1999). For all populations, comparisons with norms and anniversaries were found to trigger chronic sorrow. Both family caregivers and persons with chronic conditions experienced triggering with management crises. One trigger unique for family caregivers was the requirement of unending caregiving. The bereaved population reported that memories and role change were unique triggers.

Management Strategies

The NCRCS posited that chronic sorrow is not debilitating when individuals effectively manage feelings. The management strategies were categorized as internal or external. Self-care management strategies were designated as internal coping strategies. The NCRCS further designated internal coping strategies as action, cognitive, interpersonal, and emotional.

Action coping mechanisms were used across all subjects—individuals with chronic conditions and their caregivers (Eakes, 1993, 1995; Eakes et al., 1993, 1999; Hainsworth, 1994, 1995; Hainsworth et al., 1995; Lindgren, 1996). The examples are like distraction methods commonly used to cope with pain. For instance, "keeping busy" and "doing something fun" are given as examples of action-oriented coping (Eakes, 1995; Lindgren et al., 1992). It was found that cognitive coping was used frequently, and examples included "thinking positively," "making the most of it," and "not trying to fight it" (Eakes, 1995; Hainsworth, 1994; Lindgren, 1996). Interpersonal coping examples included "going to a psychiatrist," "joined a support group," and "talking to others" (Eakes, 1993; Hainsworth, 1994, 1995). Emotional strategy examples included "having a good cry" and expressing emotions (Eakes et al., 1998; Hainsworth, 1995). A management strategy was labeled effective when a subject described it as helpful in decreasing feelings of re-grief.

External management was described initially by Burke as interventions provided by health professionals (Eakes et al., 1998). Healthcare professionals assist affected populations to increase their comfort through roles of empathetic presence, teacher-expert, and caring and competent professional (Eakes, 1993, 1995; Eakes et al., 1993, 1999;

Hainsworth, 1994, 1995; Hainsworth et al., 1995; Lindgren, 1996).

In summary, an impressive total of 196 interviews resulted in the middle range Theory of Chronic Sorrow. The theorists summarized a decade of research with individuals with chronic sorrow and found that this phenomenon frequently occurs in persons with chronic conditions, in family caregivers, and in bereaved persons (Burke et al., 1999; Eakes et al., 1998).

MAJOR ASSUMPTIONS

Nursing

Diagnosing chronic sorrow and providing interventions are within the scope of nursing practice. Nurses can provide anticipatory guidance to individuals at risk. The primary roles of nurses include empathetic presence, teacher-expert, and caring and competent caregiver (Eakes et al., 1998).

Person

Humans have an idealized perception of life processes and health. People compare their experiences both with the ideal and with others around them. Although each person's experience with loss is unique, there are common and predictable features of the loss experience (Eakes et al., 1998).

Health

There is a normality of functioning. A person's health is dependent upon adaptation to disparities associated with loss. Effective coping results in a normal response to life losses (Eakes et al., 1998).

Environment

Interactions occur within a social context, which includes family, social, work, and healthcare environments. Individuals respond to their assessment of themselves in relation to social norms (Eakes et al., 1998).

THEORETICAL ASSERTIONS

1. Chronic sorrow is a normal human response related to ongoing disparity created by a loss situation.
2. Chronic sorrow is cyclical in nature.
3. Predictable internal and external triggers of heightened grief can be categorized and anticipated.
4. Humans have inherent and learned coping strategies that may or may not be effective in regaining normal equilibrium when experiencing chronic sorrow.
5. Health care professionals' interventions may or may not be effective in assisting the individual to regain normal equilibrium.
6. A human who experiences a single or an ongoing loss will perceive a disparity between the ideal and reality.
7. The disparity between the real and the ideal leads to feelings of pervasive sadness and grief (Eakes et al., 1998).

LOGICAL FORM

This theory is based on a series of qualitative studies. Through the analysis of 196 interviews, the middle range Theory of Chronic Sorrow evolved. With the empirical evidence, the NCRCS theorists described the phenomenon of chronic sorrow, identified common triggers of re-grief, and described internal coping mechanisms and the role of nurses in the external management of chronic sorrow. The theoretical assumptions are evidenced clearly in the empirical data.

ACCEPTANCE BY THE NURSING COMMUNITY

Practice

The series of studies by the NCRCS, which form the foundation of the middle range Theory of Chronic Sorrow (Eakes et al., 1998), are replete with implications for practice. Each article included a section that related the findings to clinical nursing practice

(Burke et al., 1999; Eakes, 1993, 1995; Hainsworth, 1994, 1995; Hainsworth et al., 1993, 1994, 1995; Lindgren, 1996; Lindgren et al., 1992). In addition, the NCRCS work has provided other authors a basis for publications that are directed to a practice-focused audience.

NCRCS Nursing Practice Implications

The major practice implications are suggestions for nurses in assisting individuals and family caregivers to effectively manage the milestones or triggering events. Roles outlined for nurses included empathetic presence, teacher-expert, and caring and competent professional (Eakes et al., 1993).

Other Practice-Focused Literature

Several non-NCRCS nurse authors have written and published articles for nurses or physicians (Gedaly-Duff, Stoger, & Shelton, 2000; Krafft & Krafft, 1998; Scornaienchi, 2003). Other practice-focused literature, although not nurse authored, provided practice guidance that nurses would find useful (Doka, 2004; Miller, 1996).

Although the work listed here is described as relating to practice, it also can be considered educationally related. The next section presents additional evidence supporting NCRCS's work on chronic sorrow's relevance for the educational community.

EDUCATION

Two aspects of the use of the middle range Theory of Chronic Sorrow are outlined here. One is its use as a nursing diagnosis by the North American Nursing Diagnosis Association (NANDA) (NANDA International, 2003). The other is the use of the work of NCRCS in continuing education.

Chronic Sorrow: A Nursing Diagnosis

Review of the literature on chronic sorrow revealed that it was accepted as a nursing diagnosis by NANDA in 1998 (NANDA International, 2003). Comparison of the definitions used by NANDA and NCRCS (Eakes et al., 1998) revealed essentially similar dimensions. Moreover, several widely used nursing diagnosis textbooks (Ackley & Ladwig, 2008; Carpenito, 2006) and undergraduate specialty textbooks have cited the work of NCRCS (Lewis, Heitkemper, & Dirksen, 2007; Wong, Hockenberry-Eaton, Wilson, Winkelstein, & Schwartz, 2001).

Educational Implications

In addition to chronic sorrow's inclusion in the NANDA listing, more recent work by the research team at the University of Iowa in developing the Nursing Intervention Classification and the Nursing Outcome Classification has included linkages among chronic sorrow and diagnostic category, interventions, and outcomes (Johnson, Bulechek, McCloskey Dochterman, Maas, & Moorhead, 2001). The linkages hold educational implications, because they provide guidance to nurse educators in teaching clinical decision making and designing curricula. Moreover, they refocus care planning to include attention to outcomes, an essential step in teaching evidence-based practice (Pesut & Herman, 1998).

Graduate Research Education

The work of NCRCS provided a theoretical basis for several master's theses and doctoral dissertations. The unpublished master's theses of Golden (1994) and Shumaker (1995) on chronic sorrow in mothers of chronically ill children and the doctoral dissertation–based articles of Hobdell (2004; Hobdell & Deatrick, 1996), Mallow (Mallow & Bechtel, 1999), and Northington (2000) attest to the use of the theoretical work of the NCRCS in graduate nursing education.

Continuing Education

Three continuing education articles used the consortium's work on chronic sorrow. Meleski (2002) and Melnyk, Feinstein, Moldenhouer, and Small (2001) published continuing education courses designed for clinicians who work with families with chronically ill children. Drench's (2003) course for physical therapists and physical therapy assistants presented content on loss and grief that included NCRCS's work.

RESEARCH

A review of published research that has used NCRCS's work revealed that most articles were an extension of this work. They involved representatives of populations previously studied, as follows:

- Individuals with cancer (Eakes, 1993) multiple sclerosis (Hainsworth et al., 1993; Isaksson, Gunnarsson & Ahlstrom, 2007) infertility (Eakes et al., 1998), and Parkinson's disease (Lindgren, 1996)
- Caregivers of children with developmental delays (Burke et al., 1999), adults with chronic mental illness (Eakes, 1995), and children with epilepsy (Hobdell, Grant, Valencia, Kothare, Legido, & Khurana, 2007)
- Bereaved individuals (Eakes et al., 1999)

Several studies extended the work to new populations, individuals with human immunodeficiency virus (Lichtenstein, Laska, & Clair, 2002), mothers with human immunodeficiency virus (Ingram & Hutchinson, 1999), and caregivers of children with sickle cell disease (Northington, 2000), asthma (Matby, Kristjanson, & Coleman, 2003), and diabetes (Lowes & Lyne, 2000).

Although most of the authors were nurses from the United States, the literature indicates an international influence as reflected in publications by nurses from Australia (Matby et al., 2003), New Zealand (Carter, McKenna, MacLeod, & Green, 1998), Sweden (Ahlstrom, 2007; Pejlert, 2001), and the United Kingdom (Lowes & Lyne, 2000). Several studies were written by occupational therapists, and one by sociologists, thereby providing support for the assertion that the NCRCS work is the basis for international and interdisciplinary research. Application of this middle range theory to research is seen in current nursing literature (Eakes, 2004; Eakes, 2008).

FURTHER DEVELOPMENT

One area for further development is the variation in intensity of chronic sorrow. As suggested in a study of caregivers of adults with mental or chronic illness and children with chronic disabilities, role changes impact the intensity of chronic sorrow (Lee, Strauss, Wittman, Jackson, & Carstens, 2001). With a measurement of intensity, the middle range Theory of Chronic Sorrow would be useful as a framework for studies of the effectiveness of interventions. Some other possible nursing outcomes suggested by Ackley and Ladwig (2008) include acceptance, health status, and depression and mood equilibrium. Ackley and Ladwig suggested nursing interventions for clients with chronic sorrow. Through research, empirical support for these nursing interventions would add to evidence-based nursing practice.

Kendall (2005) developed the Kendall Chronic Sorrow Instrument (KCSI) and used a sample of 98 females who were experiencing ongoing significant losses for validity and reliability testing. The KCSI, a quantitative uni-dimensional instrument, consists of 18 Likert scale items. With further instrument development research, the KCSI will facilitate further tests of the theory and clinical screening for chronic sorrow.

CRITIQUE

Clarity

This theory clearly describes a phenomenon that is observed in the clinical area when loss occurs, and it is clearly evident that it is accepted in nursing practice. As indicated previously, a nursing diagnosis of chronic sorrow appears in nursing textbooks and is defined as cyclical, recurrent, and potentially progressive and, as such, is consistent with the definition of these theorists. In each of the published works of these theorists, key concepts are defined, and this middle range theory describes the proposed relationship between these concepts. The relationship between concepts makes intuitive sense. For example, it is clear that effective management, whether internal or external, will lead to increased comfort, and, conversely, ineffective management will lead to increased discomfort and intensity of chronic sorrow. As a middle range theory, the scope is limited to explanation of a single phenomenon, that of response to loss, and is congruent with clinical practice experience. As Eakes has stated, the beauty of this middle range theory is that it rings true with practitioners, students, and educators, as is evident from the continued communication nationally and internationally (G. Eakes, personal communication, December 2004).

One unclear aspect of the theory is an explanation for why not all individuals with unresolved losses experience chronic sorrow. Some, albeit few, of the NCRCS's interviewees did not experience the symptoms labeled as chronic sorrow. No further data have been provided about these individuals. Do individuals who do not experience chronic sorrow have different personality characteristics, such as resiliency, or receive different healthcare interventions at the time of the loss? What would the data from these individuals suggest about coping with ongoing loss?

Another concept that needs clarification is the progression of chronic sorrow. Although chronic sorrow is described as potentially progressive, what is the progression, and is this progression pathological in nature?

Clarification of the categories of internal management strategies is warranted. It is unclear to these reviewers how problem-oriented and cognitive strategies are different. Likewise, the emotive-cognitive, emotional, and interpersonal strategies are not clearly described. There is some obvious overlap between external versus internal management when the word *interpersonal* is used to describe seeking professional help.

Simplicity

The Theoretical Model of Chronic Sorrow (Figure 31-1) enhances the understanding of the relationship between the variables. With this model, it is clear that chronic sorrow is cyclical in nature, pervasive, and potentially progressive. Further, with the subconcepts of internal versus external management

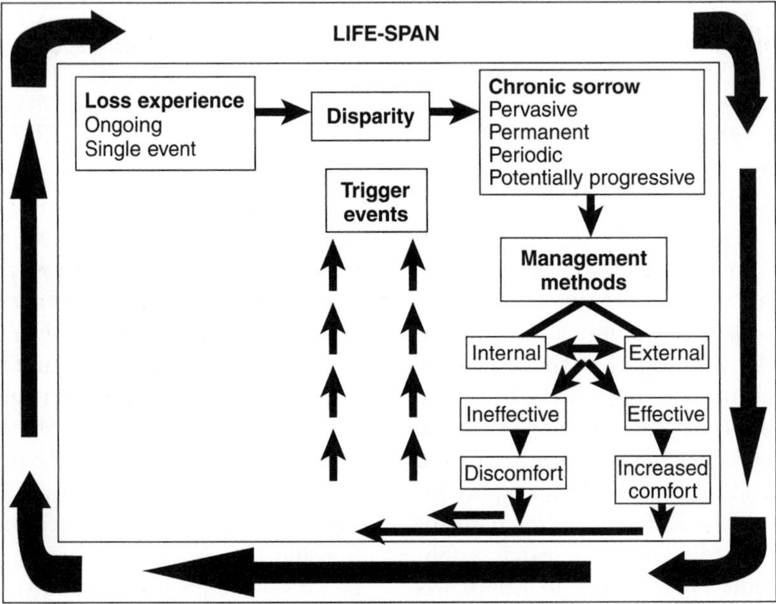

Figure 31-1 Theoretical Model of Chronic Sorrow. (From Eakes, G. G., Burke, M. L., & Hainsworth, M. A. [1998]. Middle range theory of chronic sorrow. *Image: The Journal of Nursing Scholarship, 30*[2], 180.)

and ineffective versus effective management, it is clear what type of assessment and at what point appropriate intervention by nurses and other healthcare providers would be best to prevent chronic sorrow from becoming progressive. With a limited number of defined variables, the theory is succinct and readily understood. As a middle range theory, it is useful for research design and practice guidance.

Generality

The concept of chronic sorrow began with the study of parents of children with a physical or cognitive defect. Through the empirical evidence, the theory was expanded to include a variety of loss experiences. The theory clearly applies to a wide range of losses and is applicable to the affected individual as well as to the caregivers and the bereaved. In addition, the theory is useful to a variety of healthcare practitioners. With these concepts, the unique nature of the experience is captured with the broadness of the concepts such as triggers. The triggers and the management strategies are unique to the individual situation and thus allow the application to a wide variety of situations.

Empirical Precision

As is characteristic of middle range theory, the limited scope readily allows researchers to study the phenomenon. With a limited number of variables and defined relationships among the variables, researchers are able to generate hypotheses related to the study of nursing interventions that promote effective management strategies for chronic sorrow. These outcome studies provide and add to the foundation of evidence-based practice.

Because the theory was derived from empirical evidence, it has clear utility for further research. The clear definition of chronic sorrow allows the study of individuals with a variety of losses and those loss situations that commonly result in chronic sorrow. In their study of bereaved individuals, Eakes and colleagues (1999) identified symptoms of chronic sorrow in most subjects. Through further study, researchers can devise assessment tools for clinical practice.

Derivable Consequences

As a consequence of this rich body of research, chronic sorrow is a widely accepted phenomenon, as is evident by its inclusion in NANDA diagnoses. Nurses and other healthcare professionals have found validity for their experiences with loss in the clinical arena. Subsequently, healthcare practitioners are able to normalize the experience. As Eakes stated, "chronic sorrow is like the pregnancy experience, it is a normal process in which clients can benefit from guidance and support of healthcare professionals" (G. Eakes, personal communication, December 2004). Eakes further stated that this experience is unique to each individual and to each situation.

SUMMARY

Loss is an experience common to all individuals. This middle range theory describes the phenomenon of chronic sorrow as a normal response to the ongoing disparity created by the loss. The major concepts are described and include disparity, triggers, and management strategies (internal and external). The theoretical sources and empirical evidence are described. The chapter presents evidence that the theory is accepted and used in practice, education, and research. It is referenced internationally by nurses and by providers in other disciplines. Suggestions for further development and research are presented. A thorough critique describes the clarity of concepts, and the simplicity and the usefulness of the theory for evidence-based research.

Case Study

Susan Jones is a 21-year-old woman who sustained a spinal cord injury at the age of 14 as a result of a diving accident. She is quadriplegic and attends a local college. Her mother, Mary Jones, is her primary caregiver. Mrs. Jones complains of difficulty sleeping and has frequent headaches. As the nurse, you suspect that Mrs. Jones may be experiencing chronic sorrow.

Using the Burke/NCRCS Chronic Sorrow Questionnaire (caregiver version) as an interview guide, you find evidence of chronic sorrow (Eakes, 1995). Mrs. Jones describes frequent feelings of being overwhelmed. She expresses that she feels both angry at times and heartbroken that her daughter will never have a normal life. She indicates that she has had these feelings off and on since her daughter's accident. Further, she tells you that she sees no end to her caregiving responsibilities. These feelings are strongest when her friend's children get married and get jobs away from home. She copes with these feelings by trying to focus on the positive (her daughter is alive and her sons are doing well) and talking with a few close friends.

You reassure Mrs. Jones that she is not alone in her situation, and that it is normal to have these feelings. In the course of the interview, you find that Mrs. Jones has not sought professional counseling help. Mrs. Jones tells you that she feels better, because this is the first time a health professional has asked her about her feelings. With Mrs. Jones, you begin to strategize on finding respite care and a regular mental health counselor to assist her in coping with chronic sorrow.

CRITICAL THINKING *Activities*

1. Using the middle range Theory of Chronic Sorrow as a framework, devise one or more hypotheses about parents of children with diabetes who do or do not attend a support group.
2. Providing a support group is only one possible intervention strategy to assist individuals experiencing chronic sorrow. What outcome measures or objective evaluation would you use to validate the effectiveness of interventions?
3. Compare and contrast the middle range Theory of Chronic Sorrow to Kubler-Ross' stages of grief or to Bowlby's theory of loss.
4. Describe the experience of three individuals with a chronic condition such as multiple sclerosis. Do you think that the theoretical assertions of the middle range Theory of Chronic Sorrow apply in these situations? State your rationale.

POINTS FOR *Further Study*

- Eakes, G. G. (2004). Chronic sorrow. In S. J. Peterson & T. S. Bredow (Eds.), *Middle range theories: Application to nursing research* (pp. 165–175). Philadelphia: Lippincott Williams & Wilkins.
- Eakes, G. G., & Burke, M. L. (2002). Development and validation of the Burke/Eakes chronic sorrow assessment tool. Unpublished raw data (eakesg@ecu.edu).
- Kendall, L. C. (2005). *The experience of living with ongoing loss: Testing the Kendall Chronic Sorrow Instrument.* Unpublished dissertation, Virginia Commonwealth University, Richmond.

REFERENCES

Ackley, B. J., & Ladwig, G. B. (2008). *Nursing diagnosis handbook: A guide to planning care* (7th ed.). St. Louis: Mosby. pp. 772-777.

Ahlstrom, G. (2007). Experiences of loss and chronic sorrow in persons with severe chronic illness. *Journal of Nursing and Healthcare of Chronic Illness 16*(3a), 76-83.

Burke, M. L., Eakes, G. G., & Hainsworth, M. A. (1999). Milestones of chronic sorrow: Perspectives of chronically ill and bereaved persons and family caregivers. *Journal of Family Nursing, 5*(4), 374-387.

Carpenito, L. J. (2006). *Handbook of Nursing Diagnosis, 11th Edition.* Philadelphia: Lippincott Williams & Wilkins. pp. 446-448.

Carter, H., McKenna, C., MacLeod, R., & Green, R. (1998). Health professionals' responses to multiple sclerosis and motor neuron disease. *Palliative Medicine, 12*(5), 383-394.

Doka, K. J. (2004). Grief and dementia. In K. J. Doka (Ed.), *Living with grief: Alzheimer's disease.* Washington DC: Hospice Foundation of America.

Drench, M. E. (2003). Loss, grief, and adjustment: A primer for physical therapy. Part I. *PT, 11*(6), 50-62.

Eakes, G. G. (1993). Chronic sorrow: A response to living with cancer. *Oncology Nursing Forum, 20*(9), 1327-1334.

Eakes, G. G. (1995). Chronic sorrow: The lived experience of parents of chronically mentally ill individuals. *Archives of Psychiatric Nursing, 9*(2), 77-84.

Eakes, G. G. (2004). Chronic sorrow. In S. J. Peterson & T. S. Bredow (Eds.), *Middle range theories: Application to nursing research* (pp. 165-175). Philadelphia: Lippincott Williams & Wilkins.

Eakes, G. G. (2008). Chronic sorrow. In S. J. Peterson & T. S. Bredow (Eds.), *Middle range theories: Application to nursing research,* 2nd ed. (pp. 170-185). Philadelphia: Lippincott Williams & Wilkins.

Eakes, G. G., Burke, M. L., & Hainsworth, M. A. (1998). Middle-range theory of chronic sorrow. *Image: The Journal of Nursing Scholarship, 30*(2), 179-184.

Eakes, G. G., Burke, M. L., & Hainsworth, M. A. (1999). Chronic sorrow: The lived experience of bereaved individuals. *Illness, Crisis, and Loss, 7*(1), 172-182.

Eakes, G. G., Burke, M. L., Hainsworth, M. A., & Lindgren, C. (1993). Chronic sorrow: An examination of nursing roles. In S. G. Funk, E. Tornquist, & M. T. Champagne (Eds.), *Key aspects of caring for the chronically ill: Hospital and home* (pp. 231-236). New York: Springer.

Gedaly-Duff, V., Stoger, S., & Shelton, K. (2000). Working with families. In R. E. Nickel & L. W. Desch (Eds.), *The physicians' guide to caring for children with disabilities and chronic conditions* (pp. 31-75). Baltimore: Paul H. Brooks.

Golden, B. A. (1994). *The presence of chronic sorrow in mothers of children with cerebral palsy.* Unpublished master's thesis, University of Arizona, Tempe.

Hainsworth, M. A. (1994). Living with multiple sclerosis: The experience of chronic sorrow. *Journal of Neuroscience Nursing, 26*(4), 237-240.

Hainsworth, M. A. (1995). Helping spouses with chronic sorrow related to multiple sclerosis. *Journal of Gerontological Nursing, 21*(7), 29-33.

Hainsworth, M. A., Burke, M. L., Lindgren, C. L., & Eakes, G. G. (1993). Chronic sorrow in multiple sclerosis: A case study. *Home Healthcare Nurse, 11*(2), 9-13.

Hainsworth, M. A., Busch, P. V., Eakes, G. G., & Burke, M. L. (1995). Chronic sorrow in women with chronically mentally disabled husbands. *Journal of the American Psychiatric Nurses Association, 1*(4), 120-124.

Hainsworth, M. A., Eakes, G., & Burke, M. L. (1994). Coping with chronic sorrow. *Issues in Mental Health Nursing, 15*(1), 59-66.

Hobdell, E. (2004). Chronic sorrow and depression in parents of children with neural tube defects. *Journal of Neuroscience Nursing, 36*(2), 82-88.

Hobdell, E., Grant, M. L., Valencia, J. M., Kothare, S., Legido, A., & Khurana D. S. (2007). Chronic sorrow and coping in families of children with epilepsy. *Journal of Neuroscience Nursing 39*(2), 76-82.

Hobdell, E. F., & Deatrick, J. A. (1996). Chronic sorrow: A content analysis of parental differences. *Journal of Genetic Counseling, 5*(2), 57-68.

Ingram, D., & Hutchinson, S. A. (1999). Defensive mothering in HIV-positive mothers. *Qualitative Health Research, 9*(2), 243-258.

Isaksson, A., Gunnarsson, L. & Ahlstrom, G. (2007). The presence of meaning of chronic sorrow in patients with multiple sclerosis. *Journal of Clinical Nursing 16*(11), 315-324.

Johnson, M., Bulechek, G., McCloskey Dochterman, J., Maas, M., & Moorhead, S. E. (2001). *Nursing diagnoses, outcomes, and interventions: NANDA, NOC and NIC linkages.* St. Louis: Mosby.

Kendall, L. C. (2005). *The experience of living with ongoing loss: Testing the Kendall Chronic Sorrow Instrument.* Unpublished dissertation, Virginia Commonwealth University, Richmond.

Krafft, S. K., & Krafft, L. J. (1998). Chronic sorrow: Parents' lived experience. *Holistic Nursing Practice, 13*(1), 59-67.

Lazarus, R. S., & Folkman, S. (1984). *Stress, appraisal, and coping.* New York: Springer.

Lee, A. L., Strauss, L., Wittman, P., Jackson, B., & Carstens, A. (2001). The effects of chronic illness on roles and emotions of caregivers. *Occupational Therapy in Health Care, 14*(1), 47-60.

Lewis, S. M., Heitkemper, M. L., & Dirksen, S. R. (2007). *Medical surgical nursing: Assessment and management of clinical problems* (7th ed.). St. Louis: Mosby.

Lichtenstein, B., Laska, M. K., & Clair, J. M. (2002). Chronic sorrow in the HIV-positive patient: Issues of race, gender, and social support. *AIDS Patient Care and STDs, 16*(1), 27-38.

Lindgren, C. L. (1996). Chronic sorrow in persons with Parkinson's and their spouses. *Scholarly Inquiry for Nursing Practice, 10*(4), 351-370.

Lindgren, C. L., Burke, M. L., Hainsworth, M. A., & Eakes, G. G. (1992). Chronic sorrow: A lifespan concept. *Scholarly Inquiry for Nursing Practice, 6*(1), 27-42.

Lowes, L., & Lyne, P. (2000). Chronic sorrow in parents of children with newly diagnosed diabetes: A review of the literature and discussion of the implications for nursing practice. *Journal of Advanced Nursing, 32*(1), 41-48.

Mallow, G. E., & Bechtel, G. A. (1999). Chronic sorrow: The experience of parents with children who are developmentally disabled. *Journal of Psychosocial Nursing and Mental Health Services, 37*(7), 31-35.

Matby, H. J., Kristjanson, L., & Coleman, M. (2003). The parenting competency framework: Learning to be a parent of a child with asthma. *International Journal of Nursing Practice, 9*(6), 368-373.

Meleski, D. D. (2002). Families with chronically ill children. *American Journal of Nursing, 102*(5), 47-54.

Melnyk, B. M., Feinstein, N. F., Moldenhouer, Z., & Small, L. (2001). Coping in parents of children who are chronically ill: Strategies for assessment and intervention. *Pediatric Nursing, 27*(6), 548-558.

Miller, F. E. (1996). Grief therapy for relatives of persons with serious mental illness. *Psychiatric Services, 47*(6), 633-636.

NANDA International. (2003). NANDA: Nursing diagnoses: Definitions & classification 2003-2004. Philadelphia: NANDA International.

Northington, L. (2000). Chronic sorrow in caregivers of school age children with sickle cell disease: A grounded theory approach. *Issues in Comprehensive Pediatric Nursing, 23*(3), 141-154.

Olshanky, S. (1962). Chronic sorrow: A response to a mentally defective child. *Social casework, 43*, 191-193.

Pejlert, A. (2001). Being a parent of an adult son or daughter with severe mental illness receiving professional care: Parents' narratives. *Health and Social Care in the Community, 9*(4), 194-204.

Pesut, D., & Herman, J. (1998). OPT: Transformation of nursing process for contemporary practice. Outcome-Present State-Test. *Nursing Outlook, 46*(1), 29-36.

Scornaienchi, J. M. (2003). Chronic sorrow: One mother's experience with two children with lissencephaly. *Journal of Pediatric Health Care, 17*(6), 290-294.

Shumaker, D. (1995). *Chronic sorrow in mothers of children with cystic fibrosis.* Unpublished master's thesis, University of Tennessee, Memphis.

Wong, D. L., Hockenberry-Eaton, M., Wilson, D., Winkelstein, M. L., & Schwartz, P. (2001). *Wong's essentials of pediatric nursing* (6th ed.). St. Louis: Mosby.

BIBLIOGRAPHY

Primary Sources

Book Chapters

Eakes, G. G. (2004). Chronic sorrow. In S. J. Peterson & T. S. Bredow (Eds.), *Middle range theories: Application to nursing research* (pp. 165-175). Philadelphia: Lippincott Williams & Wilkins.

Eakes, G. G., Burke, M. L., Hainsworth, M. A., & Lindgren, C. (1993). Chronic sorrow: An examination of nursing roles. In S. G. Funk, E. Tornquist, & M. T. Champagne (Eds.), *Key aspects of caring for the chronically ill: Hospital and home* (pp. 231-236). New York: Springer.

Journal Articles

Burke, M. L., Eakes, G. G., & Hainsworth, M. A. (1999). Milestones of chronic sorrow: Perspectives of chronically ill and bereaved persons and family caregivers. *Journal of Family Nursing, 5*(4), 374-387.

Burke, M. L., Hainsworth, M. A., Eakes, G. G., & Lindgren, C. L. (1992). Current knowledge and research on chronic sorrow: A foundation for inquiry. *Death Studies, 16*(3), 231-245.

Eakes, G. G. (1993). Chronic sorrow: A response to living with cancer. *Oncology Nursing Forum, 20*(9), 1327-1334.

Eakes, G. G. (1995). Chronic sorrow: The lived experience of parents of chronically mentally ill individuals. *Archives of Psychiatric Nursing, 9*(2), 77-84.

Eakes, G. G., Burke, M. L., & Hainsworth, M. A. (1998). The middle-range theory of chronic sorrow. *Image: The Journal of Nursing Scholarship, 30*(2), 179-184.

Eakes, G. G., Burke, M. L., & Hainsworth, M. A. (1999). Chronic sorrow: The lived experience of bereaved individuals. *Illness, Crisis, and Loss, 7*(1), 172-182.

Eakes, G. G., Hainsworth, M. E., Lindgren, C. L., & Burke, M. L. (1991). Establishing a long-distance research consortium. *Nursing Connections, 4*(1), 51-57.

Hainsworth, M. A. (1994). Living with multiple sclerosis: The experience of chronic sorrow. *Journal of Neuroscience Nursing, 26*(4), 237-240.

Hainsworth, M. A. (1995). Helping spouses with chronic sorrow related to multiple sclerosis. *Journal of Gerontological Nursing, 21*(7), 29-33.

Hainsworth, M. A., Burke, M. L., Lindgren, C. L., & Eakes, G. G. (1993). Chronic sorrow in multiple sclerosis: A case study. *Home Healthcare Nurse, 11*(2), 9-13.

Hainsworth, M. A., Busch, P. V., Eakes, G. G., & Burke, M. L. (1995). Chronic sorrow in women with chronically mentally disabled husbands. *Journal of the American Psychiatric Nurses Association, 1*(4), 120-124.

Hainsworth, M. A., Eakes, G., & Burke, M. L. (1994). Coping with chronic sorrow. *Issues in Mental Health Nursing, 15*(1), 59-66.

Lindgren, C. L. (1996). Chronic sorrow in persons with Parkinson's and their spouses. *Scholarly Inquiry for Nursing Practice, 10*(4), 351-370.

Lindgren, C. L., Burke, M. L., Hainsworth, M. A., & Eakes, G. G. (1992). Chronic sorrow: A lifespan concept. *Scholarly Inquiry for Nursing Practice, 6*(1), 27-42.

Dissertation

Burke, M. L. (1989). Chronic sorrow in mothers of school age children with a myelomeningocele disability (Doctoral dissertation, Boston University, 1989). *Dissertation Abstracts International, 50*, 233-234B.

Secondary Sources

Books

Ackley, B. J., & Ladwig, G. B. (2008). *Nursing diagnosis handbook: A guide to planning care* (8th ed.). St. Louis: Mosby.

Carpenito, L. J. (2006). *Nursing diagnosis: Application to clinical practice.* Philadelphia: Lippincott Williams & Wilkins.

Johnson, M., Bulechek, G., McCloskey Dochterman, J., Maas, M., & Moorhead, S. E. (2001). *Nursing diagnoses, outcomes, and interventions: NANDA, NOC and NIC linkages.* St. Louis: Mosby.

Lazarus, R. S., & Folkman, S. (1984). *Stress, appraisal, and coping.* New York: Springer.

Lewis, S. M., Heitkemper, M. L., & Dirksen, S. R. (2007). *Medical surgical nursing: Assessment and management of clinical problems* (7th ed.). St. Louis: Mosby.

NANDA International. (2003). *NANDA: Nursing diagnoses: Definitions & classification 2003-2004.* Philadelphia: NANDA International.

Walker, L. O., & Avant, K. C. (2005). *Strategies for theory construction in nursing.* Upper Saddle River, NJ: Pearson Prentice-Hall.

Wong, D. L., Hockenberry-Eaton, M., Wilson, D., Winkelstein, M. L., & Schwartz, P. (2001). *Wong's essentials of pediatric nursing.* St. Louis: Mosby.

Book Chapters

Doka, K. J. (2004). Grief and dementia. In K. J. Doka (Ed.), *Living with grief: Alzheimer's disease.* Washington DC: Hospice Foundation of America.

Gedaly-Duff, V., Stoger, S., & Shelton, K. (2000). Working with families. In R. E. Nickel & L. W. Desch (Eds.), *The physicians' guide to caring for children with disabilities and chronic conditions* (pp. 31-75). Baltimore: Paul H. Brooks.

Lindgren, C. L. (2000). Chronic sorrow in long-term illness across the life span. In J. M. Miller (Ed.), *Coping with chronic illness: Overcoming powerlessness* (3rd ed., pp. 125-143). Philadelphia: F. A. Davis.

Smith, M. J., & Liehr, P. (2003). Introduction: Middle range theory and the ladder of abstraction. In M. J. Smith & P. Liehr (Eds.), *Middle range theory for nursing* (pp. 1-23). New York: Springer.

Journal Articles

Carter, H., McKenna, C., MacLeod, R., & Green, R. (1998). Health professionals' responses to multiple sclerosis and motor neuron disease. *Palliative Medicine, 12*(5), 383-394.

Charles, K., Sellick, S. M., Montesanto, B., & Mohide, E. A. (1996). Priorities of cancer survivors regarding psychosocial needs. *Journal of Psychosocial Oncology, 14*(2), 57-72.

Dewar, A. L., & Lee, E. A. (2000). Bearing illness and injury. *Western Journal of Nursing Research, 22*(8), 912-926.

Doornbos, M. M. (1997). The problems and coping methods of caregivers of young adults with mental illness. *Journal of Psychosocial Nursing and Mental Health Services, 35*(9), 22-26.

Doornbos, M. M. (2000). King's systems framework and family health: The derivation and testing of a theory. *Journal of Theory Construction & Testing, 4*(1), 20-26.

Drench, M. E. (2003). Loss, grief, and adjustment: A primer for physical therapy. Part I. *PT, 11*(6), 50-62.

Gordon, M. (1998, September 30). Nursing nomenclature and classification system development. *Online Journal of Issues in Nursing.* Retrieved December 20, 2004, from http://www.nursingworld.org/ojin/tpc7/tpc7_1.htm

Hewson, D. (1997). Coping with loss of ability: "Good grief" or episodic stress responses. *Social Science & Medicine, 44*(8), 1129-1139.

Hobdell, E. (2004). Chronic sorrow and depression in parents of children with neural tube defects. *Journal of Neuroscience Nursing, 36*(2), 82-88.

Hobdell, E. F., & Deatrick, J. A. (1996). Chronic sorrow: A content analysis of parental differences. *Journal of Genetic Counseling, 5*(2), 57-68.

Howard, P. B. (1998). The experience of fathers of adult children with schizophrenia. *Issues in Mental Health Nursing, 19*(4), 399-413.

Ingram, D., & Hutchinson, S. A. (1999). Defensive mothering in HIV-positive mothers. *Qualitative Health Research, 9*(2), 243-258.

Johnsonius, J. R. (1996). Lived experiences that reflect embodied themes of chronic sorrow: A phenomenological pilot study. *Journal of Nursing Science, 1*(5/6), 165-173.

Kearney, P. M., & Griffin, T. (2001). Between joy and sorrow: Being a parent of a child with developmental disability. *Journal of Advanced Nursing, 34*(5), 582-592.

Krafft, S. K., & Krafft, L. J. (1998). Chronic sorrow: Parents' lived experience. *Holistic Nursing Practice, 13*(1), 59-67.

Langridge, P. (2002). Reduction of chronic sorrow: A health promotion role for children's community nurses. *Journal of Child Health Care, 6*(3), 157-217.

Lee, A. L., Strauss, L., Wittman, P., Jackson, B., & Carstens, A. (2001). The effects of chronic illness on roles and emotions of caregivers. *Occupational Therapy in Health Care, 14*(1), 47-60.

Lichtenstein, B., Laska, M. K., & Clair, J. M. (2002). Chronic sorrow in the HIV-positive patient: Issues of race, gender, and social support. *AIDS Patient Care and STDs, 16*(1), 27-38

Liehr, P., & Smith, M. J. (1999). Middle range theory: Spinning research and practice to create knowledge for the new millennium. *ANS Advances in Nursing Science, 21*(4), 81-91.

Lindgren, C. L., Connelly, C. T., & Gaspar, H. L. (1999). Grief in spouse and children caregivers of dementia patients. *Western Journal of Nursing Research, 21*(4), 521-537.

Lowes, L., & Lyne, P. (2000). Chronic sorrow in parents of children with newly diagnosed diabetes: A review of the literature and discussion of the implications for nursing practice. *Journal of Advanced Nursing, 32*(1), 41-48.

Mallow, G. E., & Bechtel, G. A. (1999). Chronic sorrow: The experience of parents with children who are developmentally disabled. *Journal of Psychosocial Nursing and Mental Health Services, 37*(7), 31-35.

Matby, H. J., Kristjanson, L., & Coleman, M. (2003). The parenting competency framework: Learning to be a parent of a child with asthma. *International Journal of Nursing Practice, 9*(6), 368-373.

Meleski, D. D. (2002). Families with chronically ill children. *American Journal of Nursing, 102*(5), 47-54.

Melnyk, B. M., Feinstein, N. F., Moldenhouer, Z., & Small, L. (2001). Coping in parents of children who are chronically ill: Strategies for assessment and intervention. *Pediatric Nursing, 27*(6), 548-558.

Miller, F. E. (1996). Grief therapy for relatives of persons with serious mental illness. *Psychiatric Services, 47*(6), 633-636.

Northington, L. (2000). Chronic sorrow in caregivers of school age children with sickle cell disease: A grounded theory approach. *Issues in Comprehensive Pediatric Nursing, 23*(3), 141-154.

Parse, R. R. (1997). Joy-sorrow: A study using the Parse research method. *Nursing Science Quarterly, 10*(2), 80-87.

Pejlert, A. (2001). Being a parent of an adult son or daughter with severe mental illness receiving professional care: Parents' narratives. *Health and Social Care in the Community, 9*(4), 194-204.

Pesut, D. J., & Herman, J. (1998). OPT: Transformation of nursing process for contemporary practice. *Nursing Outlook, 46*(1), 29-36.

Phillips, M. (1991). Chronic sorrow in mothers of chronically ill and disabled children. *Issues in Comprehensive Pediatric Nursing, 14*(2), 111-120.

Scornaienchi, J. M. (2003). Chronic sorrow: One mother's experience with two children with lissencephaly. *Journal of Pediatric Health Care, 17*(6), 290-294.

Sumner, J. (2001). Caring in nursing: A different interpretation. *Journal of Advanced Nursing, 35*(6), 926-932.

Thorne, S., Paterson, B., Acorn, S., Canam, C., Joachim, G., & Jillings, C. (2002). Chronic illness experience: Insights from a metastudy. *Qualitative Health Research, 12*(4), 437-452.

Dissertations

Hobdell, E. F. (1993). The relationship between chronic sorrow and accuracy of perception of cognitive development in parents of children with neural tube defect (Doctoral dissertation, University of Pennsylvania, 1993). *Dissertation Abstracts International, B 54/03*, 1333.

Kendall, L. C. (2005). *The experience of living with ongoing loss: Testing the Kendall Chronic Sorrow Instrument.* Unpublished dissertation, Virginia Commonwealth University, Richmond.

Northington, L. K. (1999). Chronic sorrow in caregivers of school age children with sickle cell disease: A grounded theory approach (Doctoral dissertation, Louisiana State University, Health Science Center, 1999). *Dissertation Abstracts International, B 59/10*, 5313.

Master's Theses

Golden, B. A. (1994). *The presence of chronic sorrow in mothers of children with cerebral palsy.* Unpublished master's thesis, University of Arizona, Tempe.

Shumaker, D. (1995). *Chronic sorrow in mothers of children with cystic fibrosis.* Unpublished master's thesis, University of Tennessee, Memphis.

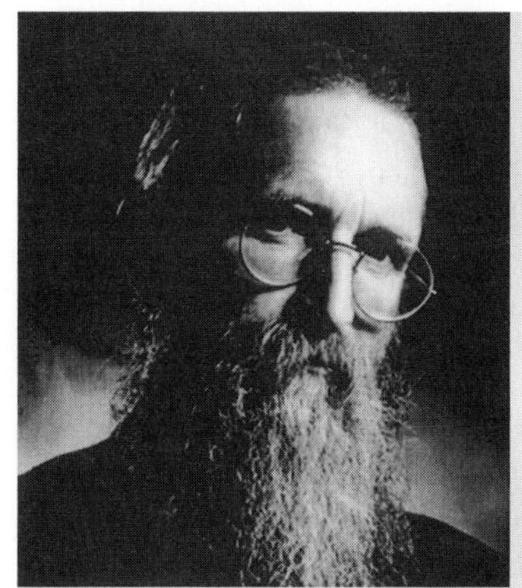

CHAPTER

32

Phil Barker

The Tidal Model of Mental Health Recovery

Nancy Brookes

"Mental illnesses or psychiatric disorders are 'problems of human living': people find it difficult to live with themselves or to live with others in the social world. A simple idea that becomes complicated when we try to engage with it. Nurses try to help people address these problems of living, in an effort to live through them. Another simple idea, that becomes complicated at the level of practice. All is paradox." (Personal communication, February 23, 2008)

CREDENTIALS OF THEORIST

Phil Barker was born in Scotland by the sea, and thus began the influence of and interest in water, the ultimate metaphor of life (Barker, 1996a, p. 239). He credits his father and grandfather with "the warmth of nurture and the discipline of boundaries," who helped him to appreciate that "life was an answer waiting for the right question," and he, like them, became a philosopher (Barker, 1999b, p. xii). Life in this context also contributed to his enduring curiosity and the philosophy of the everyday, which resonate throughout the Tidal Model.

Barker trained as a painter and sculptor in the mid-1960s, and won the prestigious Pernod Award for Young Painters in 1974, by which time he had already become a psychiatric nurse. He continues to paint word pictures in metaphor. Barker credits art school with introducing him to 'learning from Reality,' the reality of experience, which became the focus of his philosophical inquiries. His fascination with Eastern philosophies, which began at art school, flows through the Tidal Model with echoes of chaos, uncertainty, change, and the Chinese idea of crisis as opportunity. This early involvement in the arts also helps to explain Barker's view of nursing as "the craft of caring" (Barker, 2000c, 2000e; Barker & Whitehill, 1997).

Following art school, Barker worked as a commercial artist and mural painter, supplementing his income with laboring work on the railroads and in factories. His "ocean of experience" surged in a new direction in 1970, when he took a position as an "attendant at the local asylum." His fascination with the human dimension, the lived experience, and the stories of people challenged by mental distress prompted him to transfer his interest in the arts and humanities to nursing.

Barker's early progress through nursing, although unusual, was typical of the times and the context. Nursing *per se* was temporarily submerged when he began to study and practice various psychotherapies such as cognitive behavioural therapy and family and group therapy. Barker's doctoral research featured cognitive behavioral work with a group of women living with depression (Barker, 1987). However, around this time, Barker became uncomfortable with the application of therapies to people experiencing problems in living, and the "uncertainty principle" resurfaced for him. His curiosity about life and persons provoked questions about the people with whom he was working and their resilience and integrity. He was learning from them what it meant to experience distress, and he wondered what recovery meant to people? Questions re-emerged around:

- What it is to be a person
- What is the proper focus of nursing, and
- What are nurses needed for?

During his tenure as Professor of Psychiatric Nursing Practice at the University of Newcastle, these questions framed his research agenda and culminated in the development of the Tidal Model.

As the UK's first Professor of Psychiatric Nursing Practice, Barker continued to maintain a practice and develop the Tidal Model. Throughout his nursing career, Barker has wondered about the proper focus of psychiatric nursing and the role of care, compassion, understanding, and courage in helping people experiencing extreme distress or loss of self, or in spiritual crisis (Barker, 1999b). The Tidal Model was developed within this context and history. The narrative knowledge base for the Tidal Model, although particular, is not exclusive and it leaves room both for development and for other viewpoints.

Barker has published in the area of psychiatric and mental health nursing since 1978. A prolific writer, he has written 14 books, over 50 book chapters, and more than 150 academic papers. He was assistant editor for the *Journal of Psychiatric and Mental Health Nursing* for a decade. Barker was made a Fellow of the Royal College of Nursing (UK) in 1995, only the fourth psychiatric nurse to be so honored. He received the Red Gate Award for Distinguished Professors at the University of Tokyo in 2000. In 2001, he received an Honorary Doctorate from Oxford Brookes University in England, and a room was named in his honor at the Health Care Studies Faculty at Homerton College, Cambridge. He has held visiting professorships at several international universities, for example, Australia (Sydney), European (Barcelona), and Japan (Tokyo). He was visiting professor at Trinity College Dublin from 2002 to 2007. In 2006, he received the inaugural "Lifetime Achievement Award" from Blackwell journals, publishers of the *Journal of Psychiatric and Mental Health Nursing.*

Barker has travelled widely with his wife and professional partner Poppy Buchanan-Barker, in response to interest in the recovery paradigm underlying the Tidal Model, conducting workshops and seminars in Australia, Canada, New Zealand, Japan, Finland, Denmark, Turkey, Germany, and Ireland as well as the United Kingdom. A popular commentator on the human condition, he brings to radio, television, and the popular press his passion for and curiosity about the recovery process and personhood.

Currently, Barker is an Honorary Professor at the University of Dundee, Scotland, where he maintains a private psychotherapy practice. He and his wife have developed the recovery paradigm at Clan Unity, an international mental health recovery and reclamation consultancy in Scotland.

THEORETICAL SOURCES

The Tidal Model is focused on the fundamental care processes of nursing, is universally applicable, and is a practical guide for psychiatric and mental health nursing (Barker, 2001b). The theory is radical in its re-conceptualization of mental health problems and needs as unequivocally *human*, rather than psychological, social, or physical (Barker, 2002b, p. 233). The Tidal Model "emphasizes the central importance of: developing understanding of the person's needs through collaborative working, developing a therapeutic relationship through discrete methods of active empowerment, establishing nursing as an educative element at the heart of interdisciplinary intervention" (Barker, 2000e, p. 4) and seeking to resolve problems and promote mental health through narrative approaches (Stevenson, Barker & Fletcher, 2002, p. 272).

The Tidal Model is a philosophical approach to recovery of mental health. It is not a model of care or treatment of mental illness, although people described as mentally ill do need and receive care. The Tidal Model represents a specific worldview. It helps the nurse begin to understand what mental health might mean for the particular person in care, and how that person might be helped to begin the complex voyage of recovery.

The Tidal Model is not prescriptive, rather, a set of principles—the Ten Commitments—serve as the metaphorical compass for the practitioner (Buchanan-Barker & Barker, 2006, 2008). They guide the nurse in developing responses to meet the individual and contextual needs of the person who has become the patient. The experience of mental distress is invariably described in metaphorical terms. The Tidal Model employs the universal and culturally significant metaphors associated with the power of water and the sea, to represent the known aspects of human distress. Water is "the core metaphor for both the lived experience of the person . . . and the care system that attempts to mould itself around a person's need for nursing" (Barker, 2000e, p. 10).

Barker describes an "early interest in the human content of mental distress . . . and an interest in the human (phenomenological) experience of distress," which is viewed in contexts and wholes rather than isolated parts (Barker, 1999b, p. 13). The "whole" nature of being human is "re-presented on physical, emotional, intellectual, social and spiritual planes" (Barker, 2002b, p. 233). This phenomenological interest pervades the Tidal Model with an emphasis on the lived experience of persons, their stories (replete with metaphors) and narrative interventions. Nurses carefully and sensitively meet and interact with people in a "sacred space" (Barker, 2003a, p. 613).

A feature of Barker's nursing practice has been his exploration of the possibilities of genuine collaborative relationships with users of mental health services. In the 1980s, he developed the concept of "caring with" people, learning that the professional-person relationship could be more "mutual" than the original nurse-patient relationship defined by Peplau (1969). Barker further developed this concept during the 1990s in a working relationship with Dr. Irene Whitehill and others who used mental health services (Barker & Whitehill, 1997). This work led to the "need for nursing" and "empowerment" studies as well as a commitment to publish the stories of people's experience of madness, and their voyage of recovery, complete with personal and spiritual meanings (Barker, Jackson, & Stevenson, 1999a; Barker & Buchanan-Barker, 2004b). Barker enlisted the support of Dr. Whitehill and other "user/consumer consultants," to evaluate how "user friendly" were the original processes of the Tidal Model. The involvement of "user/consumer consultants" is seen in several ongoing projects, and presents a distinctive feature of continued development of the Tidal Model.

Barker's longstanding appreciation of Eastern philosophies pervades his work. The work of Shoma Morita is a specific example of how the philosophical assumptions of Zen Buddhism were integrated with psychotherapy (Morita, Kondo, Levine, & Morita, 1998). Morita's dictum—"Do what needs to be done"—resonates in many of the practical activities of the Tidal Model. In contrast to the zealous "problem-solving" attitude embraced by much of Western psychiatry and psychology, Morita believed that it was futile to try to "change" oneself or one's "problems," which come and go like the weather. Instead, the focus should be on answering the questions:

- What is my purpose in living?
- What needs to be done now?

People have the capacity to live and grow through distress, by doing what needs to be done. For people who are in acute distress—especially when they are at risk to self or others—it is vital that nurses relate directly to the person's ongoing experience. Originally Barker called this process engagement, but has now redefined the specific interpersonal process as "bridging." This term emphasizes the need to build, creatively, a means of reaching the person; crossing in the process, the murky waters of mental distress (Barker & Buchanan-Barker, 2004b).

The Tidal Model can also be viewed through the lens of social constructivism, recognizing that there are multiple ways of understanding the world. Meaning emerges through the complex webs of interaction, relationships, and social processes. Knowledge does not exist independently of the knower, and all knowledge is situated (Stevenson, 1996). Change is the only constant, as meaning and social realities are constantly renegotiated or constructed through language and interaction. Barker believes that "all I am is story; all I can ever be is story." As people try to explain to others "who" they are, they tell stories about themselves and their world of experience—revising, editing, and rewriting these stories through dialogue with another. Barker first discussed this idea with his mentor, Hilde Peplau, in 1994, who agreed by saying "people make themselves up as they talk" (Barker, 2003a; Barker & Buchanan-Barker, 2007b).

Barker credits many thinkers with influencing his work, beginning with Annie Altschul and Thomas Szasz. His view of mental health problems as *problems of living* popularized by Szasz (1961, 2000) and later Podvoll (1990) is a perspective that he prefers to diagnostic labeling and the biomedical construction of people and illness (Barker, 2001c, p. 215). He agrees with Szasz that it is futile to try to "solve problems in living." Life is not a problem to be solved. Life is something to be lived, as intelligently, as competently, as well as we can, day in and day out (Miller, 1983, p. 290). The challenge for nursing is to help persons live "intelligently" and "competently."

Travelbee's (1969) concept of the Therapeutic Use of Self flows through the Tidal Model and provides an anchor for the "proper focus of nursing." Three main theoretical frameworks underpin the Tidal Model:

1. Peplau's (1969; 1952) Interpersonal Relations Theory
2. Theory of Psychiatric and Mental Health Nursing derived from the Need for Nursing studies
3. Empowerment within Interpersonal Relationships

The pragmatic emphasis on strength-based, solution-focused approaches acknowledges the important influence of Steve de Shazer and solution-focused therapy.

The Tidal Model draws its core philosophical metaphor from chaos theory, where the unpredictable—yet bounded—nature of human behavior and experience can be compared to the flow and power of water (Barker, 2000b, p. 54). In constant flux, the tides ebb and flow; they exhibit non-repeating patterns yet stay within bounded parameters (Vicenzi, 1994). Barker (2000b) acknowledges the "complexity [of] both the internal universe of human experience and the external universe, which is, paradoxically, within and beyond the individual, at one and the same time" (p. 52). Within this complex, nonlinear perspective, small changes can create later unpredictable changes. This hopeful message directs nurses and persons to identify small changes and variations. Chaos theory suggests that there are limits to what we can know, and Barker invites nurses to cease the search for certainty, embracing instead the reality of uncertainty. Know that "change is constant," one of the Tidal commitments identifies and celebrates change in people, circumstances, relationships, and organizations (Barker, 2003b; Buchanan-Barker & Barker, 2008). This perspective also presents challenges in trying to understand people, relationships, and situations. It directs inquiry in qualitative, non-linear ways, such as action research, grounded theory, phenomenology, and critical theory (Barker, 1999a).

Annie Altschul, the *Grande Dame* of British psychiatric nursing (Barker, 2003a, p. 12), along with

Hilda Peplau, was one of Barker's mentors. Altschul's influence—especially her early appreciation of system theory—is evident in the Tidal Model, as is her interest in understanding rather than explaining mental distress and her belief that people need more straightforward help than many of the psychiatric theories suggest.

Barker credits Peplau, the mother of psychiatric nursing, with his becoming "an advocate for nursing as a therapeutic activity in its own right" (Barker, 2000a, p. 617). Peplau introduced her interpersonal paradigm for the study and practice of nursing in the early 1950s and defined nursing as "a significant, therapeutic, interpersonal process" (Peplau, 1952, p. 16). A defining characteristic of the Tidal Model is an emphasis on the narrative in the person's own voice.

The empirically derived Empowering Interactions framework suggests that improvement in the person's situation and lifestyle is possible, building on strengths is better than focusing on problems, collaboration is key, participation is the way, and self-determination is the ultimate goal (Barker & Buchanan-Barker, 2004a; Barker, Stevenson & Leamy, 2000, p. 8). Eight respectful, empowering interactions also bring generally invisible nursing interactions into the practice arena (Michael, 1994). De Shazer's (1994) influence is evident as he asserts that change and intervention "boils down to stories about the telling of stories, the shaping and reshaping of stories so that troubled people change their story" (p. xvii).

The strength base of the Tidal Model emphasizes searching for and revealing solutions, and identifying resources. The theory integrates the need for nursing studies, collaboration, empowerment, interpersonal relationships, narrative, strength-based, and solution-seeking approaches, and is systemic. The solution-focus, a model of questions, provides specific direction for nurses. In the Holistic Assessment, nurses explore the person's present "problems" or "needs," the scale of these problems/needs, what is currently part of a person's life that might help to resolve problems or meet needs, and what needs to happen to bring about change (Barker, 2000e; Barker & Buchanan-Barker, 2007a). Nurses help identify and mobilize persons' strengths and resources, and the person's goals direct the work of the healthcare team (Barker, 2000e; Stevenson, Jackson, & Barker, 2003). The 10 Commitments (Box 32-1) also support this perspective and direction. This is a significant re-framing of the view of the person-in-care and the proper focus of nursing.

Box 32-1 *The Ten Tidal Commitments: Essential Values of the Tidal Model*

The **Tidal Model** draws on our values about *relating* to people. These frame our efforts to help others in their moment of distress.

The values of the **Tidal Model** reflect a philosophy of how we would hope to be treated should we experience distress or difficulty in our lives.

As more people around the world have become involved in exploring the **Tidal Model** for their work, in different settings, the need to re-affirm the core values of the Tidal Model has become more apparent. We have come to appreciate how *both* the "helper" (whether professional, friend, or fellow traveller) *and* the person need to make a *commitment* to change. This commitment binds them together.

The Ten Commitments distils the essence of the value base of the **Tidal Model.**

These *Ten Commitments* need to be firmly in place in any team or individual practitioner who wishes to say it is developing the practice of the **Tidal Model.**

1. **Value the voice:** The person's story is the beginning and end point of the whole helping encounter, embracing not only the account of the person's distress, but also the hope for its resolution. The story is spoken by the voice of experience. We seek to encourage the true voice of the person—rather than reinforce the voice of authority.

Traditionally, the person's story is 'translated' into a third person, professional account, by different

Continued

Box 32-1 The Ten Tidal Commitments: Essential Values of the Tidal Model—cont'd

health or social care practitioners. This becomes not so much the person's story (*my* story) but the professional team's view of that story *(history)*. Tidal seeks to help people develop their own unique narrative accounts into a formalized version of '*my story*,' through ensuring that all assessments and records of care are written in the person's own "voice." If the person is unable or unwilling to write in his or her own hand, then the nurse acts as secretary, recording what has been agreed, conjointly, is important—writing this in the "voice" of the person.

2. **Respect the language:** People develop unique ways of expressing their life stories, representing to others that which the person alone can know. The language of the story—complete with its unusual grammar and personal metaphors—is the ideal medium for illuminating the way to recovery. We encourage people to speak their own words in their distinctive voice.

Stories written about patients by professionals are traditionally framed by arcane technical language of psychiatric medicine or psychology. Regrettably, many service users and consumers often come to describe themselves in the colonial language of the professionals who have diagnosed them. By valuing—and using—the person's natural language, the Tidal practitioner conveys the simplest, yet most powerful, respect for the person.

3. **Develop genuine curiosity:** The person is writing a life story but is in no sense an "open book." No one can know another person's experience. Consequently, professionals need to express genuine interest in the story so that they can better understand the storyteller and the story.

Often professionals are interested only in "what is wrong" with the person, or in pursuing particular lines of professional inquiry—for example, seeking "signs and symptoms." Genuine curiosity reflects an interest in the person and the person's unique experience, as opposed to merely classifying and categorizing features, which might be common to many other "patients."

4. **Become the apprentice:** The person is the world expert on the life story. Professionals may learn something of the power of that story, but only if they apply themselves diligently and respectfully to the task by becoming apprentice-minded. We need to learn from the person what needs to be done, rather than leading.

No one can ever know a person's experience. Professionals often talk "as if" they might even know the person better than they know themselves. As Szasz noted: "How can you know more about a person after seeing him for a few hours, a few days, or even a few months, than he knows about himself? He has known himself a lot longer!" The idea that the person remains entirely in charge of himself is a fundamental premise" (Szasz, 2000).

5. **Use the available toolkit:** The story contains examples of "what has worked" for the person in the past, or beliefs about "what might work" for this person in the future. These represent the main tools that need to be used to unlock or build the story of recovery. The professional toolkit—commonly expressed through ideas such as "evidence-based practice"—describes what has "worked" for other people. Although potentially useful, this should be used only if the person's available toolkit is found wanting.
6. **Craft the step beyond:** The professional helper and the person work together to construct an appreciation of what needs to be done "now." Any "first step" is a crucial step, revealing the power of change and potentially pointing toward the ultimate goal of recovery. Lao Tzu said that the journey of a thousand miles begins with a single step. We would go further: Any journey begins in our *imagination*. It is important to imagine—or envision—moving forward. Crafting the step beyond reminds us of the importance of working with the person in the "me now": addressing what needs to be done now, to help advance to the next step.
7. **Give the gift of time:** Although time is largely illusionary, nothing is more valuable. Often, professionals complain about not having enough time to

Box 32-1 *The Ten Tidal Commitments: Essential Values of the Tidal Model—cont'd*

work constructively with the person. Although they may not actually "make" time, through creative attention to their work, professionals often find the time to do "what needs to be done." Here, it is the professional's relationship with the concept of time which is at issue, rather than time itself (Jonsson, 2005). Ultimately, any time spent in constructive interpersonal communication, is a gift—for both parties). There is nothing more valuable than the time the helper and the person spend together.

8. **Reveal personal wisdom:** Only the person can know himself or herself. The person develops a powerful storehouse of wisdom through living the writing of the life story. Often, people cannot find the words to express fully the multitude, complexity, or ineffability of their experience, invoking powerful personal metaphors to convey something of their experience (Barker, 2002b). A key task for the professional is to help the person reveal and come to value that wisdom, so that it might be used to sustain the person throughout the voyage of recovery.
9. **Know that change is constant:** Change is inevitable because change is constant. This is the common story for all people. However, although change is inevitable, growth is optional. Decisions and choices have to be made if growth is to occur. The tasks of the professional helper are to develop awareness of how change is happening and to support the person in making decisions regarding the course of the recovery voyage. In particular, we help the person to steer out of danger and distress, keeping on the course of reclamation and recovery.
10. **Be transparent:** If the professional and the person are to become a team, then each must put down their "weapons." In the story-writing process, the professional's pen can all too often become a weapon: writing a story that risks inhibiting, restricting, and delimiting the person's life choices. Professionals are in a privileged position and should model confidence by being transparent at all times, helping the person understand exactly what is being done and why. By retaining the use of the person's own language, and by completing all assessments and care plan records together (in vivo), the collaborative nature of the professional-person relationship becomes even more transparent.

Barker, P. J. (2003b). *The 10 Commitments: Essential Values of the Tidal Model.* Retrieved February 23, 2008, from http://www.tidal-model.com/Ten%20Commitments.htm

MAJOR CONCEPTS & DEFINITIONS

THE THEORETICAL BASIS OF THE TIDAL MODEL*

The Tidal Model begins from four simple, yet important starting points:

1. The primary therapeutic focus in mental health care lies in the community. A person's natural life is an "ocean of experience." The psychiatric crisis is only one thing, among many, that might threaten to "drown" them. Ultimately, the aim of mental health care is to return people to that "ocean of experience," so that they might continue with their life voyage.
2. Change is a constant, ongoing process. However, although people are constantly changing, this may be beyond their awareness. One of the main aims of the approaches used within the **Tidal Model** is to help people develop their awareness of the small changes that, ultimately, will have a big effect on their lives.

Continued

MAJOR CONCEPTS & DEFINITIONS—cont'd

3. Empowerment lies at the heart of the caring process. However, people already have their own "power." We need to help people "power up," so they can use their own personal power to take greater charge of their lives, using this in constructive ways.
4. The nurse and the person are united (albeit temporarily) like dancers in a dance. When effective nursing happens, as W. B. Yeats (1928) might have remarked, "How do we tell the dancer from the dance?" This reminds us that genuine caring encounters involve "caring with" the person, not just "caring about" the person, or doing things that suggest we are "caring for" them.

THE THREE DOMAINS: A MODEL OF THE PERSON*

In the Tidal Model, the person is represented by three personal domains: Self, World, and Others. A domain is a sphere of control or influence, a place where the person experiences or acts out aspects of private or public life. More simply, a domain is a place where someone lives.

The domains are like the person's home address. Their house or flat has several rooms, but the person is not to be found in each of these rooms all the time. Sometimes the person is in one room, and sometimes in another. The personal domains are similar. Sometimes the person is mainly spending time in the Self Domain, and at other times is mainly spending time in the World or Others domains.

The **Self Domain** is the private place where the person lives. Here the person experiences thoughts, feelings, beliefs, values, and ideas, etc., that are known only to the person. In this private world, the distress called "mental illness" is first experienced. All people keep much of their private world secret, only revealing to others what they wish them to know. This is why people are often such a "mystery" to us, even when they are close friends or relatives.

In the Tidal Model, the **Self Domain** becomes the focus of our attempts to help the person feel more "safe" and "secure," where we try to help the person address and begin to deal with the private fears, anxieties, and other threats to emotional stability, which are related to specific problems of living. The main focus is to develop a "bridging" relationship and to help the person develop a meaningful **Personal Security Plan.** This work becomes the basis of the development of the person's "self-help" program, which will sustain the person on return to everyday life. The World Domain is the place where the person shares some of the experiences from the Self Domain, with other people, in the person's social world.

When people talk to others about their private thoughts, feelings, beliefs, or other experiences known only to them, they go to the **World Domain.**

In the Tidal Model, the **World Domain** becomes the focus of our efforts to understand the person and the person's problems of living. This is done through the use of the Holistic Assessment. At the **World Domain,** we also try to help the person begin to identify and address specific problems of living, on an everyday basis. This is done through use of dedicated **One-to-One Sessions.**

The **Others Domain** is the place where the person acts out everyday life with other people—family, friends, neighbors, work colleagues, professionals, etc. Here the person engages in different interpersonal and social encounters, within which the person may be influenced by others, and may—in turn—influence others.

The organization and delivery of professional care and other forms of support is located in

*Barker, P. J., & Buchanan-Barker, P. (2007a). *The Tidal Model: Mental health, recovery and reclamation.* Newport-on-Tay: Clan Unity International.

MAJOR CONCEPTS & DEFINITIONS—cont'd

the **Others Domain.** However, the key focus of the Tidal Model is dedicated forms of group work—*Discovery, Information-Sharing, and Solution-Finding.*

By participating in these groups, the person develops awareness of the value of social support, which (s)he can both receive from and give to others. This becomes the basis of the person's appreciation of the value of mutual support, which can be accessed in everyday life.

WATER—A METAPHOR*

The *Tidal Model* emphasizes the unpredictability of human experience through the core metaphor of water.

> Life is a journey taken on an ocean of experience. All human development—including the experience of health and illness—involves discoveries made on that journey across the ocean of experience. At critical points in the journey, people may experience storms or piracy. The ship may begin to take in water, and the person may face the prospect of drowning or shipwreck. The person may need to be guided to a safe haven, to undertake repairs, or to recover from the trauma. Once the ship is made intact or the person has regained their sea legs, the journey may begin again, as the person sets again their course on the ocean of experience.

This metaphor illustrates many of the elements of the psychiatric crisis and the necessary responses to this human predicament. "Storms at sea" is a metaphor for problems of living; "piracy" evokes the experience of rape or the "robbery of the self" that severe distress can produce. Many users describe the overwhelming nature of their experience of distress as akin to "drowning," and this often ends in a metaphorical "shipwreck" on the shores of the acute psychiatric unit. A proper "psychiatric rescue" should be akin to "lifesaving" and should lead the person to a genuine "safe haven," where the necessary human repair work can take place.

GUIDING PRINCIPLES†

1. A belief in the *virtue of curiosity:* the person is the world authority on their life and its problems. By expressing genuine curiosity, the professional can learn something of the "mystery" of the person's story.
2. Recognition of the *power of resourcefulness:* Rather than focusing on problems, deficits, and weaknesses, Tidal seeks to reveal the many resources available to the person—both personal and interpersonal—that might help on the voyage of recovery.
3. Respect for the *person's wishes*, rather than being paternalistic, and suggesting that we might "know what is best" for the person.
4. Acceptance of the *paradox of crisis* as opportunity: Challenging events in our lives signal that something "needs to be done." This might become an opportunity for change in life direction.
5. Acknowledging that all goals must, obviously, *belong to the person.* These will represent the small steps on the road to recovery.
6. The virtue in *pursuing elegance:* Psychiatric care and treatment are often complex and bewildering. The simplest possible means should be sought, which might bring about the changes needed for the person to move forward.

*From Barker, P. J. (2000d). *The Tidal Model—Humility in mental health care.* Retrieved March 12, 2008, from http://www.tidal-model.com/Humility%20in%20mental%20health%20care.htm

†Retrieved March 11, 2008, from www.tidal-model.com/Clarifying%20the%20value%20base%20of%20the%20Tidal%29Model.htm

Continued

GETTING IN THE SWIM—ENGAGEMENT BELIEFS*

When people are in serious distress, they often feel as if they are drowning. In such circumstances, they need a "lifesaver." Of course, lifesavers need to engage with the person—they need to get close—to begin the rescue process. To get in the swim and to begin the engagement process, we need to believe:

- That recovery is possible
- That change is inevitable—nothing lasts
- That ultimately, people know what is best for them
- That the person possesses all the resources they need to begin the recovery journey
- That the person is the teacher, and we, the helpers, are the pupils
- That we need to be creatively curious, to learn what needs to be done to help the person, **now!**

THERAPEUTIC PHILOSOPHY†

1. **Why this—why now?** We need to consider, first of all, why the person is experiencing this particular life difficulty *now?* The focus of care is very much on what the person is experiencing *now,* and what needs to be done *now* to address, and hopefully resolve, this problem.
2. **What works?** We need to ask "what works" (or might work) for the person under the present circumstances? This represents the "person-centered" focus of care. Rather than use standardized techniques or therapeutic approaches, which may have general value, we aim to identify either what has worked for the person in the past, or what might work for the person in the immediate future—given their history, personality, and general life circumstances?
3. **What is the person's personal theory?** Finally, we need to consider how this person understands her or his problems. What "sense" does the person "make" of her or his problems? Rather than giving the person a professionalized explanation of her or his difficulties—in the form of some theory or diagnosis—we try to understand how the person understands their experience. What is the person's personal theory?
4. **How to limit restrictions?** We should aim also to use the least restrictive means of helping the person to address and resolve their difficulties. Although this is often taken as read, the Tidal Model tried to identify how *little* the nurse might do to help the person, and *how much* the person might do to help bring about meaningful change. Together, these might represent the least restrictive intervention.

CONTINUUM OF CARE‡

As needs flow with the person across artificial boundaries, care is seamless, always with the intention of the person returning his or her "ocean of experience" within his or her own community. Across the care continuum, people may need critical or immediate, transitional or developmental care. Practical immediate care addresses searching for solutions to the person's problems, generally in the short term, and focuses upon "what needs to be done, now." People enter the care continuum for immediate care when experiencing an initial mental health crisis, possibly entering the mental health system for the first time, or with people already familiar to the system when a crisis occurs. Transitional care addresses the smooth passage from one setting to another, when the person is moving from one form of care to another. Here, nursing responsibilities include liaising with colleagues and ensuring the person's participation in the transfer of care. The other end of the continuum is developmental care, where the focus is on more intensive and longer-term support or therapeutic intervention.

*Barker, P. J. (n.d.). *A beginner's guide to the Tidal Model.* Retrieved March 12, 2008, from http://www.tidal-model.co.uk/New%20beginner's%20Guide.htm

†From Barker, P. J., & Buchanan-Barker, P. (2007a). *The Tidal Model: Mental health recovery and reclamation* (pp. 30-31). Newport-on-Tay: Clan Unity International.

‡From Barker, P. J. (2000e). *The Tidal Model Theory and practice* (pp. 22-24). Newcastle: University of Newcastle.

USE OF EMPIRICAL EVIDENCE

Barker's longstanding curiosity about the nature and focus of psychiatric nursing and the stories of persons-in-care led to the development of a theoretical construction of psychiatric nursing, or a meta-theory, that could be further explored through empirical inquiry (Barker, Reynolds, & Stevenson, 1997, p. 663). Over five years, from 1995, the Newcastle and North Tyneside research team developed an understanding of what people experiencing problems in living might need from nurses. They began to use their emergent findings in 1997 as the basis for the development of the Tidal Model.

Barker supports learning from, using, and integrating extant theory and research, as well as the experience of reality—"evidence from the most 'real' of real worlds" (Barker & Jackson, 1997). An example is the "need adapted" approach to caring with people in schizophrenia developed from Alanen's studies. One understanding that underpins Alanen's work and flows through the Tidal Model is that people and their families need to think of psychiatric admission to a psychiatric facility as a result of problems of living they have encountered and not as a mysterious illness that is within the patient (Alanen, Lehtinen, & Aaltonen, 1997).

The power of the nurse-patient relationship demonstrated through Altschul's pioneering research in the early 1960s and Peplau's paradigm of interpersonal relationships contribute to the empirical base of the Tidal Model. Altschul's study of nurse-patient interaction in the 1960s provides empirical support for "the complex, yet paradoxically 'ordinary' nature of the relationship" (Barker, 2002a). Altschul's study of community teams in the 1980s raised questions about the "proper focus of nursing" and the "need for nursing," and both Altschul and Peplau provided evidence related to interprofessional teamwork.

Two of Barker's theory-generating studies provide an empirical base for the Tidal Model. The "need for nursing" studies (Barker, Jackson, & Stevenson, 1999a, 1999b) examined the perceptions of service users, significant others, members of multidisciplinary teams, and nurses and sought to clarify discrete roles and functions of nursing within a multidisciplinary care and treatment process and to learn what people value in nurses (Barker, 2001c, p. 215). They demonstrated that professionals and persons-in-care wanted nurses to relate to people in ordinary, everyday ways. There was universal acceptance of special interpersonal relationships between nurses and persons, echoing Peplau's (1952) work. "Knowing you, knowing me" emerged as the core concept in these studies. The nurse is expected to know what the person wants even if it is not verbalized or is not clear, and needs are constantly changing (Jackson & Stevenson, 2004, p. 35). Professional nursing performance is described in three roles identified as (1) ordinary-me, (2) pseudo-ordinary/engineered-me, and (3) professional-me. The relationships are fluid, requiring nurses to "toggle" or switch back and forth from highly professional to distinctly ordinary presentations of self, and relationships differ depending upon the role (Jackson & Stevenson, 1998, 2000). The pseudo-ordinary or engineered-me is likened to a see-saw (Jackson & Stevenson, 2004, p. 41). Sometimes people need someone to take care of them, other times someone to take care with them (Barker et al., 1999a, 1999b). The studies suggested that nurses respond sensitively to persons' and their families' rapidly fluctuating human needs. They need to "tune in to what needs to be done now," to meet the person's needs (Barker, 2000e). Nurses are translators for the person to the treatment team and the "glue" that holds the system together (Stevenson & Fletcher, 2002, p. 30).

The second study focused on the nature of empowerment and how this is enacted in relationship between nurses and persons-in-care. It resulted in the Empowering Interactions Model (Barker, Stevenson, & Leamy, 2000). This was developed with Flanagan's Critical Incident Technique (Flannagan, 1954) within a cooperative inquiry method (Heron, 1996), using a modified grounded theory approach (Glaser & Strauss, 1967). It developed Peplau's assumptions about the importance of specific interpersonal transactions, and provided guidance and strategies for nurses within collaborative nurse-person relationships. Strategies include:

- Being respectful of people's knowledge and expertise about their own health and illness
- Putting the person in the driver's seat in relation to the interaction
- Seeking permission to explore the person's experience
- Valuing the person's contributing
- Being curious as a way of validating the person's experience
- Finding common language to describe the situation
- Taking stock
- Reviewing collaboratively and inspiring hope through designing a realistic future together

MAJOR ASSUMPTIONS

Nurses are involved in the process of working with people, their environments, their health status *and* their need for nursing (Barker, 1996a, p. 242). The Tidal Model rests on the assumptions that:

- There are such "things" as psychiatric needs.
- Nursing might in some way meet those needs (Barker & Whitehill, 1997, p. 15).
- Persons and those around them already possess the solutions to their life problems.
- Nursing is about drawing out these solutions (Barker, 1995, p. 12).

Two basic assumptions underpin the Tidal Model. First, "change is the only constant," nothing lasts. All human experience involves flux and people are constantly changing. This suggests the value of helping people become more aware of how change is happening within and around them in the "now" (Barker & Buchanan-Barker, 2004a). Second, people are their stories. They are no more and no less than the complex story of their lived experience. The person's story is framed in the first person, and the story of how they came to be here experiencing this "problem of living" contains raw material for solutions (Barker & Buchanan-Barker, 2004a).

The Tidal Model assumes that when people are caught in the psychic storm of "madness," it is "as if" they risk drowning in their distress or foundering on the rocks; it is "as if" they have been boarded by pirates and have been robbed of some of their human identity; it is "as if" they have been washed ashore on some remote beach, far from home and alienated from all that they know and understand.

Nursing

Nursing is continuously changing, internally and in relation to other professions, in response to changing needs and changing social structures. The nature of Barker's relationship with users of services confirms his appreciation of nursing as a social, rather than professional, construct. "If any one thing defines nursing, globally, it is the social construction of the nurse's role" (Barker, Reynolds, & Ward, 1995, p. 390). Nursing as nurturing exists only when the conditions necessary for the promotion of growth or development are being put in place (Buchanan-Barker & Barker, 2008). Nursing is an enduring human interpersonal activity and involves a focus on the promotion of growth and development (Barker & Whitehill, 1997, p. 17) and present and future direction (Barker & Buchanan-Barker, 2007a). Barker tried to extend Peplau's original definition, by defining the purpose of nursing as *trephotaxis*—from the Greek, meaning "the provision of the necessary conditions for the promotion of growth and development" (Barker, 1989). More recently, he has distinguished psychiatric nursing from mental health nursing. "When nurses help people *explore* their distress, in an attempt to discover ways of *remedying* or *ameliorating* it, they are practicing *psychiatric nursing*. When nurses help the same people *explore* ways of *growing and developing*, as persons, exploring how they presently *live with* and might move *beyond* their problems of living, they are practicing *mental health nursing*" (Barker, in press).

Nursing is a human service offered by one group of human beings to another. There is a power dynamic in the "craft of caring," one person has a duty to care for another (Barker, 1996b, p. 4). Nursing is a practical endeavor focused on identifying what people need *now;* collaboratively exploring ways of meeting those needs; and developing appropriate systems of human care (Barker, 1995, 2003a). The proper focus of nursing is the "need" expressed by the person-in-care, which "can only be defined as a function of the relationship between a *person-with-a-need-for-nursing* and a *person-who-has-met-that-need*" (Barker, 1996a, p. 241; Barker et al., 1995, p. 389). These responses are the phenomenological focus of nursing (Barker et al., 1995, p. 394; Peplau, 1987). This focus is on human responses to actual or potential health problems (American Nurses Association, 1980). These may range across behavior, emotions, beliefs, identity, capability, spirituality, and the person's relationship with the environment (Barker, 1998a).

Nursing's exploration of the human context of being and caring suggests nursing as a form of human inquiry. Being with and caring with people is the process that underpins all psychiatric and mental health nursing, and this process distinguishes nurses from all other health and social care disciplines (Barker, 1997). Nursing complements other services and is congruent with the roles and functions of other disciplines in relation to the person's needs (Barker, 2001c, p. 216).

Person

Within the Tidal Model, interest is directed toward a phenomenological view of the person's lived experience, and his or her story or narrative. Persons are natural philosophers and meaning makers, devoting much of their lives to establishing the meaning and value of their experience and to constructing explanatory models of the world and their place in it (Barker, 1996b, p. 4). Nurses are able to see and appreciate the world from the person's perspective and share this with the person. People are their stories. "The person's sense of self and the world of experience—including the experience of others—is inextricably tied to their life stories and the various meanings they have generated" (Barker, 2001c, p. 219). People are in a constant state of flux, with great capacity for change (Buchanan-Barker & Barker, 2008) and engaged in the process of becoming (Barker, 2000c, p. 330). They live within their world of experience represented in three dimensions: (1) world, (2) self, and (3) others.

Life is a developmental voyage and people travel across their "ocean of experience." This voyage of discovery and exploration can be risky, and people have both a fundamental need for security and capacity to adapt to changing circumstances. The journey across our ocean of experience depends on our physical body on which we roll out the story of our lives (Barker & Buchanan-Barker, 2007a, p. 21). The Tidal Model "holds few assumptions about the proper course of a person's life" (Barker, 2001a, p. 235). Persons are defined in relations, as for example, someone's mother, father, daughter, son, sister, brother, friend. They are also in relation with nurses.

Health

Barker provides the provocative definition of health put forth by Illich (1976) as "the result of an autonomous yet culturally shaped reaction to socially-created reality. It designates the ability to adapt to changing environments, to growing up . . . to healing when damaged, to suffering and to the peaceful expectation of death. Health embraces the future . . . includes the inner resources to live with it (p. 273). Health is a personal task where success is "in large part the result of self-awareness, self-discipline, and inner resources by which each person regulates his/her own daily rhythms and actions, his/her diet, and his/her sexuality" (Illich, 1976, p. 274). Our personhood, connections, and fragility "make the experience of pain, of sickness, and of death an integral part of life" (Illich, 1976, p. 274). Illich's (1976) description illustrates both the *chaotic* and *Zen* sense of "reality." "Health is not 'out-there,' it is not something to be pursued, gained or delivered (health-care). It is a part of the whole task of being and living" (Barker, 1999b, p. 240).

"Health means whole . . . and is likely linked to the way we live our lives, in the broadest sense. This 'living' includes the social, economic, cultural and spiritual context of our lives" (Barker, 1999b, p. 48).

The experience of health and illness is fluid. Within a holistic view, people have their own individual meanings of health and illness that we value and accept. Nurses engage with people to learn their stories and their understanding of their current situation, including relationships with health and illness within their worldview (Barker, 2001c). Ill health or illness almost always involves a spiritual crisis or a loss of self (Barker, 1996a). A state of disease is a human problem with social, psychological, and medical relations—a whole life crisis. Nursing in the Tidal Model is pragmatic and focused upon persons' strengths, resources, and possibilities, maintaining a health orientation; the Tidal Model is a healthy theory.

Environment

The environment is largely social in nature, the context in which persons travel within their ocean of experience, and nurses create "space" for growth and development. "Therapeutic relationships are used in ways that enhance persons' relationships with their environment" (Montgomery & Webster, 1993, p. 7). Human problems may derive from complex person-environment interactions in the organized chaos of the everyday world (Barker, 1998b, p. 215). "Persons live in a social and material world where their interaction with the environment includes other people, groups, and organizations" (Barker, 2003a, p. 67). Family, culture, and relationships are integral to this environment. Within the environment are vital areas of everyday living, including housing, financing, occupation, leisure, a sense of place, and of belonging (Barker, 2001c, p. 218).

The divide between community and institution is artificial and rejected as needs flow with the person across these boundaries. Much psychiatric and mental health nursing takes place in the most mundane of settings, from day rooms of hospital wards to the living room or kitchen of the person's own home (Barker, 1996b, p. 5). With critical interventions, nurses make the person and the environment safe and secure. Engagement is critical, and the social environment is critical for engagement. When people are deemed to be at risk, they may need to be detained in a safe and supportive environment, a safe harbor until they return to their ocean of experience in the community (Barker, 2003a, p. 6). "Nurses organize the kind of conditions that help to alleviate distress and begin the longer term process of recuperation, resolution or learning. They help persons to feel the 'whole' of their experience . . . and engender the potential for healing" (Barker, 2003a, p. 9).

THEORETICAL ASSERTIONS

The Tidal Model is based upon four premises concerning practice, which were developed by Barker in the mid-1990s with the "expert nurse" focus group (Barker, 1997). These premises were validated by a group of former psychiatric patients, led by Barker's colleague of many years, the mental health service user and activist, Dr. Irene Whitehill.

- Psychiatric nursing is an interactive, developmental human activity, more concerned with the future development of the person than the origins or cause of their present mental distress.
- The experience of mental distress associated with psychiatric disorder is represented through public disturbance or reports of private events that are known only to the person concerned. Nurses help people access, review, and re-author these experiences.
- Nurses and the people-in-care are engaged in a relationship based upon mutual influence. Change is constant, and within relationships there are changes in the relationship and within the participants in the relationship.
- The experience of mental illness is translated into a variety of disturbances of everyday living and human responses to problems in living (Barker & Whitehill, 1997).

These premises are framed within the wider philosophical and theoretical perspective, especially the phenomenological assertion that people own their experience; only persons can know their experience and what it means. Mental illness is a symbolic force, which is known only—in phenomenological terms—to the person involved. The lived experience is the medium through which we receive important messages about our life and its meaning (Barker, 2001c). Barker views mental distress as part of the whole that is the person, not something split off from their "normal" being.

The Tidal Model assumes and asserts that people know what their needs are, or can be helped to recognize or acknowledge them over time. From that minimally empowered position, people may be helped to meet these needs in the "short" term. What nurses and everyone else in the person's social world relate to is the expressed behavior. Mental illness is disempowering, and "people who experience any of the myriad threats to their personal or social identities, commonly called *mental illness* or *mental health problems,* experience a human threat that renders them vulnerable." However, "most people are sufficiently healthy to be able to act for themselves and to influence constructively the direction of their lives" (Barker, 2003a, pp. 6-7). Recovery is possible, and people have the personal and interpersonal resources that enable this recovery process (Barker, 2001c, p. 215).

LOGICAL FORM

The Tidal Model is logically adequate, the structure of relationships is clear, and concepts are precise, developed and developing. It contains broad ideas, addresses many situations of persons with problems in living, follows the "logic of experience" (Barker, 1996b), and develops "practice-based evidence" (Barker & Buchanan-Barker, 2005).

Barker and colleagues have constructed a metatheory of psychiatric and mental health nursing. Questions about the nature of persons, problems in living, and nursing were followed with systematic inquiry. The theory informs and is shaped by research. The Tidal Model flows from a particular philosophical perspective and worldview that provides a context for beliefs about persons and nursing.

The theory identifies the core of nursing practice in "knowing you, knowing me." It specifies a nursing focus of inquiry, identifies phenomena of particular interest to nurses, and provides a broad perspective for nursing research, practice, education, and policy. The theory classifies a body of nursing knowledge that is largely narrative. The components are clearly presented and logically derived from clinical observation, practice, theory, research, and philosophy.

The emergent evidence from users of the theory in the UK, Ireland, Canada, and New Zealand confirms the importance of the simple affirmation of the personal narrative, with its emphasis on understanding what is happening for and to the person, and what this means for persons, in their own language. Stories generated within the caring context are written in the person's own voice, signifying that the person is helped to "take back" the personal story, which has been lost from view by becoming a "patient" or "client." Even when the person is severely disabled by problems of living, the nurse keeps the focus on helping the person determine "what needs to be done," and on finding the personal and interpersonal resources necessary to be empowered.

The attempt to understand persons' constructions of their world is expressed through the holistic assessment that provides the means of helping persons relate their story and exploring what needs to be done. Care planning is a collaborative exercise with emphasis on developing an awareness of change and revealing solutions. The celebration of personhood and the holistic, narrative approach creates a style of practice that works collaboratively with people. It emphasizes persons' inherent resources and acknowledges change as an enduring characteristic.

ACCEPTANCE BY NURSING COMMUNITY

The Tidal Model has appeal for those interested in person-centered care and research-based practice. The literature illustrates the wide acceptance and use of the theory in practice and in research. Acceptance of the theory is facilitated by the philosophical, theoretical, research, and practical base, along with clearly stated values and principles.

Practice

The Tidal Model was originally developed in practice between 1995 and 1997 and was introduced formally on two acute psychiatric wards in Newcastle, England, in 1998. It was subsequently adopted by the Mental Health Program, and in 2000 rolled out across nine acute psychiatric wards, their associated community support teams, and one 24-hour facility in the community (Barker & Buchanan-Barker, 2005, p. 211). The Tidal Model is international in scope as interest spread from the United Kingdom to Ireland, then throughout the world.

Most of the early Tidal Model developmental work was undertaken in the UK, with projects ranging across hospital and community services, from acute through rehabilitation, to specialist forensic services and community care. These projects also range from metropolitan services in cities like central London and Birmingham, where the clinical populations are socially, culturally, and ethnically diverse, to Cornwall, Glamorgan, and Norfolk, where people from more traditional English and Welsh towns and villages in the wide-ranging rural community are served. The biggest project to date is in Scotland, where the Glasgow mental health services operate a series of Tidal projects across the city, embracing acute, rehabilitation, adolescent, and elder care, in the largest mental health trust in the UK (Lafferty & Davidson, 2006). By the beginning of 2008, the Glasgow projects had extended to include Greenrock, Invercycle, Paisley, and Ayrshire, representing a third of the overall population of Scotland.

The Republic of Ireland has over 30 projects, most of these situated in County Cork, with other projects in County Mayo and Dublin, ranging across hospital and community settings. Cork City, Ireland, was the first to introduce and develop the Tidal Model within community mental health care at Tosnu—Gaelic for a "fresh start"—and now there are almost 20 projects bridging hospital and community services.

At the Royal Ottawa Mental Health Centre in Canada, three programs implemented the Tidal Model in September 2002. The Forensic and Mood programs include inpatient wards and outpatient components. The Substance Use and Concurrent Disorders Program includes an inpatient ward, outpatient nursing, a day hospital, and a residential program in the community and is the first program of its kind to implement the Tidal Model. In February 2004, the Tidal Model was introduced to the remaining inpatient wards, including geriatric, crisis and evaluation, general psychiatry in transition, psychosocial rehabilitation, and schizophrenia and youth (adolescents). In 2005, Tidal was introduced and implemented in the Forensic Program at the Brockville Campus of the Royal Ottawa Health Care Group. The Tidal Model has also been introduced to the Royal Ottawa Place, a long-term care facility (nursing home), and is practiced by a Tidal Champion in consultation to another nursing home. Across Canada also there has been much interest in the Tidal Model. It has been implemented or is in progress in facilities from coast to coast.

In Australia, the Model was first introduced in Sydney followed by Townsville, Queensland. More recently, new projects have been established in child and adolescent care in Sydney, with a new development in the area of "justice health." In New Zealand, nurses at the *Rangipapa* forensic service in Porirua have been developing their care around the Tidal Model for over three years and were the first forensic service in the world to adopt the model (Cook, Phillips, & Sadler, 2005). The Tidal Model's emphasis on narrative has proven particularly attractive to the indigenous Maori and Pacific Islands people, who greatly value the power of storytelling. This is reflected in a recent evaluation of the perceptions of Tidal care by some of the unit's residents.

In Japan, the Model has been the focus of a major development program at the Kanto Medical Center, the largest private psychiatric facility in Tokyo, over the past five years. There, Dr. Tsuyoshi Akayama, the lead psychiatrist, translated all the Tidal Model training materials into Japanese and then taught his medical and nursing colleagues how to use the Model, following his short study tour in Newcastle with Dr. Barker. This was the first example of a formal collaboration between psychiatrists and nurses—in all of the earlier projects, nurses had led the implementation alone. Dr. Akayama has also promoted consideration of the Tidal Model within the "developing nations" program of the World Psychiatric Association. The Japanese have set a trend for greater interprofessional collaboration, albeit with nursing taking the lead role.

Education

Barker provides a multi-media education package for those implementing the Tidal Model, and all sites use this program to prepare for implementation. This ensures a common perspective among and fidelity to the values, principles, and processes of the Tidal Model, yet it allows creative, locally relevant implementation. Nurses within the Tidal community have the opportunity to learn about the model before, during, and following its implementation.

The Tidal Model is integrated into the diploma, graduate, and post-graduate nursing programs in most UK universities. Ian Beech, a mental health nurse and lecturer at the University of Glamorgan, developed the first educational program for practitioners in Wales. At University College Cork, the Tidal Model is linked between the university and various practice settings. At the University of Ottawa, Canada, the Tidal Model is included in the undergraduate theories and concepts course; it also frames the Community Mental Health Nursing course, as well as the post-graduate Mental Health Nursing certificate program at Algonquin College. The Tidal Model anchors the mental health nursing residency program being developed collaboratively by five tertiary mental health centres in Ontario. The post-graduate mental health nursing course at Dalhousie University in Halifax, Nova Scotia, is also framed by the Tidal Model. The Tidal Model is included in the Mount Royal College community mental health course in Calgary, Canada. The holistic, strength-based, narrative Tidal Model holds great promise for inclusion in educational programs concerned with research-based practice and person-centered care.

Research

The Tidal Model developed from a clinical research program. All International Tidal Model network members are encouraged to evaluate the model in practice. A research and development consultancy was established as a loose network for Tidal Model implementation and development projects. The consultancy provides a framework for evaluation of the Tidal Model in action from the perspective of organizational outcome, professional experience, and user/consumer experience (Barker & Buchanan-Barker, 2005). The important task of evaluating the implementation, processes, and outcomes of the Tidal Model in practice is ongoing in Canada, Ireland, Japan, and New Zealand and across the United Kingdom.

Two evaluation studies (Fletcher & Stevenson, 2001; Stevenson & Fletcher, 2002) explored outcome measures that could be important in evaluating the Tidal Model and evaluated the impact of the Tidal Model assessment in practice (Stevenson & Fletcher, 2002). Results of both studies indicate an increase in the number of admissions and a decrease in the length of stay. There were decreases in the need for the highest level of observation that correlated with the speed of assessment, decreased incidents of violence, self-harm, and the use of restraints. Nurses themselves reported that the Tidal Model enhanced professional practice, and encouraged fuller engagement with persons-in-care. It was useful in helping persons to fulfill care plans and enabled nurses to focus their interactions on persons' needs. Support workers were more able to help persons identify goals and targets for the day and carry them out; they described the Tidal Model as a way of raising their profile and professional esteem (Stevenson & Fletcher, 2002, p. 35). Similar findings, using the same method, were reported in Birmingham, the second city in England to implement the Tidal Model (Gordon, Morton, & Brooks, 2005), Glasgow, the largest city in Scotland (Laffferty & Davidson, 2006), and Dublin, the capital of Ireland (Collins, Maxwell, & Lynch, 2004). These studies provide support for the implementation of this person-centered theory in practice.

Barker and Walker (2000) studied senior nurses' views of multidisciplinary teamwork in 26 acute psychiatric admission units and the relationship to the care of persons and their families. While nurses face challenges in implementing "working in partnership," the study provides some direction for further inquiry around the interprofessional nature of the theory.

The transition for nurses to a solution focus in interactions was the subject of study by the Newcastle team (Stevenson, Jackson, & Barker, 2003). Nurses participated in a specially tailored solution education initiative, and the impact was assessed for both nurses and persons-in-care using multiple data sources. This study provides strong evidence of a significant improvement in nurses' solution-focused knowledge, performance, and use in practice. Persons-in-care also found the approach helpful.

The Royal Ottawa Mental Health Centre Tidal team replicated the Newcastle study and assessed the impact of implementation of Tidal on selected outcome measures at four time periods in the three pioneer programs, with similar results particularly with the Mood program. They also replicated the Newcastle study over four time periods in the Forensic Program at the Brockville site. The Tosnu team completed a user-focused evaluation of the Tidal Model implementation. In Birmingham, on the Tolkien ward, a four-month evaluation has been completed and published (Gordon, Morton, & Brooks, 2005). Evaluation work is ongoing at St. Tydfil Hospital in Wales

In New Zealand a qualitative, hermeneutic phenomenological study followed the implementation of the Tidal Model in a secure treatment unit (Cook, Phillips, & Sadler, 2005). The study explored the lived experience of four inpatients and four nurses. Five themes that reflected meanings attached to providing and receiving care emerged: relationships, hope, human face, levelling, and working together. This suggests positive experiences and outcomes with the implementation of the Tidal Model. The Tidal Model is set in a research base that provides the possibility of research utilization or the more contemporary knowledge transfer. Nurses practicing within the Tidal Model are actively using research in practice as well as contributing to the development of nursing practice. The Tidal Model has potential for participatory action research, uncovering knowledge embedded in practice, and developing new knowledge and understandings.

Barker and Buchanan-Barker have recently problematized the research agenda. "People often ask us: Does the Tidal Model work? We do not believe that the Tidal Model can be shown to work any more than the sheet music for a Mozart Concerto can be said to "work." To make great music, we need great musicians. Consequently, we believe that any realistic study of the Tidal Model *in practice* must focus on the "workings" of the team—both individually and collectively. It must also take account of the organizational context, the support available to the team, the quality of the environment, and a range of other physical, social, and interpersonal factors.

FURTHER DEVELOPMENT

The Tidal Model is clear, concepts are defined, and relationships identified. This enables the identification of areas for further theory development. For example, Barker is reframing his original notion of the "logic of experience" as "practice-based evidence." "Practice-based evidence" represents the knowledge of what *is* possible in this particular situation *and* which might contribute further to our shared understanding of human helping (Barker & Buchanan-Barker, 2005).

Several other developments characterize the Tidal Model. It has evolved from the initial acute, inpatient use across the continuum of care, with critical, transitional, and developmental components. The theory has evolved to the Tidal Model of Mental Health Recovery and Reclamation, broadening both its scope and utility. Colleagues in other fields such as palliative care have expressed appreciation of the model and the desire to bring it into their practice settings. Other professions also support the values, philosophy, and utility of the Tidal Model. Mental health user/consumer/survivor communities around the world are involved in the continuing development of this mental health recovery theory (Barker & Buchanan-Barker, 2005).

Since its inception, the Tidal Model has gained national and international attention. It continues to be implemented, taught, and studied internationally, with new sites joining from around the world. In November 2003, the Tidal Model was launched in North America. As new sites implement and study the Tidal Model, the practical, theoretical, and research base will be enriched. While psychiatric and mental health care is considered a specialty, it has almost limitless possibilities in geography, settings, and clinical populations.

In 2003, Barker reaffirmed the values underlying the Tidal Model in the ten commitments (see Box 32-1). They provide the necessary guidance to pursue and develop the philosophy of the Tidal Model. Although Barker expects fidelity to the principles and values of the Tidal Model (ten commitments) in its implementation, he cautions against slavish importation. Implementation needs to be tailored to fit the local context, with the result that each implementation will be unique and will contribute to the theory's development. This reflects Barker's appreciation of the concept of "practice-based evidence"—what he called the "art of the possible," that is, developing philosophically and theoretically sound forms of practice, which are based on considerations of what is appropriate, meaningful, and potentially effective in any given practice context.

The Tidal Model is developing across cultures, with different clinical populations, in a variety of settings. The body of knowledge framed within the Tidal Model continues to develop, acknowledging the wide range of complex factors which define people and their human needs—personal history, personal preferences, values and beliefs, social status, cultural background, family affiliations, community membership (Barker, 2003a).

CRITIQUE

The Tidal Model of Mental Health Recovery is directed toward understanding and explaining further the human condition. Central to this effort is helping people use their voices as the key instrument for charting their recovery from mental distress. The Tidal Model is a genuine person-centred model of mental health care delivery, which also is respectful of culture and creed (Barker & Buchanan-Barker, 2005). This practical theory identifies concepts necessary to understand the human needs of people with problems in living, and how and what nurses might do to address those needs. The theory systematically explains specific phenomena and suggests the nature of relationships within a particular worldview. Barker, however, has consistently asserted that the theory is "no more than words on paper." It is not a reified work or recipe for practice, but a practical and evolving guide for delivering collaborative, person-centered, strength-based, and empowering care through relationship.

Clarity

The concepts, subconcepts, and relationships are logically developed and clear, and the assumptions are consistent with the theory's goals. Words have multiple meanings; however, these major concepts, subconcepts, and relationships are described carefully, specifically, and metaphorically, though not necessarily concisely. The careful selection of the term "problems in living" or mental distress and the view of people experiencing these problems as "persons" direct nurses to their proper focus. The identification of "human needs" rather than psychological, social, or physical needs also provides clarity and focus. How nurses see persons and how persons want to be nursed are clearly illustrated through the core category of "knowing you, knowing me." Three subcategories—ordinary me, pseudo-ordinary or engineered-me, and professional me—each have four dimensions: depth of knowing, power, time, and translation (Barker et al., 1999a; Jackson & Stevenson, 2004).

In practice, using the person's own language, not translating into jargon or professional language, contributes to the theory's success and its clarity. Major concepts—collaboration, empowerment, relationships, solution focus—empowering through relationships, narrative, and the use of "problems in living" are sufficiently clear and open the theory for use in other areas of nursing and health care.

A number of concepts and relationships are presented elegantly and schematically within the Tidal Model. The person's unique lived experience is synergistic and reciprocal among the world, self, and others domains. This is represented as a triangle (Figure 32-1). The Holistic Assessment—the person's story is at the heart of care planning, and is represented as a heart. The circle of security assessment and plan surrounds the heart, all of which is surrounded by the interprofessional team circle (Figure 32-2) The continuum of care (immediate, transitional, and developmental) intersects with the focus of care (Barker, 2000e; Barker & Buchanan-Barker, 2007a) (Figure 32-3). This clear, easily understood theory is accessible both conceptually

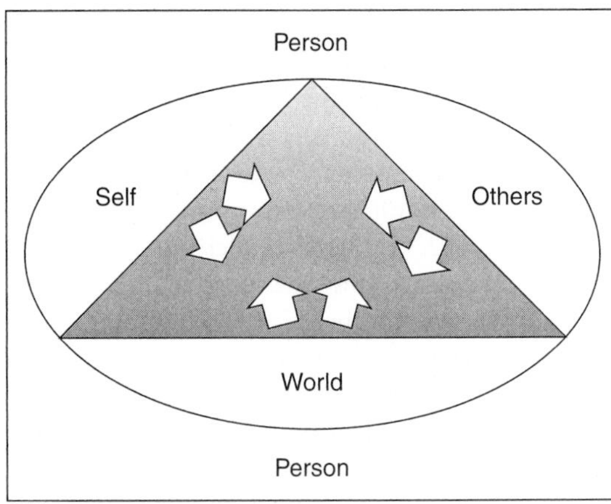

Figure 32-1 Three dimensions of personhood. (From Barker, P. J. [2000]. *The Tidal Model theory and practice* [pp. 29-31]. Newcastle, UK: University of Newcastle. Copyright Phil Barker, 2000.)

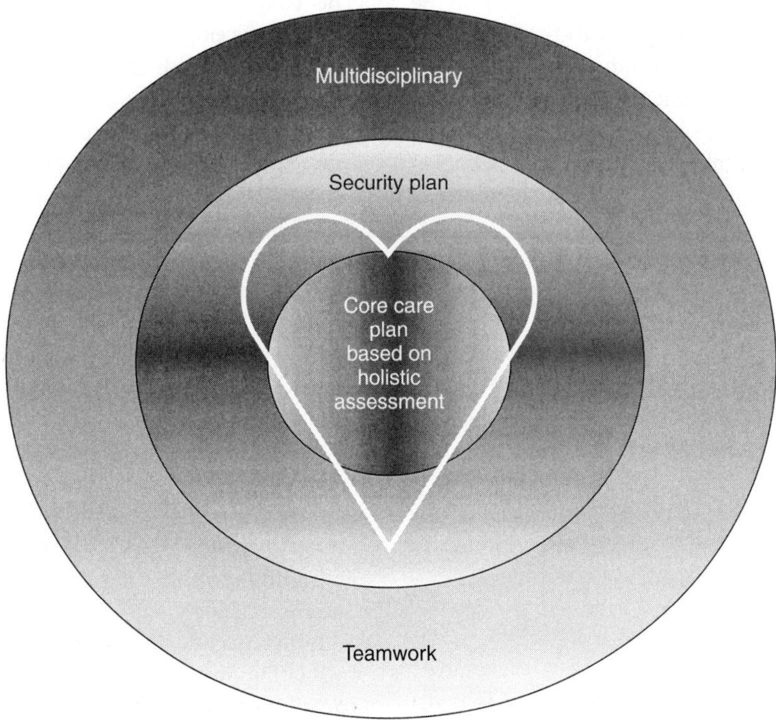

Figure 32-2 Structure of care. (From Barker, P. J. [2000]. *The Tidal Model theory and practice* [p. 27]. Newcastle, UK: University of Newcastle. Copyright Phil Barker, 2000.)

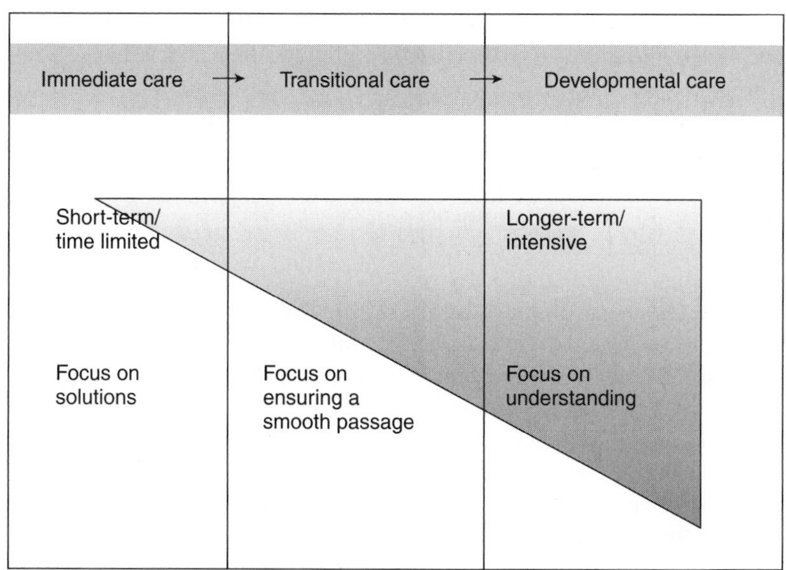

Figure 33-3 Tidal Model care continuum. (From Barker, P. J. [2000]. *The Tidal Model theory and practice* [p. 22]. Newcastle, UK: University of Newcastle. Copyright Phil Barker, 2000.)

and linguistically through the use of everyday language.

Simplicity

The Tidal Model is based upon a few simple ideas about "being human" and "helping one another" (Barker, 2000e). It is comprehensive, elegant in its simplicity, and at a level of abstraction to guide practice, education, research, and policy. However, the concepts themselves are complex, and the broad relationships among the concepts add to the complexity of the Tidal Model—people and relationships are inherently complex.

Assumptions, concepts, and relationships are described in everyday language and illuminated through metaphor. For example, simply being respectful of the persons' knowledge and expertise about their own health and illness and listening to persons' stories is empowering. Abstract and complex concepts or relationships, for example, chaos theory, are expressed metaphorically as in the ebb and flow of the tide. Practical and philosophical, the Tidal Model provides some direction in operationalizing or using some of the concepts, although it does not prescribe practice.

Generality

The Tidal Model is international in scope, suggesting its relevance cross-culturally and cross-nationally. By the beginning of 2004, there were almost 100 Tidal Model projects in progress in different clinical settings in a variety of countries around the world—Australia, Canada, England, Ireland, Japan, New Zealand, Scotland, and Wales (Barker, 2004; Barker & Buchanan-Barker, 2005). A wide range of settings and clinical populations are represented in the Tidal Model projects: rural and urban, acute, crisis and longer term care wards, private and public facilities, community programs, rehabilitation, forensic, youth, adults and older adults. The Tidal Model has been successful across the continuum of psychiatric and mental health care and in a range of practice situations. Universal characteristics of collaboration, empowerment, relationships, stories, and strengths appeal to nurses, service users, and colleagues in other disciplines and support general applicability.

The Tidal Model is also consistent with the Ottawa Charter for Health Promotion, where the process of empowerment and participation is seen as fundamental to good health (World Health Organization, 1986). The Tidal Model parallels the process of enabling people to increase control over and improve their health. The 10 tidal commitments (Barker, 2003b) provide guidance, direction, and support in using the theory. In Scotland, Lafferty and Davidson (2006) observed that the practice of the Tidal Model helped nurses to fulfill the person-centered requirements of the new Scottish Mental Health Act. In Canada, the Best Practice Guideline for Client-Centred Care (Registered Nurses' Association of Ontario, 2006), echoes the Tidal Model, even using some of the same language.

Barker acknowledges that in order to practice within the Tidal Model, we need to believe that recovery is possible and change is inevitable. "The Tidal Model *per se* does not work. The practitioner is the instrument or medium of change" (Buchanan-Barker, 2004, p. 8). Practitioners with different worldviews would not be comfortable with or accept the Tidal Model, and such diversity is respected. As the Tidal Model was developed specifically for psychiatry and mental health care, the criterion of generality is met.

Empirical Precision

This substantive theory is grounded in the data that emerged inductively from the studies of the need for nursing. Studies guided by the Tidal Model suggest its utility and precision and provide confidence that the theory is useful, practical, and accessible. Studies of the impact of the implementation of the theory in practice also support its utility and precision. The "need for nursing," the proper focus of nursing, and the empowering interactions framework provide a strong empirical base for the Tidal Model.

Nurses working with different clinical populations and in a variety of settings are testing out the Tidal Model in practice. The focus of inquiry is person-centered outcomes and the lived experience of persons collaborating in care. Studies addressing the solution orientation in empowering interactions contribute to the empirical adequacy of and confidence in this shared solution-oriented perspective. Some theoretical underpinnings such as chaos theory are not amenable to study, although they contribute to the theoretical and conceptual base of the model.

Derivable Consequences

The Tidal Model provides direction and focus for nursing. The theory is accessible conceptually and linguistically and lends itself to research. This research, relevant to nurses' work, contributes knowledge to guide and inform practice. Studies guided by the Tidal Model also explore its impact and a variety of outcomes. The narrative knowledge derived from the theory advances the practice of nursing, nursing education, nursing research, and policy. The Tidal Model is represented by a range of holistic (exploratory) and focused (risk) assessments which generate person-centered interventions that emphasize the person's extant resources and capacity for solution-finding (Barker, 2001b, p. 82).

Working within the Tidal Model enables nurses to articulate their practice and to surface "invisible skills" (Michael, 1994). For example, empowerment strategies such as respecting the person and inspiring hope also give voice to nurses themselves. Nurses gain confidence in working among interprofessional team members as their contribution and focus is more clearly articulated.

Challenges exist at a practical, personal, and system level with any change, and these are anticipated and addressed. However, the Tidal Model is an important and essential theory to develop and guide practice in psychiatry and mental health care. It is also an important theoretical context for facilities committed to person-centered care and offers practical methods for its implementation.

SUMMARY

The Tidal Model developed from a discrete focus on psychiatric nursing in acute settings to a more flexible mental health recovery and reclamation model for any setting, relevant to any discipline. It emphasizes empowering forms of engagement or bridging, the importance of the lived experience, and an appreciation of the potential for healing that lies within the re-authoring of the narrative (Barker & Buchanan-Barker, 2004a).

The Tidal Model provides an orientation to practice that is research-based, holistic, and person-centered. Keen (in Barker & Buchanan-Barker, 2005, pp. 231-241) describes a deeply collaborative, person-centered, solution-focused (McAllister, 2003), narrative-based, pragmatic, and systemic theory. The theory describes various assumptions about people, their inherent value, and the value of relating to people in particular ways. It describes how people might come to appreciate differently, perhaps better, their own value and the unique value of their experience. The Tidal Model opens possibilities of new ways of being with people in relation. Perhaps some of its appeal is that it harkens back to "our roots" and values which brought us into nursing in the first place. While the theory provides direction for practice, education, research, and policy, it is not easy. Nurses are aware of the challenge in making the shift to commit to change and to grow and develop in enacting the essence of the Tidal Model, the ten tidal commitments.

Case Study

Scott was a young man described as having a first episode psychosis. He had beaten his father, who subsequently died. Scott was transferred to a secure unit, where his primary nurse began to explore his story with him through a holistic assessment, which represents Scott's world of experience at this moment in time.

How this began: "It all started when my father punched my mother again, he was totally drunk that night. It was so noisy in that room, the T.V., the banging, and those voices in my head, they kept yelling at me to do something fast to save my mother. I don't remember exactly what had happened after. I was so confused."

How this affected me: "I don't know. I have been in jail for 4 months before coming here. They told me I killed my father, I don't remember much except that I kept hammering his head, I just remember I was standing in a pool of blood." "They told me my mother is still in the hospital, I haven't seen her since." "I'm scared. I can't sleep."

How I felt in the beginning: It "just devastated me, turned me upside down." "I felt awful even though I hated him so much, he never listened to me, no one ever listened to me or believes me." "I hate him because I watched him beating my mother all my life."

How things have changed over time: "It got worse when my stepbrother ran away. My father was a sinner, a drunk, wife beater, even conspired with the Communists. I was not allowed to leave the house except school, my mother stayed in all day to do farm work, he was the only one that ran errands outside the house." "I've always been a bit scared and angry too."

The effect on my relationships: "I don't have any relationships with anyone; I don't like people because nobody likes me."

How do I feel now? "Well, I feel nervous, very shaky and scared. I don't know what to expect, I don't know what is going to happen." "Confused, I guess, and I'm tired."

What do I think this means? "I don't know, that was my question, maybe I will go back to jail, maybe it means I needed help." "It means I have a lot of challenges to meet."

What does all this say about me as a person? "I just want to be a better person, I want to be well, and I want to take care of my mother."

What needs to happen now? "Well, I suppose I'm here for an assessment."

What do I expect the nurse to do for me? "Continue to talk to me the way you are talking to me. No one ever talks to me like this. You are listening, and it seems like you believe me. This is so different from jail and anywhere else."

The people who are important: "My mother is the only important person in this world, my stepbrother came back only for the money."

Things that are important: "Well, able to share with others." "My dog—Pepper, but he is at the Humane Society right now." "I have a really nice picture of me and my mom."

Ideas about life that are important: "Able to fit in."

Evaluating the problems: "My main problems are loneliness and what's going to happen in my future. My whole life is complex!" I would rate my loneliness as an 8 for distress, an 8 for disturbance, and a 2 for control. My future and what's going to happen would be a 10 for distress, a 10 for disturbance, and I have no control, a zero."

How will I know the problem has been solved? "I'll know the problem has been solved maybe when the voices stop talking to me, when I get out of jail and out of the hospital."

What needs to change for this to happen? "Maybe I need to take medication, maybe I just have to start talking to real people, not the voices."

The nurse recognized that Scott needed some help to feel more emotionally secure. She engaged him in a security assessment and they developed a personal security plan together.

Later in the week, the nurses noted that Scott was spending a lot of time in his room. Instead of encouraging Scott to participate in ward activities, his primary nurse shared her observation and asked Scott how it was helpful to him to spend so much time lying on his bed, alone in the room. Scott's reply was, "The voices don't bother me so much." This opened a conversation, helping the nurse begin to understand what this was like for Scott, and what might be helpful for him.

In another conversation, the primary nurse asked "the miracle question." 'Suppose that tonight, while you are asleep, the problem you have was miraculously solved. How would you know? What would be the first difference you noticed when you woke up? Scott's unexpected reply—"I'd have a friend." By exploring—rather than closing down—the narrative, the nurse began to involve Scott in "what needed to be done" to help him.

What questions might be asked in a security assessment? The security plan has two questions: What can I do that will help me to deal with my present problems? And what help can others offer that I might find valuable? What might Scott's security plan look like?

CRITICAL THINKING Activities

1. There are ten tidal commitments. Select three or four and consider how these might be realized in practice.
2. Where would you find support for each of the tidal commitments within your workplace?
3. What is the key Tidal question?

POINTS FOR Further Study

- The Tidal Model website at www.tidal-model.com enables accessibility to and connection with the international Tidal community.
- Barker, P. J. (n.d.). *A beginner's guide to the Tidal Model.* Retrieved March 12, 2008, from http://www.tidal-model.co.uk/New%20beginner's%20Guide.htm
- Barker, P. J. (2003b). *The 10 Commitments: Essential values of the Tidal Model.* Retrieved February 23, 2008, from http://www.tidal-model.com/Ten%20Commitments.htm
- Barker, P. J. (2001b). The Tidal Model: Developing a person-centerd approach to psychiatric and mental health nursing. *Perspectives in Psychiatric Care, 37*(3), 79-87.
- Barker, P. J., & Buchanan-Barker, P. (2005). *The Tidal Model: A guide for mental health professionals.* London: Brunner-Routledge.
- Barker, P. J., & Buchanan-Barker, P. (2007a). The Tidal Model—*Mental health recovery and reclamation.* Newport-on-Tay: Clan Unity International.
- Buchanan-Barker, P., & Barker, P. (2008). The Tidal Commitments: Extending the value base of mental health recovery. *Journal of Psychiatric and Mental Health Nursing, 15*, 93-100.

REFERENCES

Alanen, Y., Lehtinen, K., & Aaltonen, J. (1997). Need-adapted treatment of new schizophrenic patients: Experience and results of the Turku project. *Acta Psychiatrica Scandanavica 83*, 363-372.

American Nurses' Association. (1980). *Nursing. A social policy statement.* Kansas City, Missouri: American Nurses' Association.

Barker, P. J. (1987). *An evaluation of specific nursing interventions in the management of patients suffering from manic-depressive psychosis.* Unpublished PhD thesis, Dundee Institute of Technology (University of Abertay), Scotland.

Barker, P. J. (1989). Reflections on the philosophy of caring in mental health. *International Journal of Nursing Studies, 26*(2), 131-141.

Barker, P. J. (1995). Promoting growth through community mental health nursing. *Mental Health Nursing, 15*(3), 12-15.

Barker, P. J. (1996a). Chaos and the way of Zen: Psychiatric nursing and the 'uncertainty principle.' *Journal of Psychiatric and Mental Health Nursing, 3*, 235-243.

Barker, P. J. (1996b). The logic of experience: Developing appropriate care through effective collaboration. *Australian and New Zealand Journal of Mental Health Nursing, 5*, 3-12.

Barker, P. J. (1997). Towards a meta-theory of psychiatric nursing. *Mental Health Practice, 1*(4), 18-21.

Barker, P. J. (1998a). It's time to turn the tide. *Nursing Times, 94*(46), 11-12.

Barker, P. J. (1998b). The future of the Theory of Interpersonal Relations? A personal reflection on Peplau's legacy. *Journal of Psychiatric and Mental Health Nursing, 5*, 213-220.

Barker, P. J. (1999a). Qualitative research in nursing and health care. London: NT Books.

Barker, P. J. (Ed.). (1999b). *The philosophy and practice of psychiatric nursing.* Edinburgh: Churchill Livingstone.

Barker, P. J. (2000a). Commentaries and reflections on mental health nursing in the UK at the dawn of the new millennium: Commentary 1. *Journal of Mental Health, 9*(6), 617-619.

Barker, P. J. (2000b). From chaos to complex order: Personal values and resources in the process of psychotherapy. *Perspectives in Psychiatric Care, 36*(2), 51-57.

Barker, P. J. (2000c). Reflections on caring as a virtue ethic within an evidence-based culture. *International Journal of Nursing Studies, 37*, 329-336.

Barker, P. J. (2000d). *The Tidal Model—Humility in mental health care.* Retrieved March 8, 2008 from http://www.tidal-model.com/Humility%20in%20mental%20health%20care.htm

Barker, P. J. (2000e). *The Tidal Model: Theory and practice.* Newcastle, UK: University of Newcastle.

Barker, P. J. (2001a). The Tidal Model: Developing an empowering, person-centred approach to recovery within psychiatric and mental health nursing. *Journal of Psychiatric and Mental Health Nursing, 8*, 233-240.

Barker, P. J. (2001b). The Tidal Model: Developing a person-centered approach to psychiatric and mental health nursing. *Perspectives in Psychiatric Care, 37*(3), 79-87.

Barker, P. J. (2001c). The Tidal Model: The lived experience in person-centred mental health nursing. *Nursing Philosophy, 2*, 213-223.

Barker, P. J. (2002a). Annie Altschul—An appreciation. *Journal of Psychiatric and Mental Health Nursing, 9*, 127-128.

Barker, P. J. (2002b). Doing what needs to be done: A respectful response to Burnard and Grant. *Journal of Psychiatric and Mental Health Nursing, 9*, 232-236.

Barker, P. J. (Ed.). (2003a). *Psychiatric and mental health nursing. The craft of caring.* London: Arnold.

Barker, P. J. (2003). *Psychiatric and mental health nursing: The craft of caring.* London: Arnold.

Barker, P. J. (2003b). *The 10 Commitments: Essential values of the Tidal Model.* Retrieved 23 February, 2008 from http://www.tidal-model.com/Ten%20Commitments.htm

Barker, P. J. (2004). Uncommon sense—The Tidal Model of mental health recovery. *The New Therapist, 33*(Sept/Oct), 14-19.

Barker, P. J. (n.d.). *A beginner's guide to the Tidal Model.* Retrieved March 12, 2008 from http://www.tidal-model.co.uk/New%20beginner's%20Guide.htm

Barker, P., & Buchanan-Barker, P. (2004a). Beyond empowerment: Revering the storyteller. *Mental Health Practice, 7*(5), 18-20.

Barker, P. J., & Buchanan-Barker, P. (2004b). *Spirituality and mental health: Breakthrough.* London: Whurr.

Barker, P. J., & Buchanan-Barker, P. (2005). *The Tidal Model: A guide for mental health professionals.* London: Brunner-Routledge.

Barker, P. J., & Buchanan-Barker, P. (2007a). *The Tidal Model—Mental health recovery and reclamation.* Newport-on-Tay: Clan Unity International.

Barker, P. J., & Buchanan-Barker, P. (2007b). Words of wisdom. *Nursing Standard, 21*(37), 24-25.

Barker, P. J., & Jackson, S. (1997). No apologies for 'imperialist' view [Letter]. *Nursing Standard, 11*(20), 10.

Barker, P., Jackson, S., & Stevenson, C. (1999a). The need for psychiatric nursing: Toward a multidimensional theory of caring. *Nursing Inquiry, 6*, 103-111.

Barker, P. J., Jackson, S., & Stevenson, C. (1999b). What are psychiatric nurses needed for? Developing a theory of essential practice. *Journal of Psychiatric and Mental Health Nursing, 6*, 273-282.

Barker, P. J., Reynolds, W., & Stevenson, C. (1997). The human science basis of psychiatric nursing: Theory and practice. *Journal of Advanced Nursing, 25*, 660-667.

Barker, P. J., Reynolds, W., & Ward, T. (1995). The proper focus of nursing: A critique of the caring ideology. *International Journal of Nursing Studies, 32*(4), 386-397.

Barker, P. J., Stevenson, C., & Leamy, M. (2000). The philosophy of empowerment. *Mental Health Practice, 20*(9), 8-12.

Barker, P. J., & Walker, L. (2000). Nurses' perceptions of multidisciplinary teamwork in acute psychiatric settings. *Journal of Psychiatric and Mental Health Nursing, 7*, 539-546.

Barker, P. J., & Whitehill, I. (1997). The craft of care: Towards collaborative caring in psychiatric nursing. In S. Tilley, (Ed.). *The mental health nurse. Views of practice and education.* (pp. 15-27). Oxford: Blackwell Science.

Buchanan-Barker, P. (2004) The Tidal Model: Uncommon sense. *Mental Health Nursing, 24*(3), 6-10.

Buchanan-Barker, P., & Barker, P. (2005). The ten commitments: A value base for mental health recovery. *Journal of Psychosocial & Mental Health Nursing, 44*(9), 29-33.

Buchanan-Barker, P., & Barker, P. (2008). The Tidal Commitments: Extending the value base of mental health recovery. *Journal of Psychiatric and Mental Health Nursing, 15*, 93-100.

Collins, R, Maxwell, J, Lynch, J. (2004). Evaluation of the holistic nursing assessment of the Tidal Model. Retrieved April 11, 2009 from http://rms.ucd.ie/ufrs/W_RMS_CONFERENCE.POPUP_DETAILS?p_object_id=159734.

Cook, N., Phillips, B., & Sadler, D. (2005). The Tidal Model as experienced by patients and nurses in a regional forensic unit. *Journal of Psychiatric and Mental Health Nursing, 12*, 536-540.

De Shazer, S. (1994). *Words were originally magic.* New York: Norton.

Flannagan, J. C. (1954). The critical incident technique. *Psychological Bulletin, 51*, 327-358.

Fletcher, E., & Stevenson, C. (2001). Launching the Tidal Model in an adult mental health programme. *Nursing Standard, 15*(49), 33-36.

Glaser, B. G., & Strauss, A. L. (1967). The discovery of grounded theory: Strategies for qualitative research. Chicago: Aldine/Atherton.

Gordon, W., Morton, T., & Brooks, G. (2005). Launching the Tidal Model: Evaluating the evidence. *Journal of Psychiatric and Mental Health Nursing, 12*, 703-712.

Heron, J. (1996). *Cooperative inquiry: Research into the human condition.* London: Sage.

Illich, I. (1976). *Limits to medicine: Medical nemesis—The expropriation of health.* London: Marion Boyars.

Jackson, S., & Stevenson, C. (1998). The gift of time from the friendly professional. *Nursing Standard, 12*, 31-33.

Jackson, S., & Stevenson, C. (2000). What do people need psychiatric and mental health nurses for? *Journal of Advanced Nursing, 31*(2), 378-388.

Jackson, S., & Stevenson, C. (2004). How can nurses meet the needs of mental health clients. In D. Kirby, D. Hart, D. Cross, & G. Mitchell (Eds). *Mental health nursing—Competencies for practice* (Chapter 3, pp. 32-45). Hampshire, UK: Palgrave MacMillan.

Jonsson, B. (2005). *Ten thoughts about time.* London: Constable and Robinson.

Lafferty, S., & Davidson, R. (2006). Putting the person first. *Mental Health Today,* (March), 31-33.

McAllister, M. (2003). Doing practice differently: Solution-focused nursing. *Journal of Advanced Nursing, 41*(6), 528-535.

Michael, S. P. (1994). Invisible skills: How recognition and value need to be given to the 'invisible skills' frequently used by mental health nurses, but often unrecognized by those unfamiliar with mental health nursing. *Journal of Psychiatric and Mental Health Nursing, 1*, 56-57.

Miller, J. (Ed.). (1983). Objections to psychiatry: Dialogue with Thomas Szasz. In J. Miller (Ed). *States of mind: Conversations with psychological investigators.* London: British Broadcasting Corporation.

Montgomery, C., & Webster, D. (1993). Caring and nursing's metaparadigm: Can they survive the era of managed care. *Perspectives in Psychiatric Care, 29*(4), 5-12.

Morita, M., Kondo, A., Levine, P., & Morita, S. (1998). *Morita Therapy and the true nature of anxiety-based disorders (Shinkeishitsu).* Princeton, NJ: University of New York Press.

Peplau, H. E. (1952). *Interpersonal relations in nursing.* New York: Putman (reissued 1988. London: MacMillan.)

Peplau, H. E. (1969). Theory: The professional dimension. In C. M. Norris (Ed.). *Proceedings of the first nursing theory conference* (pp. 33-46). Kansas City, KS: University of Kansas University.

Peplau, H. (1987). Interpersonal constructs for nursing practice. *Nurse Education Today, 7*, 201-208.

Podvoll, E. M. (1990). *The seduction of madness: Revolutionary insights into the world of psychosis and a compassionate approach to recovery at home.* New York, NY: Harper Collins Publishers.

Registered Nurses' Association of Ontario. (2006). *Best practice guideline: Client-Centred Care.* Toronto: Author.

Stevenson, C. (1996). The Tao, social constructivism and psychiatric nursing practice and research. *Journal of Psychiatric and Mental Health Nursing, 3*, 217-224.

Stevenson, C., Barker, P., & Fletcher, E. (2002). Judgement days: Developing an evaluation for an innovative nursing model. *Journal of Psychiatric and Mental Health Nursing, 9*, 271-276.

Stevenson, C., & Fletcher, E. (2002). The Tidal Model: The questions answered. *Mental Health Practice, 5*(8), 29-38.

Stevenson, C., Jackson, S., & Barker, P. (2003). Finding solutions through empowerment: A preliminary study of a solution-oriented approach to nursing in acute psychiatric settings. *Journal of Psychiatric and Mental Health Nursing, 10*, 688-696.

Szasz, T. S. (1961). *The myth of mental illness: Foundations of a theory of personal conduct.* New York: Hoeber-Harper

Szasz, T. S. (2000). The case against psychiatric power. In. P. J. Barker & C. (Eds.). *The construction of power and authority in psychiatry.* Oxford: Butterworth Heinemann.

Travelbee, J. (1969). *Intervention in psychiatric nursing: Process in the one-to-one relationship.* Philadelphia: F. A. Davis Company.

Vicenzi, A. E. (1994). Chaos theory and some nursing considerations. *Nursing Science Quarterly, 7,* 32-44.

World Health Organization. (1986). *The Ottawa charter for health promotion.* Geneva; Author.

Yeats, W. B. (1928). *The tower.* New York: Macmillan.

BIBLIOGRAPHY

Primary Sources

Books

Barker, P. J. (1985). Patient assessment in psychiatric nursing. London: Croom Helm

Barker, P. J. (1997). Assessment in psychiatric and mental health nursing: In search of the whole person. Cheltenham: Stanley Thornes.

Barker, P. J. (1999). The philosophy and practice of psychiatric and mental health nursing. Edinburgh: Churchill Livingstone.

Barker, P. J. (1999). The talking cures: A guide to the psychotherapies for health care professionals. London: NT Books.

Barker, P. (2000). Qualitative research in nursing and health care. Nursing Times Clinical Monographs (No 13). London: NT Books.

Barker, P. J. (2000). The Tidal Model: Theory and practice. Newcastle: University of Newcastle.

Barker, P. J. (2003). Psychiatric and mental health nursing: The craft of caring. London: Arnold.

Barker, P. J. (2004). Assessment in psychiatric and mental health nursing: In search of the whole person (2nd Edition). London: Nelson-Thornes.

Barker, P. J., & Baldwin, S. (Eds.). (1991). Ethical issues in mental health. London: Croom Helm.

Barker, P. J., & Buchanan-Barker, P. (2004). Spirituality and mental health: Breakthrough. London: Whurr:

Barker, P. J., & Buchanan-Barker, P. (2005). The Tidal Model: A guide for mental health professionals. London: Brunner-Routledge.

Barker, P. J., Campbell, P., & Davidson, B. (1999). From the ashes of experience: The experience of recovery from psychosis. London: Whurr Publications.

Barker, P. J., & Davidson, B. (1998). Psychiatric nursing: Ethical strife. London: Edward Arnold.

Barker, P. J., & Kerr, B. (2001). The process of psychotherapy. Oxford: Butterworth-Heinemann.

Barker, P. J., & Stevenson, C. (1999). The construction of power and authority in psychiatry. Oxford: Butterworth-Heinemann.

Book Chapters

Barker, P. J. (1990). Cognitive therapy model: Principles and general applications. In W. Reynolds & D. F. S. Cormack (Eds.). Psychiatric and mental health nursing: Theory and practice. London: Chapman & Hall.

Barker, P. J. (1990). Professional stress. In D. F. S. Cormack (Ed.). Developing your career in nursing. London: Chapman & Hall.

Barker P. J. (1992). Professional and practice perspectives: Psychiatric nursing. In T. Butterworth & J. Faugier (Eds.). Clinical supervision and mentorship in nursing. London: Chapman & Hall.

Barker, P. J. (1992). Understanding people—Problems of development: Stress and distress. In H. Wright & M. Giddey (Eds.). Mental health nursing: From first Principles to professional practice (Chapter 11). London: Chapman & Hall.

Barker, P. J. (1993). Foreword. In D. Milne (Ed.). Psychology and mental health nursing. London: BPS Books.

Barker, P. J. (1996). The Interview. In D. F. S. Cormack (Ed.). The research process in nursing. 3rd Ed. Oxford: Blackwell Scientific Publications.

Barker, P. J. (1997). Counselling for behavioural change. In P. Burnard & I. Hulatt (Eds.). Nurses counseling: The view from the practitioners. Oxford: Butterworth-Heinemann.

Barker, P. J. (1998). Advanced practice in mental health nursing: developing the core. In G. Rolfe & P. Fulbrook (Eds.). Advanced nursing practice. Oxford: Butterworth Heinemann.

Barker, P. J. (1998). Depression. In M. Clinton & S. Nelson (Eds.). Advanced practice in mental health nursing. Oxford: Blackwell.

Barker, P. J. (1998). Psychiatric nursing. In A. C. Butterworth, J. Faugier, & P. Burnard (Eds.). Clinical supervision and mentorship in nursing. Cheltenham: Stanley Thornes.

Barker, P. J. (1999). History, truth and the politics of madness. In P. J. Barker & C. Stevenson (Eds.). The construction of power and authority in psychiatry. Oxford: Butterworth-Heinemann.

Barker, P. J. (1999). The construction of mind and madness: From Leonardo to the Hearing Voices Network. In P. J. Barker & C. Stevenson (Eds.). The construction of power and authority in psychiatry. Oxford: Butterworth-Heinemann.

Barker, P. J. (2001). Working with the metaphor of life and death. In D. Kirklin & R. Richardson (Eds.). Medical humanities: A practical introduction. London: Royal College of Physicians.

Barker, P. J. (2002). Realizing the promise of liaison mental health care. In S. Regel & D. Roberts (Eds.). Mental health liaison: A handbook for nurses and health professionals. London: Baillière Tindall.

Barker, P. J. (2004). Who cares any more, anyway? In S. Wilshaw (Ed.). Consultant nursing in mental health. Sussex: Kingsham Press.

Barker, P. (2008). Foreword in J. Morrissey, B. Keogh, & L. Doyle (Eds.). Psychiatric/mental health nursing—Concepts, application, challenges and reflections: An Irish perspective. Dublin: Gill & MacMillan.

Barker, P. J., & Baldwin, S. (1991). Change not adjustment: The ethics of psychotherapy. In: P. J. Barker & S. Baldwin (Eds.). Ethical issues in mental health. London: Chapman & Hall.

Barker, P. J., & Buchanan-Barker, P. (2004). Spirituality and mental health: An integrated dimension. In S. Ramon & J. Williams (Eds.). Mental health at the crossroads: The promise of the psychosocial approach. Sussex: Ashgate.

Barker, P. J., & Buchanan-Barker, P. (2006). The psychological impact of serious illness. In J. Cooper (Ed.). Stepping into palliative care 1: Relationships and responses. Oxford: Radcliffe Publishing.

Barker, P. J., & Buchanan-Barker, P. (2008). Patiently, telling the story. In T. Warne & S. McAndrew (Eds.). Creative approaches in health and social care education and practice: Knowing me, understanding you. Basingstoke, UK: Palgrave Macmillan.

Barker, P. J., & Buchanan-Barker, P. (2008). Spirituality and mental health. In T. Turner & R. Tumney (Eds.). Critical issues in mental health. Basingstoke, UK: Palgrave Macmillan.

Barker, P. J., & Buchanan-Barker, P. (2008). [tr m. Kayama]. The Tidal Model of Mental Health Recovery. In Kayama, Noda, Myamoto, & Ohyama (Eds.). Textbook of psychiatric nursing. Tokyo: Nankodo Co. (Japanese).

Barker, P. J., & Davidson, B. (1998). Epilogue: The heart of the ethical matter. In P. J. Barker & B. Davidson (Eds.). Psychiatric nursing: Ethical strife. London: Arnold.

Barker, P. J., Manos, E., Novak, V., & Reynolds, B. (1998). The wounded healer and the myth of mental well-being: Ethical issues concerning the mental health status of psychiatric nurses. In P. J. Barker & B. Davidson (Eds.). Psychiatric nursing: Ethical strife. London: Arnold.

Barker, P. J., & Whitehill, I. (1997). The craft of care: Towards collaborative caring in psychiatric nursing. In S. Tilley (Ed.). The mental health nurse: Views of practice and education. Oxford: Blackwell Science.

Stevenson, C., & Barker, P. J. (1996). Negotiating boundaries: Reconciling differences in mental health teamwork. In N. Cooper, C. Stevenson & G. Hale (Eds.). Integrating Perspectives on Health (pp. 47-56). Buckingham: Open University Press.

Published Papers

Barker, P. J. (1988). Reasoning about madness: the long search for the vanishing horizon (Part 2). *Community Psychiatric Nursing Journal, 8*(5), 14-19.

Barker, P. J. (1989). Reflections on the philosophy of caring in mental health. *International Journal of Nursing Studies, 26*(2), 131-141.

Barker, P. J. (1990). Needs and wants and fairy-tale wishes: A Scottish impression of care in the community. *Architecture and Comportment: Architecture and Behaviour, 6*(3), 233-244.

Barker, P. J. (1990). The conceptual basis of mental health nursing. *Nurse Education Today, 10*, 339-348

Barker, P. J. (1990). The philosophy of psychiatric nursing. *Nursing Standard 3*(12), 28-33.

Barker, P. J. (1990). Training to meet the new agenda. *Nursing Times, 86*(39), 71.

Barker, P. J. (1993). The Peplau Legacy . . . Hildegard Peplau. *Nursing Times, 89*(11), 48-51.

Barker, P. J. (1995). Seriously misguided. *Nursing Times 92*(34), 56-57.

Barker, P. J. (1996). Chaos and the way of Zen: Psychiatric nursing and the 'uncertainty principle.' *Journal of Psychiatric and Mental Health Nursing, 3*, 235-344.

Barker, P. J. (1996). The logic of experience: Developing appropriate care through effective collaboration. *Australian and New Zealand Journal of Mental Health Nursing, 5*, 3-12.

Barker, P. J. (1997). Towards a meta theory of psychiatric nursing. *Mental Health Practice, 1*(4), 18-21.

Barker, P. J. (1998). Creativity and psychic distress in writers, artists and scientists. *Journal of Psychiatric and Mental Health Nursing, 5*(2), 109-118.

Barker, P. J. (1998). Different approaches to family therapy. *Nursing Times, 94*(14), 60-62.

Barker, P. J. (1998). It's time to turn the tide. *Nursing Times, 18*(94), 70-72.

Barker, P. J. (1998). La Funcion Psicoterapeutica de la Enfermera en la Cuidado del Paciente Psicotico. *Avances en Salud Mental, 2*, 4-7.

Barker, P. J. (1998). Psychodynamic psychotherapy in nursing. *Nursing Times 94*(2), 54-56.

Barker, P. J. (1998). Sharpening the focus of mental health nursing: Primary health care. *Mental Health Practice, 1*(7), 14-15.

Barker, P. J. (1998). Solution-focused therapies. *Nursing Times, 94*(19), 53-55.

Barker, P. J. (1998). The behavioural psychotherapies. *Nursing Times, 94*(10), 44-46.

Barker, P. J. (1998). The future of Interpersonal Relations Theory: A personal reflection on Peplau's legacy. *Journal of Psychiatric and Mental Health Nursing, 5*(3), 213-220.

Barker, P. J. (1998). The humanistic therapies. *Nursing Times, 94*(6), 52-53.

Barker, P. J. (2000). Commentaries and reflections on mental health nursing in the UK at the dawn of the new millennium. *Journal of Mental Health, 9*(6), 617-619.

Barker, P. J. (2000). The Tidal Model of mental health care: Personal caring within the chaos paradigm. *Mental Health Care, 4*(2) 59-63.

Barker, P. J. (2000). The Tidal Model: The lived experience in person-centred mental health care. *Nursing Philosophy, 2*(3), 213-223.

Barker, P. J. (2000). The virtue of caring. *International Journal of Nursing Studies, 37*, 329-336.

Barker, P. J. (2000). Turning the tide. *Open Mind, 106* (Nov/Dec), 10-11.

Barker, P. J. (2000). Working with the metaphor of life and death. *Journal of Medical Ethics, 26*, 97-102.

Barker, P. J. (2001). Psychiatric caring. *Nursing Times, 97*(10), 38-39.

Barker, P. J. (2001). Response to Duncan-Grant. *Journal of Psychiatric and Mental Health Nursing, 8*, 180-183.

Barker, P. J. (2001). The ripples of knowledge and the boundaries of practice. *International Journal of Psychotherapy, 6*(1), 11-23.

Barker, P. J. (2001). The Tidal Model: Developing an empowering, person-centred approach to recovery within psychiatric and mental health nursing. *Journal of Psychiatric and Mental Health Nursing, 8*(3), 233-240.

Barker, P. J. (2001). The Tidal Model: Developing a person-centred approach to psychiatric and mental health nursing. *Perspectives in Psychiatric Care, 37*(3), 79-87.

Barker, P. J. (2002). Annie Altschul: An appreciation. *Journal of Psychiatric and Mental Health Nursing, 9*(2), 127-128.

Barker, P. J. (2002). Doing what needs to be done: A respectful response to Burnard and Grant. *Journal of Psychiatric and Mental Health Nursing, 9*, 232-236.

Barker, P. J. (2002). End of an era? *Mental Health Practice, 5*(5), 26-27.

Barker, P. J. (2002). Inspiration: My cousin Vinnie. Pendulum: *The Journal of the Manic Depression Fellowship, 18*(4), 11, 180-193.

Barker, P. J. (2002). The Tidal Model: The healing potential of metaphor within the patient's narrative. *Journal of Psychosocial Nursing and Mental Health Services, 40*(7), 42-50, 54-55.

Barker, P. J. (2002). Update: Acute care guidelines. *Openmind, 116*, July/Aug, 24.

Barker, P. J. (2003). Putting acute care in its place. *Mental Health Nursing, 23*(1), 12-15.

Barker, P. J. (2003). The Tidal Model: Psychiatric colonization, recovery and the paradigm shift in mental health care. *International Journal of Mental Health Nursing, 12*(2), 96-102.

Barker, P. J. (2004). Commentary: Mental health recovery and occupational therapy in Australia and New Zealand. *International Journal of Therapy and Rehabilitation, 11*(2) 70.

Barker, P. (2004). Uncommon sense: The Tidal Model of Mental Health Recovery: *The New Therapist, 33*, Sept/Oct, 14-19.

Barker, P. J. (2005). Missing pieces. *Nursing Standard, 19*(24), 26.

Barker, P. (2005). People make change happen. *Mental Health Practice, 8*(5), 10-11.

Barker, P. (2005). Voices. *Mental Health Practice, 9*(3), 46.

Barker, P. (2005). Voices. *Mental Health Practice, 8*(8), 46.

Barker, P. (2006). 30th anniversary on Crowe, M. (2000). Psychiatric Diagnosis: Some implications for mental health nursing care. *Journal of Advanced Nursing, 31*(3), 580-589. *Journal of Advanced Nursing, 53*, 132-133.

Barker, P. (2006). Book reviews. *Journal of Psychiatric and Mental Health Nursing, 13*, 468-472.

Barker, P. (2006). More harm than good. *Nursing Standard, 20*(30), 28-29.

Barker, P. (2006). Voices. *Mental Health Practice*, 9(8), 38.

Barker, P. (2006). Voices. *Mental Health Practice, 10*(4), 39.

Barker, P. (2007). Voices. *Mental Health Practice, 10*(10), 38.

Barker, P. J., & Baldwin, S. (1993). Speaking Out. *Nursing Times* Feb. 24th, *89*(8), 62.

Barker, P. J., Baldwin, S., & Ulas, M. (1989). Medical expansionism: some implications for psychiatric nursing practice. *Nurse Education Today, 9*, 192-202.

Barker, P. J., & Buchanan-Barker, P. (2001). Apologizing for our colonial past. *Openmind, 112*, (Nov/Dec), 10.

Barker, P. J., & Buchanan-Barker, P. J. (2003). Banning 'bonkers'. *Openmind, 124*, Nov/Dec, 26.

Barker, P. J., & Buchanan-Barker, P. (2003). Beyond empowerment: Revering the storyteller. *Mental Health Practice, 7*(5), 18-20.

Barker, P. J., & Buchanan-Barker, P. J. (2003). Death by assimilation. *Asylum, 13*(3), 10-13.

Barker, P. J., & Buchanan-Barker, P. J. (2003). Not so NICE guidelines. *Openmind, 121*, May/June, 14.

Barker, P. J., & Buchanan-Barker, P. (2003). Schizophrenia: The 'not-so-nice' guidelines [commentary]. *Journal of Psychiatric and Mental Health Nursing, 10*, 372-378.

Barker, P., & Buchanan-Barker, P. (2004). Beyond empowerment: Revering the storyteller. *Mental Health Practice, 7*(5), 18-20.

Barker, P., & Buchanan-Barker, P. (2004). Bridging: Talking meaningfully about the care of people at risk. *Mental Health Practice, 8*(3), 12-15.

Barker, P., & Buchanan-Barker, P. (2004). Caring as craft. *Nursing Standard, 19*(9), 17-18.

Barker, P., & Buchanan-Barker, P. (2004). Does the gold standard have feet of clay? *Mental Health Nursing, 23*(3), 9-11.

Barker, P., & Buchanan-Barker, P. (2004). Experts without a voice. *Nursing Standard, 18*(50), 22-23.

Barker, P., & Buchanan-Barker, P. (2004). Guidelines miss the reality of self harm. *Mental Health Nursing, 24*(6), 4-6.

Barker, P., & Buchanan-Barker, P. (2005). Still invisible after all these years: Mental health nursing on the margins. *Journal of Psychiatric and Mental Health Nursing, 12,* 252-256.

Barker, P., & Buchanan-Barker, P. (2006). More harm than good. *Nursing Standard, 20*(30), 28.

Barker, P., & Buchanan-Barker, P. (2006). Post-psychiatry: Good ideas, bad language and getting out of the box. *Journal of Psychiatric and Mental Health Nursing, 13,* 619-625.

Barker, P., & Buchanan-Barker, P. (2006). Staying in touch. *Nursing Standard, 21*(1), 16-18.

Barker, P., & Buchanan-Barker, P. (2007). Words of wisdom. *Nursing Standard, 21*(37), 24-25.

Barker, P., Buchanan-Barker, P., Freshwater, D., Stevenson, C., Fuagier, J., Wright, S., Rolfe, G. et al. (2005). Dear CNO . . . *Nursing Standard, 19*(30), 36-37.

Barker, P. J. & Cutcliffe, J. (1999). Clinical risk: A need for engagement not observation. *Mental Health Practice, 2*(8), 8-12.

Barker, P., & Cutcliffe, J. (2000). Creating a hopeline for suicidal people: A new model for acute sector mental health nursing. *Mental Health Care, 3*(4), 190-192.

Barker, P. J., Glenister, D., Jackson, S., Parkes, T., Parson, S., Ryan, D., Stevenson, C., Tilley, S., & Walker, L. (1998). End of the old pier show? *Mental Health Practice, 1*(7), 22.

Barker, P. J., & Jackson, S. (1996). No apology for 'imperialist' views. *Nursing Standard, 11*(20), 10.

Barker, P. J., & Jackson, S. (1997). Mental health nursing: making it a primary concern. *Nursing Standard, 11*(17), 39-41.

Barker, P. J., Jackson, S., & Stevenson, C. (1999). The need for psychiatric nursing: Towards a multidimensional theory of caring. *Nursing Inquiry, 6,* 103-111.

Barker, P. J., Jackson, S., & Stevenson, C. (1999). What are psychiatric nurses needed for? Developing a theory of essential nursing practice. *Journal of Psychiatric and Mental Health Nursing, 6*(4), 273-282.

Barker, P. J., Keady, J., Croom, S., Stevenson, C., Adams, T., & Reynolds, B. (1998). The concept of serious mental illness: Modern myths and grim realities. *Journal of Psychiatric and Mental Health Nursing, 5*(4), 247-254.

Barker, P. J., Leamy, M., & Stevenson, C. (2000). The philosophy of empowerment. *Mental Health Nursing, 20*(9), 8-12.

Barker, P. J., & Reynolds, W. (1994). A critique: Watson's caring ideology, the proper focus of psychiatric nursing. *Journal of Psychosocial Nursing and Mental Health Services, 32*(5), 17-22.

Barker, P. J., & Reynolds, B. (1996). Rediscovering the proper focus of nursing: a critique of Gournay's position on nursing theory and models. *Journal of Psychiatric and Mental Health Nursing, 3,* 75-80.

Barker, P. J., Reynolds, B., & Stevenson, C. (1998). The human science basis of psychiatric nursing: Theory and practice. *Perspectives in Psychiatric Care, 34,* 5-14.

Barker, P. J., Reynolds, B., Whitehill, I., Delaval, S., & Novak, V. (1996) Working with mental distress. *Nursing Times 92*(2), 25-27

Barker, P. J., & Stevenson, C. (2002). Reply to Gamble and Wellman. *Journal of Psychiatric and Mental Health Nursing, 9*(6), 743-745.

Barker, P. J., & Walker, L. (2000). Nurses' perceptions of multidisciplinary teamwork in acute psychiatric settings. *Journal of Psychiatric and Mental Health Nursing, 7,* 539-546.

Barker, P. J., Walker, L., & Pearson, P. (1998). Extending the role of the community mental health nurse. *British Journal of Community Nursing, 3*(10), 496-500.

Buchanan-Barker, P., & Barker, P. J. (2002). Lunatic language. *Openmind, 115,* 23.

Buchanan-Barker, P. J., & Barker, P. J. (2003). NICE: Does the gold standard have feet of clay? *Mental Health Nursing, 23,* 9-11.

Buchanan-Barker, P. J., & Barker, P. J. (2004). More than a feeling. *Nursing Standard, 19*(11), 18-19.

Buchanan-Barker, P. J., & Barker, P. (2005). Observation: The original sin of mental health nursing? *Journal of Psychiatric and Mental Health Nursing, 12,* 541-549.

Buchanan-Barker, P. J., & Barker, P. J. (2008). The Tidal Commitments: Extending the value base of mental health recovery. *Journal of Psychiatric and Mental Health Nursing, 15,* 93-100.

Cutcliffe, J., & Barker, P. J. (2002). Considering the care of the suicidal client and the case for 'engagement and inspiring hope' or 'observations'. *Journal of Psychiatric and Mental Health Nursing, 9*(5), 611-621.

Higgins, A., Barker, P. J., & Begley, C. M. (2005). Neuroleptic medication and sexuality: The forgotten aspect of education and care. *Journal of Psychiatric and Mental Health Nursing, 12,* 439-446.

Higgins, A., Barker, P. J., & Begley, C. M. (2006). Iatrogenic sexual dysfunction and the protective withholding of information: In whose interest? *Journal of Psychiatric and Mental Health Nursing, 13,* 437-446.

Higgins, A., Barker, P. J., & Begley, C. M. (2006). Sexual health education for people with mental problems: What can we learn from the literature? *Journal of Psychiatric and Mental Health Nursing, 13,* 687-297.

Higgins, A., Barker, P. J., & Begley, C. M. (2006). Sexuality and the challenge to espoused holistic care. *International Journal of Nursing Practice, 12*(6), 345-351.

Parsons, S., & Barker, P. J. (2001). The Phil Hearne Course: An evaluation of a multidisciplinary mental health education programme. *Journal of Psychiatric and Mental Health Nursing, 7*(2), 101-108.

Simpson, A., & Barker, P. J. (2007). The persistence of memory: Using narrative picturing to co-operatively explore life stories in qualitative inquiry. *Nursing Inquiry, 14*(1), 35-41.

Stevenson, C., Barker, P. J., & Fletcher, E. (2002). Judgement days: Developing an evaluation for an innovative nursing model. *Journal of Psychiatric and Mental Health Nursing, 9*(3), 271-276.

Stevenson, C., Jackson, S., & Barker, P. (2003). Finding solutions through empowerment: A preliminary study of a solution-oriented approach to nursing in acute psychiatric settings. *Journal of Psychiatric and Mental Health Nursing, 10*(6), 688-696.

Walker, L., & Barker, P. J. (1998). The required role of the CPN: Uniformity or flexibility? *Clinical Effectiveness in Nursing, 2*, 21-29.

Wilkin, P., & Barker, P. (2002). A conversation with Phil Barker. Sacred Space: *International Journal of Spirituality and Health, 3*(4), 15-23.

Dissertation

Barker, P. J. (1987). An evaluation of specific nursing interventions in the management of patients suffering from manic depressive psychosis. Unpublished PhD thesis. Dundee Institute of Technology (University of Abertay), Scotland.

Secondary References

Adam, R., Tilley, S., & Pollock, L. (2003). Person first: What people with enduring mental disorders value about community psychiatric nurses and CPN services. *Journal of Psychiatric and Mental Health Nursing, 10*, 203-212.

Allott, P., Loganathan, L., & Fulford, K. W. M. (2002). Discovering hope for recovery. *Canadian Journal of Community Mental Health, 21*(2), 13-34.

Anthony, P., & Crawford, P. (2000). Service user involvement in care planning: The mental health nurse's perspective. *Journal of Psychiatric and Mental Health Nursing, 7*, 425-434.

Barry, K. J. (2007). Collective inquiry: Understanding the essence of best practice construction in mental health. *Journal of Psychiatric and Mental Health Nursing, 14*, 558-565.

Beech, P., & Norman, I. J. (1995). Patients' perceptions of the quality of psychiatric nursing care: Findings from a small study. *Journal of Clinical Nursing, 4*, 117-123.

Brookes, N. L. (2006). The Tidal Model of Mental Health Recovery. In A. M. Tomey & M. R. Alligood (Eds.). *Nurse theorists and their work*, 6th Edition (Chapter 32, pp. 696-725). St. Louis: Mosby.

Brookes, N., Tansey, M., & Murata, L. (2006). Guiding practice development using the Tidal commitments. *Journal of Psychiatric and Mental Health Nursing, 13*, 460-463.

Buchanan-Barker, P. (2004). The Tidal Model: Uncommon sense. *Mental Health Nursing, 24*(3), 6-10.

Burnard, P. (2002). Not waving but drowning: A personal response to Barker and Grant. *Journal of Psychiatric and Mental Health Nursing, 9*, 221-232.

Bowles, A. (2000). Therapeutic nursing care in acute psychiatric wards: Engagement over control. *Journal of Psychiatric and Mental Health Nursing, 7*, 179-184.

Cameron, D., Kapur, R., & Campbell, P. (2005). Releasing the therapeutic potential of the psychiatric nurse: A human relations perspective of the nurse-patient relationship. *Journal of Psychiatric and Mental Health Nursing, 12*, 64-74.

Casey, B., & Long, A. (2003). Meanings of madness: A literature review. *Journal of Psychiatric and Mental Health Nursing, 10*, 89-99.

Cleary, M., Horsfall, J., & Hunt, G. (2003). Consumer feedback on nursing care and discharge planning. *Journal of Advanced Nursing, 42*(3), 269-277.

Collins, S., & Cutcliffe, J. (2003). Addressing hopelessness in people with suicidal ideation: Building upon the therapeutic relationship utilizing a cognitive behavioural approach. *Journal of Psychiatric and Mental Health Nursing, 10*, 175-185.

Cutcliffe, J. R., Black, C., Hanson, E., & Goward, P. (2001). The commonality and synchronicity of mental health nurses and palliative care nurses: Closer than you think? Part one. *Journal of Psychiatric and Mental Health Nursing, 8*, 53-59.

Cutcliffe, J. R., Black, C., Hanson, E., & Goward, P. (2001). The commonality and synchronicity of mental health nurses and palliative care nurses: Closer than you think? Part two. *Journal of Psychiatric and Mental Health Nursing, 8*, 61-66.

Cutcliffe, J. R., & Goward, P. (2000). Mental health nurses and qualitative research methods: A mutual attraction? *Journal of Advanced Nursing, 31*(3), 590-598.

Cutcliffe, J. R., & Grant, G. (2001). What are the principles and processes of inspiring hope in cognitively impaired older adults within a continuing care environment? *Journal of Psychiatric and Mental Health Nursing, 8*, 427-436.

Davidson, L. (2005). Recovery, self-management and the expert patient—Changing the culture of mental health from a UK perspective. *Journal of Mental Health, 14*(1), 25-35.

Deacon, M. (2003). Caring for people in the 'virtual ward:' *Journal of Psychiatric and Mental Health Nursing, 10*, 465-471.

Dodds, P., & Bowles, N. (2001). Dismantling formal observation and refocusing nursing activity in acute inpatient psychiatry: A case study. *Journal of Psychiatric and Mental Health Nursing, 8,* 183-188.

Fiddler, M., Borglin, G., Galloway, A., Jackson, C., & Lovell, K. (2007). Developing a framework for admission and discharge: A nurse-led initiative within a mental health setting. *Journal of Psychiatric and Mental Health Nursing, 14,* 705-712.

Flood, C., Brennan, G., Bowers, L., Hamilton, B., Li-pang, M., & Oladapo, P. (2006). Reflections on the process of change on acute psychiatric wards during the City Nurse Project. *Journal of Psychiatric and Mental Health Nursing, 13,* 260-268.

Forchuk, C., Jewell, J., Tweedell, D., & Steinnagel, L. (2003). Reconnecting: The client experience of recovery from psychosis. *Perspectives in Psychiatric Care, 39*(4), 141-150.

Gamble, C., & Wellman, N. (2002). Judgement impossible. *Journal of Psychiatric and Mental Health Nursing, 9,* 741-742.

Grant, A. (2001). Knowing me knowing you: Towards a new relational politics in 21st century mental health nursing [commentary]. *Journal of Psychiatric and Mental Health Nursing, 8,* 269-275.

Grant, A. (2001). Psychiatric nursing and organizational power: Rescuing the hidden dynamic [commentary]. *Journal of Psychiatric and Mental Health Nursing, 8,* 173-177.

Grant, A. (2001). Rejoinder to Barker and Clarke. *Journal of Psychiatric and Mental Health Nursing, 8,* 463-465.

Hannigan, B., & Cutcliffe, J. (2002). Challenging contemporary mental health policy: Time to assuage the coercion? *Journal of Advanced Nursing, 37*(5), 477-484.

Harnett, P. J., & Greaney, A. M. (2008). Operationalizing autonomy: Solutions for mental health nursing practice. *Journal of Psychiatric and Mental Health Nursing, 15,* 2-9.

Hayne, Y. M. (2003). Experiencing psychiatric diagnosis: Client perspectives on being named mentally ill. *Journal of Psychiatric and Mental Health Nursing, 10,* 722-729.

Holst, H., & Severinsson, E. (2003). A study of collaboration inpatient treatment between the community psychiatric health services and a psychiatric hospital in Norway. *Journal of Psychiatric and Mental Health Nursing, 10,* 650-658.

Hopton, J. (1996). Reconceptualizing the theory-practice gap in mental health nursing. *Nurse Education Today, 16,* 227-232.

Hosany, Z., Wellman, N., & Lowe, T. (2007). Fostering a culture of engagement: A pilot study of the outcomes of training mental health nurses working in two UK acute admission units in brief solution-focused therapy techniques. *Journal of Psychiatric and Mental Health Nursing, 14,* 688-695.

Hostick, T., & McClelland, F. (2002). 'Partnership:' A cooperative inquiry between community mental health nurses and their clients. 2. The nurse-client relationship. *Journal of Psychiatric and Mental Health Nursing, 9,* 111-117.

Hummelvoll, J., & Severinsson, E. (2001). Coping with everyday reality: Mental health professionals' reflections on the care provided in an acute psychiatric ward. *Australian and New Zealand Journal of Mental Health Nursing, 10,* 156-166.

Hurley, J., & Linsley, P. (2007). Expanding roles within mental health legislation: An opportunity for professional growth or a missed opportunity. *Journal of Psychiatric and Mental Health Nursing, 14,* 535-541.

Jackson, S., & Stevenson, C. (1998). The gift of time from the friendly professional. *Nursing Standard, 12*(51), 31-33.

Jackson, S., & Stevenson, C. (2000). What do people need psychiatric and mental health nurses for? *Journal of Advanced Nursing, 31*(2), 378-388.

Jackson, S., & Stevenson, C. (2004). How can nurses meet the needs of mental health clients? In D. Kirby, D. Hart, D. Cross, & G. Mitchell (Eds.). *Mental health nursing—Competencies for practice* (Chapter 3, pp. 32-45). Hampshire, UK: Palgrave MacMillan.

Jones, A. (1996). The value of Peplau's theory for mental health nursing. *British Journal of Nursing, 5*(14), 877-881.

Keen, T. M. (2003). Post-psychiatry: paradigm shift or wishful thinking? A speculative review of future possibles for psychiatry. *Journal of Psychiatric and Mental Health Nursing, 10,* 29-37.

Kilkku, N., Munnukka, T., & Lehtinen, K. (2003). From information to knowledge: The meaning of information-giving to patients who had experienced first-episode psychosis. *Journal of Psychiatric and Mental Health Nursing, 10,* 57-64.

Kirby, D., Hart, D., Cross, D., & Mitchell, G. (Eds.). *Mental health nursing—Competencies for practice.* Hampshire, UK: Palgrave MacMillan.

Kitson, A. (2004). The state of the art and science of evidence-based nursing in UK and Europe. *Worldviews on Evidence-Based Nursing, 1*(1), 6-8.

Koivisto, K., Janhonen, S., & Vaisanen, L. (2003). Patients' experiences of psychosis in an inpatient setting. *Journal of Psychiatric and Mental Health Nursing, 10,* 221-229.

Lacey, D. (1993). Discovering theory from psychiatric nursing practice. *British Journal of Nursing, 2*(15), 763-766.

Lakeman, R. (1998). Beyond glass houses in the desert: A case for a mental health 'care' system. *Journal of Psychiatric and Mental Health Nursing, 5,* 324-328.

Mason, T., Lovell, A., & Coyle, D. (2008). Forensic psychiatric nursing: Skills and competencies: 1 role dimensions. *Journal of Psychiatric and Mental Health Nursing, 15,* 118-130.

McAllister, M. (2007). *Solution focused nursing: Rethinking practice.* Bassingstoke: Palgrave MacMillan.

McAllister, M., & Moyle, W. (2008). An exploration of mental health nursing models of care in a Queensland psychiatric hospital. *International Journal of Mental Health Nursing, 17,* 18-26.

McAllister, M., & Walsh, S. (2003). CARE: A framework for mental health practice. *Journal of Psychiatric and Mental Health Nursing, 10*, 39-48.

McCann, T., & Hemingway, S. (2003). Models of prescriptive authority for mental health nurse practitioners [Commentary]. *Journal of Psychiatric and Mental Health Nursing, 10*, 743-749.

Morita, M., Kondo, A., Levine, P., & Morita, S. (1998). *Morita Therapy and the true nature of anxiety-based disorders (Shinkeishitsu)*. Princeton NJ: University of New York Press.

Moyle, W. (2003). Nurse-patient relationship: Anatomy of expectations. *International Journal of Mental Health Nursing, 12*, 105-109.

Murata, L. (2005). The Tidal Model continues to make waves. Worth the change. *Mental Health Practice, 9*(8), 10.

Musker, M. (1997). Applying empowerment in mental health practice. *Nursing Standard, 11*(31), 45-47.

Newnes, C., Holmes, G., & Dunn, C. (Eds.). (2000). *This is madness. A critical look at psychiatry and the future of mental health services*. Ross-on-Wye: PCCS Books.

Noak, J. (2001). Do we need another model for mental health care? *Nursing Standard, 16*(8), 33-35.

O'Donovan, A. (2007). Patient-centred care in acute psychiatric admission units: Reality or rhetoric? *Journal of Psychiatric and Mental Health Nursing, 14*, 542-548.

Perraud, S., Delaney, K., Carlson-Sabelli, Johnson, M., Shepard, R., & Paun, O. (2006). Advanced practice psychiatric mental health nursing, finding our core: The therapeutic relationship in the 21st century. *Perspectives in Psychiatric Care, 42*, 215-226.

Repper, J. (2000). Adjusting the focus of mental health nursing: Incorporating service users' experiences of recovery. *Journal of Mental Health, 9*(6), 575-587.

Rolfe, G. (1999). What to do with psychiatric nursing [commentary]. *Journal of Psychiatric and Mental Health Nursing, 3*, 330-333.

Saunders, J. (1997). Walking a mile in their shoes . . . Symbolic interactionism for families living with severe mental illness. *Journal of Psychosocial Nursing, 35*(6), 8-13.

Stevenson, C., & Fletcher, E. (2002). The Tidal Model: The questions answered. *Mental Health Practice, 5*(8), 29-38.

Stickley, T. (2002). Counseling and mental health nursing: A qualitative study. *Journal of Psychiatric and Mental Health Nursing, 9*, 301-308.

Tee, S., Lathlean, J., Hebert, L., Coldham, T., East, B., & Johnson, T. (2007). User participation in mental health nurse decision-making: A co-operative inquiry. *Journal of Advanced Nursing, 60*, 135-145.

Tilley, S. (1995). Notes on narrative knowledge in psychiatric nursing. *Journal of Psychiatric and Mental Health Nursing, 2*, 217-226.

Tilley, S. (1999). Altschul's legacy in mediating British and American psychiatric nursing discourses: Common sense and the 'absence' of the accountable practitioner. *Journal of Psychiatric and Mental Health Nursing, 6*, 283-295.

Wand, T., & White, K. (2007). Progression of the mental health nurse practitioner role. *Journal of Psychiatric and Mental Health Nursing, 14*, 644-651.

Warne, T., & McAndrew, S. (2007). Passive patient or engaged expert? Using a Ptolemaic approach to enhance mental health nurse education and practice. *International Journal of Mental Health Nursing, 16*, 224-229.

Wilkin, P. (2006). In search of the True Self: A clinical journey through the vale of the soul. *Journal of Psychiatric and Mental Health Nursing, 13*, 12-18.

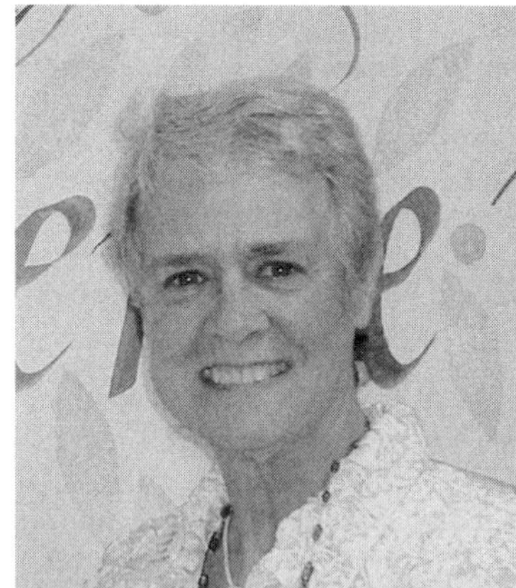
Photo credit: Barker's Camera Shop, Chagrin Falls, OH.

CHAPTER 33

Katharine Kolcaba

1944-present

Theory of Comfort

Thérèse Dowd

"In today's technological world nursing's historic mission of providing comfort to patients and family members is even more important. Comfort is an antidote to the stressors inherent in health care situations today, and when comfort is enhanced, patients and families are strengthened for the tasks ahead. In addition, nurses feel more satisfied with the care they are giving." K. Kolcaba (personal communication, March 7, 2008)

CREDENTIALS AND BACKGROUND OF THE THEORIST

Katharine Kolcaba was born and educated in Cleveland, Ohio. In 1965, she received a diploma in nursing and practiced part time for many years in medical-surgical nursing, long-term care, and home care before returning to school. In 1987, she graduated in the first R.N. to M.S.N. class at the Frances Payne Bolton School of Nursing, Case Western Reserve University (CWRU), with a specialty in gerontology. While in school, she jobshared in a head nurse position on a dementia unit. It was in the context of that experience that she began theorizing about the outcome of comfort.

After graduating with her master's degree in nursing, Kolcaba joined the faculty at The University of Akron College of Nursing. She acquired and maintains American Nurses Association (ANA) certification in gerontology. She returned to CWRU to pursue her doctorate in nursing on a part-time basis while continuing to teach. Over the next 10 years, she used course work in her doctoral program to develop and explicate her theory. She published a concept analysis of comfort with her philosopher-husband (Kolcaba & Kolcaba, 1991), diagrammed aspects of comfort (Kolcaba, 1991), operationalized

The author wishes to thank Katharine Kolcaba for her assistance with this chapter.

comfort as an outcome of care (Kolcaba, 1992a), contextualized comfort in a middle range theory (Kolcaba, 1994), and tested the theory in an intervention study (Kolcaba & Fox, 1999).

Currently, Kolcaba is an emeritus associate professor of nursing at The University of Akron College of Nursing, where she continues to teach nursing theory part time. Her areas of interest include interventions for and measurements of comfort for evidence-based practice. She continues to reside in the Cleveland area with her husband, where she enjoys being near her grandchildren and her mother. She represents her own company known as The Comfort Line, to assist healthcare agencies implement Comfort Theory on an institutional-wide basis. She is founder and coordinator of a local parish nurse program and a member of ANA and Sigma Theta Tau International. Kolcaba continues to work with students conducting comfort studies.

THEORETICAL SOURCES

Kolcaba began her theoretical work as she diagrammed her nursing practice early in her doctoral studies. When Kolcaba presented her framework for dementia care (Kolcaba, 1992b), a member of the audience asked, "Have you done a concept analysis of comfort?" Kolcaba replied that she had not but that would be her next step. That question began her long investigation into the concept of comfort.

The first step, the promised concept analysis, began with an extensive review of the literature about comfort from the disciplines of nursing, medicine, psychology, psychiatry, ergonomics, and English (specifically Shakespeare's use of comfort and the *Oxford English Dictionary* [OED]). From the OED, Kolcaba learned that the original definition of comfort was "to strengthen greatly." This definition provided a wonderful rationale for nurses to comfort patients since the patients would do better and the nurses would feel more satisfied.

Historical accounts of comfort in nursing are numerous. For example, Nightingale (1859) exhorted, "It must never be lost sight of what observation is for. It is not for the sake of piling up miscellaneous information or curious facts, but for the sake of saving life and increasing health and comfort" (p. 70).

From 1900 to 1929, comfort was the central goal of nursing and medicine because, through comfort, recovery was achieved (McIlveen & Morse, 1995). The nurse was duty bound to attend to details influencing patient comfort. Aikens (1908) proposed that nothing concerning the comfort of the patient was small enough to ignore. Comfort of the patient was the nurse's first and last consideration. A good nurse made patients comfortable, and the provision of comfort was a primary determining factor of a nurse's ability and character (Aikens, 1908).

Harmer (1926) stated that nursing care was concerned with providing a "general atmosphere of comfort," and that personal care of patients included attention to "happiness, comfort, and ease, physical and mental," in addition to "rest and sleep, nutrition, cleanliness, and elimination" (p. 26). Goodnow (1935) devoted a chapter in her book, *The Technique of Nursing*, to the patient's comfort. She wrote, "A nurse is judged always by her ability to make her patient comfortable. Comfort is both physical and mental, and a nurse's responsibility does not end with physical care" (p. 95). In textbooks dated 1904, 1914, and 1919, emotional comfort was called *mental comfort* and was achieved mostly by providing physical comfort and modifying the environment for patients (McIlveen & Morse, 1995).

In these examples, comfort is positive and achieved with the help of nurses and, in some cases, indicates improvement from a previous state or condition. Intuitively, comfort is associated with a nurturing activity. From its word origins, Kolcaba explicated its strengthening features, and from ergonomics, its direct link to job performance. However, often its meaning is implicit, hidden in context, and ambiguous. The concept varies semantically as a verb, noun, adjective, adverb, process, and outcome.

Three early nursing theorists' ideas were used by Kolcaba to synthesize or derive the types of comfort in the concept analysis (Kolcaba & Kolcaba, 1991). Relief was synthesized from the work of Orlando (1961), who posited that nurses relieved the needs expressed by patients. Ease was synthesized from the work of Henderson (1966), who described 13 basic functions of human beings to be maintained during care. Transcendence was derived from Paterson and Zderad (1975), who proposed that patients rise above their difficulties with the help of nurses.

Four contexts of comfort, as experienced by those receiving care, came from the review of nursing literature (Kolcaba, 2003). The contexts are physical, psychospiritual, sociocultural, and environmental. When these four contexts are juxtaposed with the three types of comfort, a taxonomic structure is created from which to consider the complexities of comfort as an outcome (Figure 33-1).

The taxonomic structure provides a map of the content domain of comfort. It is anticipated that future researchers will design instruments using the structure such as the questionnaire developed from the taxonomy for the end-of-life instrument (Novak, Kolcaba, Steiner, & Dowd, 2001). Kolcaba includes the steps for adapting the General Comfort Questionnaire on her website for future researchers.

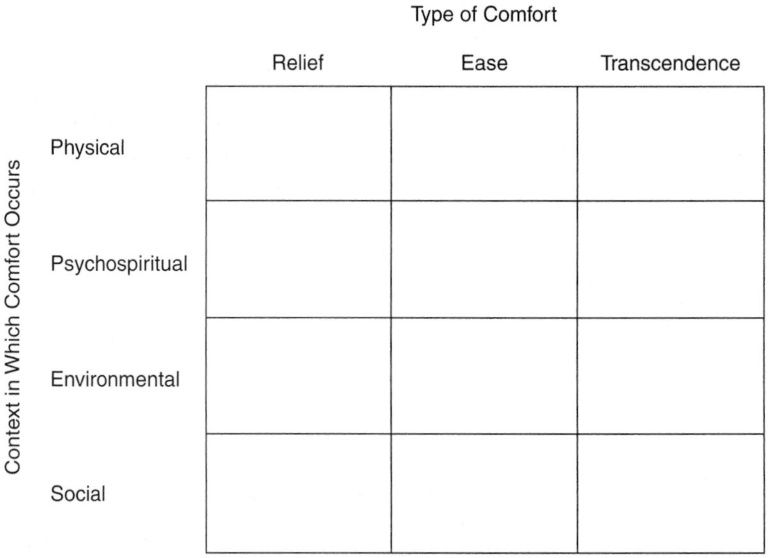

Type of Comfort

Context in Which Comfort Occurs	Relief	Ease	Transcendence
Physical			
Psychospiritual			
Environmental			
Social			

Type of Comfort:
Relief: The state of a patient who has had a specific need met
Ease: The state of calm or contentment
Transcendence: The state in which one rises above one's problems or pain

Context in Which Comfort Occurs:
Physical: Pertaining to bodily sensations
Psychospiritual: Pertaining to internal awareness of self, including esteem, concept, sexuality, and meaning in one's life; one's relationship to a higher order or being
Environmental: Pertaining to the external surroundings, conditions, and influences
Social: Pertaining to interpersonal, family, and societal relationships

Figure 33-1 Taxonomic structure of comfort. (From Kolcaba, K., & Fisher, E. [1996]. A holistic perspective on comfort care as an advance directive. *Critical Care Nursing Quarterly, 18*[4], 66-76.)

MAJOR CONCEPTS & DEFINITIONS

Those receiving comfort measures are referred to as recipients, patients, students, prisoners, workers, older adults, communities, and institutions in Kolcaba's theory.

HEALTH CARE NEEDS

Health care needs are needs for comfort arising from stressful health care situations that cannot be met by recipients' traditional support systems. These needs may be physical, psychospiritual, sociocultural, and environmental. The needs become apparent through monitoring, verbal or nonverbal reports, pathophysiological parameters, education and support, and financial counseling and intervention (Kolcaba, 1994).

COMFORT INTERVENTIONS

Comfort interventions are nursing actions designed to address specific comfort needs of recipients, including physiological, social, cultural, financial, psychological, spiritual, environmental, and physical interventions (Kolcaba, 2003).

INTERVENING VARIABLES

Intervening variables are interacting forces that influence recipients' perceptions of total comfort. They consist of past experiences, age, attitude, emotional state, support system, prognosis, finances, education, cultural background, and the totality of elements in the recipients' experience (Kolcaba, 1994).

COMFORT

Comfort is the state experienced by recipients of comfort interventions. It is the immediate and holistic experience of being strengthened when needs are addressed for three types of comfort (relief, ease, and transcendence) in four contexts (physical, psychospiritual, sociocultural, and environmental) (Kolcaba, 2003). Types and contexts are defined in Figure 33-1.

HEALTH-SEEKING BEHAVIORS

A broad category of outcomes related to the pursuit of health as defined by recipient(s) in consultation with the nurse Health-Seeking Behaviors (HSBs) was synthesized by Schlotfeldt (1975) and proposed to be internal, external, or a peaceful death.

INSTITUTIONAL INTEGRITY

Corporations, communities, schools, hospitals, regions, states, and countries that possess qualities of being complete, whole, sound, upright, appealing, ethical, and sincere. When an institution displays this type of integrity, it produces evidence for best practices and best policies (Kolcaba, 2001).

BEST PRACTICES

Use health care interventions based on evidence to produce best possible patient and family outcome.

BEST POLICIES

Institutional or regional policies ranging from protocols for procedures and medical conditions to access and delivery of health care. Figure 33-2 depicts the relationship of these last three concepts.

USE OF EMPIRICAL EVIDENCE

The seeds of modern inquiry about the outcome of comfort were sown in the late 1980s, marking a period of collective, but separate, awareness about the concept of holistic comfort. Hamilton (1989) made a leap forward by exploring the meaning of comfort from the patient's perspective. She used interviews to ascertain how each patient in a

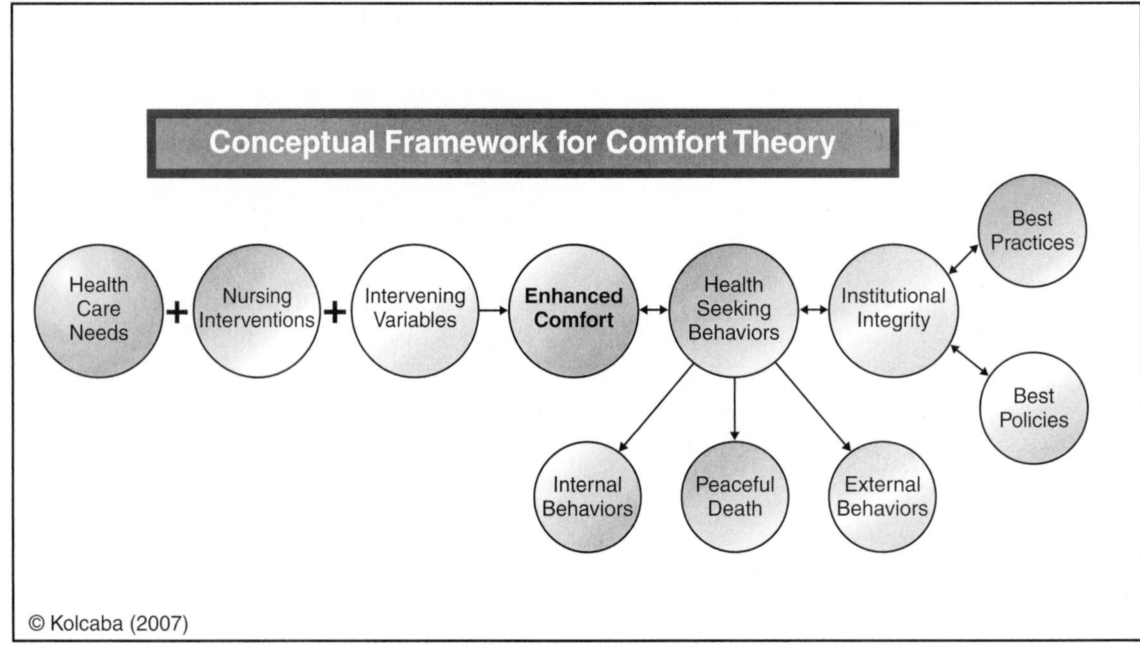

Figure 33-2 Conceptual Framework for Comfort Theory. (Copyright Kolcaba, 2007. Retrieved from www.thecomfortline.com, February 25, 2008.)

long-term care facility defined comfort. The theme that emerged most frequently was relief from pain, but patients also identified good position in well-fitting furniture and a feeling of being independent, encouraged, worthwhile, and useful. Hamilton (1989) concluded, "The clear message is that comfort is multi-dimensional, meaning different things to different people" (p. 32).

After Kolcaba developed her theory, she tested it using an experimental design in her dissertation (Kolcaba & Fox, 1999). In that study, health care needs were those (comfort needs) associated with a diagnosis of early breast cancer. The holistic intervention was guided imagery, designed specifically for this patient population to meet their comfort needs, and the desired outcome was their comfort. The findings revealed a significant difference in comfort over time between women receiving guided imagery and the usual care group (Kolcaba & Fox, 1999). Additional empirical testing of the Comfort Theory has been conducted by Kolcaba and associates. They are detailed in her book (Kolcaba, 2003, pp. 113-124) and cited on her website. These comfort studies demonstrated significant differences between treatment and comparison groups on comfort over time. The following interventions have been tested:

- Types of immobilization for persons after coronary angiography
- Cognitive strategies for persons with urinary frequency and incontinence
- Reducing stress in college students
- Hand massage for hospice patients and residents in long-term care (Kolcaba, Dowd, Steiner, & Mitzel, 2004)

In each study, interventions were targeted to all attributes of comfort relevant to the research settings, comfort instruments were adapted from the General Comfort Questionnaire (Kolcaba,

1997, 2003) using the taxonomic structure (TS) of comfort as a guide, and there were at least two measurement points, usually three, to capture change in comfort over time. The evidence for efficacy of hand massage as an intervention to enhance comfort is published in *Evidence-Based Nursing Care Guidelines: Medical-Surgical Interventions* (Kolcaba & Mitzel, 2008).

Further support for the Theory of Comfort has been found in a study of the following four major theoretical propositions about the nature of holistic comfort (Kolcaba & Steiner, 2000):

1. Comfort is generally state specific.
2. The outcome of comfort is sensitive to changes over time.
3. Any consistently applied holistic nursing intervention with an established history for effectiveness enhances comfort over time.
4. Total comfort is greater than the sum of its parts.

The results of tests with data from Kolcaba and Fox's (1999) earlier study of women with breast cancer supported each proposition. Other areas of study included in the Kolcaba website are burn units, labor and delivery, infertility, nursing homes, home care, chronic pain, pediatrics, oncology, dental hygiene, transport, prisons, deaf patients, and those with mental disabilities.

MAJOR ASSUMPTIONS

Metaparadigm Concepts

Nursing

Nursing is the intentional assessment of comfort needs, the design of comfort interventions to address those needs, and reassessment of comfort levels after implementation compared with a baseline. Assessment and reassessment may be intuitive or subjective or both, such as when a nurse asks if the patient is comfortable, or objective, such as in observations of wound healing, changes in laboratory values, or changes in behavior. Assessment is achieved through the administration of verbal rating scales (clinical) or comfort questionnaires (research), using instruments developed by Kolcaba (2003).

Patient

Recipients of care may be individuals, families, institutions, or communities in need of health care. Nurses may be recipients of enhanced work-place comfort when initiatives to improve working conditions are undertaken, such as those to gain Magnet Status (Kolcaba, Tilton, & Drouin, 2006).

Environment

The environment is any aspect of patient, family, or institutional settings that can be manipulated by nurse(s), loved one(s), or the institution to enhance comfort.

Health

Health is optimal functioning of a patient, family, health care provider, or community as defined by the patient or group.

Assumptions

1. Human beings have holistic responses to complex stimuli (Kolcaba, 1994).
2. Comfort is a desirable holistic outcome that is germane to the discipline of nursing (Kolcaba, 1994).
3. Comfort is a basic human need which persons strive to meet or have met. It is an active endeavor (Kolcaba, 1994).
4. Enhanced comfort strengthens patients to engage in health-seeking behaviors (HSBs) of their choice (Kolcaba & Kolcaba, 1991).
5. Patients who are empowered to actively engage in HSBs are satisfied with their health care (Kolcaba, 1997, 2001).
6. Institutional integrity is based on a value system oriented to the recipients of care (Kolcaba, 1997, 2001). Of equal importance is an orientation to a health promoting, holistic setting for families and providers of care.

THEORETICAL ASSERTIONS

The Theory of Comfort contains three parts (assertions) to be tested separately or as a whole.

Part I states that comforting interventions, when effective, result in increased comfort for recipients (patients and families), compared to a pre-intervention baseline. Care providers may also be considered recipients if the institution makes a commitment to the comfort of their work setting. Comfort interventions address basic human needs, such as rest, homeostasis, therapeutic communication, and treatment as holistic beings. These comfort interventions are usually non-technical and complement delivery of technical care.

Part II states that increased comfort of recipients of care results in increased engagement in health-seeking behaviors (HSBs) that are negotiated with the recipients.

Part III states that increased engagement in HSBs results in increased quality of care, benefiting the institution and its ability to gather evidence for best practices and best policies.

Kolcaba believes that nurses want to practice comforting care and that it can be easily incorporated with every nursing action. She proposes that this type of comfort practice promotes greater nurse creativity and satisfaction, as well as high patient satisfaction. In order to enhance comfort, the nurse must deliver the appropriate intervention in a caring manner. However, when the appropriate intervention is delivered in an intentional and comforting manner, comfort still may not be enhanced sufficiently. When comfort is not yet enhanced to its fullest, nurses then consider intervening variables to explain why comfort management did not work. Such variables may be abusive homes, lack of financial resources, devastating diagnoses, or cognitive impairments that render the most appropriate interventions and comforting actions ineffective. Comfort management or comforting care includes interventions, comforting actions, the goal of enhanced comfort, and the selection of appropriate HSBs by patients, families, and their nurses. Thus, comfort management is proposed to be proactive, energized, intentional, and longed for by recipients of care in all settings.

LOGICAL FORM

Kolcaba (2003) used the following three types of logical reasoning: (1) induction, (2) deduction, and (3) retroduction (Bishop & Hardin, 2006) in the development of the Theory of Comfort.

Induction

Induction occurs when generalizations are built from a number of specific observed instances (Bishop & Hardin, 2006). When nurses are earnest about their practice and earnest about nursing as a discipline, they become familiar with implicit or explicit concepts, terms, propositions, and assumptions that underpin their practice. Nurses in graduate school may be asked to diagram their practice (as Dr. Rosemary Ellis asked Kolcaba to do), and it is a deceptively easy-sounding assignment.

Such was the scenario during the late 1980s. Kolcaba was head nurse on an Alzheimer's unit at the time and knew some of the terms then used to describe the practice of dementia care, such as *facilitative environment, excess disabilities,* and *optimum function.* When she drew relationships among them, she recognized that these three terms did not fully describe her practice. An important nursing piece was missing, and she pondered about what nurses were doing to prevent excess disabilities (later naming those actions *interventions*) and how to judge if the interventions were working. Optimum function had been conceptualized as the ability to engage in special activities on the unit, such as setting the table, preparing a salad, or going to a program and sitting through it. These activities made the residents feel good about themselves, as if it were the right activity at the right time. These activities did not happen more than twice a day, because the residents couldn't tolerate much more than that. What were they doing in the meantime? What behaviors did the staff hope they would exhibit that would indicate an absence of excess disabilities? Should the term *excess disabilities* be delineated further for clarity?

Partial solutions to these questions were to (1) divide excess disabilities into physical and mental, (2) introduce the concept of comfort to the original diagram, because this word seemed to convey the desired state for patients when they were not engaging in special activities, and (3) note the non-recursive relationship between comfort and optimum functioning. These efforts marked the first steps toward a theory of comfort and thinking about the complexities of the concept (Kolcaba, 1992a).

Deduction

Deduction occurs when specific conclusions are inferred from more general premises or principles; it proceeds from the general to the specific (Bishop & Hardin, 2006). The deductive stage of theory development resulted in relating comfort to other concepts to produce a theory. The work of three nursing theorists was entailed in the definition of comfort; therefore Kolcaba looked elsewhere for the common ground needed to unify relief, ease, and transcendence (three major concepts). What was needed was a more abstract and general conceptual framework that was congruent with comfort and contained a manageable number of highly abstract constructs.

The work of psychologist Henry Murray (1938) met these criteria for a framework upon which to hang Kolcaba's nursing concepts. His theory was about human needs; therefore it was applicable to patients who experience multiple stimuli in stressful health care situations. Furthermore, Murray's idea about unitary trends gave Kolcaba the idea that, although comfort was state specific, if comforting interventions were implemented over time, the overall comfort of patients could be enhanced over time. In this deductive stage of theory development, she began with abstract, general theoretical construction and used the sociological process of substruction to identify the more specific (less abstract) levels of concepts for nursing practice.

Retroduction

Retroduction is useful for selecting phenomena that can be developed further and tested. This type of reasoning is applied in fields that have few available theories (Bishop & Hardin, 2006). Such was the case with outcomes research, which now is centered on collecting databases for measuring selected outcomes and relating those outcomes to types of nursing, medical, institutional, or community protocols. Murray's twentieth-century framework could not account for the twenty-first–century emphasis on institutional and community outcomes. Therefore using retroduction, Kolcaba added the concept of institutional integrity to the middle range Theory of Comfort. Adding that term to the Theory of Comfort extended the theory for consideration of relationships between HSBs and institutional integrity. In 2007, the concepts of *best practices* and *best policies* were linked to Institutional Integrity. Theory-based evidence organizes the knowledge base for best practices and policies (see Figure 33-2).

ACCEPTANCE BY THE NURSING COMMUNITY

Practice

This theory has been selected frequently by students and nurse researchers as a guiding frame for their studies in such areas as nurse midwifery (Schuiling & Sampselle, 1999), labor and delivery (Koehn, 2000), cardiac catheterization (Hogan-Miller, Rustad, Sendelbach, & Goldenberg, 1995), critical care (Jenny & Logon, 1996; Kolcaba & Fisher, 1996), hospice (Vendlinski & Kolcaba, 1997), infertility (Schoerner & Krysa, 1996), radiation therapy (Cox, 1998; Kolcaba & Fox, 1999), orthopedic nursing (Panno, Kolcaba, & Holder, 2000), perioperative nursing (Wilson & Kolcaba, 2004), hospitalized elderly (Robinson & Benton, 2002), urinary bladder control (Dowd, Kolcaba, & Steiner, 2000), and stressed college students (Dowd, Kolcaba, Steiner, & Fashinpaur, 2007).

For clinical practice, Kolcaba recommends asking patients or family members to rate their comfort from 0 to 10, with 10 being the highest possible comfort in their situation. This verbal rating scale is sensitive to changes in comfort over time (Dowd, Kolcaba, Steiner, & Fashinpaur, 2007). This may be done along with pain assessment or for documentation purposes. A list of effective comforting interventions for each patient/family member should be readily available and communicated.

Comfort Theory has been incorporated by perianesthesia nurses into their Clinical Practice Guidelines for management of patient comfort. In this setting, comfort management specifies (1) assessing patients' comfort needs related to current surgery, chronic pain issues, and co-morbidities; (2) creating a comfort contract with patients prior to surgery, which specifies comfort interventions that are effective, comfort measurement that is understandable and efficient, and the type of post-surgical analgesia preferred; (3) facilitating comfortable positioning, body temperature, and other factors related to comfort during surgery; and (4) continuing with comfort management and measurement in the post-surgical period (Kolcaba & Wilson, 2002; Wilson & Kolcaba, 2004).

Education

Following the guidelines for teaching comfort in baccalaureate nursing programs, the Theory of Comfort was applied to the nursing care of patients receiving radiation therapy and reported by Cox (1998). The theory proved easy for student nurses to understand and apply and provided an effective method to assess and address holistic comfort needs in elders in an acute care setting. Comfort Theory is included in *Core Concepts in Advanced Nursing Practice* (Robinson & Kish, 2001). The theory is appropriate for students to use in any clinical setting, and its application can be facilitated by the use of Comfort Care Plans available on Kolcaba's website.

Recently, Goodwin, Sener, and Steiner (2007) utilized Comfort Theory as a teaching philosophy in a fast-track nursing education program for students who had baccalaureate degrees in other disciplines. The taxonomic structure and conceptual framework guided ways of being a comforting faculty member. The theory also provided ways for students to obtain *relief* from their heavy course work (by knowing where to find answers to their questions and clinical problems), to maintain *ease* with their curriculum (through trusting their faculty members), and to achieve *transcendence* from their stressors (with the use of self-comforting techniques). The authors anticipate "that this adaptation may assist students to transform into professional nurses who are comfortable and comforting in their roles and who are committed to the goal of lifelong learning" (p. 278).

Research

An entry in *The Encyclopedia of Nursing Research* speaks to the importance of measuring comfort as a nursing-sensitive outcome (Kolcaba, 1992a). Nurses can provide evidence to influence decision making at institutional, community, and legislative levels through comfort studies that demonstrate the effectiveness of holistic comforting care. Measurement of comfort in large hospital and home care data sets is essential to add to the literature on outcomes research (Kolcaba, 1997, 2001).

Using the taxonomic structure of comfort (see Figure 33-1) as a guide, Kolcaba (1992a) developed the General Comfort Questionnaire to measure holistic comfort in a sample of hospital and community participants. To do this, positive and negative items were generated for each cell in the grid. Twenty-four positive items and twenty-four negative items were compiled with a Likert-type format ranging from strongly agree to strongly disagree. Higher scores indicated higher comfort. At the end of the instrumentation study with 206 one-time participants from all types of units in two hospitals and 50 people from the community, the General Comfort Questionnaire demonstrated a Cronbach alpha of 0.88 (Kolcaba, 1992a).

Researchers are welcome to generate comfort questionnaires specific to their areas of research. The verbal rating scales and other traditionally formatted questionnaires may be downloaded from Kolcaba's website, where she responds to inquiries in an effort to enhance the use of her theory. In addition, instructions for the use of the questionnaires is available on her website. The popularity of the theory seems to be associated with universal recognition of comfort as a desirable outcome of nursing care for patients and their families.

Qualitative approaches have been used for research designed to describe comfort from the perspective of the outcome of holistic nursing strategies in the emergency room (Hawley, 2000), orthopedics (Santy, 2001), postsurgical areas (McCaffrey & Good, 2000), postpartum (Collins, McCoy, Sale, & Weber, 1994), critical care (Walters, 1994), and infertility (Schoerner & Krysa, 1996).

FURTHER DEVELOPMENT

Kolcaba has persisted in the development of her theory from the original conception as the root of her practice, to the concept analysis that provided taxonomic structure of comfort, to the development of ways to measure the concept, and currently in its use for practice, education, and research. She used a full array of approaches to build her theory.

The methodical development of the concept resulted in a strong, clearly organized, and logical theory that is readily applied in many settings for education, practice, and research. Kolcaba has developed templates for instrument development to facilitate measures of comfort in additional new settings. She provides comfort management templates for use in practice settings that have been useful to students and faculty members. Research outcomes have demonstrated the appropriateness of her theory for measuring whole-person changes that had been less effectively captured with other types of instruments, as was noted in studies of urinary incontinence (Dowd, Kolcaba, & Steiner, 2000; Dowd, Kolcaba, & Steiner, 2006).

The original theoretical assertion (Part 1) of the Theory of Comfort has stood up to empirical testing. When a comfort intervention is targeted to meet the holistic comfort needs of patients in specific health care situations, patients' comfort is enhanced over a baseline measurement. Furthermore, enhanced comfort has been correlated with engagement in HSBs (Schlotfeldt, 1975). Path analysis of comfort and HSB variables is planned for future studies.

Empirical tests of the theoretical assertions for the second and third parts of Theory of Comfort should be conducted. Outcomes for desirable HSBs could include increased functional status, faster progress during rehabilitation, faster healing, or peaceful death when appropriate. HSBs should be negotiated among the patient, family members, and care providers. Institutional outcomes might include decreased length of stay for hospitalized patients, smaller number of readmissions, and achievement of national awards such as Magnet Status or the Beacon Award. Kolcaba has consulted with hospital administrators who want to enhance quality of care. She views quality care as comforting actions delivered in an intentional manner in order to create an environment that leads to engagement in health-seeking behaviors.

Kolcaba postulates that intentional emphasis on and support for comfort management by an institution or community will increase patient/family satisfaction, because persons are healed, strengthened, and motivated to be healthier. An important proposition yet to be tested is that comfort management matters for recipients of care and for the viability of institutions. Extending the Theory of Comfort to the community is of current interest. It is well known that some communities are more comfortable to live in, grow old in, and go to school in than are others.

An area of interest for further development is the universal nature of comfort. Currently, the General Comfort Questionnaire has been translated into Taiwanese, Spanish, Iranian, Portuguese, and Italian (see Kolcaba website), and translation into Turkish is pending. Comfort of children has been accurately observed and documented in perioperative settings (personal communication, Nancy Laurelberry, February 16, 2008), and the use of Comfort Daisies by children who self-report (see website) was tested in a hospital setting (personal communication, Carrie Majka, February 28, 2008).

Comfort Theory has been included in electronic nursing classification systems such as NANDA

(2007-2008), NIC (2001), and NOC (2004). Kolcaba consults with hospitals to include comfort management in their documentation systems. Use of the Theory of Comfort has made significant contributions to nursing and practice and the discipline. Kolcaba has time and energy for developing and disseminating the theory through presentations, publications, and discussions since her retirement from full-time teaching.

CRITIQUE

Clarity

Some of the early articles such as the concept analysis (Kolcaba, 1991) may lack clarity but are consistent in terms of definitions, derivations, assumptions, and propositions. Clarity is much improved in the article explicating the theory and subsequent articles. Kolcaba applies the theory to specific practices using academic, but understandable, language. All research concepts are defined theoretically and operationally.

Simplicity

The Theory of Comfort is simple because it is basic to nursing care and the traditional mission of nursing. Its language and application are of low technology, but this does not preclude its use in highly technological settings. There are few variables in the theory, and selected variables may be used for research or educational projects. The main thrust of the theory is for nurses to return to a practice focused on holistic needs of patients inside or outside institutional walls. It is its simplicity that allows students and nurses to learn and practice the theory easily (Kolcaba, 1995; Panno et al., 2000).

Generality

Kolcaba's theory has been applied in numerous research settings, cultures, and age groups. The only limiting factor for its application is how well nurses and administrators value it to meet the comfort needs of patients. If nurses, institutions, and communities are committed to this type of nursing care, the Theory of Comfort enables efficient, individualized, holistic practice. The taxonomic structure of comfort facilitates researchers' development of comfort instruments for new settings (Kolcaba, 1991).

Empirical Precision

The first part of the theory, asserting that effective nursing interventions offered over time will demonstrate enhanced comfort, has been tested and supported with women with breast cancer (Kolcaba & Fox, 1999), persons with UI (Dowd et al., 2000), persons in hospice (Kolcaba, Dowd, Steiner, & Mitzel, 2004), and stressed college students (Dowd, Kolcaba, Steiner, & Fashinpaur, 2007). In the UI study, enhanced comfort was a strong predictor of increased HSBs, supporting the second part of the comfort theory. The comfort instruments have demonstrated strong psychometric properties, supporting the validity of these questionnaires as measures of comfort that reveal changes in comfort over time and support of the taxonomic structure (see website).

Derivable Consequences

The Theory of Comfort describes patient-centered practice and explains how to determine if comfort measures matter to patients, their health, and the viability of institutions. The theory predicts the benefit of effective comfort measures (interventions) for enhancing comfort and engagement in HSBs. The Theory of Comfort is dedicated to sustaining nursing by bringing the discipline back to its roots.

SUMMARY

From its inception, the Theory of Comfort has focused on what the discipline of nursing does for patients. As the theory has evolved, the definition that was derived from a concept analysis has expanded to include broader aspects of the patient such as cultural and spiritual, but the basic format remains the same. The development of the General Comfort Questionnaire was important to validate that the concept can be measured, and that it measures an outcome that is unique and separate from other outcomes of nursing care.

The concept has relevancy for practice and easily guides nurses in the planning and designing of nursing care in any setting. Its usefulness in education has been described as providing a framework that enables students to organize their assessments and plans of care and yet to learn about the art of nursing as well as the science. It is also useful for expert nurses in the delivery of care and as they explain what they do beyond the technical aspects of nursing.

In research, the theory provides a way to validate improvement in patient comfort after receiving comforting interventions. The concept of comfort accounts for that aspect of quality that the patient describes as "feeling better." Kolcaba has made consistent and persistent efforts to develop and expand the concept into all realms of nursing. Through her own thinking and in interaction with nurses and other person-oriented professionals, the concept has continually evolved into patient and nurse care techniques. Institutions have recognized the value of designing comfort environments for both their patients and their staff. Through Kolcaba's publications and Internet activities (see website), the Theory of Comfort is known worldwide.

Case Study

A 32-year-old African-American mother of three toddlers who is 28 weeks pregnant is admitted to the high-risk pregnancy unit with regular contractions. She is concerned because plans for her family are not finalized. She has many comfort needs that are diagrammed in Table 33-1. When nurses assess for comfort needs in any of their patients, they can use the taxonomic structure, or comfort grid, to identify and organize all known needs. Using the comfort grid (see Figure 33-1) as a mental guide, nurses can design interrelated comforting interventions that can be implemented in one or two nurse-patient-family interactions. For this case, some suggestions to individualize the types of comfort interventions that might be considered are presented in Table 33-2.

For clinical use, the nurse could ask the patient to rate her comfort before and after receiving the interventions on a scale from 0 to 10, with 10 being the highest level possible. To determine through research if a specific comforting intervention enhanced the comfort of a group of patients, a comfort questionnaire could be developed and administered, assessing each cell in the comfort grid (see Figure 33-1). A Likert-type scale with responses ranging from 1 to 6

Table 33-1 *Taxonomic Structure of Comfort Needs for Case Study*

Context of Comfort	Relief	Ease	Transcendence
Physical	Aching back Early strong contractions	Restlessness and anxiety	Patient thinking, "What will happen to my family and to my babies?"
Psychospiritual	Anxiety and tension	Uncertainty about prognosis	Need for emotional and spiritual support
Environmental	Roommate is a primigravida Room small, clean, and pleasant	Lack of privacy Phone in room Feeling of confinement with bed rest	Need for calm, familiar environmental elements and accessibility of distraction
Sociocultural	Absence of family and culturally sensitive care	Family not present Language barriers	Need for support from family or significant other Need for information, consultation

Table 33-2 Comfort Care Actions and Interventions

Type of Comfort Care Action or Intervention	Example
Standard comfort interventions	Vital signs
	Laboratory test results
	Patient assessment
	Medications and treatments
	Social worker
Coaching	Emotional support
	Reassurance
	Education
	Listening
	Clergy
Comfort food for the soul	Energy therapy such as healing touch if it is culturally acceptable
	Music therapy or guided imagery (patient's choice of music)
	Spending time
	Personal connections
	Reduction of environmental stimuli

would facilitate a total comfort score. Such a questionnaire could be given to the patient before and after the interventions are implemented to demonstrate the level of effectiveness for the comfort interventions.

CRITICAL THINKING *Activities*

1. If you were asked to diagram your practice, what concepts would you include as desirable outcomes? As intervening variables? Where is comfort in your diagram?
2. Does the Theory of Comfort offer a framework you could use in your nursing practice? Why or why not?
3. There is some evidence that comfort is a universal need. Can you identify a way to meet a comfort need for someone you cared for recently? Would this comfort intervention work in another culture? What is the context of that comfort need in the Taxonomic Structure? (see Figure 33-1).
4. How would you apply comfort theory in a community setting? What interventions could you use to enhance comfort in an aggregate group? How could you assess to see if your intervention was effective?
5. Identify an area of nursing practice for comfort research and explain why it is needed.
6. How might comfort theory influence policy change?

POINTS FOR *Further Study*

- Kolcaba, K. (1997). TheComfortLine.com. Retrieved February 25, 2007, from http://www.thecomfortline.com (the Kolcaba website).
- American Society of Perianesthesia Nurses, www.ASPAN.org, retrieved at http://www.aspan.org/PDFfiles/pain&comfort.pdf on 3/3/08.
- Kolcaba, K. (1991). A taxonomic structure for the concept comfort. Image: *The Journal of Nursing Scholarship, 23*(4), 237–240.

- Kolcaba, K. (2008). The theory of comfort. In S. J. Peterson & T. S. Brednow (Eds.), Middle range theories: Application to nursing research, 2nd edition (pp. 255-273). Philadelphia: Lippincott Williams & Wilkins.
- Kolcaba, K. (2006). Comfort (including definition, theory of comfort, relevance to nursing, review of comfort studies, and future directions.) In J. Fitzpatrick (Ed.), The encyclopedia of nursing research (2nd ed.). New York: Springer.

REFERENCES

Aikens, C. (1908). Making the patient comfortable. *The Canadian Nurse, 4*(9), 422-424.

Bishop, S. & Hardin, S. (2006). Logical reasoning. In A. Marriner Tomey & M. R. Alligood (Eds.), *Nursing theorists and their work* (6th ed., pp. 25-34). St. Louis: Mosby-Elsevier.

Collins, B. A., McCoy, S.A., Sale, S., & Weber, S. E. (1994). Descriptions of comfort by substance-using and no using postpartum women. *Journal of Obstetric, Gynecologic, and Neonatal Nursing, 23*(4), 293-300.

Cox, J. (1998). Assessing patient comfort in radiation therapy. *Radiation Therapist, 5*(2), 119-125.

Dowd, T., Kolcaba, K., & Steiner, R. (2000). Using cognitive strategies to enhance bladder control and comfort. *Holistic Nursing Practice, 14*(2), 91-103.

Dowd, T., Kolcaba, K., & Steiner, R. (2006). Development of an instrument to measure holistic client comfort as an outcome of healing touch. *Holistic Nursing Practice, 20*(3), 122-129.

Dowd, T., Kolcaba, K., Steiner, R., & Fashinpaur, D. (2007). Comparison of healing touch and coaching on stress and comfort in young college students. *Holistic Nursing Practice, 21*(4), 194-202.

Goodnow, M. (1935). *The technique of nursing* (p. 95). Philadelphia: W. B. Saunders.

Goodwin, M., Sener, I., & Steiner, S. (2007). A novel theory for nursing education: Holistic comfort. *Journal of Holistic Nursing,* 278-285.

Hamilton, J. (1989). Comfort and the hospitalized chronically ill. *Journal of Gerontological Nursing, 15*(4), 28-33.

Harmer, B. (1926). *Methods and principles of teaching the principles and practice of nursing,* (p. 26). New York: Macmillan.

Hawley, M. P. (2000). Nurse comforting strategies: Perceptions of emergency department patients. *Clinical Nursing Research, 9*(4), 441-459.

Henderson, V. (1966). *The nature of nursing.* New York: Macmillan.

Hogan-Miller, E., Rustad, D., Sendelbach, S., & Goldenberg, I. (1995). Effects of three methods of femoral site immobilization on bleeding and comfort after coronary angiogram. *American Journal of Critical Care, 4*(2), 143-148.

Jenny, J., & Logon, J. (1996). Caring and comfort metaphors used by patients in critical care. *Image: The Journal of Nursing Scholarship, 28*(4), 349-352.

Koehn, M. L. (2000). Alternative and complementary therapies for labor and birth: An application of Kolcaba's theory of holistic comfort. *Holistic Nursing Practice, 15*(1), 66-77.

Kolcaba, K. (1991). A taxonomic structure for the concept comfort. *Image: The Journal of Nursing Scholarship, 23*(4), 237-240.

Kolcaba, K. (1992a). Holistic comfort: Operationalizing the construct as a nurse-sensitive outcome. *ANS Advances in Nursing Science, 15*(1), 1-10.

Kolcaba, K. (1992b). The concept of comfort in an environmental framework. *Journal of Gerontological Nursing, 18*(6), 33-38.

Kolcaba, K. (1994). A theory of holistic comfort for nursing. *Journal of Advanced Nursing, 19,* 1178-1184.

Kolcaba, K. (1995). The art of comfort care. *Image: The Journal of Nursing Scholarship, 27*(4), 287-289.

Kolcaba, K. (1997). *TheComfortLine.com. Akron, OH: The University of Akron College of Nursing.*

Kolcaba, K. (2001). Evolution of the mid range theory of comfort for outcomes research. *Nursing Outlook, 49*(2), 86-92.

Kolcaba, K. (2003). *Comfort theory and practice: A vision for holistic health care and research* (pp. 113–124). New York: Springer.

Kolcaba, K., Dowd, T., Steiner, R., & Mitzel, A. (2004). Hand massage to enhance comfort for hospice patients. *Journal of Hospice and Palliative Care, 6*(2), 91-102.

Kolcaba, K., & Fisher, E. (1996). A holistic perspective on comfort care as an advance directive. *Critical Care Nursing Quarterly, 18*(4), 66-76.

Kolcaba, K., & Fox, C. (1999). The effects of guided imagery on comfort of women with early stage breast cancer undergoing radiation therapy. *Oncology Nursing Forum, 26*(1), 67-92.

Kolcaba, K., & Kolcaba, R. (1991). An analysis of the concept of comfort. *Journal of Advanced Nursing, 16,* 1301-1310.

Kolcaba, K., & Mitzel, A. (2008). Two chapters: Hand Massage; Simple Massage. In B. J. Ackley, G. B. Ladwig, B. A. Swan, & S. J. Tucker (Eds.), Evidence-*based nursing care guidelines: Medical-surgical interventions* (pp. 402-407, 504-508). Mosby.

Kolcaba, K., & Steiner, R. (2000). Empirical evidence for the nature of holistic comfort. *Journal of Holistic Nursing, 18*(1), 46–62.

Kolcaba, K., Tilton, C., & Drouin, C. (2006). Comfort Theory: A unifying framework to enhance the practice environment. *Journal of Nursing Administration, 36*(11), 538-544.

Kolcaba, K., & Wilson, L. (2002). The framework of comfort care for Perianesthesia Nursing. *Journal of Perianesthesia Nursing, 17*(2), 102-114. With post-test for 1.2 contact hours.

McCaffrey, R. G., & Good, M. (2000). The lived experience of listening to music while recovering from surgery. *Journal of Holistic Nursing, 18*(4), 378-390.

McIlveen, K., & Morse, J. (1995). The role of comfort in nursing care: 1900-1980. *Clinical Nursing Research, 4*(2), 127-148.

Murray, H. (1938). *Explorations in personality*. New York: Oxford Press.

NANDA: Herdman, T. H., Heath, C., Meyer, G., Scroggins, L., & Vassallo, B. (2007-2008). *Nursing Diagnoses: Definitions & Classification*. St. Louis: Mosby, 34.

NIC: Johnson, M., Bulechek, G., Dochterman, J., Maas, M., & Moorhead, S. (2001). *Nursing Diagnoses, Outcomes, & Interventions*. St. Louis: Mosby, 221.

Nightingale, F. (1859). *Notes on nursing*. London: Harrison, 70.

NOC: Moorhead, S., Johnson, M., & Mass, M. (2004). *Nursing Outcomes Classification*. St. Louis: Mosby, 228.

Novak, B., Kolcaba, K., Steiner, R., & Dowd, T. (2001). Instrumentation study for end-of-life comfort questionnaires. *American Journal of Palliative Care, 18*(3), 170-180.

Orlando, I. (1961). *The dynamic nurse-patient relationship: Function, process, and principles.* New York: Putnam.

Panno, J., Kolcaba, K., & Holder, C. (2000). Acute care for elders (ACE): A holistic model for geriatric orthopedic nursing care. *Journal of Orthopedic Nursing, 19*(6), 53-60.

Paterson, J., & Zderad, L. (1975). *Humanistic nursing* (2nd ed.). New York: National League for Nursing. [Reprinted in 1988.]

Robinson, D., & Kish, C. (2001). *Core concepts in advanced nursing practice.* St. Louis: Mosby.

Robinson, S., & Benton, G. (2002) Warmed blankets: An intervention to promote comfort for elderly hospitalized patients. *Geriatric Nursing, 23*(6), 320-323.

Santy, J. (2001). An investigation of the reality of nursing work with orthopedic patients. *Journal of Orthopedic Nursing, 5*(1), 22-29.

Schlotfeldt, R. (1975). The need for a conceptual framework. In P. Verhovic (Ed.), *Nursing research* (pp. 3-25). Boston: Little & Brown.

Schoerner, C., & Krysa, L. (1996). The comfort and discomfort of infertility. *Journal of Obstetrical, Gynecological, & Neonatal Nurses, 25*(2), 167-172.

Schuiling, K., & Sampselle, C. (1999). Comfort in labor and midwifery art. *Image: The Journal of Nursing Scholarship, 31*(1), 77-81.

Vendlinski, S., & Kolcaba, K. (1997). Comfort care: A framework for hospice nursing. *The American Journal of Hospice and Palliative Care, 14*(6), 271-276.

Walters, A. (1994). The comforting role in critical care nursing practice: A phenomenological interpretation. *International Journal of Nursing Studies, 31*(6), 607-616.

Wilson, L., & Kolcaba, K. (2004). Practical application of comfort theory in the perianesthesia setting (Invited article). *Journal of PeriAnesthesia Nursing, 19*(3), 164-173.

BIBLIOGRAPHY

Primary Sources

Book Chapters

Kolcaba, K. (2001). Holistic care: Is it feasible in today's health care environment? In H. Feldman (Ed.), *Nursing leaders speak out* (pp. 49–54). New York: Springer.

Kolcaba, K. (2001). Kolcaba's theory of comfort. In D. Robinson & C. Kish (Eds.), *Core concepts for advanced nursing practice* (pp. 418–422). St. Louis: Mosby.

Kolcaba, K. (2003). The theory of comfort. In S. J. Peterson & T. S. Brednow (Eds.), *Middle range theories: Application to nursing research* (pp. 255-273). Philadelphia: Lippincott Williams & Wilkins.

Kolcaba, K. (2006). Comfort (including definition, theory of comfort, relevance to nursing, review of comfort studies, and future directions.) In J. Fitzpatrick (Ed.), *The encyclopedia of nursing research* (2nd ed.). New York: Springer.

Journal Articles

Dowd, T., & Kolcaba, K. (2007). Two interventions to relieve stress in college students. *AHNA Beginnings*, Winter 2007.

Dowd, T., Kolcaba, K., & Steiner, R. (2003). The addition of coaching to cognitive strategies. *Journal of Ostomy and Wound Management, 30*(2), 90-99.

Dowd, T., Kolcaba, K., & Steiner, R. (2002). Correlations among six measures of bladder function. *Journal of Nursing Measurement, 10*(1), 27-38.

Fox, C., & Kolcaba, K. (1995). Unsafe practice: A lack of strategies for effective decision making. *Nurse Educator, 20*(5), 3-4.

Fox, C., & Kolcaba, K. (1996, Spring). Decision making in unsafe practice situations. *Revolution: The Journal of Nurse Empowerment, 6*(1/2), 68-69.

Kolcaba, K. (1987). Reaching optimum function is realistic goal for elderly (Letter to the editor). *Journal of Gerontological Nursing, 13*(12), 36.

Kolcaba, K. (1988). A framework for the nursing care of demented patients. *Mainlines, 9*(6), 12-13.

Kolcaba, K. (1995). Process and product of comfort care, merged in holistic nursing art. *Journal of Holistic Nursing, 13*(2), 117-131.

Kolcaba, K. (1995). The art of comfort care. *Image: The Journal of Nursing Scholarship, 27*, 293-295.

Kolcaba, K., & DiMarco, M. (2005). Comfort Theory and Its Application to Pediatric Nursing. *Pediatric Nursing, 31*(3), 187-194.

Kolcaba, K., & Dowd, T. (2000). Kegel exercises: Strengthening the weak pelvic floor muscles that cause urinary incontinence. *American Journal of Nursing, 100*(11), 59.

Kolcaba, K., & Kolcaba, R. (2003). Fiduciary decision-making using comfort care. *Philosophy in the Contemporary World, 10*(1), 81-86.

Kolcaba, K., & Miller, C. (1989). Geropharmacology: A nursing intervention. *Journal of Gerontological Nursing, 15*(5), 29-35.

Kolcaba, K., Panno, J., & Holder, C. (2000) Acute care for elders (ACE): A holistic model for geriatric orthopedic nursing care. *Journal of Orthopedic Nursing, 19*(6), 53-60.

Kolcaba, K., Schirm, V., & Steiner, R. (2006). Effects of Hand Massage on Comfort of Nursing Home Residents. *Geriatric Nursing, 27*(2), 85-91.

Kolcaba, K., & Wykle, M. (1996). Comfort research: Spreading comfort around the world. *Reflections: Sigma Theta Tau International, 23*(2), 12-13.

Schirm, V., Baumgardner, J., Dowd, T., Gregor, S., & Kolcaba, K. (2004). Development of a healthy bladder education program for older adults. *Geriatric Nursing, 25*(5), 301-306.

Wagner, D., Byrne, M., & Kolcaba, K. (2006). Effect of Comfort Warming on Preoperative Patients. *AORN Journal, 84*(3), 1-13.

Secondary Source

Book Chapter

Sitzman, K., & Eichelberger, L. (2004). *Understanding the work of nurse theorists: A creative beginning* (pp. 117-122). Sudbury, MA: Jones & Bartlett.

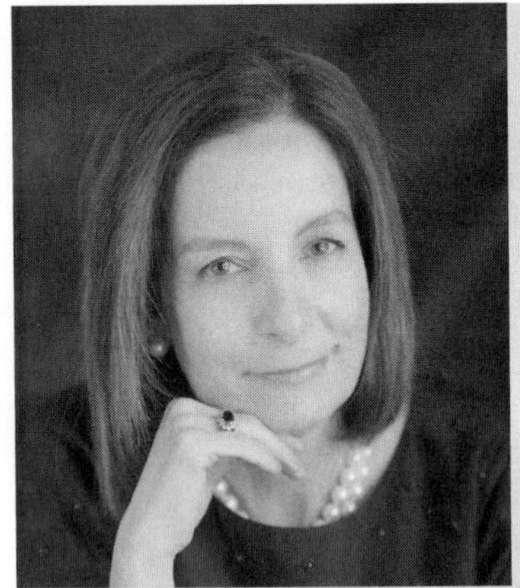

CHAPTER 34

Cheryl Tatano Beck

Postpartum Depression Theory

M. Katherine Maeve

"The birth of a baby is an occasion for joy—or so the saying goes . . . But for some women, joy is not an option." (Beck, 2006b, p. 40)

CREDENTIALS AND BACKGROUND OF THE THEORIST

Cheryl Tatano Beck graduated from the Western Connecticut State University with a baccalaureate in nursing in 1970. She recognized during her first clinical rotation that obstetrical nursing was to be her lifelong specialty. After graduation, Beck worked as a registered nurse at the Yale New Haven Hospital on the postpartum and normal newborn nursery unit. By 1972, Beck had graduated from Yale University with a master's degree in maternal-newborn nursing and a certificate in nurse midwifery. In 1982, she received a doctorate in nursing science from Boston University.

Beginning at the rank of instructor in 1973, Beck has held academic appointments with increasing rank at several major universities, including University of Maryland, University of Michigan, Florida Atlantic University, University of Rhode Island, and Yale University, and as professor at the University of Connecticut, where she holds a joint appointment in the School of Nursing and the School of Medicine. Beck has served as consultant on numerous research projects for universities and state agencies in the northeastern United States. During her career,

The author wishes to thank Dr. Cheryl Tatano Beck for her generosity of spirit in allowing me liberties with the interpretation of her life's work. Dr. Beck's work represents an enormous contribution to nursing, made even more remarkable because it did not depend on boatloads of NIH funding. That alone is an inspiration. Thanks are also extended to Dr. Peggy L. Chinn, who happily has not retired as a mentor or friend.

Beck has received more than 30 awards, including Distinguished Researcher of the Year from the Eastern Nursing Research Society in 1999. She was inducted as a fellow in the American Academy of Nursing in 1993.

A prolific author and disseminator of her research, Beck has authored more than 100 journal articles and given scores of research presentations locally, nationally, and internationally. She has served on the editorial boards of many nursing journals, including *Advances in Nursing Science, Nursing Research*, and the *Journal of Nursing Education.* Beck served on the executive board for the Marce Society, an international society for the understanding, prevention, and treatment of mental illness associated with childbirth, and on the advisory committee of the Donaghue Medical Research Foundation in Connecticut.

Beck has written several articles regarding statistical analysis strategies and approaches to qualitative analysis strategies. Many in nursing will recognize the classic Polit and Hungler research text, a fixture in countless graduate nursing programs. Beck became coauthor of Polit's seventh edition (Polit & Beck, 2003), reflecting Beck's research expertise.

Although Beck conducted seven major studies regarding educational and caring issues with undergraduate nursing students, for over three decades she has contributed to knowledge development in obstetrical nursing. Fittingly, her research career began by studying women in labor, examining their responses to fetal monitoring (Beck, 1980). Beck's research focus eventually became the postpartum period and specific studies of postpartum mood disorders.

This body of work has resulted in a substantive theory of postpartum depression (Beck, 1993) and the development of the Postpartum Depression Screening Scale (PDSS) (Beck, 2002c; Beck & Gable, 2000) and the Postpartum Depression Predictors Inventory (PDPI) (Beck, 1998, 2001, 2002b). A time line of Beck's research is outlined in Table 34-1, demonstrating the logical progression of her work.

THEORETICAL AND PHILOSOPHICAL SOURCES

Although Beck does not address caring as a theoretical or philosophical construct specific to her research, she has conducted several studies that evidence her belief that "caring is the essence of nursing" (Beck, 1999, p. 629). Beck's use of the ideas of Jean Watson with regard to caring theory endorses caring as central to nursing, while acknowledging Watson's concern that quantitative methodologies may not reflect adequately the ideal of transpersonal caring. It is obvious throughout Beck's writings, including research reports using both quantitative and qualitative methods, that advancing nursing as a caring profession is desirable and achievable in practice, research, and education.

Because many of the studies used to develop Beck's Postpartum Depression Theory were qualitative in nature, various theoretical sources have been cited by Beck reflecting the philosophical and theoretical roots of methodologies that were important for the kind of knowledge developed in each study. Phenomenology was used in the first major study of how women experienced postpartum depression, using Colaizzi's (1978) approach. In her next study, Beck used grounded theory as influenced by the theoretical and philosophical ideas of Glaser (1978), Glaser and Strauss (1967), and Hutchinson (1986). Throughout all of Beck's work and consistent with feminist theory, there is explicit valuing of the importance of understanding pregnancy, birth, and motherhood through "the eyes of women" (Beck, 2002a). Furthermore, Beck acknowledges that childbirth occurs in many simultaneous contexts (medical, social, economic), and that mothers' reactions to childbirth and motherhood are shaped by their responses to these contexts.

An unusual theoretical source came from the work of Sichel and Driscoll (1999), who developed an earthquake model to conceptualize how interactions between biology and life result in what they term *biochemical loading.* Over time, with constant chemical challenges related to stressors, women's brains may develop a kind of "fault line" that is less

Table 34-1 Time Line of Beck's Perinatal Research

Year	Focus of Research
1972	Women's cognitive and emotional responses to fetal monitoring (master's thesis)
1977	Replication of master's thesis
1982	Parturients' temporal experiences during labor (doctoral dissertation)
1985	Mothers' temporal experiences in postpartum period after vaginal and cesarean deliveries
1988	Postpartum temporal experiences of primiparas
1989	Incidence of maternity blues in primiparas and length of hospital stay
1990	Teetering on the edge: a grounded theory study of PPD
1992	The lived experience of PPD
1994	Nurses' caring with postpartum depressed mothers
1995	Screening methods for PPD
1995	PPD and maternal-infant interaction
1995	Mothers with PPD perceptions of nurses' caring
1996	The relationship between PPD and infant temperament
1996	Predictors of PPD meta-analysis
1996	Mothers with PPD and their experiences interacting with children
1996	Concept analysis of panic
1997	Developing research programs using qualitative and quantitative approaches
1998	Effects of PPD on child development
1998	Checklist to identify women at risk for PPD
1999	Maternal depression and child behavioral problems
2000	PDSS: development and psychometric testing
2001	Comparative analysis between PDSS and two other depression instruments
2001	Item response theory in affective instrument development
2001	Ensuring content validity
2002	PPD—metasynthesis
2002	Revision of PDPI
2002	Mothering multiples
2003	PPD in mothers of babies in NICU
2003	PDSS—Spanish version
2004	Birth trauma
2004	Posttraumatic stress disorder after childbirth
2004	Benefits of internet interviews
2005	DHA in pregnancy
2005	Birth trauma and breastfeeding
2005	Mapping birth trauma narratives
2007	PDSS-Internet
In progress	Subsequent childbirth after previous birth trauma
In progress	Mother's caring for child with brachial plexus injury
In progress	PDSS—telephone version

NICU, Neonatal intensive care unit; *PDPI*, Postpartum Depression Predictors Inventory; *PDSS*, Postpartum Depression Screening Scale; *PPD*, postpartum depression.

likely to remain intact during critical moments in women's lives, such as the challenges women face around childbirth, resulting in a kind of "earthquake." Beck understood Sichel and Driscoll's model to "suggest that a woman's genetic makeup, hormonal and reproductive history, and life experiences all combine to predict her risk of 'an earthquake' which occurs when her brain cannot stabilize and mood problems erupt" (Beck, 2001, p. 276). Although it is easy to understand the physiological and hormonal challenges of pregnancies for women, Sichel and Driscoll's earthquake model was important in helping Beck holistically conceptualize the phenomena that might affect the development of postpartum depression for women. Although Beck states that she never experienced postpartum depression after the birth of her own children, those who have may relate to the earthquake metaphor complete with tremors culminating in postpartum depression or, worse, postpartum psychosis.

Beck has identified Robert Gable as a particularly important source in her work. Now Professor Emeritus at the Neag School of Education, University of Connecticut, Gable coauthored an important text called *Instrument Development in the Affective Domain* (Gable & Wolf, 1993). After developing a wealth of knowledge about postpartum depression, the next logical steps for Beck became developing instruments that could predict and screen for postpartum depression. Gable assisted Beck with theoretical operationalization of her theory for practical use. Gable has remained directly involved through the step-by-step development of the PDSS, including the Spanish version (Beck & Gable, 2003).

MAJOR CONCEPTS & DEFINITIONS

Beck's major concepts have undergone refinement and clarification over years of work on postpartum depression. The first two concepts, postpartum mood disorders and loss of control, are conceptualizations that Beck developed utilizing phenomenology and grounded theory methods.

CONCEPTS 1 THROUGH 2

1. Postpartum Mood Disorders

Postpartum depression and maternity blues have become better delineated over time, as has the understanding of postpartum psychosis. Two other perinatal mood disorders, postpartum obsessive-compulsive disorder and postpartum-onset panic disorder, have been identified, as has how these disorders are different and how they are interrelated (Beck, 2002c).

Postpartum Depression. A non-psychotic major depressive disorder with distinguishing diagnostic criteria that often begins as early as 4 weeks after birth. It may also occur anytime within the first year after childbirth. Postpartum depression is not self-limiting and is more difficult to treat than simple depression. Prevalence rates are 13% to 25%, with more women affected who are poor, live in the inner city, or are adolescents. Approximately 50% of all women suffering from postpartum depression have episodes lasting 6 months or longer.

Maternity Blues. Also known as postpartum blues and baby blues, it is a relatively transient and self-limited period of melancholy and mood swings during the early postpartum period. Maternity blues affects up to 75% of all women in all cultures.

Postpartum Psychosis. A psychotic disorder characterized by hallucinations, delusions, agitation, and inability to sleep, along with bizarre and irrational behavior. Although postpartum psychosis is relatively rare (1 to 2 women per 1000 births), it represents a true psychiatric emergency because both mother and baby (and perhaps

Continued

MAJOR CONCEPTS & DEFINITIONS—cont'd

other children) are in grave danger of harm. Although postpartum psychosis often begins to appear during the first week postpartum, it is frequently not detected until serious harm has occurred.

Postpartum Obsessive-Compulsive Disorder. Only recently identified, the prevalence rates have not been reported. Symptoms include repetitive, intrusive thoughts of harming the baby, a fear of being left alone with the infant, and hypervigilance in protecting the infant.

Postpartum-Onset Panic Disorder. This disorder has been identified only recently and is also without reported prevalence rates. It is characterized by acute onset of anxiety, fear, rapid breathing, heart palpitations, and a sense of impending doom.

2. Loss of Control

It was identified as the basic psychosocial problem in the 1993 substantive theory of Beck's early work. This descriptive theory captured a process women go through with postpartum depression. Loss of control was experienced in all areas of women's lives, although the particulars of the circumstances may be different. The concept of loss of control fit with extant literature and left women with feelings of "teetering on the edge" (Beck, 1993). The process identified consisted of the following four stages:

1. Encountering terror: consisted of horrifying anxiety attacks, enveloping fogginess, and relentless obsessive thinking
2. Dying of self: consisted of alarming unrealness, contemplating and attempting self-destruction, isolating oneself
3. Struggling to survive: consisted of battling the system, seeking solace at support groups, and praying for relief
4. Regaining control: consisted of unpredictable transitioning, guarded recovery, and mourning lost time

CONCEPTS 3 THROUGH 9

The conceptual ideas and definitions described above were used to develop specific foci for testing. Initially, Beck (1998) identified eight risk factors for postpartum depression. Many studies have expanded areas where Beck determined that more conceptual clarity was needed. For example, through her own study and meta-analysis of other studies, infant temperament was identified as a separate risk factor and predictor for postpartum depression (Beck, 1996b).

Another important change is marriage. Through subsequent research, it was noted that there were two marital factors of concern: marital status and the nature of the marital relationship satisfaction (Beck, 2002b). Two other risk factors identified were socioeconomic status and issues of unplanned and unwanted pregnancies.

CONCEPTS 3 THROUGH 15

These are major concepts found to be significant predictors or risk factors for postpartum depression (Beck, 2002b). The most current interpretation of effect size was assigned from a meta-analysis of 138 extant studies and is at the end of each concept definition (Beck, 2002b).

3. Prenatal Depression

Depression during any or all of the trimesters of pregnancy has been found to be the strongest predictor of postpartum depression. (Effect size = Medium)

4. Child Care Stress

Stressful events related to childcare such as infant health problems and difficulty in infant care pertaining to feeding and sleeping. (Effect size = Medium)

MAJOR CONCEPTS & DEFINITIONS—cont'd

5. Life Stress

An index of stressful life events during pregnancy and postpartum. The number of life experiences and the amount of stress created by each of the life events are combined to determine the amount of life stress a woman is experiencing. Stressful life events can be either negative or positive and can include experiences such as the following:

- Marital changes (e.g., divorce, remarriage)
- Occupational changes (e.g., job change)
- Crises (e.g., accidents, burglaries, financial crises, illness requiring hospitalization)

(Effect size = Medium)

6. Social Support

Instrumental support (e.g., babysitting, help with household chores) and emotional support. Structural features of a woman's social network (husband or mate, family, and friends) include proximity of its members, frequency of contact, and number of confidants with whom the woman can share personal matters. Lack of social support is when a woman perceives she is not receiving the amount of instrumental or emotional support she expects. (Effect size = Medium)

7. Prenatal Anxiety

Occurs during any trimester or throughout the pregnancy. Anxiety refers to feelings of uneasiness or apprehension concerning a vague, nonspecific threat. (Effect size = Medium)

8. Marital Satisfaction

The degree of satisfaction with a marital relationship is assessed and includes how happy or satisfied the woman is with certain aspects of her marriage, such as communication, affection, similarity of values (e.g., finances, child care), mutual activity and decision making, and global well-being. (Effect size = Medium)

9. History of Depression

A report of having had a bout of depression before this pregnancy. (Effect size = Medium)

10. Infant Temperament

The infant's disposition and personality. Difficult temperament describes an infant who is irritable, fussy, unpredictable, and difficult to console. (Effect size = Medium)

11. Maternity Blues

Previously defined as a non-pathological condition after giving birth. Prolonged episodes of maternity blues (lasting more than 10 days) may predict postpartum depression. (Effect size = Small to medium)

12. Self-Esteem

A woman's global feelings of self-worth and self-acceptance. It is her confidence and satisfaction in self. Low self-esteem reflects a negative self-evaluation and feelings about oneself or one's capabilities. (Effect size = Medium)

13. Socioeconomic Status

A person's rank or status in society involving a combination of social and economic factors such as income, education, and occupation. (Effect size = Small)

14. Marital Status

A woman's standing in regard to marriage; denotes whether a woman is single, married or cohabiting, divorced, widowed, separated, or partnered. (Effect size = Small)

15. Unplanned or Unwanted Pregnancy

Refers to a pregnancy that was not planned or wanted. Of particular note is the issue of pregnancies that remain unwanted after initial ambivalence. (Effect size = Small)

CONCEPTS 16 THROUGH 22

These final concepts represent the distillation of all predictor and risk factors that are used to screen women for symptoms of postpartum depression in the PDSS (Beck, 2002c).

Continued

MAJOR CONCEPTS & DEFINITIONS—cont'd

16. Sleeping and Eating Disturbances

Inability to sleep even when the baby is asleep, tossing and turning before actually falling asleep, waking up in the middle of the night, and difficulty going back to sleep. Loss of appetite, consciously being aware of the need to eat, and still unable to eat.

17. Anxiety and Insecurity

Overattentive to relatively minor issues, feelings of jumping out of one's skin, feeling the need to keep moving, or pacing. An ever-present feeling of insecurity and a sense of being overwhelmed in the new role of mother.

18. Emotional Lability

A woman's sense that her emotions are unstable and out of her control, commonly characterized as crying for no particular reason, irritability, explosive anger, and fear of never being happy again.

19. Mental Confusion

Marked inability to concentrate, focus on a task, or make a decision. There is a general feeling of being unable to regulate one's own thought processes.

20. Loss of Self

Women sense that those aspects of self that reflected their personal identity have changed since birth of their infant, so they cannot identify who they really are and are fearful that they might never be able to be their real selves again.

21. Guilt and Shame

A woman's perception that she is performing poorly as a mother and has negative thoughts regarding her infant. Results in an inability to be open with others about how she feels, and this contributes to a delay in diagnosis and intervention.

22. Suicidal Thoughts

Women's frequent thoughts of harming themselves or ending their lives to escape the living nightmare of postpartum depression.

USE OF EMPIRICAL EVIDENCE

When Beck began to examine postpartum depression in 1993, she noted that only two qualitative studies contributed to the knowledge base of the disorder. Most studies were based upon knowledge developed in disciplines other than nursing. Beck's background as a nurse midwife undoubtedly gave her a view of women throughout the postpartum period not commonly available to those in other disciplines involved with women during the perinatal period.

In 1993, after four major studies regarding women in the postpartum period (see Table 34-1), Beck developed a substantive theory of postpartum depression using grounded theory methodology. The substantive theory developed was entitled "teetering on the edge," with the basic psychosocial problem identified as loss of control (Beck, 1993). Since development of the substantive theory, Beck has designed 14 other studies to refine the theory by examining the experiences of postpartum depression on mother-child interactions, postpartum panic, posttraumatic stress disorder (PTSD), and birth trauma to tease out differences among postpartum mood disorders (postpartum depression, maternity blues, postpartum psychosis, postpartum obsessive-compulsive disorder, postpartum-onset panic disorder). Meta-analyses were conducted on predictors of postpartum depression, the relationship between postpartum depression and infant temperament, and the effects of postpartum depression on mother-infant interaction. In addition, two qualitative meta-syntheses were conducted on postpartum depression and mothering multiples.

Beck used ten qualitative studies of PPD in women from a wide variety of geographic locations and cultures. Women represented in these studies included Black Caribbean women, Irish women, Indian women, Hong Kong Chinese women, Hmong women, middle eastern women (living in the UK), Asian women, Portuguese women, Australian women, Canadian women, and African American women. These new data were used to compare Beck's original teetering on the edge grounded theory with women in other cultures. Beck found that the theory's modifiability was in keeping with theoretical expectations of a relevant substantive grounded theory. Therefore, the theory of "teetering on the edge," with "loss of control" as the basic psychosocial process, has functionally expanded to women in other cultures (Beck, 2006a, 2007).

MAJOR ASSUMPTIONS

Nursing

Beck describes nursing as a caring profession with caring obligations to persons we care for, students, and each other. In addition, interpersonal interactions between nurses and those for whom we care are the primary ways nursing accomplishes goals of health and wholeness.

Person

Persons are described in terms of wholeness with biological, sociological, and psychological components. Further there is a strong commitment to the idea that persons or personhood is understood within the context of family and community.

Health

Beck does not define health explicitly. However, her writings include traditional ideas of physical and mental health. Health is the consequence of women's responses to the contexts of their lives and their environments. Contexts of health are vital to understanding any singular issue of health.

Environment

Beck writes about the environment in broad terms that include individual factors as well as the world outside of each person. The outside environment includes events, situations, culture, physicality ecosystems, and sociopolitical systems. In addition, there is an acknowledgment that women in the childbearing period receive care within a health care environment structured in the medical model and permeated with patriarchal ideology.

THEORETICAL ASSERTIONS

The theoretical assertions within Beck's theory are well represented throughout her writings. She acknowledges the importance of Sichel and Driscoll's (1999) work related to the biological factors involved in postpartum depression in the following assertions:

- The brain can biochemically accommodate various stressors, whether related to internal biology or external events.
- Stressful events (internal or external), particularly over long periods, cause disruption of the biochemical regulation in the brain. The more insults to the brain, the more chronically deregulated the brain becomes. Because an already deregulated brain is again challenged with new stressors (internal or external), it is likely that serious mood and psychiatric disorders will result.
- Women's unique and normal brain and hormonal chemistry result in a vulnerability to mood disorders at critical times in their lives, including after giving birth.
- Postpartum depression is caused by a combination of biological (including genetic), psychological, social, relational, economic, and situational life stressors.
- Postpartum depression is not a homogenous disorder. Women may express postpartum depression with a single symptom but are more likely to have a constellation of varying symptoms. This

is related to varying life histories of internal and external stressors.

- Culturally, women are expected to feel happy, look happy, act happy, understand how to be a mother naturally, and experience motherhood with a sense of fulfillment. These expectations make it difficult for women to express genuine feelings of distress.
- The stigma attached to mental illness increases dramatically when a mental illness is related to the birth of a child, leading women to suffer in silence.
- Within a level of prevention framework, postpartum depression can be prevented through identification and mitigation of risk factors during the prepartum period. Postpartum depression can be identified early with careful screening and can be treated effectively. Prevention can alleviate months of suffering and decrease the harmful effects on women, their infants, and their families.
- A number of biological, sociological, and psychological issues and challenges are entirely normal in all pregnancies. These may include fatigue, sleep alterations, questioning one's abilities, and the like. Comprehensive prenatal and postnatal care can eliminate troublesome pathological symptoms and help women normalize expected symptoms, thus reducing the degree of stress they actually experience.

LOGICAL FORM

Chinn and Kramer (2004) identify inductive logic as foundational to qualitative methods, with reasoning from the particular to the general. In contrast, deductive reasoning moves from the general to the particular, drawing conclusions that represent the general. Beck's Postpartum Depression Theory, as described in previous sections of this chapter, identifies how both inductive and deductive logic significantly contributed to the development of the theory.

Because Beck's theory reflects a very complex and focused path in its evolution, it is helpful to be clear about what criteria were used to understand and present the theory. The definition of theory currently used is "a creative and rigorous structuring of ideas that projects a tentative, purposeful, and systematic view of phenomena" (Chinn & Kramer, 2004, p. 91). Middle range theories may be derived using grounded theory approaches, and they identify social processes that may occur in various social events. For example, Beck's substantive theory of postpartum depression found that loss of control was the basic psychosocial problem facing women, but this problem could also occur in contexts other than the postpartum period.

The evolution of Beck's theory is instructional for several reasons. First, Beck's unceasing, linear, and logical efforts to develop the theory for pragmatic practice concerns led to a theory that addresses a specific practice problem. Because her theory is relatively new, there are few contributors to the substance of the theory. Therefore, there is opportunity to follow a very clear and focused process of theory development by a scholar who began the work as a young woman. Beck has tested her theory, used it with various populations, tested instruments, and developed a work in which other scholars can join her to contribute to the science. Second, Beck's theory of postpartum depression is remarkable as an example of extensive inductive theory development in a specific area of nursing practice addressing a specific patient problem. Although Beck began her work with a global understanding of caring, her focused work on postpartum depression was advanced through the development of a substantive middle range theory and continues to advance. From the beginning, Beck's goal has been to understand postpartum depression in a way that would allow professionals to develop adequate prevention strategies, develop screening programs for early intervention, and develop adequate treatment strategies to prevent harm to women, their children, and their families. True to her research aims, what began as a descriptive substantive theory of postpartum depression has now evolved into an extensive program of research. What follows is the story of this evolution of Beck's Postpartum Depression Theory, uniquely approached, and uniquely understood by me.

ACCEPTANCE BY THE NURSING COMMUNITY

Practice

As Beck's research findings have been disseminated more widely, the theory and the instruments based on the theory have been utilized increasingly throughout the United States. In addition, the PDSS is in use and translated as appropriate in Canada, Australia, New Zealand, Ireland, South Africa, Germany, Russia, Turkey, and Israel.

The PDSS became a standard of care for women in the high-risk obstetrical clinic of the Medical University of South Carolina Hospital (A. Raney, personal communication, April 28, 2004). The clients in this clinic vary in age across the spectrum, come from various ethnic backgrounds, and have a wide range of medical risk factors. She has noted that the tool is a vehicle for opening discussions with women that had not occurred prior to implementation of the tool. High scores on the PDSS have given physicians evidence to understand how postpartum depression is expressed in their patients, increasing their sensitivity and awareness. Predictably, marshaling of community resources to meet the specific needs of individual clients has been a challenge; however, the landscape for the Charleston community in understanding and responding to the special needs of women during this time has occurred.

Public health initiatives that involve working with new mothers and babies are also utilizing Beck's theory of postpartum depression via the PDSS. For example, the Healthy Start CORPS: Inter-Conceptual Care Case Management Project in North Carolina begins to follow women when they are 6 weeks postpartum. All new clients, many of whom are Native American, are given the PDSS so that intervention and management strategies can be built into plans of care for individual women and their families (L. Baker, personal communication, April 29, 2004). The director of the program emphasizes the ease with which women are able to discuss symptoms of postpartum depression after completing the tool.

Beck's work has also been instrumental in community intervention and education projects such as the Ruth Rhoden Craven Foundation for Postpartum Depression Awareness located in South Carolina. Helena Bradford founded this organization because of a tragic postpartum mood disorder within her own family. Ms. Bradford advocates for postpartum awareness within her community and conducts support groups (H. Bradford, personal communication, April 28, 2004).

Education

Beck is a frequently invited speaker for professional educational conferences and workshops. Her work is cited frequently in nursing texts concerning maternal and newborn nursing, such as that of Ladewig, London, and Olds (2001). At both undergraduate and graduate levels, Beck's work sets the standard for knowledge and understanding about postpartum depression. In addition, Beck's work has been used to educate members of other disciplines, such as physicians, mental health workers, public health professionals, social workers, and those who work in social service agencies that provide protective care for women and children. Beck also brings her work to the general public and policy makers through active community involvement at the local, state, national, and international levels.

Research

The long research development of Beck's theory is evident in Table 34-1. As previously noted, she has received numerous awards recognizing the importance of her research. Nurses increasingly are using Beck's work for master's and doctoral level research. In addition, Beck facilitates practice implementation research for academic and nonacademic sites.

FURTHER DEVELOPMENT

Beck has identified what will likely become another major concept in her theory, as well as a restructuring of postpartum mood disorder definitions (Beck, 2004a, 2004b). Because of increasing reports of PTSD after childbirth, she examined women's experiences of traumatic births (Beck, 2004a). In this beginning work, birth trauma was defined as "an event occurring during the labor and delivery process that involves actual or threatened serious injury or death to the mother or her infant. The birthing woman experiences intense fear, helplessness, loss of control, and horror" (Beck, 2004a, p. 28). Beck noted that women who actually had been suffering from PTSD were misdiagnosed as having postpartum depression and were treated incorrectly with antidepressant medications. She has recommended that postpartum mood disorders be changed to postpartum mood and anxiety disorders (Beck, 2004b). PTSD would then be differentiated as a distinct diagnosis with different treatment approaches. Birth trauma, as a concept, will be examined empirically and included in predictor and screening instruments as appropriate. Beck (2006c) examined women's experience of the anniversary of their birth trauma, noting that the birthday of a woman's child might represent a time of re-experiencing the trauma all over again. Current research by Beck and co-investigator, Carol Lammi-Keefe, focuses on docasahexaenoic acid in pregnancy and its effect on PPD.

Recently completed research utilized the PDSS to screen for PPD in a sample acquired on the Internet compared with a community based sample (Le, Perry, & Sheng, 2008). Initial results indicated a high degree of internal consistency and construct validity between the two groups. Findings suggested that the Internet group included greater numbers of participation among Hispanic and Asian women, and in general, the Internet group evidenced more risk factors for a PPD diagnosis. Future research will focus on successful ways to connect women screened on the Internet with appropriate services for intervention for prevention and treatment.

CRITIQUE

Clarity

Beck's theory evidences a semantic clarity as concepts are defined clearly and consistently. Within and between research reports, Beck uses terms, ideas, definitions, and concepts in a way that reflects growth, yet they are defined and easily understood. Her research and writings use both inductive and deductive language, and her verbiage is both economical and clear.

Simplicity

Postpartum depression is a complex phenomenon, experientially and theoretically. Yet Beck's theory of postpartum depression follows a logical progression specific to observations made in nursing practice. It is accessible empirically and theoretically. Importantly, concepts and definitions used for predicting a woman's risk for postpartum depression and concepts and definitions used to screen women for symptoms of postpartum depression are directly meaningful for women, the lay public, and practitioners from nursing and other related disciplines.

Generality

Chinn and Kramer (2004) note that generality refers to a theory's ability to remain conceptually simple, yet account for a broad range of empirical experiences. Postpartum depression is a relatively narrow experience; however, its causation is especially complex. Beck has accounted for the complexity of postpartum depression within the expansion of the concepts within the theory. Generality issues relate to how broadly the theory describes human experience, and this is supported by applicability of the theory in different cultural contexts. Importantly, Beck (2007) has used research from numerous sources that address postpartum depression in various geographical and cultural groups. Her use of data from these studies to compare and contrast within the extant theory gives new breadth to the theory and significantly impacts its generality.

Empirical Precision

The PDSS (Postpartum Depression Screening Scale) has been subjected to rigorous statistical processes for development and standardization. Beck and Gable (2000) examined psychometric properties of the scale with regard to reliability of the measure within developmental and diagnostic samples.

Validity analyses were conducted with the two samples, as were procedures used to establish cutoff scores for clinical interpretations. These studies indicated that the PDSS is a reliable and valid screening instrument for detection of postpartum depression (Beck & Gable, 2000, 2001a, 2001b, 2001c, 2001d). As previously noted, the theory and the PDSS are relatively new and have therefore not been critiqued empirically by a wide variety of scholars. Beck has two instruments: the PDSS that is well established, and the Postpartum Depression Prediction Inventory (PDPI) that has more recently been found valid and reliable in studies (Beck, 2002b; Hanna, Jarman, Savage, & Layton, 2004).

Derivable Consequences

The value of Beck's work is of growing importance within nursing and within other disciplines. The sequence of events in the life of our fellow nurse, Andrea Yates (along with too many others) (Meier, 2002), points to the extraordinary need for a greater awareness and use of Beck's Postpartum Depression Theory for prevention, identification, early intervention, and treatment. Perinatal mood disorders are obviously more than transient inconveniences for women and their families.

There is a growing awareness that identification and early intervention of postpartum depression belong to more than those who are primarily responsible for caring for women during pregnancy and immediately after birth (Beck, 2003; Kennedy, Beck, & Driscoll, 2002). Because of consistent interactions with mothers, pediatric and neonatal nurses can make valuable contributions to successful interventions with mothers suffering from postpartum depression. Psychiatric nurses might also be able to identify problems in women (or their children) that do not immediately indicate postpartum depression.

However, knowledge about postpartum depression is developing in a way that sheds light on less obvious consequences. Recently, postpartum depression has been linked to adverse effects on children's cognitive and emotional development and behavior problems of older children in school (Beck, 1996a, 1996b, 1999). Postpartum depression could have a negative effect upon situations such as substance use, traffic accidents, criminal behaviors, domestic violence, progress in school, employment and income, and many others. A growing awareness within nursing, other health care professionals, and the general public will allow greater identification of the influence of postpartum depression on the many contexts within which people live their lives.

SUMMARY

The development of Beck's Postpartum Depression Theory is the quintessential example of how nursing knowledge is developed from nursing problems, utilizing multiple methods with rigorous testing. The theory was influenced by various theoretical and philosophical stances, adding breadth and texture. The most important features of Beck's theory are its immediate accessibility and its dynamic nature. Most maternity nurses are able to read the theory and understand how to apply it in their own practice. Beck and others continue to expand the theory by exploring its applicability to different cultures and exploring ways of reaching women who have potential for its benefit.

Increasingly, nurses and the wider society are recognizing that issues of postpartum depression have not been adequately understood or acknowledged. Nursing, like other health care professions, has been shocked by unanticipated events when postpartum depression leads to untoward outcomes that appear in the evening news. These events point out the importance of this theory. Dr. Cheryl Tatano Beck's work has demonstrated how nursing research provides evidence to understand phenomena and prevent postpartum depression. Her research and instruments facilitate detection, early intervention, and treatment.

Case Study

At the tender age of 11, Kim was "sold" by her mother to three adult men for an evening of sex and drugs. Kim related that as her mother went out

the door, she advised her to "do what they tell you and I'll be back in the morning." Kim was never OK again. Although Kim did relatively well during the sporadic times she went to school, her life was a series of drug and sex binges. At 17, Kim was in jail and pregnant. Kim had been arrested several times and released, but the judge insisted that this time she stay incarcerated until after the baby was born to guarantee the baby would be crack-free at birth. Kim's prenatal records, however, did not indicate drug or alcohol use, and neither did her jail records. She adamantly insisted that she never used drugs or alcohol once she found out she was pregnant (late in the first trimester). Through a series of misunderstandings, she was released 2 weeks before the baby's birth. However, Kim did well, continued to stay drug-free, even refused medication during labor, and delivered a beautiful healthy baby—a baby whose blood test results were negative for drugs.

Kim recalls that she began motherhood believing this would be the event that would turn her own life around. It did for several weeks, but slowly Kim became involved in her old life. She received money to buy clothes and food for her baby. In spite of that help, however, Kim had no place to live and no money to support herself. She never held a legal job in her life. She qualified for postpartum medical care for 6 weeks, but after that she was on her own.

When the baby was 7 months old, Kim called a nurse who had once cared for her during her pregnancy and asked for help to give her daughter up for adoption. She believed she would simply never be able to give her baby the life she knew all babies deserved. Kim was using drugs again, and the baby was being kept by whoever was in the mood to do so. Kim absolutely loved this baby, and the choice for adoption came from this love. Kim chose a local Christian adoption agency. Staff there gave her the opportunity to read the profiles of potential families, see pictures of them, and actually choose the family who would raise her baby. Though she did not know the family's name or address, the family and the agency committed to regular photographs and updates about her daughter.

Without resources or support, and without her baby, Kim returned to the only life she had ever known among the only people she really knew. Eighteen months later, Kim gave birth to another baby. This time, she swore things would be different. When this new baby was also about 7 months old, Kim found herself deeply involved in crack use, with her baby being passed around from relative to relative and from friend to friend. Unfortunately, Kim was present during the commission of a violent crime with a predictably tragic outcome. Although Kim did not actually commit this crime, she was present and was ultimately sent to prison.

Kim once remarked that she loved being pregnant, loved giving birth, and loved the idea of being a mother. She said, "It would be great in the beginning, but after a couple of months I'd start feeling bad. It seems like with both my babies that around 6 or 7 months, I just couldn't handle anything."

Although Kim took the baby to a pediatrician for follow-up care, none of those care providers knew her or knew her history—they were primarily concerned with her son's health. Kim's affect is usually very upbeat; she smiles easily. It is not likely that anyone ever asked her any important questions about her life or her experience of being a mother. Kim was, for all intents and purposes, "lost to follow-up."

Kim's story illustrates the kinds of complexities that can make postpartum depression especially challenging for women who live amid drugs and chaos. In the midst of this life, women still want to be good mothers and have the same hopes and same dreams we all have. Drugs, alcohol, crimes, and all the other ways Kim's life was chaotic were the only avenues by which she received services—after-the-fact services.

Interventions by others could have made a difference at many points in Kim's life. One of those points was during her prenatal period. She clearly evidenced most of the risk factors for postpartum depression, despite her cheerful attitude toward the pregnancy. If you had been one of Kim's nurses during her prenatal care and identified her to be at risk for postpartum depression, what kind of care plan would you have developed before or after her baby's birth? Would you have been willing to

intervene on Kim's behalf, or on her baby's behalf, even when their needs occurred deep within the community and not within the confines of a hospital or office?

CRITICAL THINKING *Activities*

1. Interview a friend or family member about her prenatal and postnatal experiences.
2. Did she have feelings that you expected? Any that surprised you?
3. Might she have been at risk for postpartum depression?
4. What resources are available in your community for a woman with postpartum depression?

POINTS FOR *Further Study*

- Beck, C.T. (in press). State of the science on postpartum depression: What nurse researchers have contributed. Part 1. *MCN: American Journal of Maternal Child Nursing.*
- Beck, C.T. (in press). State of the science on postpartum depression: What nurse researchers have contributed. Part 2. *MCN: American Journal of Maternal Child Nursing.*
- Polit, D. & Beck, C.T. (2007). *Nursing research: Generating and assessing evidence for nursing practice* (8th Ed.). Philadelphia: Lippincott Williams & Wilkins.

Beck Instruments

- Beck, C.T. (1998). Postpartum Depression Predictors Inventory (PDPI). Available from *Journal of Obstetric, Gynecologic, & Neonatal Nursing*, published on behalf of the Association of Women's Health, Obstetrics and Neonatal Nurses, by Sage Science Press, an imprint of Sage Publications; Print ISSN: 0884–2175.
- Beck, C.T., & Gable, R. K. (2002). *Postpartum Depression Screening Scale (PDSS)*. Available through Western Psychological Services, 12031 Wilshire Blvd., Los Angeles, CA 90025-1251.

REFERENCES

Beck, C. T. (1980). Patient acceptance of fetal monitoring as a helpful tool. *Journal of Obstetric, Gynecologic, & Neonatal Nursing, 9*, 350-353.

Beck, C. T. (1993). Teetering on the edge: A substantive theory of postpartum depression. *Nursing Research, 42*, 42-48.

Beck, C. T. (1996a). Postpartum depressed mothers' experiences interacting with their children. *Nursing Research, 45*(2), 98-104.

Beck, C. T. (1996b). The relationship between postpartum depression and infant temperament: A meta-analysis. *Nursing Research, 45*, 225-230.

Beck, C. T. (1998). A checklist to identify women at risk for developing postpartum depression. *Journal of Obstetric, Gynecologic, & Neonatal Nursing, 27*, 39-46.

Beck, C. T. (1999). Quantitative measurement of caring. *Journal of Advanced Nursing, 30*, 24-32.

Beck, C. T. (2001). Predictors of postpartum depression: An update. *Nursing Research, 50*(5), 275-285.

Beck, C. T. (2002a). A meta-synthesis of qualitative research. *MCN: The American Journal of Maternal Child Nursing, 27*(4), 214-221.

Beck, C. T. (2002b). Revision of the Postpartum Depression Predictors Inventory. *Journal of Obstetric, Gynecologic, & Neonatal Nursing, 31*(4), 394-402.

Beck, C. T. (2002c). *Postpartum depression screening scale (PDSS): Manual.* Los Angeles: Western Psychological Services.

Beck, C. T. (2003). Recognizing and screening for postpartum depression in mothers of NICU infants. *Advances in Neonatal Care, 3*, 37-46.

Beck, C. T. (2004a). Birth trauma: In the eye of the beholder. *Nursing Research, 53*, 28-35.

Beck, C. T. (2004b). Post traumatic stress disorder due to childbirth: The aftermath. *Nursing Research, 53*(4), 216-224.

Beck, C. T. (2006a). Acculturation: Implications for perinatal research. *Maternal Child Nursing, 31*(2), 114-120.

Beck, C. T. (2006b). Postpartum depression: It isn't just the blues. *American Journal of Nursing, 106*(5), 40-50.

Beck, C. T. (2006c). The anniversary of birth trauma: Failure to rescue. *Nursing Research, 55*(6), 381-390.

Beck, C. T. (2007). Exemplar: Teetering on the edge: A continually emerging theory of postpartum depression. In P. Munhall (Eds.). *Nursing research: A qualitative perspective* (4th Ed.) (pp. 273-292). Boston: Jones & Bartlett.

Beck, C. T., & Gable, R. K. (2000). Postpartum depression screening scale: Development and psychometric testing. *Nursing Research, 49*(5), 272-282.

Beck, C. T., & Gable, R. K. (2001a). Item response theory in affective instrument development: An illustration. *Journal of Nursing Measurement, 9*, 5-22.

Beck, C. T., & Gable, R. K. (2001b). Comparative analysis of the performance of the Postpartum Depression Screening Scale with two other depression instruments. *Nursing Research, 50*, 242-250.

Beck, C. T., & Gable, R. K. (2001c). Further validation of the postpartum depression screening scale. *Nursing Research, 50*(3), 155-164.

Beck, C. T., & Gable, R. K. (2001d). Ensuring content validity: An illustration of the process. *Journal of Nursing Measurement, 9*(2), 201-215.

Beck, C. T., & Gable, R. K. (2003). Postpartum Depression Screening Scale—Spanish version. *Nursing Research, 52*, 296-306.

Chinn, P., & Kramer, M. (2004). *Integrated knowledge development in nursing* (6th ed.). St. Louis: Mosby.

Colaizzi, P. (1978). Psychological research as the phenomenologist views it. In R. Valle & M. King (Eds.), *Existential phenomenological alternative for psychology* (pp. 48-71). New York: Oxford University Press.

Gable, R., & Wolf, M. (1993). *Instrument development in the affective domain.* Boston: Kluwer Academic.

Glaser, B. (1978). *Theoretical sensitivity: Advances in the methodology of grounded theory.* Mill Valley, CA: Sociology Press.

Glaser, B., & Strauss, A. (1967). *The discovery of grounded theory.* Chicago: Aldine.

Hanna, B., Jarman, H., Savage, S., & Layton, K. (2004). The early detection of postpartum depression: Midwives and nurses trial a checklist. *Journal of Obstetric, Gynecologic, & Neonatal Nursing, 33*, 191-197.

Hutchinson, S. (1986). Grounded theory: The method. In P. Munhall & C. Oiler (Eds.), *Nursing research: A qualitative perspective* (pp. 111-130). Norwalk, CT: Appleton-Century-Crofts.

Kennedy, H., Beck, C., & Driscoll, J. (2002). A light in the fog: Caring for women with postpartum depression. *Journal of Midwifery & Women's Health, 47*(5), 318-330.

Ladewig, P., London, M., & Olds, S. (2001). *Contemporary maternal-newborn nursing care* (5th ed.). Philadelphia: Prentice Hall.

Le, H.-N., Perry, D., & Sheng, X. (2008). Using the internet to screen for postpartum depression. *Maternal and Child Health Journal,* Springer Netherlands: SpringerLink, February 16, 2008.

Meier, E. (2002). Pediatric ethics, issues & commentary. Andrea Yates: where did we go wrong? *Pediatric Nursing, 28*(3), 299.

Polit, D., & Beck, C. T. (2003). *Nursing research: Principles and methods* (7th ed.). Philadelphia: Lippincott Williams & Wilkins.

Sichel, D., & Driscoll, J. (1999). *Women's moods.* New York: Harper Collins.

BIBLIOGRAPHY

Primary Sources

Books

Beck, C. T. (1999). *Postpartum depression: Case studies, research, and nursing care.* Washington, DC: Association of Women's Health, Obstetric and Neonatal Nurses.

Beck, C. T. (2008). *Postpartum mood and anxiety disorders: Case studies, research, and nursing care.* Washington, D.C.: Association of Women's Health, Obstetrics, and Neonatal Nursing.

Beck, C. T., & Driscoll, J. W. (2006). *Postpartum mood and anxiety disorders: A clinician's guide.* Sudbury, MA: Jones & Bartlett Publishers.

Beck, C. T., & Gable, R. K. (2002). *Postpartum Depression Screening Scale manual.* Los Angeles: Western Psychological Services.

Cesario, S. K., Beck, C. T., Creehan, P., Watts, N. & Santa-Donato, A. (2006). *Compendium of postpartum care* (2nd Ed.). Washington, D.C.: Association of Women's Health, Obstetric, and Neonatal Nursing.

Loiselle, C., & Profetto-McGrath, J., Polit, D. F., & Beck, C. T. (2004). *Canadian essentials of nursing research.* Philadelphia: Lippincott Williams & Wilkins.

Loiselle, C., & Profetto-McGrath, J., Polit, D. F., & Beck, C. T. (2007). *Canadian essentials of nursing research* (2nd Ed.). Philadelphia: Lippincott Williams & Wilkins.

Polit, D. & Beck, C. T. (2004). *Instructor's resource CD-ROM to accompany nursing research: Principles and methods.* Philadelphia: Lippincott.

Polit, D., & Beck, C. T. (2004). *Nursing research: Principles and methods* (7th ed.). Philadelphia: Lippincott Williams & Wilkins.

Polit, D., & Beck, C. T. (2004). *Study guide to accompany nursing research: Principles and methods.* Philadelphia: Lippincott Williams & Wilkins.

Polit, D. F., & Beck, C. T. (2006). *Essentials of nursing research: Methods, appraisal, and utilization* (6th Ed.). Philadelphia: Lippincott Williams & Wilkins.

Polit, D. F., & Beck, C. T. (2006). *Instructor's resource manual and textbook to accompany essentials of nursing research: Methods, appraisal, and utilization.* Philadelphia: Lippincott Williams & Wilkins.

Polit, D. F., & Beck, C. T. (2006). *Study guide to accompany essentials of nursing research: Methods, appraisal, and utilization.* Philadelphia: Lippincott Williams & Wilkins.

Polit, D. F., & Beck, C. T. (2007). *Instructor's Resource CD-ROM to accompany nursing research: Generating and assessing evidence for nursing practice.* Philadelphia: Lippincott Williams & Wilkins.

Polit, D. F., & Beck, C. T. (2007). *Resource manual to accompany nursing research: Generating and assessing evidence for nursing practice.* Philadelphia: Lippincott Williams and Wilkins.

Polit, D. F., Beck, C. T., & Hungler, B. P. (2001). *Essentials of nursing research: Methods, appraisal, and utilization.* Philadelphia: Lippincott.

Polit, D. F., Beck, C. T., & Hungler, B. P. (2001). *Instructor's resource manual and textbook to accompany essentials of nursing research:* Methods, appraisal, and utilization. Philadelphia: Lippincott.

Polit, D. F., Beck, C. T., & Hungler, B. P. (2001). *Study guide to accompany essentials of nursing research:* Methods, appraisal, and utilization. Philadelphia: Lippincott.

Book Chapters

Beck, C. T. (1994). Researching the lived experience of caring. In A. Boykin (Ed.), *Living a caring based program* (pp. 93-126). New York: National League for Nursing Publications.

Beck, C. T. (1998). Meta-analysis. In J. Fitzpatrick (Ed.), *Encyclopedia of nursing research* (pp. 308-310). New York: Springer.

Beck, C. T. (1998). Phenomenology. In J. Fitzpatrick (Ed.), *Encyclopedia of nursing research* (pp. 431-433). New York: Springer.

Beck, C. T. (1998). Replication research. In J. Fitzpatrick (Ed.), *Encyclopedia of nursing research* (pp. 485-486). New York: Springer.

Beck, C. T. (1999). Grounded theory research. In J. Fain (Ed.), *Reading, understanding, and applying nursing research* (pp. 205-225). Philadelphia: F. A. Davis.

Beck, C. T. (2004). Grounded theory research. In J. Fain, *Reading, understanding, and applying nursing research* (pp. 205-225). Philadelphia: F. A. Davis Company.

Beck, C. T. (2006). Chapter 6. Postpartum mood and anxiety disorders. In *The Compendium of Postpartum Care.* Association of Women's Health, Obstetric, and Neonatal Nursing: Washington D.C.

Beck, C. T. (2007). Exemplar: Teetering on the edge: A continually emerging theory of postpartum depression (pp. 273-292). In P. L. Munhall (Ed.). *Nursing research: A qualitative perspective* (4th edition). Sudbury, MA: Jones & Bartlett.

Beck, C. T. (in press). Postpartum mood and anxiety disorders. In S. Cesario, K. Morin, & D. Hobbins (Eds.). *Nursing care of women and newborns.* Upper Saddle River, NJ: Pearson-Prentice-Hall.

Beck, C. T., & Gable, R. K. (2005). The Postpartum Depression Screening Scale (PDSS). In C. Henshaw & S. Elliott (Eds.). *Screening for perinatal depression* (pp. 133-140). London: Jessica Kingley Publishers.

Judge, M. P., & Beck, C. T. (in press). Postpartum depression and the role of nutritional factors. In C. J. Lammi-Keefe, S. C. Couch & E. Philipson (Eds.). *Nutrition and health: Handbook of nutrition and pregnancy.* Totoway, NJ: Humana Press.

Journal Articles

Beck, C. T. (1979). The occurrence of depression in women and the effect of the women's movement. *Journal of Psychiatric Nursing and Mental Health Services, 17*, 14-16.

Beck, C. T. (1980). Patient acceptance of fetal monitoring as a helpful tool. *Journal of Obstetric, Gynecologic, & Neonatal Nursing, 9*, 350-353.

Beck, C. T. (1982). The conceptualization of power. *ANS Advances in Nursing Science, 4*, 1-17.

Beck, C. T. (1983). Parturients' temporal experiences during the phases of labor. *Western Journal of Nursing Research, 5*, 283-295.

Beck, C. T. (1984). Subject mortality: It is inevitable? *Western Journal of Nursing Research, 6*, 331-339.

Beck, C. T. (1985). Teaching strategy for an undergraduate research course: Student exercises. *Nurse Educator, 10*, 6.

Beck, C. T. (1985). Theoretical frameworks cited in *Nursing Research* from 1974-1985. *Nurse Educator, 10*, 36-39.

Beck, C. T. (1986). Research attitudes in baccalaureate nursing students. *Nurse Educator, 11*, 6-7.

Beck, C. T. (1986). Strategies for teaching nursing research: Small group games. *Western Journal of Nursing Research, 8*, 233-238.

Beck, C. T. (1986). Teaching practicum with an educational nurse specialist. *Nurse Educator, 11*, 5.

Beck, C. T. (1986). Use of nonparametric statistics in graduate student research projects. *Journal of Nursing Education, 25*, 41-42.

Beck, C. T. (1987). Vaginal and cesarean birth mothers' temporal experiences during the postpartum period. *Journal of Obstetric, Gynecologic, & Neonatal Nursing, 16*, 366-367.

Beck, C. T. (1988). Creating a research atmosphere for the student body of a nursing department: The use of small group projects. *Nurse Educator, 13*, 5-6.

Beck, C. T. (1988). Norm setting for the verbal estimation of a 40-second interval by women of childbearing age. *Perceptual and Motor Skills, 67*, 557-578.

Beck, C. T. (1988). Pediatric nursing research published from 1977-1986. *Issues in Comprehensive Pediatric Nursing, 11*, 261-270.

Beck, C. T. (1988). Review of strategies for teaching nursing research 1979-1986. *Western Journal of Nursing Research, 10*, 222-225.

Beck, C. T. (1989). A teaching strategy: Mini publication workshop. *Nurse Educator, 14*, 28.

Beck, C. T. (1989). Fundamentals of obstetric, gynecologic, and neonatal nursing research. Part I. *Journal of Obstetric, Gynecologic, & Neonatal Nursing, 18*, 216-221.

Beck, C. T. (1989). Fundamentals of obstetric, gynecologic, and neonatal nursing research. Part II. *Journal of Obstetric, Gynecologic, & Neonatal Nursing, 18*, 288-294.

Beck, C. T. (1989). Fundamentals of obstetric, gynecologic, and neonatal nursing research. Part III. *Journal of Obstetric, Gynecologic, & Neonatal Nursing, 18*, 385-389.

Beck, C. T. (1989). Maternal newborn nursing research published from 1977-1986. *Western Journal of Nursing Research, 11*, 621-626.

Beck, C. T. (1990). The research critique: General criteria for evaluating a research project. *Journal of Obstetric, Gynecologic, & Neonatal Nursing, 19*, 18-22.

Beck, C. T. (1990). Qualitative research: Methodologies and use in pediatric nursing. *Issues in Comprehensive Pediatric Nursing, 13*(3), 193-201.

Beck, C. T. (1991). Early postpartum discharge: Literature review and critique. *Women and Health, 17*, 125-138.

Beck, C. T. (1991). How students perceive faculty caring: A phenomenological study. *Nurse Educator, 16*(5), 18-22.

Beck, C. T. (1991). Maternity blues research: A critical review. *Issues in Mental Health Nursing, 12*, 291-300.

Beck, C. T. (1991). Nursing students' lived experience of health: A phenomenological study. *Journal of Nursing Education, 30*(8), 371-374.

Beck, C. T. (1992). Caring among nursing students: A phenomenological study. *Nurse Educator, 17*, 22-27.

Beck, C. T. (1992). Caring between nursing students and physically/mentally handicapped children: A phenomenological study. *Journal of Nursing Education, 31*, 361-366.

Beck, C. T. (1992). The lived experience of postpartum depression: A phenomenological study. *Nursing Research, 41*, 166-170.

Beck, C. T. (1993). Caring relationships between nursing students and their patients. *Nurse Educator, 18*, 28-32.

Beck, C. T. (1993). Integrating research into an RN to BSN clinical course, a phenomenological method. *Western Journal of Nursing Research, 15*, 118-121.

Beck, C. T. (1993). Nursing students' initial clinical experience: A phenomenological study. *International Journal of Nursing Studies, 30*, 489-497.

Beck, C. T. (1993). Qualitative research: The evaluation of its credibility, fittingness and auditability. *Western Journal of Nursing Research, 15*, 263-266.

Beck, C. T. (1993). Teetering on the edge: A substantive theory of postpartum depression. *Nursing Research, 42*, 42-48.

Beck, C. T. (1994). Achieving statistical power through design sensitivity. *Journal of Advanced Nursing, 20*, 912-916.

Beck, C. T. (1994). Phenomenology: Its use in nursing research. *International Journal of Nursing Studies, 31*, 499-510.

Beck, C. T. (1994). Reliability and validity issues in phenomenological research. *Western Journal of Nursing Research, 16*, 254-267.

Beck, C. T. (1994). Replication strategies and their use in nursing research. *Image: The Journal of Nursing Scholarship, 26*, 191-194.

Beck, C. T. (1994). Statistical power analysis in pediatric nursing research. *Issues in Comprehensive Pediatric Nursing, 17*, 73-80.

Beck, C. T. (1994). Women's temporal experiences during the delivery process: A phenomenological study. *International Journal of Nursing Studies, 31*, 245-252.

Beck, C. T. (1995). Burnout in undergraduate nursing students. *Nurse Educator, 20*, 19-23.

Beck, C. T. (1995). Meta-analysis: Overview and application to clinical nursing research. *Journal of Obstetric, Gynecologic, & Neonatal Nursing, 27*, 39-46.

Beck, C. T. (1995). Perceptions of nurses' caring by mothers experiencing postpartum depression, *Journal of Obstetric, Gynecologic, & Neonatal Nursing, 24*, 819-825.

Beck, C. T. (1995). Screening methods for postpartum depression. *Journal of Obstetric, Gynecologic, & Neonatal Nursing, 24*, 308-312.

Beck, C. T. (1995). The effect of postpartum depression of maternal-infant interaction: A meta-analysis. *Nursing Research, 44*, 298-304.

Beck, C. T. (1996). A concept analysis of panic. *Archives of Psychiatric Nursing, 10*, 265-275.

Beck, C. T. (1996). Nursing students' experiences caring for cognitively impaired elders. *Journal of Advanced Nursing, 23*, 992-998.

Beck, C. T. (1996). Postpartum depressed mothers' experiences interacting with their children. *Nursing Research, 45*, 98-104.

Beck, C. T. (1996). Predictors of postpartum depression: A meta-analysis. *Nursing Research, 45*, 297-303.

Beck, C. T. (1996). The relationship between postpartum depression and infant temperament: A meta-analysis. *Nursing Research, 45*, 225-230.

Beck, C. T. (1996). Use of a meta-analytic database management system. *Nursing Research, 45*, 181-184.

Beck, C. T. (1997). Developing a research program using qualitative and quantitative approaches. *Nursing Outlook, 45*, 265-269.

Beck, C. T. (1997). Humor in nursing practice: A phenomenological study. *International Journal of Nursing Studies, 34*, 346-352.

Beck, C. T. (1997). Nursing students' experiences caring for dying patients. *Journal of Nursing Education, 36*, 408-415.

Beck, C. T. (1997). Use of meta-analysis as a teaching strategy in nursing research courses. *Journal of Nursing Education, 36*, 87-90.

Beck, C. T. (1998). A checklist to identify women at risk for developing postpartum depression. *Journal of Obstetric, Gynecologic, & Neonatal Nursing, 27*, 39-46.

Beck, C. T. (1998). A review of research instruments for use during the postpartum period. *MCN: The American Journal of Maternal Child Nursing, 23*, 254-261.

Beck, C. T. (1998). Effects of postpartum depression on child development: A meta-analysis. *Archives of Psychiatric Nursing, 12*, 12-20.

Beck, C. T. (1998). Intuition in nursing practice. Sharing graduate students' exemplars with undergraduate students. *Journal of Nursing Education, 37*, 169-172.

Beck, C. T. (1998). Postpartum onset of panic disorder. *Image: The Journal of Nursing Scholarship, 30*, 131-135.

Beck, C. T. (1998). Screening for postpartum depression. *OB/GYN Nursing Forum, 6*, 1-8.

Beck, C. T. (1999). Available instruments for research on prenatal attachment and adaptation to pregnancy. *MCN: The American Journal of Maternal Child Nursing, 24*, 25-32.

Beck, C. T. (1999). Content validity exercises for nursing students. *Journal of Nursing Education, 38*, 133-135.

Beck, C. T. (1999). Facilitating the work of a meta-analyst. *Research in Nursing and Health, 22*, 523-530.

Beck, C. T. (1999). Maternal depression and child behavioral problems: A meta-analysis. *Journal of Advanced Nursing, 29*, 623-629.

Beck, C. T. (1999). Opening students' eyes: The process of selecting a research instrument. *Nurse Educator, 24*, 21-23.

Beck, C. T. (1999). Postpartum depression: Stopping the thief that steals motherhood. *AWHONN Lifelines, 3*, 41-44.

Beck, C. T. (1999). Quantitative measurement of caring. *Journal of Advanced Nursing, 30*, 24-32.

Beck, C. T. (2000). Choosing nursing as a career. *Journal of Nursing Education, 39*, 320-322.

Beck, C. T. (2000). Trends in nursing education since 1976. *MCN: The American Journal of Maternal Child Nursing, 25*, 290-295.

Beck, C. T. (2001). Caring within nursing education: A meta-synthesis. *Journal of Nursing Education, 40*, 101-109.

Beck, C. T. (2001). Comparative analysis of the performance of the Postpartum Depression Screening Scale with two other depression instruments. *Nursing Research, 50*(4), 242-250.

Beck, C. T. (2001). Maternal depression and problematic behavior in children. *Understanding Mental Health* (Online journal). Accessed January 12, 2004, at: *http://www.depression.org.uk*

Beck, C. T. (2001). Predictors of postpartum depression: An update. *Nursing Research, 50*, 275-285.

Beck, C. T. (2002). Mothering multiples: A meta-synthesis of the qualitative research. *MCN: The American Journal of Maternal Child Nursing, 27*, 214-221.

Beck, C. T. (2002). Postpartum depression: A metasynthesis of qualitative research. *Qualitative Health Research, 12*, 453-472.

Beck, C. T. (2002). Releasing the pause button: Mothering twins during the first year of life. *Qualitative Health Research, 12*, 593-608.

Beck, C. T. (2002). Revision of the Postpartum Depression Predictors Inventory. *Journal of the Obstetric, Gynecologic, & Neonatal Nursing, 31*, 394-402.

Beck, C. T. (2002). Theoretical perspectives of postpartum depression. *MCN: The American Journal of Maternal Child Nursing, 27*, 282-287.

Beck, C. T. (2003). Initiation into qualitative data analysis. *Journal of Nursing Education, 42*, 231-234.

Beck, C. T. (2003). Recognizing and screening for postpartum depression in mothers of NICU infants. *Advances in Neonatal Care, 3*, 37-46.

Beck, C. T. (2003). Seeing the forest for the trees: A qualitative synthesis exercise. *Journal of Nursing Education, 42*, 231-234.

Beck, C. T. (2004). Birth trauma: In the eye of the beholder. *Nursing Research, 53*, 28-35.

Beck, C. T. (2004). Post traumatic stress disorder due to childbirth: The aftermath. *Nursing Research, 53*(4), 216-224.

Beck, C. T. (2005). Benefits of participating in internet interviews: Women helping women. *Qualitative Health Research, 15*, 411-422.

Beck, C. T. (2006a). Acculturation: Implications for perinatal research. *Maternal Child Nursing, 31*(2), 114-120.

Beck, C. T. (2006b). Postpartum depression: It isn't just the blues. *American Journal of Nursing, 106*(5), 40-50.

Beck, C. T. (2006c). The anniversary of birth trauma: Failure to rescue. *Nursing Research, 55*(6), 381-390.

Beck, C. T. (2006d). Pentadic cartography: Mapping birth trauma narratives. *Qualitative Health Research, 16*, 453-466.

Beck, C. T. (in press). The impact of birth trauma on breastfeeding: A tale of two pathways. *Nursing Research.*

Beck, C. T. (in press). An adult survivor of childhood sexual abuse and her breastfeeding experience: A case study. *MCN: American Journal of Maternal Child Nursing.*

Beck, C. T., & Barnes, D. L. (2006). Post-traumatic stress disorder in pregnancy. *Annals of the American Psychotherapy Association,* Summer, 4-9.

Beck, C. T., Bernal, H., & Froman, R. D. (2003). Methods to document the semantic equivalence of a translated scale. *Research in Nursing & Health, 26*, 64-73.

Beck, C. T., Froman, R. D., & Bernal, H. (2005). Acculturation level and postpartum depression in Hispanic mothers. *MCN: The American Journal of Maternal Child Nursing, 30*, 299-304.

Beck, C. T., & Gable, R. K. (2000). Postpartum Depression Screening Scale: Development and psychometric testing. *Nursing Research, 49*, 272-282.

Beck, C. T., & Gable, R. K. (2001). Comparative analysis of the performance of the Postpartum Depression Screening Scale with two other depression instruments. *Nursing Research, 50*, 242-250.

Beck, C. T., & Gable, R. K. (2001). Ensuring content validity: An illustration of the process. *Journal of Nursing Measurement, 9*, 201-215.

Beck, C. T., & Gable, R. K. (2001). Further validation of the Postpartum Depression Screening Scale. *Nursing Research, 50*, 155-164.

Beck, C. T., & Gable, R. K. (2001). Item response theory in affective instrument development: An illustration. *Journal of Nursing Measurement, 9*, 5-22.

Beck, C. T., & Gable, R. K. (2003). Postpartum Depression Screening Scale—Spanish version, *Nursing Research, 52*, 296-306.

Beck, C. T., & Gable, R. K. (2005). Screening performance of the Postpartum Depression Screening Scale—Spanish Version. *Journal of Transcultural Nursing, 16*, 331-338.

Beck, C. T., & Indman, P. (2005). The many faces of postpartum depression. *Journal of Obstetric, Gynecologic, and Neonatal Nursing, 34*, 569-576.

Beck, C. T., Records, K., & Rice, M. (2006). Further validation of the Postpartum Depression Predictors Inventory—Revised. *Research in Nursing & Health, 29*, 489-497.

Beck, C. T., Reynolds, M., & Rutowski, P. (1992). Maternity blues and postpartum depression. *Journal of Obstetric, Gynecologic, & Neonatal Nursing, 21*, 287-293.

Beck, C. T., Reynolds, M., & Rutowski, P. (1992). Women's verbal estimation of a 40-second interval during the first week postpartum: A replication. *Perceptual and Motor Skills, 74*, 321-322.

Clemmens, D., Driscoll, J., & Beck, C. T. (2004). Postpartum depression as profiled through the Postpartum Depression Screening Scale. *MCN: The American Journal of Maternal Child Nursing, 29*(3), 180-185.

Kennedy, H., Beck, C. T., & Driscoll, J. (2002). A light in the fog: Caring for women with postpartum depression. *Journal of Midwifery & Women's Health, 47*, 318-330.

Le, H., Perry, D., & Sheng, X. (2009). Using the internet to screen for postpartum depression. *Maternal Child Health Journal, 13*, 213-221.

Polit, D., & Beck, C. T. (2006). The content validity index: Are you sure you know what's being reported? *Research in Nursing & Health, 29*, 489-497.

Polit, C., & Beck, C. T. (2007). Is the CVI an acceptable indicator of content validity? Appraisal and recommendations. *Research in Nursing & Health, 30*, 459-467.

Polit, D., & Beck, C. T. (2008). Is there gender bias in nursing research? *Research in Nursing & Health,* 31(5),417-427.

Records, K., Rice, M., & Beck, C. T. (2007). Psychometric assessment of the Postpartum Depression Predictors Inventory—Revised. *Journal of Nursing Measurement, 15*, 189-202.

Rychnovsky, J. D., & Beck, C. T. (2006). Screening for postpartum depression in military women using the Postpartum Depression Screening Scale, *Military Medicine, 171*, 1100-1104.

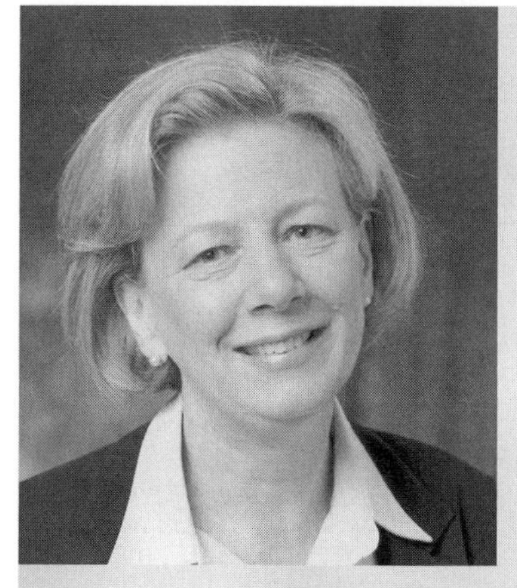

CHAPTER 35

Kristen M. Swanson

1953-present

Theory of Caring

Danuta M. Wojnar

"Caring is a nurturing way of relating to a valued other toward whom one feels a personal sense of commitment and responsibility."(Swanson, 1991, p. 162)

CREDENTIALS AND BACKGROUND OF THE THEORIST

Kristen M. Swanson, R.N., Ph.D., F.A.A.N., was born on January 13, 1953, in Providence, Rhode Island. She earned her baccalaureate degree (magna cum laude) from the University of Rhode Island College of Nursing in 1975. After graduation, Swanson began her career as a registered nurse at the University of Massachusetts Medical Center in Worcester. She was drawn to that institution because the founding nursing administration clearly articulated a vision for professional nursing practice and actively worked with nurses to apply these ideals while working with clients (Swanson, 2001).

As a novice nurse, more than anything Swanson wanted to become a knowledgeable and technically skillful practitioner with an ultimate goal of teaching these skills to others. Thus, she pursued graduate studies in Adult Health and Illness Nursing Program at the University of Pennsylvania in Philadelphia. After receiving a master's degree in nursing (1978), Swanson worked for a year as a clinical instructor of medical-surgical nursing at the University of Pennsylvania School of Nursing and subsequently enrolled in the Ph.D. in nursing program at the University of Colorado in Denver, Colorado. There she studied psychosocial nursing with an emphasis on exploring the concepts of loss, stress, coping, interpersonal relationships, person and personhood, environments, and caring.

While a doctoral student, as part of a hands-on experience with a self-selected health promotion activity, Swanson participated in a cesarean birth support group. At one of the meetings, which focused on miscarriage, she observed that while the guest speaker, a physician, focused on pathophysiology and health problems prevalent after miscarriage, women who attended the meeting were more interested in talking about their personal experiences with pregnancy loss. From that day on, Swanson decided to learn more about the human experience and responses to miscarrying. Caring and miscarriage became the focus of her doctoral dissertation and, subsequently, her program of research.

After earning a Ph.D. in nursing science, Swanson received an individually awarded National Research Service postdoctoral fellowship from the National Center for Nursing Research, which she completed under the direction of Dr. Kathryn E. Barnard at the University of Washington in Seattle. Afterward, she joined the faculty at University of Washington School of Nursing, where she continues scholarly work to this day as a professor and chairperson of the Department of Family Child Nursing. In addition to teaching and administrative responsibilities, Swanson conducts research funded by the National Institutes of Health and National Institutes of Nursing Research, publishes, mentors faculty and students, and serves as a consultant at national and international levels. In recognition of the many outstanding contributions to the development of nursing discipline, among other honors, Swanson was inducted as a fellow in the American Academy of Nursing (1991) and received a Distinguished Alumnus Award from the University of Rhode Island (2002).

THEORETICAL SOURCES

Swanson has drawn on various theoretical sources while developing her Theory of Caring. She recalls that from the beginning of her nursing career, knowledge obtained from book learning and clinical experience made her acutely aware of the profound difference caring made in the lives of people she served:

> Watching patients move into a space of total dependency and come out the other side restored was like witnessing miracles unfold. Sitting with spouses in the waiting room while they entrusted the heart (and lives) of their partner to the surgical team was awe inspiring. It was encouraging to observe the inner reserves family members could call upon in order to hand over that which they could not control. It warmed my heart to be so privileged as to be invited into the spaces that patients and families created in order to endure their transitions through illness, recovery, and, in some instances, death (Swanson, 2001, p. 412).

In addition, Swanson credits several nursing scholars for the insights that shaped her beliefs about the nursing discipline and influenced her program of research. She acknowledges that taking Dr. Jacqueline Fawcett's course on the conceptual basis of nursing practice as a master's-prepared nurse not only made her better understand the differences between the goals of nursing and other health disciplines, but also made her realize that caring for others as they go through life transitions of health, illness, healing, and dying was congruent with her personal values (Swanson, 2001). Hence, Swanson chose Dr. Jean Watson as a mentor during her doctoral studies. She attributes the emphasis on exploring the concept of caring in her doctoral dissertation to Dr. Watson's influence. However, despite the close working relationship and emphasis on caring in Swanson's dissertation work, neither Swanson nor Watson has ever seen Swanson's program of research as application of Watson's Theory of Human Caring (Watson, 1979, 1988, 1999). Instead, both Swanson and Watson assert that compatibility of findings on caring in their individual programs of research adds credibility to their theoretical assertions (Swanson, 2001). Swanson also acknowledges Dr. Kathryn E. Barnard for encouraging her to make the transition from the interpretive to contemporary empiricist paradigm, to transfer what she learned and postulated about caring through several phenomenological investigations to guide intervention research and, hopefully, clinical practice with women who have miscarried.

MAJOR CONCEPTS & DEFINITIONS

CARING

Caring is a nurturing way of relating to a valued other toward whom one feels a personal sense of commitment and responsibility (Swanson, 1991).

KNOWING

Knowing is striving to understand the meaning of an event in the life of the other, avoiding assumptions, focusing on the person cared for, seeking cues, assessing meticulously, and engaging both the one caring and the one cared for in the process of knowing (Swanson, 1991).

BEING WITH

Being with means being emotionally present to the other. It includes being there in person, conveying availability, and sharing feelings without burdening the one cared for (Swanson, 1991).

DOING FOR

Doing for means to do for others what one would do for self if at all possible, including anticipating needs, comforting, performing skillfully and competently, and protecting the one cared for while preserving his or her dignity (Swanson, 1991).

ENABLING

Enabling is facilitating the other's passage through life transitions and unfamiliar events by focusing on the event, informing, explaining, supporting, validating feelings, generating alternatives, thinking things through, and giving feedback (Swanson, 1991).

MAINTAINING BELIEF

Maintaining belief is sustaining faith in the other's capacity to get through an event or transition and face a future with meaning, believing in other's capacity and holding him or her in high esteem, maintaining a hope-filled attitude, offering realistic optimism, helping to find meaning, and standing by the one cared for no matter what the situation (Swanson, 1991).

USE OF EMPIRICAL EVIDENCE

Swanson formulated her Theory of Caring inductively, as a result of several investigations. For her doctoral dissertation, using descriptive phenomenology, Swanson analyzed data obtained from in-depth interviews with 20 women who had recently miscarried. As a result of this phenomenological investigation, Swanson proposed two models:

1. The Caring Model
2. The Human Experience of Miscarriage Model

The Caring Model, in which Swanson proposed that five basic processes (knowing, being with, doing for, enabling, and maintaining belief) give meaning to acts labeled as caring (Swanson-Kauffman, 1986, 1988a, 1988b), later became the foundation for Swanson's (1991) middle range Theory of Caring.

While a postdoctoral fellow, Swanson conducted another phenomenological study, which explored what it was like to be a provider of care to vulnerable infants in the neonatal intensive care unit (NICU). As a result of this investigation, Swanson (1990) discovered that the caring processes she identified with women who miscarried were also applicable to mothers, fathers, physicians, and nurses who were responsible for taking care of infants in the NICU. Hence, she decided to retain the wording that described the acts of caring and proposed all-inclusive care in a complex environment embraces balance among caring (for self and the one cared for), attaching (to others and roles), managing responsibilities (assigned by self, others, and society), and avoiding bad outcomes (Swanson, 1990).

In a subsequent phenomenological investigation conducted with socially at-risk mothers, Swanson (1991) explored what it had been like for these mothers to receive an intense, long-term nursing intervention. Swanson recalls that after this study, she was finally able to define caring and further refine the understanding of caring processes. Collectively, phenomenological inquiries with women who miscarried, with caregivers in the NICU, and with socially at-risk mothers provided the basis for expanding the Caring Model into the middle range Theory of Caring (Swanson, 1991, 1993).

Later, Swanson tested her Theory of Caring with women who miscarried in several investigations funded by the National Institutes of Health, National Institutes of Nursing Research, and other funding sources. Swanson's (1999a, 1999b) intervention research ($N = 242$) focused on examining the effects of caring-based counseling sessions on the women's coming to terms with loss and emotional well-being during the first year after miscarrying. Additional aims of the project were to examine the effects of the passage of time on healing during that first year and to develop strategies to monitor caring interventions. This study established that although passing of time had positive effects on women's healing after miscarriage, caring interventions had a positive impact on decreasing the overall disturbed mood, anger, and level of depression. The second aim of this investigation was to monitor the caring variable and identify whether caring was delivered as intended. To do so, caring was monitored in the following three ways:

1. Approximately 10% of counseling sessions were transcribed and data were analyzed using inductive and deductive content analysis.
2. Before each caring session, the counselor completed McNair, Lorr, and Droppleman's (1981) Profile of Mood States to monitor whether the counselor's mood was associated with women's ratings of caring after each session, using an investigator-developed Caring Professional Scale.
3. After each session, the counselor completed an investigator-developed Counselor Rating Scale and took narrative notes about her own counseling.

The most noteworthy finding of monitoring caring was that, overall, the clients were highly satisfied with caring received during counseling sessions, suggesting that caring was delivered and received as intended.

Swanson's (1999c) subsequent investigation was a literary meta-analysis on caring. An in-depth review of 130 investigations on caring led Swanson to propose that knowledge about caring may be categorized into five hierarchical domains (levels) and that research conducted in any one domain assumes the presence of all previous domains (Swanson, 1999c). The first domain refers to the persons' capacities to deliver caring; the second domain refers to individuals' concerns and commitments that lead to caring actions; the third domain refers to the conditions (nurse, client, organizational) that enhance or diminish likelihood of delivering caring; the fourth domain refers to actions of caring; and the fifth domain refers to the consequences or the intentional and unintentional outcomes of caring for both the client and the provider (Swanson, 1999c). Conducting the literary meta-analysis clarified the meaning of the concept of caring as it is used in nursing discipline and validated transferability of Swanson's middle range Theory of Caring beyond the perinatal context.

Most recently, Swanson conducted an intervention study funded by the National Institutes of Health called Couples Miscarriage Healing Project. The purposes of this investigation were to better understand the effects of miscarriage on men and women as individuals and as couples, to explore the effects of miscarriage on couple relationships, and to identify best ways of helping men and women heal as individuals and as couples after unexpected pregnancy loss. Study participants (341 heterosexual couples) were randomly assigned to control or one of the following three treatment groups: (1) nurse caring, which entailed attending three counseling sessions with a nurse, (2) self-caring, which involved completing three videos and workbooks, or (3) combined caring, which involved attending one nurse caring session and three videos and workbooks, to determine the most effective way of supporting couples after miscarriage. All interventions were designed and delivered within Swanson's Theory of Caring framework. Ongoing data analysis has shown that while both genders are affected by early-unexpected pregnancy loss, women experience more pure grief and depression than men. Moreover, Swanson found that caring interventions were effective in facilitating couples' healing. Currently, articles discussing study findings are being prepared for publication.

MAJOR ASSUMPTIONS

In 1993, Swanson further developed her theory of informed caring by making explicit her major assumptions about the four main phenomena of concern to the nursing discipline: nursing, person/client, health, and environment.

Nursing

Swanson (1991, 1993) defines nursing as informed caring for the well-being of others. She asserts that the nursing discipline is informed by empirical knowledge from nursing and other related disciplines, as well as "ethical, personal and aesthetic knowledge derived from the humanities, clinical experience, and personal and societal values and expectations" (Swanson, 1993, p. 352).

Person

Swanson (1993) defines persons as "unique beings who are in the midst of becoming and whose wholeness is made manifest in thoughts, feelings, and behaviors" (p. 352). She posits that the life experiences of each individual are influenced by a complex interplay of "a genetic heritage, spiritual endowment and the capacity to exercise free will" (Swanson, 1993, p. 352). Hence, persons both shape and are shaped by the environment in which they live.

Swanson (1993) views persons as dynamic, growing, self-reflecting, yearning to be connected with others, and spiritual beings. She suggests the following: " . . . spiritual endowment connects each being to an eternal and universal source of goodness, mystery, life, creativity, and serenity. The spiritual endowment may be a soul, higher power/Holy Spirit, positive energy, or, simply grace. Free will equates with choice and the capacity to decide how to act when confronted with a range of possibilities" (p. 352). Swanson (1993) noted, however, that limitations set by race, class, gender, or access to care might prevent individuals from exercising free will. Hence, acknowledging free will mandates the nursing discipline to honor individuality and to consider a whole range of possibilities that are acceptable or desirable for those whom nurses attend.

Moreover, Swanson posits that the other, whose personhood nursing discipline serves, refers to families, groups, and societies. Thus, with this understanding of personhood, nurses are mandated to take on leadership roles in fighting for human rights, equal access to health care, and other humanitarian causes. Lastly, when nurses think about the other to whom they direct their caring, they also need to think of self and other nurses and their care as that cared-for other.

Health

According to Swanson (1993), to experience health and well-being is:

> " . . . to live the subjective, meaning-filled experience of wholeness. Wholeness involves a sense of integration and becoming wherein all facets of being are free to be expressed. The facets of being include the many selves that make us a human: our spirituality, thoughts, feelings, intelligence, creativity, relatedness, femininity, masculinity, and sexuality, to name just a few" (p. 353).

Thus, Swanson sees reestablishing well-being as a complex process of curing and healing that includes "releasing inner pain, establishing new meanings, restoring integration, and emerging into a sense of renewed wholeness" (Swanson, 1993, p. 353).

Environment

Swanson (1993) defines environment situationally. She maintains that for nursing, it is "any context that influences or is influenced by the designated client" (p. 353). Swanson states that there are many kinds of influences on environment, such as the cultural, social, biophysical, political, and economic realms, to name only a few. According to Swanson (1993), the terms *environment* and *person-client* in nursing may be viewed interchangeably. For example, Swanson posits, "for heuristic purposes the lens on environment/designated client may be specified to the intra-individual level, wherein the 'client' may be at the cellular level and the environment may be the organs, tissues or body of which the cell is a component" (p. 353). Therefore, what is considered an environment in one situation may be considered client in another.

THEORETICAL ASSERTIONS

Swanson's Theory of Caring (Swanson, 1991, 1993, 1999b) was empirically derived through phenomenological inquiry. It offers a clear explanation of what it means for nurses to practice in a caring manner. It emphasizes that the goal of nursing is to promote the well-being of others. Swanson (1991) defines caring as "a nurturing way of relating to a valued other toward whom one feels a personal sense of commitment and responsibility" (p. 162).

According to Swanson, a fundamental and universal component of good nursing is caring for the client's biopsychosocial and spiritual well-being. Swanson (1993) asserts that caring is grounded in maintenance of a basic belief in human beings, supported by knowing the client's reality, conveyed by being emotionally and physically present, and enacted by doing for and enabling the client. The caring processes are overlapping and may not exist in separation from each other. Each of them is an integral component of the overarching structure of caring (Figure 35-1). In summarizing the caring relationships between nurses and clients, Swanson (1993) noted that the repertoire of caring therapeutics of novice nurses might be somewhat limited and restricted by inexperience. Conversely, the techniques and knowledge imbedded in the caring of experienced nurses are so elaborate and subtle that caring might go unnoticed by an uninformed observer.

Yet, Swanson (1993) asserts that, regardless of the years of nursing experience, caring is delivered as a set of sequential processes (subconcepts) that are

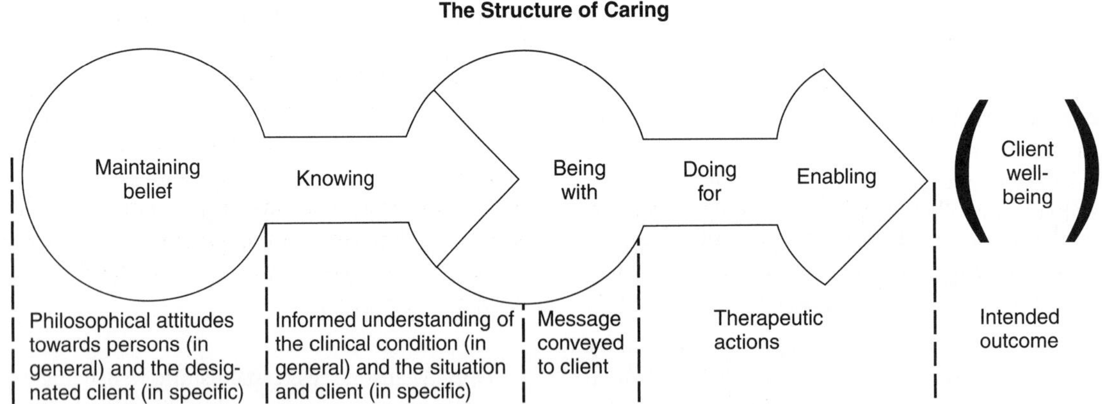

Figure 35-1 The structure of caring as linked to the nurse's philosophical attitude, informed understandings, message conveyed, therapeutic actions, and intended outcome. (From Swanson, K. M. [1993]. Nursing as informed caring for the well-being of others. *Image: The Journal of Nursing Scholarship, 25*[4], 352-357.)

created by the nurse's own philosophical attitude (maintaining belief), understanding (knowing), verbal and nonverbal messages conveyed to the client (being with), and therapeutic actions (doing for and enabling), and the consequences of caring (intended client outcome).

LOGICAL FORM

Swanson's middle range Theory of Caring was developed empirically using inductive methodology. Chinn and Kramer (2004, 2008) have proposed that with inductive reasoning, hypotheses and relationships are induced by experiencing or observing phenomena and reaching conclusions. Swanson's theory was generated from phenomenological investigations with women who experienced unexpected pregnancy loss, caregivers to premature and ill babies in the newborn intensive care unit (NICU), and socially at-risk mothers who received long-term care from master's-prepared nurses. Swanson (1991) posits that caring, as a nurturing way of relating to another human being, is not the sole domain of perinatal nursing. In fact, she purports that knowing, being with, doing for, enabling, and maintaining belief are essential components of any nurse-client relationship. She claims that her in-depth meta-analysis of research on caring supports the generality of her theory beyond perinatal context (Swanson, 1999c).

ACCEPTANCE BY THE NURSING COMMUNITY

Practice

The usefulness of Swanson's Theory of Caring has been demonstrated in research, education, and clinical practice. The proposition that caring is central to nursing practice had its beginning in the theorist's own insights into the importance of caring in professional nursing practice and in the findings from Swanson's phenomenological investigations. Her subsequent investigations demonstrated applicability of the Theory of Caring in clinical nursing practice and research. Hence, Swanson's theory has been embraced as a framework for professional nursing practice by various organizations in the United States, Canada, and Sweden. An example is the Dalhousie University School of Nursing in Halifax, Nova Scotia, Canada, which selected Swanson's Theory of Caring to guide development of future generations of nurses as caring professionals. Likewise, nurses at IWK (Izaak Walton Killam) Health Centre, a tertiary care hospital for women, children, and families in Halifax, Nova Scotia, recognized the traditional legacy of nursing as a caring-healing discipline and the concepts in Swanson's theory as applicable in practice. Thus, since 1998, Nursing Practice Council at IWK used Swanson's Theory of Caring as their framework for professional nursing practice.

Reynolds (1971) has proposed that theory provides a sense of understanding and applicability in practice. Nurse caring may be manifested in a variety of ways and in many practice contexts. For example, in a postpartum context, demonstrating how to do a baby bath to new parents with competence and sensitivity incorporates all five caring processes. The act involves doing for (demonstrating bathing the newborn as parents would otherwise have done if they had the skill); the unrushed timing of the bath to make sure that infant is in an awake state and parents are present conveys willingness to be with; and the observing, querying, and involving parents in the task engages them in their own infant's care (enabling) while acknowledging that they are perfectly capable of caring for their new child and that their preferences matter (maintaining belief and knowing). In carrying out this seemingly simple act, the nurse can create an optimal environment for learning and enabling new parents to make decisions about infant care, while leveraging the task as an opportunity to engage in a meaningful social encounter and developing a trusting relationship.

Education

Caring is a concept difficult to embrace without understanding. Humane and altruistic caring that occurs when the theory is used in practice ranges from the simplicity of feeding or grooming an incapacitated elder, to the complexity of monitoring and managing the recovery of a patient who suffered a stroke, to enhancing infant care skills of new parents. Nurse caring, as demonstrated by Swanson in research with women who miscarried, caregivers in the NICU, and socially at-risk mothers, recognizes the importance of attending to the wholeness of humans in their everyday lives. Thus Swanson's theory offers teachers of modern day nursing a simple way of initiating students into the profession by immersing them in the language of what it means to be caring and cared for to promote, restore, or maintain optimal wellness of individuals.

Research

Swanson has persisted in the development of her theory, from describing and defining the concept of caring and basic caring processes, to instrument development and testing in intervention research with women and men who experienced unexpected pregnancy loss. Recent review of computerized databases (MEDLINE, CINHAL, and Digital Dissertations) indicated that Swanson's work on caring and miscarriage has been cited or otherwise utilized in over 160 data-based publications. Latest examples of application of Swanson's Theory of Caring in clinical research include exploration of clinical scholarship in practice (Kish & Holder, 1996), guidelines for nurses working with patients diagnosed with multiple sclerosis (Yorkston, Klasner, & Swanson, 2001), assessing impact of caring in work with vulnerable populations (Kavanaugh, Moro, Savage, & Mehendale, 2006), the importance of creating a caring environment in work with the elderly (Sikma, 2006), and Wojnar's (2007) study of lesbian couples who miscarried, to name only a few.

FURTHER DEVELOPMENT

Swanson implies that she is more interested in testing and applying her theory in clinical practice than in its further development. Yet, there is much potential for further development and testing of Swanson's Theory of Caring in diverse contexts of health and illness. Conceivably, her claim about what constitutes caring may be applicable in other helping disciplines such as teaching, social work, and medicine, and in various life situations beyond nursing.

CRITIQUE

Clarity

Clarity refers to how well the theory can be understood and how clearly and consistently the concepts are presented and conceptualized (Chinn & Kramer, 2004, 2008). Meleis (2007) states, "it denotes precision of boundaries, a communication of a sense of orderliness, vividness of meaning and consistency throughout the theory" (p. 258). The concept of caring, central to the theory, and caring processes (knowing, being with, doing for, enabling, and maintaining belief) are clearly defined and arranged in a logical sequence that describes how caring is delivered. Moreover, Swanson's theory offers clear definitions of the main domains of nursing discipline (person, nurse, environment, and health) and describes them indirectly in various contexts in which nurse-client interactions take place. By doing so, Swanson further explicates the definitions.

Simplicity

A simple theory has a minimal number of concepts. Swanson's Theory of Caring is simple yet elegant. It brings to the forefront the importance of caring, which exemplifies the discipline's traditional and modern values. Its main purpose is to help practitioners deliver nursing care that focuses on the needs of individuals in a way that fosters their dignity, respect, and empowerment. Simplicity and consistency of language used to define the concepts allows students and nurses to understand and apply Swanson's theory in practice.

Generality

Swanson's Theory of Caring may be applied in research and clinical work with diverse populations. The conditions essential for delivering caring that promotes individuals' wholeness across the life span have been described clearly (Swanson, 1999c). Hence, the theory is generalizable to any nurse-client relationship and any clinical setting.

Empirical Precision

Swanson's Theory of Caring assumes that applying caring processes in therapeutic communication with clients enhances comfort and accelerates healing. The concepts and assumptions are grounded in clinical nursing practice and research and are congruent. The completeness and simplicity of operational definitions strengthen the empirical precision of this theory. Swanson (1999a, 1999b) has successfully applied and continues testing her Theory of Caring in a clinical trial with women and couples. Furthermore, she has developed self-report measures to measure caring as delivered by health care professionals and by couples to each other. Both the template for delivering caring-based interventions and the development of research-based measures open possibilities for use and further testing with other populations.

Derivable Consequences

Fawcett (1984) suggests that nursing theories differentiate the focus of nursing from other helping disciplines. Swanson's theory of caring describes nurse-client relationships that promote wholeness and healing. Hence, the theory offers a framework for enhancing contemporary nursing practice while bringing the discipline to its traditional caring-healing roots. However, as Swanson purports, the Theory of Caring may be applied to caring relationships beyond nurse-client encounters, therefore, it does not meet the criterion of differentiating caring as solely within the domain of nursing.

Case Study

The birth of a child is one of the most memorable experiences in a woman's life. You are a birth unit nurse, and at the change of a shift, you are assigned to care for a teen mother who came to hospital alone and is now in active labor. When you arrive in her room, you notice that she is teary and appears frightened. Describe how you would apply Swanson's theory to connect emotionally and deliver caring in your work with this young mother.

CRITICAL THINKING Activities

1. Consider Swanson's caring theory as a framework for your own nursing practice. In what ways is it applicable?
2. Think about a time when you felt that someone cared about you deeply. What was it like for you to experience caring? What was most special in your interactions with that person?
3. Think about an interaction with a client-family in your clinical practice that you wish you could change or improve. Use the processes of the Theory of Caring to think critically about where you might have made more appropriate choices. If it were possible to improve this interaction, what would you change and why?

POINTS FOR Further Study

- Swanson, K. M. (1993). Nursing as informed caring for the well-being of others. *Image: The Journal of Nursing Scholarship, 25*(4), 352-357.
- Swanson, K. M. (1998). Caring made visible. *Creative Nursing, 4*(4), 8-11, 16.
- Swanson, K. M. (1999a). Research-based practice with women who have had miscarriages. *Image: The Journal of Nursing Scholarship, 31*(4), 339-345.
- Swanson, K. M. (1999b). The effects of caring, measurement, and time on miscarriage impact and women's well-being in the first year subsequent to loss. *Nursing Research, 48*(6), 288-298.
- Swanson, K. M. (1999c). What's known about caring in nursing: A literary meta-analysis. In A. S. Hinshaw, J. Shaver,

& S. Feetham (Eds.), *Handbook of clinical nursing research* (pp. 31-60). Thousand Oaks, CA: Sage.

- Swanson, K. M., & Wojnar, D. (2004). Optimal healing environments in nursing. *Journal of Alternative and Complementary Medicine, 10*(1), 43-48.

REFERENCES

Chinn, P. L., & Kramer, M. (2004). *Integrated knowledge development in nursing* (6th ed.). St. Louis: Mosby.

Chinn, P. L., & Kramer, M. (2008). *Integrated knowledge development in nursing* (7th ed.). St. Louis: Mosby-Elsevier

Fawcett, J. (1984). The metaparadigm of nursing: Current status and future refinements. *Image: The Journal of Nursing Scholarship, 16*, 84-87.

Kavanaugh, K., Moro, T. T., Savage, T., & Mehendale, R. (2006). Enacting a theory of caring to recruit and retain vulnerable populations for sensitive research. *Research in Nursing and Health. 29*(3), 244-252.

Kish, C. P., & Holder, L. M. (1996). Helping to say goodbye: merging clinical scholarship with community service. *Holistic Nursing Practice, 10*(3), 74-82.

McNair, D. M., Lorr, M., & Droppleman, L. F. (1981). *Profile of mood states: Manual.* San Diego: Educational and Industrial Testing Service.

Meleis, A. I. (2007). *Theoretical nursing: Development and progress.* Philadelphia: Lippincott Williams & Wilkins.

Reynolds, P. D. (1971). *A primer of theory construction.* Indianapolis: Bobbs-Merrill.

Sikma, S. (2006). Staff perceptions of caring. The importance of a supportive environment. *Journal of Gerontological Nursing, 32*(6), 22-29.

Swanson, K. M. (1990). Providing care in the NICU: Sometimes an act of love. *ANS Advances in Nursing Science, 13*(1), 60-73.

Swanson, K. M. (1991). Empirical development of a middle range theory of caring. *Nursing Research, 40*(3), 161-166.

Swanson, K. M. (1993). Nursing as informed caring for the well-being of others. *Image: The Journal of Nursing Scholarship, 25*(4), 352-357.

Swanson, K. M. (1999a). Research-based practice with women who have had miscarriages. *Image: The Journal of Nursing Scholarship, 31*(4), 339-345.

Swanson, K. M. (1999b). The effects of caring, measurement, and time on miscarriage impact and women's well-being in the first year subsequent to loss. *Nursing Research, 48*(6), 288-298.

Swanson, K. M. (1999c). What's known about caring in nursing: A literary meta-analysis. In A. S. Hinshaw, J. Shaver, & S. Feetham (Eds.), *Handbook of clinical nursing research* (pp. 31-60). Thousand Oaks, CA: Sage.

Swanson, K. M. (2001). A program of research on caring. In M. E. Parker (Ed.), *Nursing theories and nursing practice* (pp. 411-420). Philadelphia: F. A. Davis.

Swanson-Kauffman, K. M. (1986). Caring in the instance of unexpected early pregnancy loss. *Topics in Clinical Nursing, 8*(2), 37-46.

Swanson-Kauffman, K. M. (1988a). The caring needs of women who miscarry. In M. M. Leininger (Ed.), *Care, discovery and uses in clinical and community nursing* (pp. 55-71). Detroit: Wayne State University Press.

Swanson-Kauffman, K. M. (1988b). There should have been two: Nursing care of parents experiencing the perinatal death of a twin. *Journal of Perinatal and Neonatal Nursing, 2*(2), 78-86.

Watson, J. (1979). *Nursing: The philosophy and science of caring.* Boston: Little & Brown.

Watson, J. (1988). New dimensions of human caring theory. *Nursing Science Quarterly, 1*, 175-181.

Watson, J. (1999). *Nursing: Human science and human care: A theory of nursing.* Sudbury, MA: Jones & Bartlett.

Wojnar, D. M. (2007). Miscarriage Experiences of Lesbian Birth and Social Mothers: Couples' perspective: *Journal of Midwifery and Women's Health, 52*(5), 479-485.

Yorkston, K. M., Klasner, E. R., & Swanson, K. M. (2001). Communication in multiple sclerosis: Understanding the insider's perspective. *American Journal of Speech Language Pathology, 10*, 126-137.

BIBLIOGRAPHY
Primary Sources
Book Chapters

Swanson, K. M. (1992). Foreword. In S. Wheeler & M. Pike (Eds.), *Grief ltd. manual.* Covington, IN: Grief Limited.

Swanson, K. M. (1999c). What's known about caring in nursing: A literary meta-analysis. In A. S. Hinshaw, J. Shaver, & S. Feetham (Eds.), *Handbook of clinical nursing research* (pp. 31-60). Thousand Oaks, CA: Sage.

Swanson, K. M. (2001). A program of research on caring. In M. E. Parker (Ed.), *Nursing theories and nursing practice* (pp. 411-420). Philadelphia: Davis.

Swanson, K. M. (2002). Caring Professional Scale. In J. Watson (Ed.), *Assessing and measuring caring in nursing and health science* (pp. 203-206). New York: Springer.

Swanson-Kauffman, K. M. (1987). Overview of the balancing act: Having it all. In K. Swanson-Kauffman (Ed.), *Women's work, families and health.* New York: Hemisphere. (Reprint of Swanson-Kauffman, K. M. [1987]. Overview of the balancing act: Having it all. *Health Care of Women International, 8*[2-3], 101-108.)

Swanson-Kauffman, K. M. (1988). The caring needs of women who miscarry. In M. M. Leininger (Ed.), *Care, discovery and uses in clinical and community nursing* (pp. 55-71). Detroit: Wayne State University Press.

Swanson-Kauffman, K. M., & Roberts, J. (1990). Caring in parent and child nursing. In *Knowledge about care and caring: State of the art and future development.* Washington, D.C.: American Academy of Nursing.

Swanson-Kauffman, K. M., & Schonwald, E. (1988). Phenomenology. In B. Sarter (Ed.), *Paths to knowledge: Innovative research methods for nursing* (pp. 97-105). New York: National League for Nursing Publications.

Yorkston, K. M., Klasner, E. R., & Swanson, K. M. (2001). Communication in multiple sclerosis: Understanding the insider's perspective. *American Journal of Speech Language Pathology, 10*, 126-137.

Journal Articles

Grant, S. & Swanson, K. M. (2006). Steaming the tide of the nursing shortage. *The CERNER Quarterly, 2*(2), 34-35.

Jennings, B. M., Heiner, S. L., Loan, L. A., Hemman, E. A., & Swanson, K. M (2005). What really matters to health care consumers. *Journal of Nursing Administration, 35*(4), 173-180.

Jennings, B. M., Loan, L. A., Heiner, S. L., Hemman, E. A., & Swanson, K. M. (2005). Soldiers' experiences with military health care. *Military Medicine, 170*(12), 999-1004.

Quinn, J., Smith, M., Ritenbaugh, C., & Swanson, K. M. (2003). Research guidelines for assessing the impact of the healing relationship in clinical nursing. *Alternative Therapies, 9*(31), 69-79.

Swanson, K. M. (1990). Providing care in the NICU: Sometimes an act of love. *ANS Advances in Nursing Science, 13*(1), 60-73.

Swanson, K. M. (1991). Empirical development of a middle range theory of caring. *Nursing Research, 40*(3), 161-166.

Swanson, K. M. (1993). Commentary: The phenomena of doing well in people with AIDS. *Western Journal of Nursing Research, 15*(1), 56.

Swanson, K. M. (1993). Nursing as informed caring for the well-being of others. *Image: The Journal of Nursing Scholarship, 25*(4), 352-357.

Swanson, K. M. (1995). Commentary, the power of human caring: Early recognition of patient problems. *Scholarly Inquiry for Nursing Practice, 9*(4), 319-321.

Swanson, K. M. (1998). Caring made visible. *Creative Nursing, 4*(4), 8-11, 16.

Swanson, K. M. (1999). Research-based practice with women who have had miscarriages. *Image: The Journal of Nursing Scholarship, 31*(4) 339-345.

Swanson, K. M. (1999). The effects of caring, measurement, and time on miscarriage impact and women's well-being in the first year subsequent to loss. *Nursing Research, 48*(6), 288-298.

Swanson, K. M. (2000). Predicting depressive symptoms after miscarriage: A path analysis based on Lazarus' paradigm. *Journal of Women's Health & Gender-Based Medicine, 9* (2), 191-206.

Swanson, K. M., Connor, S., Jolley, S., Pettinato, M., & Wang, T. J. (2007). Context and evolution of women's responses to miscarriage during the first year after loss. *Research in Nursing and Health, 30*(1), 2-16.

Swanson, K. M., Karmali, Z., Powell, S., & Pulvermakher, F. (2003). Miscarriage effects on couples' interpersonal and sexual relationships during the first year after loss: Women's perceptions. *Psychosomatic Medicine, 65*(5), 902-910.

Swanson, K. M., & Wojnar, D. (2004). Optimal healing environments in nursing. *Journal of Alternative and Complementary Medicine, 10*(1), 43-48.

Swanson-Kauffman, K. M. (1981). Echocardiography: An access route to the heart. *Critical Care Nurse, 1*(6), 20-26.

Swanson-Kauffman, K. M. (1986). A combined qualitative methodology for nursing research. *ANS Advances in Nursing Science, 8*(3), 58-69.

Swanson-Kauffman, K. M. (1986). Caring in the instance of unexpected early pregnancy loss. *Topics in Clinical Nursing, 8*(2), 37-46.

Swanson-Kauffman, K. M. (1987). Overview of the balancing act: Having it all. *Health Care for Women International, 8*(2-3), 1-8.

Swanson-Kauffman, K. M. (1988). There should have been two: Nursing care of parents experiencing the perinatal death of a twin. *Journal of Perinatal and Neonatal Nursing, 2*(2), 78-86.

Wojnar, D. M., & Swanson, K. M. (2006). Why shouldn't lesbian miscarriage receive special consideration? A viewpoint. *Journal of GLTB Family Studies, 2*(1), 1-12.

Wojnar, D. M., & Swanson, K. M. (2007). Phenomenology: an exploration. *Journal of Holistic Nursing, 25*(3), 172-180; discussion 181-182, quiz 183-185.

Yorkston, K. M., Klasner, E. R., & Swanson, K. M. (2001). Communication in multiple sclerosis: Understanding the insider's perspective. *American Journal of Speech Language Pathology, 10*, 126-137.

Dissertation

Swanson-Kauffman, K. M. (1983). *The unborn one: A profile of the human experience of miscarriage.* Unpublished doctoral dissertation, University of Colorado, Denver.

Newsletters and Reprints

Swanson-Kauffman, K. M. (1984, Spring). A methodology for the study of nursing as a human science. *Alpha Kappa Chapter at Large News*, 3.

Swanson-Kauffman, K. M. (1987). Caring in the instance of unexpected early pregnancy loss. *Counselor Connection, 3*(2), 2-5. (Reprint of Swanson-Kauffman, K. M. [1986]. Caring in the instance of unexpected early pregnancy loss. *Topics in Clinical Nursing, 8*[2], 37-46.)

Swanson-Kauffman, K. M. (1988). Miscarriage: An often-overlooked maternal loss. *Perinatal Newsletter, 2*(3), 1.

Published Abstracts

Swanson, K. M. (1993). Caring as intervention (Abstract). *Communicating Nursing Research, 26*, 299.

Swanson, K. M. (1993). Caring theory: Structure and assumptions (Abstract). *Communicating Nursing Research, 26*, 255.

Swanson, K. M. (1995). Effects of caring on healing post miscarriage (Abstract). *Communicating Nursing Research, 28*, 281.

Swanson, K. M., Kieckhefer, G., Henderson, D., Powers, P., Leppa, C., & Carr, K. (1991). Miscarriage: Patterns of meaning (Abstract). *Communicating Nursing Research, 24*, 110.

Swanson, K. M., Kieckhefer, G., Powers, P., & Carr, K. (1990). Meaning of miscarriage scale: Establishment of psychometric properties (Abstract). *Communicating Nursing Research, 23*, 89.

Swanson, K. M., Klaich, K., & Leppa, C. (1992). A caring intervention to promote well-being in women who miscarry (Abstract). *Communicating Nursing Research, 25*, 365.

Swanson, K. M., Pulvermakher, F., Karmali, Z., & Powell, S. (2001). Effects of miscarriage on couple relationships (Abstract). *Communicating Nursing Research, 34*, 339.

Swanson, K. M., Taylor, G., Shipman, L., Spoor K., & Zillyet, K. (2002). Miscarriage and healing amongst the Shoalwater (Abstract). *Communicating Nursing Research, 35*, 135.

Swanson, K. M., Wojnar, D. M., Petras, A., Chen, H., & Graham, C. (2008). Effects of caring on couples' grief after miscarriage. *Communicating Nursing Research, 40*, 162.

Swanson-Kauffman, K. M. (1984). A profile of the human experience of miscarriage (Abstract). *Communicating Nursing Research, 6*(3), 46.

Swanson-Kauffman, K. M. (1985). A combined qualitative methodology for nursing research (Abstract). *Communicating Nursing Research, 18*, 57.

Swanson-Kauffman, K. M. (1986). Work and family: The delicate balance. Symposium (Abstract). *Communicating Nursing Research, 19*, 153-156.

Swanson-Kauffman, K. M. (1988). Empirical development and refinement of a model of caring (Abstract). *Communicating Nursing Research, 21*, 80.

Swanson-Kauffman, K. M. (1989). From phenomenological to experimental design: Qualitative inquiry as a framework for the intervention (Abstract). *Communicating Nursing Research, 22*, 147.

Swanson-Kauffman, K. M., Powers, P., Klaich, K., Lethbridge, D., & Jarrett, M. (1990). Success: As women view it (Abstract). *Communicating Nursing Research, 23*, 59.

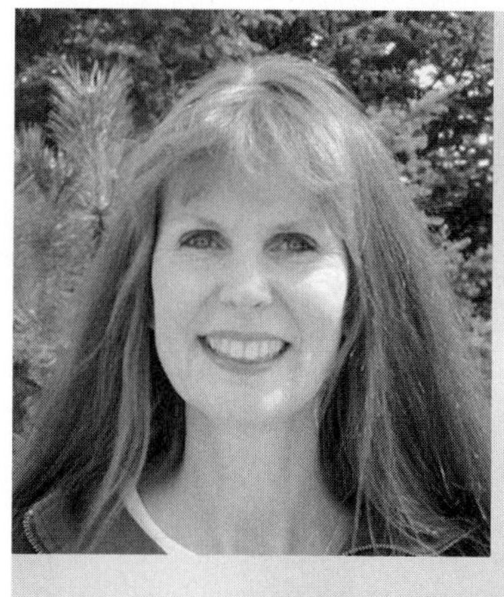

CHAPTER

36

Cornelia M. Ruland

1954-present

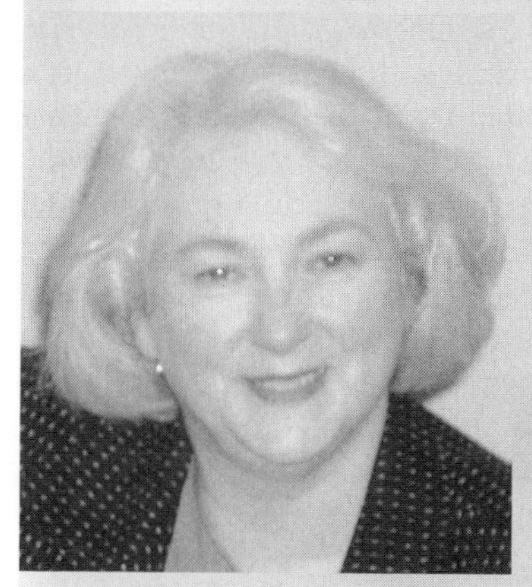

Shirley M. Moore

1948-present

Peaceful End of Life Theory

Patricia A. Higgins

"Standards of care offer a promising approach for the development of middle-range prescriptive theories because of their empirical base in clinical practice and their focus on linkages between interventions and outcomes." (Ruland & Moore, 1998, p. 169)

CREDENTIALS AND BACKGROUND OF THE THEORISTS

Cornelia M. Ruland

Cornelia M. Ruland received her Ph.D. in nursing from Case Western Reserve University, Cleveland, Ohio, in 1998. She is now the Director of the Center for Shared Decision Making and Nursing Research at Rikshospitalet University Hospital in Oslo, Norway. She also holds an appointment as adjunct faculty at the Department of Biomedical Informatics, Columbia University, in New York. Ruland has established an extensive research program on improving shared decision making and patient-provider partnerships in health care, and the development, implementation, and evaluation of information systems to support it. Her focus is on aspects of and tools for shared decision making in clinically challenging situations: (1) when patients are confronted with difficult treatment or screening decisions for which they need help to understand the potential benefits and harms of alternative options and to elicit their values and preferences, and (2) preference-adjusted management of chronic or serious long-term illness over time. Ruland has been the primary investigator on a number of research projects and has received several awards for her work.

The author wishes to express her appreciation to Cornelia Ruland and Shirley Moore for their contributions to the chapter.

Shirley M. Moore

Shirley M. Moore is Associate Dean for Research and Professor, School of Nursing, Case Western Reserve University. She received her diploma in nursing from the Youngstown Hospital Association School of Nursing (1969) and her bachelor's degree in nursing from Kent State University (1974). At Case Western Reserve University, she earned a master's degree in psychiatric and mental health nursing (1990), as well as a Ph.D. in nursing science (1993). She has taught nursing theory and nursing science to all levels of nursing students and conducts a program of research and theory development that addresses recovery after cardiac events. Early in her own doctoral study, Moore was encouraged by nurse theorists Joyce J. Fitzpatrick, Jean Johnson, and Elizabeth Lenz to not only use theory but to develop it as well. The Rosemary Ellis Theory Conference, held annually for several years at Case Western Reserve University, offered Moore another opportunity to explore theory as a practical tool for practitioners, researchers, and teachers. Influenced by these experiences, Moore has assisted in the development and publication of several theories (Good & Moore, 1996; Huth & Moore, 1998; Ruland & Moore, 1998) and has considered theory construction a skill essential to doctoral students.

THEORETICAL SOURCES

The Peaceful End of Life (EOL) Theory is informed by a number of theoretical frameworks (Ruland & Moore, 1998). It is based primarily on Donabedian's model of structure, process, and outcomes, which in part was developed from general system theory. The influence of general system theory is pervasive in other types of nursing theory, from conceptual models to middle and microrange theories—an indicator of its usefulness in explaining the complexity of health care interactions and organizations. In the EOL theory, the structure-setting is the family system (terminally ill patient and all significant others) that is receiving care from professionals on an acute care hospital unit, and process is defined as those actions (nursing interventions) designed to promote the positive outcomes of the following: (1) being free from pain, (2) experiencing comfort, (3) experiencing dignity and respect, (4) being at peace, and (5) experiencing a closeness to significant others and those who care.

A second theoretical underpinning is preference theory (Brandt, 1979), which has been used by philosophers to explain and define quality of life (Sandoe, 1999), a concept that is significant in EOL research and practice. In preference theory, the good life is defined as getting what one wants, an approach that seems particularly appropriate in EOL care. It can be applied to both sentient persons and incapacitated persons who have previously provided documentation related to EOL decision making. Quality of life, therefore, is defined and evaluated as a manifestation of satisfaction through empirical assessment of such outcomes as symptom relief and satisfaction with interpersonal relationships. Incorporating patient preferences into health care decisions is considered both appropriate (Ruland & Bakken, 2001; Ruland, Kresevic, & Lorensen, 1997) and necessary for successful processes and outcomes (Ruland & Moore, 2001).

This theory was derived in a doctoral theory course in which Ruland was a student and Moore was the faculty. Middle range theories were just emerging, and there were few good definitions or examples. The class was challenged to think about the future use and development of middle range theory for nursing science and practice. The students discussed knowledge sources from which they could derive middle range theory, such as empirical knowledge, clinical practice knowledge, and synthesized knowledge. Each student was asked to derive a middle range theory from a knowledge source of choice. Ruland had just completed a major project to develop a clinical practice standard for peaceful EOL with a group of cancer nurses in Norway. The standard was synthesized into the theory of peaceful EOL by Ruland and later was refined with Moore's assistance. This is an example of middle range theory developed by doctoral nursing students as they study knowledge development methods. This theory is also an example of early middle range theory development using a standard of practice as a source.

MAJOR CONCEPTS & DEFINITIONS

NOT BEING IN PAIN

Being free of the suffering or symptom distress is the central part of many patients' EOL experience. Pain is considered an unpleasant sensory or emotional experience associated with actual or potential tissue damage (Lenz, Suppe, Gift, Pugh, & Milligan, 1995; Pain terms, 1979).

EXPERIENCE OF COMFORT

Comfort is defined inclusively, using Kolcaba and Kolcaba's (1991) work as "relief from discomfort, the state of ease and peaceful contentment, and whatever makes life easy or pleasurable" (Ruland & Moore, 1998, p. 172).

Continued

MAJOR CONCEPTS & DEFINITIONS—cont'd

EXPERIENCE OF DIGNITY AND RESPECT

Each terminally ill patient is "respected and valued as a human being" (Ruland & Moore, 1998, p. 172). This concept incorporates the idea of personal worth, as expressed by the ethical principle of autonomy or respect for persons, which states that individuals should be treated as autonomous agents, and persons with diminished autonomy are entitled to protection (United States, 1978).

BEING AT PEACE

Peace is a "feeling of calmness, harmony, and contentment, (free of) anxiety, restlessness, worries, and fear" (Ruland & Moore, 1998, p. 172). A peaceful state includes physical, psychological, and spiritual dimensions.

CLOSENESS TO SIGNIFICANT OTHERS

Closeness is "the feeling of connectedness to other human beings who care" (Ruland & Moore, 1998, p. 172). It involves a physical or emotional nearness that is expressed through warm, intimate relationships.

USE OF EMPIRICAL EVIDENCE

The theory of peaceful EOL is based on empirical evidence from both direct experience of expert nurses and a thorough review of the literature addressing several components of the theory. The group of expert practitioners who developed the standard of care for peaceful EOL had at least 5 years of clinical experience caring for terminally ill patients. The standard of care consisted of best practices based on research-derived evidence in the areas of pain management, comfort, nutrition, and relaxation. This prescriptive theory comprises several proposed relational statements for which more empirical evidence is needed as well. Importantly, explicit hypotheses can be derived easily from these relational statements to be tested for their usefulness. It should be noted that the authors of the standard of care and the theory attempted to incorporate clearly described, observable concepts and relationships that expressed the notion of caring.

MAJOR ASSUMPTIONS

Nursing, Person, Environment, and Health

Because the theory of peaceful EOL was derived from standards of care written by a team of expert nurses who were addressing a practice problem, the metaparadigm concepts were inherent in the nursing phenomena addressed, the complex and holistic care required to support peaceful EOL.

Two assumptions of Ruland and Moore's (1998) theory are identified as follows:

1. The occurrences and feelings at the EOL experience are personal and individualized.
2. Nursing care is crucial for creating a peaceful EOL experience. Nurses assess and interpret cues that reflect the person's EOL experience and intervene appropriately to attain or maintain a peaceful experience, even when the dying person cannot communicate verbally.

Two additional assumptions are implicit:

1. Family, a term that includes all significant others, is an important part of EOL care.

2. The goal of EOL care is not to optimize care, in the sense that it must be the best, most technologically advanced treatment, a type of care that frequently results in overtreatment. Rather, the goal in EOL care is to maximize treatment, that is, the best possible care will be provided through the judicious use of technology and comfort measures, in order to enhance quality of life and achieve a peaceful death.

THEORETICAL ASSERTIONS

Six explicit relational statements were identified (Ruland and Moore, 1998) as theoretical assertions for the theory, as follows:

1. Monitoring and administering pain relief and applying pharmacologic and nonpharmacologic interventions contribute to the patient's experience of not being in pain.
2. Preventing, monitoring and relieving physical discomfort, facilitating rest, relaxation, and contentment, and preventing complications contribute to the patient's experience of comfort.
3. Including the patient and significant others in decision making regarding patient care, treating the patient with dignity, empathy and respect, and being attentive to the patient's expressed needs, wishes, and preferences contribute to the patient's experience of dignity and respect.
4. Providing emotional support, monitoring and meeting the patient's expressed needs for antianxiety medications, inspiring trust, providing the patient and significant others with guidance in practical issues, and providing physical presence of another caring person if desired contribute to the patient's experience of being at peace.
5. Facilitating participation of significant others in patient care, attending to significant others' grief, worries, and questions, and facilitating opportunities for family closeness contribute to the patient's experience of closeness to significant others or persons who care.
6. The patient's experiences of not being in pain, comfort, dignity, and respect, being at peace, closeness to significant others or persons who care contribute to the peaceful end of life (p. 174).

LOGICAL FORM

The Peaceful EOL Theory was developed using both inductive and deductive logic. A unique feature of the theory is its development from a standard of care. The peaceful EOL standard was created by expert nurses in response to a lack of direction for managing the complex care of terminally ill patients. The standard was developed for the surgical gastroenterological care unit in a university hospital in Norway. Thus, the standard served as a logical intermediary step linking practice and theory. Standards of care are intended to serve as credible, authoritative statements that describe a practitioner's roles and responsibilities and an expected performance or level of nursing care by which the quality of practice can be evaluated (American Association of Critical Care Nurses, 1998). In this instance of knowledge development, the standard of care can be considered an interim step that effectively links clinical practice to theory.

Ruland and Moore (2001) detailed the steps they followed in the development of the standard for peaceful EOL, which included review of the relevant literature, clarification of important concepts, and the incorporation of knowledge of clinical practice. Each of these steps is analogous to those used in theory development. Thus, the logic used for the development of this theory is straightforward, and their process is clearly stated.

ACCEPTANCE BY THE NURSING COMMUNITY

Practice

A small but growing number of articles cite the Peaceful EOL Theory. It is included on Clayton State University School of Nursing Theory Link page with a link to *American Journal of Critical Care*, End of

Life Care (Kirchhoff, Spuhler, Walker, Hutton, Cole, & Clemmer, 2000). Liehr and Smith (1999) refer to the theory's development of a practice standard as a foundation for developing theory, Kehl (2006) cites it in her concept analysis of a "good death," and Baggs and Schmitt (2000) discuss the potential usefulness of the theory as a means to improve EOL decision making for critically ill adults. Kirchoff (2002) continued the discussion on creating an environment of care in the intensive care unit that promotes a peaceful death by synthesizing information from three sources (the Peaceful EOL Theory [Ruland & Moore, 1998], the Institute of Medicine's definition of peaceful death [Field & Cassell, 1997], and precepts from the American Association Colleges of Nursing's "Peaceful Death: Recommended Competencies and Curricular Guidelines for End of Life Nursing Care," 1997).

Education

Peaceful end of life has been integrated into nursing courses for generations with a focus on care of the patient and family care at that time. More recently, that content has become more standardized in the form of theory, competencies, and curricular guidelines. Ruland and Moore (1998) is an example of an early end of life theory as attention to hospice and palliative care has developed. Ruland and Moore (1998) was cited by Kirchoff and colleagues (2000) when End of Life was a featured topic of a CE (continuing education) offering for critical care nurses in their online journal.

Research

A descriptive study using the Peaceful EOL Theory by Beckstrand, Callister, and Kirchoff (2006) surveyed critical care nurses on how to improve end-of-life care. Providing for a "good death" was the number one theme. The EOL theory's relatively recent publication may partially explain this gap in the literature. Both theorists (Ruland and Moore) report that they routinely receive inquires about using the theory from graduate students, and Ruland plans to begin testing the theory in her program of research.

FURTHER DEVELOPMENT

Since Peaceful EOL Theory is relatively new, Ruland and Moore acknowledge the need for further refinement and development. There are a number of potential ideas to advance its development, and testing the theory is in the planning stage. Testing the relationships among the five major concepts is a possibility. Another idea is to consider merging some of the process criteria from the three concepts of pain, comfort, and peace to explore outcomes related to physical-psychological symptom management. Concept analysis or mapping might be used to determine if the process criteria associated with the three concepts are different or sufficiently alike to allow merging. For instance, for the concept of pain, two process criteria (monitoring and administering pain relief and applying pharmacological and nonpharmacological interventions) are closely related to the comfort process criterion (preventing, monitoring, and relieving physical discomfort) and the peace process criterion (monitoring and meeting patient's needs for antianxiety medication). Nonpharmacological interventions (e.g., music, humor, relaxation) that serve to distract a dying patient are useful for the relief of pain, anxiety, and general physical discomfort. Future studies are suggested to explore linkages of the Peaceful EOL Theory to other middle range theories such as one for acute pain based on practice guidelines (Good and Moore, 1996), pain management (Good, 1998), and unpleasant symptoms (Lenz, Pugh, Milligan, Gift, & Suppe, 1997; Lenz, Suppe, Gift, Pugh, & Milligan, 1995).

CRITIQUE

Clarity

All elements of the theory are stated clearly, including the setting, assumptions, and concepts and relational statements. These concepts vary considerably in their level of abstraction, from more concrete (pain and comfort) to more abstract (dignity).

Simplicity

Despite its uncomplicated terms and clear expression of ideas, the theory has been described as one of a higher level middle range theories (Higgins & Moore, 2000), primarily because of the level of abstraction of the outcome criteria and the multidimensional complexity expressed in its relational statements.

Generality

The Peaceful EOL Theory has specific boundaries related to time, setting, and patient population. It was developed for use with terminally ill adults and their families who are receiving care in an acute care setting. The concept of peaceful EOL came from a Norwegian context and thus may not be appropriate for all cultures. Nevertheless, its concepts and relationships resonate with many nurses, and it comprehensively addresses the multidimensional aspects of EOL care. For example, the outcome indicators associated with the five concepts address the technical aspect of care (providing both pharmacological and nonpharmacological interventions for the relief of symptoms), communication (decision making), the psychological aspect (emotional support), and dignity and respect (treating the patient with dignity, empathy, and respect) (Figure 36-1).

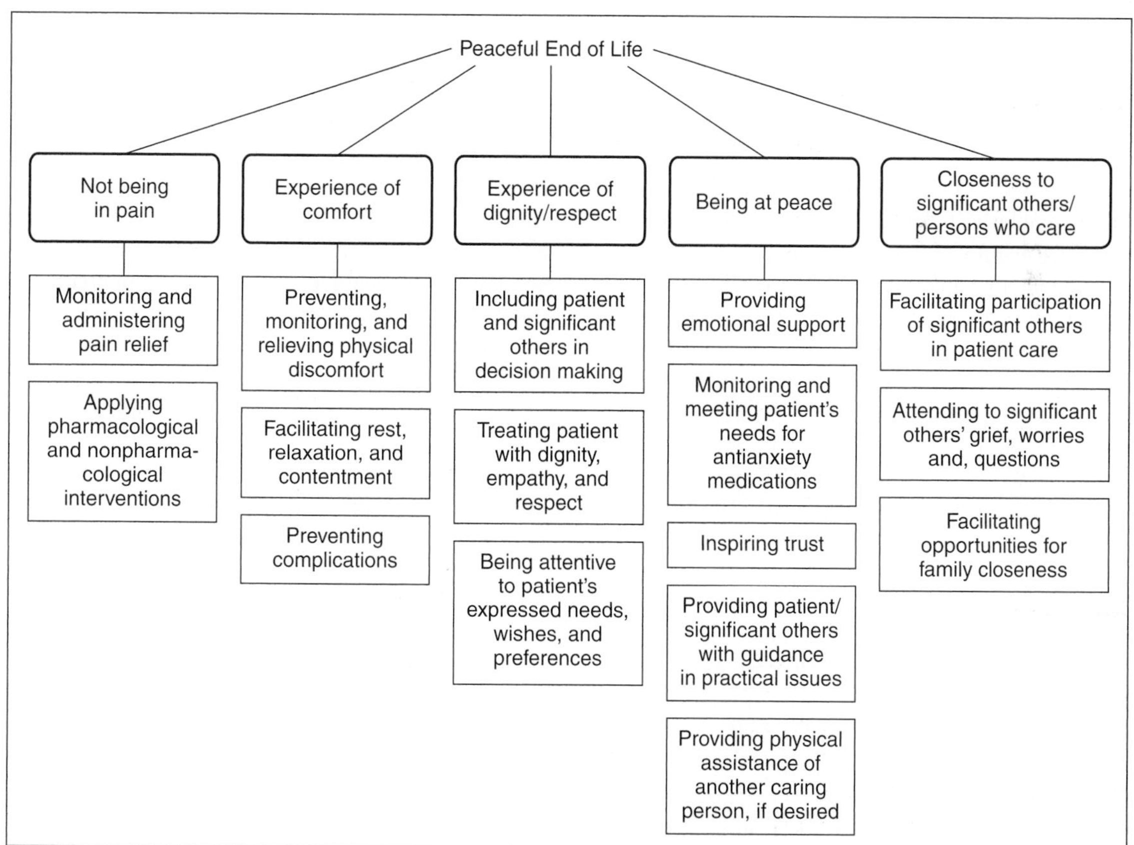

Figure 36-1 Relationships among the concepts of the Peaceful End of Life Theory. (From Ruland, C. M., & Moore, S. M. [1998]. Theory construction based on standards of care: A proposed theory of the peaceful end of life. *Nursing Outlook, 46*(4), 174.)

Empirical Precision

The deductive and inductive logic used to develop this theory provides a solid basis for developing testable hypotheses among the five concepts of the theory. Theoretical congruency is demonstrated through the outcome indicators, all of which are conceptualized from the perspective of the patients and their families.

Derivable Consequences

As a successful synthesis of clinical practice and scholarly theory development, the Peaceful EOL Theory is a framework that illustrates one way to bridge the theory-practice-research continuum. In addition to addressing an identified need for a comprehensive middle range theory to guide care of patients in the EOL experience, Ruland and Moore's (2001) work clearly illustrates the richness of practice and standards as a source for the development of theory.

All of the outcome indicators are measurable, using qualitative or quantitative methodology or both (see Figure 36-1). Unlike some middle range theories, that have a specific instrument to measure a particular concept, no instrument was developed for Peaceful EOL Theory. Therefore, for future studies among the five concepts, instruments would be needed to measure hypothesized relationships. Mixed method (Tashakkori & Teddlie, 2003) has been described as a particularly appealing approach for measuring the concepts. For example, phenomenological methodology could be used to investigate patient and family perceptions of their opportunities for and satisfaction with family closeness or decision making or both. On the other hand, a number of existing instruments could be used to measure the outcome indicators associated with the five concepts (see Figure 36-1), for example, perception of symptoms with the Memorial Symptom Assessment Scale (Portenoy, Thaler, Kornblith, Lepore, Friedlander-Klar et al., 1994) or the General Comfort Questionnaire developed by Kolcaba (2003).

Case Study

Mr. Kelley is a retired 85-year-old engineer with advanced dementia. His large, extended family includes his wife, children, and grandchildren, and their families. Mr. Kelley has been a resident in a nursing home for six months; his family visits frequently, and his friendly, easy-going personality makes him a favorite with staff members. In the past month, Mr. Kelley has become increasingly confused, withdrawn, and nonverbal; he takes food and fluids sparingly and only with much urging. He did not leave any written instructions about end-of-life measures although he told his wife that he did not want extraordinary measures, and she has signed a DNR order. There is discussion about starting intravenous fluids and tube feeding, and family and staff members differ in their opinions on the best options for Mr. Kelley's care. The Peaceful EOL Theory has been adapted for patients who do not have a cancer diagnosis, and Mr. Kelley represents a growing patient population that is both similar yet very different from the oncology patient population. Describe how the Peaceful EOL Theory will help you develop, implement, and evaluate appropriate nursing interventions for patients with end-stage dementia.

CRITICAL THINKING *Activities*

1. Using professional practice standards from a national nursing organization, evaluate the correspondence of the concept "experience of dignity and respect" with the organization's standard(s) related to ethics. Discuss both similarities and differences related to relevance, significance, scope, usefulness, and adequacy.
2. Describe how the concepts of the Peaceful EOL Theory apply to patients with end-stage congestive heart failure. How might the theory help you develop, implement, and evaluate appropriate nursing interventions? What limitations of the theory do you see?

3. Focusing on the concept "closeness to significant others," develop an evaluation plan to assess the quality and effectiveness of care.
4. Identify applications of end-of-life concepts in your clinical practice with patients and families.

POINTS FOR *Further Study*

- Kirchoff, K.T. (2002). Promoting a peaceful death in the ICU. *Critical Care Nursing Clinics of North America, 14*(2), 201-206.
- Ruland, C. M., & Moore, S. M. (1998). Theory construction based on standards of care: A proposed theory of the peaceful end of life. *Nursing Outlook, 46*(4), 169-175.
- Higgins, P. A., & Moore, S. M. (2000). Levels of theoretical thinking in nursing. *Nursing Outlook, 48*(4), 179-183.

REFERENCES

American Association of Critical Care Nurses (AACN). (1998). Standards for acute and critical care nursing practice. Aliso Viejo, CA: AACN. Retrieved August 1, 2008, from http://www.aacn.org/AACN/practice.nsf/ad0ca3b3bdb4f33288256981006fa692/5e3c9805e57b3b0888256a6b00791f35

Baggs, J. G., & Schmitt, M. H. (2000). End-of-life decisions in adult intensive care: Current research base 158 and directions for the future. *Nursing Outlook, 48*(4), 158-164.

Beckstrand, R. L. Callister, L. C., & Kirchoff, K. T. (2006). Providing a "Good Death": Critical care nurses' suggestions for improving end-of-life care. *American Journal of Critical Care, 15*(1), 38-45.

Brandt, R. B. (1979). A theory of the good and the right. Oxford: Clarendon Press.

Field, M. J., Cassell, C. K. (1997). Approaching death: Improving care at the end of life (IOM report). Washington D.C.: National Academy Press.

Good, M. (1998). A middle-range theory of acute pain management: Use in research. *Nursing Outlook, 46*(3), 120-124.

Good, M., & Moore, S. M. (1996). Clinical practice guidelines as a new source of middle-range theory: Focus on acute pain. *Nursing Outlook, 44*(2), 74-79.

Higgins, P. A., & Moore, S. M. (2000). Levels of theoretical thinking in nursing. *Nursing* Outlook, 48(4), 179-183.

Huth, M. M., & Moore, S. M. (1998). Prescriptive theory of acute pain management in infants and children. *Journal of the Society of Pediatric Nurses, 3*(1), 23-32.

Kehl, K. A. (2006). Moving toward a peace: An analysis of the concept of the good death. *American Journal of Hospice and Palliative Medicine, 23*(4), 277-286.

Kirchoff, K. T. (2002). Promoting a peaceful death in the ICU. *Critical Care Nursing Clinics of North America, 14*(2), 201-206.

Kirchhoff, K. T., Spuhler, V., Walker, L., Hutton, A., Cole, B., and Clemmer, T. (2000). End-of-Life Care: Intensive care nurses' experiences with end-of-life care, *American Journal of Critical Care, 9*(1) retrieved August, 6, 2008. http://classic.aacn.org/AACN/jrnlajcc.nsf/bd5ca01ff707c8948825653f000cd2b6/479f8ee84

Kolcaba, K. (2003). Comfort theory and practice: A vision for holistic health care and research. New York: Springer.

Kolcaba, K. Y., & Kolcaba, R. J. (1991). An analysis of the concept of comfort. *Journal of Advanced Nursing, 16*(11), 1301-1310.

Lenz, E. R., Pugh, L. C., Milligan, R. A., Gift, A., & Suppe, F. (1997). The middle-range theory of unpleasant symptoms: An update. *ANS Advances in Nursing Science, 19*(3), 14-27.

Lenz, E. R., Suppe, F., Gift, A. G., Pugh, L. C., & Milligan, R. A. (1995). Collaborative development of middle-range nursing theories: Toward a theory of unpleasant symptoms. *ANS Advances in Nursing Science, 17*(3), 1-13.

Liehr, P., & Smith, M. J. (1999). Middle range theory: Spinning research and practice to create knowledge for the new millennium. *ANS Advances in Nursing Science, 21*(4), 81-91.

Pain terms: A list with definitions and notes on usage. Recommended by the IASP Subcommittee on Taxonomy. (1979). *Pain, 6*(3), 249.

Portenoy, R. K., Thaler, H. T., Kornblith, A. B., Lepore, J. M., Friedlander-Klar, H., Coyle, N., et al. (1994). The Memorial Symptom Assessment Scale: An instrument for the evaluation of symptom prevalence, characteristics and distress. *European Journal of Cancer, 30A*(9), 1326-1336.

Ruland, C. M., & Bakken, S. (2001). Representing patient preference-related concepts for inclusion in electronic health records. *Journal of Biomedical Informatics, 34*(6), 415-422.

Ruland, C. M., Kresevic, D., & Lorensen, M. (1997). Including patient preferences in nurses' assessment of older patients. *Journal of Clinical Nursing, 6*(6), 495-504.

Ruland, C. M., & Moore, S. M. (1998). Theory construction based on standards of care: A proposed theory of the peaceful end of life. *Nursing Outlook, 46*(4), 169-175.

Ruland, C. M., & Moore, S. M. (2001). Eliciting exercise preferences in cardiac rehabilitation: Initial evaluation of a new strategy. *Patient Education and Counseling, 44*(3), 283-291.

Sandoe, P. (1999). Quality of life—Three competing views. *Ethical Theory and Moral Practice, 2*(1), 11-23.

Tashakkori, A., & Teddlie, C., (2003). Handbook of mixed methods in social & behavioral research. Thousand Oaks, CA: Sage.

United States, National Commission for the Protection of Human Subjects of Biomedical and Behavioral Research. (1978). *The Belmont report: Ethical principles and guidelines for the protection of human subjects of research (Bethesda, MD)*, Washington, DC: For Sale by the Commission. Superintendent of Documents, U.S. Government Printing Office.

UNIT

VI

Future of Nursing Theory

- *Theoretical systems are active and give direction to future research and administrative, educational, and practice applications.*
- *Theoretical works developed in a discipline affect the nature of the questions asked, the frameworks used to seek answers, and the scope of knowledge that is produced.*
- *Nursing models and theories exhibit Kuhn's criteria for normal science, that is, a scientific community with research based on scientific achievements as a foundation of practice.*
- *Expansion of the philosophy of nursing science has increased qualitative theory development approaches as well as quantitative methods and has greatly increased the development and use of middle range theories.*
- *Expanded communication opportunities on the Internet have contributed to global communities of nurse scholars.*

CHAPTER

37

State of the Art and Science of Nursing Theory

Martha Raile Alligood

"In this seventh edition, the goal is to clarify the relevance of nursing theoretical works, facilitate their recognition as systematic presentations of nursing substance, and stimulate their use as frameworks for nursing scholarship in practice, research, education, and administration." Martha Raile Alligood

From studying this text, it becomes obvious that nursing theoretical works are active and growing as they point the way to new knowledge through research, education, administration, and practice applications. Each successive edition goes through reviews by the publisher in addition to published reviews that are given careful consideration in the production of new editions (Burns, 1999; Malinski, 1999; Paley, 2006; Reed, 1999). In this seventh edition, you will find updates of the chapters and the addition of a new theory chapter (Meleis's Transitions in Chapter 20). Middle range theories continue to be a very important unit as more nurses recognize their utility and applicability in nursing practice (Sieloff & Frey, 2007; Peterson & Bredow, 2008; Smith & Liehr, 2008). As Burns (1999) noted, middle range theory fosters "theoretic thought and the growing recognition of the potential impact of theory on nursing practice" (p. 263).

The references and bibliography are consistently noted as a major strength of the text. As Malinski (1999) observed, "they provide a valuable resource for students" (p. 265). The chapters are updated in this seventh edition, as in previous editions, with literature written by those using the various theoretical works in their professional practice and research. More and more nurses are recognizing that the theoretical works are vital for them to know, apply and guide practice, research, education, and administration (Alligood & Marriner Tomey, 1997, 2002, 2006; Alligood 2004; 2006c; 2010, in press). In the sixth edition, to deal with the growing body of nursing theoretical works and not eliminate those in earlier editions, a chapter was created to chronicle their historical significance. In this seventh edition, the work of Orlando has been added to this chapter (see Chapter 5).

Reed (1999) observed in her review that "the book supports the momentum building within nursing to transcend the tired debate about the relevance of nursing models and apply this field of knowledge as a basis for understanding the substance and scholarship of nursing" (p. 268). In this seventh edition, the goal is to clarify the relevance of nursing theoretical works, facilitate their recognition as systematic presentations of nursing substance, and stimulate their use as frameworks for nursing scholarship in practice, research, education, and administration. The theoretical works developed within a discipline determine the nature of the questions asked, the research methods used to answer questions, and the scope of knowledge the questions address. Simply put, the framing of an issue determines the outcome. How might we as nurses explore the state of the art and science of nursing theory? That question is answered in the nursing literature that documents the use of nursing theoretical works around the world.

This chapter presents the growth of nursing theory from three perspectives. First, the impact of the shift in philosophy of science on the development of theoretical works, changes that have informed qualitative approaches and quantitative methods (Carper, 1978; Kuhn, 1962, 1970). Second, nursing theory is viewed in the context of its new growth in this postmodern period that encourages reframing knowledge in present day understanding. Morris (2000) suggests, "the postmodern era often co-opts or revises rather than reject outright the achievements of modernism . . . " (p. 8). Finally, and third, the global nature of development and the use of nursing theoretical works call attention to the growing communities of scholars, highlight significant growth in theoretical organizations, and remind the reader of the transient but vital nature of theory for the profession, discipline, and science.

NATURE OF NORMAL SCIENCE

Many nursing models and theories included in this text have developed such that they now exhibit characteristics of Kuhn's (1970) criteria for normal science (Wood & Alligood, 2006). Increasingly, over the past 30 years, the conceptual models of nursing and nursing theories as presented by Alligood and Marriner Tomey (1997, 2002, 2006), Fawcett (1984a, 1989, 1993, 1995, 2000, 2005), Fitzpatrick and Whall (1984, 1989, 1996), George (1985, 1986, 1989, 1995, 2002), Marriner Tomey (1986, 1989, 1994), Marriner Tomey and Alligood (1998, 2002, 2006), McEwen and Wills (2002, 2006), Meleis (1985, 1991, 1997, 2005, 2007), and Parker (2001, 2006) have led to theory-based education, administration, research, and practice. Communities of scholars continue to grow, become more formally organized, address deeper questions, and share knowledge from their research and practice in newsletters and journals. Nursing models and theories provide nurses with perspectives of the central concepts of the discipline: person, environment, health, and nursing, the metaparadigm of nursing as set forth by Fawcett (1984b); concepts with wide acceptance as discipline boundaries are often noted without an author reference.

The theoretical works generate scholarship as frameworks for research and theory-based nursing practice. Work within the communities of scholars around the nursing models has led to research instruments unique to that paradigm. Kuhn (1970) stated, "paradigms gain their status by being more successful than their competitors in solving a few problems that the group of practitioners have come to recognize as acute" (p. 23). Kuhn (1970) defines normal science as "research firmly based upon one or more past scientific achievements, achievements that some particular scientific community acknowledges for a time as supplying the foundation for its further practice" (p. 10). The characteristics of paradigms that evidence their nature and lead to normal science include:

- A community of scholars who base their research and practice on the paradigm
- The formation of specialized journals
- The foundation of specialists' societies
- The claim for a special place in curricula (Kuhn, 1970)

Rodgers (2005) describes normal science as ". . . the highly cumulative process of puzzle solving in which the paradigm guides scientific activity and the paradigm is, in turn, articulated and expanded"

(p. 100). Rodgers (2005) cites Kuhn's premise that research in normal science "is directed to the articulation of those phenomena and theories that the paradigm supplies" (p. 100).

The conceptual models of nursing in this text exhibit these characteristics. Each model is unique and has ranges of development in these characteristics. Rogers' Science of Unitary Human Beings (see Chapter 13) is an excellent example, having generated hundreds of research studies, 13 research instruments, and 12 nursing process clinical tools for practice (Fawcett, 2005; Fawcett & Alligood, 2001). The Society of Rogerian Scholars, founded in 1988, publishes a refereed journal, *Visions: The Journal of Rogerian Nursing Science,* which facilitates communication and fosters development of the science among the community of scholars. Rogerian science is the basis of award winning texts and is used to structure curricula for undergraduate and graduate nursing programs (Fawcett, 2005). In 2008, at the Society of Rogerian Scholars fall conference at Case Western University, they celebrated twenty-five years of Rogerian conferences, the twentieth anniversary of the society, and fifteen years of the journal.

Other conceptual models of nursing, such as Orem's Self-Care Deficit Theory (see Chapter 14), the Neuman Systems Model (see Chapter 16), and Roy's Adaptation Model (see Chapter 17), have experienced similar growth. Examples of nursing theories that exhibit characteristics of normal science are Erickson, Tomlin, and Swain's Theory of Modeling and Role-Modeling (see Chapter 25), Leininger's Theory of Culture Care (see Chapter 22), Parse's Theory of Human Becoming (see Chapter 24), and Margaret Newman's Theory of Health as Expanding Consciousness (see Chapter 23). As these societies of nursing scholars grow, the volume of publications increases, and research and practice grow exponentially.

EXPANSION OF THEORY DEVELOPMENT

Theoretical works provide ways to think about nursing. Johnson and Webber (2001, 2004) addressed the future of nursing in questions about the importance of theory development for recognition of nursing as a profession, as a discipline, and as a science. They identify three significant areas affected by nursing knowledge and dependent on its continued development. Although theory affects recognition of nursing as a profession, a discipline, and a science, the future existence of nursing depends on use of substantive nursing knowledge not only for recognition, but also, to improve the quality of care to the patients whom we serve. Moving the practice of nursing to a professional delivery model requires transposing from the vocational style that many nurses have been taught and to which many cling to a professional style of delivery. This requires a systematic presentation of nursing. As knowledge is transferred to those coming into the profession, it is also done so with a style of practice. Substance is the requirement in any field of learning to be recognized as a discipline in academe. Although there are different views about nursing knowledge development, as nurses shift to a professional style of nursing, they move beyond "the tired debate about the relevance of nursing models and apply this field of knowledge as a basis for understanding the substance and scholarship of nursing" (Reed, 1999, p. 268). Most agree that "nursing knowledge arises from inquiry and guides practice" (Parse, 2008, p. 101).

Dialogue also continues about the myriad of ways scholars classify nursing theoretical works. It is important to remember that each work is unique and therefore any classification is arbitrary at best and is based on the judgment of the one doing the classifying. Most importantly, rather than focusing on classification of the works, it is more useful to emphasize knowing the individual works, teaching them to students, and using them for a professional style of practice to improve quality of care.

Nursing eagerly embraced qualitative research approaches to explore questions that quantitative research methods could not answer, and this expanded philosophy of nursing science resulted in qualitative theory development and many new middle range theories (Alligood, 2002; Alligood & May, 2000; Liehr & Smith, 1999; Peterson & Bredow, 2008;

Sieloff & Frey, 2007; Smith & Liehr, 2003, 2008; Thorne, Kirkham, & MacDonald-Emes, 1997; Thorne, Kirkham, & O'Flynn-Magee, 2004). These new theories expand the volume that continues to be developed with conceptual models of nursing and nursing theories as middle range or practice theory applications noted in these few examples: Orem (Biggs, 2008), Neuman (Casalenuovo, 2002; Gigliotti, 2003), Roy (DeSanto-Madeya, 2007; Dunn, 2005; Hamilton & Bowers, 2007), Rogers (Kim, Kim, Park, Park, & Lee, 2008), Newman (Pharris & Endo, 2007), King (Sieloff & Frey, 2007), and Parse (Wang, 2008). There is also a wealth of knowledge in early nursing theoretical writings (Alligood, 2002; Alligood & Fawcett, 1999; 2004; Butcher, 1999, 2002) that are rich resources for discovery of new theory, such as empathy in King's Interacting Systems Framework (Alligood & May, 2000). Middle range theory is "the least abstract set of related concepts that propose a truth specific to the details of nursing practice" (Alligood & Marriner Tomey, 2006, p. 522).

Expansive growth has occurred with nursing texts exclusively devoted to the presentation of middle range theories (Peterson & Bredow 2008; Sieloff & Frey, 2007; Smith & Liehr, 2003, 2008). This development is especially exciting as it closes the gap between research and practice (Alligood, 2006b). Liehr and Smith (1999) explored the nature of middle range theories in the nursing literature from 1988 to 1998 and identified 24 middle range theories. They noted that theory-generating approaches used in the 24 middle range theories were both quantitative and qualitative methods. Smith and Liehr (2003, 2008) subsequently published their method of middle range theory development and selected theories. Sieloff and Frey (2007) is middle range theory using King's conceptual system. Other middle range theories are developed exploring aspects of people's lived experiences to understand the meaning of life events.

Application of middle range theories in nursing practice is encouraged for improving nursing practice quality, whether developed quantitatively or qualitatively. Both approaches are at the level of practice and develop useful nursing knowledge. Consideration of development of middle range theory in relation to a generic structure of knowledge reveals that theory from the hypothetical-deductive method and theory from qualitative approaches arrive at a similar level of abstraction. In spite of the fact of their different philosophical basis and different methods and approaches, they produce knowledge at a similar level of abstraction (Figure 37-1).

Considering nursing knowledge in a generic structure as presented in Figure 37-1 moves discussions beyond dichotomous research method and philosophy debates to focus on the knowledge and content within nursing science. Actually, middle range theories vary in range and levels of abstraction as the name suggests. This is true for the theoretical works in other classifications (philosophies, models, and theories) as they have similarities and differences in their levels of abstraction (Fawcett, 2005).

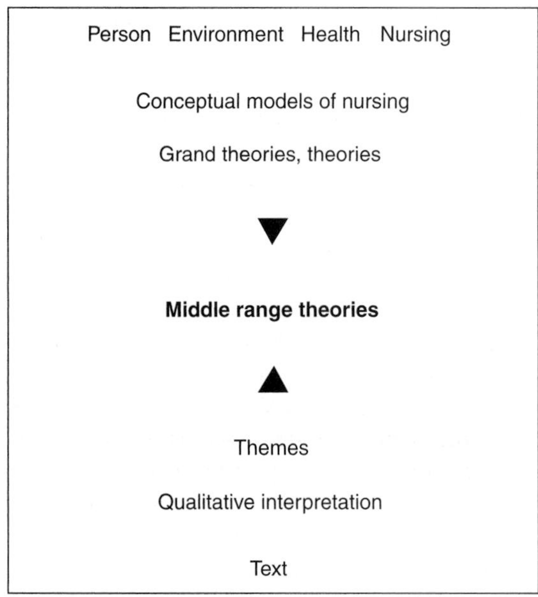

Figure 37-1 Middle range theory in a generic structure of nursing knowledge from quantitative research methods and qualitative research approaches. (Data from Fawcett, J. [2000]. *Contemporary nursing knowledge: Nursing models and theories.* Philadelphia: F. A. Davis.)

Middle range theories are recognizable because they include details that are specific to practice. Items such as:

- The situation or health condition of the patient
- Patient population or age group
- Location of the patient or area of practice
- Action of the nurse or intervention
- The proposed outcome (Alligood, 2006a, p. 488)

GLOBAL COMMUNITIES OF NURSING SCHOLARS

In addition to the growth stimulated by a broader philosophy of nursing science, expansion of research methods and approaches, and the emergence of middle range theories, another major contribution to the state of the art and science of nursing theory is the globalization of communities of nurse scholars and expanded communication possibilities via the Internet. Most of the nursing conceptual model and theory organizations have international members. The International Orem Society, founded in 1990, sponsors biennial conferences alternating between the United States and other countries. The tenth conference in Vancouver, Canada, in 2008 included attendees from eight countries. Their 2010 conference is planned for Thailand. The *International Orem Society* has an active website, where you can access abstracts from the last conference and an online journal, *Self-Care, Deficit Care, and Nursing.*

Similarly, the theme for the 12th International Biennial Neuman Systems Model Symposium in 2009 is "Enhancing Global Health with Nursing Theories—NSM." This conference routinely has a global theme and includes attendees from Holland, where the Neuman Systems Model is used widely. This has come about largely through global communication, increased world travel, and translation of nursing theory textbooks into other languages.

Nurses around the world are embracing nursing theory as they experience its utility in their practice. Numerous nursing journals such as *Journal of Nursing Scholarship, Nursing Science Quarterly, Journal of Advanced Nursing, Visions: The Journal of Rogerian Nursing Science,* and *International Journal for Human Caring,* to name a few, publish articles by international scholars. Various editions of *Nursing Theorists and Their Work* (Marriner Tomey, 1989, 1994; Marriner Tomey & Alligood, 1998, 2002, 2006) and *Nursing Theory: Utilization and Application* (Alligood & Marriner Tomey, 1997, 2002, 2006) have been published in classical Chinese, which is Taiwanese, Finnish, German, Italian, Japanese, Korean, Spanish, and Portuguese. Both texts have consistent international circulation to English speaking countries. In relation to global interest in conceptual models of nursing and nursing theory, publications in journals also demonstrate interest among nurses globally. Publication of nursing theory articles verifies international use of nursing models and theories by theorists from the United States and theory development contributions from other countries.

A PubMed search conducted on October 23, 2008, listed the following number of nursing theory publications when limited to individual languages (Table 37-1):

A nursing model, developed by Kappeli (1999), Department of Health of the State of Zurich in Switzerland, was introduced in five Swiss hospitals (Anderregg-Tschudin, 1999). Kappeli (1999) presented at the University of Basel, examining requirements for nursing science at a university hospital, and concluded nursing science is compatible with the ethos and goals of the nursing profession. The theoretical works of the following international theorists is included in this text: Evelyn Adam, Canada (see Chapter 5), Roper, Logan, and Tierney, Scotland (see Chapter 5), Katie Eriksson, Finland (see Chapter 11), Phil Barker, Ireland (see Chapter 32), Kari Martinsen, Norway (see Chapter 10), and Nightingale, England (see Chapter 6).

Global consciousness has arrived, as is evidenced by nursing theory articles from around the world in nursing journals in the United States and those from other countries (Shamsudin, 2002). The expansion of Sigma Theta Tau International contributed through worldwide membership and publications. The Internet facilitates global communication among nurses, and nurses share nursing theoretical

Table 37-1 Number of Nursing Theory Publications Retrieved When Limited by Each Language Possible in a PubMed Search October 23, 2008

Languages Searched	Nursing Theory Publications	Languages Searched	Nursing Theory Publications
English	10,144	Finnish	24
Japanese	409	Polish	13
Portuguese	298	Afrikaan	7
German	295	Russian	3
French	214	Greek	2
Korean	79	Thai	1
Chinese	59	Turkish	1
Dutch	56	Hebrew	1
Danish	54	Hungarian	1
Spanish	41	Czech	1
Norwegian	41	All other possible languages	0
Italian	33		
Swedish	28		

knowledge in research and for professional practice. *Nursing Science Quarterly* has a regular global feature in each issue on countries such as Canada, Australia, New Zealand, England, Japan, Sweden, Korea, Germany, Turkey, Taiwan, Hong Kong, Ireland, and Israel.

Several general nursing theory websites, such as the Nursing Theory Page offered by Valdosta State University, College of Nursing; the Nursing Theory Link Page maintained by Clayton College and State University Department of Nursing; and the Nursing Theory Page maintained by the school of nursing at the University of San Diego in California. These outstanding websites link to home pages or websites for most theorists and their work.

In conclusion, the state of the art and science of nursing theory is one of mushrooming growth. First, nursing theoretical works are used by communities of scholars who collaborate to develop nursing science with a particular paradigm in the mode of normal science (Kuhn, 1970). Secondly, theory develops along with an expanded philosophy of nursing science and maturing of qualitative research approaches that address unanswered nursing questions. The most exciting development in recent years is middle range theory and its relevance to nursing practice. Whether developed quantitatively or qualitatively, it is at a level of abstraction that facilitates practice (see Figure 37-1). Third, and finally, global communities of nursing scholars are sharing nursing theoretical works and contributing to the development of nursing knowledge. Using the Internet, nurses of the world share ideas and knowledge using the earlier theoretical works and new theories. It is vital that nursing knowledge be taught, learned, used, and applied in practice for the profession, and that nursing research continue knowledge development for the discipline. Because it remains true, "Theory without practice is empty and practice without theory is blind" (Cross, 1981, p. 110).

REFERENCES

Alligood, M. R. (2002). A theory of the art of nursing discovered in Rogers' science of unitary human beings. *International Journal for Human Caring, 6*(2), 55-60.

Alligood, M. R. (2004). The theoretical basis of professional nursing. In K. K. Chitty (Ed.), *Professional nursing* (3rd ed., pp. 271-298). Philadelphia: W. B. Saunders.

Alligood, M. R. (2006a). Areas for further development of theory-based nursing practice. In M. Alligood & A. Marriner Tomey (Eds.), *Nursing theory: Utilization & application* (3rd ed., pp. 487-497). St. Louis: Mosby.
Alligood, M. R. (2006b). Philosophies, models, and theories: Critical thinking structures. In M. Alligood & A. Marriner Tomey (Eds.), *Nursing theory: Utilization & application* (3rd ed., pp. 43-65). St. Louis: Mosby.
Alligood, M. R. (2006c). The nature of knowledge needed for nursing practice. In M. Alligood & A. Marriner Tomey (Eds.), *Nursing theory: Utilization & application* (3rd ed., pp. 3-15). St. Louis: Mosby.
Alligood, M. R. (2010 in press). *Nursing theory: Utilization & application,* (4th ed.). St. Louis: Mosby-Elsevier.
Alligood, M. R., & Fawcett, J. (1999). Acceptance of the invitation to dialogue: Examination of an interpretive approach for the science of unitary human beings. *Visions: The Journal of Rogerian Nursing Science, 7*(1), 5-13.
Alligood, M.R. & Fawcett, J. (2004). An interpretive study of Martha Rogers' conception of pattern. *Visions: The Journal of Rogerian Nursing Science, 12* (1), 8-13.
Alligood, M. R., & Marriner Tomey, A. (1997). *Nursing theory: Utilization & application*. St. Louis: Mosby.
Alligood, M. R., & Marriner Tomey, A. (2002). *Nursing theory: Utilization & application* (2nd ed.). St. Louis: Mosby.
Alligood, M. R., & Marriner Tomey, A. (2006). *Nursing theory: Utilization & application* (3rd ed.). St. Louis: Mosby.
Alligood, M. R., & May, B. A. (2000). A nursing theory of personal system empathy: Interpreting a conceptualization of empathy in King's interacting systems. *Nursing Science Quarterly, 13*(3), 243-247.
Anderregg-Tschudin, H. (1999). The complex interrelations between nursing diagnostic and nursing management [German]. *Pflege, 12*(4), 216-222.
Biggs, A. (2008). Orem's self-care deficit nursing theory: Update on the state of the art and the science, *Nursing Science Quarterly, 21*, 200-206.
Burns, N. (1999). [Review of the book *Nursing theorists and their work* (4th ed.)]. *Nursing Science Quarterly, 12*(3), 263-264.
Butcher, H. K. (1999). Rogerian ethics: An ethical inquiry into Rogers' life and science. *Nursing Science Quarterly, 12*(2), 111-118.
Butcher, H. K. (2002). Living in the heart of helicy: An inquiry into the meaning of compassion and unpredictability within Rogers' nursing science, *Visions: The Journal of Rogerian Nursing Science, 10(1)*, 6-22.
Carper, B. (1978). Fundamental patterns of knowing. *Advances in Nursing Science, 1(1)*, 13-23.
Casalenuovo, G. A. (2002). Fatigue in diabetes mellitus: Testing a middle range theory of optimal client system stability and the Neuman Systems Model. *Dissertation Abstracts International, 63, 2301B.*
Cross, P. (1981). *Adults as learners.* Washington, D.C.: Jossey-Bass.
DeSanto-Madeya, S. (2007). Using case studies based on a nursing conceptual model to teach medical-surgical nursing, *Nursing Science Quarterly, 20*, 324-329.
Dunn, K. S. (2005). Testing a middle-range theoretical mode of adaptation to chronic pain, *Nursing Science Quarterly, 18*, 146-156.
Fawcett, J. (1984a). *Analysis and evaluation of conceptual models of nursing.* Philadelphia: F. A. Davis.
Fawcett, J. (1984b). The metaparadigm of nursing, Current status and future refinements. *Image: The Journal of Nursing Scholarship, 16*, 84-87.
Fawcett, J. (1989). *Analysis and evaluation of conceptual models of nursing* (2nd ed.). Philadelphia: F. A. Davis.
Fawcett, J. (1993). *Analysis and evaluation of nursing theories.* Philadelphia: F. A. Davis.
Fawcett, J. (1995). *Analysis and evaluation of conceptual models of nursing* (3rd ed.). Philadelphia: F. A. Davis.
Fawcett, J. (2000). *Analysis and evaluation of contemporary nursing knowledge: Nursing models and theories.* Philadelphia: F. A. Davis.
Fawcett, J. (2005). *Analysis and evaluation of contemporary nursing knowledge: Nursing models and theories,*(2nd ed.). Philadelphia: F. A. Davis.
Fawcett, J., & Alligood, M. (2001). SUHB INSTRUMENTS: An overview of research instruments and clinical tools derived from the science of unitary human beings. *Theoria: Journal of Nursing Theory, 10*(2), 5-12.
Fitzpatrick, J. J., & Whall, A. L. (1984). *Conceptual models of nursing: Analysis and application.* Norwalk, CT: Appleton & Lange.
Fitzpatrick, J. J., & Whall, A. L. (1989). *Conceptual models of nursing: Analysis and application* (2nd ed.). Norwalk, CT: Appleton & Lange.
Fitzpatrick, J. J., & Whall, A. L. (1996). *Conceptual models of nursing: Analysis and application* (3rd ed.). Stamford, CT: Appleton & Lange.
George, J. B. (1985). *Nursing theories.* Norwalk, CT: Appleton & Lange.
George, J. B. (1986). *Nursing theories* (2nd ed.). Norwalk, CT: Appleton & Lange.
George, J. B. (1989). *Nursing theories* (3rd ed.). Norwalk, CT: Appleton & Lange.
George, J. B. (1995). *Nursing theories* (4th ed.). Upper Saddle River, NJ: Prentice Hall.
George, J. B. (2002). *Nursing theories* (5th ed.). Upper Saddle River, NJ: Prentice Hall.
Gigliotti, E. (2003). The Neuman Systems Model Institute: Testing middle-range theories. *Nursing Science Quarterly, 16*, 201-206.
Hamilton, R. J., & Bowers, B.J. (2007). The theory of genetic vulnerability: A Roy model exemplar, *Nursing Science Quarterly, 20*, 254-264.

Johnson, B., & Webber, P. (2001). *An introduction to theory and reasoning in nursing.* Philadelphia: Lippincott.

Johnson, B., & Webber, P. (2004). *An introduction to theory and reasoning in nursing* (2nd ed.). Philadelphia: Lippincott.

Kappeli, S. (1999). What sort of science does nursing require? [German]. *Pflege, 12*(3), 153-157.

Kim, T. S., Kim, C., Park, K. M., Park, Y. C., Lee, B. S. (2008). The relation of power and well-being in Korean adults, *Nursing Science Quarterly, 21,* 247-254.

Kuhn, T. S. (1962). *The structure of scientific revolutions.* Chicago: University of Chicago Press.

Kuhn, T. S. (1970). *The structure of scientific revolutions* (2nd ed.). Chicago: University of Chicago Press.

Liehr, P., & Smith, M. J. (1999). Middle range theory: Spinning research and practice to create knowledge for the new millennium. *ANS Advances in Nursing Science, 21*(4), 81-91.

Malinski, V. (1999). [Review of the book *Nursing theorists and their work* (4th ed.)]. *Nursing Science Quarterly, 12*(3), 264-266.

Marriner Tomey, A. (1986). *Nursing theorists and their work.* St. Louis: Mosby.

Marriner Tomey, A. (1989). *Nursing theorists and their work* (2nd ed.). St. Louis: Mosby.

Marriner Tomey, A. (1994). *Nursing theorists and their work* (3rd ed.). St. Louis: Mosby.

Marriner Tomey, A., & Alligood, M. (1998). *Nursing theorists and their work* (4th ed.). St. Louis: Mosby.

Marriner Tomey, A., & Alligood, M. R. (2002). *Nursing theorists and their work* (5th ed.). St. Louis: Mosby.

Marriner Tomey, A., & Alligood, M. R. (2006). *Nursing theorists and their work (*6th ed.). St. Louis: Mosby-Elsevier.

McEwen, M., & Wills, E. (2002). *Theoretical basis for nursing.* Philadelphia: Lippincott Williams & Wilkins.

McEwen, M., & Wills, E. (2006). *Theoretical basis for nursing* (2nd ed.). Philadelphia: Lippincott Williams & Wilkins.

Meleis, A. I. (1985). *Theoretical nursing: Development and progress.* Philadelphia: Lippincott.

Meleis, A. I. (1991). *Theoretical nursing: Development and progress.* Philadelphia: Lippincott.

Meleis, A. I. (1997). *Theoretical nursing: Development and progress* (2nd ed.). Philadelphia: Lippincott.

Meleis, A. I. (2005). *Theoretical nursing: Development and progress* (3rd ed.). Philadelphia: Lippincott.

Meleis, A. I. (2007). *Theoretical nursing: Development and progress* (4th ed.). Philadelphia: Lippincott.

Morris, D. B. (2000). How to speak postmodern: Medicine, illness, and cultural change. *Hastings Center Report, 30*(6), 7-16.

Paley, J. (2006). Nursing theorists and their work. Book review. *Nursing Philosophy, 7*(4), 275-280.

Parker, M. (2001). *Nursing theories and nursing practice.* Philadelphia: F. A. Davis.

Parker, M. (2006). *Nursing theories and nursing practice* (2nd ed.). Philadelphia: F. A. Davis.

Parse, R. R. (2008). Nursing knowledge development: Who's to say how? *Nursing Science Quarterly, 21,* 101.

Peterson, S. J., & Bredow, T. S. (2008). *Middle range theories, (*2nd ed.). Philadelphia: Lippincott Williams & Wilkins.

Pharris, M. D., & Endo, E. (2007). Flying free: The evolving nature of nursing practice guided by the theory of health as expanding consciousness, *Nursing Science Quarterly, 20,* 136-143.

Reed, P. G. (1999). [Review of the book *Nursing theorists and their work* (4th ed.)]. *Nursing Science Quarterly, 12*(3), 266-268.

Rodgers, B. L. (2005). *Developing nursing knowledge: Philosophical traditions and influences.* Philadelphia: Lippincott Williams & Wilkins.

Shamsudin, N. (2002). Can the Neuman Systems Model be adapted to the Malaysian nursing context? *International Journal of Nursing Practice, 8*(2), 99-105.

Sieloff, C. L., & Frey, M. A. (Eds.) (2007). *Middle range theory development using King's conceptual system.* New York: Springer.

Smith, M. J., & Liehr, P. (2003). *Middle range theory for nursing.* New York: Springer.

Smith, M. J., & Liehr, P. (2008). *Middle range theory for nursing.* New York: Springer.

Thorne, S., Kirkham, S. R., & MacDonald-Emes, J. (1997). Interpretive description: A noncategorical qualitative alternative for developing nursing knowledge. *Research in Nursing and Health, 20,* 169-177.

Thorne, S., Kirkham, S. R., & O'Flynn-Magee, K. (2004). The analytic challenge in interpretive description. *International Journal of Qualitative Methods, 3*(1), article 1. Retrieved May 21, 2004, from http://www.ualberta.ca/aiiqm/backissues/3_1/pdf/thorneetal.pdf

Wang, C. H. (2008). Working with older adults: A nurse practitioner's experience from a humanbecoming perspective. *Nursing Science Quarterly, 21,* 218-221.

Wood, A., & Alligood, M. (2006). Nursing models: Normal science for nursing practice. In M. R. Alligood & A. M. Tomey (Eds.), *Nursing theory: Utilization & application* (3rd ed., pp. 17-42). St. Louis: Mosby.

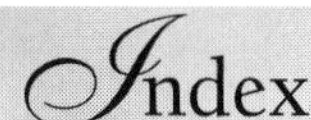

Index

A

Abdellah, Faye G., 50
  theory and influence of, 57
  website for, 57
Abductive reasoning, 31, 568–569
Achievement subsystem, in Johnson Behavioral System Model, 369
Achieving Methods of Intraprofessional Consensus, Assessment and Evaluation (AMICAE), 145–146, 150–151
Activity-related affect, in Health Promotion Model, 438
Adam, Evelyn, 52, 62
Adaptation
  in Conservation Model, 227
  in Modeling and Role-Modeling Theory, 543
  in Roy's Adaptation Model, 337–338, 341
  in Uncertainty in Illness Theory, 602
Adaptation Model, Roy, 7, 27, 335–365, 767
  case study based on, 356–357
  critique of, 352–354
  empirical evidence for, 340–341
  example of, 27
  further development of, 352
  logical form of, 344–345
  major assumptions of, 341–343, 341b
  major concepts and definitions in, 337–340
  nursing community's acceptance of, 345–352
  overview of adaptive modes in, 355t–356
  sources for, 336–337
  subsystems of, 343, 343f
  summary of, 354–356
  theoretical assertions of, 343–344, 343f, 344f
Adaptive Potential Assessment Model (APAM), 541, 543–544, 544f
Administration, nursing service. *See also* Health care administration
Adolescent empowerment, Frame theory of, 351
Affect, in Health Promotion Model, 439
Agency, in Symphonological Bioethical Theory, 563
Aggressive-protective subsystem, in Johnson Behavioral System Model, 369
Akayama, Tsuyoshi, 688–689
Alanen, Y., 683
Alexander, J. W., 377
Altschul, Annie, 676–677, 683
Alzheimer's disease, in Humanbecoming Theory, 520
AMICAE (Achieving Methods of Intraprofessional Consensus, Assessment and Evaluation) Project, 145–146, 150–151
Anthropology, 455
Anxiety
  In Maternal Role Attainment Theory, 584
  as risk factor for postpartum depression, 727, 728
Aquilina, Donna, 309
Araich, M., 347
Arendt, Hannah, 168
Argument, in logical reasoning, 26, 27–28
Aristotle, 16–17, 18, 562–563
Articulation research, 139
Assessment tools, in Johnson Behavioral System Model, 376–377
Attachment, in Maternal Role Attainment Theory, 585
Attachment-affiliative subsystem, in Johnson Behavioral System Model, 369
Attending Nurse Caring Model (ANCM), 100
Attention deficit-hyperactivity disorder (ADHD), in Frame theory of adolescent empowerment, 351
Awareness
  in Conservation Model, 228
  in transition experience, 420
Axioms
  defined, 26
  in theory development, 42, 43f, 44

B

Baccalaureate programs, 3–4, 8–9
Bacon, Frances, 17, 18
Baiardi, J., 351
Bandura, Albert, 436–437
Barker, Phil, 673–705
  background of, 673–674
  publications by, 674
  Tidal Model of Mental Health Recovery of, 33, 673–705
Barnard, Kathryn E., 52, 742
  background of, 61–62
  Child Health Assessment Interaction Theory of, 62, 63f
Barnum, B. S., 138
Basic Needs Satisfaction Inventory, 546
Bates, M., 227
Beck, Cheryl Tatano, 722–740
  background of, 722–723
  honors and awards, 723

Page numbers followed by *f*, *t*, and *b* indicate figures, tables, boxes, respectively.

Beck, Cheryl Tatano, *(Continued)*
Postpartum Depression Theory of, 722–735
and time line of perinatal research, 724t
Beech, Ian, 689
Behavior
In Health Promotion Model, 440, 442
In Johnson's Behavioral System Model, 368
Behavioral System Model, Johnson, 366–390
case study based on, 382–384
critique of, 381–382
disorders in, 376
empirical evidence for, 370–371
further development of, 379–381
logical form of, 375
major assumptions of, 371–373
major concepts and definitions in, 368–370
nursing community's acceptance of, 375–379
subsystems in, 368–369, 371–373, 374f, 378
summary of, 382
theoretical assertions of, 373–375
theoretical sources, 367–368
Being with, in Theory of Caring, 743
Beland, Irene, 227
Belief, in Theory of Caring, 743
Benner, Patricia, 137, 168
background of, 137–139
theory of
case study based on, 154–156
critique of, 152–154
empirical evidence in, 145–147
further development of, 151–152
logical form of, 149
major assumptions of, 147–149
major concepts and definitions in, 142–145
nursing community's acceptance of, 150–151
philosophical sources for, 139–145
summary of, 154
theoretical assertions of, 149
Benson, S., 377
Bentov, I., 482, 485
Bereavement, NCRCS studies of, 662, 665. *See also* Chronic Sorrow Theory
Berry, T., 337, 341
Best practices, in Theory of Comfort, 709
Biochemical loading, 723, 725
Bioethical standards, 567b. *See also* Symphonological Bioethical Theory
Bioethics, concerns of, 562. *See also* Symphonological Bioethical Theory
Biographical work, in Illness Trajectory Theory, 642. *See also* Story
Birth experience, perception of, 584
Bixenstine, E., 18
Blom, I., 167
Boca Raton Community Hospital, Nursing as Care Theory at, 405
Body
in Illness Trajectory Theory, 642, 643t
as natural attitude, 170
Body temperature, theoretical *versus* operational definition of, 40t
Bohm, David, 117, 482
Boundaries, in philosophy of caring, 174–175
Bourdieu, P., 169
Bournaki, M. C., 350
Boykin, Anne, 115, 393
background of, 394
co-authoship with S.Schoenhofer of, 395
and Nursing as Caring Theory, 395–415
Boyle, Joyceen, 114
Bradford, Helena, 731
Breast cancer, adaptation to, 348
Brecht, M., 378
Bronfenbrenner, U., 588, 590
Brown, H., 16, 18–20
Brown, Martha, 19–20
Bureaucratic Caring Theory
assertions of, 122–123
case study based on, 130–131
critique of, 129–130
empirical evidence for, 119–121
further development of, 126–129
holographic, 121, 121f
logical form of, 123
major assumptions of, 121–122
major concepts and definitions in, 118–119
nursing community's acceptance of, 123–126
original grounded, 120, 120f
research publications related to, 127t–128t
sources for, 116–119
Burke, Mary Lermann, 656–672. *See also* Chronic Sorrow Theory
background of, 658–659
Chronic Sorrow Theory of, 659–672
Burke Chronic Sorrow Questionnaire, 659
Burr, H. S., 245

C

California, University of, Neuropsychiatric Institute and Hospital at, 377
Cancer
  NCRCS studies of, 662, 665
  in Roy Adaptation Model, 348
  trajectory of living with, 643–646
Cancer patients, chronic sorrow and, 657–658. *See also* Chronic Sorrow Theory
Caplan, G., 310–311
Carative factors in Transpersonal Caring Theory, 94–96, 97t
Care
  culturally congruent, 466f
  in K. Martinsen's philosophy of caring, 173–174
  In Self-Care Deficit Theory, 269
  in transcultural nursing, 463
Care continuum, in Tidal Model of Mental Health Recovery, 682, 693f
Caregivers
  environmental stimuli and, 350
  NCRCS studies of, 662, 665
  of NICU infants, 743
  self-transcendence and, 626
Caregiving, adaptation to, 352
Caring. *See also* Bureaucratic Caring Theory; Caring, Theory of; Caritative Caring Theory; Culture Care Theory; Nursing as Caring Theory; Transpersonal Caring Theory
  as basis of moral nursing practice, 167–168
  P. Benner's examination of, 151–152
  Caring from the heart model, 406
  in Caritative Caring Theory, 198–199
  M. Heidegger's theory of, 170–171
  K. Martinsen's trinity of, 176
  in Postpartum Depression Theory, 723
  science of, 152
  K. M. Swanson's concept of, 743.
Caring, K. Martinsen's philosophy of
  case study based on, 181
  critique of, 180–181
  empirical evidence for, 175
  further development of, 179–180
  logical form of, 177–178
  major assumptions of, 176–177
  nursing community's applications of, 178–179
  sources for, 169–175
  theoretical assertions in, 177
Caring, Theory of
  Caring Model in, 743
  case study based on, 749
  critique of, 748–749
  empirical evidence for, 743–745
  further development of, 748
  Human Experience of Miscarriage in, 743
  logical form of, 747
  major assumptions of, 745–746
  major concepts and definitions of, 743
  nursing community's acceptance of, 747–748
  structure of caring in, 746, 746f
  theoretical assertions of, 746–747, 746f
  theoretical sources for, 742
Caritas, meaning of, 198
Caritas processes, in Transpersonal Caring Theory, 94, 97t, 101
Caritative Caring Theory, 190–221
  case study based on, 206–207
  critique of, 205–206
  empirical evidence for, 196–197
  further development of, 204–205
  logical form of, 201–202
  major assumptions of, 197–200
  major concepts and definitions in, 195–196
  nursing community's acceptance of, 202–204
  sources for, 193–194
  theoretical assertions in, 200–201
Causal process approach, to theory building, 42, 44, 45f
Center for Human Caring, Univ. of Colorado, 92
Certainty, in Symphonological Bioethical Theory, 567–568. *See also* Uncertainty in Illness Theory
Chadwick, E., 74
Chaos theory, 116, 245
  In Tidal Model of Mental Health Recovery, 676
  in Uncertainty in Illness Theory, 604–605
Chick, Norma, 418
Childbirth, PTSD after, 731–732. *See also* Postpartum Depression Theory
Child Health Assessment Interaction Theory, 61–62, 63f
Childrearing attitudes, in Maternal Role Attainment Theory, 584
Children
  assessment tool for hospitalized, 376
  caring for visually impaired, 378
Chiou, C. P., 349
Chronic sorrow
  management strategies for, 667–668
  theoretical model of, 666f
  triggers of, 662

Chronic Sorrow Theory, 656–672
  case study based on, 667–668
  critique of, 665–667
  empirical evidence for, 661–663
  further development of, 665
  logical form of, 663
  major assumptions of, 663
  major concepts and definitions in, 661
  model of, 666f
  nursing community acceptance of, 663–665
  summary of, 667
  theoretical assertions of, 663
  theoretical sources for, 660–661
  versus time-bound concept of grief, 660–661
Circle of Caring model, in advanced practice nursing, 407
Clarity
  in analysis of nursing theory, 12
  in Bureaucratic Theory, 129
  in Caring Theory, 748
  in Caritative Caring Theory, 205
  in Chronic Sorrow Theory, 665–666
  in Comfort Theory, 716
  in Conservation Model, 233
  in Health as Expanding Consciousness Theory, 493
  in Illness Trajectory Theory, 648
  in K. Martinson's philosophy of caring, 180
  in Maternal Attainment Role Theory, 593–594
  in Modeling and Remodeling Theory, 549
  in Neuman Systems Model, 321
  in Nursing as Caring Theory, 321, 407–408
  in Peaceful End of Life Theory, 758–759
  in Postpartum Depression Theory, 732
  in Roy Aaptation Model, 352–353
  in Self-care Deficit Theory, 276
  in Self-Transcendence Theory, 627
  in Symphonological Bioethical Theory, 572
  in Tidal Model of Mental Health Recovery, 691–693, 692f
  in Transition Theory, 425
  in Transpersonal Caring Theory, 101
  in Uncertainty in Illness Theory, 608–609
Client system, in Neuman Systems Model, 312–313
Clifford, J., 138
Clinical nurse specialist, skilled performance areas of, 150–151
Clinical nursing, helping art of, 57–58, 59f
Clinical practice. *See also* Practice, nursing
  In Culture Care Theory of Diversity and Universality, 469–470
  In Johnson's behavioral system model, 379
Coconstitution in Humanbecoming Theory, 505
Cody, W., 47
Coexistence in Humanbecoming Theory, 505–506
Coffman, S., 115
Cognator subsystem, in Roy's Adaptation Model, 338, 343–344, 343f, 355t
Cognition, Piaget's theory of, 20
Cognitive capacities, in Uncertainty in Illness Theory, 602
Cognitive schema, in Uncertainty in Illness Theory, 601
Colorado, University of, Center for Human Caring of, 92
Comfort
  historical accounts of, 707
  K. Kolcaba's concept of, 709
  in Peaceful End of Life Theory, 755
  taxonomic structure of, 708, 708f
  in Theory of Caring, 755
Comfort Theory, 706–719
  case study based on, 717–718
  comfort questionnaires based on, 714–715
  conceptual framework for, 710f
  critique of, 716
  empirical evidence for, 709–710
  further development of, 715–716
  logical form of, 712–713
  major assumptions of, 711
  major concepts and definitions in, 709, 710f
  nursing community's acceptance of, 713–715
  Peaceful End of Life Theory and, 755
  summary of, 716–717
  taxonomic structure of comfort needs for, 717t
  taxonomy in, 708, 708f, 714
  theoretical assertions of, 712
  theoretical sources for, 707–708, 708f
Communication, in Goal Attainment Theory, 297–298
Community, in Humanbecoming Theory, 506
Competence
  in P. Benner's philosophy, 143, 144
  in Dreyfus model, 143
Computers, in modern science, 18
Comte, A., 18
Concept analysis, 39, 39t
Concepts
  abstract *versus* concrete, 37–38
  discrete *versus* continuous, 38–39
  nonvariable, 38
  variable, 38–39
Conceptual models, 7, 7b, 63, 335
Conditioning factors, in Self-Care Deficit Theory, 272
Conditions, necessary/sufficient, 40–41

Connecting-separating concept in Humanbecoming Theory, 509, 515, 515f
Consciousness
movement as reflection of, 487
M. Newman's definition of, 482–483, 485
Consensus, scientific, 21–22
Conservation, concept of, 228–229
Conservation Model
case study based on, 234
critique of, 233
empirical evidence for, 230
further development of, 233
logical form of, 231
major assumptions of, 230–231
major concepts and definitions in, 227–229
nursing community's applications of, 231–233
sources for, 227
theoretical assertions of, 231
Consistency, in Self-Transcendence Theory, 627
Context, in Symphonological Bioethical Theory, 563
Contextual stimuli, in Roy's Adaptation Model, 338
Continuum of care, in Tidal Model of Mental Health Recovery, 682
Control, in Johnson Behavioral System Model, 370
Cook, E. T., 73
Cooley, M. E., 349
Coping
causal model of, 44, 45f
in Illness Trajectory Theory, 641, 643–645
Coping strategies
for chronic sorrow, 662–663
in Roy's Adaptation Model, 338
Corbin, J., 646
Core, Care, and Cure Model, of L. Hall, 60–61, 60f
Core self, in Maternal Role Attainment Theory, 587
Coronary artery bypass surgery, in Roy Adaptation Model, 348
Cotranscendence, in Humanbecoming Theory, 508–509
Ruth Rhoden Craven Foundation for Postpartum Depression Awareness, 731
Creation spirituality in Roy Adaptation Model, 341
Crisis, in Tidal Model of Mental Health Recovery, 681
Critical hermeneutics, P. Ricoeur's, 173
Critical Incident Technique, 684
Cross-cultural nursing, transcultural nursing compared with, 458
Cultural applications, of Neuman Systems Model, 319–320
Cultural blindness, nursing care and, 463
Cultural factors. *See also* Leininger's Culture Care Theory of Diversity and Universality; Transcultural nursing
P. Benner's assumptions about, 147
in Bureaucratic Caring Theory, 118
in expectations about pregnancy, 730
in Transition Theory, 418–419, 421, 423
Western *versus* non-Western, 455
Culturally competent nursing care, in Leininger's Culture Care Theory of Diversity and Universality, 461, 463
Cultural studies, Ray's theory and, 113–114
Culture
defined, 459
in Leininger's Culture Care Theory of Diversity and Universality, 460
Culture care, 460
accommodation in, 461
diversity in, 460
maintenance of, 461
preservation of, 461
repatterning/restructuring in, 461
universality in, 460
Culture Care Theory of Diversity and Universality, 454–479, 767
case study based on, 472
clinical application of, 469–470
critique of, 470–472
empirical evidence for, 461–463
enablers in, 467
further development of, 470
logical form of, 464–467
major assumptions of, 463–464
major concepts and definitions in, 460–461
nursing community's acceptance of, 467–469
summary of, 472
Sunrise Enabler in, 465, 466f, 467
theoretical assertions of, 464
theoretical sources for, 458–460
unique features of, 459–460
Curriculum, standardized, 4

D

Damus, K., 379
Dance of Caring Persons, 400–401, 401f
Data, P. Benner's assumptions about, 147
Davidson, A., 115
Death/dying. *See* Peaceful End of Life Theory
De Chardin, Pierre Teilhard, 94, 310, 337

Decision making
  of case manager, 117
  in Symphonological Bioethical Theory, 568, 569f
  triadic collaborative, 33
Deduction
  basic characteristics of, 33t
  examples of, 27, 33t
  in logical reasoning, 26–29
Dee, V., 378
Definitions
  theoretical *versus* operational, 40t
  in theory development, 37–39
Degree of reaction, in Neuman Systems Model, 313
Dependency subsystem, in Johnson Behavioral System Model, 369
Dependent care, in Self Care Deficit Theory, 269, 271
Depression. *See also* Postpartum Depression Theory
  in Maternal Role Attainment Theory, 584
  as risk factor for postpartum depression, 726
  and Self-Transcendence Theory, 621, 625
Derdiarian Behavioral System Model, 376–377
Derivable consequences
  in analysis of nursing theory, 13
  in P. Benner's account of nursing practice, 153–154
  in Bureaucratic Theory, 130
  in Caring Theory, 749
  in Caritative Caring Theory, 206
  in Chronic Sorrow Theory, 667
  in Comfort Theory, 716
  in Conservation Model, 233
  in Culture Care Theory, 471–472
  in Goal Attainment Theory, 298–299
  in Health as Expanding Consciousness Theory, 493
  in Health Promotion Model, 443–444
  in Humanbecoming Theory, 519–520
  in Illness Trajectory Theory, 648
  in Johnson Behavioral System Model, 382
  in K. Martinson's philosophy of caring, 180–181
  in Maternal Attainment Role Theory, 594–595
  in Modeling and Remodeling Theory, 550
  in Neuman Systems Model, 322
  in Nursing as Caring Theory, 426
  in Peaceful End of Life Theory, 760
  in Postpartum Depression Theory, 733
  in Roy Aaptation Model, 354
  in Science of Unitary Human Beings, 251
  in Self-Care Deficit Theory, 277–278
  in Self-Transcendence Theory, 628
  in Symphonological Bioethical Theory, 573
  in Tidal Model of Mental Health Recovery, 694
Derivable consequences *(Continued)*
  in Transition Theory, 426
  in Transpersonal Caring Theory, 102
  in Uncertainty in Illness Theory, 609–610
Developmental Resources of Later Adulthood (DRLA) Scale, 621
DeVillers, M. J., 346
Diagnoses, nursing
  chronic sorrow as, 664
  and Roy Adaptation Model, 345
Dickens, Charles, 74
Differential diagnosis, as empirical strategy, 17
Dignity, in Peaceful End of Life Theory, 756
DiMattio, M. J., 348
Discernment, professional, 173–174
Discipline
  defined, 8–10
  profession *versus,* 8
Diversity, in Culture Care Theory, 460
Dobratz, M. C., 347
Doctoral programs, 5, 9
  transcultural, 114–115
  in Transpersonal Caring Theory, 92
Dodd, Marylin J., 638–655
  background of, 639–640
  honors and awards, 640
  Illness Trajectory Theory of, 641–655
  and Johnson's behavioral system model, 378
Doing for, in Theory of Caring, 743
Domain, in Dreyfus Model, 144
Dossey, B. M., 73
Dreyfus, Hubert, 140, 148
Dreyfus, Stuart, 140
Dreyfus Model of Skill Acquisition, 150
  in P. Benner's philosophy, 140–141
  clinical application of, 149
  major concepts and definitions in, 142–145
Driscoll, J., 723, 725, 729
Droesbeke, J. L., 115
Dubin, R., 44
Dunlop, M. J., 152
Dunn, Halpert, 435
Dunne, Joseph, 140
Dunphy, L. H., 407

E

Eakes, Georgene Gaskill, 656
  background of, 657–658
  Chronic Sorrow Theory of, 660–672
  honors and awards, 658

Eating disturbances, as risk for postpartum depression, 728
Economics, in Bureaucratic Caring Theory, 119
Education, nursing
  baccalaureate and higher degree programs in, 3–4, 8–9
  P. Benner's theory in, 150–151
  Bureaucratic Caring Theory in, 125–126, 125f
  Caritative Caring Theory in, 202–203
  Chronic Sorrow Theory and, 664–665
  Comfort Theory in, 714
  Conservation Model in, 232
  Culture Care Theory in, 468–469
  doctoral programs, 5, 92, 114–115
  Goal Attainment Theory in, 296
  Health as Expanding Consciousness Theory in, 492–493
  Health Promotion Model in, 442–443
  Humanbecoming Theory in, 516–517
  Illness Trajectory Theory in, 647
  Johnson Behavioral System Model in, 378
  K. Martinsen's philosophy of caring in, 178–179
  master's programs, 4, 5, 9
  Maternal Role Attainment Theory in, 592
  Modeling and Role-modeling Theory in, 548
  B. Neuman's Systems Model applications in, 318–319
  F. Nightingale's role in, 4, 78–81
  Norwegian debate over, 166–167
  Nursing as Caring Theory in, 403–404
  Peaceful End of Life Theory in, 758
  Roy Adaptation Model and, 347
  Symphonological Bioethical Theory in, 570–571
  Theory of Caring in, 747–748
  Tidal Model of Mental Health Recovery in, 689
  Transition Theory and, 425
  Transpersonal Caring Theory in, 100–101
  Uncertainty in Illness Theory in, 606–607
  and Unitary Human Beings Theory, 249
Einstein, Albert, 17, 245
Eipperle, M. K., 470
Eliminative subsystem, in Johnson Behavioral System Model, 369
Embodiment, definition of, 148
Emic beliefs, in Culture Care Theory, 461, 462
Emic culture care
  health and illness outcomes and, 464
  study of, 469–470
Emotional lability, as risk for postpartum depression, 728
Empirical precision
  in analysis of nursing theory, 13
  in P. Benner's account of nursing practice, 153
  in Bureaucratic Theory, 129–130
  in Caring Theory, 749
  in Caritative Caring Theory, 206
  in Chronic Sorrow Theory, 667
  in Comfort Theory, 716
  in Conservation Model, 233
  in Culture Care Theory, 471
  in Goal Attainment Theory, 298
  in Health as Expanding Consciousness Theory, 493
  in Health Promotion Model, 443
  in Humanbecoming Theory, 519
  in Illness Trajectory Theory, 648
  in Johnson Behavioral System Model, 381–382
  in K. Martinson's philosophy of caring, 180
  in Maternal Attainment Role Theory, 594
  in Modeling and Remodeling Theory, 550
  in Neuman Systems Model, 321
  in Nursing as Caring Theory, 426
  in Peaceful End of Life Theory, 760
  in Postpartum Depression Theory, 732–733
  in Roy Aaptation Model, 353–354
  in Science of Unitary Human Beings, 251
  in Self-care Deficit Theory, 277
  in Self-Transcendence Theory, 628
  in Symphonological Bioethical Theory, 572–573
  in Tidal Model of Mental Health Recovery, 694
  in Transition Theory, 426
  in Transpersonal Caring Theory, 102
  in Uncertainty in Illness Theory, 609
Empiricism, 16–18
Empowerment
  in Health as Expanding Consciousness Theory, 490
  in Tidal Model of Mental Health Recovery, 683–684
Enabling, in Theory of Caring, 743
Enabling-limiting concept, in Humanbecoming Theory, 508–509, 515, 515f
End-of-life decisions, self-transcendence and, 626–627. *See also* Peaceful End of Life Theory
Energy, in Conservation Model, 229
Energy field, M. Rogers' concept of, 244
Engagement, in transition experience, 420–421
Environment
  in Bureaucratic Caring Theory, 122
  in Caring Theory, 746
  in Chronic Sorrow Theory, 663
  in Comfort Theory, 711, 746

Environment *(Continued)*
in Conservation Model, 227–228, 231
in Culture Care Theory, 460
F. Nightingale's emphasis on, 75–79, 81, 82
in Goal Attainment Theory, 292
in Health as Expanding Consciousness Theory, 483
in Johnson Behavioral System Model, 372–373
in Maternal Role Attainment Theory, 587–588
in Modeling and Role-Modeling Theory, 547
in Neuman's Systems Model, 312, 316
in Peace at End of Life Theory, 756–757
in philosophy of caring, 177
in Postpartum Depression Theory, 729
Roy Adaptation Model in, 342–343
in Self-Transcendence Theory, 622–623
in Tidal Model of Mental Health Recovery, 686
in Transpersonal Caring Theory, 99
in Unitary Human Beings Theory, 246
Environment-agreement, in Symphonological Bioethical Theory, 563, 565–566
Epistemology
defined, 16
rationalist, 17
recent approaches to, 18–19
Equilibrium, in Johnson Behavioral System Model, 369, 373
Erickson, Helen C.
background of, 537–538
honors and awards, 538
Modeling and Role-Modeling Paradigm of, 540–559
Erickson, Milton H., and Modeling and Role-Modeling Paradigm, 541
Erickson Maternal Bonding-Attachment Tool, 546
Erikson, Erik, 94, 99, 227, 540
Erikson Psychosocial Stage Inventory, 546
Eriksson, Katie, 179
background of of, 190–193
Caritative Caring Theory of, 190–221
and K. Martinsen's philosophy of caring, 168
Ethical health care, deficiency of, 562
Ethics
in Dreyfus Model of Skill Acquisition, 144–145
G. L. Husteds' definition of, 562
as primary, 171
in Symphonological Bioethical Theory, 566–567, 567b
Ethnohistory, in Culture Care Theory, 460
Ethnonursing research, 455, 460, 462, 463, 464–465, 471
Etic beliefs, in Culture Care Theory, 461–462
Etic culture care
and health and illness outcomes, 464
study of, 469–470
Everyday-life work, in Illness Trajectory Theory, 642
Exemplar, Dreyfus Model definition of, 144
Exercise, in Roy Adaptation Model, 348
Exercise Benefits-Barrier Scale, 440–441
Exosystem, *versus* mesosystem, 588
Experience, Dreyfus Model definition of, 144
Expert, Dreyfus Model definition of, 143–144
Eye, registering, in philosophy of caring, 175
Eye of the heart, in philosophy of caring, 175

F

Family, in Role Attainment Theory, 585
Family therapy, 19
Father/intimate partner, in Maternal Role Attainment Theory, 585, 588f
Fawcett, Jacqueline, 45, 278, 346, 349, 742
metaparadigm concepts of, 44–45
and Roy Adaptation Model, 346
and Science of Unitary Human Beings, 251
Feminism, F. Nightingale and, 80
Feshbach, S., 369
Fight or flight response, in Conservation Model, 228
Fitzpatrick, Joyce J., 618, 619
Flexibility, in Maternal Role Attainment Theory, 584
Focal stimulus, in Roy's Adaptation Model, 338
Folkman, S., 601, 660–661
Foucault, Michel, 18, 169, 172–173
Frame theory of adolescent empowerment, 351
Frankl, Viktor, 61, 623
Frank-Stromborg, Marilyn, 435
Freedom, in Humanbecoming Theory, 506
Freud, Sigmund, 32
Fry, S., 23
Functional requirements, in Johnson Behavioral System Model, 370

G

Gable, Robert K., 725
Gadsup people, M. Leininger's study of, 455
Gale, G., 16–17, 19, 24
Gallagher, M. S., 350
General Comfort Questionnaire, 714–715
Generality
in analysis of nursing theory, 12–13
in P. Benner's account of nursing practice, 152–153
in Bureaucratic Theory, 129

Generality *(Continued)*
in Caring Theory, 748–749
in Caritative Caring Theory, 205–206
in Chronic Sorrow Theory, 667
in Comfort Theory, 716
in Conservation Model, 233
in Culture Care Theory, 471
in Goal Attainment Theory, 297–298
in Health as Expanding Consciousness Theory, 493
in Health Promotion Model, 443
in Humanbecoming Theory, 518–519
in Illness Trajectory Theory, 648
in Johnson Behavioral System Model, 381
in K. Martinson's philosophy of caring, 180
in Maternal Attainment Role Theory, 594
in Modeling and Remodeling Theory, 550
in Neuman Systems Model, 321
in Nursing as Caring Theory, 425–426
in Peaceful End of Life Theory, 759
in Postpartum Depression Theory, 732
in Roy Aaptation Model, 353
in Science of Unitary Human Beings, 251
in Self-care Deficit Theory, 277
in Self-Transcendence Theory, 628
in Symphonological Bioethical Theory, 572
in Tidal Model of Mental Health Recovery, 693–694
in Transition Theory, 425–426
in Transpersonal Caring Theory, 102
in Uncertainty in Illness Theory, 609
General system theory. *See also* Systems theory
in Johnson Behavioral System Model, 370–371
in Maternal Role Attainment Theory, 583
in Neuman Systems Model, 310, 317–318
Peaceful End of Life Theory and, 755
Unitary Human Beings Theory and, 245
Gestalt theory, in Neuman Systems Model, 310
Gibson, J. E., 227
Giere, R. N., 40, 41
Glaser, B., 114, 723
Goal Attainment Theory
case study based on, 299
critique of, 297–299
empirical evidence for, 289–291
further development of, 297
logical form of, 294
major assumptions of, 292
major concepts and definitions in, 288–289
middle range, 291, 294, 298–299
nursing community's acceptance of, 294–297
Goal Attainment Theory *(Continued)*
propositions within, 293b
relationship table for, 293t
theoretical assertions of, 292, 293b, 293f, 294
Goal-Oriented Nursing Record (GONR), 295
Gomez, O. J., 124
Goodnow, M., 707
Gratification-satisfaction, in Maternal Role Attainment Theory, 584
Grice, S. L., 377
Grief, time-bound concept of, 660–661
Grieving and loss, and Humanbecoming Theory, 517, 520. *See also* Chronic Sorrow Theory
Grounded theory, of bureaucratic caring, 120, 120f
Growth Through Uncertainty Scale, 607
Guilt, as risk for postpartum depression, 728

H

Hage, J., 36–37, 39, 41–42, 44
Hainsworth, Margaret A., 656
background of, 659–660
Chronic Sorrow Theory of, 656–672
Hall, James, 435
Hall, John, 73
Hall, Lydia, 51
background of, 60
Core, Care, and Cure Model of, 60–61, 60f
Hardy, M. E., 81
Harmer, B., 707
Healing, self-transcendence and, 625
Healing web model, 492
Health
P. Benner on, 149
in Bureaucratic Caring Theory, 122
in Caring Theory, 745
in Caritative Caring Theory, 200
in Chronic Sorrow Theory, 663
in Comfort Theory, 711
in Conservation Model, 231
in Culture Care Theory, 461
in Goal Attainment Theory, 288, 292
in Health as Expanding Consciousness Theory, 483–484
in Humanbecoming Theory, 514
in Johnson Behavioral System Model, 372
in Maternal Role Attainment Theory, 587
in Modeling and Role-Modeling Theory, 546
in Neuman Systems Model, 313, 314, 316
F. Nightingale's definition of, 77

Health (Continued)
in Peace at End of Life Theory, 756–757
in philosophy of caring, 176–177
in Postpartum Depression Theory, 729
in Roy's Adaptation Model, 342
in Self-Transcendance Theory, 622
in Symphonological Bioethical Theory, 563–564, 565
in Tidal Model of Mental Health Recovery, 685–686
in Transition Theory, 418
in Transpersonal Caring Theory, 99
in Unitary Human Beings Theory, 246
Health as Expanding Consciousness Theory, 480–502, 767
case study based on, 494–495
client populations used with, 490–491
cooperative inquiry/integrative participation in, 491–492
empirical evidence for, 486
further development of, 493
influence of M. Rogers on, 250
logical form of, 489
major assumptions of, 486
major concepts and definitions in, 484–485
nursing community's acceptance of, 489–493
relationship to metaparadigm concepts, 481–484
summary of, 493–494
theoretical assertions and development of, 486–489
theoretical sources for, 484
Health care administration
and Bureaucratic Theory, 124
Husted Symphonological model and, 571
and Transpersonal Caring Theory, 100
Health care needs, in Comfort Theory, 709
Health care professionals, in Symphonological Bioethical Theory, 562–563
Health care system, and bioethical dilemmas, 562
Health Promoting Lifestyle Profile, 435, 440–441
Health Promotion Model (HPM), 434–453, 437f
action in, 439, 440, 442
case study based on, 444–445
critique of, 443–444
empirical evidence for, 439–441
further development of, 443
logical form of, 442
major assumptions of, 441
major concepts and definitions in, 438–439
nursing community's acceptance of, 442–443
revised, 439–440, 440f
summary of, 444
theoretical assertions of, 441–442
theoretical sources of, 436–437, 437f
Health-seeking behaviors, in Comfort Theory, 709
Health status, in Maternal Role Attainment Theory, 584
Healthy Start CORPS: Inter-Conceptual Care Case Management Project, 731
Heart, eye of, in K. Martinsen's philosophy of caring, 175
Heart failure, theoretical *versus* operational definition of, 40t
Hegel, G. W. F., 116, 482
Heidegger, Martin, 94, 140, 149, 168, 170–171, 504, 512
Helicy principle, 19, 247t, 248
Helping methods, in Self-Care Deficit Theory, 271
Helson, Harry
adaptation-level theory of, 27
and Roy Adaptation Model, 336, 344–345
Henderson, Virginia, 50, 138
Comfort Theory and, 708
theory and influence of, 55–57
Herbert, S., 72, 74
Hermeneutic phenomenology
P. Ricoeur on, 173
Hermeneutics
P. Benner on, 147, 152
in Dreyfus Model, 145
in Nursing as Caring Theory, 406
Holaday, B., 376
Holism
in Conservation Model, 227
in Modeling and Role-Modeling Theory, 542–543
Hologram, universe as, 117
Holographic Theory, of Bureaucratic Caring, 121. *See also* Bureaucratic Caring Theory
Holonomy, defined, 116–117
Home health nursing, Schoenhofer-Boykin study of, 406
Homeodynamic principles, in Science of Unitary Human Beings, 246, 247t, 248
Hope Study, R. R. Parse's, 504
Humanbecoming
concepts of, 514–515
R. R. Parse's concept of, 506, 514
postulates of, 506
Humanbecoming hermeneutic model, 511–512, 517
Humanbecoming teaching-learning model, 516–517
Humanbecoming Theory, 504–535, 515f, 767
applications of, 519–520
case study based on, 521
critique of, 518–520
empirical evidence for, 510–512
logical form of, 515, 515f

Humanbecoming Theory, *(Continued)*
major assumptions of, 512–514
major concepts and definitions in, 507–510
nursing community's acceptance of, 515–518
summary of, 520–521
theoretical assertions in, 514–515
theoretical sources for, 504–506
Human being. *See also* Person; Personhood
in Caritative Caring Theory, 195–198
D. E. Orem's view of, 267–268
Human care, in Culture Care Theory, 460. *See also* Care; Caregivers; Caring
Human development, in Self-Transcendence Theory, 19
Human evolution, A. M. Young's stages of, 488, 488f
Humanism, in Roy Adaptation Model, 341
Human needs
V. Henderson on, 14, 56, 56b
in Transpersonal Caring Theory, 96
E. Wiedenbach's identification of, 58, 59f, 60f
Human subjectivity, in Humanbecoming Theory, 505
Human-to-Human Relationship Model, of J. Travelbee, 62, 63f
Humanuniverse, in Humanbecoming Theory, 506, 514
Husserl, E., 19, 168, 170, 175
Husted, Gladys L., 560
background of, 561–562
Symphonological Bioethical Theory of, 562–578
Husted, James H., 560
background of, 561–562
Symphonological Bioethical Theory of, 562–578
Hutchinson, S., 723
Hypochondriasis, in Unitarian Human Beings Theory, 246

I

Iatrogenesis, in Science of Unitary Human Beings, 246
Identity
in Illness Trajectory Theory, 642, 643t
in Maternal Role Attainment Theory, 584
Illich, Ivan, 685
Illness
and chronic sorrow, 656–672
in Neuman Systems Model, 313
in Uncertainty in Illness Theory, 602–603, 605f
Illness Trajectory Theory, 642
case study based on, 649–650
critique of, 648–649
empirical evidence for, 643–645
further development of, 647–648
Illness Trajectory Theory, *(Continued)*
logical form of, 646
major assumptions of, 645–646
major concepts and definitions in, 642–643, 643t, 644t
status of uncertainty in, 643f
theoretical assertions of, 646
theoretical sources for, 641
Illusion, in Uncertainty in Illness Theory, 602
Imaging concept, in Humanbecoming Theory, 507, 514–515, 515f
Immigrants, Transition Theory and, 418–419, 423
Induction
basic characteristics of, 29–31, 33t–34t
in clinical practice, 30–31
degrees of strength and probability of, 30
examples of, 29
method, 17
F. Nightingale's use of, 79
Ineffective responses, in Roy's Adaptation Model, 338
Infant, in Maternal Role Attainment Theory, 585
Infant nursing, E. Wiedenbach's contributions to, 57–58, 59f
Infant temperament, as risk for postpartum depression, 727
Inference
defined, 26
statistical, 30
in Uncertainty in Illness Theory, 602
Inflammatory response, in Conservation Model, 228
Ingestive subsystem, in Johnson Behavioral System Model, 369
Institutional integrity, in Comfort Theory, 709
Integrality, in Unitary Human Beings Theory, 248
Integrated life process, in Roy's Adaptation Model, 339
Integrity, in Conservation Model, 229, 230
Interactionist perspective, in history of science, 20
Interdependence mode, in Roy's Adaptation Model, 340
International Association for Human Caring, 115
International Orem Society for Nursing Science and Scholarship, 276, 769
Interpersonal influences, in Health Promotion Model, 439
Interpersonal relations, H. E. Peplau's theory of, 54–55, 54f, 55f
Interpersonal systems, in Goal Attainment Theory, 290–292
Interpretive paradigm, and development of knowledge in nursing, 23
Isenberg, M. A., 349, 351

J

Jenkins, J., 351
JFK Medical Center, Nursing as Caring Theory at, 405
Jirovec, M. M., 351
Johnson, Dorothy E., 63, 335
  background of, 366–367
  Behavioral System Model of, 367–390
  honors and awards, 366–367
Johnson, Jean, 754
Journals
  Nursing Research, 9
  on nursing theory, 769
  Visions: The Journal of Rogerian Nursing Science, 767
Jowett, B., 74

K

Kalish, B. J., 73
Kalish, P. A., 73
Keenan, J., 40
Kendall Chronic Sorrow Instrument, 665
Kennedy, M., 73
Kierkegaard, Søren, 94, 140
King, Imogene M., 286
  background of, 286–288
  Goal Attainment Theory of, 286–308
  honors and awards, 287–288
  Nightingale tribute to, 286–288
  publications by, 286–288
King International Nursing Group, 288
Kirkevold, M., 178
Kiser-Larson, N., story and caring study of, 406
Knowing, in Theory of Caring, 743
Knowledge
  nursing, 767, 767f
  self-care, 544–546
  structural levels for, 8, 8t
  and theory-based evidence, 11
Knowledge development, P. Benner's approach to, 141–142
Kolcaba, Katharine, 706
  background of, 706–707
  Theory of Comfort of, 707–721
Kuhn, T. S., 6, 10, 766

L

Lachicotte, J. L., 377
Languaging concept, in Humanbecoming Theory, 507–508, 514–515, 515f
Lanouette, M., 377
Lazarus, Richard S., 140, 141, 601, 660–661
Leadership, in Transpersonal Caring Theory, 100
Leininger, Madeleine M., 454
  background of, 454–458
  Culture Care Theory of Diversity and Universality of, 454–479, 767
  honors and awards, 457–458
  influence on M. A. Ray of, 113–114
Lenz, Elizabeth, 754
Levine, Myra Estrin, 225
  background of, 225–226
  Conservation Model of, 227–241
  honors and awards, 226
  publications by, 230, 232
Life, in Uncertainty in Illness Theory, 602
Life process, in Roy's Adaptation Model, 339
Life utterances
  in K. E. Løgstrup's ethics, 174
  in K. M. Martinsen's philosophy of caring, 171
Lindgren, Carolyn, 657, 659
Linkages, in theory development, 41–42, 44
Lipscomb, J. A., 80
Living, activities of, Roper-Logan-Tierney model based on, 63, 64f, 65f, 66t
Locsin, R. C., 407
Loeb Center for Nursing and Rehabilitation, 60
Logan, Winifred W., 53, 62–64, 63
Logic, discipline of, 26
Logical empiricists, 18
Logical positivism, 18
Logical reasoning, 26–35
  deduction, 26–29, 33t–34t
  induction, 29–31, 33t–34t
  retroduction, 31–33, 33t–34t
Løgstrup, Knud E., 140, 168, 171–172
Løgstrup, R., 168
Lorentzon, M., 73, 80
Lorenz, Konrad, 369
Loss, in Chronic Sorrow Theory, 661
Lovejoy, N, 378
Luther, M., 172
Lynaugh, J., 138

M

MacIntyre, Alistair, 140
Macrae, J. A., 73
Macrosystem, in Maternal Role Attainment Theory, 588, 588f
Maintaining belief, in Theory of Caring, 743

Managed health care, patient outcomes from, 378
Management strategies, in Chronic Sorrow Theory, 661–663
Marchione, J. M., 490
Marineau, H., 74
Maritain, J., 268
Martinsen, Kari, 140, 165
  background of, 165–169
  philosophy of caring of, 169–189
Marx, Karl, 169–170, 310
Maslow, Abraham, 94, 99, 540, 623
Master's degree programs, 4, 5, 9
Maternal identity, in Maternal Role Attainment Theory, 584
Maternal role attainment, *versus* becoming a mother, 586
Maternal Role Attainment Theory, 581–598, 583f, 584
  case study based on, 594
  critique of, 593–594
  empirical evidence for, 586
  further development of, 592–593
  logical form of, 590–591
  major assumptions of, 586–587
  major concepts and definitions of, 584–585
  maternal and infant traits and, 589
  microsystem, mesosystem, and macrosystem in, 588, 588f
  nursing community's acceptance of, 591–592
  original model, 583f, 588–589
  revised model, 588f, 589–590
  role acquisition stages in, 589
  summary of, 594
  theoretical assertions of, 587–590, 591f
  theoretical sources for, 583
Maternity blues, 725, 727. *See also* Postpartum Depression Theory
Maxim, Dreyfus Model definition of, 144
May, R., 61
Mayeroff, M., 396
McCance, K., 114
McCorkle, R., 349
McCray-Stewart, D., 123
McDonald, L., 73
McElmurry, Beverly, 435
McFarland, M. R., 470
McPhaul, K. M., 80
Mead, Margaret, 455, 583
Meaning
  P. Benner's concept of, 147
  in Humanbecoming Theory, 507–508, 513
Meleis, Afaf Ibrahim, 416
  background of, 416–419
  honors and awards, 417
  Transition Theory of, 416–433
Memory, P. Benner's concept of, 152
Mental confusion, as risk for postpartum depression, 728
Mental health services, collaborative relationships in, 675
Mental illness, in Tidal Model, 686. *See also* Tidal Model of Mental Health Recovery
Mercer, Ramona T., 581
  background of, 581–582
  honors and awards, 582
  Maternal Role Attainment Theory of, 582–598
  publications by, 582, 593
Merleau-Ponty, Maurice, 140, 148, 149, 170, 504, 512
Mesosystem, *versus* exosystem, 588
Metaparadigm, 8t, 45, 47
Microsystem, in Maternal Role Attainment Theory, 588, 588f
Middle range theory, 7–8, 7b. *See also specific theories*
  of adaptation, 351–352
  Caring, Theory of, 741–752
  characteristics of, 425–426, 579, 769
  Chronic Sorrow Theory, 657–672
  Comfort Theory, 706–721
  development of, 46
  examples of, 8t, 768
  in generic structure, 768, 768f
  Goal Attainment Theory, 286–308
  growth of, 770
  Illness Trajectory Theory, 638–655
  Maternal Role Attainment Theory, 581–598
  nursing practice applications of, 768
  Peaceful End of Life Theory, 753–762
  Postpartum Depression Theory, 722–740
  role of, 765
  Self-Transcendence Theory, 618–637
  texts on, 768
  theorists producing, 7–8, 7b
  Tidal Model of Mental Health Recovery, 673–705
  Transition Theory, 417–433
  Uncertainty in Illness Theory, 599–617
Mill, John Stuart, 74, 80
Mind-body relationships in Modeling and Role-Modeling Theory, 543
Miscarriage, in Theory of Caring, 742, 744–745
Mishel, Merle H., 599
  background of, 599–600
  honors and awards, 600
  Uncertainty in Illness Theory of, 601–617, 604f

Mishel Uncertainty in Illness Scale, 599, 602
Model for Nursing Education Grounded in Caring, 407
Modeling, concept of, 541
Modeling and Role-Modeling Theory, 32–33, 536–559, 767
  assessment tool based on, 558–559
  case study based on, 551
  critique of, 549–550
  empirical evidence for, 543–546
  further development of, 549
  logical form of, 547
  major assumptions of, 546–547
  major concepts and definitions in, 541–543
  nursing community's acceptance of, 547–549
  and Reed Self-Transcendence Theory, 625
  retroductive reasoning in, 32
  summary of, 550
  theoretical assertions of, 547
  theoretical sources for, 540–541
Models, conceptual, 7, 7b
Modrcin-Talbott, M. A., Roy Adaptation Model and, 349–350
Montag, Mildred, 286
Mood disorders, in Postpartum Depression Theory, 725–726
Moore, C., 352
Moore, Shirley M., 753
  background of, 754
  Peaceful End of Life Theory of, 755–762
Moral practice, and K. Martinsen's philosophy of caring, 174
Morita, Shoma, 675–676
Morse, J., 114
Moss, I., 482
Mother-father relationship, in Maternal Role Attainment Theory, 585
Mothers, at-risk, in Caring Theory, 744
Motivational drives, in Johnson Behavioral System Model, 368
Movement-space-time, in Health as Expanding Consciousness Theory, 485, 487
Mubarak, H., 417
Mullins, N., 44
Multiple sclerosis, and chronic sorrow, 660
Murdaugh, Carolyn L., 435
Murray, Henry, 713

N

NANDA (North American Nursing Diagnosis Association), 664
Narrative memory, P. Benner's concept of, 152
National League for Nursing (NLN), higher education accreditation criteria of, 5
National Transcultural Nursing Society, 456
Needs. *See* Human needs
Negentropy
  in general system theory, 245
  in Neuman Systems Model, 312
Neuman, Betty, 309
  background of, 309–310
  Systems Model of, 309–334, 315f, 767
Neuman Nursing Process Format, steps in, 317
Neuman Systems Model-Based Nursing Research, 319
Neuman Systems Model Symposium, 320, 769
Newman, D. M., Roy Adaptation Model and, 346–347
Newman, Margaret A., 31, 480
  background of, 480–481
  Health as Expanding Consciousness Theory of, 481–502, 767
  honors and awards, 480–481
  publications by, 481, 486
New view of life, Mishel's concept of, 602
Nhat Hanh, Thich, 94
Nightingale, Florence, 9, 71–90
  and acceptance by nursing community, 79–81
  biographies of, 73
  case study using approach of, 84
  on comfort, 707
  Conservation Model and, 227
  credentials and background of, 71–73
  in Crimean War, 72
  critique of, 82–83
  and empirical evidence, 76–77
  environmental emphasis of, 75–79
  and feminism, 80
  as founder of modern nursing, 4
  germ theory and, 78
  influence on Dorothy E. Johnson of, 367
  logical form of, 79
  major assumptions of, 77–78
  major concepts and definitions of, 75–76
  mentoring by, 80
  religious influences on, 74–75
  retrospective analyses of work of, 72–73
  schools established by, 72

Nightingale, Florence, *(Continued)*
suffrage movement and, 80
theory of, 73–75, 78–79, 81–83
vision of, 5
Northrup, F. S.C., 245
Nosocomial conditions, in Science of Unitary Human Beings, 246
Notes on Nursing (Nightingale), 75, 77–78, 81, 83
Nowack, S., 44
Nuamah, I. F., 349
Nurse Educator Nursing Theory Conference, 9
Nurse-patient interactions, in Goal Attainment Theory, 291, 291f, 297–298
Nurse-patient relationship
A. Altschul's research on, 683
changing aspects of, 55
in Health as Expanding Consciousness Theory, 482–483, 483f
in Neuman Systems Model, 316
in F. Nightingale's writings, 82
in Nursing as Caring Theory, 398
overlapping phases in, 54f
H. E. Peplau's theory of, 54–55, 54f, 55f, 675
in Tidal Model of Mental Health Recovery, 683–684, 686
Nurse-Patient Relationship Resource Analysis Tool, 128
Nurse practitioners, caring relationships of, 406
Nursing
in Behavioral Systems Model, 371
in Bureaucratic Caring Theory, 121
changing paradigms of, 23
Chronic Sorrow Theory in, 663
in Comfort Theory, 711
conceptual models in, 7, 7b, 8t, 9
in Conservation Model, 230
as discipline, 8–10
in Goal Attainment Theory, 288, 292
Health as Expanding Consciousness Theory in, 482
V. Henderson's definition of, 55–57
in Humanbecoming Theory, 513–514
knowledge base of, 3, 5, 23, 767
Maternal Role Attainment Theory in, 586–587
Modeling and Role-Modeling Theory in, 542, 546
B. Neuman's Systems Model in, 314
in Novice to Expert Skill Acquisition Model, 148
in Nursing as Caring Theory, 396–398, 400
philosophy and philosophical shifts of, 23–24
in Postpartum Depression Theory, 729
professional status of, 4, 5, 8, 10–12
Nursing *(Continued)*
Roy Adaptation Model in, 341–342
Science of Unitary Human Beings in, 245
Self-Transcendence Theory in, 622
shared interests with anthropology of, 455
in Symphonological Bioethical Theory, 564, 565
Theory of Caring in, 745
Tidal Model of Mental Health Recovery in, 684–685
transcultural (*see* Culture Care Theory; Transcultural nursing)
Transpersonal Caring Theory in, 98
Nursing agency, in Self-Care Deficit Theory, 271
Nursing assessment, in Johnson Behavioral System Model, 375–376
Nursing care
comparative systems of, 456
cultural blindness and, 463
culturally competent, 461, 463
Nursing as Caring Theory, 395–415
case study based on, 409–410
critique of, 407–408
Dance of Caring Persons in, 400–401, 401f
empirical evidence for, 398–399
further development of, 407
logical form of, 401
major assumptions of, 399–400
major concepts and definitions in, 396–398
research studies in, 404–407
summary of, 408–409
theoretical assertions of, 400–401
theoretical sources for, 395–396
Nursing Child Assessment Satellite Training Project, 62
Nursing clinician-case manager, 117, 489
Nursing community's acceptance of, 401–407, 663–665, 713–715
Nursing Consortium for Research on Chronic Sorrow, 657–658, 662
Nursing frameworks
significance of, 10
types of, 6–8, 7b
Nursing interventions
in Johnson Behavioral System Model, 375
outcomes and, 545
Roy Adaptation Model and, 345–346
Nursing knowledge
generic structure of, 767f
role of, 767
Nursing problems, F. G. Abdellah's typology of, 57, 58b

Nursing process
in Johnson Behavioral System Model, 375–376
I. J. Orlando's theory of, 65–66, 66t
Nursing programs
master's degree, 4, 5, 9
PhD, 5, 9, 92, 114–115
Nursing record, goal-oriented, 295
Nursing response, in Nursing as Caring Theory, 398
Nursing scholars, global communities of, 769–770, 770t. *See also* Nursing theorists; *specific theorists*
Nursing science, D. E. Orem's sets of, 268, 268b. *See also* Science
Nursing service administration, in Nursing as Caring Theory, 402–403
Nursing situation, in Nursing as Caring Theory, 397
Nursing systems in Self-Care Deficit Theory, 271, 273f
Nursing theorists, 54–68
Abdellah, F. G., 57
Adam, E., 62
Barnard, K., 61-62
Hall, L., 60-61
Henderson, V., 55-57
international, 769
Logan, W. W., 62-64
Orlando (Pellitier), I. J., 65-66
Peplau, H. E., 54-55
Roper, N., 62-64
Tierney, A. J., 62-64
Travelbee, J., 61
Weidenbach, E., 57-60
Nursing therapeutics, in Transition Theory, 422
Nurturance, in Modeling and Role-Modeling Paradigm, 542
Nyberg, J. J., 124

O

O'Brien, K., 124
Obsessive-compulsive disorder, postpartum, 726. *See also* Postpartum Depression Theory
O'Donnell, Michael, 436
Older adults, Self-Transcendence Theory and, 621, 625
Olshansky, S., 659, 660
O'Malley, I. B., 73
O'Neill, Onora, 140
Open system
in Neuman Systems Model, 311–312
in Science of Unitary Human Beings, 244
Ordering, in theory development, 41–42, 44
Orem, Dorothea E., 265
background of, 265–266
honors and awards of, 266
Self-Care Deficit Theory of, 266–285, 767
Organismic response, in Conservation Model, 228
Originating concept, in Humanbecoming Theory, 509–510, 515, 515f
Orlando (Pelletier), Ida Jean, 9, 53, 57
background of, 65
Comfort Theory and, 708
theory and influence of, 65–66

P

Pain
middle range theory of, 352
in Peaceful End of Life Theory, 755
in Theory of Caring, 748
Pain control behaviors, research on, 378–379
Palencia, I., 352
Pandimensionality, in Science of Unitary Human Beings, 244
Panic disorder, postpartum-onset, 726
Paradigm case, Dreyfus Model definition of, 144
Parse, Rosemarie Rizzo, 503
background of, 503–504
honors and awards, 504
Humanbecoming Theory of, 504–535
publications by, 503–504
M. Rogers' theory and, 250
Parsons, Mary Ann, 435
Parsons, Talcott, 367
Paterson, J. G., 395, 708
Patient. *See also* Nurse–patient relationship
in Comfort Theory, 711
E. Wiedenbach's approach to, 58, 59f, 60f
Patterns
in Health as Expanding Consciousness Theory, 482–484, 483f, 485
in Science of Unitary Human Beings, 244
Peace, experience of, 756
Peaceful End of Life Theory
case study based on, 760
critique of, 758–760, 759f
empirical evidence for, 756
further development of, 758
logical form of, 757
major assumptions of, 756–757
major concepts and definitions in, 755–756
nursing community's acceptance of, 757–758

Peaceful End of Life Theory *(Continued)*
theoretical assertions of, 757
theoretical sources for, 755
Pelletier (Orlando), Ida Jean. *See* Orlando (Pelletier), Ida Jean
Pender, Nola J., 434
awards and honors, 435–436
background of, 434–436
Health Promotion Model of, 436–453
Penhale, Helen, 434
Peplau, Hildegard E., 50
and P. Barker's work, 675–677, 683
theory and influence of, 54–55
Perceived Enactment of Autonomy Tool, 546
Perception, in Roy's Adaptation Model, 340, 344, 344f
Perceptual awareness, in Conservation Model, 228
Person. *See also* Human beings
P. Benner and J. Wrubel's concept of, 121
in Bureaucratic Caring Theory, 121
in Caring Theory, 745
in Chronic Sorrow Theory, 663
in Conservation Model, 230
in Goal Attainment Theory, 292
in Health as Expanding Consciousness Theory, 482–483
in Humanbecoming Theory, 505–506, 510
in Johnson Behavioral System Model, 371–372
in K. Martinsen's philosophy of caring, 176
in Maternal Role Attainment Theory, 587
in Modeling and Role-Modeling Theory, 542, 546
in B. Neuman's Systems Model, 314
in Nursing as Caring Theory, 399
in Peaceful End of Life Theory, 756–757
in Postpartum Depression Theory, 729
in Roy's Adaptation Model, 342, 343f, 344
in Science of Unitary Human Beings, 245
in Self-Transcendence Theory, 622
in Theory of Caring, 745
in Tidal Model of Mental Health Recovery, 680–681, 685
Personal factors, in Health Promotion Model, 438, 439
Personal integrity, in Conservation Model, 229
Person-as-agent, in Self-deficit Theory, 267–268
Person-client, in Theory of Caring, 746
Person-environment interactions
in Health as Expanding Consciousness Theory, 483
in Self-Transcendence Theory, 623
Personhood
P. Benner's assumptions about, 148
in Bureaucratic Caring Theory, 121
in Nursing as Caring Theory, 395, 397, 400
in Tidal Model of Mental Health Recovery, 692f
in Transpersonal Caring Theory, 99
Person-patient, in Symphonological Bioethical Theory, 564, 565
Phenomenology, 19
M. Foucault and, 172–173
fracture and difference in, 172
hermeneutic, 173
K. E. Logstrup's, 171
as natural attitude, 170
Philosophy, nursing, 6, 7, 7b. *See also* Nightingale, F., Ray, M. A., Watson, J.
P. Benner's, 137–164
characteristics and contributions of, 69
K. Eriksson's, 190–221
example of, 8t
K. Martinsen's, 165–189
F. Ray's, 113–136
J. Watson's, 91–112
Philosophy, 20th-century assumptions in, 341b
Piaget, Jean, 20, 540
Podvoll, E. M., 676
Polanyi, Michael, 562
Politics, in Bureaucratic Caring Theory, 119
Popper, K., 17, 22–23
Positivism, origins of and challenges to, 18
Postpartum Depression Predictors Inventory (PDPI), 723, 733
Postpartum Depression Screening Scale, 723, 725, 727, 731–744
Postpartum Depression Theory, 722–723
case study based on, 733–735
critique of, 732–733
empirical evidence for, 728–729
further development of, 731–732
logical form of, 730
major assumptions of, 729
major concepts and definitions in, 725–728
nursing community's acceptance of, 731
prevention in, 730
risk factors in, 726–728
summary of, 733
theoretical assertions of, 729–730
theoretical and philosophical sources for, 723, 725

Postpositivism, 23
Posttraumatic stress disorder, postpartum, 731–732
Powering concept, in Humanbecoming Theory, 509, 515, 515f
Practice, nursing
  apprenticeship model of, 5
  P. Benner on, 150–151
  and Bureaucratic Caring Theory, 123–124
  Caring Theory in, 747
  Caritative Caring Theory in, 202
  Chronic Sorrow Theory in, 663–664
  Comfort Theory in, 713–714
  Conservation Model in, 231–232
  critical analysis in, 169–170
  Culture Care Theory in, 467–468
  Goal Attainment Theory in, 294–296
  Health as Expanding Consciousness Theory in, 489–492
  Health Promotion Model in, 442
  Humanbecoming Theory in, 515–516
  Illness Trajectory Theory in, 646–647
  D. E. Johnson's Behavioral System Model in, 375–378
  knowledge base for, 3, 23
  K. Martinsen's philosophy of caring in, 178
  Maternal Role Attainment Theory in, 591–592
  Modeling and Role-Modeling Theory in, 547–548
  B. Neuman's Systems Model applications in, 317–318
  F. Nightingale's influence on, 79–80
  Nursing as Caring Theory in, 401–402
  nursing theory's role in, 11
  and Peaceful End of Life Theory, 757–758
  Postpartum Depression Theory in, 731
  research and, 32
  and Rogerian model, 248–249
  Roy Adaptation Model in, 345–347
  Self-Transcendence Theory in, 624–625
  Symphonological Bioethical Theory in, 570
  and theory development, 46–47
  Tidal Model of Mental Health Recovery in, 688–689
  Transition Theory in, 424–425
  Transpersonal Caring Theory in, 100
  Uncertainty in Illness Theory in, 606
Practice tools, in Science of Unitary Human Beings, 252t–254t
Preference theory, 755
Pregnancy, unwanted/unplanned, 727
Premature infants, families of, 377
Premise
  in deductive reasoning, 27–28
  in inductive reasoning, 29–30
Prevention, in Neuman Systems Model, 313–314
Preventive nursing *versus* preventive medicine, 379–380
Prigogine, I., 482
Primary nursing, 60
Probabilistic thinking, in Uncertainty in Illness Theory, 602
Profession
  criteria for, 10–11
  defined, 8
  nursing as, 4, 8, 10–12
Professionalism, person-oriented, 174
Proficiency, Dreyfus Model definition of, 143
PRO-SELF: Pain Control Program, 640
Psychiatric disorder, in Tidal Model of Mental Health Recovery, 686
Psychiatric nursing, in Tidal Model of Mental Health Recovery, 686
Psychiatric patients, in Goal Attainment Theory, 298
Psychosis, postpartum, 725–726. *See also* Postpartum Depression Theory
Purnell, M. J., 407
Pythagoras, 16–17

Q

Qualitative research, nursing's acceptance of, 468
Quality of life, in Peaceful End of Life Theory, 755

R

Rapoport, A., 368
Rationalism, 16–17
Ray, Marilyn Anne, 113
  Air Force service of, 114
  background of, 113–116
  Bureaucratic Caring Theory of, 116–136
Reaction, in Neuman Systems Model, 313
Reasoning. *See also* Logical reasoning
  abductive, 31, 568–569
  a priori, 17
  retroductive, 31–33, 33t–34t
Reciprocity, in homeodynamics, 247t, 250f
Reconstitution, in Neuman Systems Model, 314
Reed, Pamela G., 618
  background of, 618–619
  Self-Transcendence Theory of, 619–637
Reeder, F., 115
Regulation, in Johnson Behavioral System Model, 370

Regulator, in Roy Adaptation Model, 338, 343–344, 343f, 355t
Rehabilitation nursing, L. Hall's contributions to, 60–61, 60f
Relational Caring Questionnaires, 128–129
Relational statements, in theory development, 39–41
Relationships. *See also* Nurse-patient relationship
in Humanbecoming Theory, 505
in mental health services, 675
in Transpersonal Caring Theory, 94, 95
Research
F. G. Abdellah's contributions to, 57
articulation, 139
P. Benner on, 151
in Bureaucratic Caring Theory, 126, 127t–128t
in Caritative Caring Theory, 203
in Chronic Sorrow Theory, 665
Comfort Theory and, 714–715
Conservation Model in, 232–233
critique of methods and assumptions of, 22
Culture Care Theory in, 469
ethnonursing, 455, 460, 462–465, 471
Goal Attainment Theory in, 296–297
Health as Expanding Consciousness Theory in, 489–492
Health Promotion Model in, 443
V. Henderson's contribution to, 56
Humanbecoming Theory in, 511–512, 517–518
interdependence with theory of, 21–24
Johnson Behavioral System Model in, 378–379
Maternal Role Attainment Theory in, 592
Modeling and Role-Modeling in, 548–549
Neuman Systems Model applications, 319–320
and F. Nightingale, 76–77, 81
nurses' participation in, 4
in Nursing as Caring Theory, 404–407
and nursing practice, 32
Peaceful End of Life Theory in, 758
and philosophy of caring, 179
in Postpartum Depression Theory, 724t
qualitative, 468, 767–768
reviews of, 9
M. Rogers' theory and, 249–251
role of theory in, 4–5
Roy Adaptation Model in, 348–352
Self-Transcendence Theory and, 625–626
Symphonological Bioethical Theory in, 571
Theory of Caring in, 748
theory-testing, 46–47
Research *(Continued)*
Tidal Model of Mental Health Recovery in, 689–690
Transition Theory in, 425
Transpersonal Caring Theory in, 101
Uncertainty in Illness Theory in, 607
and Wiener-Dodd Theory of Illness Trajectory, 647
Research instruments
and Roy Adaptation Model, 350–351
and Science of Unitary Human Beings, 252t–254t
Research-then-theory strategy, 17
Residual stimuli, in Roy's Adaptation Model, 338
Resonancy, in Science of Unitary Human Beings, 247t, 248
Resourcefulness in Tidal Model of Mental Health Recovery, 681
The Resource Manual for Women with Breast Cancer, 346
Respect, In Peaceful End of Life Theory, 756
Retroductive reasoning, 31–33, 33t–34t
Revealing-concealing concept, in Humanbecoming Theory, 508, 515, 515f
Reynolds, P., 17, 42, 44
Rhythmical patterns, in Humanbecoming Theory, 508
Rhythmicity, in Humanbecoming Theory, 513
Ricoeur, P., 173
Riegel, K., 619
Rights, in Symphonological Bioethical Theory, 564, 566
Roach, M. S., 395
Robbins, Lorraine, 436
Robinson Self-Appraisal Inventory, 546
Rogers, Carl, 94, 99
Rogers, Martha E., 242, 287
background of, 242–243
Conservation Model and, 227
and Health as Expanding Consciousness Theory, 250, 482, 486
honors and awards, 243
Humanbecoming Theory and, 504–505, 512
normal science defined by, 766–767
Self-Transcendence Theory and, 619, 622–623
Unitary Human Beings Theory of, 244–264
Role attainment, maternal, 584. *See also* Maternal Role Attainment Theory
Role function mode, in Roy's Adaptation Model, 339–340
Role insufficiency, 417–418
Role-modeling, in Modeling and Role-Modeling Paradigm, 541
Role strain-role conflict, in Maternal Role Attainment Theory, 584
Role supplementation, in Transition Theory, 417–418, 424

Roper, N., 52, 62–64
Roper–Logan–Tierney Model of Nursing, 63–65, 64f, 65f
Roy, Sister Callista, 335
  Adaptation Model of, 7, 27, 336–365, 767
  background of, 335–336
  honors and awards, 336
Rubin, Jane, 140
Rubin, Reva, Mercer's theory and, 583
Ruland, Cornelia M., 753
  background of, 754
  Peaceful End of Life Theory of, 755–762
Rumi, 94
Russell, B., 18
Ruth Rhoden Craven Foundation for Postpartum Depression Awareness, 731

S

Salience, Dreyfus Model definition of, 144
Salmon, W. D., 44
Samarel, N., 346, 349
Sample size, in inductive arguments, 30
Sartre, Jean-Paul, 94, 504, 512
Schoenhofer, Savina O., 393
  background of, 394–395
  Nursing as Caring Theory of, 395–415
Schumacher, K., 418
Schutz, A., 18–19
Science
  commonalities in, 23
  historical views of, 16–21
  history and philosophy of, 16–25
  interactionist perspective in, 20
  normal, 6, 766–767
  philosophical foundations of, 16–17
  presuppositions in, 20–21
  as social enterprise, 24
  stages of development of, 23
  20th-century assumptions in, 341b
Scientific consensus, 21–22
Scientific theory. *See also* Theory, nursing
  data-driven (bottom-up) *versus* concept-driven (top-down), 20
  derivation strategy of, 32
  interdependence with research, 21–24
  observation and, 20
  phases of, 21
  refutation of, 22–23
  revolutionary, 22
Scott, J. M., 287
Sechrist, Karen, 435
Seip, A. L., 167
Self
  in Goal Attainment Theory, 288–289
  in Maternal Role Attainment Theory, 587
  in Postpartum Depression Theory, 728
Self-care
  in Modeling and Role-Modeling Paradigm, 543
  in Self-Care Deficit Theory, 269–270, 274, 276
Self-care agency, in Self-Care Deficit Theory, 271
Self-care deficit, in Orem's Self-Care Deficit Theory, 271, 274
Self-Care Deficit Theory, 265–285, 767
  case study based on, 278–280
  conceptual framework for, 274, 275f
  critique of, 276–278
  curricula using framework of, 275
  empirical evidence for, 272
  further development of, 275–276
  logical form of, 274
  major assumptions of, 272–273
  major concepts and definitions in, 269–272
  moderate realism position of, 267
  nursing community's acceptance of, 274–275
  nursing systems theory in, 273–274, 273f
  sources for, 266–269
  theoretical assertions in, 273–274
Self-care demand, therapeutic, 270–271
Self-care knowledge, in Modeling and Role-Modeling Theory, 544–546
Self-Care Resource Inventory, 546
Self-care resources, operationalized, studies of, 545
Self-concept, in Maternal Role Attainment Theory, 584
Self-concept-group identity mode, in Roy's Adaptation Model, 339
Self-efficacy, in Health Promotion Model, 438, 439, 442
Self-esteem
  in Maternal Role Attainment Theory, 584
  in Postpartum Depression Theory, 727
  in Roy Adaptation Model, 348–349
Self-transcendence
  mental health and, 621–622
  moderating-mediating factors in, 620
  P. G. Reed's concept of, 620, 625
Self-Transcendence Theory, 618–637
  case study based on, 629–630
  critique of, 627–628
  empirical evidence for, 621–622

Self-Transcendence Theory, *(Continued)*
further development of, 626–627
logical form of, 624
major assumptions of, 622–623
major concepts and definitions in, 620–621
Modeling and Role-Modeling Theory and, 625
model of, 624f
nursing community's acceptance of, 624–626
points of intervention in, 621
summary of, 628–629
theoretical assertions of, 623, 624f
theoretical sources for, 619–620
Selye, Hans, 94, 227, 310, 371, 540
Set-of-laws approach, to theory building, 42, 43f
Sexual subsystem, in Johnson Behavioral System Model, 369
Shame, in Postpartum Depression Theory, 728
Sichel, D., 723, 725, 729
Significant others, in Peaceful End of Life Theory, 756
Simplicity
in analysis of nursing theory, 12
in P. Benner's account of nursing practice, 152
in Bureaucratic Theory, 129
in Caring Theory, 748
in Caritative Caring Theory, 205
in Chronic Sorrow Theory, 666–667
in Comfort Theory, 716
in Conservation Model, 233
in Culture Care Theory, 470–471
in Goal Attainment Theory, 297
in Health as Expanding Consciousness Theory, 493
in Health Promotion Model, 443
in Humanbecoming Theory, 518
in Illness Trajectory Theory, 648
in Johnson Behavioral System Model, 381
in K. Martinson's philosophy of caring, 180
in Maternal Attainment Role Theory, 594
in Modeling and Remodeling Theory, 550
in Nursing as Caring Theory, 425
in Peaceful End of Life Theory, 759
in Postpartum Depression Theory, 732
in Roy Aaptation Model, 353
in Science of Unitary Human Beings, 251
in Self-care Deficit Theory, 276
in Self-Transcendence Theory, 627
in Symphonological Bioethical Theory, 572
in Tidal Model of Mental Health Recovery, 693
in Transition Theory, 425
in Transpersonal Caring Theory, 101–102
in Uncertainty in Illness Theory, 609
Situation, P. Benner's assumptions about, 149
Situational influences, in Health Promotion Model, 438, 439–440
Situation-specific theory, 46
Skinner, B. F., 17–18
Sleeping disturbances, as risk for postpartum depression, 728
Small, B., 378
Small, H., 73, 78
Smith, F. B., 73
Social integrity, in Conservation Model, 229
Social interaction theory, 337
Social support
lack of as risk for postpartum depression, 727
in Maternal Role Attainment Theory, 585
uncertainty and, 603
Society of Rogerian Scholars, 243
Socioeconomic conditions, in transition experience, 421–422
Sorrow. *See* Chronic Sorrow Theory
Source theory, 31–32
Sovereign life utterances
in K. Martinsen's philosophy of caring, 174
K. E. Logstrup's concept of, 171
Spinoza, Benedict, 561, 562–563
Spirituality, theoretical *versus* operational definition of, 40t
Spouse abuse, in Roy Adaptation Model, 348
Statistical inference, 30
Steiner, E., 31
Stimuli frame, in Uncertainty in Illness Theory, 601, 602
St-Jacques, A., 377
Story
in Nursing as Caring Theory, 398, 403, 405
in Tidal Model of Mental Health Recovery, 677–678, 688–689
Strachey, L., 73
Strauss, Anselm, 114, 639, 646, 723
Stress
biochemical disruption due to, 729
in Johnson's Behavioral System Model, 371
in Maternal Role Attainment Theory, 585
and postpartum depression, 727
Roy Adaptation Model in study of, 348
Stress and coping theory, of R. S. Lazarus, 141
Stressors
in Johnson Behavioral System Model, 370
in Neuman Systems Model, 313

Stress response, in Conservation Model, 228
Structural integrity, in Conservation Model, 229
Structure providers in Uncertainty in Illness Theory, 601–602, 605
Suffering, in Caritative Caring Theory, 195, 199
Suicidal thoughts, as risk for postpartum depression, 728
Sunrise Enabler, in Culture Care Theory of Diversity and Universality, 465, 466f, 467
Sustenal imperatives, in Johnson Behavioral System Model, 370
Swain, Mary Ann P., 536
  background of, 539–540
  honors and awards, 540
  Modeling and Role-Modeling Theory of, 540–559
Swanson, Kristen M., 741
  background of, 741–742
  honors and awards, 742
  Theory of Caring of, 742–752
Swimme, Brian, 337, 341
Symphonological Bioethical Theory
  case study based on, 573
  critique of, 572–573
  empirical evidence for, 564–565
  further development of, 571–572
  logical form of, 568–569
  major assumptions in, 565–566
  major concepts and definitions in, 563–564
  nursing community's acceptance of, 570–571
  retroductive reasoning in, 32
  summary of, 573
  theoretical assertions of, 566–568, 569f
  theoretic sources for, 562–563
Symphonology, defined, 562
Synchrony, in homeodynamics, 247t, 250f
Systems
  in Johnson's Behavioral System Model, 368
  nursing, 273–274, 273f
  in Roy's Adaptation Model, 337
Systems Model, B. Neuman's, 309–334, 315f, 767
  case study based on, 322–323
  critique of, 321–322
  cross-cultural applications of, 319–320
  empirical evidence for, 314, 315f
  further development of, 320–321
  logical form of, 316
  major assumptions of, 314, 316
  major concepts and definitions in, 311–314
  nursing community's applications for, 316–320
  sources for, 310–311
  theoretical assertions in, 316
Systems theory. *See also* General system theory
  in Goal Attainment Theory, 290–291, 290f
  in Roy Adaptation Model, 341
Szasz, Thomas, 676

T

Tak, S., 352
Taylor, Charles, 140
Taylor, V., 103–104
Temperament, infant, in Maternal Role Attainment, 585
Temporality, in Illness Trajectory Theory, 642, 643t
Ten Commitments of Tidal Model of Mental Health Recovery, 675, 691, 694
Tension, in Johnson Behavioral System Model, 370
Tesler, M., 378
Theory, nursing. *See also* Middle range theories; Nursing theorists; Scientific theory; *specific theory*
  analysis of, 12–13
  characteristics of, 391
  clarifying role of, 766
  clarity of, 12
  classification of, 6–8, 767
  components of, 36–44, 37t
  derivable consequences of, 13
  development of, 26
  empirical precision of, 13
  era of, 6
  example of, 8t
  future of, 763–771
  generality of, 12–13
  and global communities of nursing scholars, 769–770, 770t
  growth of, 766
  history of, 4–8
  introduction to, 3–15
  journals on, 769
  knowledge structure levels and examples of, 8t
  M. Leininger's definition of, 459
  and nature of normal science, 766–767
  paradigm period of, 5–6
  publications in, 769–770t
  role in research of, 4–5
  significance of, 8–12
  simplicity of, 12
  situation-specific, 46
  source, 31–32
  state of the art and science of, 765–771
  theorists producing, 7, 7b
  wanted, 31
  J. Watson's definition of, 93–94
  websites for, 770

Theory development, 36–49. *See also* Middle Range theories
analogy in, 32
axiomatic approach to, 42, 43f, 44
causal process approach to, 42, 44, 45f
completeness of, 42
components of, 36–44, 37t–40t, 43f
concept analysis in, 39, 39t
concepts and definitions in, 37–39
contemporary issues in, 44–47
linkages and ordering in, 41–42, 44
middle range, 46
relational statements in, 39–41
set-of-laws approach to, 42, 43f
systematic, 36
typologies and, 38
Theory models, 31–32
Theory-then-research strategy, for theory construction, 17
Thinking, probabilistic, 602
Tidal Model of Mental Health Recovery
bridging concept in, 676
care continuum in, 682, 693f
case study based on, 695–696
critique of, 691–694
Eastern philosophical influences on, 675–676
empirical evidence for, 683–684
engagement beliefs of, 682
essential values of, 677b–679b
further development of, 690–691
guiding principles of, 681
logical form of, 687
major assumptions of, 684–686
nursing community's acceptance of, 687–690
personhood dimensions in, 692f
social constructivism and, 676
story in, 677–678
structure of care in, 692f
summary of, 694–695
ten commitments of, 675, 677b–679b, 691, 694
theoretical assertions of, 686–687
theoretical basis of, 679–680
theoretical sources for, 675–677
therapeutic philosophy of, 682
three domains of, 680–681
Tidal Model of Mental Health Recovery, 33
water metaphor in, 681
Tidal Model of Mental Health Recovery and Reclamation, 690
Tierney, Alison J., 53, 62–64
Time span, in transition experience, 421
Tomlin, Evelyn M., 536
background of, 538–539
Modeling and Role-Modeling Theory of, 540–559
Touch, preterm infant response to, 350
Transaction, in Goal Attainment Theory, 291, 291f
Transcendence, in Humanbecoming Theory, 513
Transcultural nursing. *See also* Culture Care Theory of Diversity and Universality
versus cross-cultural nursing, 458
founding and development of, 454–457
M. Leininger's definition of, 458
programs in, 114–115, 455–456, 468–469
Transforming concept, in Humanbecoming Theory, 510, 515, 515f
Transition experience
conditions of, 421–422
properties of, 420–421
Transitions, types and pattern of, 420
Transition Theory, 7, 419–433, 419f
case study based on, 426–427
critique of, 425–426
cultural factors in, 418–419, 421, 423
empirical evidence for, 422
further development of, 425
logical form of, 424
major assumptions of, 422–424
major concepts and definitions in, 420–422
nursing community's acceptance of, 424–425
sources for, 419
summary of, 426
theoretical assertions of, 424
Transparency, in Tidal Model of Mental Health Recovery, 679
Transpersonal Caring Relationship, postmodern paradigm shift in, 94, 96–98
Transpersonal Caring Theory, 91–112
assertions of, 98–99
and carative factors and caritas process, 97t
case study based on, 103–104
critique of, 101–102
empirical evidence in, 96
further development of, 101
logical form of, 99–100
major assumptions of, 96–98
major concepts and definitions, 94–96
nursing community's application of, 100–101
sources for, 93–94
summary of, 102

Travelbee, Joyce, 51, 179
theory and influence of, 61
Therapeutic Use of Self concept of, 676
Trephotaxis, in Tidal Model of Mental Health Recovery, 684
Triadic collaborative decision making, 33
Trigger events, in Chronic Sorrow Theory, 661, 662
Trophicognosis, in Conservation Model, 228
Trust, role in client involvement of, 545
Tsai, P. F., 352
Tulman, L., 346, 348
Turkel, M., 115–116, 126, 129–130
Typologies, 38

U

Uhl-Pierce, J., 114
Uncertainty
M. H. Mishel's concept of, 601, 603–604
sources and impacts of, 602–603
Uncertainty abatement work, in Illness Trajectory Theory, 642–643, 643t
Uncertainty in Illness Theory, 599–617, 604f
case study based on, 610
coping with uncertainty in, 608
critique of, 608–610
empirical evidence for, 602–603
further development of, 607–608
logical form of, 605–606
major assumptions of, 603–605, 605f
major concepts and definitions in, 601–602
nursing community's acceptance of, 606–607
reconceptualization of, 604–605, 607, 608
summary of, 610
theoretical assertions of, 605
theoretical sources for, 601
uncertainty antecedents in, 608
uncertainty appraisal in, 608
Uncertainty principle, P. Barker's work and, 674
Unconditional acceptance, in Modeling and Role-Modeling Paradigm, 542
Unitary Human Beings Theory, 244–264, 767
case study based on, 255
critique of, 251, 254
empirical evidence for, 245
evolution of principles of homeodynamics in, 247t
further development of, 251
homeodynamic principles in, 247t
logical form of, 248
major assumptions of, 245–246
Unitary Human Beings Theory, *(Continued)*
major concepts and definitions in, 243–244
nursing community's acceptance of, 248–251
research instruments and practice tools derived from, 252t–254t
sources for, 243
theoretical assertions of, 246, 248
Universal experiences, in Humanbecoming Theory, 511
Universality, in Culture Care Theory, 460
Universe of open systems, M. Rogers' concept of, 244
Untouchable zone, in K. Martinsen's philosophy of caring, 174–175
Urine control theory, Roy Adaptation Model and, 350–352

V

Validity, assessment of, 27–28
Valuing concept, in Humanbecoming Theory, 507, 514–515, 515f
Van Manen, M., 115
Van Servellen, G., 378
Variables, relational statements of, 40
Venipuncture, pain-related responses to, 350
Villareal, E., Roy Adaptation Model and, 346
Visions: The Journal of Rogerian Nursing Science, 767
Vocation
in K. Martinsen's philoosophy of caring, 175
N.A. Weber's philosophy of, 172
Von Bertalanffy, L., 245, 583
Vulnerability,in Self-Transcendence Theory, 620, 623

W

Walker, Susan, 435
Wallace, W. A., 268
Wanted theory, 31
Wærness, K., 167
Watson, Jean, 91
background of, 91–93
influence on K. M. Swanson of, 742
Postpartum Depression Theory and, 723
Transpersonal Caring Theory of, 93–112, 115
Weber, M., 169, 172
Well-being
self-transcendence and, 620, 623, 626
in Theory of Caring, 746
Wellness, in Neuman Systems Model, 313
Whall, Ann, 619
Whitehead, Alfred North, 18, 94
Whitehill, Irene, 675, 686

Whittemore, R., 352
Wholeness (holism), in Conservation Model, 227
Wholistic approach, in Neuman Systems Model, 311, 318
Wiedenbach, E., 51
  background of, 57–58
  on clinical nursing background of, 58
  on ministration of help, 58, 59f
  theory and influence of, 57–60
  on validation of meeting needs, 60f
Wiener, Carolyn L., 639
  background of, 639
  honors and awards, 639
  Illness Trajectory Theory of, 641–655
Wilkie, D. J., 378
Williams, R., 80
Winland-Brown, 407
Woods, S. J., 349
Work, categories of, in Illness Trajectory Theory, 642, 645–646
Worldview
  in Culture Care Theory, 460, 464
  holographic, 117
  in Tidal Model of Mental Health Recovery, 675
Wrubel, Judith, 140, 146, 148–149

Y

Yeh, C. H., Roy Adaptation Model and, 348
Young, A. M., Newman's theory and, 482
Young-McCaughan, S., Roy Adaptation Model and, 348

Z

Zderad, L. T., 395, 708
Zetterberg, H. L., 17, 40